The APhA Complete Review for Pharmacy

Notices

The authors, editors, and publisher have made every effort to ensure the accuracy and completeness of the information presented in this book. However, the authors, editors, and publisher cannot be held responsible for the continued currency of the information, any inadvertent errors or omissions, or the application of this information. Therefore, the authors, editors, and publisher shall have no liability to any person or entity with regard to claims, loss, or damage caused or alleged to be caused, directly or indirectly, by the use of information contained herein.

The inclusion in this book of any product in respect to which patent or trademark rights may exist shall not be deemed, and is not intended as, a grant of or authority to exercise any right or privilege protected by such patent or trademark. All such rights or trademarks are vested in the patent or trademark owner, and no other person may exercise the same without express permission, authority, or license secured from such patent or trademark owner.

The inclusion of a brand name does not mean the authors, the editors, or the publisher has any particular knowledge that the brand listed has properties different from other brands of the same product, nor should its inclusion be interpreted as an endorsement by the authors, the editors, or the publisher. Similarly, the fact that a particular brand has not been included does not indicate the product has been judged to be in any way unsatisfactory or unacceptable. Further, no official support or endorsement of this book by any federal or state agency or pharmaceutical company is intended or inferred.

NAPLEX® is a trademark of the National Association of Boards of Pharmacy® (NABP®), and NABP® in no way endorses, authorizes, or sponsors this guide.

The APhA Complete Review for Pharmacy

Eleventh Edition

Peter A. Chyka, PharmD
Editor-in-Chief
Professor of Clinical Pharmacy
Executive Associate Dean
College of Pharmacy, University of Tennessee Health Science Center
Knoxville, Tennessee

Bradley A. Boucher, PharmD
Associate Editor
Professor of Clinical Pharmacy
Associate Dean, Strategic Initiatives and Operations
College of Pharmacy, University of Tennessee Health Science Center
Memphis, Tennessee

Andrea S. Franks, PharmD
Associate Editor
Associate Professor of Clinical Pharmacy and Family Medicine
Clinical Pharmacy Specialist, Family Medicine
College of Pharmacy, University of Tennessee Health Science Center
Knoxville, Tennessee

J. Aubrey Waddell, PharmD
Associate Editor
Professor of Clinical Pharmacy
Oncology Pharmacist
College of Pharmacy, University of Tennessee Health Science Center
Knoxville, Tennessee

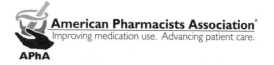

American Pharmacists Association®
Improving medication use. Advancing patient care.
APhA

Washington, D.C.

Acquiring Editor: Julian I. Graubart
Managing Editors: Mary-Ann Moalli and Rachel Ledbetter, Publications Professionals LLC
Copyeditors: Wendi Russell, Christine Stinson, Sharlette Visaya, and Liesl Wiederkehr, Publications Professionals LLC
Proofreaders: Frances Kalavritinos, Sarah LaCourse, and Jennifer Thompson, Publications Professionals LLC
Composition: Circle Graphics
Cover Design: Scott Neitzke, APhA Creative Services

©2015 by the American Pharmacists Association
Published by the American Pharmacists Association
2215 Constitution Avenue, NW
Washington, DC 20037-2985
www.pharmacist.com www.pharmacylibrary.com

APhA was founded in 1852 as the American Pharmaceutical Association.

To comment on this book via e-mail, send your message to the publisher at aphabooks@aphanet.org

Library of Congress Cataloging-in-Publication Data

The APhA complete review for pharmacy / Peter A. Chyka, editor-in-chief ; associate
editor[s], Bradley A. Boucher, Andrea S. Franks, J. Aubrey Waddell. — 11th edition.
    p. ; cm.
Includes bibliographical references and index.
ISBN 978-1-58212-217-5 (alk. paper)
    I. Chyka, Peter A., editor. II. Boucher, Bradley A., editor. III. Franks, Andrea S., editor. IV.
Waddell, J. Aubrey., editor. V. American Pharmacists Association.
    [DNLM: 1. Pharmacy—Examination Questions. 2. Pharmaceutical Preparations—
Examination Questions. QV 18.2]
    RS98
    615.1076—dc23
                        2014041049

Dedication

We dedicate this publication to three important groups in our lives. We are thankful for the constant support and patience of our families throughout our careers for projects like this publication. Our teachers and mentors at the Universities of Arkansas, Minnesota, Tennessee, and Utah set us on a path to become the pharmacists we are today. Every day our students, colleagues, and patients stimulate us to rethink our ideas and to discover new knowledge.

PETER, BRAD, ANDREA, AND AUBREY

Contents

Preface

In this publication, the 11th edition of *The APhA Complete Review for Pharmacy*, several new features have been introduced. All 42 chapters have been reviewed and revised by the authors and editorial team to provide up-to-date information and concepts. The tables that list medications now have the top 100 drugs indicated in bold to alert the reader of medicines in frequent use. A summary of a chapter's concepts, Key Points, has been moved from the back of the chapter to the very front. This repositioning should give the reader a quick and ready snapshot of some important points discussed in the chapter. The Key Points section is followed by a new feature—the Study Guide Checklist. The Checklist should serve as a guide in preparation for the NAPLEX as part of a self-assessment. The Checklist covers broad areas of information, including concepts and skills that are not necessarily covered fully in *The APhA Complete Review for Pharmacy* but should be considered in the overall preparation for the exam. This information can be found in comprehensive textbooks and references that are typically used in a pharmacy curriculum and can be easily retrieved. Although *The APhA Complete Review for Pharmacy* is complete in covering key topics, no single reference can fully condense the entire curriculum and body of knowledge into a review. The items in the Checklist should stimulate the reader to seek supplemental information to fill in any gaps in a self-assessment. This edition contains an index, which should assist the reader in finding specific information and in locating information that may be cross-covered in more than one chapter or therapeutic area.

These enhancements would not have been possible without the talents and cooperation of the authors.

The 11th edition includes the work of 9 new and 38 returning authors. All authors have a strong pharmacy tie to the College of Pharmacy at The University of Tennessee Health Science Center at its locations in Knoxville, Memphis, and Nashville. They are faculty members, alumni, fellows, or residents (past or present) of the College, and many have more than one of those University of Tennessee (UT) ties. A common core of education and training at UT has served as a strong baseline and framework for this publication that has been diversified and complemented through experiences in clinical care, teaching, community outreach, professional service, and research in or outside of Tennessee.

After 10 editions of this publication, Drs. Dick Gourley and James Eoff III have turned over the editorial leadership to a new team. The editor-in-chief and the associate editors only now fully appreciate the effort and organization needed to assemble a publication such as *The APhA Complete Review for Pharmacy*. We are also aware of the responsibility to bring relevant and contemporary information to readers in their preparation for the NAPLEX. We each bring 25–35 years of experience as educators, clinicians, and scholars to the editorial process. Our efforts have been supported by Ms. Rhonda Green at the College and by the staff at the American Pharmacists Association (APhA) to whom we owe much gratitude.

Although this edition includes changes, it also is a product of the steady support of APhA. The guidance, ideas, and encouragement of Mr. Julian Graubart, Associate Vice President, Books and Electronic Products, and his staff are invaluable contributors to this work. Their wisdom has been developed through many years in the publishing business, and Mr. Graubart has served as APhA's responsible party for *The APhA Complete Review for Pharmacy* through the years. The copyeditors and proofreaders of Publications Professionals LLC have also been involved with this publication for several years and bring important items to the attention of authors and editors from their unique point of view.

We, the editorial team for *The APhA Complete Review for Pharmacy*, hope you find this publication in printed or electronic form to be an asset to your successful preparation and passing of the NAPLEX. We have often found that by globally reviewing a topic, we gain new insights and understanding that reinforce and build on previous knowledge. As a health care professional, you in your role of a pharmacist will be challenged out of necessity to continue your education as a life-long learner for the benefit of your patients and profession. We look forward to you joining the profession of pharmacists and making contributions throughout your career.

PETER A. CHYKA, PHARMD
EDITOR-IN-CHIEF

BRADLEY A. BOUCHER, PHARMD
ASSOCIATE EDITOR

ANDREA S. FRANKS, PHARMD
ASSOCIATE EDITOR

J. AUBREY WADDELL, PHARMD
ASSOCIATE EDITOR

Contributors

Anita Airee, PharmD, BCPS
Associate Professor of Clinical Pharmacy
Clinical Pharmacy Specialist, Ambulatory Care
University of Tennessee Health Science Center
Knoxville, Tennessee

Elizabeth L. Alford, PharmD
PGY2 Pharmacy Resident, Academia and
    Pediatric Pharmacotherapy
University of Tennessee Health Science Center
Memphis, Tennessee

Hassan Almoazen, PhD
Assistant Professor of Pharmaceutical Sciences
Assistant Professor of Clinical Pharmacy
University of Tennessee Health Science Center
Affiliated Assistant Professor of Biomedical
    Engineering
University of Tennessee, Knoxville
Memphis, Tennessee

W. Andrew Bell, PharmD, BCPS
Associate Chief, Clinical Pharmacy Section
Veterans Affairs Health Care System
Phoenix, Arizona

Bradley A. Boucher, PharmD, BCPS,
    FCCP, FCCM
Professor of Clinical Pharmacy
Associate Dean, Strategic Initiatives and Operations
University of Tennessee Health Science Center
Clinical Pharmacy Specialist, Critical Care
Regional Medical Center
Memphis, Tennessee

Joyce E. Broyles, PharmD, MHA, BCNSP
Associate Professor of Clinical Pharmacy
University of Tennessee Health Science Center
Manager, Pharmacy Services
Clinical Specialist, Infectious Disease/Nutrition
Methodist University Hospital
Memphis, Tennessee

Jason Carter, PharmD
Associate Professor of Clinical Pharmacy
University of Tennessee Health Science Center
Chief Pharmacist
Tennessee Department of Mental Health and
    Substance Abuse Services
State Opioid Treatment Authority
Nashville, Tennessee

Michael L. Christensen, PharmD, BCNSP, FPPAG
Professor of Clinical Pharmacy and Pediatrics
University of Tennessee Health Science Center
Clinical Pharmacy Specialist, Pediatrics
Le Bonheur Children's Hospital
Memphis, Tennessee

Peter A. Chyka, PharmD, DABAT, DPNAP, FACCT
Professor of Clinical Pharmacy
Executive Associate Dean
University of Tennessee Health Science Center
Knoxville, Tennessee

Catherine M. Crill, PharmD, FCCP, BCPS, BCNSP
Associate Professor of Clinical Pharmacy
    and Pediatrics
University of Tennessee Health Science Center
Clinical Pharmacy Specialist and Director, Parenteral
    Nutrition Service
Le Bonheur Children's Hospital
Memphis, Tennessee

Benjamin Duhart, Jr, MS, PharmD
Assistant Professor of Clinical Pharmacy
University of Tennessee Health Science Center
Memphis, Tennessee

Michelle Z. Farland, PharmD, BCPS, CDE
Associate Professor of Clinical Pharmacy
Clinical Pharmacy Specialist, Ambulatory Care
University of Tennessee Health Science Center
Knoxville, Tennessee

Glen E. Farr, PharmD, FAPhA
Professor of Clinical Pharmacy
Associate Dean for Continuing Education
University of Tennessee Health Science Center
Knoxville, Tennessee

Shannon W. Finks, PharmD, FCCP, BCPS (AQ Cardiology)
Associate Professor of Clinical Pharmacy
University of Tennessee Health Science Center
Clinical Pharmacy Specialist
Veterans Affairs Medical Center
Memphis, Tennessee

Stephanie A. Flowers, PharmD, PhD
Infectious Diseases Pharmacotherapy Fellow
University of Tennessee Health Science Center
Memphis, Tennessee

Stephan L. Foster, PharmD, FAPhA, FNAP
Professor of Clinical Pharmacy
University of Tennessee Health Science Center
Memphis, Tennessee

Andrea S. Franks, PharmD, BCPS
Associate Professor of Clinical Pharmacy and Family Medicine
Clinical Pharmacy Specialist, Family Medicine
University of Tennessee Health Science Center
Knoxville, Tennessee

Fred P. Gattas, PharmD, BCNP
Assistant Professor of Clinical Pharmacy
University of Tennessee Health Science Center
Pharmacy Quality Manger, Triad Isotopes
St. Louis, Missouri

Christa M. George, PharmD, BCPS, CDE
Assistant Professor of Clinical Pharmacy and Family Medicine
University of Tennessee Health Science Center
Clinical Pharmacist, Ambulatory Care
University of Tennessee Family Practice Center
Memphis, Tennessee

Benjamin N. Gross, PharmD, BCPS, BCACP, CDE, BC-ADM
Associate Professor of Pharmacy Practice
Clinical Pharmacist, Ambulatory Care
Lipscomb University College of Pharmacy
Nashville, Tennessee

Anthony J. Guarascio, PharmD, BCPS
Assistant Professor of Pharmacy Practice
Duquesne University College of Pharmacy
Pittsburgh, Pennsylvania

Gale L. Hamann, PharmD, BCPS, CDE
Professor of Clinical Pharmacy
Associate Professor, College of Medicine
University of Tennessee Health Science Center
Clinical Pharmacy Specialist, Ambulatory Care
Regional Medical Center
Memphis, Tennessee

Amanda Howard-Thompson, PharmD, BCPS
Associate Professor of Clinical Pharmacy and Family Medicine
University of Tennessee Health Science Center
Clinical Pharmacy Specialist, Family Medicine
University of Tennessee Family Practice Center
Memphis, Tennessee

Joanna Q. Hudson, PharmD, BCPS, FASN, FCCP, FNKF
Associate Professor of Clinical Pharmacy and Medicine
University of Tennessee Health Science Center
Clinical Specialist, Nephrology
Methodist University Hospital
Memphis, Tennessee

Jessica N. Lee, PharmD
Clinical Specialist, Hematology/Oncology
University of Tennessee Medical Center
Knoxville, Tennessee

Vivian S. Loveless, PharmD, BCNP, FAPhA
Associate Professor of Pharmaceutical Sciences
University of Tennessee Health Science Center
Memphis, Tennessee

Bernd Meibohm, PhD, FCP
Professor of Pharmaceutical Sciences
Associate Dean of Graduate Programs and Research
University of Tennessee Health Science Center
Memphis, Tennessee

Elizabeth S. Miller, PharmD
Senior Director, Medical Communications
Med Communications Inc.
Memphis, Tennessee

Robert J. Nolly, BSPh, MS
Professor of Pharmaceutical Sciences
University of Tennessee Health Science Center
Memphis, Tennessee

Carrie S. Oliphant, PharmD, BCPS (AQ Cardiology)
Associate Professor of Clinical Pharmacy
University of Tennessee Health Science Center
Clinical Pharmacy Specialist, Cardiology/Anticoagulation
Methodist University Hospital
Memphis, Tennessee

Robert B. Parker, PharmD, FCCP
Professor of Clinical Pharmacy
University of Tennessee Health Science Center
Memphis, Tennessee

Stephanie J. Phelps, BSPharm, PharmD, BCPS, FCCP, FAPhA, FPPG, DPNAP
Professor of Clinical Pharmacy and Pediatrics
Associate Dean of Academic Affairs
University of Tennessee Health Science Center
Memphis, Tennessee

William Nathan Rawls, BSPharm, PharmD
Professor of Clinical Pharmacy
University of Tennessee Health Science Center
Clinical Pharmacy Specialist
Veterans Affairs Medical Center
Memphis, Tennessee

Shaunta' M. Ray, PharmD, BCPS
Assistant Professor of Clinical Pharmacy and Family
  Medicine
Clinical Pharmacy Specialist, Family Medicine
University of Tennessee Health Science Center
Knoxville, Tennessee

Kelly C. Rogers, PharmD, FCCP
Professor of Clinical Pharmacy
University of Tennessee Health Science Center
Memphis, Tennessee

P. David Rogers, PharmD, PhD, FCCP
First Tennessee Endowed Chair of Excellence
  in Clinical Pharmacy
Professor of Clinical Pharmacy and Pediatrics
Director of Division of Clinical and Experimental
  Therapeutics
University of Tennessee Health Science Center
Memphis, Tennessee

Carol A. Schwab, JD, LLM
Professor of Clinical Pharmacy
Director of Medical/Legal Education
Office of Academic, Faculty, and Student Affairs
University of Tennessee Health Science Center
Memphis, Tennessee

Timothy H. Self, PharmD
Professor of Clinical Pharmacy
University of Tennessee Health Science Center
Clinical Specialist, Internal Medicine
Methodist University Hospital
Memphis, Tennessee

Sarah T. Stapleton, PharmD, MEd
Medical Information Specialist
Med Communications Inc.
Memphis, Tennessee

Joseph M. Swanson, PharmD, BCPS
Associate Professor of Clinical Pharmacy and
  Pharmacology

University of Tennessee Health Science Center
Clinical Specialist, Critical Care and Nutrition
  Support
Regional Medical Center
Memphis, Tennessee

Melanie P. Swims, PharmD, BCPS
Associate Professor of Clinical Pharmacy
University of Tennessee Health Science Center
Clinical Pharmacy Specialist, Ambulatory Care
Veterans Affairs Medical Center
Memphis, Tennessee

Laura A. Thoma, PharmD
Professor of Pharmaceutical Sciences
University of Tennessee Health Science Center
Memphis, Tennessee

Camille W. Thornton, PharmD
Associate Professor of Clinical Pharmacy
University of Tennessee Health Science Center
Clinical Pharmacy Specialist, Primary
  Care–HIV
Regional Medical Center
Memphis, Tennessee

J. Aubrey Waddell, PharmD, BCOP, FAPhA
Professor of Clinical Pharmacy
University of Tennessee Health Science Center
Oncology Pharmacist
Blount Memorial Hospital
Maryville, Tennessee

Junling Wang, PhD
Associate Professor of Clinical Pharmacy
University of Tennessee Health Science Center
Memphis, Tennessee

G. Christopher Wood, PharmD, FCCP,
  FCCM, BCPS
Associate Professor of Clinical Pharmacy
University of Tennessee Health Science Center
Memphis, Tennessee

Charles R. Yates, PharmD, PhD
Professor of Pharmaceutical Sciences and
  Ophthalmology
University of Tennessee Health Science Center
Memphis, Tennessee

+63,000 Strong!

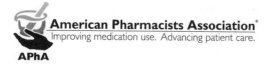

American Pharmacists Association®
Improving medication use. Advancing patient care.

APhA

Being A Pharmacist Means Being A Member of APhA

At every stage of your career or practice, membership in the American Pharmacists Association is a wise investment!

Membership in the American Pharmacists Association (APhA) is the simplest way to gain access to a solid support system to help you meet even the toughest career challenges. For more than 150 years, APhA has supported tens of thousands of pharmacists in their professional goals. Whether you're a current member or thinking of joining, we're here to support you today, so you'll be prepared for tomorrow!

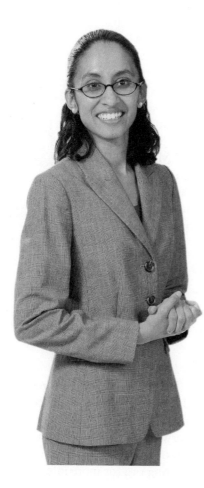

"As a student I learned of all APhA can offer its members, which led me to become more passionate about my profession and about getting involved. These opportunities have helped me grow as a participating pharmacist..."

—Sheena Patel, PharmD
Community Chain Pharmacist
Carlisle, Pennsylvania
APhA Member Since 2010

APhA has all the resources you need to succeed!

APhA supports you every step of the way as you begin your career in pharmacy. From programs and benefits to help you find the perfect job and become more marketable to potential employers to management and leadership information, training programs, and the latest in pharmacy news, APhA wants to be your primary resource!

Look to APhA to help you with the issues you face every day: new perspectives on drug therapy and disease state management, changing laws and regulations, and pressing decisions related to clinical and practice management. Membership in APhA gives you easy access to the tools you need to connect with like-minded pharmacists from across the country—working to improve medication use and advance patient care.

Strengthen Your Career

Through the **New Practitioners Network**, pharmacists in their first three years of practice enjoy discounted dues and special programming and information to help them get started in their careers. APhA members enjoy opportunities designed to increase professional knowledge and keep up with the latest information. You can take advantage of extensive benefits—to name just a few:

- APhA provides a variety of **Career Development Tools** to help you navigate your career—the **Pathway Program**; career development publications; and access to **APhA's Career Center**, an online resource featuring hundreds of job listings.
- **APhA Community-based Pharmacy Residency Program** fosters the development of formal postgraduate education and training experiences for pharmacists in innovative pharmacy practice to meet the challenges presented by the rapidly changing health care system, the implementation of pharmaceutical care, the explosion of drug and therapeutics information, and the needs of society for improving patient care and monitoring therapeutic outcomes.
- **APhA's Educational Library** links you to more than 80 CPE opportunities, all free to members. **Advanced training programs** include Pharmacy-Based Travel Health Services and APhA Advanced Preceptor Training, publications, drug information resources, and more.
- **Student loan refinancing through Credible.** Get instant offers for student loan refinancing from top lenders. Members receive an $86 credit toward APhA membership when they activate a loan through Credible.
- **APhA Certificate Training Programs** such as Delivering Medication Therapy Management Services, Pharmacy-Based Cardiovascular Disease Risk Management and more, provide nationally and regionally conducted practice-based education and training sessions designed to promote quality pharmaceutical care services and expand the pharmacist's role as a health care provider.
- A 20% discount for APhA members is available when ordering APhA books and electronic products at **Shop APhA**. Members also receive discounts

on education training, and APhA's Annual Meeting. Visit www.pharmacist.com for more details!

Advance Patient Care

The more you learn about drug and treatment updates, the better equipped you are to help your patients. APhA is a vital source of information, delivering resources to you in a variety of convenient ways:

- **Pharmacist.com**, the one-stop online resource, fulfills your information needs
- *Journal of the American Pharmacists Association (JAPhA)* in print or online AND the online *Journal of Pharmaceutical Sciences (JPharmSci)*
- *Pharmacy Today*, the monthly medication therapy management (MTM) magazine, *Pharmacy Today* daily newsletter, or select *Pharmacy Today* Health System Edition

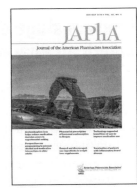

- *DrugInfoLine* delivers the latest in drug therapy developments in a digital format
- *Transitions* is a special e-newsletter for new practitioners, postgraduate students, and residents

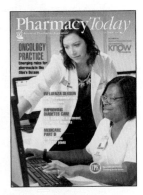

- **MTM Central** puts comprehensive information on the clinical and business aspects of MTM within easy reach online and allows access to our **MTM e-Community**, as a benefit of membership

Engage With the Community of Pharmacists

Through your membership in APhA, you can network with others in your field. No one understands your professional life better than your APhA colleagues. There are many ways to connect with your peers:

- **APhA's Annual Meeting & Exposition**, where attendees take advantage of more than 80 core education sessions, a state-of-the-art exposition, and the opportunity to network with 7,000 of your peers. Join us annually at our Annual Meeting & Exposition, visit aphameeting.org for more information.

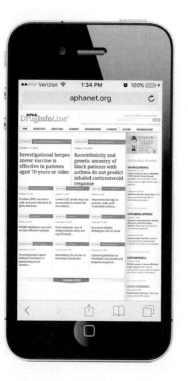

- APhA's networking sites on **LinkedIn, Facebook,** and **Pharmacist.com** to meet members online from your state or from across the country. ENGAGE, a members' exclusive online community featuring the APhA New Practitioner Network Community and nine APhA-APPM Special Interest Groups (SIGs).
- **APhA's Academies** provide invigorating networking opportunities through the **APhA Academy of Pharmacy Practice and Management (APhA-APPM)** and the **APhA Academy of Pharmaceutical Research and Science (APhA-APRS).** Most likely you are currently or have been a member of APhA's **Academy of Student Pharmacists (APhA-ASP)** and are acquainted with the many valuable benefits of belonging to a like-minded group of dedicated professionals.

Advocate for Your Profession

APhA serves as the unified voice of pharmacists and is the only organization representing pharmacists in all practice settings. APhA works to do the following:

- Through the **APhA Pharmacists Provide Care** initiative, APhA promotes patient access to pharmacists' services. Achieving "provider status" recognition is crucial to the pharmacy profession and the key to expanding professional opportunities for pharmacists. Visit PharmacistsProvideCare.com for more details.

Did You Receive This Book for FREE?

Congratulations—you are receiving this publication as a benefit of your membership in the American Pharmacists Association (APhA)!* *APhA is proud to provide* The APhA Complete Review for Pharmacy *to you.* Over the years, thousands of student pharmacist members have used earlier editions of this publication to study for and pass their NAPLEX exams.

"*The APhA Complete Review for Pharmacy* is fantastic because it is a review of everything that I learned in pharmacy school, *all in one place,*" said APhA Member Gretchen Kreckel Garofoli, PharmD, BCACP, Clinical Assistant Professor, Department of Clinical Pharmacy, West Virginia University School of Pharmacy. "The questions at the end of each chapter prepared me for the types of questions that I encountered on the NAPLEX exam."

"I still go back and reference the book today because I know that the information is easy to find and accurate. I always emphasize the book as **just one of the many benefits of APhA membership** to my students when we discuss the boards and prepare for them. **This resource is second to none!**"

APhA is there for you at every stage of your pharmacy career, offering you valuable member benefits just like this one. If you haven't yet renewed your membership, do so today by logging into your member profile at **www.pharmacist.com**.

If you aren't an APhA member, what else are you missing out on? Find out by visiting www.pharmacist.com/JoinAPhA.

*APhA offers *The APhA Complete Review for Pharmacy* to eligible final-year student pharmacist members who joined APhA prior to October 31st, and ordered and paid a shipping/handling fee prior to December 31st.

- Keep pharmacists informed of new developments in health care legislation and regulation including the steps necessary to implement recognition and reform through the **Get Involved** section of pharmacist.com and the members-only newsletter *APhA Legislative and Regulatory Update.*
- Enhance pharmacists' professional development through the **APhA Advocacy Key Contact Network**. To ensure our voices are heard, APhA provides support to volunteer leaders to help spread the word on pharmacy issues and get the attention of legislators.

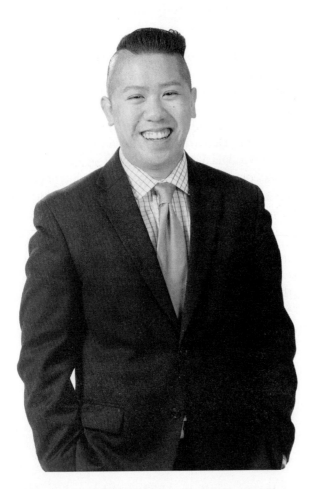

"Whether I am developing connections with new colleagues, taking advantage of CE and learning resources, or participating in advocacy work, APhA constantly provides me with avenues in which to better myself and the profession as a whole. Because I was able to benefit from leadership and training opportunities at APhA, I am a better pharmacist and better health care provider."

—Jonathan Lee, PharmD
Pharmacy Manager
Southampton, New York
APhA Member Since 2011

Proclaim Your Professionalism

As a member of APhA, you'll join more than 63,000 pharmacy professionals, declaring your pride in pharmacy's activities and achievements. Your membership dues help to support work that benefits the entire profession such as

- APhA's **advocacy efforts** on health care reform and other pending legislation and regulations that affect the profession. APhA works hard to increase policy makers' understanding of how pharmacists are integral to patients' continued health and well-being.
- APhA's concerted activities to promote the **importance of pharmacists** and the professional role you play in improving medication use and advancing patient care.

We are here to serve you! Whenever you have a question about your membership or want more information about any of APhA's many benefits, please contact an APhA Member Services representative by phone at 800-237-2742 x2 or e-mail at infocenter@aphanet.org.

If you're not currently a member of APhA, what are you waiting for?

Join APhA today, and take the first step toward a successful and rewarding career tomorrow! Whether you're looking to interact with other like-minded professionals, explore additional topics in pharmacy, or keep up with the latest pharmacy news, information, and trends, be sure to visit us online to *renew or activate* your membership. If you've never had a membership with APhA, *join now* so that you, too, can have the quality resources necessary to stay competitive with those who already enjoy being a part of APhA.

4 Easy Ways to Join

Web:	www.pharmacist.com/Join
Toll-free:	800-237-2742 x2
Fax:	1-240-554-2367
Mail:	Fill out the application found online and return it to **Membership Department American Pharmacists Association 9050 Junction Drive Annapolis Junction, MD, 20701-0411**

If you are reinstating your membership, please include your member number on the application.

Study Guide for the Exams

Peter A. Chyka

1-1. Key Points

■ The NAPLEX and MPJE are comprehensive exams that are based on competencies established by the National Association of Boards of Pharmacy for licensure to practice as a pharmacist.

■ Establish a routine of a positive attitude, steady preparation, and adequate practice in studying for the exams during a period of several months before the exam date.

■ Use the opportunity to take the Pre-NAPLEX exam to become familiar with navigating in the computerized format, experience the type of questions, and assess your stamina for a 6-hour exam.

■ In reviewing the chapters of *The APhA Complete Review for Pharmacy*, perform a self-assessment of your knowledge.

■ Be mindful of distractions and stress, and maintain your focus on the exams.

1-2. Introduction

Think of yourself as an elite athlete or an accomplished musician for a moment. Would you wait until the week before a competition or performance to begin training or practicing? Would you focus only on your mind and not include your body? Would you neglect knowing the rule book or the sheet music? Would you check your smartphone periodically while

Editor's Note: This chapter is based on the 10th edition study guide written by James C. Eoff III. Information about the exams was updated in August 2016 for this printing.

practicing? Would you rely only on what you remember to do without the benefit of a coach or trainer? Successful athletes and musicians train for months, focus on mind and body, avoid distractions, and look to coaches to find strengths and weaknesses. You might still be competitive and accomplished with your natural abilities, but the odds are working against you without a proper conditioning and training period. This same attitude should translate to your preparation for the NAPLEX and MPJE. Throughout your pharmacy curriculum, you have already been road tested and have not only learned facts and skills, but you should have developed learning and study habits that were successful for you. Now is the time to apply what you have learned about yourself to successfully pass the NAPLEX and MPJE by considering attitude, preparation, and practice.

1-3. Attitude

Begin with and maintain a positive attitude. Nearly 90% of first-time test takers pass the NAPLEX, but they don't just show up and pass. Unlike most tests in a single course that are like sprints of a discrete collection of knowledge, the NAPLEX is akin to a marathon covering years of a large body of knowledge. Adjust your attitude and habits accordingly. Consider creating a schedule for study at least 4–5 months before the exam date. Devote some of your best time of the day to studying; do not just fit your studying in whenever. Some of us are morning people, others are night people, and some can adjust to any time. Like an athlete or musician, focus on the material during your study time, because studying is more efficient and effective without distractions or multitasking.

Distractions and lack of focus make it easy to procrastinate. Develop a personal system and routine leading up to the exam. There is no doubt that the months leading up to the NAPLEX will be stressful at times for all sorts of reasons. Be sure to routinely use relaxation techniques that you find helpful, such as exercise, listening to music, playing a musical instrument, working on a hobby, playing electronic games, or watching a TV show. Write down your goal for the next study session the night before; this practice may help relieve anxiety and allow you to relax. Just don't fall victim to stress-relief time eclipsing study time—you might just exacerbate your stress level. Positively look forward to reviewing material for the NAPLEX and MPJE. You might be surprised by what you remember from your curriculum that just needs some reinforcement. Your self-confidence will be also be reinforced to move on to the next topic. Admittedly, the scope and breadth of information and skills are broad and deep, but these are things that you will need to know in varying degrees as you start your career as a pharmacist. It can also be a time of discovery of things that were not quite clear the first time; but now you have an opportunity to put the pieces of the puzzle together. By keeping to a schedule to review 3–4 chapters a week and by maintaining a list of things to go over again, you will have time to address problem areas. Don't kid yourself and foolishly fail to adequately prepare for the NAPLEX. If self-study isn't sufficient to clear up a concept, ask a colleague or instructor for advice. Consider the Key Points, Study Guide Checklist, and practice questions as a self-assessment and guide to focus your follow-up of the material.

1-4. Preparation

The Rule Books

Before you start studying, take some time to review the guidance, rules, and description of the NAPLEX provided by the organization conducting the exam—the National Association of Boards of Pharmacy (NABP). The NABP Web site's section on the NAPLEX and MPJE (www.nabp.net/programs/examination/naplex) has critical information about exam procedures and policies, content areas, question format, and other important information. Each year, NABP produces the *NAPLEX/MPJE Candidate Registration Bulletin,* which is essential for you to download (www.nabp.net/programs/examination/naplex) and review. This publication will help you focus your attention on the exam and describe essential procedures from start to finish. Be sure to know the rules and follow the guidance provided by the NABP. With a metaphor to an athletic competition, an athlete may be the fastest and strongest, but if he or she fails to know and follow the rules then that athlete will not successfully finish or even compete.

The Playing Fields

Effective November 1, 2016, the NAPLEX consists of 250 (previously 185) multiple-choice questions of which 50 (previously 35) questions are evaluated for future use, distributed throughout the exam, and not used in exam scoring. The exam is administered as a linear form exam, which means the questions are pre-assembled prior to the start of the exam. Each exam is unique and comprised of questions from varying levels of difficulty. Recent past exams used a computer adaptive format, which ceased November 1, 2016. The exam lasts 6 (previously 4.25) hours, which averages about 1.5 minutes per question. Some questions will take more or less time, but the time period is sufficient for you to answer all questions. Preparation and practice will allow you to answer the easier questions in less time so you may devote more time to more challenging ones.

There are several question formats on the NAPLEX. *You cannot skip a question nor can you return to it later.*

1. Multiple-choice question with a single answer out of 4–5 possible responses, for example:

   Which of the following is the agent of choice for the initial treatment of contact dermatitis, whether irritant or allergic?

   A. Topical antihistamine
   B. Oral antihistamine
   C. Topical corticosteroid
   D. Local anesthetic
   E. Coal tar product

2. Multiple-response question, which is followed by a phrase similar to "Select ALL that apply," for which there is no partial credit, for example:

   Isotretinoin adverse effects may include which of the following?

   (Select ALL that apply.)

   A. Cheilitis
   B. Hypertriglyceridemia
   C. Photosensitivity
   D. Muscle and joint pain
   E. Cardiac arrhythmias

3. Constructed-response question where a value is typically entered, for example:

   How much dextrose is required to prepare 500 mL of an aqueous 10% solution? (Answer must be numeric: Round the final answer to the nearest WHOLE number.)

   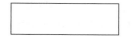

4. Ordered-response question, where the choices are ranked by dragging an option to the appropriate rank position, for example:

   Rank the following β-blockers from shortest to longest half-life. (ALL options must be used.)

Unordered options	Ordered response
Betaxolol	
Carteolol	
Bisoprolol	
Acebutolol	

5. Hot-spot question where the response is marked on a location of a diagram using the cursor to mark the spot following the directions for doing so, for example:

   Using the diagram below, identify the site of action of furosemide in the nephron.

   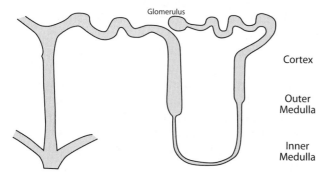

6. Scenario-based questions are typically associated with a patient profile or medical record. The scenario will be in a separate window on the same screen for one or more questions. The questions refer to the scenario or are stand-alone questions related to the scenario. Because the entire scenario may not be fully displayed in the window, the image can be moved within the window with the cursor to review the complete scenario. Use the scrap paper provided to write down significant points from the scenario, such as allergies, age, preexisting diseases, pregnancy, nursing, and age for the likelihood of pregnancy. Review the scenario first to also look for the potential of a drug allergy, duplicate therapy, contraindication, or adverse drug effect. Medications may appear with trade or generic names.

The MPJE is a 2.5-hour, computer-based exam composed of 120 multiple-choice questions where 20 questions are evaluated for future use. Each exam is individualized on the basis of the candidate's responses to questions using computer-adaptive technology to select questions from a question bank. Three exam formats are used in the MPJE, as follows.

1. Multiple-choice question with a single answer typically out of 4 possible responses, for example:

   How many times may a Schedule III controlled substance be refilled if authorized?

   A. No refills allowed
   B. Five refills within six months from the date the prescription was issued
   C. Five refills within six months from the date the prescription was originally filled
   D. Five refills within one year from the date the prescription was issued

2. Multiple-response question, which is followed by a phrase similar to "Select ALL that apply," for example:

   Who must be notified if your pharmacy had a robbery of controlled substances? (Select ALL that apply.)

   A. State board of pharmacy
   B. Drug Enforcement Administration (DEA)
   C. County health department
   D. Local law enforcement

3. Ordered-response question where the choices are ranked by dragging an option to the appropriate rank position, for example:

   Rank the penalties for unlawful sale of the following drugs from the most severe to the least severe as in length of jail time and amount of fine. (ALL options must be used. Left-click the mouse to highlight, drag, and order the answer options.)

Unordered options	Ordered response
Heroin	
Propranolol	
Demerol	
Alprazolam	

The Play Book

The NAPLEX tests for two general domains of competency, referred to as *The NAPLEX Blueprint,* which is included in the *NAPLEX/MPJE Candidate Registration Bulletin* (www.nabp.net/programs/examination/naplex). The 2016 *Candidate Registration Bulletin* describes the competency domains as follows:

■ Area 1: Ensure Safe and Effective Pharmacotherapy and Health Outcomes (approximately 67% of test)
■ Area 2: Safe and Accurate Preparation, Compounding, Dispensing, and Administration of Medications and Provision of Health Care Products (approximately 33% of test)

The MPJE is based on competencies related to the following three domains as described in the 2016 *NAPLEX/MPJE Candidate Registration Bulletin:*

■ Area 1: Pharmacy Practice (approximately 83% of test)
■ Area 2: Licensure, Registration, Certification, and Operational Requirements (approximately 15% of test)
■ Area 3: General Regulatory Process (approximately 2% of test)

The distribution of the domains should guide your emphasis for review and study. The content of *The APhA Complete Review for Pharmacy* reflects these areas of emphasis.

Priorities for Review

The following suggested strategies provide some guidance on priorities for review. Several areas are not high priorities for review because they are not emphasized in the current NAPLEX, such as the manufacturer of a drug product, chemical structures, and identification or physical descriptions (e.g., color, shape) of the drug product. The emphasis is greater on patient-oriented competencies.

Generic and trade names: Although generic products are widely used, there are many drugs with trade names in practice and in the NAPLEX. Generic or trade names can appear in the scenarios, questions, and response options for the different question formats. It is critical to review the generic and trade names for commonly used or unique medications. If you are not familiar with these names, it could be impossible to comprehend the question or responses.

Math: Pharmacy math is another critical area to review. Must-know information includes conversion factors among the systems of measurement, math for compounding typical dosage forms such as topical, solutions and intravenous preparations, and basic elements of statistics. Be careful to take notice of the units of measure and decimal points in any math problem and calculations. By making this area a high priority for study, the calculations on the exam should be second nature and unambiguous. With care, the questions can be answered confidently straightaway, thereby conserving time for more complicated questions.

Dosage schedules: The frequency of use has greater emphasis in the competencies than specific dosages. Be able to recognize that a medication is administered in a divided schedule during the day, once a day, or at greater intervals such as monthly or yearly.

Classes of drugs: Focus on a review of medications within a class of drugs, such as β-adrenergic blockers, calcium-channel antagonists, angiotensin-converting enzyme inhibitors and angiotensin II receptor blockers, benzodiazepines, cephalosporins, quinolones, aminoglycosides, nonsteroidal anti-inflammatory drugs, histamine-2 blockers, protease inhibitors, oral diabetic medications, and statins. Be able to recognize drugs within these categories, the general indications, contraindications, adverse effects, and drug interactions for the class, and the different characteristics of a drug within the category, such as duration of action, dosage schedules, unique adverse effects, and preference for certain diseases.

Patient counseling and warning labels: In the review of drug classes, recognize specific points for patient counseling, particularly about possible untoward effects, duration of therapy, and special handling, in addition to the general counseling advice. Also consider if warning labels may be necessary, such as refrigerate, avoid hazardous activities, or shake well.

Chronic and common diseases: Focus on the more common and chronic diseases and their therapy. A general knowledge of the disease process is important, but avoid focusing the majority of study time on detailed disease characteristics, such as etiology, pathophysiology, diagnosis, and signs and symptoms at the expense of drug and nondrug therapy. To evaluate a patient scenario, knowledge of basic laboratory tests and their normal values is important. The NAPLEX is heavily weighted toward drug therapy as indicated by the competencies, but also be aware of the effects of healthy lifestyle habits on disease prevention and management.

General guidance on content: The NAPLEX is heavily weighted toward drug therapy as indicated by the competencies. As a general guide, you should be familiar with the following information regarding drug therapy and should focus your study time on areas of weakness or unfamiliarity.

- What is the therapeutic category or categories of this drug?
- What is the basic mechanism of action?
- What type of patient counseling information should be provided?
- What are the major adverse effects (side effects and toxic effects)?
- What is the dosage schedule (frequency)?
- What are the major drug interactions and disease contraindications?

Exam-Taking Advice

The following list contains suggestions for test taking that after years of college coursework should be second nature.

1. Read directions carefully, and read questions at least twice to be sure of the nature of the question. Note any modifying terms such as *always, all, never, most,* or *usually;* any double negatives; and anything else about the way the question is worded that may change the meaning of the question and your response.
2. Review the case scenario first (briefly, but fully) and then refer back to scenario for specific facts for each question associated with the scenario.
3. Read all the answer options thoroughly, and eliminate the obvious distractors or incorrect answers. Typically two to three options can be eliminated for one or more reasons, and the final choice is between two answers. Select the *single best answer* for the multiple-choice format. Be cautious about reading multiple possibilities into questions, because most questions should be straightforward. If you simply do not know the answer, eliminate any distractors and guess intelligently from the remaining options.
4. Pace yourself, but do not rush through the exam. The 6 hours scheduled for the NAPLEX should be more than adequate for most candidates to complete the exam. Proceed at a reasonable pace, and answer approximately 40–45 questions per hour to finish comfortably

in the time available. A timer is displayed on the computer screen for your information. If only 25–35 questions are completed in the first hour, you should increase your speed.
5. If you feel that you have made a mistake on a previous question, don't dwell on it, but move on to the next question. As it relates to the musician metaphor, all musicians make mistakes in a performance, but they don't stop. They continue to the end of the song. A performance will not be judged by a few errors nor will that be the case for your performance on the NAPLEX or MPJE. Since the NAPLEX contains 50 unscored questions being tested for suitability on a future exam and 200 scored questions, there is no way to determine if you made a mistake on a scored or unscored question.

The Venue

Testing center location: If you are not familiar with or have never been to the exact location of the testing center, locate it (better to actually visit) at least the day before the exam. Arrive at the testing site at least 30 minutes before the scheduled time so you can comfortably register and get settled. You do not want to be caught in traffic or get lost on the way to the testing center and panic before taking the exam.

Hours before the exam: Avoid studying the day and evening before the exam—last-minute cramming may cause anxiety and affect your performance. On the evening before the exam, do something relaxing. Like an athlete, keep to your regular sleeping schedule and eating habits. On the day of the exam, eat breakfast (a healthy one). If your exam is scheduled in the afternoon, be on guard against fatigue by having a light lunch and adequate, but not excessive, hydration. (Hint: If you find that you are becoming tired during the exam, check your posture to assure that you are sitting up straight—you may become more alert as your lungs can more effectively ventilate and oxygenate when you are not slouching.) Then go to the testing center like an athlete and musician, and perform at your best.

1-5. Practice

As any athlete or musician will tell you, "practice, practice, practice leads to good performance." The same is true for the NAPLEX and MPJE. Earlier general practices such as devote your best time, start early, create a routine, avoid distractions, keep a steady pace of studying, and self-assess your weaknesses and strengths in the competencies tested in the exams will serve you well.

Weekly Review

In *The APhA Complete Review for Pharmacy,* review the tables of the major categories of drugs, including the table of antidotes. Look for the generic and trade names, commonly available dosage forms, and frequency of use. Develop a method to review generic and trade names. If you work in a pharmacy or are on a pharmacy rotation, ask the pharmacist or pharmacy technician to quiz you on the generic or trade name of medications in a section of the pharmacy stock of medications. Perhaps even reverse the roles and be the quizzer. Look at the container before and after the quiz. On a computer, smartphone, or tablet, perform a Web or app search with a term like *generic and brand name drug quiz* and find a program that allows you to quiz yourself during a spare moment throughout the day and week. Just be sure you are using a U.S. site that is relatively current, because trade names may change (often for drug safety reasons) and can be different in another country.

Pre-NAPLEX

The NABP offers a tremendous opportunity to take two practice exams that simulate the NAPLEX testing experience (see www.nabp.net/programs/examination/pre-naplex). It is well worth the small fee to take the 100-question, 140-minute practice exam to become familiar with navigating in the computerized format, experience the type of questions, and assess your stamina to be able to sit in front of a computer for 2 hours for test taking. The content is not in the current version of the NAPLEX, so the score is not particularly relevant to success in the NAPLEX. The Pre-NAPLEX can be taken on any computer with an Internet connection. Take one version early in your preparation for the NAPLEX, and consider taking the other version a month before the NAPLEX exam date.

Self-assessment

As you review the chapters of *The APhA Complete Review for Pharmacy,* perform a self-assessment of your knowledge by responding to the questions at the end of each chapter. These questions can be supplemented by additional questions found in the NAPLEX Review section of the APhA Pharmacy Library (http://pharmacylibrary.com). To make your learning experience more effective, study the expla-

nations for the correct response. Also note the distractors, and learn why they are incorrect.

1-6. Conclusion

The NAPLEX and MPJE are comprehensive in scope and are not easy exams. By adopting and maintaining a positive attitude, steady preparation, and adequate practice, the exam will be less stressful and the likelihood of your success on first attempt will be improved. Consider some principles about how your brain works from John Medina's book, *Brain Rules.*

Rule #1: Exercise boosts brain power.
Rule #3: Every brain is wired differently.
Rule #5: Repeat to remember (short-term memory).
Rule #6: Remember to repeat (long-term memory).
Rule #7: Sleep well, think well.
Rule #8: Stressed brains don't learn the same way.
Rule #9: Stimulate more of the senses (multisensory learning).

Review all 12 of the principles on the *Brain Rules* Web site (http://brainrules.net/about-brain-rules).

In conclusion, the contributors to *The APhA Complete Review for Pharmacy* hope that this publication will assist in your preparation for and your successful completion of the licensure exams to practice as a pharmacist. By imagining yourself as an elite athlete or accomplished musician preparing for a competition or a performance, you will become an accomplished professional—a pharmacist ready to perform at the highest level of practice.

1-7. References

Barker, E. 6 things the most productive people do every day. Barking Up the Wrong Tree (blog), June 1, 2014. Available at: www.bakadesuyo.com/2014/06/most-productive-people.

Medina J. *Brain Rules: 12 Principles for Surviving and Thriving at Work, Home, and School.* Seattle: Pear Press; 2008.

National Association of Boards of Pharmacy. *NAPLEX/MPJE 2016 Candidate Registration Bulletin.* Mount Prospect, IL.: National Association of Boards of Pharmacy; 2016. Available at: http://www.nabp.net/programs/examination/naplex/registration-bulletin.

NABP Newsletter. *New NAPLEX to launch in November 2016* Mount Prospect, IL: National Association of Boards of Pharmacy; March 2016. Available at: https://www.nabp.net/system/rich/rich_files/rich_files/000/001/302/original/march2016nabpnewsletter.pdf

Pharmacy Math 2

Michael L. Christensen

2-1. Key Points

- Pharmacy math is used daily for preparing prescriptions, determining required doses, and measuring the weight or volume of a drug.
- Pay close attention to units: the dose of a drug may be mcg/kg/min, the drug concentration in mg/mL, and the infusion rate in ml/h.
- Know the International System of Units (SI) and the relative value of the prefixes.

2-2. Study Guide Checklist

The following topics may guide your study of this subject area:

- Math calculations include ratio and proportion, enlarging, reducing, alligation, aliquot, dilution, and concentration.
- Dosing can be based on body weight or body surface area, especially in children.
- Conversion of drug concentrations may be among percentage strength, ratio strength, and weight per volume (e.g., mg/mL or mcg/dL).
- Use specific gravity to measure volume by weighing a solution.
- Calculate doses using SI and other systems of measure such as the apothecary system and common household measures.
- Perform calculations of isotonicity, osmolarity, milliequivalents, and milliosmoles.

Editor's Note: This chapter is based on the 10th edition chapter written by Hassan Almoazen.

2-3. Units of Measure

Calculations in pharmacy may involve four different systems of measure: the metric system, the apothecaries' system, the avoirdupois system, and the household system.

Metric System

The fundamental units of the metric system are the gram, the liter, and the meter. Prefixes are used extensively to express quantities much greater and much less than the fundamental units. Some of the most commonly used prefixes are provided in Table 2-1.

Apothecaries' System

Although the metric system is the official system of measure for pharmacy today, the apothecaries' system is the traditional system, and some elements might be found in prescriptions. Units of the apothecaries' system are presented in Table 2-2.

Avoirdupois System

The avoirdupois system of measure for weight is used in ordinary commerce. Here, the ounce corresponds to 437.5 grains. The avoirdupois grain unit is equal to the apothecaries' grain unit. Sixteen ounces (7,000 grains) correspond to 1 pound. Note that the avoirdupois ounce (437.5 grains) and pound (7,000 grains) measures are not equal to the apothecaries' ounce (480 grains) and pound (5,760 grains) measures.

Table 2-1. Metric System Prefixes

Prefix	Meaning
mega-	one million times the base unit (10^6)
kilo-	one thousand times the base unit (10^3)
deci-	one-tenth the base unit (10^{-1})
centi-	one-hundredth the base unit (10^{-2})
milli-	one-thousandth the base unit (10^{-3})
micro-	one-millionth the base unit (10^{-6})
nano-	one-billionth the base unit (10^{-9})
pico-	one-trillionth the base unit (10^{-12})

(handwritten annotations: "1 mg/1000 Km" near mega-; "1 mL/1000 μm, 1000, 1 μm/100" near milli-/micro-; "mm, μm, nm, pico" in left margin)

Table 2-2. Apothecaries' System of Measure

Weight	Volume
20 grains = 1 scruple	60 minims = 1 fluid dram
3 scruples = 1 dram	8 fluid drams = 1 fluid ounce
8 drams = 1 ounce	16 fluid ounces = 1 pint
12 ounces = 1 pound	2 pints = 1 quart
	4 quarts = 1 gallon

Household Measures

A tablespoon is equivalent to 15 mL, and a teaspoon is equivalent to 5 mL.

Conversion Factors

A short list of convenient conversion factors follows:

1 inch = 2.54 cm
1 fl oz = 29.57 mL
1 g = 15.4 grains
1 kg = 2.20 lb (avoirdupois)
1 lb (avoirdupois) = 454 g
1 gal (U.S.) = 3,785 mL

2-4. Significant Figures

All measured quantities are approximations. The accuracy of a given measurement is conveyed by the number of figures that are recorded. The number of significant figures in a measurement includes the first approximate figure. The last recorded digit to the right of a measured quantity is taken to be an approximation. For example, the weight 13.24 g has four significant figures, and the final digit, 4, is approximate. Calculations should be conducted to carry the correct numbers of significant figures.

Frequently, the different quantities in a given calculation have different numbers of significant figures. When that occurs, the following rules apply.

Addition and Subtraction

When adding or subtracting decimal numbers, round all measurements so that they have the same number of decimal places as the least in the set. For example, 13.78 mL and 53.5 mL would be added as 13.8 mL + 53.5 mL = 67.3 mL, using and retaining only one decimal place.

Multiplication and Division

When multiplying or dividing decimal numbers, round the measurements to include the number of significant figures contained in the least accurate number. For example, 25.678 mL × 1.24 g/mL would be multiplied as 25.7 mL × 1.24 g/mL = 31.9 g, using and retaining three significant figures in each number.

Handling Zero

The digit zero may or may not be counted as a significant figure, depending on where it appears in the measured number. If zero occurs at an interior position in the number (e.g., 3,052 or 2.031), it is significant. If zero occurs as the last digit to the right of the decimal (e.g., 44.50), it is significant. If zero occurs as the first digit to the right of the decimal in a number that is less than 1, it is not significant. For example, in 0.078 there are only two significant figures. If zero occurs as the last digit, or digits, in a whole number (i.e., no decimal is expressed), its significance is unknown without further information. For example, 3,500 might have two, three, or four significant figures.

From a medication safety perspective, never use trailing zeros for drug doses expressed as a whole number (1.0 mg can be mistaken as 10 mg: use 1 mg). Always use a zero before the decimal point when the drug dose is less than 1 (.1 mg may be mistaken as 1 mg: use 0.1 mg).

2-5. Ratios and Proportions

Most dosage calculations in pharmacy use ratios and proportions. A ratio is used to convey the relationship between two quantities, and a proportion involves a relationship among four quantities. You can always solve for one of those quantities when the other three are known. If the ratio x/y is equal to the ratio a/b, then the proportion $x/y = a/b$ exists, and x can be obtained by algebraic manipulation ($x = ay/b$). Such problems are frequently encountered when calculating doses.

One common source of error in proportion problems involves writing one of the ratios upside down (e.g., writing $x/y = b/a$, when it should be written $x/y = a/b$). A disciplined approach to setting up such problems can help. For example, you might establish a rule in which you express each ratio as the quotient of like quantities. If the numerator of one ratio is smaller (or larger) than its denominator, the same should be true of the other ratio.

Another source of error involves using mixed units (e.g., using one number expressed in grams and the other in milligrams). To guard against that kind of error, always write the units into the equation along with the numbers. All unit expressions should cancel except those required for the quantity being solved for (dimensional analysis).

Example: If 300 mL of a preparation contains 250 mg of drug, what weight of drug (x) is contained in 1,800 mL of the preparation?

Equate the ratios x: 250 mg and 1,800 mL: 300 mL to solve for x:

$$\frac{x}{250 \text{ mg}} = \frac{1,800 \text{ mL}}{300 \text{ mL}}$$

$$x = \frac{250 \text{ mg} \times 1,800 \text{ mL}}{300 \text{ mL}} = 1,500 \text{ mg}$$

Note that because the new volume is six times greater, the new weight should be six times greater as well.

2-6. Specific Gravity and Density

At times, you will be required to convert a volume measure to a weight measure, or vice versa. This process is used by parenteral nutrition–compounding devices that prepare multicomponent intravenous solutions. To convert a measure, you will need to use either the specific gravity or the density of the material. The specific gravity (SpGr) is a ratio of the weight of the material to the weight of the same volume of a standard material. For liquids, the standard material is water, which has a density of 1 g/mL. Specific gravity is unitless. Density is the quotient of any

measure of the weight of a sample of the material divided by any measure of the volume of the sample. The units must be explicitly expressed (e.g., g/mL, lb/gal, etc.). When density is expressed in grams per milliliter, it is numerically equal to specific gravity. Algebraically, density (weight/volume) is easier to work with than the corresponding expression for specific gravity.

Example: What are the volume and weight of 70% dextrose (D70) (SpGr = 1.24) that are required to prepare a parenteral nutrition solution that contains 210 g of dextrose?

$$\text{Volume D70} = 210 \text{ g} \div 0.7 \text{ g/mL} = 300 \text{ mL}$$

$$\text{Weight D70} = 300 \text{ mL} \times 1.24 = 372 \text{ g}$$

Thus, the parenteral nutrition compounder would weigh 372 g D70 to add 300 mL of D70 to provide 210 g of dextrose.

2-7. Percentage Error

Because all measurements are approximations, one must characterize the extent of error involved, or *percentage of error,* which is defined as

$$\% \text{ error} = \frac{(\text{error} \times 100\%)}{(\text{quantity desired})}$$

The term *error* in the numerator indicates the maximum potential error in the measurement (error = larger quantity − smaller quantity), while the term *quantity desired* in the denominator represents the total amount measured. Percentage of error may be calculated for either a weight or a volume measurement.

Example: A quantity of material weighs 5.81 g on a prescription balance. Using a much more accurate analytical balance, the quantity weighs 5.893 g. What is the percentage of error for the original weighing?

$$\text{error} = 5.893 \text{ g} - 5.810 \text{ g} = 0.083 \text{ g}$$

The quantity desired is 5.81 g. Thus,

$$\% \text{ error} = 0.083 \text{ g} \times \frac{100\%}{5.81} = 1.4\%$$

Example: Suppose you wish to weigh out 75 mg of an ingredient but mistakenly weigh 65 mg instead.

Based on the quantity desired, what is the percentage of error?

$$\% \text{ error} = \frac{(\text{error} \times 100\%)}{(\text{quantity desired})}$$

$$= \frac{(10 \text{ mg} \times 100\%)}{75 \text{ mg}} = 13\%$$

2-8. Minimum Measurable

By United States Pharmacopeia (USP) standards, weighing by a pharmacist cannot exceed a percentage of error greater than 5%, which requires that the sensitivity of the balance be known and limits the smallest quantity that can be weighed. *Balance sensitivity* is defined in terms of the *sensitivity requirement* (SR), which is the weight of material that will move the indicator one marked unit on the index plate of the balance. For a class A prescription balance, SR = 6 mg. The minimum weighable quantity for a given balance can be calculated using the percentage of error formula: replace the "error" term with the SR (e.g., 6 mg), replace the percentage of error term with 5%, and replace the "quantity desired" term with "minimum weighable quantity" as follows:

$$5\% = \frac{(\text{SR} \times 100\%)}{\text{minimum weighable quantity}}, \text{ or}$$

$$\text{minimum weighable quantity} = \frac{(\text{SR} \times 100\%)}{5\%}$$

$$120 \text{ mg} = \frac{(6 \text{ mg} \times 100\%)}{5\%}$$

Example: For a balance that has an SR of 4 mg, what is the minimum weighable quantity to ensure a percentage of error no greater than 2%?

$$\% \text{ error} = \frac{(\text{error} \times 100\%)}{\text{quantity desired}}$$

$$= \frac{\text{SR} \times 100\%}{\text{minimum weighable quantity}}$$

$$\text{minimum weighable quantity} = \frac{(\text{SR} \times 100\%)}{\% \text{ error}}$$

$$= 4 \text{ mg} \times \frac{100\%}{2\%}$$

$$= 200 \text{ mg}$$

Example: What is the SR for a balance with a percentage of error of 5% when weighing 120 mg?

$$\% \text{ error} = \frac{(\text{SR} \times 100\%)}{\text{quantity desired}}$$

$$\text{SR} = \frac{(\% \text{ error} \times \text{quantity desired})}{100\%}$$

$$= \frac{(5\% \times 120 \text{ mg})}{100\%} = 6 \text{ mg}$$

2-9. Patient-Specific Dosage Calculations

Drugs with a narrow therapeutic range often are dosed on the basis of patient weight or body surface area. For patients with renal impairment, some drugs are dosed on the basis of creatinine clearance.

Dosing Based on Body Weight

Weight-based dosing might involve using the patient's actual body weight (ABW), ideal body weight (IBW), or perhaps an adjusted ideal body weight that is a function of IBW and ABW. Those weights are invariably expressed in kilograms.

Example: A patient weighing 180 lb is to receive 0.25 mg/kg per day amphotericin B (reconstituted and diluted to 0.1 mg/mL) by intravenous (IV) infusion. What volume of solution is required to deliver the daily dose?

$$\text{patient weight} = \frac{180 \text{ lb}}{2.2} = 82 \text{ kg}$$

$$\text{daily dose} = 82 \text{ kg} \times 0.25 \text{ mg/kg}$$

$$= 20.5 \text{ mg}$$

$$= \frac{20.5 \text{ mg}}{0.1 \text{ mg/mL}} = 205 \text{ mL}$$

A commonly used equation for calculating IBW is

$$\text{IBW (kg)} = (\text{sex factor})$$

$$+ (2.3 \times \text{height in inches over 5 feet}),$$

where the sex factor for males is 50 and the sex factor for females is 45.5.

Example: The recommended adult daily dosage for patients with normal renal function for tobramycin is 3 mg/kg IBW given in three evenly divided doses. What would the dose of each injection be for a male patient who weighs 185 lb and is 5 feet 9 inches tall?

$$IBW\,(kg) = 50 + (2.3 \times 9) = 50 + 21$$
$$= 71\ kg\ (ignore\ ABW\ of\ 84\ kg)$$

$$daily\ dose\,(tid) = 71\ kg \times 3\ mg/kg = 213\ mg\,(per\ day)$$

Thus, each injection $= 213\ mg/3 = 71\ mg$

In the absence of other information, the usual drug doses are considered generally suitable for 70-kg individuals. Thus, in the absence of more specific information, an adjusted dosage for a notably larger or smaller individual may be obtained by multiplying the usual dose by the ratio of patient weight to 70 kg (Clark's rule).

Example: If the adult dose of a drug is 100 mg and no child-specific dosing information is available, what would the weight-adjusted dose be for a child who weighs 40 kg?

$$child\ dose = 100\ mg \times \frac{40\ kg}{70\ kg} = 57\ mg$$

Dosing Based on Body Surface Area

Dosing based on body surface area requires an estimation of the patient's body surface area (BSA) expressed in square meters (m^2). That parameter might be estimated from a nomogram using height and weight or, for adults, by using one of several equations such as the Mosteller equation:

$$BSA\,(m^2) = \left[\frac{height\,(cm) \times weight\,(kg)}{3,600} \right]^{1/2}$$

Example: What is the computed BSA for an adult who weighs 194 lb and is 5 feet 10 inches tall?

$$Height = 70\ inches \times 2.54\ cm/inch = 178\ cm$$

$$Weight = 194\ lb/2.2\ lb/kg = 88\ kg$$

$$BSA = \sqrt{\frac{178 \times 88}{3,600}} = 2.09\ m^2$$

The average adult BSA is taken to be 1.73 m^2. That value can be used to obtain an approximate child's dose, given the usual dose for an adult and the child's estimated BSA.

Example: If the adult dose of a drug is 50 mg, what would the BSA-adjusted dose be for a child having an estimated BSA of 0.55 m^2?

$$child\ dose = 50\ mg \times \frac{0.55\ m^2}{1.73\ m^2} = 16\ mg$$

Dosing Based on Creatinine Clearance

For many drugs, the rate of elimination depends on kidney function. With a decline in kidney function, there is a decrease in drug clearance. Creatinine clearance (CrCl) estimates kidney function as a measure of the volume of blood plasma that is cleared of creatinine by kidney filtration per minute, and it is expressed in milliliters per minute. CrCl can be calculated as a function of patient sex, age, body weight, and serum creatinine using the Cockcroft–Gault equation for adults and the Schwartz equation for children.

The Cockcroft–Gault equation for males:

$$CrCl\,(mL/min) = \frac{(140 - age\,[years]) \times body\ weight\,(kg)}{72 \times serum\ creatinine\,(mg/dL)}$$

For females:

$$CrCl = 0.85 \times CrCl\ for\ males$$

Example: Using the Cockcroft–Gault equation, calculate the creatinine clearance rate for a 76-year-old female weighing 65 kg and having a serum creatinine of 0.52 mg/dL.

$$CrCl = 0.85 \times (140 - 76\ years) \times \frac{65\ kg}{(72 \times 0.52\ mg/dL)}$$
$$= 94\ mL/min$$

The Schwartz equation:

$$CrCl\,(mL/min) = \frac{k \times height\,(cm)}{serum\ creatinine\,(mg/dL)}$$

Age	k
Premature infant < 1 year	0.33
Term infant < 1 year	0.45
Child or adolescent girl	0.55
Adolescent boy	0.7

The maintenance dose for some drugs is based on IBW and CrCl. See Chapter 7 for more detailed information.

2-10. Use of Batch Preparation Formulas

The relative amounts of ingredients in a pharmaceutical product are specified in a formula. A pharmacist may be required to reduce or enlarge the formula to prepare a lesser or greater amount of product. A given formula might specify either the actual amount (weight or volume) of each ingredient for a specified total amount of product or just the relative amount (part) of each ingredient. In the latter case, the ingredients must all be of the same measure (e.g., weight in grams).

Example: From the following lotion formula, calculate the quantity of triethanolamine required to make 200 mL of lotion.

Triethanolamine	10 mL
Oleic acid	25 mL
Benzyl benzoate	250 mL
Water ad	1,000 mL

$$\frac{x}{10 \text{ mL}} = \frac{200 \text{ mL}}{1,000 \text{ mL}}$$

$$x = \frac{200 \text{ mL}}{1,000 \text{ mL}} = 2 \text{ mL}$$

Example: From the following formula, calculate the quantity of chlorpheniramine maleate required to make 500 g of product.

Chlorpheniramine maleate	6 parts
Phenindamine	20 parts
Phenylpropanolamine HCl	55 parts

Note that the formula will give a total of 81 parts, which will correspond to the desired quantity of 500 g. Then,

$$\frac{x}{500 \text{ g}} = \frac{6 \text{ parts}}{81 \text{ parts}}$$

$$x = 500 \text{ g} \times \frac{6 \text{ parts}}{81 \text{ parts}} = 37 \text{ g}$$

2-11. Conventions in Expression of Concentration

Drug concentrations can be expressed in a variety of units. One must be prepared to calculate drug concentration units directly from their definitions and to interconvert among them.

Percentage Strength

Percentage, strictly speaking, specifies the number of parts per 100 parts. In pharmacy, percentage comes in three varieties:

- Percent weight-in-weight = % (w/w) = grams of ingredient in 100 grams of product (assumed for mixtures of solids and semisolids, e.g., ointment base)
- Percent volume-in-volume = % (v/v) = milliliters of ingredient in 100 milliliters of product (assumed for solutions or mixtures of liquids)
- Percent weight-in-volume = % (w/v) = grams of ingredient in 100 milliliters of product (assumed for solutions of solids in liquids)

Example: What is the concentration in % (w/v) for a preparation containing 250 mg of drug in 50 mL of solution? Note that % (w/v) is defined as g/100 mL. Thus,

$$\text{concentration} = 0.25 \text{ g} \times \frac{100}{50 \text{ mL}} = 0.5\% \text{ (w/v)}$$

Parts (Ratio Strength)

Concentrations may be expressed in "parts" or ratio strength when the active ingredient is highly diluted. Assumptions concerning (w/w), (v/v), and (w/v) ratios are identical to those for percentages.

Example: What is the concentration in % (v/v) of a solution that has a ratio strength of 1:2,500 (v/v)?

$$\frac{1 \text{ part}}{2,500 \text{ parts}} = \frac{x}{100\%}$$

$$x\% = \frac{100 \text{ parts}}{2,500 \text{ parts}} = 0.04\% \text{ (v/v)}$$

Millimoles

By definition, a 1 molar solution contains the molecular weight (MW) of the substance in grams per liter of solution. The molarity expresses the number of moles per liter. The millimolarity (millimoles/liter) is 1,000 times the molarity of a solution.

Example: What is the millimolar concentration of a solution consisting of 0.9 g of sodium chloride (MW = 58.5) in 100 mL of water? The quantity of 0.9 g in 100 mL corresponds to 9 g in 1,000 mL.

$$\text{molarity} = \frac{1 \text{ mole}}{1,000 \text{ mL}} = \left(9 \text{ g}/58.5 \text{ g/mole}\right)$$

$$= 0.154$$

$$\text{millimolarity} = 1,000 \times \text{molarity} = 154$$

Milliequivalents

A milliequivalent is a measure of the total number of ionic charges in a solution. The equivalent weight of an ion is the molecular weight of the ion divided by the valence. Thus, the equivalent weight of sodium ion, Na^+ (MW = 23, valence = 1), is 23 and for ferric ion, Fe^{3+} (MW = 55.9, valence = 3), 18.6. A milliequivalent is 1,000th of an equivalent weight (i.e., 1,000 milliequivalent weights equal 1 equivalent weight). For a molecule, the equivalent weight is obtained by dividing the molecular weight by the total valence of the positive or negative ion. For example, the equivalent weight of $MgCl_2$ (MW Mg^{++} = 24.3, valence = 2; MW Cl^- = 35.5, valence = 1) is (24.3 + 2 × 35.5)/2 = 47.7 g. Its milliequivalent weight is 0.0477 g, or 47.7 mg.

Example: What is the concentration, in milliequivalents per liter, of a solution containing 14.9 g of KCl (MW = 74.5 g) in 1 liter? Note that the valence of potassium is 1, so the equivalent weight equals the molecular weight. Accordingly,

$$\text{Equivalent weight KCl} = 74.5$$

$$1 \text{ mEq} = 74.5 \text{ mg}$$

$$14.9 \text{ g KCl} = 14,900 \text{ mg}$$

$$\frac{14,900 \text{ mg/L}}{74.5 \text{ mg/mEq}} = 200 \text{ mEq}$$

Example: What weight of $MgSO_4$ (MW = 120) is required to prepare 1 liter of a solution that is 25 mEq/L? The valence of Mg is 2+; therefore, the equivalent weight of $MgSO_4$ is 120/2 = 60 g. Accordingly, 60 mg corresponds to 1 mEq of $MgSO_4$. Then,

$$\frac{x}{60 \text{ mg}} = \frac{25 \text{ mEq}}{1 \text{ mEq}}$$

$$x = 25 \text{ mEq}/1 \text{ mEq} \times 60 \text{ mg}$$

$$x = 1,500 \text{ mg} = 1.5 \text{ g}$$

Example: How many milliequivalents of $CaCl_2$ are contained in 100 mL of a solution that is 5.0% (w/v)

(MW = 111, atomic weight of Ca^{2+} = 40, atomic weight of Cl^- = 35.5)? Note that the valence of calcium is 2+; therefore, the milliequivalent weight of $CaCl_2$ is 55.5 mg. The solution contains 5 g $CaCl_2$ per 100 mL, which corresponds to 5,000 mg/100 mL and 5,000 mg/55.5 mg/mEq = 90 mEq. Thus, 100 mL of the 5% $CaCl_2$ solution contains 90 mEq of Ca^{2+}.

Milliosmoles

Osmotic concentration is a measure of the total number of particles in solution and is expressed in milliosmoles (mOsm). The number of milliosmoles is based on the total number of cations *and* the total number of anions. The milliosmolarity of a solution is the number of milliosmoles per liter of solution (mOsm/L), where

$$\text{mOsm/L} = \text{moles/L} \times \text{number of species}$$

$$\times 1,000 \text{ mOsm/moles}$$

$$\text{number of species} = \text{number of ionic species}$$

$$\text{upon complete dissociation}$$

$$\text{dextrose} = 1 \text{ specie}$$

$$\text{NaCl} = 2 \text{ species}$$

$$\text{CaCl}_2 = 3 \text{ species}$$

The total osmolarity of a solution is the sum of the osmolarities of the solute components of the solution. When calculating osmolarities, in the absence of other information, assume that salts (e.g., NaCl, etc.) dissociate completely (referred to as the *ideal osmolarity*). You should be aware of the distinction between the terms *milliosmolarity* (milliosmoles per liter of solution) and *milliosmolality* (milliosmoles per kilogram of solution).

Example: What is the concentration, in milliosmoles per liter, of a solution that contains 224 mg of KCl (MW = 74.6 g) and 234 mg of NaCl (MW = 58.5) in 500 mL? What is the number of milliosmoles per liter of K^+ alone?

$$\frac{\text{mOsm KCl}}{500 \text{ mL}} = \left(\frac{0.224 \text{ g}}{74.6}\right) \times 2 \times 1,000$$

$$= 6 \text{ for } 500 \text{ mL}$$

$$\frac{\text{mOsm NaCl}}{500 \text{ mL}} = \left(\frac{0.234 \text{ g}}{58.5}\right) \times 2 \times 1,000$$

$$= 8 \text{ for } 500 \text{ mL}$$

$$\text{total mOsm/L} = 2 \times (6 \text{ mOsm KCl} + 8 \text{ mOsm NaCl})$$

$$= 28 \text{ mOsm/L}$$

$$\text{mOsm/L of K}^+ = \text{mOsm/L of } \frac{\text{KCl}}{2} = \frac{12}{2} = 6$$

Milligrams per 100 Milliliters and Milligrams per Deciliter

Certain laboratory test values are reported as the number of milligrams per deciliter (mg/dL) or milligrams percent (mg%), which is the same as milligrams per 100 milliliters (mg/100 mL)

Example: What is the % (w/v) concentration of glucose in a patient with a blood glucose reading of 230 mg/dL? Note that 1 dL = 100 mL and that 230 mg = 0.23 g. Then,

$$\text{glucose concentration} = \frac{0.23 \text{ g}}{100 \text{ mL}} = 0.23\% \, (\text{w/v})$$

"Units" and Micrograms per Milligram

The concentrations for some drugs, e.g., antibiotics and vitamins, are expressed as "units" of activity or micrograms per milligram (mcg/mg) as determined by a standardized bioassay.

Example: A preparation of penicillin G sodium contains 2.2 mEq of sodium (atomic weight = 23, valence = 1) per 1 million units of penicillin. How many milligrams of sodium are contained in an IV infusion of 5 million units? The 5 million unit dose will contain 5×2.2 mEq = 11 mEq.

Weight of sodium = 23 mg/mEq × 11 mEq = 253 mg

Parts per Million and Parts per Billion

Very low concentrations often are expressed in terms of parts per million (ppm, or the number of parts of ingredient per million parts of mixture or solution) or parts per billion (ppb, or the number of parts of ingredient per billion parts of mixture or solution). Thus, ppm and ppb are special cases of ratio strength concentrations.

Example: Express 1:25,000 as parts per million.

$$\frac{1}{x} = \frac{25,000}{1,000,000}$$

$$x = 40 \text{ ppm}$$

2-12. Dilutions and Concentrations

Simple Dilutions

In simple dilutions, a desired drug concentration is obtained by adding more solvent (diluent) to an existing solution or mixture. Mathematically, the key feature of this process is that the initial and final amounts of drug present remain unchanged. The amount of drug in any solution is proportional to the concentration times the quantity of the solution. Thus, taking the initial concentration as C_1, the initial quantity of solution as Q_1, the final concentration as C_2, and the final quantity of solution as Q_2, one has the relationship:

$$C_1 \times Q_1 = C_2 \times Q_2$$

When the values for any three of those variables are provided, the fourth variable can be calculated. (Because the equation can be rearranged to $C_1/C_2 = Q_2/Q_1$, it sometimes is referred to as an *inverse proportionality*.)

Example: How much water should be added to 250 mL of a solution of 0.2% (w/v) benzalkonium chloride to make a 0.05% (w/v) solution?

$$C_1 = 0.2\% \, (\text{w/v})$$

$$Q_1 = 250 \text{ mL}$$

$$C_2 = 0.05\% \, (\text{w/v})$$

$$Q_2 = x$$

$$x = Q_2 - 250 \text{ mL}$$

$$C_1 \times Q_1 = C_2 \times Q_2$$

$$Q_2 = \frac{C_1 \times Q_1}{C_2} = 0.2\% \times \frac{250 \text{ mL}}{0.05\%} = 1,000 \text{ mL}$$

$$x = Q_2 - 250 \text{ mL} = 1,000 \text{ mL} - 250 \text{ mL}$$

$$= 750 \text{ mL of water to be added}$$

Alcohol Solutions

The preceding treatment of dilutions assumes that solution and solvent volumes are reasonably additive. For dilutions of concentrated ethyl alcohol in water, that is not the case, because a contraction in volume occurs on mixing. Consequently, you cannot extend the calculation to determine the exact volume of water to add to the initial alcohol solution. That is, the volume of water to be added cannot be obtained simply as $Q_2 - Q_1$. Rather, you can specify only that sufficient water be added to the initial concentrated alcohol solution (Q_1) to reach the specified or calculated final volume (Q_2) of the diluted alcohol solution.

Example: How much water should be added to 100 mL of 95% (v/v) ethanol to make 50% (v/v) ethanol?

$$C_1 = 95\% \, (v/v)$$
$$Q_1 = 100 \text{ mL}$$
$$C_2 = 50\% \, (v/v)$$
$$Q_2 = x$$
$$C_1 \times Q_1 = C_2 \times Q_2$$
$$Q_2 = \frac{C_1 \times Q_1}{C_2} = 95\% \times \frac{100 \text{ mL}}{50\%}$$
$$= 190 \text{ mL (the final total volume)}$$

Thus, to the 100 mL of 95% (v/v) ethanol, add sufficient water to make 190 mL. The sufficient quantity of water will be more than 90 mL because of the contraction that occurs when concentrated alcohol is mixed with water.

Concentrated Acids

Concentrated mineral acids (hydrochloric, sulfuric, nitric, and phosphoric) are manufactured by bubbling the pure acid gas into water to produce a saturated solution. The manufacturer specifies the concentration as a % (w/w). However, when preparing diluted acids for compounding, the pharmacist must express the concentration as a % (w/v), which requires use of the specific gravity of the concentrated acid.

Example: What volume of 35% (w/w) concentrated HCl (SpGr 1.20) is required to make 500 mL of 5% (w/v) solution?

First, determine the weight of HCl required for the dilute solution. Because the dilute solution is 5% (w/v), it will contain 5 g in each 100 mL, or 25 g in 500 mL.

Next, determine what weight, x, of the 35% (w/w) solution contains 25 g of HCl. By proportion,

$$x : 100 \text{ g} = 25 \text{ g} : 35 \text{ g}$$
$$x = 100 \text{ g} \times \frac{25 \text{ g}}{35 \text{ g}}$$
$$x = 71.4 \text{ g of the concentrated solution}$$

Finally, use the specific gravity of the concentrated solution to convert the weight to volume. Here, recall that specific gravity is numerically equal to density when the latter is expressed in grams per milliliter. Thus,

$$\text{density} = 1.2 \text{ g/mL} = \text{weight/volume}$$

Rearranging,

$$\text{volume} = \text{weight/density} = \frac{71.4 \text{ g}}{1.2 \text{ g/mL}} = 59.5 \text{ mL}$$

Triturations

Triturations are simply 10% (w/w) dilutions of finely powdered (triturated) mixtures of a drug in an inert substance.

Example: What weight of colchicine trituration is required to prepare 30 doses of 0.25 mg each of colchicine?

For the trituration, 10 mg of the mixture contains 1 mg of drug. Thus,

$$x \text{ mg of trituration} : 10 \text{ mg of trituration}$$
$$= (30 \times 0.25 \text{ mg drug}) : 1 \text{ mg drug}$$
$$x = 10 \text{ mg trituration} \times \frac{(30 \times 0.25 \text{ mg drug})}{1 \text{ mg drug}}$$
$$= 75 \text{ mg trituration}$$

Simple Concentrations

In simple concentrations, a desired drug concentration is obtained by adding more pure drug to an existing solution or mixture. Mathematically, the key feature of this process is that the initial and final amounts of the base or diluent present remain unchanged. As opposed to dilution, the amount of base or diluent in any solution or mixture is proportional to the concentration times the quantity of the solution or mixture. Thus, taking the initial base concentration as C_1, the initial quantity of mixture as Q_1, the final base concentration as C_2, and the final quantity of mixture as Q_2, one has the relationship:

$$C_1 \times Q_1 = C_2 \times Q_2$$

When the values for any three of those variables are provided, the fourth variable can be calculated.

Example: How many grams of zinc oxide should be added to 3,200 g of 5% (w/w) zinc oxide ointment to prepare an ointment containing 20% (w/w) zinc oxide?

$$C_1 = 95\% \left(\begin{array}{c} \text{concentration of} \\ \text{the initial base} \end{array}\right)$$

$$Q_1 = 3,200 \text{ g}$$

$$C_2 = 80\% \,(\text{concentration of final base})$$

$$Q_2 = x$$

$$C_1 \times Q_1 = C_2 \times Q_2$$

$$95\% \times 3,200 \text{ g} = 80\% \times x$$

$$x = 3,800 \text{ g}$$

$$3,800 \text{ g} - 3,200 \text{ g} = 600 \text{ g}$$

600 g of zinc oxide is added

Alligation Alternate Method

Sometimes a drug concentration is required that is between the concentrations of two (or more) stock solutions (or available drug products). In that case, the alligation alternate method may be used to quickly obtain the relative parts of each of the stock solutions needed to yield the desired concentration. If stock solutions of concentrations A% and B% (A% > B%) are to be used to make a solution of concentration C%, set up the following diagram to obtain the relative parts of solutions A and B.

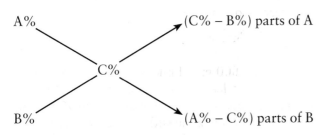

Example: In what proportion should 20% (w/v) dextrose be mixed with 5% (w/v) dextrose to obtain 15% (w/v) dextrose? How much of each is required to make 75 mL of 15% (w/v) solution?

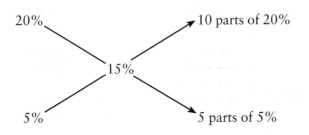

Thus, combine the stock solutions in the ratio of 10 parts of 20% (w/v) dextrose and 5 parts of 5% (w/v) dextrose (total of 15 parts). Accordingly, to make 75 mL of 15% solution (75 mL/15 parts = 5 mL/part), mix 50 mL (10 parts × 5 mL/part) of 20% solution with 25 mL (5 parts × 5 mL/part) of 5% solution.

Alligation Medial Method

Sometimes one may need to know the final concentration of a solution obtained by mixing specified volumes of two or more stock solutions. In that case, the alligation medial method may be used.

Example: What is the concentration of a solution prepared by combining 100 mL of a 10% solution, 200 mL of a 20% solution, and 300 mL of a 30% solution? Proceed as follows:

$$0.1 \times 100 \text{ mL} = 10 \text{ mL}$$

$$0.2 \times 200 \text{ mL} = 40 \text{ mL}$$

$$\underline{0.3 \times 300 \text{ mL} = 90 \text{ mL}}$$

$$600 \text{ mL} \quad 140 \text{ mL}$$

$$140 \text{ mL}/600 \text{ mL} \times 100 = 23.3\%$$

2-13. Isotonic Solutions

The preparation of many solutions requires attention to tonicity, a property that is based on the osmotic pressure that different concentrations of solutes exert as the solvent passes through a semipermeable membrane from a dilute solution to a more concentrated solution. Here, the term *solute* corresponds to cations, anions, and neutral undissociated molecules. A solution that has the same osmotic pressure as bodily fluids (blood or tears) is said to be *isotonic* (and *isosmotic*). As a point of reference, 0.9% (w/v) sodium chloride is isotonic.

Dissociating Solutes

Preparing solutions of specific tonicities requires knowledge of the dissociation properties of the solutes involved. One must know if the solute in question dissociates and, if so, to what extent and into how many particles. For example, in aqueous solutions, sodium chloride dissociates about 80% into two particles, yielding a solution containing Na^+ ions, Cl^- ions, and undissociated NaCl molecules. A measure of the extent of dissociation is provided by the dissociation factor, *i*, which is defined as the ratio of the total number of particles following dissociation to the number of molecules prior to dissociation. For example, 100 molecules of sodium chloride (prior to dissociation) will dissociate 80% to produce 80 particles of Na^+, 80 particles of Cl^-, and 20 particles of NaCl, or 180 particles in all. The dissociation factor, *i*, for NaCl, then, is 180/100 = 1.8. A nondissociating molecule (such as dextrose or tobramycin) is assigned a dissociation constant of 1. If measured dissociation information is not available, one can assume approximately 80% dissociation for aqueous solutions of salts. In that case, salts (including drugs) that dissociate into two ions (such as sodium chloride and ephedrine hydrochloride) will have a dissociation factor of 1.8; salts that dissociate into three ions (such as ephedrine sulfate) will have a dissociation factor of 2.6; and salts that dissociate into four ions (such as sodium citrate) will have a dissociation factor of 3.4.

Example: What is the dissociation factor (*i*) for a compound that dissociates 60% into three ions?

For each 100 undissolved molecules, one will obtain the following on dissolution:

$60 \times 3 = 180$ particles of ions + 40 particles of

undissociated molecules = a total of 220 particles

Thus, the dissociation factor (*i*) = 220/100 = 2.2.

Example: What is the dissociation factor for dextrose, a nondissociating compound?

For each 100 undissolved molecules, one will obtain the following on dissolution:

0 particles of ions + 100 particles of

undissociated molecules = a total of 100 particles

Thus, the dissociation factor (*i*) = 100/100 = 1.

Sodium Chloride Equivalents

When preparing isotonic drug solutions, one must take the tonicity contribution of the drug into consideration. That can be accomplished by using the *sodium chloride equivalent* (E value) for the drug, which is defined as the number of grams of sodium chloride that would produce the same tonicity effect as 1 gram of the drug. If the value of the sodium chloride equivalent is not provided, it can be calculated using the molecular weights (MWs) and dissociation factors of sodium chloride and the drug in question:

$$\text{sodium chloride equivalent} = (\text{MW of NaCL})$$

$$\times \frac{(\text{drug dissociation factor})}{(\text{MW of drug}) \times \left(\begin{array}{c}\text{sodium chloride} \\ \text{dissociation factor}\end{array}\right)}$$

$$= \frac{(58.5)(i)}{(\text{MW of drug})(1.8)}$$

Example: What is the sodium chloride equivalent of demecarium bromide (MW = 717, *i* = 2.6)?

$$\text{sodium chloride equivalent} = \frac{(58.5 \times 2.6)}{(717 \times 1.8)} = 0.12$$

Thus, each gram of demecarium bromide is equivalent to 0.12 g sodium chloride. So how does one proceed to prepare a drug solution that must be made isotonic? Using the total volume of isotonic solution to be prepared, first calculate the hypothetical weight, *x*, of sodium chloride (alone) that would be required to make that volume of water isotonic (0.9%). Next, using the weight of drug to be incorporated in the solution and its sodium chloride equivalent, calculate the weight of sodium chloride, *y*, that would correspond to the weight of the drug. Then, calculate the true weight of sodium chloride, *z*, to be added to the preparation as $z = x - y$.

Example: What weight of sodium chloride would be required to prepare 50 mL of an isotonic solution containing 1,000 mg of pilocarpine nitrate (sodium chloride equivalent = 0.23)?

Because isotonic saline requires 0.9 g/100 mL, 50 mL of isotonic saline will require 0.45 g (*x*). The 1,000 mg of pilocarpine nitrate will correspond to 1 g × 0.23 = 0.23 mg sodium chloride (*y*). Thus, the weight of sodium chloride (*z*) needed to make an isotonic solution:

$$0.45\,g - 0.23\,g = 0.22\,g$$

Example: Fluorescein sodium (MW = 376, dissociation factor *i* = 2.6), is to be provided as 500 mg in 60 mL of solution made isotonic with sodium chloride. What is the required weight of sodium chloride?

Here, the sodium chloride equivalent of the drug is not given and must be calculated from the information provided.

sodium chloride equivalent fluorescein sodium

$$= \frac{58.5 \times 2.6}{376 \times 1.8} = 0.22$$

Because isotonic saline requires 0.9 g/100 mL, 60 mL of isotonic saline will require 0.54 g (*x*). The 500 mg of fluorescein sodium will correspond to 0.5 g × 0.22 = 0.11 g of sodium chloride (*y*). Thus, the weight of sodium chloride (*z*) needed to make an isotonic solution:

$$0.54\,g - 0.11\,g = 0.43\,g$$

2-14. Intravenous Infusion Flow Rates

A physician may specify the rate of flow of IV fluids in drops per minute, amount of drug per hour, or the duration of time of administration of the total volume of the infusion. Therefore, to program an infusion pump to give the medication at the correct rate, one may need to calculate the infusion rate in per minute or per hour increments.

Example: If 250 mg of a drug is added to a 500 mL D_5W bag, what should the flow rate be, in milliliters per hour, to deliver 50 mg of drug per hour? The amount per hour is divided by the drug concentration to calculate the infusion rate.

$$250\,mg/500\,mL = 0.5\,mg/mL$$

$$50\,mg/h \div 0.5\,mg/mL = 100\,mL/h$$

Example: If an infusion flow rate is 100 mL/h and the infusion set delivers 15 drops/mL, what is the rate of flow in drops per minute?

$$15\,drops/mL \times 100\,mL/h = 1{,}500\,drops/h$$

$$\frac{1{,}500\,drops/h}{60\,min} = 25\,drops/min$$

Example: If 500 mL of an infusion is to be delivered at a flow rate of 1.25 mL/min, how long will it take to deliver the 500 mL in hours?

$$Total\ time\ of\ delivery = \frac{500\,mL}{1.25\,mL/min} = 400\,min$$

$$= 6.7\,h$$

2-15. Buffers

Buffer solutions are used to reduce pH fluctuations associated with the introduction of small amounts of strong acids or bases. Typical buffer solutions are composed of a weak acid or weak base plus a salt of the acid or base. Solution pH in the presence of a buffer can be calculated using the Henderson–Hasselbalch equations.

For weak acids, $pH = pK_a + \log(salt/acid)$

For weak bases, $pH = pK_w - pK_b + \log(base/salt)$

where $pK_w = 14$

Example: What is the pH of a buffer solution prepared to be 0.5 moles (M) in sodium acetate and 0.05 M in acetic acid (pK_a of acetic acid = 4.76)?

For weak acids, $pH = pK_a + \log(salt/acid)$

$$Thus,\ pH = 4.76 + \log\left(\frac{0.5}{0.05}\right) = 4.76 + \log(10)$$

$$= 4.76 + 1 = 5.76$$

Example: What is the pH of a buffer solution prepared to be 0.5 M in ammonia (pK_b = 4.74) and 0.05 M in ammonium chloride?

Ammonia forms a base in aqueous solution.

$$pH = pK_w - pK_b + \log(base/salt) = 14 - 4.74$$

$$+ \log(0.5/0.05) = 14 - 4.74 + 1 = 10.26$$

2-16. Temperature

Frequently, one must convert temperature from Fahrenheit (F) to Centigrade (C), and vice versa. The following formula can be used: 9°C = 5°F − 160.

Example: A patient has an oral temperature of 100°F. What is that temperature in °C?

$$9°C = 5°F - 160$$

$$C = \frac{(5°F - 160)}{9} = \frac{(5 \times 100 - 160)}{9} = 37.8°C$$

2-17. Questions

1. If 100 capsules contain 340 mg of active ingredient, what is the weight of active ingredient in 75 capsules?

   A. 453 mg
   B. 340 mg
   C. 255 mg
   D. 128 mg
   E. 75 mg

   100 cap = 75 cap
   340 mg

2. What is the weight of 500 mL of a liquid whose specific gravity is 1.13? *g/mL*

   A. 442 mg
   B. 565 g
   C. 442 g
   D. 885 mg
   E. 221 g

   $1.13 g/mL = \dfrac{x \, g}{500 mL}$

3. A pharmacist weighs out 325 mg of a substance on her class A prescription balance. When she subsequently checks the weight on a more sensitive analytical balance, she finds it to be only 312 mg. What is the percentage of error in the original weighing?

   A. 4%
   B. 5%
   C. 6%
   D. 10%
   E. 12%

   $MWQ = SR \dfrac{100}{\%}$

   $\dfrac{(325-312) \times 100}{325}$

   $312 = 6 \cdot \dfrac{100}{x}$

   $52 = \dfrac{100}{x}$

4. What is the minimum weighable quantity for a maximum of 5% error using a balance with a sensitivity requirement of 6 mg?

   A. 80 mcg
   B. 100 mg
   C. 120 mg
   D. 150 mg
   E. 240 mg

5. A patient weighing 175 lb is to receive an initial daily IM dosage of procainamide HCl (500 mg/mL vial) of 50 mg/kg (ABW) to be given in divided doses every 3 hours. How many milliliters should each injection contain?

   A. 3.98 mL
   B. 0.49 mL
   C. 8.23 mL

   $175 lb \times \dfrac{1 kg}{2.2 lb} \times \dfrac{50 mg}{1 kg} \times \dfrac{1 mL}{500 mg} = 7.95 mL$

   D. 1.87 mL
   E. 0.99 mL

6. What is the IBW of a female patient whose height is 5 feet 8 inches?

   A. 68 kg
   B. 64 kg
   C. 150 lb
   D. 121 lb
   E. 53 kg

   $45.5 + 2.3(8)$

7. What is the approximate BSA of an adult patient who weighs 154 lb and is 6 feet tall?

   A. 1.73 m²
   B. 3.15 m²
   C. 1.89 m²
   D. 0.70 m²
   E. 2.67 m²

   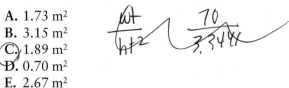

8. If the adult dose of a drug is 125 mg, what is the dose for a child whose BSA is estimated to be 0.68 m²?

   A. 485 mcg
   B. 318 mg
   C. 85 mg
   D. 49 mg
   E. 33 mg

   $\dfrac{125 mg}{2 m^2}$

   $\dfrac{0.68 \times 25}{1.73}$

   0.5

9. What is the CrCl for a 65-year-old female who weighs 50 kg and has a serum creatinine level of 1.3 mg/dL?

   A. 34 mL/min
   B. 40 mL/min
   C. 26 mL/min
   D. 82 mL/min
   E. 100 mL/min

   50

   $\dfrac{(140-65)(50)}{72 \cdot 1.3} \times 1.85$

   $\dfrac{3750}{93.6} \times 0.85$

10. Using the formula that follows, determine how much zinc oxide is required to make 750 g of mixture:

Zinc oxide	150 g
Starch	250 g
Petrolatum	550 g
Coal tar	50 g

    A. 200 g
    B. 188 g
    C. 413 g
    D. 113 g
    E. 38 g

    $\dfrac{150 g}{1000 g} = 750$

    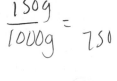
    $\dfrac{58.5(i)}{MW(1.8)}$

11. Using the formula that follows, determine the weight of kaolin that would be required to produce 500 g of mixture:

    Kaolin   12 parts
    Magnesium oxide   3 parts
    Bismuth subcarbonate   5 parts

    A. 83 g
    B. 300 g
    C. 208 g
    D. 333 g
    E. 250 g

12. How much dextrose is required to prepare 500 mL of an aqueous 10% solution?

    A. 250 mg
    B. 500 mg
    C. 10 g
    D. 25 g
    E. 50 g

    $0.1 = \dfrac{}{500mL}$

13. What weight of hexachlorophene should be used in compounding 20 g of an ointment containing hexachlorophene at a concentration of 1:400?

    A. 25 mcg
    B. 50 mcg
    C. 50 mg
    D. 80 mg
    E. 5 g

    $\dfrac{1\,part}{400\,part} = \dfrac{x}{100}\;\dfrac{0.25}{100} = 20$

    $0.25\% \quad 0.05\,g \times \dfrac{}{\text{in }1000mL}$

14. What weight of magnesium chloride ($MgCl_2$, formula weight = 95.3) is required to prepare 200 mL of a solution that is 5 mmol?

    A. 191 mg
    B. 95.3 mg
    C. 19.1 mg
    D. 477 mcg
    E. 95 g

    $5\,mmol \times \dfrac{9530\,mg}{1\,mmol}$

    $5\,mmol \times \dfrac{95.3}{1\,mmol}$

15. What weight of magnesium chloride ($MgCl_2$, formula weight = 95.3; Mg^{2+}, atomic weight = 24.3; Cl^{1-}, atomic weight = 35.5) is required to prepare 1,000 mL of a solution that contains 5 mEq of magnesium?

    A. 238 mg
    B. 4.76 g
    C. 1.19 g
    D. 60.7 mg
    E. 476 mcg

    $5\,mEQ\,Mg \times \dfrac{12150\,mg}{1\,mEQ\,Mg}$

    $5\,mEQ\,Mg \times \dfrac{}{1\,mEQ\,Mg}$

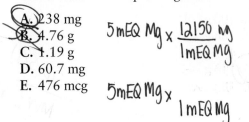

16. What is the milliosmolarity (ideal) of normal saline (NaCl, formula weight = 58.5)?

    A. 100 mOsm/L
    B. 154 mOsm/L
    C. 254 mOsm/L
    D. 287 mOsm/L
    E. 308 mOsm/L

17. How much water for injection should be added to 250 mL of 20% dextrose to obtain 15% dextrose?

    A. 333 mL
    B. 83 mL
    C. 250 mL
    D. 166 mL
    E. 58 mL

18. What volume of a 5% dextrose solution should be mixed with 200 mL of a 20% dextrose solution to prepare 300 mL of a 15% dextrose solution?

    A. 150 mL
    B. 200 mL
    C. 100 mL
    D. 50 mL
    E. 250 mL

19. What is the final concentration obtained by mixing 200 mL of 20% dextrose with 100 mL of 5% dextrose?

    A. 10%
    B. 15%
    C. 7.5%
    D. 12.5%
    E. 17.5%

    $(200 \cdot 20) + (100 \cdot 5) = 300 \cdot \%$

    300

20. Magnesium chloride ($MgCl_2$) is a 3-ion electrolyte that dissociates 80% at the relevant concentration. Calculate its dissociation factor (i).

    A. 1.8
    B. 2.2
    C. 2.4
    D. 2.6
    E. 3.2

21. Tobramycin (formula weight = 468) has a dissociation factor of 1. What is its sodium chloride equivalent?

    A. 0.069
    B. 0.0092

C. 0.117
D. 0.286
E. 0.782

(handwritten)
1 1.8
2 2.6
3 3.4
4 4.2
5

C. 45.95 g
D. 65.25 g
E. 35 g

22. What weight of sodium chloride should be used in compounding the following prescription for ephedrine sulfate (formula weight = 429, dissociation factor = 2.6, sodium chloride equivalent = 0.23)?

Ephedrine sulfate   0.25 g
Sodium chloride   qs
Purified water ad   30 mL
Make isotonic solution

(handwritten) $\frac{0.9g}{100mL} = \frac{x}{30m}$ 0.27 g

A. 1.22 g
B. 784 mcg
C. 212 mg *(circled)*
D. 527 mcg
E. 429 mg

(handwritten)
$$\frac{58.5(2.6)}{429(1.8)} = \frac{152.1}{772.2} \quad \frac{1g}{?} = 0.21$$
$= E = 0.197$ 0.23E
$= 0.0421$

23. A patient is to receive an infusion of 2 g of lidocaine in 500 mL D_5W at a rate of 2 mg/min. What is the flow rate in milliliters per hour?

A. 2 mL/h
B. 6.5 mL/h
C. 15 mL/h
D. 30 mL/h *(circled)*
E. 150 mL/h

(handwritten)
$$\frac{2mg}{1min} \times \frac{1g}{1000mg} \times \frac{60min}{1hr} =$$
$$\frac{0.12g}{1hr} \times \frac{500mL}{2g}$$

24. What is the pH of a buffer solution prepared with 0.05 M disodium phosphate and 0.05 M sodium acid phosphate (pK$_a$ = 7.21)?

A. 4.55
B. 5.23
C. 6.18
D. 7.05
E. 7.21 *(circled)*

(handwritten) pH = pKa + log

25. Convert 104°F to Centigrade.

A. 22°C
B. 34°C
C. 40°C *(circled)*
D. 46°C
E. 54°C

(handwritten) F = 1.8 C + 32

26. Calculate the amount of water (in grams) in 100 mL of 65% (w/w) syrup that has a density of 1.313. g/mL

A. 30 g
B. 75 g

(handwritten) 65g   1.313 g/mL = 65

27. How much boric acid will be needed to prepare an isotonic solution of the following prescription?

Phenacaine HCl	1%	E value for phenacaine HCl is 0.2
Chlorobutanol	0.5%	E value for chlorobutanol is 0.24
Boric acid	qs	E value for boric acid is 0.52
Purified water ad	60 mL	

(handwritten) $\frac{0.5}{100} = \frac{x}{60}$ 0.192

A. 0.55 g
B. 0.67 g *(circled)*
C. 0.75 g
D. 1.2 g
E. 2.2 g

(handwritten)
$\frac{0.9g}{100mL} = \frac{x g}{60}$ $\frac{1g}{0.24ECh} = \frac{0.3}{x}$
x = 0.54 g NaCl   x = 0.072 E
$\frac{1g}{0.2EPh} = \frac{0.09}{x}$ $\frac{1g}{0.52E} = \frac{y}{0.34E}$
x = 0.12 E ✓

28. How many milligrams of sodium chloride are required to make 30 mL of a solution of 1% dibucaine HCl isotonic with tears?

Note: The freezing point depression of 1% dibucaine HCl solution is −0.08°C, and the freezing point depression of an isotonic solution is −0.52°C.

A. 1.2 g
B. 0.950 g
C. 0.450 g
D. 0.228 g
E. 0.850 g

(handwritten) MEQ

29. How many milliequivalents of Na$^+$ are contained in a 30 mL dose of the following solution?

Disodium hydrogen phosphate	18 g	Na$_2$HPO$_4$ 7H$_2$O (MW 268)
Sodium biphosphate	48 g	NaH$_2$PO$_4$ 4H$_2$O (MW 138)
Purified water ad	100 mL	

A. 144.63 mEq *(circled)*
B. 104.34 mEq
C. 40.29 mEq
D. 100 mEq
E. 52 mEq

(handwritten) $48 g \times \frac{1mEQ}{138g}$ 18g

30. How many milliequivalents of magnesium sulfate are represented in 1 g of anhydrous magnesium sulfate ($MgSO_4$) (MW 120)?

    A. 122 mEq
    B. 16.67 mEq
    C. 12 mEq
    D. 10 mEq
    E. 19 mEq

    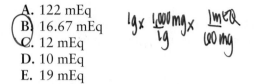

31. What is the concentration (g/mL) of a solution containing 4 mEq of $CaCl_2$ $2H_2O$ per milliliter (MW 147)?

    A. 0.345 g/mL
    B. 0.986 g/mL
    C. 0.389 g/mL
    D. 0.294 g/mL
    E. 0.545 g/mL

Use the following problem to answer Questions 32 through 36:

An IV infusion for a patient weighing 132 lb calls for 7.5 mg of drug/kg of body weight to be added to 250 mL of 5% dextrose injection solution.

32. What is the patient's weight in kilograms?

    A. 75 kg
    B. 25 kg
    C. 120 kg
    D. 55 kg
    E. 60 kg

33. How much drug is needed?

    A. 250 mg
    B. 350 mg
    C. 150 mg
    D. 450 mg
    E. 900 mg

34. What is the total number of milliliters the patient receives per day if the IV solution runs at 52 mL/h?

    A. 1,350 mL
    B. 1,248 mL
    C. 256 mL
    D. 1,000 mL
    E. 1,500 mL

35. What is the infusion rate in drops per minute (1 mL = 20 drops)?

    A. 25 drops/min
    B. 22 drops/min

    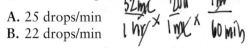

C. 17 drops/min
D. 30 drops/min
E. 15 drops/min

36. How many IV bags does the patient receive per day?

    A. 10 bags
    B. 12 bags
    C. 2 bags
    D. 5 bags
    E. 8 bags

37. If 50 mg of drug X is mixed with enough ointment base to obtain 20 g of mixture, what is the concentration of drug X in ointment (expressed as a ratio)?

    A. 1:300
    B. 1:400
    C. 1:200
    D. 1:600
    E. 1:100

    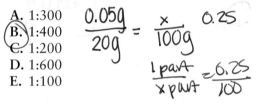

38. When 23 mL of water for injection are added to drug-lyophilized powder, the resulting concentration is 200,000 units/mL. What is the volume of the dry powder if the amount of drug in the vial was 5,000,000 units?

    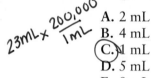

    A. 2 mL
    B. 4 mL
    C. 1 mL
    D. 5 mL
    E. 9 mL

39. If 20 g of salicylic acid are mixed with enough hydrophilic petrolatum to obtain a concentration of 5%, how much ointment was used to prepare the prescription?

    A. 400 g
    B. 380 g
    C. 250 g
    D. 480 g
    E. 280 g

    $$\frac{20}{x} = \frac{5}{100}$$

2-18. Answers

1. C. 255 mg

   x mg : 340 mg = 75 cap : 100 cap

   x = 340 mg × 75 cap/100 cap

   = 255 mg

2. **B.** 565 g, because a specific gravity of 1.13 corresponds to a density of 1.13 g/mL.

   density = weight/volume; thus, weight

   $$= \text{density} \times \text{volume} = 1.13 \text{ g/mL}$$

   $$\times 500 \text{ mL} = 565 \text{ g}$$

3. **A.** 4%

   error × 100
   quant

   $$\% \text{ error} = \frac{(\text{error} \times 100\%)}{\text{quantity desired}}$$

   $$= (325 - 312) \times \frac{100}{325} = 4\%$$

4. **C.** 120 mg

   $$\text{minimum weighable quantity} = \frac{\text{SR} \times 100\%}{5\%}$$

   $$= 6 \text{ mg} \times \frac{100\%}{5\%}$$

   $$= 120 \text{ mg}$$

5. **E.** 0.99 mL

   $$\text{daily dosage} = 50 \text{ mg/kg} \times \frac{175 \text{ lb}}{2.2 \text{ lb/kg}}$$

   $$= 3,977 \text{ mg}$$

   $$\text{single IM injection} = (3,977/8) \text{ mg} \times \frac{1}{500 \text{ mg/mL}}$$

   $$= 0.99 \text{ mL}$$

6. **B.** 64 kg

   $$\text{IBW} = 45.5 + (2.3 \times 8) = 64 \text{ kg}$$

7. **C.** 1.89 m²

   $$\text{weight} = \frac{154 \text{ lb}}{2.2 \text{ lb/kg}} = 70 \text{ kg}$$

   $$\text{height} = 6 \text{ ft} \times 12 \text{ in/ft} \times 2.54 \text{ cm/in} = 183 \text{ cm}$$

   $$\text{BSA} = \text{square root} \left[70 \times \frac{183}{3,600} \right]$$

   $$= \text{square root} [3.56] = 1.89 \text{ m}^2$$

8. **D.** 49 mg

   $$\text{child dose} = \text{adult dose} \times \frac{\text{child BSA}}{1.73} = 125 \text{ mg}$$

   $$\times \frac{0.68 \text{ m}^2}{1.73 \text{ m}^2} = 49 \text{ mg}$$

9. **A.** 34 mL/min

   $$\text{CrCl} = 0.85 \times (140 - 65) \times \frac{50}{(72 \times 1.3)}$$

   $$= 34 \text{ mL/min}$$

10. **D.** Note that the formula is designed to produce a total of 1,000 g of the mixture. Then, by proportions:

    $$x \text{ g ZnO} : 150 \text{ g ZnO} = 750 \text{ g mix} : 1,000 \text{ g}$$

    $$x = 150 \text{ g} \times \frac{750 \text{ g}}{1,000 \text{ g}} = 113 \text{ g}$$

11. **B.** Note that the formula will produce a total of 20 parts of the mixture. Then, by proportions:

    $$x \text{ g kaolin} : 500 \text{ g mix}$$

    $$= 12 \text{ parts kaolin} : 20 \text{ parts mix}$$

    $$x = 500 \text{ g} \times \frac{12 \text{ parts}}{20 \text{ parts}} = 300 \text{ g}$$

12. **E.** Note that this will be a solution of a solid in a liquid; thus, the concentration will be % (w/v).

    $$10\% (\text{w/v}) = x \text{ g dextrose} \times \frac{100}{500}$$

    $$x = 10 \times \frac{500}{100} = 50 \text{ g}$$

13. **C.** By proportions,

    $$x \text{ g hexachlorophene} : 20 \text{ g ung} = 1 \text{ part}$$

    $$\text{hexachlorophene} : 400 \text{ parts ung}$$

    $$x = 20 \text{ g} \times \frac{1 \text{ part}}{400 \text{ parts}} = 0.05 \text{ g} = 50 \text{ mg}$$

14. **B.** A 1 M solution will contain 95.3 g in 1,000 mL. A 5 M solution will contain 95.3 g × 5 = 477 g in 1,000 mL. A 5 mmol solution will contain

477 mg in 1,000 mL. Thus, 200 mL of a 5 mmol solution will contain 477 mg/5 = 95.3 mg in 200 mL.

15. **A.** Because magnesium has a valence of 2, a formula weight of $MgCl_2$ will contain two equivalent weights of magnesium (and chloride, for that matter). Thus, 5 equivalents of magnesium are contained in $5 \times 95.3/2$ g = 238 g $MgCl_2$. Accordingly, 5 mEq of magnesium are contained in 238 mg $MgCl_2$.

16. **E.** Normal saline is 0.9% (w/v), or 0.9 g/100 mL = 9 g/1,000 mL.

$$\text{milliosmolarity} = \left(\frac{9 \text{ g}}{58.5}\right) \times 2 \times 1,000$$

$$= 308 \text{ mOsm/L}$$

17. **B.** 83 mL

$$C_1 = 20\%, Q_1 = 250 \text{ mL}$$
$$C_2 = 15\%, Q_2 = x$$
$$C_1 \times Q_1 = C_2 \times Q_2$$
$$Q_2 = C_1 \times \frac{Q_1}{C_2} = 20\% \times \frac{250 \text{ mL}}{15\%}$$
$$= 333 \text{ mL}$$

added water = 333 mL − 250 mL = 83 mL

18. **C.** 100 mL

20% (concentration of stock A)	15 − 5 = 10 = parts of A
15% (desired concentration)	
5% (concentration of stock B)	20 − 15 = 5 = parts of B

Relative volumes are 10:5, or 2:1. Thus, 200 mL of a 20% dextrose solution (A) will require 100 mL of a 5% dextrose solution (B) to produce 300 mL of a 15% dextrose solution.

19. **B.** 15%

$$20\% \times 200 \text{ mL} = 4,000\% \text{ mL}$$
$$5\% \times 100 \text{ mL} = 500\% \text{ mL}$$
$$300 \text{ mL} = 4,500\% \text{ mL}$$
$$\text{Mixture concentration} = \frac{4,500\% \text{ mL}}{300 \text{ mL}} = 15\%$$

20. **D.** Each 100 molecules will provide

80 Mg ions
160 Cl ions
20 undissociated molecules
260 particles total

Thus, the dissociation factor = 260/100 = 2.6

21. **A.** 0.069

$$\text{sodium chloride equivalent} = \frac{(58.5)(1)}{(468)(1.8)}$$
$$= 0.069$$

22. **C.** Because 900 mg of sodium chloride in 100 mL is isotonic,

$$x : 900 \text{ mg} = 30 \text{ mL} : 100 \text{ mL}$$
$$x = 900 \times \frac{30}{100} = 270 \text{ mg}$$

which is the amount of sodium chloride alone needed to make 30 mL isotonic. But 1 g of ephedrine sulfate is equivalent to 0.23 g of sodium, thus:

$$y = 0.25 \text{ g} \times 0.23 = 0.058 \text{ g}$$
$$= 58 \text{ mg of sodium chloride}$$

Accordingly, the amount of sodium chloride to add ($z = x - y$) is (270 mg − 58 mg) = 212 mg.

23. **D.** The bag contains 2,000 mg in 500 mL, or 4 mg/mL. Therefore, a rate of 2 mg/min corresponds to 0.5 mL/min, which corresponds to 30 mL/h.

24. **E.** 7.21

$$pH = pK_a + \log\left(\frac{\text{salt}}{\text{acid}}\right)$$
$$= 7.21 + \log\left(\frac{0.05}{0.05}\right) = 7.21 + \log(1) = 7.21$$

25. **C.** 40°C

$$9°C = 5°F - 160$$
$$9°C = 5 \times 104 - 160 = 520 - 160 = 360$$
$$C = \frac{360}{9} = 40°C$$

26. **C.** Note that 65% w/w means 65 g in 100 g syrup. The total weight of the 100 mL syrup is 100 mL × 1.313 (density) = 131.3 g. Every 100 g of syrup contains 35 g of water, so

$$\frac{100\ g}{131.3\ g} = \frac{35\ g}{x}$$

$$x = \frac{(131.3 \times 35)}{100}$$

$$= 45.95\ g\ \text{(amount of water in the syrup)}$$

[handwritten: 1.313 g/mL   100 mL × 1.313 g/1 mL = 131.3 g]

27. **B.** The 1% phenacaine HCl equals 0.6 g, and the 0.5% chlorobutanol equals 0.3 g. Because we know the E value of phenacaine HCl, we can write the ratio:

$$\frac{0.6\ g\ drug}{1\ g\ drug} = \frac{x\ g\ NaCl}{0.2\ g\ NaCl}$$

$$x = \frac{(0.2 \times 0.6)}{1}$$

$$= 0.12\ g\ NaCl\ \text{(amount of sodium chloride that is equivalent to 0.6 g drug)}$$

Because we know the E value of chlorobutanol, we can write the ratio:

$$\frac{0.3\ g}{1\ g} = \frac{x\ g\ NaCl}{0.24\ g\ NaCl}$$

$$x = \frac{(0.3 \times 0.24)}{1}$$

$$= 0.072\ g\ NaCl\ \text{(amount of sodium chloride that is equivalent to 0.3 g chlorobutanol)}$$

The amount of sodium chloride needed to make 60 mL of solution isotonic is calculated as follows:

$$\frac{0.9\ g\ NaCl}{x\ g\ NaCl} = \frac{100\ mL}{60\ mL}$$

$$x = \frac{(0.9 \times 60)}{100}$$

$$= 0.54\ g\ NaCl\ \text{(amount of sodium chloride needed to make 60 mL of water isotonic if no drug or preservative were present)}$$

amount of sodium chloride needed

$$= 0.54\ g - (0.12\ g + 0.072\ g)$$

$$= 0.348\ g\ NaCl$$

Because we know the E value for boric acid, we can write the ratio:

$$\frac{1\ g}{x\ g} = \frac{0.52\ g\ NaCl}{0.348\ g\ NaCl}$$

$$x = \frac{(1\ g \times 0.348\ g)}{0.52\ g}$$

$$= 0.67\ g\ \text{(boric acid needed to make the prescription isotonic)}$$

28. **D.** The weight of 1% of drug equals 0.3 g. The needed change in freezing point depression to make the solution isotonic is 0.52°C − 0.08°C = 0.44°C, so the ratio is as follows:

$$\frac{0.9\ g\%\ NaCl}{x\%\ NaCl} = \frac{0.52°C}{0.44°C}$$

$$x = \frac{(0.9\ g\% \times 0.44)}{0.52}$$

$$= 0.76\ g\%\ \text{(percentage of sodium chloride needed to make an isotonic solution based on freezing point depression)}$$

The amount of sodium chloride needed to make 30 mL of water isotonic is calculated as follows:

$$\frac{0.76}{x} = \frac{100\ mL}{30\ mL}$$

$$x = \frac{(0.76\ g \times 30\ mL)}{100\ mL}$$

$$= 0.228\ g\ \text{(amount of sodium chloride needed)}$$

29. **A.** 144.63 mEq

1 mEq of disodium hydrogen phosphate

$$= \frac{268\ mg}{2} = 134\ mg$$

1 mEq of disodium biphosphate

$$= \frac{138\ mg}{1} = 138\ mg$$

We can write the ratio as follows:

$$\frac{1 \text{ mEq}}{x \text{ mEq}} = \frac{134 \text{ mg}}{18{,}000 \text{ mg}}$$

$$x = \frac{(18{,}000 \times 1)}{134} = 134.33 \text{ mEq disodium hydrogen phosphate}$$

We can also write the ratio as follows:

$$\frac{1 \text{ mEq}}{x} = \frac{138 \text{ mg}}{48{,}000 \text{ mg}}$$

$$x = \frac{(1 \times 48{,}000)}{138} = 347.83 \text{ mEq sodium biphosphate}$$

To adjust for volumes, we can write the ratios as follows:

$$\frac{134.32 \text{ mEq}}{x_1 \text{ mEq}} = \frac{100 \text{ mL}}{30 \text{ mL}} \text{ and}$$

$$\frac{347.82 \text{ mEq}}{x_2 \text{ mEq}} = \frac{100 \text{ mL}}{30 \text{ mL}}$$

Thus, $x_1 = 40.29$ mEq disodium hydrogen phosphate, and $x_2 = 104.34$ mEq sodium biphosphate. The total Na^+ mEq $= 104.34 + 40.29 = 144.63$ mEq.

30. **B.** 16.67 mEq

$$1 \text{ mEq} = \frac{120}{2} = 60 \text{ mg}$$

$$\frac{1 \text{ mEq Mg}^{++}}{60 \text{ mg}} = \left(\frac{x}{1{,}000 \text{ mg}}\right) x = \frac{(1 \times 1{,}000)}{60}$$

$$= 16.67 \text{ mEq}$$

31. **D.** 0.294 g/mL

$$1 \text{ mEq} = \frac{147}{2} = 73.5 \text{ mg}$$

$$4 \text{ mEq} = 4 \times 73.5 \text{ mg} = 294 \text{ mg/mL}$$

$$= 0.294 \text{ g/mL}$$

32. **E.** 60 kg

$$\frac{132}{2.2} = 60 \text{ kg}$$

33. **D.** 450 mg

$$7.5 \text{ mg/kg} \times 60 \text{ kg} = 450 \text{ mg}$$

34. **B.** 1,248 mL

$$52 \text{ mL/h} \times 1 \text{ h} \times 24 = 1{,}248 \text{ mL}$$

35. **C.** 17 drops/min

$$\frac{(52 \times 20)}{60} = \frac{x}{1 \text{ min}} = 17 \text{ drops/min}$$

36. **D.** 5 bags

$$\frac{1{,}248 \text{ mL}}{250 \text{ mL/bag}} = 5 \text{ bags}$$

37. **B.** 1:400

$$\frac{0.05 \text{ g}}{20 \text{ g}} = \frac{1}{X}, \text{ so } X = 400$$

38. **A.** 2 mL

$$\frac{200{,}000 \text{ units/mL}}{1 \text{ mL}} = \frac{5{,}000{,}000}{x},$$

so $x = 25$ mL, and the volume of powder is $25 - 23 = 2$ mL

39. **B.** 380 g

$$\frac{5}{100} = \frac{20}{x}, \text{ so } x = 400 \text{ g,}$$

and the amount of ointment is $400 - 20 = 380$ g

2-19. References

Ansel HC. *Pharmaceutical Calculations.* 12th ed. Philadelphia, PA: Wolters Kluwer and Lippincott Williams & Wilkins; 2010.

Khan MA, Reddy IK. *Pharmaceutical and Clinical Calculations.* 2nd ed. Lancaster, PA: Technomic Publishing Co; 2000.

O'Sullivan TA, Albrecht L. *Understanding Pharmacy Calculations.* 2nd ed. Washington, DC: American Pharmacists Association; 2012.

Pharmaceutics and Drug Delivery Systems

Hassan Almoazen

3-1. Key Points

- Drug absorption depends not only on the fraction of the un-ionized form of the drug but also on the surface area available for absorption.
- The Noyes–Whitney equation can be used for determining the dissolution rate of a drug from its dosage form.
- Surfactants consist of hydrophilic and hydrophobic groups and can be used as emulsifying agents to reduce interfacial tensions.
- The pharmaceutical dosage form contains the active drug ingredient in association with non-drug (usually inert) ingredients (excipients). Together they form the vehicle, or formulation matrix.
- Water-soluble drugs are often formulated as sustained-release tablets so that their release and dissolution rates can be controlled, whereas enteric-coated tablets are used to protect drugs from gastric degradation.
- Capsules are solid dosage forms with hard or soft gelatin shells that contain drugs and excipients.
- Aerosols are pressurized dosage forms designed to deliver drugs to pulmonary tissues with the aid of a liquefied or propelled gas.
- Inserts, implants, and devices allow slow release of the drug into a variety of cavities (e.g., vagina, buccal cavity, cul de sac of the eye, and skin).
- Transdermal patches deliver drugs directly through the skin and into the bloodstream.

- The drug delivery system deals with the pharmaceutical formulation and the dynamic interactions among the drug, its formulation matrix, its container, and the physiologic milieu of the patient. These dynamic interactions are the subject of pharmaceutics.
- Macromolecular drug carriers, such as protein–polymer conjugates, and particulate delivery systems, such as microspheres and liposomes, are commonly used for delivery of drugs with low molecular weight, such as peptides and proteins, to different disease targets.
- Targeted (or site-specific) drug delivery systems are used for drug delivery to the target or receptor site in a manner that provides maximum therapeutic activity by preventing degradation during transit to the target site while avoiding delivery to nontarget sites.

3-2. Study Guide Checklist

The following topics may guide your study of the subject area:

- The relationship between the pH and the dissociation constant (pK_a) for a weak acid or a weak base drug and how this relationship affects drug absorption
- The relationship between solubility and dissolution rate for any drug and the major factors that affect both
- Rheology and evaluation of selected parameters that are used to describe the rheological behavior of different pharmaceutical systems

Editor's Note: This chapter is based on the 10th edition chapter written by Ram I. Mahato.

- Surfactants and the factors that affect the formation of micelles
- Hydrophilic-lipophilic balance and the way it influences the formation of emulsions
- Dispersed systems and different colloidal systems
- Excipients and their functions in different dosage forms
- Basic knowledge about each individual dosage form

3-3. Introduction

Basic pharmaceutics includes the physicochemical properties of the drug such as solubility and dissolution rate, hydrophilicity and hydrophobicity as characterized by oil-to-water partition coefficient ($K_{o/w}$), dissociation constant (pK_a), viscosity, and solid-state chemistry (amorphous and crystalline forms). A pharmaceutical *dosage form* is the delivery system that is administered to the patient so that an effective dose of the drug is delivered. Typical examples of dosage forms are tablets, capsules, suppositories, parenterals, oral and nasal solutions, oral suspensions, metered dose inhalers, and transdermal patches. Achieving an optimal dose-response curve requires delivery of the drug to its site of action at a rate and a concentration that minimizes its side effects and maximizes its therapeutic effects. The development of safe and effective pharmaceutical dosage forms and delivery systems requires a thorough understanding of the basic pharmaceutics concepts that enable the drug to be formulated into a pharmaceutical dosage form. The successful design of a delivery system depends on the following:

- Dose of the drug
- Route of administration
- Desired drug delivery system
- Drug release from the delivery system
- Bioavailability of the drug

The pH Partition Theory and Dissociation Constant pK_a

The *pH partition theory* states that drugs are absorbed from the biological membranes by passive diffusion depending on the fraction of the un-ionized form of the drug at the pH of the fluids close to that of the biological membrane. The degree of ionization of the drug depends on both the pK_a and the pH of the drug solution. The gastrointestinal (GI) tract acts as a lipophilic barrier, and thus ionized drugs are more hydrophilic than un-ionized ones and have minimal membrane transport. The solution pH affects the overall partition coefficient of an ionizable substance. The pK_a of a molecule is the pH at which a 50:50 mixture of acid and conjugated base coexists in equilibrium. For an acidic drug, the acid form predominates at a pH lower than the pK_a, and the conjugated base form dominates at a pH higher than the pK_a. For a basic drug, the base form (un-ionized) dominates at pH values higher than the pK_a, and the conjugated acidic form (ionized) dominates at pH values below the pK_a. The extent of ionization of a drug molecule is given by the following Henderson–Hasselbalch equations, which describe a relationship between ionized and un-ionized species of a weak acid or base:

Weakly acidic drugs	Weakly basic drugs
$pH = pK_a + \log\dfrac{[A^-]}{[HA]}$	$pH = pK_a + \log\dfrac{[B]}{[BH^+]}$

where [HA] is the concentration of un-ionized acid, [A$^-$] is the concentration of ionized base, [B] is the concentration of un-ionized base, and [BH$^+$] is the concentration of ionized base. Although pH partition theory is useful, it often does not hold true. For example, most weak acids are well absorbed from the small intestine, which is contrary to the prediction of the pH partition hypothesis. Similarly, quaternary ammonium compounds are ionized at all pH levels but are readily absorbed from the GI tract. These discrepancies arise because pH partition theory does not take into consideration the following factors, among others:

- Large epithelial surface areas of the small intestine compensate for ionization effects.
- Long residence time in the small intestine also compensates for ionization effects.
- Charged drugs, such as quaternary ammonium compounds and tetracyclines, may interact with opposite-charged organic ions, resulting in a neutral species that is absorbable.
- Some drugs are absorbed by means of active transport.

Solubility and the Noyes–Whitney Equation of Dissolution

Drug solubility is the maximum amount of the drug that is soluble in unit volume of the solvent. For most drugs, the rate at which the solid drug dissolves in a solvent (dissolution) is often the rate-limiting step in the drug's bioavailability. The rate at which a solid drug of limited water solubility dissolves in a solvent can be determined using the Noyes–Whitney equation:

$$\frac{dM}{dt} = k \cdot S \cdot (C_s - C)$$

where dM/dt is the rate of dissolution (in mass/time), k is the dissolution rate constant (in cm/s) ($k = D/h$), S is the surface area of exposed solid (in cm²), D is the diffusion coefficient of solute in solution (in cm²/s), h is the thickness of the diffusion layer (in cm), C_s is the drug solubility (in mass/mL), and C is the drug concentration in bulk solution at time t (in mass/mL).

Under sink conditions, when C is much less than C_s, the Noyes–Whitney equation can be simplified as follows:

$$\frac{dM}{dt} = k\,S\,C_s \quad \text{or} \quad \frac{dC}{dt} = \frac{kSC_s}{V}$$

where dC/dt is the dissolution rate (in concentration/time) and V is the volume of the dissolution medium (in mL).

The following factors influence the dissolution rate:

- The conditions in the GI tract affect the dissolution rate. For example, the presence of foods that increase the viscosity of GI fluids decreases the diffusion coefficient, D, of a drug and its dissolution rate.
- The thickness of the diffusion layer, h, is influenced by the degree of agitation experienced by each drug particle in the GI tract. Hence, an increase in gastric or intestinal motility may increase the dissolution rate of poorly soluble drugs.
- The dissolution rate of a weakly acidic drug in GI fluids is influenced by the drug solubility in the diffusion layer surrounding each dissolving drug particle. The pH of the diffusion layer significantly affects the solubility of a drug and its subsequent dissolution rate. The dissolution rate of a weakly acidic drug in GI fluid (pH 1–3) is relatively low because of its low solubility in the diffusion layer. If the pH in the diffusion layer could be increased, the solubility (C_s) exhibited by the weak acidic drug in this layer (and hence the dissolution rate of the drug in GI fluids) could be increased. The potassium or sodium salt form of the weakly acidic drug has a relatively high solubility at the elevated pH in the diffusion layer. Thus, the dissolution of the drug particles takes place at a faster rate. The reverse is true for weakly basic drugs; a reduction in pH of

the diffusion layer would increase its solubility in the GI tract.

- Particle size and the surface area of the drug significantly influence the drug dissolution rate. An increase in the total effective surface area of the drug in contact with GI fluids causes an increase in its dissolution rate. The smaller the particle size is, the greater will be the effective surface area exhibited by a given mass of drug and the higher will be the dissolution rate. However, particle size reduction is not always helpful and may fail to increase the bioavailability of a drug. In the case of certain hydrophobic drugs, excessive particle size reduction tends to cause aggregation into larger particles. Preventing the formation of aggregates requires the dispersion of small drug particles in polyethylene glycol (PEG), polyvinylpyrrolidone (PVP), dextrose, or other agents. For example, a dispersion of griseofulvin in PEG 4,000 enhances its dissolution rate and bioavailability. Certain drugs, such as penicillin G and erythromycin, are unstable in gastric fluids and do not dissolve readily in them. For such drugs, particle size reduction yields an increased rate of drug dissolution in gastric fluid and also increases the extent of drug degradation.
- Amorphous or noncrystalline forms of a drug may have faster dissolution rates than crystalline forms.
- Surface-active agents will increase dissolution rates by lowering interfacial tension, which allows better wetting and penetration by the solvent. Weakly acidic and basic drugs may be brought into solution by the solubilizing action of surfactants.

Rheology

Rheology is the study of flow properties of liquids under the influence of stress. The flow of simple liquids can be described by viscosity, an expression of the resistance to flow. Liquids are divided into two general categories, Newtonian and non-Newtonian, depending on their characteristics. Rheological properties are useful for the formulation and analysis of emulsions, suspensions, and lotions. Pourability, spreadability, and syringeability of an emulsion or a suspension are determined by its rheological properties.

According to Newton's law of viscous flow, the rate of flow (D) is directly proportional to the applied stress (τ). That is, $\tau = \eta \cdot D$, where η is the viscosity. Fluids that obey Newton's law of flow are referred to as *Newtonian fluids*, and fluids that deviate are known as *non-Newtonian fluids*. The force per unit area (F'/A) required to bring about flow is called the shearing stress (F):

$$F = \frac{F'}{A} = \eta \frac{dv}{dr}$$

where η is the viscosity, dv/dr is the rate of shear = G (s^{-1}), and F'/A units are in dynes per cm². For simple Newtonian fluids, a plot of the rate of shear against shearing stress gives a straight line (Figure 3-1A); thus, η is a constant. In the case of Newtonian fluids, viscosity does not change with increasing shear rate. Various types of water and pharmaceutical dosage forms that contain a high percentage of water are examples of liquid dosage forms that have Newtonian flow properties.

Most pharmaceutical fluids (including colloidal dispersions, emulsions, and liquid suspensions) do not follow Newton's law of flow, and the viscosity of the fluid varies with the rate of shear. There are three types of non-Newtonian flow: plastic, pseudoplastic, and dilatant (Figure 3-1B, C, and D).

Plastic flow

Fluids that undergo plastic flow are called *Bingham bodies*; these materials are defined as fluids that exhibit a yield value (Figure 3-1B). Plastic flow is associated with the presence of flocculated particles in concentrated suspensions. *Flocculated solids* are light, fluffy conglomerates of adjacent particles held together by weak van der Waals forces. The yield value exists because a certain shearing stress must be exceeded to break up van der Waals forces. A plastic system resembles a Newtonian system at shear stresses above the yield value. Yield value, f, is an indicator of flocculation (the higher the yield value, the greater the degree of flocculation). The characteristics of plastic flow materials can be summarized as follows:

- Plastic flow does not begin until a shearing stress, corresponding to a yield value, f, is exceeded.
- The curve intersects the shearing stress axis but does not cross through the origin.
- The materials are said to be "elastic" at shear stresses below the yield value.
- Viscosity decreases with increasing shear rate at shear stress below the yield value.

Pseudoplastic flow

Pseudoplastic flow is exhibited by polymers in solution. A large number of pharmaceutical products, including natural and synthetic gums (e.g., liquid dispersions of tragacanth, sodium alginate, methyl

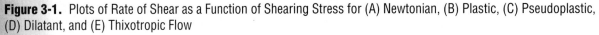

Figure 3-1. Plots of Rate of Shear as a Function of Shearing Stress for (A) Newtonian, (B) Plastic, (C) Pseudoplastic, (D) Dilatant, and (E) Thixotropic Flow

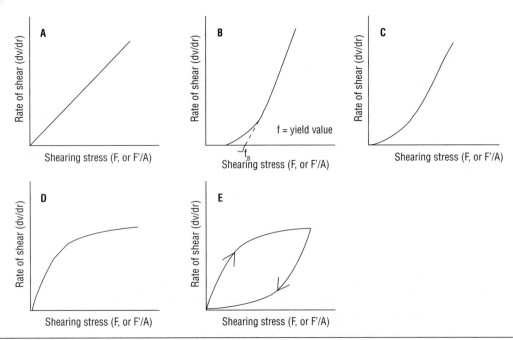

cellulose, and sodium carboxymethylcellulose), exhibit pseudoplastic flow properties. The characteristics of pseudoplastic flow materials can be summarized as follows:

- Pseudoplastic substances begin to flow when a shearing stress is applied: that is, there is no yield value (it does cross the origin).
- The viscosity of a pseudoplastic substance decreases with increasing shear rate.
- With increasing shearing stress, the rate of shear increases; these materials are called *shear-thinning* systems.
- Shear thinning occurs when molecules (polymers) align themselves along their long axes and slip and slide past each other.

Dilatant flow

Certain suspensions with a high percentage of dispersed solids exhibit an increase in resistance to flow with increasing rates of shear. Dilatant systems are usually suspensions with a high percentage of dispersed solids that exhibit an increase in resistance to flow with increasing rates of shear. Dispersions containing a high percentage ($\geq 50\%$) of small, defloculated particles may exhibit this type of behavior. The characteristics of dilatant flow materials can be summarized as follows:

- Dilatant materials increase in volume when sheared.
- They are also known as *shear-thickening systems* (the opposite of pseudoplastic systems).
- When the stress is removed, the dilatant system returns to its original state of fluidity.
- Viscosity increases with increasing shear rate.
- Dilatant materials may solidify under conditions of high shear.

Thixotropy

Thixotropy is a nonchemical isothermal gel–sol–gel transformation. If a thixotropic gel is sheared (by simple shaking), the weak bonds are broken, and a lyophobic solution is formed (Figure 3-1E). On standing, the particles collide, leading to flocculation and formation of gel. Thixotropy is a desirable property in liquid pharmaceutical preparations. The advantage associated with thixotropic preparations is that the particles remain in suspension during storage, but when required for use, the gels are readily made fluid by tapping or shaking. The shearing force on the injection as it is pushed through the needle ensures that it is fluid when injected; however, the rapid resumption of the gel structure prevents excessive spreading in the tissues, and consequently a more compact depot is produced than with nonthixotropic suspensions. A well-formulated thixotropic suspension will not settle out readily in the container and will become fluid on shaking. Flow curves (rheograms) for thixotropic materials are highly dependent on the rate at which shear is increased or decreased and the length of time a sample is subjected to any one rate of shear.

Negative thixotropy

Negative thixotropy is also known as *antithixotropy*, which represents an increase rather than a decrease in consistency on the down curve (an increase in thickness or resistance to flow with an increased time of shear). It may result from an increased collision frequency of dispersed particles (or polymer molecules) in suspension, which causes increased interparticle bonding with time.

3-4. Surfactants and Micelles

Surface-active agents, or *surfactants*, are substances that adsorb to surfaces or interfaces to reduce surface or interfacial tension. They may be used as emulsifying agents, solubilizing agents, detergents, and wetting agents. Surfactants have two distinct regions in one chemical structure. One area is hydrophilic (water loving); another is hydrophobic (water repelling). The existence of two such moieties in a molecule is known as *amphipathy*, and the molecules are consequently referred to as *amphipathic molecules* or *amphiphiles*. Depending on the number and nature of the polar and nonpolar groups present, the amphiphile may be predominantly hydrophilic, lipophilic, or somewhere in between. For example, alkyl chain alcohols, amines, and acids are amphiphiles that change from being predominantly hydrophilic to lipophilic as the number of carbon atoms in the alkyl chain is increased. The hydrophobic portions are usually saturated or unsaturated hydrocarbon chains or, less commonly, heterocyclic or aromatic ring systems.

Surfactants are classified according to the nature of the hydrophilic or hydrophobic groups. In addition, some surfactants possess both positively and negatively charged groups and can exist as either anionic or cationic, depending on the pH of the solution. These surfactants are known as *ampholytic compounds*.

At low concentrations in solutions, amphiphiles exist as monomers. As the concentration is increased, aggregation occurs over a narrow concentration range. These aggregates, which may contain 50 or more monomers, are called *micelles*. Therefore, micelles are small spherical structures composed of both hydrophilic and hydrophobic regions. The polar head groups of the surfactant molecules are arranged in an outer shell while their hydrocarbon chains are oriented toward the center, forming a hydrophobic core. The concentration of monomer at which micelles are formed is called the *critical micellization concentration*, or CMC. Surface tension decreases up to the CMC but remains constant above the CMC. The longer the hydrophobic chain or the lower the polarity of the polar group, the greater the tendency for monomers to "escape" from the water to form micelles and hence lower the CMC.

Types of Micelles

In the case of amphiphiles in water, in dilute solution (still above but close to the CMC), the micelles are considered to be spherical in shape. At higher concentrations, they become more asymmetric and eventually assume cylindrical or lamellar structures. Oil-soluble surfactants have a tendency to self-associate into *reverse micelles* in nonpolar solvents, with their polar groups oriented away from the solvent.

Factors Affecting CMC and Micellar Size

- *Structure of hydrophobic group:* An increase in the hydrocarbon chain length causes a logarithmic decrease in the CMC.
- *Nature of hydrophilic group:* An increase in chain length increases hydrophilicity and the CMC. In general, nonionic surfactants have very low CMC values and high aggregation numbers compared with their ionic counterparts with similar hydrocarbon chains.
- *Nature of counterions:* Note that $Cl^- < Br^- < I^-$ for cationic surfactants, and $Na^+ < K^+$ for anionic surfactants.
- *Electrolytes:* The addition of electrolytes to ionic surfactants decreases the CMC and increases the micellar size. In contrast, micellar properties of nonionic surfactants are affected only minimally by the addition of electrolytes.
- *Temperature:* At temperatures up to the cloud point, an increase in micellar size and a decrease in CMC is noted for many nonionic surfactants but has little effect on that of ionic surfactants.
- *Alcohol:* CMCs are increased by the addition of alcohols.

Hydrophilic–Lipophilic Balance Systems

Griffin's method of selecting emulsifying agents is based on the balance between the hydrophilic and lipophilic portions of the emulsifying agent, now widely known as the *hydrophilic–lipophilic balance (HLB) system*. The higher the HLB value of an emulsifying agent, the more hydrophilic it is. The emulsifying agents with lower HLB values are less polar and more lipophilic. The Spans (i.e., sorbitan esters) are lipophilic and have low HLB values (1.8–8.6); the Tweens (polyoxyethylene derivatives of the Spans) are hydrophilic and have high HLB values (9.6–16.7). Surfactants with the proper balance of hydrophilic and lipophilic affinities are effective emulsifying agents because they concentrate at the oil-in-water (o/w) interface. The type of an emulsion that is produced depends primarily on the property of the emulsifying agent. The HLB of an emulsifier or a combination of emulsifiers determines whether an o/w or water-in-oil (w/o) emulsion results. In general, o/w emulsions are formed when the HLB of the emulsifier is within the range of about 9 to 12; w/o emulsions are formed when the range is about 3 to 6. The type of emulsion is a function of the relative solubility of the supernatant. An emulsifying agent with high HLB is preferentially soluble in water and results in the formation of an o/w emulsion. The reverse situation is true with surfactants of low HLB value, which tend to form w/o emulsions.

Micellar Solubilization

Micelles can be used to increase the solubility of materials that are normally insoluble or poorly soluble in the dispersion medium used. The interior of micelles is composed of a hydrophobic core in which compounds that are poorly soluble in the dispersion medium can be dissolved. For example, surfactants are often used to increase the solubility of poorly soluble steroids. The factors affecting micellar solubilization are the nature of surfactants, the nature of solubilizates, and the temperature.

3-5. Dispersed Systems

Dispersed systems consist of particulate matter, known as the *dispersed phase*, distributed throughout a continuous or dispersion medium. The particulate matter, or dispersed phase, consists of particles that range from 1 nanometer (nm) to 0.5 micrometer

$(10^{-9}$ m to 5×10^{-7} m$)$. Depending on the dispersed phase, dispersed systems are classified as follows:

- *Molecular dispersions:* Less than 1 nm, invisible under electron microscopy. Examples are oxygen molecules, ions, and glucose.
- *Colloidal dispersions:* From 1 nm to 0.5 micrometer, visible under electron microscopy. Examples are colloidal silver sols and natural and synthetic polymers.
- *Coarse dispersions:* Greater than 0.5 micrometer, visible under light microscopy. Examples are grains of sand, activated charcoal, emulsions, suspensions, and red blood cells.

Types of Colloidal Systems

On the basis of the interaction of the particles, molecules, or ions of the dispersed phase with the molecules of dispersion medium, colloidal systems are classified into three groups: lyophilic, lyophobic, and association colloids.

Lyophilic or hydrophilic colloids

Systems containing colloidal particles that interact with the dispersion medium are referred to as *lyophilic colloids*. In the case of lipophilic colloids, organic solvent is the dispersion medium, whereas water is used as the dispersion medium for hydrophilic colloids. Because of their affinity for the dispersion medium, such materials form colloidal dispersions with relative ease. For example, the dissolution of acacia or gelatin in water, or celluloid in amyl acetate, leads to the formation of a solution. Most lyophilic colloids are polymers (e.g., gelatin, acacia, povidone, albumin, rubber, and polystyrene).

Lyophobic or hydrophobic colloids

Lyophobic colloids are composed of materials that have little attraction for the dispersion medium. Lyophobic colloids are intrinsically unstable and irreversible. Hydrophobic colloids are generally composed of inorganic particles dispersed in water.

Association colloids

Association colloids (referring to amphiphilic colloids) are formed by the grouping or association of amphiphiles (i.e., molecules that exhibit both lyophilic and lyophobic properties). At low concentrations, amphiphiles exist separately and do not form a colloid. At higher concentrations, aggregation occurs at around 50 or more monomers, leading to micelle formation. As with lyophilic colloids, formation of association colloids is spontaneous if the concentration of the amphiphile in solution exceeds the CMC.

Zeta Potential and Its Effect on Colloidal Stability

Zeta (ζ) potential is defined as the difference in potential between the surface of the tightly bound layer (shear plane) and the electroneutral region of the solution. The zeta potential governs the degree of repulsion between adjacent, similarly charged, dispersed particles. If the zeta potential is reduced below a certain value, the attractive forces exceed the repulsive forces, and the particles come together. This phenomenon is known as *flocculation*.

Stabilization is accomplished by providing the dispersed particles with an electric charge and a protective solvent sheath surrounding each particle to prevent mutual adherence attributable to collision. This second effect is significant only in the case of lyophilic colloids. Lyophilic and association colloids are thermodynamically stable and exist in a true solution so that the system constitutes a single phase. In contrast, lyophobic colloids are thermodynamically unstable but can be stabilized by preventing aggregation or coagulation by providing the dispersed particles with an electric charge, which can prevent coagulation through repulsion of like particles.

3-6. Pharmaceutical Ingredients

Turning a drug into a pharmaceutical dosage form or a drug delivery system requires pharmaceutical ingredients. For example, in the preparation of tablets, the addition of diluents or fillers increases the bulk of the formulation. Binders are added to promote adhesion of the powdered drug to other ingredients. Lubricants assist the smooth tableting process. Disintegrants promote tablet breakup after administration. Coatings improve stability, control disintegration, or enhance appearance. In the preparation of pharmaceutical solutions, preservatives are added to prevent microbial growth, stabilizers are added to prevent drug decomposition, and colorants and flavorants are added to ensure product appeal. Thus, for each dosage form, the pharmaceutical ingredients establish the primary features of the product and control the physicochemical properties, drug-release profiles, and bioavailability of the product. Table 3-1 lists some typical pharmaceutical ingredients used in different dosage forms.

Table 3-1. Typical Pharmaceutical Ingredients

Ingredient type	Definition	Examples
Antifungal preservative	Used in liquid and semisolid formulations to prevent growth of fungi	Benzoic acid, butylparaben, ethylparaben, sodium benzoate, sodium propionate
Antimicrobial preservative	Used in liquid and semisolid formulations to prevent growth of microorganisms	Benzalkonium chloride, benzyl alcohol, cetylpyridinium chloride, phenyl ethyl alcohol
Antioxidant	Used to prevent oxidation	Ascorbic acid, ascorbyl palmitate, sodium ascorbate, sodium bisulfite sodium metabisulfite
Binder	Used to cause adhesion of powder particles in tablet granulations	Acacia, alginic acid, ethylcellulose, starch, povidone
Diluent	Used as fillers to create desired bulk, flow properties, and compression characteristics in tablet and capsule preparations	Kaolin, lactose, mannitol, cellulose, sorbitol, starch
Disintegrant	Used to promote disruption of solid mass into small particles	Microcrystalline cellulose, carboxymethylcellulose calcium, sodium alginate, sodium starch glycolate, alginic acid
Emulsifying agent	Used to promote and maintain dispersion of finely divided droplets of a liquid in a vehicle in which it is immiscible	Acacia, cetyl alcohol, glyceryl monostearate, sorbitan monostearate
Glidant	Used to improve flow properties of powder mixture	Colloidal silica, cornstarch, talc
Humectant	Used for prevention of dryness of ointments and creams	Glycerin, propylene glycol, sorbitol
Lubricant	Used to reduce friction during tablet compression and to facilitate ejection of tablets from the die cavity	Calcium stearate, magnesium stearate, mineral oil, stearic acid, zinc stearate
Plasticizer	Used to enhance coat spread over tablets, beads, and granules	Glycerin, diethyl palmitate
Surfactant	Used to reduce surface or interfacial tension	Polysorbate 80, sodium lauryl sulfate, sorbitan monopalmitate
Suspending agent	Used to reduce sedimentation rate of drug particles dispersed throughout a vehicle in which they are not soluble	Carbopol, hydroxymethylcellulose, hydroxypropyl cellulose, methylcellulose, tragacanth

3-7. Types of Commonly Used Dosage Forms

Solutions

Solutions are homogeneous mixtures of one or more solutes dispersed in a dissolving medium (solvent). Aqueous solutions containing a sugar or sugar substitute with or without added flavoring agents and drugs are classified as *syrups*. Sweetened hydroalcoholic (combinations of water and ethanol) solutions are termed *elixirs*. Hydroalcoholic solutions of aromatic materials are termed *spirits*. *Tinctures* are alcoholic or hydroalcoholic solutions of chemical or soluble constituents of vegetable drugs. Most tinctures are prepared by an extraction process. *Mouthwashes* are solutions used to cleanse the mouth or treat diseases of the oral membrane. *Antibacterial topical solutions* (e.g., benzalkonium chloride and strong iodine) will kill bacteria when applied to the skin or mucous membrane.

Solutions intended for oral administration usually contain flavorants and colorants to make the medication more attractive and palatable to the patient. They may contain stabilizers to maintain the physicochemical stability of the drug and preservatives to prevent the growth of microorganisms in the solution. A drug dissolved in an aqueous solution is in the solution; no dissolution step is necessary before systemic absorption occurs. Solutions that are prepared to be sterile, that are pyrogen free, and that are intended for parenteral administration are classified as *injectables*.

Some drugs, particularly certain antibiotics, have insufficient stability in aqueous solution to withstand long shelf lives. These drugs are formulated as dry powder or granule dosage forms for reconstitution with purified water immediately before dispensing to the patient. The dry powder mixture contains all of the formulation components—that is, drug, flavorant, colorant, buffers, and others—except for the solvent. Examples of dry powder mixtures intended for reconstitution to make oral solutions include cloxacillin sodium, nafcillin sodium, oxacillin sodium, and penicillin V potassium.

Sucrose is the sugar most frequently used in syrups; in special circumstances, it may be replaced in whole or in part by other sugars (e.g., dextrose) or nonsugars (e.g., sorbitol, glycerin, and propylene glycol). Most syrups consist of between 60% and 80% sucrose. Sucrose not only provides sweetness and viscosity to the solution, but also renders the solution inherently stable (unlike dilute sucrose solutions, which are unstable).

Compared with syrups, elixirs are usually less sweet and less viscous because they contain a lower proportion of sugar, and they are consequently less effective than syrups in masking the taste of drugs. In contrast to aqueous syrups, elixirs are better able to maintain both water-soluble and alcohol-soluble components in solution because of their hydroalcoholic properties. These stable characteristics often make elixirs preferable to syrups. All elixirs contain flavoring and coloring agents to enhance their palatability and appearance. Elixirs containing over 10% to 12% ethanol are usually self-preserving and do not require the addition of antimicrobial agents for preservation. Alcohols precipitate tragacanth, acacia, agar, and inorganic salts from aqueous solutions; therefore, such substances should either be absent from the aqueous phase or be present in such low concentrations as not to promote precipitation on standing. Examples of some commonly used elixirs include dexamethasone elixir U.S. Pharmacopeia (USP), pentobarbital elixir USP, diphenhydramine hydrochloride elixir, and digoxin elixir.

Tablets

Depending on the physicochemical properties of the drug, site and extent of drug absorption in the GI tract, stability to heat or moisture, biocompatibility with other ingredients, solubility, and dose, the following types of tablets are commonly formulated:

- *Swallowable tablets* are intended to be swallowed whole and then disintegrate and release their medicaments in the GI tract.

- *Effervescent tablets* are dissolved in water before administration. In addition to the drug substance, these tablets contain sodium bicarbonate and an organic acid such as tartaric acid. These additives react in the presence of water, liberating carbon dioxide, which acts as a disintegrator and produces effervescence.
- *Chewable tablets* are used when a faster rate of dissolution or buccal absorption is desired. Chewable tablets consist of a mild effervescent drug complex dispersed throughout a gum base. The drug is released from the dosage form by physical disruption associated with chewing, chemical disruption caused by the interaction with the fluids in the oral cavity, and the presence of effervescent material. For example, antacid tablets should be chewed to obtain quick relief of indigestion.
- *Buccal* and *sublingual tablets* dissolve slowly in the mouth, cheek pouch (buccal), or under the tongue (sublingual). Buccal or sublingual absorption is often desirable for drugs subject to extensive hepatic metabolism, often referred to as the *first-pass effect*. Examples are isoprenaline sulfate (a bronchodilator), glyceryl trinitrate (a vasodilator), nitroglycerin, and testosterone tablets. These tablets do not contain a disintegrant and are compressed lightly to produce a fairly soft tablet.
- *Lozenges* are compressed tablets that do not contain a disintegrant. Some lozenges contain antiseptics (e.g., benzalkonium) or antibiotics for local effects in the mouth.
- *Controlled-release tablets* are used to improve patient compliance and to reduce side effects. Some water-soluble drugs are formulated as sustained-release tablets so that their release and dissolution are controlled over a long period. The combination of high- and low-viscosity grades of hydroxypropyl methylcellulose (HPMC) was used as the matrix base to prepare zileuton sustained-release tablets. A ternary polymeric matrix system composed of protein, HPMC, and highly water-soluble drugs such as diltiazem hydrochloride was developed by the direct compression method. Sustained-release tablets can also be prepared by formulating inert polymers such as polyvinyl chloride, polyvinyl acetate, and methyl methacrylate. These polymers protect the tablet from disintegration and reduce the dissolution rate of the drug inside the tablet. Examples of commonly used sustained-release drug delivery products are listed in Table 3-2.

Table 3-2. Examples of Sustained-Release Drug Delivery Products

Dosage forms	Active ingredients	Indications
Controlled-release tablets		
Abacavir (Ziagen)	Nucleoside reverse transcriptase inhibitor	HIV-1 infection
Sinemet	Carbidopa + levodopa	Parkinson's disease
Voltaren	Diclofenac sodium	Osteoarthritis and rheumatoid arthritis
Capsules		
Dexedrine Spansules	Dextroamphetamine	Narcolepsy
Adderall XL	Amphetamine + dextroamphetamine	Attention-deficit/hyperactivity disorder (ADHD)
Ritalin LA	Methylphenidate hydrochloride	ADHD
Videx EC	Didanosine	HIV-1 infection
Aerosols		
Ventolin HFA	Albuterol sulfate	Bronchodilator
Serevent	Salmeterol	Bronchodilator
Osmotic systems		
Ditropan XL	Oxybutynin chloride	Overreacting bladder
Covera-HS	Verapamil	Antihypertensive
Concerta	Methylphenidate HCl	ADHD
Inserts		
Lacrisert	Hydroxypropyl cellulose	Ophthalmic moisturizer
Atridox	Doxycycline	Periodontal disease
Transdermal patches		
Alora	Estradiol	Menopausal symptoms
CombiPatch	Estradiol/norethindrone acetate	Vasomotor symptoms associated with menopause
Androderm	Testosterone	Testosterone deficiency
Nicotine transdermal system	Nicotine	Smoking cessation
PEGylated proteins		
PEGASYS	PEGylated interferon + ribavirin	Hepatitis B, hepatitis C
Liposomes		
Doxil	Doxorubicin HCl	Kaposi's sarcoma
DaunoXome	Daunorubicin	Kaposi's sarcoma
Poly(lactic-co-glycolic acid)/polylactic acid microspheres		
Lupron Depot	Luteinizing hormone-releasing hormone agonist	Prostate cancer, endometriosis
Zoladex Depot	Goserelin acetate	Prostate cancer, endometriosis
Nutropin Depot	Recombinant human growth hormone	Growth deficiencies

Boldface indicates one of top 100 drugs for 2012 by units sold at retail outlets, www.drugs.com/stats/top100/2012/units.

■ *Coated tablets* are used to prevent decomposition or to minimize the unpleasant taste of certain drugs. Several types of coated tablets are made: film coated, sugar coated, gelatin coated (gel caps), or enteric coated. Enteric coatings are resistant to gastric juices but readily dissolve in the small intestine. These enteric coatings can protect drugs against decomposition in the acidic environment of the stomach. Commonly used polymers for enteric coating are acid-impermeable polymers such as cellulose acetate trimellitate, HPMC phthalate, polyvinyl acetate phthalate, cellulose acetate phthalate, and EUDRAGIT. Aspirin formulated as enteric-coated sustained-release tablets has been shown to produce less gastric bleeding than do conventional aspirin preparations. Film-coated tablets are compressed tablets coated with a thin layer of a water-insoluble or water-soluble polymer such as methylcellulose phthalate, ethylcellulose, povidone, or polyethylene glycol. Abacavir is a capsule-shaped film-coated tablet containing a nucleoside reverse transcriptase inhibitor, which is a potent antiviral agent for the treatment of HIV infection.

Tablet formulation

In addition to the drug, the following materials are added to make the powder system compatible with tablet formulation by the compression or granulation methods:

■ *Diluents* or bulking agents are invariably added to very-low-dose drugs to bring overall tablet weight to at least 50 mg, which is the minimum desirable tablet weight. Commonly used diluents are lactose, very low-dose, starches, microcrystalline cellulose, dextrose, sucrose, mannitol, and sodium chloride. Dicalcium phosphate absorbs less moisture than lactose and is therefore used with hygroscopic drugs such as meperidine hydrochloride.

■ *Adsorbents* are substances capable of holding quantities of fluids in an apparently dry state. Oil-soluble drugs or fluid extracts can be mixed with adsorbents and then granulated and compressed into tablets. Examples are fumed silica, microcrystalline cellulose, magnesium carbonate, kaolin, and bentonite.

■ *Moistening agents* are liquids that are used for wet granulation. Examples include water, industrial methylated spirits, and isopropanol.

■ *Binding agents (adhesives)* bind powders together in the wet granulation process. They also help bind granules together during compression. Examples include starches, gelatin, PVP, alginic acid derivatives, cellulose derivatives, glucose, and sucrose. Choice of binders affects the dissolution rate. For example, the tablet formulation of furosemide with PVP as the binder has a t_{50} (time required for 50% of the drug to be released during an in vitro dissolution study) of 3.65 minutes, but with starch mucilage as the binder, the t_{50} of the tablets was 117 minutes.

■ *Glidants* are added to tablet formulations to improve the flow properties of the granulations. They act by reducing interparticle friction. Commonly used glidants are fumed (colloidal) silica, starch, and talc.

■ *Lubricants* have a number of functions in tablet manufacture. They prevent adherence of the tablet material to the surfaces of the punch faces and dies, reduce interparticle friction, and facilitate the smooth ejection of the tablet from the die cavity. Many lubricants also enhance the flow properties of the granules. Commonly used lubricants are magnesium stearate, talc, stearic acid and its derivatives, PEG, paraffin, and sodium or magnesium lauryl sulfate. Among these lubricants, magnesium stearate is the most popular because it is effective as both a die and a punch lubricant. However, for many drugs (e.g., aspirin), magnesium stearate is chemically incompatible; therefore, talc or stearic acid is often used. Most lubricants, with the exception of talc, are used in concentrations below 1%.

■ *Disintegrating agents* are added to tablets to promote breakup or disintegration after administration, which increases the effective surface area and promotes rapid release of the drug. Disintegrants act either by bursting open the tablet or by promoting the rapid ingress of water into the center of the tablet or capsule. Examples include starches, cationic exchange resins, cross-linked PVP, celluloses, modified starches, alginic acid and alginates, magnesium aluminum silicate, and cross-linked sodium carboxymethylcellulose. Among these agents, starch is the most popular disintegrant because it has a great affinity for water and swells when moistened, thus facilitating the rupture of the tablet matrix.

Disintegration, dissolution, and absorption

A solid drug product has to disintegrate into small particles and release the drug before absorption can take place. Tablets that are intended for chewing or sustained release do not have to undergo disintegration. The various excipients for tablet formulation affect the rates of disintegration, dissolution, and absorption. Systemic absorption of most products consists of a succession of rate processes such as the following:

- Disintegration of the drug product and subsequent release of the drug
- Dissolution of the drug in an aqueous environment
- Absorption across cell membranes into the systemic circulation

In the process of tablet disintegration, dissolution, and absorption, the rate at which the drug reaches the circulatory system is determined by the slowest step in the sequence. Disintegration of a tablet is usually more rapid than drug dissolution and absorption. For the drug that has poor aqueous solubility, the rate at which the drug dissolves (dissolution) is often the slowest step, and it therefore exerts a rate-limiting effect on drug bioavailability. In contrast, for the drug that has a high aqueous solubility, the dissolution rate is rapid, and the rate at which the drug crosses or permeates cell membranes is the slowest or rate-limiting step.

Capsules

Capsules are the dosage forms in which unit doses of powder, semisolid, or liquid drugs are enclosed in a hard or soft, water-soluble container or shell of gelatin. Coating of the capsule shell or drug particles within the capsule can affect bioavailability. There are two types of capsules: hard and soft capsules. Hard gelatin capsules are more versatile for controlled drug delivery.

Hard gelatin capsules

A hard gelatin capsule consists of two pieces, a cap and a body, that fit one inside the other. They are produced empty and are then filled in a separate operation. Hard gelatin capsules are usually filled with powders, granules, or pellets containing the drug. After ingestion, the gelatin shell softens, swells, and begins to dissolve in the GI tract. Encapsulated drugs are released rapidly and dispersed easily, leading to high bioavailability. Capsules are supplied in a variety of sizes, and high-speed filling machinery capable of filling approximately 1,500 capsules per minute is available. The empty hard gelatin capsules

are numbered from 000, the largest size, to 5, which is the smallest. The approximate filling capacity of capsules ranges from 6,000 to 30 mg, depending on the types and bulk densities of powdered drug materials.

Powder formulations for encapsulation into hard gelatin capsules require careful consideration of the filling process, such as lubricity, compactibility, and fluidity. Additives present in the capsule formulations, such as the amount and choice of fillers and lubricants, the inclusion of disintegrants and surfactants, and the degree of plug compaction, can influence drug release from the capsule. Formulation factors influencing drug release and bioavailability are as follows:

- *Fillers (or diluents):* Active ingredient is mixed with a sufficient volume of a diluent—usually lactose, mannitol, starch, and dicalcium phosphate—to yield the desired amount of the drug in the capsule when the base is filled with the powder mixture.
- *Glidants:* The flow properties of the powder blend should be adequate to ensure a uniform flow rate from the hopper. Glidants such as silica, starch, talc, and magnesium stearate are used to improve the fluidity. The optimal concentration of the glidant used to improve the flow of a powder mixture is generally less than 1%.
- *Lubricants:* These ease the ejection of plugs by reducing adhesion of powder to metal surfaces and friction between sliding surfaces in contact with the powder. Typical lubricants for capsule formulations include magnesium stearate and stearic acid.
- *Surfactants:* These may be included in capsule formulations to increase wetting of the powder mass and to enhance drug dissolution. The most commonly used surfactants in capsule formulations are 0.1% to 0.5% sodium lauryl sulfate and sodium docusate.
- *Wetting agents:* Hydrophilic polymer is used as a wetting agent for improving the wettability of poorly soluble drugs. Powder wettability and dissolution rate of several drugs, including hexobarbital and phenytoin, from hard gelatin capsules have been shown to be enhanced if the drug is treated with methylcellulose or hydroxyethylcellulose.

Vancomycin hydrochloride is a highly hygroscopic antibiotic. To achieve acceptable stability, a hard gelatin capsule is filled with a PEG 6,000 matrix of vancomycin hydrochloride, which produces plasma and urine levels of the antibiotic similar to those obtained with the solution of vancomycin hydrochloride. Controlled-release beads and minitablets are often placed in gelatin capsules for convenient administration of an oral controlled-release dosage form. For example, sustained-release antihistamines, antitussives, and analgesics are first preformulated into extended-release microcapsules or microspheres and then placed inside a gelatin capsule. Another example is enteric-coated lipase minitablets, which are placed in a gelatin capsule for more effective protection and dosing of these enzymes.

Soft gelatin capsules

Soft gelatin capsules are prepared from plasticized gelatin by a rotary die process. They are formed, filled, and sealed in a single operation. Soft gelatin capsules may contain a nonaqueous solution, a powder, or a drug suspension, none of which solubilizes the gelatin shell. In contrast to hard gelatin capsules, soft gelatin capsules contain about 30% glycerol as a plasticizer in addition to gelatin and water. The moisture uptake of soft gelatin capsules plasticized with glycerol is considerably higher than that of hard gelatin capsules. Therefore, oxygen-sensitive drugs should not be inserted into soft gelatin capsules, nor should emulsions, because they are unstable and crack the shell of the capsule when water is lost in the manufacturing process. Extreme acidic and basic pH must also be avoided because a pH below 2.5 hydrolyzes gelatin, whereas a pH above 9.0 has a tanning effect on the gelatin. Insoluble drugs should be dispersed with an agent such as beeswax, paraffin, or ethylcellulose. Surfactants are also often added to promote wetting of the ingredients. Drugs that are commercially prepared in soft capsules include declomycin, vitamin A, vitamin E, and chloral hydrate.

Formulation of soft gelatin capsules involves liquid, rather than powder, technology. It requires careful consideration of the composition of the gelatin shell and filling materials. The composition of the soft capsule shell consists of two main ingredients: gelatin and a plasticizer. Water is used to form the capsule, and other additives are often added as follows:

- *Gelatin:* Properties of gelatin shells are controlled by choice of gelatin grade and by adjustment of the concentration of plasticizer in the shell.
- *Plasticizers:* The main plasticizer used for soft gelatin capsules is glycerol. Sorbitol and polypropylene glycol are also used in combination with glycerol. Compared to hard gelatin cap-

sules and tablet film coatings, a relatively large amount (~30%) of plasticizers is added in soft gelatin capsule formulation to ensure adequate flexibility.

- *Water:* The desirable water content of the gelatin solution used to produce a soft gelatin capsule shell depends on the viscosity of the gelatin used and ranges between 0.7 and 1.3 parts of water to each part of dry gelatin.
- *Other additives:* Preservatives are added to prevent mold growth in the gelatin shell. Potassium sorbate and methyl, ethyl, and propyl hydroxybenzoate are commonly used as preservatives.

Emulsions

An *emulsion* is a thermodynamically unstable system that consists of at least two immiscible liquid phases—one of which is dispersed as globules (dispersed phase) and the other, a liquid phase (continuous phase)—that are stabilized by the presence of an emulsifying agent. Emulsified systems range from lotions of relatively low viscosity to ointments and creams, which are semisolid in nature.

Types of emulsions

One liquid phase in an emulsion is essentially polar (e.g., aqueous), whereas the other is relatively nonpolar (e.g., an oil).

- *Oil-in-water emulsion:* When the oil phase is dispersed as globules throughout an aqueous continuous phase, the system is referred to as an *oil-in-water emulsion.*
- *Water-in-oil emulsion:* When the oil phase serves as the continuous phase, the emulsion is termed a *water-in-oil emulsion.*
- *Multiple (w/o/w or o/w/o) emulsions:* These are emulsions whose dispersed phase contains droplets of another phase. Multiple emulsions are of interest as delayed-action drug delivery systems.
- *Microemulsions:* These consist of homogeneous transparent systems of low viscosity that contain a high percentage of both oil and water and high concentrations of emulsifier mixture. Microemulsions form spontaneously when the components are mixed in the appropriate ratios and are thermodynamically stable.

Externally applied emulsions may be o/w or w/o. The o/w emulsions use the following emulsifiers: sodium lauryl sulfate, triethanolamine stearate, sodium oleate, and glyceryl monostearate. The w/o emulsions are used mainly for external applications and may contain one or several of the following emulsifiers: calcium palmitate, sorbitan esters (Spans), cholesterol, and wool fats.

Interfacial free energy and emulsification

Two immiscible liquids in an emulsion often fail to remain mixed because of the greater cohesive force between the molecules of each separate liquid, rather than the adhesive force between the two liquids. These forces lead to phase separation, which is the state of minimum surface free energy. When one liquid is broken into small particles, the interfacial area of the globules constitutes a surface area that is enormous compared with that of the original liquid. The adsorption of a surfactant or other emulsifying agent at the globule interface lowers the oil-to-water or water-to-oil interfacial tension. In addition, the process of emulsification is made easier, and the drug's stability may be enhanced.

Emulsifying agents

Preventing coalescence requires the introduction of an emulsifying agent that forms a film around the dispersed globules. Emulsifying agents may be divided into three groups:

- *Surface-active agents:* Surfactants are adsorbed at oil–water interfaces to form monomolecular films and to reduce interfacial tensions. Unless the interfacial tension is zero, the oil droplets have a natural tendency to coalesce to reduce the area of oil–water contact. The presence of the surfactant monolayer at the surface of the droplet reduces the possibility of collisions leading to coalescence. To retain a high surface area for the dispersed phase, surface-active agents must be used to decrease the surface free energy. Often a mixture of surfactants is used: one with hydrophilic character and the other with hydrophobic character. A hydrophilic emulsifying agent is needed for the aqueous phase, and a hydrophobic emulsifying agent is needed for the oil phase. A complex film results that produces an excellent emulsion. Nonionic surfactants are widely used in the production of stable emulsions. They are less toxic than ionic surfactants and are less sensitive to electrolytes and pH variation. Examples include sorbitan esters and polysorbates.

- *Hydrophilic colloids:* A number of hydrophilic colloids are used as emulsifying agents. They include gelatin, casein, acacia, cellulose derivatives, and alginates. These materials adsorb at the oil–water interface and form multilayer films around the dispersed droplets of oil in an o/w emulsion. Hydrated lyophilic colloids differ from surfactants because they do not appreciably lower interfacial tension. Their action is caused by the strong multimolecular film's resistance to coalescence. Additionally, they increase the viscosity of the dispersion medium. Hydrophilic colloids are used for formation of o/w emulsions because the films are hydrophilic. Most cellulose derivatives are not charged but can sterically stabilize the systems.

- *Finely divided solid particles:* These particles are adsorbed at the interface between two immiscible liquid phases and form a film of particles around the dispersed globules. Finely divided solid particles that are wetted to some degree by both oil and water can act as emulsifying agents. They are concentrated at the interface, where they produce a film of particles around the dispersed droplets that prevents coalescence. Finely divided solid particles that are wetted by water form o/w emulsions; those that are wetted by oil form w/o emulsions. Examples include bentonite, magnesium hydroxide, and aluminum hydroxide.

Types of instability in emulsions

The stability of an emulsion is characterized by the absence of coalescence of the internal phase; the absence of creaming; and the maintenance of elegance with respect to appearance, odor, color, and other physical properties. An emulsion becomes unstable because of creaming, breaking, coalescence, phase inversion, and some other factors.

Creaming and sedimentation

Creaming is the upward movement of dispersed droplets relative to the continuous phase, whereas *sedimentation*, the reverse process, is the downward movement of particles. Density differences in the two phases cause these processes, which can be reversed by shaking. Creaming is undesirable, however, because a creamed emulsion increases the likelihood of coalescence because of the proximity of the globules in the cream. Factors that influence the rate of creaming are similar to those involved in the sedimentation rate of suspension particles and are indicated by Stokes's law. The rate of creaming is decreased by the following:

- A reduction in the globule size
- A decrease in the density difference between the two phases
- An increase in the viscosity of the continuous phase

This decrease may be achieved by homogenizing the emulsion to reduce the globule size and increasing the viscosity of the continuous phase by the use of thickening agents such as tragacanth or methylcellulose.

Creaming, breaking, coalescence, and aggregation

Creaming is a reversible process, whereas breaking is irreversible. When breaking occurs, simple mixing fails to resuspend the globules in a stable emulsified form. Because the film surrounding the particles has been destroyed, the oil tends to coalesce. *Coalescence* is the process by which emulsified particles merge with each other to form large particles. The major factor preventing coalescence is the mechanical strength of the interfacial barrier. Formation of a thick interfacial film is essential for minimal coalescence. In aggregation, the dispersed droplets come together but do not fuse. Aggregation is to some extent reversible.

Phase inversion

An emulsion is said to invert when it changes from an o/w to a w/o emulsion or vice versa. Inversion can be caused by adding an electrolyte or by changing the phase-to-volume ratio. For example, an o/w emulsion stabilized with sodium stearate can be inverted to a w/o emulsion by adding calcium chloride to form calcium stearate.

Microbial growth

Growth of microorganisms in an emulsion can cause physical separation of the phases. Because bacteria can degrade nonionic and anionic emulsifying agents, preservatives must be added to the product in adequate concentrations to prevent bacterial growth.

Suspensions

Suspensions are dispersions of finely divided solid particles of a drug in a liquid medium in which the drug is not readily soluble. Suspending agents are often hydrophilic colloids (e.g., cellulose derivatives, acacia, or xanthan gum) added to suspensions to increase viscosity, inhibit agglomeration, and decrease sedimentation. Highly viscous suspensions may prolong gastric emptying time, slow drug dissolution, and decrease the absorption rate. A suspension that is thixotropic as well as pseudoplastic should prove useful because it forms a gel on standing and becomes fluid when disturbed.

Desired characteristics of suspensions

- Suspended material should settle slowly and should readily disperse on gentle shaking of the container.
- Particle size of the suspension should remain fairly constant.
- The suspension should pour readily and evenly from its container.

Flocculation

The DLVO (Derjaguin, Landau, Verwey, and Overbeek) theory is the classic explanation of stability of colloids in suspension that is based on two opposite forces: electrostatic forces of repulsion and van der Waals forces of attraction. The large surface area of the colloidal particles is associated with a surface free energy that makes the system thermodynamically unstable. This instability makes particles highly energetic; they tend to regroup, resulting in the decrease in total surface area and surface free energy. Therefore, the particles in a liquid suspension tend to flocculate. *Flocculation* is the formation of light, fluffy conglomerates held together by weak van der Waals forces. *Aggregation* occurs when crystals come together to form a compact cake (growth and fusing together of crystals in the precipitate to form a solid aggregate). Flocculating agents can prevent caking, whereas deflocculating agents increase the tendency to cake. Surfactants can reduce interfacial tension, but they cannot reduce it to zero. Thus, suspensions of insoluble particles tend to have a positive finite interfacial tension, and particles tend to flocculate.

Forces at the surface of a particle affect the degree of flocculation and agglomeration in a suspension. Forces of attraction are of the London–van der Waals type, whereas repulsive forces arise from the interaction of the electric double layers surrounding each particle. When the repulsion energy is high, collision of the particles is opposed. The system remains deflocculated, and when sedimentation is complete, the particles form a close-packed arrangement with the smaller particles filling the voids between the larger ones. Those particles that are lowest in the sediment are gradually pressed together by the weight of the ones above; the energy barrier is thus overcome, allowing the particles to come into close contact with each other. Resuspending and redispersing these particles require that the high-energy barrier be overcome. Because agitation does not easily achieve this, the particles tend to remain strongly attracted to each other and form a hard cake. When the particles are flocculated, the energy barrier is still too large to be surmounted. Thus, the approaching particles in the second energy minimum, which are at a distance of separation of perhaps 1,000 to 2,000 Å, are sufficient to form the loosely structured flocs.

Sedimentation of flocculated particles

Flocs tend to fall together, producing a distinct boundary between the sediment and the supernatant liquid. The liquid above the sediment is clear because even the small particles present in the system are associated with flocs. In deflocculated systems with variable particle sizes, by contrast, the large particles settle more rapidly than the smaller particles, and no clear boundary is formed. The supernatant remains turbid for a longer time.

Flocculation or deflocculation?

Whether a suspension is flocculated or deflocculated depends on the relative magnitudes of the electrostatic forces of repulsion and the forces of attraction between the particles. Flocculated systems form loose sediments that are easily redispersible, but the sedimentation rate is usually fast. In contrast, a suspension is deflocculated when the dispersed particles remain as discrete units and will settle slowly. This condition prevents the entrapment of liquid within the sediment, which leads to caking—a serious stability problem encountered in suspension formulation.

Flocculating agents

If the charge on the particle is neutralized, flocculation will occur. If a high charge density is imparted to the suspension particles, then deflocculation will be the result. The following flocculating agents are often used to convert the suspension from a deflocculated to a flocculated state:

- *Electrolytes:* The addition of an inorganic electrolyte to an aqueous suspension will alter the zeta potential of the dispersed particles. If this value is lowered sufficiently, then flocculation may occur. The most widely used electrolytes include sodium salts of acetates, phosphates, and citrates.

- *Surfactants:* Ionic surfactants may also cause flocculation by neutralizing the charge on each particle.

- *Polymeric flocculating agents:* Starches, alginates, cellulose derivatives, tragacanth, carbomers, and silicates are examples of polymeric flocculating agents that can be used to control the degree of flocculation. Their linear branched-chain molecules form a gel-like network within the system and become adsorbed on the surfaces of the dispersed particles, thus holding them in a flocculated state.

Formulation of suspensions

Physically stable suspensions can be formulated in two ways. One is to use a structured vehicle to maintain deflocculated particles in suspension. However, the major disadvantage of deflocculated systems is that when the particles eventually settle, they form a compact cake. The other is by production of flocs, which may settle rapidly but are easily resuspended with a minimum of agitation. Optimum physical stability is obtained when the suspension is formulated with flocculated particles in a structured vehicle of a hydrophilic colloid type.

Ointments, Creams, and Gels

Ointments, creams, and gels are semisolid preparations intended for topical applications. These semisolid formulations are designed for local or systemic drug absorption.

Ointments are typically used as follows:

- Emollients to make the skin more pliable
- Protective barriers to prevent harmful substances from coming in contact with the skin
- Vehicles in which to incorporate medication

Ointment bases are classified into four general groups: (1) hydrocarbon bases, (2) absorption bases, (3) water-removable bases, and (4) water-soluble bases.

Hydrocarbon bases

Hydrocarbon (oleaginous) bases are anhydrous and insoluble in water. They cannot absorb or contain water and are not washable in water.

Petrolatum is a good base for oil-insoluble ingredients. It forms an occlusive film on the skin and absorbs less than 5% water under normal conditions. Wax can be incorporated to stiffen the base. Synthetic esters are used as constituents of oleaginous bases. These esters include glycerol monostearate, isopropyl myristate, isopropyl palmitate, butyl stearate, and butyl palmitate.

Absorption bases

Absorption bases are of two types: (1) those that permit the incorporation of aqueous solutions, resulting in the formation of w/o emulsions (e.g., hydrophilic petrolatum and anhydrous lanolin), and (2) those that are already w/o emulsions (emulsion bases) and thus permit the incorporation of small additional quantities of aqueous solutions (e.g., lanolin and cold cream). These bases are useful as emollients although they do not provide the degree of occlusion afforded by the oleaginous bases. Absorption bases are also not easily removed from the skin with water. An aqueous solution may be first incorporated into the absorption base, and then this mixture added to the oleaginous base.

Water-removable bases

Emulsion, water-washable, or water-removable bases, commonly referred to as creams, represent the most commonly used type of ointment base. The majority of dermatologic drug products are formulated in an emulsion or cream base. Emulsion bases are washable and removed easily from skin or clothing. An emulsion base can be subdivided into three component parts: the oil phase, the emulsifier, and the aqueous phase. Drugs can be included in one of these phases or added to the formed emulsion. The oil phase, also known as the *internal phase,* is typically made up of petrolatum or liquid petrolatum together with cetyl or stearyl alcohol. Types of emulsion bases are as follows:

- *Hydrophilic ointment* is an o/w emulsion that uses sodium lauryl sulfate as an emulsifying agent. It is readily miscible with water and is removed from the skin easily. The aqueous phase of an emulsion base contains the preservatives that are included to control microbial growth. The preservatives in the emulsion include methylparaben, propylparaben, benzyl alcohol, sorbic acid, or quaternary ammonium compounds. The aqueous phase also contains the water-soluble components of the emulsion system, together with any additional stabilizers, antioxidants, and buffers that may be necessary for stability and pH control.

- *Cold cream* is a semisolid white w/o emulsion prepared with cetyl ester wax, white wax, mineral oil, sodium borate, and purified water. Sodium borate combines with free fatty acids present in the waxes to form sodium soaps that act as the emulsifiers. Cold cream is used as an emollient and ointment base. Eucerin cream is a w/o emulsion of petrolatum, mineral oil, mineral wax, wool wax, alcohol, and bronopol. It is frequently prescribed as a vehicle for delivery of lactic acid and glycerin to treat dry skin.
- *Lanolin* is a w/o emulsion that contains approximately 25% water and acts as an emollient and occlusive film on the skin, effectively preventing epidermal water loss.
- *Vanishing cream* is an o/w emulsion that contains a large percentage of water as well as a humectant (e.g., glycerin or propylene glycol) that retards surface evaporation. An excess of stearic acid in the formula helps to form a thin film when the water evaporates.

Water-soluble bases

Water-soluble bases may be anhydrous or may contain some water. They are washable in water and absorb water to the point of solubility. Polyethylene glycol ointment is a blend of water-soluble PEG that forms a semisolid base. This base can solubilize water-soluble drugs and some water-insoluble drugs. It is compatible with a wide variety of drugs. It contains 40% PEG 4,000 and 60% PEG 400. Another water-soluble base is the ointment prepared with propylene glycol and ethanol, which form a clear gel when mixed with 2% hydroxypropyl cellulose. This base is a commonly used dermatologic vehicle.

Incorporation of drugs into an ointment

Drugs may be incorporated into an ointment base by levigation and fusion. Normally, drug substances are in fine-powdered forms before being dispersed in the vehicle. Levigation of powders into a small portion of base is facilitated by the use of a melted base or a small quantity of compatible levigation aid, such as mineral oil or glycerin. Water-soluble salts are incorporated by dissolving them in a small volume of water and incorporating the aqueous solution into a compatible base. Fusion is used when the base contains solids that have higher melting points (e.g., waxes, cetyl alcohol, or glyceryl monostearate).

Suppositories

A *suppository* is a solid dosage form intended for insertion into body orifices (e.g., rectum, vagina, or urethra). Once inserted, the suppository base melts, softens, or dissolves at body temperature, distributing its medications to the tissues of the region. Suppositories are used for local or systemic effects. Rectal suppositories intended for local action are often used to relieve the pain, irritation, itching, and inflammation associated with hemorrhoids. Vaginal suppositories intended for local effects are used mainly as contraceptives, antiseptics in feminine hygiene, and methods to combat invading pathogens. The suppository base has a marked influence on the release of active constituents. Two main classes of suppository bases are in use: the glyceride-type fatty bases and the water-soluble ones. The main water-soluble and water-miscible suppository bases are glycerinated gelatin and polyethylene glycols. Polyethylene glycol suppositories do not melt at body temperature but rather dissolve slowly in the body's fluids. Examples of rectal suppositories include acetaminophen and promethazine.

Inserts, Implants, and Devices

Inserts, implants, and devices are used to control drug delivery for localized or systemic drug effects. In these systems, drugs are embedded into biodegradable or nonbiodegradable materials to allow slow release of the drug. The inserts, implants, and devices are inserted into a variety of cavities (e.g., vagina, buccal cavity, cul de sac of the eye, or subcutaneous tissue).

Degradable inserts consist of polyvinyl alcohol, hydroxypropyl cellulose, PVP, and hyaluronic acid. Nondegradable inserts are prepared from insoluble materials such as ethylene vinyl acetate copolymers and styrene–isoprene–styrene block copolymers. The initial use of contact lenses was for vision correction; however, they are becoming more useful as potential drug delivery devices by presoaking them in drug solutions. The use of contact lenses can simultaneously correct vision and release the drug.

A number of degradable and nondegradable inserts are currently available for ophthalmic delivery. These ophthalmic inserts can be insoluble, soluble, or bioerodible. Insoluble inserts are further classified as diffusional, osmotic, and contact lens (Figure 3-2). Ocular inserts are no more affected by nasolacrimal drainage and tear flow than are conventional dosage forms; they can provide slow drug release and longer residence times in the conjunctival cul de sac. A pilo ocular insert consists of a drug reservoir (pilocarpine

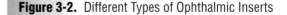

Figure 3-2. Different Types of Ophthalmic Inserts

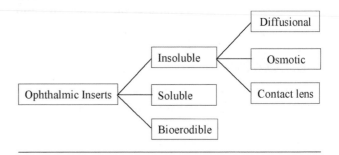

hydrochloride in an alginate gel) enclosed by two release-controlling membranes made of ethylene vinyl acetate copolymer and further enclosed by a white ring, which allows positioning of the system in the eye. It has demonstrated slow release of pilocarpine, which can effectively control the increased intraocular pressure in glaucoma. Other inserts (e.g., medicated contact lenses, collagen shields, and minidiscs) have been shown to diminish the systemic absorption of ocularly applied drugs as a result of decreased drainage into the nasal cavity. Lacrisert is a soluble insert composed of hydroxypropyl cellulose and is useful in the treatment of dry eye syndrome. The device is placed in the lower fornix, where it slowly dissolves over 6–8 hours to stabilize and thicken the tear film.

In addition to ophthalmic delivery, inserts are used for localized delivery of drugs to various other tissues. For example, the Progestasert device is designed for implantation into the uterine cavity, where it releases 65 mg progesterone per day to provide contraception for 1 year. Atridox is a product designed for controlled-release delivery of doxycycline for the treatment of periodontal disease. When injected into the periodontal cavity, the formulation sets, forming a drug delivery depot that delivers the antibiotic to the subgingival.

An *implant* is a drug delivery system designed to deliver a drug moiety at a desired rate over a prolonged period. Implants are available in many forms, including polymeric implants and minipumps. Diffusional and osmotic systems contain a reservoir that is in contact with the inner surface of a controller, to which it supplies the drug. The reservoir contains a liquid, a gel, a colloid, a semisolid, a solid matrix, or a carrier that contains the drug. Carriers consist of hydrophilic or hydrophobic polymers. Viadur is a once-yearly implant of leuprolide for the palliative treatment of advanced prostate cancer. It uses a nondegradable, osmotically driven system that delivers small amounts of drugs, peptides, proteins, and deoxyribonucleic acid (DNA) for systemic or tissue-specific therapy.

One of the more commonly used devices is the oral osmotic pump, composed of a core tablet and a semipermeable coating with a 0.3–4.0 mm diameter hole, produced by a laser beam, for drug exit. This system requires only osmotic pressure to be effective, but the drug release rate depends on the surface area, the nature of the membrane, and the diameter of the hole. When the dosage form comes in contact with water, water is imbibed because of the resultant osmotic pressure of the core, and the drug is released from the orifice at a controlled rate.

Transdermal Drug Delivery Systems

Transdermal drug delivery systems (often called *transdermal patches*) deliver drugs directly through the skin and into the bloodstream. Percutaneous absorption of a drug generally results from direct penetration of the drug through the stratum corneum. Once through the stratum corneum, drug molecules may pass through the deeper epidermal tissues and into the dermis. When the drug reaches the vascularized dermal area, it becomes available for absorption into the general circulation. Among the factors influencing percutaneous absorption are the physicochemical properties of the drug, including its molecular weight, solubility, and partition coefficient; the nature of the vehicle; and the condition of the skin. Chemical permeation enhancers or iontophoresis are often used to enhance the percutaneous absorption of a drug.

In general, patches are composed of three key compartments: a protective seal that forms the external surface and protects it from damage, a compartment that holds the medication itself and has an adhesive backing to hold the entire patch on the skin surface, and a release liner that protects the adhesive layer during storage and is removed just prior to application. Examples of transdermal patches include Estraderm (estradiol), Nicoderm (nicotine), Testoderm (testosterone), Alora (estradiol), and Androderm (testosterone). Transderm Scōp relies on the rate-limiting polymeric membranes to control drug release of scopolamine through the skin.

Aerosol Products

Aerosols are pressurized dosage forms designed to deliver drugs with the aid of a liquefied or propelled gas (propellant). Aerosol products consist of a pressurizable container, a valve that allows the pressurized product to be expelled from the container when the actuator is pressed, and a dip tube that conveys the formulation from the bottom of the container to the valve assembly. Inhalation devices broadly fall into three categories: pressurized metered dose inhalers (MDIs), nebulizers, and dry powder inhalers. The most commonly used inhalers on the market are MDIs. They contain an active ingredient as a solution or as a suspension of fine particles in a liquefied propellant held under high pressure. MDIs use special metering valves to regulate the amount of formulation dispensed with each dose. Nebulizers do not require propellants and can generate large quantities of small droplets capable of penetrating into the lung. Sustained release of drugs, such as bronchodilators and corticosteroids for the treatment of asthma and chronic obstructive pulmonary diseases, involves encapsulation of the drugs in slowly degrading particles that can be inhaled. For accumulation in the alveolar zone of the lungs, which has a very large surface area, inhaled liquid or dry powder aerosols should have particle sizes in the range of 1–5 micrometers. Inhaled drugs play a prominent role in the treatment of asthma because this route has significant advantages over oral or parenteral administration. Azmacort (triamcinolone acetonide), Ventolin HFA (albuterol sulfate), and Serevent Diskus (salmeterol) are examples of commercially available aerosols for the treatment of asthma.

3-8. Targeted Drug Delivery Systems

Targeted drug delivery systems are drug carrier systems that deliver the drug to the target or receptor site in a manner that provides maximum therapeutic activity, prevents degradation or inactivation during transit to the target sites, and protects the body from adverse reactions because of inappropriate disposition. Design of an effective delivery system requires a thorough understanding of the drug, the disease, and the target site (Figure 3-3). Examples include macromolecular drug carriers (protein drug carriers); particulate drug delivery systems (e.g., microspheres, nanospheres, and liposomes); monoclonal antibodies; and cells. Plasma clearance kinetics, tissue distribution, metabolism, and cellular interactions of a drug can be controlled by the use of a site-specific delivery system. Targeting of drugs to specific sites in the body can be achieved by linking particulate systems or macromolecular carriers to monoclonal antibodies or to cell-specific ligands (e.g., asialofetuin, glycoproteins, or immunoglobulins) or by altering the

Figure 3-3. Essential Components of Drug Delivery

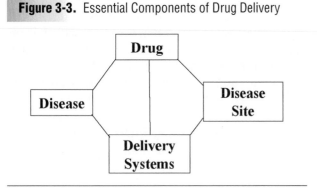

surface characteristics so that they are not recognized by the reticuloendothelial system.

Macromolecular Carrier Systems

Both natural and synthetic water-soluble polymers have been used as macromolecular drug carriers. The drug can be attached to the polymer chain either directly or via a spacer. Attachment of PEG to proteins can protect them from rapid hydrolysis or degradation within the body, increase blood circulation time, and lower the immunogenicity of proteins. For example, PEGylated forms of interferon Peg-Intron are used for treatment of hepatitis C to reduce dosing frequency from daily injections to once-weekly injection dosing. PEGylation improves macromolecule solubility and stability by minimizing the uptake by the cells of the reticuloendothelial system. Because PEG drug conjugates are not well absorbed from the gut, they are mainly used as injectables. The drug–polymer conjugate may also contain a receptor-specific ligand to achieve selective access to, and interaction with, the target cells.

Particulate Drug Delivery Systems

Many particulate carriers have been designed for drug delivery and targeting. They include liposomes, micelles, microspheres, and nanoparticles.

Liposomes

Liposomes are microscopic phospholipid vesicles composed of uni- or multilamellar lipid bilayers surrounding compartments. Multilamellar vesicles have diameters in the range of 1.0–5.0 micrometers. Sonication of multilamellar vesicles results in the production of small unilamellar vesicles with diameters in the range of 0.02–0.08 micrometers. Large unilamellar vesicles can be made by evaporation under reduced pressure, resulting in liposomes with a diameter of 0.1–1.0 micrometer. The bilayer-forming lipid is the essential part of the lamellar structure, while the other compounds are added to impart certain characteristics to the vesicles. Water-soluble drugs can be entrapped in liposomes by intercalation in the aqueous bilayers, whereas lipid-soluble drugs can be entrapped within the hydrocarbon interiors of the lipid bilayers. Liposomes can encapsulate low-molecular-weight drugs, proteins, peptides, oligonucleotides, and genes. The antifungal agent amphotericin B is formulated in liposomes in the intravenous product AmBisome. Because conventional liposomes can be recognized by the immune system as foreign bodies, stealth liposomes evade recognition by the immune system because of their unique polyethylene glycol coating. Doxil is a stealth liposome formulation of doxorubicin that is used for the treatment of AIDS-related Kaposi's sarcoma.

Microparticles and nanoparticles

Microencapsulation is a technique that involves the encapsulation of small particles or the solution of drugs in a polymer film or coat. Different methods of microencapsulation result in either microcapsules or microspheres. For example, interfacial polymerization of a monomer usually produces microcapsules, whereas solvent evaporation may result in microspheres or microcapsules, depending on the amount of drug loading. A *microcapsule* is a reservoir-type system in which the drug is located centrally within the particle, whereas a *microsphere* is a matrix-type system in which the drug is dispersed throughout the particle. Microcapsules usually release their drug at a constant rate (zero-order release), whereas microspheres typically give a first-order release of drugs. Low-molecular-weight drugs, proteins, oligonucleotides, and genes can be encapsulated into microparticles to provide their sustained release at disease sites.

The most commonly used method of microencapsulation is coacervation, which involves the addition of a hydrophilic substance to a colloidal drug dispersion. The hydrophilic substance, which acts as a coating material, may be selected from a variety of natural and synthetic polymers, including shellacs, waxes, gelatin, starches, cellulose acetate phthalate, and ethylcellulose, among others. Following dissolution of the coating materials, the drug inside the microcapsule is available for dissolution and absorption.

Biodegradable polylactide and its copolymers with glycolide—poly(lactic-co-glycolic acid), or PLGA—are commonly used for preparation of microparticles from which the drug can be released slowly over a period of a month or so. Microspheres can be used in a wide variety of dosage forms, including tablets, capsules, and suspensions. Lupron Depot is a preparation of PLGA microspheres for sustained release of leuprolide, a small peptide analog of gonadotropin-releasing hormone.

3-9. Questions

1. If the pK$_a$ of a weak acid drug is 2.5, at which pH will this drug become more ionized?

   A. pH 5
   B. pH 2.5
   C. pH 1.5
   D. pH 1

2. Which equation describes the rate of drug dissolution from a tablet?

   A. Fick's law
   B. Henderson–Hasselbalch equation
   C. Michaelis–Menten equation
   D. Noyes–Whitney equation

3. The pH of a buffer system can be calculated with

   A. the Henderson–Hasselbalch equation.
   B. the Noyes–Whitney equation.
   C. the Michaelis–Menten equation.
   D. Yong's equation.

4. If the pK$_a$ of a drug is 5, at which of the following pH values do the ionic and nonionic forms of the drug exist at equal ratio?

   A. pH 1
   B. pH 5
   C. pH 7
   D. pH 9

5. What is bioavailability?

   A. Bioavailability is the measurement of the rate and extent of active drug that reaches the systemic circulation.

   B. It is the relationship between the physical and chemical properties of a drug and its systemic absorption.
   C. It is the movement of the drug into body tissues over time.
   D. It is the dissolution of the drug in the GI tract.

6. Which of the following may be used to assess the relative bioavailability of two chemically equivalent drug products in a crossover study?

   A. Dissolution test
   B. Peak concentration
   C. Time-to-peak concentration
   D. Area under the plasma-level time curve

7. What condition usually increases the rate of drug dissolution for a tablet?

   A. Increase in the particle size of the drug
   B. Decrease in the surface area of the drug
   C. Use of the ionized, or salt, form of the drug
   D. Use of the free acid or free base form of the drug

8. If the pK$_a$ of a weak base drug is 8.3, at which of the following pH values does this drug become more ionized?

   A. pH 4
   B. pH 9
   C. pH 10
   D. pH 13

9. Which of the following dosage forms may use surface-active agents in their formulations?

   A. Emulsions
   B. Suspensions
   C. Colloidal dosage forms
   D. Creams
   E. All of the above

10. Which of the following statements about lyophilic colloidal dispersions is true?

    A. They tend to be more sensitive to the addition of electrolytes than do lyophobic systems.
    B. They tend to be more viscous than lyophobic systems.
    C. They can be precipitated by prolonged dialysis.
    D. They separate rapidly.

11. Which of the following is *not* true for tablet formulations?

    A. A disintegrating agent promotes granule flow.
    B. Lubricants prevent adherence of granules to the punch faces of the tableting machine.
    C. Glidants promote flow of the granules.
    D. Binding agents are used for adhesion of powder into granules.

12. The absorption rate of a drug is most rapid when the drug is formulated as

    A. a controlled-release product.
    B. a hard gelatin capsule.
    C. a compressed tablet.
    D. a solution.

13. According to the Noyes–Whitney equation, the drug concentration immediately at the solid surface within the diffusion layer (stagnant layer) is recognized as the

    A. drug solubility.
    B. dissolution rate.
    C. thickness layer.
    D. diffusion coefficient.

14. Adding PEG groups to large molecules will enhance their

    A. absorption through the intestine.
    B. solubility.
    C. oxidation.
    D. degradation.

15. Which of the following statements is true?

    A. Flocculation is desirable for pharmaceutical suspensions.
    B. The diffusion rate of molecules of a smaller particle size is less than that of molecules of a larger particle size.
    C. The particle size of molecular dispersions is larger than a coarse dispersion.
    D. Pseudoplastic flow is shear-thickening type, and dilatant is shear-thinning type.

16. Which of the following statements is false?

    A. The Henderson–Hasselbalch equation describes the effect of physical parameters on the stability of pharmaceutical suspensions.

    B. The passive diffusion rate of hydrophobic drugs across biological membranes is higher than that of hydrophilic compounds.
    C. When the dispersed phase in an emulsion formulation is heavier than the dispersion medium, creaming can still occur.
    D. Targeted drug delivery systems deliver the drug to the target or receptor site in a manner that provides maximum therapeutic activity.

17. Which of the following is an emulsifying agent?

    A. Sorbitan monooleate (Span 80)
    B. Polyoxyethylene sorbitan monooleate (Tween 80)
    C. Sodium lauryl sulfate
    D. Gum acacia
    E. All of the above

18. Which of the following surfactants is incompatible with bile salts?

    A. Polysorbate 80
    B. Potassium stearate
    C. Sodium lauryl sulfate
    D. Benzalkonium chloride

19. Which of the following statements is false?

    A. The partition coefficient is the ratio of drug solubility in n-octanol to that in water.
    B. Absorption of a weak electrolyte drug does not depend on the extent to which the drug exists in its un-ionized form at the absorption site.
    C. The drug dissolution rate can be determined using the Noyes–Whitney equation.
    D. Amorphous forms of drugs have faster dissolution rates than do crystalline forms.

20. Which of the following statements is true?

    A. Most substances acquire a surface charge by ionization, ion adsorption, and ion dissolution.
    B. The term *surface tension* is used for liquid-vapor and solid-vapor tensions.
    C. At the isoelectric point, the total number of positive charges is equal to the total number of negative charges.
    D. All of the above

21. Agents that may be used in the enteric coating of tablets include

    A. hydroxypropyl methylcellulose.
    B. carboxymethylcellulose.
    C. cellulose acetate phthalate.
    D. none of the above.

3-10. Answers

1. **A.** The answer is pH 5. For a weak acid, a higher pH increases ionization.

2. **D.** The Noyes–Whitney equation describes the rate of drug dissolution from a tablet. Fick's first law of diffusion is similar to the Noyes–Whitney equation in that both equations describe drug movement attributable to a concentration gradient. The Michaelis–Menten equation involves enzyme kinetics, whereas Henderson–Hasselbalch equations are used for determination of pH of the buffer and the extent of ionization of a drug molecule.

3. **A.** The Henderson–Hasselbalch equation for a weak acid and its salt is represented as pH = pK_a + log [salt]/[acid], where pK_a is the negative log of the dissolution constant of a weak acid, as [salt]/[acid] is the ratio of the molar concentration of salt and acid used to prepare a buffer.

4. **B.** The answer is pH 5. When pH equals pK_a, the ratio of ionized to un-ionized become the same.

5. **A.** Bioavailability is the measurement of the rate and extent of systemic circulation of an active drug.

6. **D.** The plasma drug concentration versus time curve measures the bioavailability of a drug from a product. The peak plasma drug concentration (C_{max}) relates to the intensity of the pharmacologic response, while the time for peak plasma drug concentration (T_{max}) relates to the rate of systemic absorption.

7. **C.** The ionized, or salt, form of a drug is generally more water soluble and therefore dissolves more rapidly than the nonionized (free acid or free base) form of the drug. According to the Noyes–Whitney equation, the dissolution rate is directly proportional to the surface area and inversely proportional to the particle size. Therefore, an increase in the particle size or a decrease in the surface area slows the dissolution rate.

8. **A.** The answer is pH 4. For a weak base, a lower pH value increases ionization of the molecule.

9. **E.** Surface-active agents facilitate emulsion formation by lowering the interfacial tension between the oil and water phases. Adsorption of surfactants on insoluble particles enables these particles to be dispersed in the form of a suspension.

10. **B.** Most lyophilic colloids are organic molecules (including gelatin and acacia); they spontaneously form colloidal solutions and tend to be viscous. Dispersion of lyophilic colloids is stable in the presence of electrolytes.

11. **A.** Disintegrating agents are added to the tablets to promote breakup of the tablets when placed in the aqueous environment. Lubricants are required to prevent adherence of the granules to the punch faces and dies. Glidants are added to tablet formulations to improve the flow properties of the granulations. Binding agents are added to bind powders together in the granulation process.

12. **D.** For a drug in solution, no dissolution is required before absorption. Consequently, compared with other drug formulations, a drug in aqueous solution has the highest bioavailability rate and is often used as the reference preparation for other formulations.

13. **A.** According to the Noyes–Whitney equation, the drug concentration in the stagnant layer is equal to the drug solubility.

14. **B.** PEG group increases the solubility of the molecule.

15. **A.** Flocculation is the formation of light, fluffy conglomerates held together by weak van der Waals forces and is a reversible process. Pseudoplastic flow is a shear-thinning process, whereas dilatant is a shear-thickening type process.

16. **A.** The Henderson–Hasselbalch equation describes the relationship between ionized and nonionized species of a weak electrolyte.

17. **E.** Sorbitan monooleate (Span 80), polyoxyethylene sorbitan monooleate (Tween 80), sodium lauryl sulfate, and gum acacia are surfactants used as emulsifiers.

18. **D.** Benzalkonium chloride is a cationic surfactant and can interact with bile salts.

19. **B.** According to pH partition theory, absorption of a weak electrolyte drug depends on the extent to which the drug exists in its un-ionized form at the absorption site. However, pH partition theory often does not hold true because most weakly acidic drugs are well absorbed from the small intestine, possibly because of the large epithelial surface areas of the organ.

20. **D.** Most substances acquire a surface charge by ionization, ion adsorption, and ion dissolution. At the isoelectric point, the total number of positive charges is equal to the total number of negative charges.

21. **C.** An enteric-coated tablet has a coating that remains intact in the stomach but dissolves in the intestine when the pH exceeds 6. Enteric-coating materials include cellulose acetate phthalate, polyvinyl acetate phthalate, and hydroxypropyl methylcellulose phthalate.

3-11. References

Ansel HC, Popovich NG, Allen LV, eds. *Pharmaceutical Dosage Forms and Drug Delivery Systems*. 6th ed. Malvern, PA: Williams & Wilkins; 1995.

Aulton ME, ed. *Pharmaceutics: The Science of Dosage Form Design*. New York, NY: Churchill Livingstone; 1988.

Banker GS, Rhodes CT, eds. *Modern Pharmaceutics*. 3rd ed. New York, NY: Marcel Dekker; 1995.

Block LH, Collins CC. Biopharmaceutics and drug delivery systems. In: Shargel L, Mutnick AH, Souney PH, Swanson LN, eds. *Comprehensive Pharmacy Review*. New York, NY: Lippincott Williams & Wilkins; 2001:78–91.

Block LH, Yu ABC. Pharmaceutical principles and drug dosage forms. In: Shargel L, Mutnick AH, Souney PH, Swanson LN, eds. *Comprehensive Pharmacy Review*. New York, NY: Lippincott Williams & Wilkins; 2001:28–77.

Florence AT, Attwood D. *Physicochemical Principles of Pharmacy*. 3rd ed. Palgrave, NY: Macmillan; 1998.

Gennaro AR, Gennaro AL, eds. *Remington: The Science and Practice of Pharmacy*. Baltimore, MD: Lippincott Williams & Wilkins; 2000.

Hillery AM. Advanced drug delivery and targeting: An introduction. In: Hillery AM, Lloyd AW, Swarbrick J, eds. *Drug Delivery and Targeting: For Pharmacists and Pharmaceutical Scientists*. New York, NY: Taylor & Francis; 2001:63–82.

Mahato RI, Narang AS. *Pharmaceutical Dosage Forms and Drug Delivery*. 2nd ed. New York, NY: Taylor & Francis; 2011.

Martin A. *Physical Pharmacy*. 4th ed. Baltimore, MD: Lippincott Williams & Wilkins; 1993.

Mathiowitz E, Kretz MR, Bannon-Peppas L. Micro-encapsulation. In: Mathiowitz E, ed. *Encyclopedia of Controlled Drug Delivery*. New York, NY: John Wiley & Sons; 1999:493–546.

Washington N, Washington C, Wilson CG. *Physiological Pharmaceutics: Barriers to Drug Absorption*. 2nd ed. New York, NY: Taylor & Francis; 2001.

Compounding

4

Robert J. Nolly

4-1. Key Points

- Each extemporaneously compounded prescription is for a specific patient.
- Three parties are involved in extemporaneous compounding: prescriber, patient, and pharmacist.
- A thorough knowledge of and proficiency in pharmacy math is required for the extemporaneous compounding of prescriptions.
- The sensitivity of the pharmacy balance must be determined, and the minimum weighable quantity must be known for that particular balance.
- All weighing and measuring must be accurate with errors of 5% or more avoided.
- Once a component is removed from a stock container, it may not be returned to the stock container.
- Trituration is used to reduce the particle size of powders to make a greater surface area available, to uniformly mix powders using geometric dilution, and to dissolve solutes in solvents.
- Levigation is the process of mixing or triturating a powder with a liquid in which it is insoluble to reduce particle size and aid in incorporating the powder into a base.
- A pharmacist must choose a levigating agent that is miscible with the base.
- Mineral oil is an appropriate levigating agent for a hydrophobic ointment base such as white petrolatum.
- Up to 5% of a levigating agent is usually sufficient unless the amount of powder is large.

- Heat should be used sparingly in compounding. Use only enough heat to melt components, make a solution, or enhance a reaction. Do not subject components to excessive heat.
- Use of a water bath normally prevents overheating of components when compounding.
- Care must be taken to not lose components during the preparation process. Doing so can alter the concentration of active pharmaceutical ingredient(s) in the finished preparation, potentially making it subpotent or superpotent.
- To promote accuracy in the compounding process, such as when weighing, place all unused stock containers on the left side of the workstation. As each one is weighed, place it on the right side.
- The dry gum or continental method of preparing an emulsion uses oil, purified water, and gum (e.g., acacia) in a ratio of 4:2:1, respectively.
- An extemporaneously compounded preparation has no National Drug Code (NDC) number.

4-2. Study Guide Checklist

The following topics may guide your study of this subject area:

- The characteristics of an extemporaneously compounded preparation compared to those of a manufactured product
- Compliance with regulatory and professional guidelines pertaining to pharmacy compounding
- Recommended equipment and supplies required for compounding
- Consideration of the grade of the components and their sources used in extemporaneous compounding

---

Editor's Note: This chapter is based on the 10th edition chapter written by Robert J. Nolly and Charles N. May.

- The achievement of accuracy in weighing and measuring
- Calculations and procedures required for compounding the variety of available compounded dosage forms
- The meaning of the following terms and their application to compounding: triturate (trituration), geometric dilution, levigate (levigation), and eutectic mixture
- Application of beyond-use date (BUD) guidelines to compounded preparations
- Knowledge of compounding quality assurance, quality control, preparation testing, and necessary recordkeeping requirements

4-3. Introduction

Pharmacists extemporaneously compound medications to provide patients and prescribers additional options for treatment and therapy than are available as commercial products. Individualized, custom-prepared medications are needed because some therapeutic agents (1) are not commercially manufactured; (2) are not available in the dosage form or size needed; (3) contain offending components, such as dyes, preservatives, fillers, and binders; (4) contain patient-averse flavors, fragrances, or colors; and (5) are necessary for patients who do not fit into the standard categories treated by manufactured products. In addition, from time to time, commercially manufactured products are unavailable for a variety of reasons, such as when (1) a drug product is recalled; (2) a manufacturing facility has closed; (3) a strike, disaster, or regulatory action has occurred; (4) the product is no longer commercially profitable; or (5) the manufacturer no longer supplies the product for other corporate reasons. Several segments of the population are not sufficiently served by pharmaceutical manufacturers, including pediatric, geriatric, and veterinary patients and patients with rare or complicated disease states. Prescribers and pharmacists working closely with patients may improve the quality of life for those patients by providing compounded medications that meet their unique needs.

4-4. Philosophy of Compounding

- Compounding is extemporaneous for an individual patient.
- It fulfills the need for unique dosage forms and sizes.

- The pharmacist works as part of a three-party team of the prescriber, patient, and pharmacist to satisfy patient needs that commercially available products cannot.
- The pharmacist follows up with the patient, the prescriber, or both to determine whether the compounded preparation needs further adjustment or refinement to be satisfactory.

4-5. Compounding versus Manufacturing

Compounded preparations are as follows:

- Extemporaneously prepared
- Patient specific in conjunction with the prescriber
- Regulated by a state board of pharmacy
- Not advertised
- Labeled with beyond-use dates (BUDs)
- Not prepared in advance except in the case of documented usage or demand
- Not given National Drug Code (NDC) numbers

Manufactured products are as follows:

- Subject to an approved New Drug Application (NDA)
- Subject to U.S. Food and Drug Administration (FDA)–approved labeling
- Manufactured in FDA-approved facilities in accordance with good manufacturing practices (GMPs)
- Often advertised and promoted
- Labeled with expiration dates
- Regulated by the FDA
- Given NDC numbers

4-6. Guidelines for Compounding

In November 2013, the Drug Quality and Security Act was enacted. The federal law consists, in part, of Sections 503A and 503B. Section 503B addresses outsourcing facilities where sterile dosage forms are compounded in the absence of the traditional compounding three-party team of the prescriber, patient, and pharmacist. These facilities compound larger quantities of such dosage forms, register voluntarily with the FDA, must be compliant with GMPs, and are subject to inspection by the FDA. Section 503A addresses traditional pharmacy compounding where the three-party team exists. It clarifies FDA involvement in compounding and recognizes that state boards of pharmacy are responsible for regulatory oversight. A new guidance addressing pharmacy compounding under Section 503A will be issued by the FDA. Following are published guidelines that pharmacists use in designing and carrying out their compounding practices.

Allen LV Jr. Extemporaneous prescription compounding. In: Allen LV Jr, Adejare A, Desselle SP, eds. *Remington: The Science and Practice of Pharmacy.* 22nd ed. Philadelphia, PA: Pharmaceutical Press; 2013:2311–28.

National Association of Boards of Pharmacy. Good compounding practices applicable to state licensed pharmacies. In: *Model State Pharmacy Act and Model Rules of the National Association of Boards of Pharmacy.* Mount Prospect, IL: National Association of Boards of Pharmacy; 2013:224–33.

U.S. Pharmacopeial Convention. Pharmaceutical calculations in prescription compounding: Chapter <1160>. In: *U.S. Pharmacopeia 35/National Formulary 30.* Rockville, MD: U.S. Pharmacopeial Convention; 2012:784–95.

U.S. Pharmacopeial Convention. Pharmaceutical compounding–nonsterile preparations: Chapter <795>. In: *U.S. Pharmacopeia 35/National Formulary 30.* Rockville, MD: U.S. Pharmacopeial Convention; 2012:344–50.

U.S. Pharmacopeial Convention. Prescription balances and volumetric apparatus: Chapter <1176>. In: *U.S. Pharmacopeia 35/National Formulary 30.* Rockville, MD: U.S. Pharmacopeial Convention; 2012:804–6.

U.S. Pharmacopeial Convention. Quality assurance in pharmaceutical compounding: Chapter <1163>. In: *U.S. Pharmacopeia 35/National Formulary 30.* Rockville, MD: U.S. Pharmacopeial Convention; 2012:795–99.

4-7. Pharmacy Requirements

Space

- An appropriate amount is required; a dedicated area is ideal.
- Space should be properly arranged and maintained, with components and equipment readily available.
- A controlled atmosphere is necessary, with limited traffic flow and appropriate lighting, temperature, humidity, and ventilation control.
- Separate areas are needed for sterile and nonsterile compounding.
- A sink with potable and purified water should be readily available.
- Materials used in the construction of a compounding area should be as nonporous and seamless as possible. A well-lighted space with bright fixtures, walls, and floors gives a clean, professional appearance.

Equipment

Appropriate equipment is required, such as the following:

- Measuring devices including graduated cylinders, pharmacy graduates, and pipettes
- Weighing equipment such as an electronic balance or Class A prescription torsion balance
- Mixing devices including Wedgwood, porcelain, and glass mortars with pestles and blenders
- Sufficient counters and shelves. Countertop space must be available to allow the compounding of a variety of dosage forms, and shelving must be appropriately located so that components are properly stored.
- Processing equipment including a hot plate, magnetic stirrer, ointment mill, electronic mortar and pestle, tablet pulverizer, and pH analyzer
- Safety and protective equipment such as gloves, face masks, hair covers, gowns, and goggles for personnel
- Devices that control the air from the work area to keep it free of component contamination, and a powder containment enclosure for personnel who are working with light, fine, and fluffy components or components that are irritating, odorous, or hazardous
- Packaging equipment including a capsule-filling machine, tube-sealing equipment, and calibrated measuring and filling devices
- Computer equipment for maintaining and processing labels, profiles, formulas, and required records

Formulas

Categories for component classification and quality include the following:

- USP/NF: United States Pharmacopeia/National Formulary (components meet official standards and are suitable for human use)

- FCC: Food Chemicals Codex (food grade)
- ACS: American Chemical Society (reagent grade)
- AR: analytical reagent (high purity)
- CP: chemically pure (uncertain quality)
- Tech: technical (industrial quality)

Note: Components are either active pharmaceutical ingredients or other added substances. USP/NF or FCC components are preferred for compounding. Always obtain the certificate of analysis for every component used, and use components manufactured in an FDA-registered facility.

Supplies

Supplies include items such as the following:

- Weigh boats, weighing paper (parchment and glassine), filter paper, ointment paper, ointment slab, water bath, spatulas (stainless steel and hard rubber), stirring rods (glass and polypropylene), rubber scrapers, beakers, flasks, funnels, casseroles, and thermometers
- Lollipop, rapid dissolve tablet, tablet triturate, troche, and suppository molds
- Containers of various types and sizes to properly package the dosage forms, such as prescription bottles, powder jars, capsule containers, ointment jars, ointment tubes, "ride-up" tubes, powder paper boxes, and suppository boxes

Records

Types of records include the following:

- A master formulation record must be in place for each preparation compounded, and it must be approved, signed, and dated by the pharmacist in charge.
- A compounding record of each compounded prescription must be made and maintained.
- A chronological record of each day's compounding activity should be made and kept for future reference and use.

Policies and Procedures

Types of policies and procedures include the following:

- Standard operating procedures
- Material safety data sheets
- Certificates of analysis
- Quality assurance and control
- Other policies and procedures

The Pharmacist

- *Interest:* A distinct interest in being creative, solving often difficult patient problems, working closely with prescribers and patients, and formulating and compounding customized medications is very important.
- *Education:* The emphasis on compounding varies among colleges of pharmacy. Even graduates of programs that require students to compound a wide variety of formulations may need additional training.
- *Training:* Additional training can be obtained through continuing education courses, seminars, professional development programs, and professional associations.
- *Experience:* Experience in compounding is perhaps the key to how effective a pharmacist can be in creating specialized formulations that can make a difference in a patient's quality of life. Such experience enables the pharmacist to suggest to the prescriber a therapeutic agent in a unique dosage form that may help solve the patient's therapeutic problem. Pharmacists who compound must be certain that they possess the appropriate requisites for the level of compounding they perform. USP Chapter <795>, *Pharmaceutical Compounding—Nonsterile Preparations*, identifies three categories of compounded preparations: simple, moderate, and complex.
- *Compounding support:* Compounding pharmacists should consider joining professional organizations that support compounding, such as the International Academy of Compounding Pharmacists. They should consider subscribing to journals that focus on compounding, such as the *International Journal of Pharmaceutical Compounding* and *U.S. Pharmacist*, and use the professional resources of companies that fulfill their compounding needs.

Professional Considerations

- Is there a commercially available product in the exact dosage, size, form, and package needed?
- Is there an alternative product that will satisfy the patient's requirements?
- Can I perform any pharmaceutical calculations required?
- Can I accurately compound and package the preparation?

Table 4-1. Nonsterile Maximum Beyond-Use Dates[a]

Beyond-Use Date	14 Days	30 Days	6 Months
Storage condition	Cold temperature (2–8°C, 36–46°F)	Room temperature (20–25°C, 68–77°F)	Room temperature (20–25°C, 68–77°F)
Preparation type	Oral preparations containing water	Liquid and semisolid topical, dermal and mucosal preparations containing water	Preparations containing no water

a. The BUD cannot be greater than the expiration date of any component used to compound the preparation. Inclusion of an antimicrobial agent should be considered, if appropriate. Dispense in a container that reduces exposure to light and moisture.

Quality Control Requirements

- Accurate calculations
- Accurate weights
- Accurate measurements
- Proper processing techniques
- Proper packaging
- Proper records
- Proper labeling, including BUDs
- Proper documentation of quality assurance, quality control, and preparation testing

Beyond-Use Dates

- Pharmacists assign BUDs to compounded preparations to guide patients in the proper use and storage of the preparation.
- The goal is to provide a BUD that will allow the patient enough time to fully use the amount of preparation dispensed but not enough time to allow the preparation to degrade, lose potency, or be stored for future use.
- If the pharmacist does not have a reference on the stability of the specific dosage form compounded or sufficient experience with it, the section "General Guidelines for Assigning Beyond-Use Dates" in USP Chapter <795> is followed. Table 4-1 summarizes beyond-use dating.

4-8. Compounded Dosage Forms

Solutions

- *Definition:* Solutions are chemically and physically homogenous mixtures of two or more substances.
- *Types:* Examples include syrups, elixirs, aromatic waters, tinctures, and spirits. Solutions can be aqueous or nonaqueous.

- *Properties:* Examples include hypertonic, isotonic, hypotonic, osmolar, and osmolal.
- *Stability:* Examples of how the stability of solutions can be enhanced include adjusting pH, adding a preservative, and adding an antioxidant.
- *Rate of dissolution:* Examples of how the rate of dissolution is enhanced include stirring, heating, and reducing particle size.
- *Beyond-use dates:* Aqueous solutions have shorter BUDs than do nonaqueous solutions.
- *Testing:* Organoleptic, pH, and other tests are performed.

An example of an isotonic *aqueous* solution follows:

Ephedrine sulfate	1%
Sodium chloride	qs
Purified water, qs ad	30 mL
M.ft. isotonic nasal solution	

Steps in compounding are as follows:

1. Calculate the required quantity of each component. The NaCl equivalent of ephedrine sulfate is 0.2.
2. Accurately weigh or measure each component.
3. Dissolve the solid components in about 25 mL of purified water.
4. Add sufficient purified water to measure 30 mL.
5. The BUD is a maximum of 30 days according to USP Chapter <795> guidelines.

An example of a *nonaqueous* solution follows:

Urea	10 g
Salicylic acid	5 g
Coal tar solution	5 mL
Propylene glycol, qs ad	100 mL

Steps in compounding are as follows:

1. Accurately weigh or measure each component.
2. Dissolve the urea and salicylic acid in about 75 mL of propylene glycol.
3. Add the coal tar solution, and mix well.

4. Add sufficient propylene glycol to measure 100 mL.
5. The BUD is a maximum of 6 months according to USP Chapter <795> guidelines.

Note: Use of a mechanical stirrer can reduce the time needed to dissolve the urea and salicylic acid.

Suspensions

- *Definition:* A suspension is a two-phased system containing a finely divided solid in a vehicle.
- *Requirement:* The drug is uniformly dispersed throughout the vehicle.
- *Concentration:* Suspending agents are typically used in a concentration of 0.5–6%.
- *Viscosity:* The vehicle has enough viscosity to keep drug particles suspended separately.
- *Insolubility:* The active pharmaceutical ingredient is insoluble in the vehicle.
- *Tip:* Wet the insoluble powder with a vehicle-miscible liquid.
- *Advantage:* A suspension allows the preparation of a liquid form of an insoluble drug.
- *Stability:* Stability is enhanced by adding a preservative.
- *Testing:* Organoleptic, pH, and other tests are performed.

Categories of suspending agents are as follows:

- *Natural hydrocolloids:* Acacia, alginic acid, gelatin, guar gum, sodium alginate, tragacanth, and xanthan gum
- *Semisynthetic hydrocolloids:* Ethylcellulose, methylcellulose, and sodium carboxymethyl-cellulose
- *Synthetic hydrocolloids:* Carbomers (Carbopol), poloxamers (Pluronic), polyvinyl alcohol, and polyvinylpyrrolidone
- *Clays:* Bentonite and magnesium aluminum silicate (Veegum)

An example of an oral suspension follows:

Progesterone, micronized	1.2 g
Glycerin	3 mL
Methylcellulose 1% solution	30 mL
Flavored syrup, qs ad	60 mL

Steps in compounding are as follows:

1. Accurately weigh or measure each component.
2. In a glass mortar, wet the progesterone with the glycerin to form a thick paste.
3. Slowly add the methylcellulose solution while triturating.

4. When mixed thoroughly, pour into a graduate.
5. Add small amounts of syrup to the mortar, mix, and add to graduate until the desired volume is reached.
6. The BUD is a maximum of 14 days refrigerated according to USP Chapter <795> guidelines.

Note: The methylcellulose 1% solution should be prepared before compounding the suspension.

The methylcellulose 1% solution can be prepared as follows:

Methylcellulose 1,500 CPS	1%
Sodium benzoate	200 mg
Purified water, qs ad	100 mL

1. Calculate the amount of each component required.
2. Accurately weigh or measure each component.
3. Add methylcellulose to 50 mL boiling purified water, and mix well.
4. Add sodium benzoate, and mix.
5. Add cold purified water to bring to final volume. Stir until thick and uniform.

Emulsions

- *Definition:* An emulsion is a two-phase system of two immiscible liquids, one of which is dispersed throughout the other as small droplets.
- *Components:* An emulsion has an external, continuous phase or dispersion medium; an internal, discontinuous or dispersed phase; and an emulsifying agent.
- *Type:* Types are oil in water (o/w) and water in oil (w/o), depending on which is the internal or external phase.
- *Emulsifying agents:* Emulsifying agents can be natural gums (acacia, agar, chondrus, pectin, and tragacanth) or hydrophilic or lipophilic agents (the esters of sorbitan).
- *Lipophilic agents:* Trade names for lipophilic agents include Arlacel and Span.
- *Hydrophilic agents:* Trade names for hydrophilic agents include Myrj and Tween.
- *Hydrophilic–lipophilic balance:* A lower hydrophilic–lipophilic balance (HLB) value favors a w/o emulsion; a higher HLB value favors an o/w emulsion. Agents with an HLB value of 1–10 are considered to be lipophilic, while agents with an HLB value of > 10 are considered to be hydrophilic. Emulsions with an HLB value of 3–8 are water in oil, while those with an HLB value of > 8 to 16 are oil in water.

- *Other agents:* Other agents include bentonite, cholesterol, gelatin, lecithin, methylcellulose, soaps of fatty acids, sodium docusate, sodium lauryl sulfate, and triethanolamine.
- *Equipment:* Equipment includes mortars and pestles, homogenizers, colloid mills, mechanical mixers, agitators, and ultrasonic vibrators.
- *Solids:* Solid components should be dissolved before they are incorporated into the emulsion, or if a sizable quantity is added, a levigating or wetting agent may be needed.
- *Flavors or fragrances:* Flavors or fragrances should generally be incorporated into the external phase.
- *Preservatives:* Preservatives should be added in the aqueous phase but may also be added in the oily phase, if necessary.
- *Stability:* Emulsions can either cream or crack.
- *Continental method:* The continental or dry gum method of preparing an emulsion nucleus involves using the oil:water:dry gum emulsifier in a 4:2:1 ratio.
- *Advantages:* An emulsion can be used to mask taste, improve palatability, increase absorption, and enhance bioavailability.
- *Testing:* Organoleptic testing is performed.

An example of preparing an emulsion by the continental, dry gum (4:2:1) method follows:

Cod liver oil	50 mL
Acacia	12.5 g
Syrup	10 mL
Methyl salicylate	0.4 mL
Purified water, qs ad	100 mL

Steps in compounding are as follows:

1. Accurately weigh or measure each component.
2. Place the cod liver oil in a dry porcelain mortar.
3. Sprinkle the acacia on the oil, and give it a very quick mix with the pestle.
4. Add 25 mL of purified water, and immediately triturate rapidly to form the thick, white, homogenous emulsion nucleus.
5. Add the methyl salicylate, and mix thoroughly.
6. Add the syrup, and mix thoroughly.
7. Add sufficient purified water to measure 100 mL.
8. The BUD is a maximum of 14 days refrigerated according to USP Chapter <795> guidelines.

Capsules

- *Definition:* This dosage form incorporates components into a shell called a *capsule.*
- *Procedure:* Determine capsule size to fit total powder weight, triturate powders to reduce particle size, mix powders by geometric dilution, incorporate the diluent by geometric dilution if required, and clean the outside of the filled capsules.
- *Advantages:* Capsules mask unpleasant taste; allow the mixture of components that could not be mixed in other vehicles; can alter the release rate of active pharmaceutical ingredients by adding hydroxypropyl methylcellulose (HPMC); allow incorporation of several components into one dosage form; provide an accurate dosage size for liquids, semisolids, and powders; and provide a dosage form that is easier to swallow and more acceptable to the patient.
- *Methods of filling:* Hand punch from powder on an ointment slab or use a capsule-filling machine.
- *Sizing:* Capsules available, listed from largest to smallest, include 000, 00, 0, 1, 2, 3, 4, and 5. Determining the size of capsule to use for a particular dosage involves assessing the density or fluffiness of the powder, comparing it to known weights of various reference powders with published capsule-size capacities, and then filling and weighing the capsule. If the requested dosage does not fill a specific size of capsule, a filler should be added.
- *Testing:* Organoleptic, weight percent error, weight variance, and other tests are performed.

An example of an altered-release capsule follows:

Progesterone, micronized	25 mg
HPMC	50%
Lactose, qs ad per capsule size	
M.ft. capsules	15 doses

Steps in compounding are as follows:

1. Select the appropriate capsule size, and calculate the required quantity of each component. The quantity of lactose needed depends on the capsule size required.
2. Accurately weigh each component.
3. If necessary, reduce particle size, and mix thoroughly by geometric dilution.
4. Fill capsules.
5. Weigh capsules.
6. The BUD is a maximum of 6 months according to USP Chapter <795> guidelines.

Tablet Triturates

- *Definition:* A tablet triturate is a small tablet that is made in a mold and intended for sublingual administration. The molded tablet usually weighs about 60 to 200 mg.

- *Advantages:* A tablet triturate rapidly dissolves under the tongue, is rapidly absorbed, avoids the first pass through the liver, and provides a rapid therapeutic response.

- *Components:* Tablet triturates consist of an active pharmaceutical ingredient and a base, which may consist of lactose, sucrose, dextrose, and mannitol.

- *Formulation:* Molds that make 50 tablets are generally available in approximate 60, 100, and 200 mg tablet sizes. Formulations must be calculated to fit the size of mold that will be used. If this capacity is not known, the capacity must be determined by filling the mold holes with the tablet triturate base and weighing the resulting tablets. On the basis of the size of the mold holes, mix the active pharmaceutical ingredient with the base, which often consists of four parts lactose and one part sucrose. Thoroughly triturate powders, mix by geometric dilution, and then moisten with a wetting solution containing four parts 95% ethyl alcohol and one part purified water until the powder mixture is adhesive. Press into mold uniformly.

- *Testing:* Organoleptic, weight percent error, weight variance, and other tests are performed.

- *Tip:* Tablets may be flavored by adding a flavor to the wetting solution. Color may be added by adding a small amount of powdered color to the powder mixture.

An example of a tablet triturate follows:

Testosterone	3 mg
Base, qs ad per mold size	
M.ft. tabs	50 doses

Steps in compounding are as follows:

1. The base may consist of a 1:4 mixture of sucrose and lactose.
2. The wetting solution may consist of a 1:4 mixture of purified water and 95% ethyl alcohol.
3. Select the size of tablet triturate mold to be used. The quantity of base needed depends on the size of the mold selected.
4. Calibrate the mold for the base being used. Based on the weight of tablets it makes, calculate the required quantity of each component.
5. Accurately weigh or measure each component.
6. Reduce particle size, and mix components by geometric dilution.
7. In a glass mortar, gradually moisten the powder mixture until it becomes adhesive. Drop the wetting solution onto the powder a few drops at a time, and triturate after each addition until the powder becomes moist and adhesive.
8. Press moist powder evenly into all holes in the tablet triturate mold plate.
9. Place the mold plate on the base plate, and press down until the tablets rest on top of the pegs.
10. Let tablets air dry.
11. Very gently remove dried tablets from pegs.
12. The BUD is a maximum of 30 days according to USP Chapter <795> guidelines.

Troches, Lozenges, and Lollipops

- *Definition:* Troches, lozenges, and lollipops or suckers are solid dosage forms intended to be slowly dissolved in the mouth for local or systemic effects.

- *Formulation:* Troches, lozenges, and lollipops are composed of an active pharmaceutical ingredient and a base that may consist of (1) sugar and other carbohydrates that produce a hard preparation, (2) polyethylene glycols (PEGs) and other components that produce a softer preparation, or (3) a glycerin–gelatin combination that produces a chewable preparation.
  - Formulations made in a mold complete with sticks are called lollipops or suckers.
  - Formulations must be calculated to fit the size of mold that will be used. If this capacity is not known, the capacity must be determined by filling the mold cavities with the base and weighing the resulting troches, lozenges, or lollipops.
  - Flavors and colors are added just before the molds are filled.

- *Advantages:* Troches, lozenges, and lollipops are easy to administer, are convenient for patients who cannot swallow oral dosage forms, maintain a constant level of drug in the oral cavity and throat, and can have a pleasant taste.

- *Testing:* Organoleptic, weight percent error, weight variance, and other tests are performed.

An example of a troche follows:

Gelatin	2.62 g
Glycerin	9.36 mL
Purified water	1.3 mL
Acacia	0.28 g
Bentonite	0.28 g
Benzocaine	0.17 g
Citric acid	0.3 g
Stevia	0.15 g

Flavor	qs
Color	qs
M. ft. troches	12 doses
Mold holds	1.4 g.

Note: With a specific gravity of 1.25, the 9.36 mL of glycerin weighs 11.7 g. The formula is written for 12 troches. Dividing the final formula weight by 12 determines the weight of a single troche.

Steps in compounding are as follows:

1. Calibrate the mold for the base composed of gelatin, glycerin, and purified water to verify a troche weight of 1.4 g per cavity. If needed, based on the actual troche weight, recalculate the required quantity of each component.
2. Accurately weigh or measure each component.
3. Triturate and thoroughly mix, using geometric dilution, the acacia, bentonite, benzocaine, citric acid, and stevia powders.
4. Heat the glycerin on a boiling water bath until warm.
5. Add the water, and heat for a few minutes.
6. While stirring, *very slowly* add the gelatin. The gelatin must be lump free; the mixture must be homogeneous.
7. Add the powders to the warm liquid and mix thoroughly.
8. Add flavor and color. Mix, pour into the mold, and let cool.
9. The BUD is a maximum of 30 days according to USP Chapter <795> guidelines.

Transdermal Gels

- *Definition:* Transdermal gels move medications through the skin in quantities sufficient to produce a therapeutic effect.
- *Components:* Transdermal gels have the following components:
  - Active pharmaceutical ingredients and other components
  - Gelling agents: for example, the carbomers (e.g., Carbopol 934P), methylcellulose, the poloxamers (e.g., Pluronic F-127), and sodium carboxymethylcellulose
  - Wetting or levigating agents: for example, propylene glycol and glycerin
  - Penetration-enhancing agents: for example, alcohol, lecithin, dimethyl sulfoxide, isopropyl myristate, isopropyl palmitate, propylene glycol, and PEG
  - Suspending or dispersing agents: for example, bentonite and silica gel

- *Testing:* Organoleptic testing is performed.
- *Advantages:* Transdermal gels are convenient, effective, and acceptable to patients. The gels avoid some problems that other dosage forms have, such as gastrointestinal irritation from oral dosages, pain from injections, and the undesirability of suppositories.
- *Formulation:* Use proper techniques for creating the gel, adjust the pH for carbomer gels, respect the temperature for poloxamer gels, use small amounts of nonaqueous solvents, and, if possible, keep electrolyte components to a minimum.
- *Tip:* Do not use transdermal gels for the systemic use of antibiotics, and do not try to get large molecules such as proteins through the skin by transdermal gels.

An example of a transdermal gel using carbomer as the base follows:

Ketoprofen	5%
Carbomer 934P	2%
Alcohol 95%	qs
Triethanolamine	2 mL
Purified water, qs ad	30 mL

Steps in compounding are as follows:

1. Calculate the required quantity of each component.
2. Accurately weigh or measure each component.
3. Triturate the carbomer 934P in a glass mortar.
4. While triturating, gradually add about 18 mL of purified water.
5. Be sure that the carbomer and water are thoroughly mixed and the mixture is homogenous.
6. Dissolve the ketoprofen in about 10 mL 95% ethyl alcohol.
7. While triturating, add the ketoprofen solution to the carbomer–water mixture and mix thoroughly.
8. If necessary, add purified water to make about 28 mL, and pour into an ointment jar.
9. Add triethanolamine, and stir quickly with a stirring rod until the gel is thoroughly formed.
10. The BUD is a maximum of 30 days according to USP Chapter <795> guidelines.

Note: A trade name for carbomer 934P is Carbopol 934P, and for triethanolamine, it is Trolamine.

An example of a transdermal gel using pluronic lecithin organogel (PLO) as the base follows:

Ketoprofen	5%
Propylene glycol	10%
Lecithin isopropyl palmitate liquid	20%
Poloxamer 407 20% gel, qs ad	100 mL

Steps in compounding are as follows:

1. Calculate the required quantity of each component.
2. Accurately weigh or measure each component.
3. In a glass mortar, triturate the ketoprofen with the propylene glycol to make a smooth paste.
4. Add the lecithin isopropyl palmitate liquid, and mix well.
5. Add sufficient poloxamer 407 20% gel to measure 100 mL.
6. Triturate until a high-quality gel is produced.
7. Package in a light-resistant container.
8. The BUD is a maximum of 30 days according to USP Chapter <795> guidelines.

Note: The lecithin isopropyl palmitate liquid and the poloxamer 407 20% gel should be prepared before compounding the gel. The lecithin isopropyl palmitate liquid may be prepared as follows:

Soy lecithin, granular	10 g
Isopropyl palmitate	10 g
Sorbic acid	0.2 g

1. Accurately weigh or measure each component.
2. Add the soy lecithin granules and the sorbic acid to the isopropyl palmitate, mix well, and allow to set overnight at room temperature.
3. The next morning, stir very gently to ensure complete mixing.

Note: Isopropyl myristate may be used in place of isopropyl palmitate.

The poloxamer 407 20% gel may be prepared as follows:

Poloxamer 407	20 g
Potassium sorbate	0.2 g
Purified water, qs ad	100 mL

1. Accurately weigh or measure each component.
2. Add the poloxamer 407 and the potassium sorbate to a portion of the water, mix well, and add water to make 100 mL.
3. Mix thoroughly, ensuring that the poloxamer 407 is completely wet.
4. Allow to set overnight in the refrigerator.
5. The next morning, stir slowly to be sure that mixing is complete.
6. Store in the refrigerator.

Note: A trade name for poloxamer 407 is Pluronic F-127.

Suppositories

- *Definition:* Suppositories are solid dosage forms for insertion into the rectum, vagina, or urethra to provide localized or systemic therapy.
- *Sizes:* Rectal suppositories are approximately 2 g, vaginal suppositories are 3–5 g, and urethral suppositories are 2 g (female) or 4 g (male). Urethral suppositories were formerly called *bougies*.
- *Formulation:* Suppositories are usually made by fusion with either a fatty or a water-miscible base. They can also be hand molded or made by compression.
  - Suppositories are usually made in a metal or plastic mold. A plastic mold is called a shell.
  - The active pharmaceutical ingredient in powder form should be triturated (comminuted) to reduce particle size and should be levigated with a wetting agent before incorporation into the melted base.
  - The melted formulation should be poured continuously into the mold to prevent layering.
- *Calculations:* The capacity in grams of the suppository mold must be known to determine the quantity of base needed. If this capacity is not known, the capacity must be determined by filling the mold with the suppository base and weighing the resulting suppositories. The space in the suppository occupied by the active pharmaceutical ingredient(s) must be calculated using the density factor of each active ingredient. If the density factor is not known, it can be calculated by making a suppository containing a known amount of the active ingredient.
- *Advantages:* Suppositories deliver medication for local or systemic effects. The systemically absorbed medication avoids the first pass through the liver. They can be used when patients cannot take medication orally or by injection.
- *Testing:* Organoleptic, weight percent error, weight variance, and other tests are performed.

An example of a rectal suppository follows:

Progesterone, micronized	25 mg
PEG base	qs
M.ft. suppositories	12 doses

The base is as follows:

PEG 300	50%
PEG 6000	50%

Steps in compounding are as follows:

1. Calibrate the mold for the base being used. Based on the weight of the suppositories made, calculate the required amount of each component.
2. Accurately weigh or measure each component.
3. Carefully heat the PEG 6000 until it melts.
4. Add the PEG 300, and mix well.
5. Very slowly add the micronized progesterone, and mix thoroughly.
6. Pour the mixture into the suppository mold.
7. The BUD is a maximum of 6 months according to USP Chapter <795> guidelines.

Note: When using the plastic molds (shells), the liquid mixture must not be too hot.

Powders

- *Definition:* Powders are fine particles that result from the comminution of dry substances. Particle sizes are usually determined by the size of sieve they will pass through and may be described as very coarse, coarse, moderately coarse, fine, and very fine.
- *Mixtures:* Mixtures of powders should have the same or similar size particles, and mixing should be accomplished by geometric dilution.
- *Preparation: Comminution* is the process of reducing particle size in powders. It is accomplished manually by trituration, levigation, or pulverization by intervention and mechanically by grinders and various types of mills.
- *Uses:* Powders taken by mouth may provide systemic effects, while powders are applied topically for local effects. Powders that contain mucoadhesive components, when insufflated into body cavities, adhere to moist body surfaces.
- *Advantages:* Because they are dry, powders often have greater stability and may not react with components that they are otherwise incompatible with, except for explosive mixtures. Once in the gastrointestinal tract, they are ready to be absorbed.
- *Testing:* Organoleptic testing is performed.

An example of a powder for external use follows:

Calamine	
Zinc oxide, of each	8%
Red mercuric oxide	1%
Magnesium oxide, heavy, qs ad	60 g
M.ft. powder	

Steps in compounding are as follows:

1. Calculate the required amount of each component.
2. Accurately weigh each component.
3. Thoroughly mix the powders by geometric dilution using a porcelain mortar.
4. To determine when the mixture is totally homogeneous, use the "spread test," which is performed by using a spatula to spread a small amount of the mixed powders into a thin layer on a sheet of weighing paper.
5. The BUD is a maximum of 6 months according to USP Chapter <795> guidelines.

Powder Papers

- *Definition:* Powders or mixtures of powders are enfolded in papers containing one dose each and dispensed in an appropriate box or container.
- *Preparation:* Powder papers or charts contain finely subdivided (comminuted) powders, mixed by geometric dilution, with a dose of the appropriate size placed on a powder paper and properly folded. The appropriate size can be obtained by weighing.
- *Advantages:* For patients who have difficulty swallowing tablets or capsules and those who have indwelling nasogastric tubes, powder papers are a useful dosage form. Several medications can be given as one dose. The medication is in powder form and ready to be absorbed once it is in the gastrointestinal tract. For patients who have many medications to take each day, they may be combined into a smaller number of powder papers.
- *Testing:* Organoleptic, weight percent error, weight variance, and other tests are performed.

An example of a powder paper follows:

Aspirin	226 mg
Acetaminophen	162 mg
Caffeine	32 mg
M.ft. charts	12 doses

Steps in compounding are as follows:

1. Determine the weight of powder to be weighed into one paper.
2. Accurately weigh each component.
3. Triturate each component separately to reduce particle size.
4. Thoroughly mix the components by geometric dilution.
5. Weigh the correct amount for each powder paper on a separate paper.

6. Properly fold each paper, and place it in a powder box.
7. The BUD is a maximum of 6 months according to USP Chapter <795> guidelines.

Ointments and Creams

■ *Definition:* Ointments and creams are semisolid dosage forms for external application. Properties are typically characteristic of the base selected (e.g., white petrolatum, hydrophilic petrolatum, cold cream, hydrophilic ointment, polyethylene glycol ointment). Ointments and creams protect the skin and mucous membranes, moisturize the skin, and provide a vehicle for various types of medications. Types and classifications include oleaginous or hydrocarbon, absorption, emulsion, and water soluble.

■ *Characteristics of an oleaginous or hydrocarbon ointment base.* Such a base is
  * Occlusive: for example, white petrolatum
  * Greasy: for example, white ointment
  * Emollient: for example, vegetable shortening
  * Not water washable
  * Not water absorbing
  * Insoluble in water

■ *Characteristics of an absorption ointment base.* Such a base is
  * Occlusive: for example, hydrophilic petrolatum
  * Greasy: for example, lanolin, USP (anhydrous)
  * Emollient: for example, Aquaphor
  * Not water washable: for example, Aquabase
  * Water absorbing
  * Insoluble in water

■ *Characteristics of an emulsion, w/o ointment base.* Such a base is
  * Occlusive: for example, cold cream
  * Greasy: for example, rose water ointment
  * Emollient: for example, Eucerin
  * Not water washable: for example, hydrous lanolin
  * Absorbs water: for example, hydrocream
  * Insoluble in water: for example, Nivea

■ *Characteristics of an emulsion, o/w ointment base.* Such a base is
  * Nonocclusive: for example, hydrophilic ointment
  * Nongreasy: for example, acid mantle cream
  * Water washable: for example, Cetaphil
  * Absorbs water: for example, Dermabase
  * Insoluble in water: for example, Keri lotion, Lubriderm, Neobase, Unibase, Velvachol, and vanishing cream

■ *Characteristics of water-soluble ointment base.* Such a base is
  * Nonocclusive: for example, polyethylene glycol ointment
  * Nongreasy: for example, Polybase
  * Water washable
  * Absorbs water
  * Water soluble

■ *Preparation:* Ointments are typically prepared by fusion or levigation. Powders should be comminuted to fine particles; some powders may be dissolved. If using the fusion method, use only enough heat to melt the component with the highest melting point. For the levigation method, an ointment slab and metal spatula usually work well. Levigating agents should be carefully selected, considering both the component(s) to be incorporated and the base. Table 4-2 shows commonly used levigating agents grouped by type and matched with the appropriate group of ointment base classifications.

■ *Uses:* Ointments or creams are an effective dosage form for treating skin and mucous membranes. On occasion, an ointment or cream will move sufficient quantities of medication through the skin to produce a systemic effect. Some formulations provide effective protection for the skin and mucous membranes.

■ *Packaging:* Typically, ointments and creams are packaged in ointment jars. The tube is often an ideal alternative package because it protects the preparation until it is squeezed out and used.

Table 4-2. Levigating Agents by Type and Ointment Base Classification

Type of agent	Ointment base classification
Aqueous	
Glycerin	Oil-in-water emulsion
Propylene glycol	Water soluble
Polyethylene glycol 400	Water washable
Oily	
Mineral oil	Oleaginous or hydrocarbon
Castor oil	Absorption
Cottonseed oil	Water-in-oil emulsion

Note: Other agents may be useful for certain preparations, such as Tween 80 for incorporating coal tar. Castor oil is useful for incorporating ichthammol and peru balsam.

■ *Testing:* Organoleptic, homogenicity, and other tests are performed.

An example of a nongreasy ointment follows:

Benzoyl peroxide	10%
Sulfur	1%
PEG base, qs ad	30 g

The base is as follows:

PEG 400	65%
PEG 3,350	35%

Steps in compounding are as follows:

1. Calculate the quantity of each component required. Benzoyl peroxide, hydrous, USP contains about 26% water. Thus, 4.05 g of benzoyl peroxide would be required because of its water content.
2. Accurately weigh or measure each component.
3. Triturate each powder to a fine particle size.
4. Melt the PEG 3,350, and remove it from the heat source.
5. Add the PEG 400, and mix thoroughly.
6. Add the powders, mix thoroughly, and stir until congealed.
7. Package in an ointment jar.
8. The BUD is a maximum of 6 months according to USP Chapter <795> guidelines.

An example of a greasy ointment follows:

Salicylic acid	3%
Mineral oil	qs
White petrolatum, qs ad	30 g

Steps in compounding are as follows:

1. Calculate the required quantity of each component.
2. Accurately weigh each component.
3. Triturate the salicylic acid, if necessary, to reduce particle size.
4. Levigate with a small quantity of mineral oil.
5. By geometric dilution, incorporate the levigated salicylic acid into the white petrolatum.
6. The BUD is a maximum of 6 months according to USP Chapter <795> guidelines.

An example of a cream follows:

Almond oil	56 g
White wax	12 g
Light mineral oil	10 g
Cetyl esters wax	2.5 g
Sodium borate	0.5 g
Purified water	19 g
M.ft. cream	

Steps in compounding are as follows:

1. Accurately weigh or measure each component.
2. Melt the white wax.
3. Add the cetyl esters wax, almond oil, and light mineral oil. Bring to a temperature of 70°C.
4. Dissolve the sodium borate in the purified water. Bring to a temperature of 70°C.
5. With both liquids at 70°C, mix and stir until the cream is completely formed.
6. Package in a tube or jar.
7. The BUD is a maximum of 30 days according to USP Chapter <795> guidelines.

Sticks

■ *Definition:* This topical dosage form is made in the shape of a rod, stick, or variation thereof and packaged in a container that allows it to be advanced upward as it is used.
■ *Advantages:* Sticks are an effective, convenient method of applying a topical agent exactly in the location desired. They are very portable and can deliver a variety of agents, including those that are therapeutic, protective, and cosmetic.
■ *Preparation:* Select a semisolid vehicle from a variety of polyethylene glycols, waxes, and oils that will produce the consistency desired. Triturate solid components, wet them with an appropriate wetting or levigating agent, and add them along with any liquid components to the melted vehicle. Mix thoroughly. Pour into an appropriate "ride-up" container.
■ *Testing:* Organoleptic testing is performed.
■ *Tip:* Sticks can usually be considered a stable dosage form.

An example of a stick follows:

Menthol	1%
Camphor	0.5%
Phenol	0.25%
Flavor	qs
Color	qs
PEG base, qs ad	10 g

The base is as follows:

PEG 400	70%
PEG 4,500	30%

Steps in compounding are as follows:

1. Calculate the required quantity of each component.
2. Accurately weigh or measure each component.

3. Melt the PEG 4,500, and remove it from the heat source.
4. Add the PEG 400, and mix thoroughly.
5. Mix the menthol, camphor, and phenol together; they will liquefy, forming a eutectic mixture.
6. Add the eutectic mixture to the other components, and mix thoroughly.
7. Pour into a "ride-up" lip balm tube, and let cool.
8. The BUD is a maximum of 6 months according to USP Chapter <795> guidelines.

4-9. Quality Assurance and Preparation Testing

The assurance of high quality influences every facet of compounding. Factors such as the compounding environment, facility design, fixtures, equipment, components, containers, personnel expertise and experience, policies, procedures, and documentation play important roles in achieving the highest quality possible in the compounding of individualized, customized preparations. Each preparation should be reviewed prior to dispensing to determine that the calculations, components, compounding process, and documentation are accurate and correct and that the preparation has the appropriate appearance. Perhaps the most important element in quality assurance is the commitment of each individual who plays any role in the compounding process to be of such intensity that the individual will not vary from the correct way of performing every function required. A program of preparation testing should be in place. USP Chapter <1163> contains a table identifying the types of tests that can be performed on various compounded preparations. The ultimate test of quality for a compounded preparation is having the preparation analyzed by a competent analytical laboratory. The typical goal is to have the contents of the preparation vary no more than plus or minus 5% of the stated label potency.

An indicator that a compounding pharmacy is committed to a high-quality practice is voluntary accreditation by the Pharmacy Compounding Accreditation Board (PCAB). As a national organization, PCAB carefully evaluates all aspects of a pharmacy's compounding operation. It ensures that policies and procedures are in place and operational for a high-quality practice. Accreditation by PCAB is currently the only benchmark available to attest to the quality of a compounding pharmacy and should be considered by pharmacies that provide compounding services.

4-10. Questions

1. Which type of water should be used when compounding a nonsterile preparation?

   A. Tap water
   B. Potable water
   C. Purified water
   D. Water for injection

2. What alcohol is used to compound a nonsterile preparation when its type and percentage are not specified?

   A. Ethyl alcohol 100%
   B. Ethyl alcohol 95%
   C. Ethyl alcohol 70%
   D. Isopropyl alcohol 70%

3. Which component is used as an antioxidant to increase the stability of potassium iodide oral solution (SSKI) by preventing the release of free iodine?

   A. Sodium alginate
   B. Sodium glycinate
   C. Sodium succinate
   D. Sodium thiosulfate

4. As an o/w type of ointment base, hydrophilic ointment, USP, possesses which property?

   A. Emollient
   B. Greasy
   C. Occlusive
   D. Water washable

5. When one compounds an o/w emulsion containing a flavoring agent, the flavor should be in which emulsion phase?

   A. External.
   B. Internal
   C. Dispersed
   D. Discontinuous

6. When the addition of an active ingredient lowers the melting point of cocoa butter used as a suppository base, what percentage of white wax can be used to replace an equal amount of the base to restore the melting point?

   A. 5
   B. 10
   C. 15
   D. 25

7. What is the emulsifier when lime water and olive oil are triturated together to form a primary emulsion?

    A. Oleic acid
    B. Calcium hydroxide
    C. Calcium oxide
    D. Calcium oleate

8. What is the ratio of lactose to sucrose when used as the base to compound tablet triturates?

    A. 4:1
    B. 3:2
    C. 1:4
    D. 2:3

9. Which process best describes how the following preparation should be compounded?

Camphor	1%
Menthol	1%
Thymol	0.5%
White petrolatum, qs ad	30 g
M.ft. ointment	

    A. Dissolve the camphor, menthol, and thymol in alcohol, and incorporate them into the white petrolatum by geometric dilution.
    B. Dissolve the camphor, menthol, and thymol in glycerin, and incorporate them into the white petrolatum by geometric dilution.
    C. Dissolve the camphor, menthol, and thymol in propylene glycol, and incorporate them into the white petrolatum by geometric dilution.
    D. Form a eutectic mixture with the camphor, menthol, and thymol, and incorporate it into the white petrolatum by geometric dilution.

10. Which process best describes how to compound the following preparation using available 2% salicylic acid ointment?

Salicylic acid	5%
White petrolatum, qs ad	30 g

    A. Weigh 0.5 g of salicylic acid powder, and qs to 30 g with 2% salicylic acid ointment, incorporating the salicylic acid powder by geometric dilution.
    B. Weigh 0.5 g of salicylic acid powder, levigate it with 5 mL of ethyl alcohol, and qs to 30 g with 2% salicylic acid ointment, incorporating the salicylic acid by geometric dilution.
    C. Weigh 1.5 g of salicylic acid powder, and qs to 30 g with 2% salicylic acid ointment, incorporating the salicylic acid powder by geometric dilution.
    D. Weigh 1 g of salicylic acid powder, levigate it with 4 g of mineral oil, and incorporate it into 25 g of 2% salicylic acid ointment by geometric dilution.

11. Which of the following is the process of using potassium iodide to increase the solubility of iodine when compounding Strong Iodine Solution, USP?

    A. Coagulation
    B. Coalescence
    C. Comminution
    D. Complexation

12. A solution containing 55% ethyl alcohol is required. Solutions of 15% and 80% ethyl alcohol are available. What volume of the 15% solution is required to make 100 mL?

    A. 64.8 mL
    B. 41.7 mL
    C. 61.5 mL
    D. 38.5 mL

13. What is the maximum BUD that can be given to powder-filled capsules according to UPS Chapter <795> guidelines?

    A. 6 months
    B. 3 months
    C. 30 days
    D. 14 days

14. Which is a characteristic of a preparation in the moderate compounding category according to USP Chapter <795>?

    A. It requires manipulation of a commercial product by adding a component.
    B. It has a USP compounding monograph.
    C. It requires special calculations to determine component quantities per preparation of individualized units.
    D. It has appeared in a peer-reviewed journal.

Use the following topical preparation to answer
Question 15:

Sulfur
Benzoyl peroxide aa   10%
PEG base, qs ad   90 g

The base is as follows:

PEG 3,350   1 part
PEG 400   1.5 parts

15. If benzoyl peroxide contains 26% water,
     what quantity should be weighed for the
     preparation?

     A. 9 g
     B. 12.2 g
     C. 6.6 g
     D. 11.34 g

Use the following topical preparation to answer
Question 16:

Sulfur
Benzoyl peroxide aa   10%
PEG base, qs ad   90 g

The base is as follows:

PEG 3,350   1 part
PEG 400   1.5 parts

16. What quantity of sulfur should be weighed
     for the preparation?

     A. 7.5 g
     B. 8.1 g
     C. 4.5 g
     D. 9 g

Use the following topical preparation to answer
Question 17:

Sulfur
Benzoyl peroxide aa   10%
PEG base, qs ad   90 g

The base is as follows:

PEG 3,350   1 part
PEG 400   1.5 parts

17. What quantity of base is required for the
     preparation?

     A. 81 g
     B. 76.2 g
     C. 68.8 g
     D. 72 g

Use the following topical preparation to answer
Question 18:

Sulfur
Benzoyl peroxide aa   10%
PEG base, qs ad   90 g

The base is as follows:

PEG 3,350   1 part
PEG 400   1.5 parts

18. What quantity of PEG 3,350 should be
     weighed for the preparation?

     A. 32.4 g
     B. 27.5 g
     C. 0.5 g
     D. 28.8 g

Use the following topical preparation to answer
Question 19:

Sulfur
Benzoyl peroxide aa   10%
PEG base, qs ad   90 g

The base is as follows:

PEG 3,350   1 part
PEG 400   1.5 parts

19. PEG 400 is a liquid with a specific gravity
     of 1.13. What volume should be measured
     for the preparation?

     A. 43 mL
     B. 40.3 mL
     C. 38.3 mL
     D. 36.5 mL

Use the following topical preparation to answer
Question 20:

Sulfur
Benzoyl peroxide aa   10%
PEG base, qs ad   90 g

The base is as follows:

PEG 3,350   1 part
PEG 400   1.5 parts

20. What would be the maximum BUD for the
     preparation according to USP Chapter <795>
     guidelines?

     A. 14 days
     B. 30 days

C. 3 months

D. 6 months

21. If the powder in a chart should weigh 350 mg, what is the acceptable weight range for dispensing?

   A. 280 to 420 mg
   B. 300 to 400 mg
   C. 315 to 385 mg
   D. 333 to 368 mg

22. Which federal legislation enacted in November 2013 amended the Food, Drug and Cosmetic Act to make a distinction between traditional pharmacy compounding regulated by a state board of pharmacy and a compounding outsourcing facility regulated by the FDA?

   A. Drug Quality and Security Act
   B. Food and Drug Administration Modernization Act
   C. Pharmacy Compounding Compliance Act
   D. American Medicinal Drug Use Clarification Act

23. If a USP component is unavailable for a compounded preparation, which chemical grade would be the next best choice to use?

   A. ACS
   B. FCC
   C. AR
   D. Tech

24. Compared to a manufactured product, a compounded preparation has which of the following characteristics?

   A. Made according to current GMP
   B. Subject to an approved NDA
   C. Patient specific in conjunction with the prescriber
   D. Has an NDC number

25. What type of cellulose is used to compound longer-acting capsules?

   A. Methylcellulose
   B. HPMC
   C. Hydroxyethylcellulose
   D. Sodium carboxymethylcellulose

4-11. Answers

1. **C.** For nonsterile compounding, the USP specifies that purified water be used. Purified water is prepared by the processes of distillation, reverse osmosis, or ion exchange. These methods remove heavy metals and other contaminants from the water. Water for injection is used in sterile compounding, and tap and potable water meet the requirements for drinking water but not for compounding.

2. **B.** When the type or percentage of alcohol is not specified in a compounded preparation, alcohol, USP, is used. It contains 95% ethyl alcohol.

3. **D.** Sodium thiosulfate is the antioxidant that prevents the iodide ion from oxidizing to form free iodine. The other choices are not antioxidants.

4. **D.** Hydrophilic ointment is water washable and does not possess the other properties listed of being an emollient that softens the skin, of being greasy because the external phase is water, and of being occlusive because it prevents water from evaporating from the skin.

5. **A.** For the flavoring agent to be tasted, it must be in the external or continuous phase. In an o/w emulsion, the oil is the internal, dispersed, or discontinuous phase.

6. **A.** Five percent cocoa butter replaced by an equal amount of white wax will overcome the lowered melting point. The higher percentages would result in a higher melting point than desired.

7. **D.** The lime water is calcium hydroxide solution, and the olive oil contains oleic acid. The two react to form calcium oleate, which is the emulsifying agent that forms the w/o emulsion. Calcium oxide is not an emulsifier.

8. **A.** The ratio of lactose to sucrose is 4:1. Lactose is used as a filler, and sucrose is the binder that holds the tablets together.

9. **D.** Camphor, menthol, and thymol are three components that liquefy when mixed together, forming a *eutectic mixture*. This liquid mixture is then gradually incorporated into the white petrolatum by geometric dilution.

10. **D.** The compounded preparation must contain 1.5 g of salicylic acid. Twenty-five grams of 2% ointment contain 500 mg, requiring an additional 1 g of salicylic acid powder. The remaining components must not contain any salicylic acid and must consist of a combination of the levigating agent mineral oil and white petrolatum. With a specific gravity of 0.89, the 4 g of mineral oil would measure 4.5 mL.

11. **D.** In solution, potassium iodide ionizes into potassium and the iodide ion. The iodide ion complexes with elemental iodine to form the soluble I^3 complex. This process is called common ion complexation.

12. **D.** Using alligation, 25 parts/65 parts = x/100 mL, and $x = 38.5$ mL.

13. **A.** USP Chapter <795> allows a maximum 6-month BUD for a nonaqueous preparation, if all conditions are met.

14. **C.** The compounding of troches is an example of a preparation in the moderate category. The cavities of the mold used to make them require calibration. The USP recognizes three compounding categories of simple, moderate, and complex.

15. **B.** A 10% concentration requires 9 g to be weighed ($90 \text{ g} \times 0.1 = 9 \text{ g}$). If benzoyl peroxide contains 26% water, it is 74% benzoyl peroxide. If, 74%/100% = 9 g/x, then $x = 12.2$ g.

16. **D.** The abbreviation "aa" means "of each." This indicates that a 10% concentration of both benzoyl peroxide and sulfur are required. Thus, $90 \text{ g} \times 0.1 = 9 \text{ g}$.

17. **C.** The combined weight of the benzoyl peroxide and sulfur is 21.2 g. Because 90 g must be compounded, 68.8 g of base is needed.

18. **B.** The base consists of 1 part PEG 3,350 and 1.5 parts PEG 400 for a total of 2.5 parts. With 68.8 g of base needed, 68.8 ÷ 2.5 parts = 27.5 g per part. Thus, 27.5 g is needed.

19. **D.** PEG 400 is 1.5 parts of the base. If 1 part is 27.5 g, then 1.5 parts are 41.3 g. To determine the volume, divide by the specific gravity of 1.13. Thus, 36.5 mL is needed.

20. **D.** The maximum BUD would be 6 months. Water is contained in the hydrous benzoyl peroxide used to compound the preparation, but that component's container should be labeled with an expiration date. If the expiration date is at least 6 months and no additional water is necessary to make the preparation, then a 6-month BUD could be used.

21. **D.** In compounding, an accuracy within +/−5% of theoretical weight is generally considered acceptable. $350 \text{ mg} \times 0.95 = 333 \text{ mg}$ and $350 \text{ mg} \times 1.05 = 368 \text{ mg}$.

22. **A.** The Drug Quality and Security Act was enacted in November 2013. The Pharmacy Compounding Compliance Act does not exist, and the other federal acts were enacted before November 2013.

23. **B.** USP/NF or FCC grade components are preferred for compounding. Always obtain the certificate of analysis (COA) for every component used, and use components manufactured in FDA-registered facilities. Other component grades may be used if the COA is reviewed to determine that they are appropriate for use.

24. **C.** Extemporaneous pharmacy compounding requires the three-party team of physician, patient, and pharmacist in which the physician writes a prescription requiring the pharmacist to compound a preparation for a specific patient. All the other characteristics are for pharmaceutical manufactured products.

25. **B.** HPMC is the cellulose used to compound longer-acting capsules.

4-12. References

The following are examples of references that should be available in a compounding pharmacy to provide assistance as the pharmacist formulates the variety of dosage forms that customized medications require:

Allen LV Jr. *The Art, Science, and Technology of Pharmaceutical Compounding*. 4th ed. Washington, DC: American Pharmacists Association; 2012.

Allen LV Jr, Ansel H. *Ansel's Pharmaceutical Dosage Forms and Drug Delivery Systems*. 10th ed. Baltimore, MD: Lippincott Williams & Wilkins; 2013.

Ansel H. *Pharmaceutical Calculations*. 14th ed. Baltimore, MD: Lippincott Williams & Wilkins; 2012.

Allen LV Jr, Adejare A, Desselle SP, Felton LA, eds. *Remington: The Science and Practice of Pharmacy*. 22nd ed. Philadelphia, PA: Pharmaceutical Press; 2013.

O'Neil M, ed. *The Merck Index*. 15th ed. London, UK: Royal Society of Chemistry; 2013.

Shrewsbury R. *Applied Pharmaceutics in Contemporary Compounding*. 2nd ed. Englewood, CO: Morton; 2009.

Sweetman S, ed. *Martindale: The Complete Drug Reference*. 38th ed. London, UK: Pharmaceutical Press; 2014.

Thompson J, Davidow L. *A Practical Guide to Contemporary Pharmacy Practice*. 3rd ed. Baltimore, MD: Lippincott Williams & Wilkins; 2009.

Trissel L. *Stability of Compounded Formulations*. 5th ed. Washington, DC: American Pharmacists Association; 2012.

United States Pharmacopeial Convention. *U.S. Pharmacopeia 37/National Formulary 32*. Rockville, MD: United States Pharmacopeial Convention; 2014.

United States Pharmacopeial Convention. *USP on Compounding: A Guide for the Compounding Practitioner*. Rockville, MD: United States Pharmacopeial Convention; 2014.

Sterile Products

Laura A. Thoma

5-1. Key Points

- A sterilizing filter (0.2 micron) is required to filter sterilize a compounded sterile preparation (CSP). The integrity of the filter used to sterilize the CSP must be verified before the preparation may be released. The test is often referred to as the *bubble point test*.
- The high-efficiency particulate air (HEPA) filter is 99.97% efficient at filtering out particles 0.3 micron in size. Certification of the HEPA filter involves testing the velocity of airflow from the filter and the integrity of the filter.
- The air in an International Organization for Standardization (ISO) class 5 area has no more than 3,520 particles 0.5 micron and larger per cubic meter of air. The laminar flow workbench provides an ISO class 5 area.
- The critical site is any opening or pathway between the CSP and the environment. The larger the critical site is and the longer it is exposed to the environment, the greater the risk of contamination of the preparation.
- The bacterial endotoxin test is designed to detect the level of bacterial endotoxin from Gram-negative organisms in the CSP. All bacterial endotoxins are pyrogens, but not all pyrogens are bacterial endotoxins.
- The sterility test and the bacterial endotoxin test (BET) should be performed on all high-risk compounded sterile preparations intended for administration by injection into the vascular or central nervous system that are prepared in groups of more than 25 identical individual single-dose packages or in multidose vials for administration to multiple patients. The BET must be performed before the CSP can be dispensed.
- Any pharmacist preparing CSPs must have training in aseptic technique. One way to validate aseptic technique is by performing media fills. The growth medium most often used is trypticase soy broth, also known as soybean-casein digest medium in the U.S. Pharmacopeia (USP).
- The laminar airflow in a horizontal laminar flow workbench flows toward the operator. The operator must never put his or her hands between the HEPA filter and the critical site. Never break first air.
- The laminar airflow in a vertical laminar flow workbench flows down onto the work surface.
- A biological safety cabinet should always be used for preparing cytotoxic drugs. All biological safety cabinets have vertical laminar airflow.
- The hot air oven is used to depyrogenate items used in compounding and to sterilize compounded preparations that cannot be sterilized by steam.
- Moist-heat sterilization is a common way to sterilize equipment used in the compounding process. Only items that can be moistened by steam can be sterilized by autoclaving.

5-2. Study Guide Checklist

The following topics may guide your study of this subject area:

- Routes of administration and the unique characteristics of each
- ISO classifications 5, 7, and 8
- Primary engineering controls and how they work

- Specification of the HEPA filter that must be met
- Requirements of the buffer area and the anteroom
- Gowning qualification requirements in order to compound CSPs
- Media fills
- Microbial risk levels and the associated beyond-use dates
- Sources of physical incompatibilities
- Chemical degradation pathways
- Quality control tests specific to sterile products

5-3. Parenteral Products

Parenteral products are products that are administered by injection and that, therefore, bypass the gastrointestinal tract. Parenteral products must be sterile and free of pyrogens and particulate matter. Drugs that are destroyed, are inactivated in the gastrointestinal tract, or are poorly absorbed can be given by a parenteral route. Parenteral routes of administration may also be used when the patient is uncooperative, unconscious, or unable to swallow. This route is also used when rapid drug absorption is essential, such as in emergency situations.

Parenteral Routes of Administration

Intravenous route

An intravenous (IV) medication is administered directly into the vein. The IV route gives a rapid effect with a predictable response. It is used for irritating medications because the medication is rapidly diluted. This route does not have as much volume restriction as other parenteral routes.

A *bolus* is an injection of solution into the vein over a short period of time. A bolus is used to administer a relatively small volume of solution and is often written as "IV push."

An *infusion* refers to the introduction of larger volumes of solution given over a longer period of time. A continuous infusion is used to administer a large volume of solution at a constant rate. Intermittent infusions are used to administer a relatively small volume of solution over a specified amount of time at specific intervals.

Intramuscular route

An intramuscular medication is injected deep into a large muscle mass, such as the upper arm, thigh, or buttocks. The medication is absorbed from the muscle tissue, acting more quickly than when given by the oral route, but not as quickly as when given by the intravenous route. Up to 2 mL may be administered intramuscularly as a solution or suspension given in the upper arm, and 5 mL may be given in the gluteal medial muscle of each buttock. A sustained-release-type action can be achieved with certain drugs that have low solubility because they are released from muscle tissue at a slow rate. Intramuscular injections are often painful, and reversing adverse effects from medications given by this route is very difficult. Antibiotics are often given by this route.

Subcutaneous route

Subcutaneous injections of solution or suspension are given beneath the surface of the skin. Medications administered by this route are not absorbed as well as and have a slower onset of action than medications given by the intravenous or intramuscular route. The volume of solution or suspension that can be injected subcutaneously is 2 mL or less. Drugs often given by this route include epinephrine, heparin, insulin, and vaccines.

Intradermal route

An intradermal injection is injected into the top layer of the skin. The injection is not as deep as a subcutaneous injection. Medications used for diagnostic purposes, such as a tuberculin test or an allergy test, are often administered by this route. The volume of solution that can be administered intradermally is limited to 0.1 mL. The onset of action and the rate of absorption of medication from this route are slow.

Intra-arterial route

An intra-arterial injection is injected directly into an artery. It delivers a high drug concentration to the target site with little dilution by the circulation. Generally, this route is used only for radiopaque materials and some antineoplastic agents.

Other routes

- *Intracardiac:* An injection is made directly into the heart.
- *Intra-articular:* Administration by injection is made into a joint space. Corticosteroids are often administered by this route for the treatment of arthritis.

- *Intrathecal:* An injection is made into the lumbar intraspinal fluid sacs. Local anesthetics are frequently administered by this route during surgical procedures. Preservative-free drugs should be used for intrathecal administration.

5-4. Definitions for Compounding of Sterile Preparations

- *Admixture:* Parenteral dosage forms that are combined for administration as a single entity.
- *Antearea:* An International Organization for Standardization (ISO) Class 8 or better area where personnel hand hygiene and garbing procedures, sanitizing of supplies, and other particulate-generating activities are performed. The area contains a line of demarcation separating the clean side from the dirty side.
- *Aseptic processing:* The separate sterilization of a product and its components, containers, and closures, which are then brought together and assembled in an aseptic environment. The primary objective of aseptic processing is to create a sterile preparation.
- *Aseptic technique:* Performance of a procedure or procedures under controlled conditions in a manner that will minimize the chance of contamination. Contaminants can be introduced from the environment, equipment and supplies, or personnel (see the section on ISO classification).
- *Buffer area:* The area where the primary engineering control is located.
- *Compounding aseptic containment isolator (CACI):* An isolator that protects workers from exposure to undesirable levels of airborne drugs while providing an aseptic environment during the compounding of sterile preparations.
- *Compounding aseptic isolator (CAI):* An isolator that maintains an aseptic compounding environment within the isolator throughout the compounding and material transfer process during the compounding of sterile preparations.
- *Critical site:* Any opening or surface that can provide a pathway between the sterile product and the environment.
- *Hypertonic:* A solution that contains a higher concentration of dissolved substances than the red blood cell, thereby causing the red blood cell to shrink.
- *Hypotonic:* A solution that contains a lower concentration of dissolved substances than the red

blood cell, thereby causing the red blood cell to swell and possibly burst.
- *Isotonic:* A solution that has an osmotic pressure close to that of bodily fluids, thus minimizing patient discomfort and damage to red blood cells. Dextrose 5% in water and sodium chloride 0.9% solutions are approximately isotonic.
- *Primary engineering control (PEC):* A device or room that provides an ISO Class 5 environment for the exposure of critical sites when producing compounded sterile preparations (CSPs). These devices could include a laminar airflow workbench, a biological safety cabinet, CAIs, and CACIs.
- *Sterilizing filter:* A filter that, when challenged with the microorganism *Brevundimonas diminuta* at a minimum concentration of 10^7 organisms per cm^2 of filter surface, will produce a sterile effluent. A sterilizing filter has a nominal pore size rating of 0.2 or 0.22 micron.
- *Tonicity:* Osmotic pressure exerted by a solution from the solutes or dissolved solids present.
- *Validation:* Establishment of documented evidence providing a high degree of assurance that a specific process will consistently produce a product meeting predetermined specifications and quality attributes.

ISO Classification

The ISO Classification of Particulate Matter in Room Air is the standard for clean rooms and associated environments. Limits are expressed in particles 0.5 micron and larger per cubic meter. In contrast, the limits from Federal Standard 209E are expressed in particles 0.5 micron and larger per cubic foot (1 cubic meter = 35.31 cubic feet).

ISO class 5 area

The air in an ISO class 5 area has a count of no more than 3,520 particles 0.5 micron or larger per cubic meter of air. This area is equivalent to a class 100 area under Federal Standard 209E, where the air has a count of no more than 100 particles 0.5 micron or larger per cubic foot of air. This class is the quality of air provided by the PEC and required for sterile product preparation.

ISO class 7 area

The air in an ISO class 7 area has a count of no more than 352,000 particles 0.5 micron or larger per cubic meter. This area is equivalent to a class 10,000 area under Federal Standard 209E, where the air has a count of no more than 10,000 particles 0.5 micron or larger per cubic foot of air. This class is the quality of air usually required in the buffer area.

ISO class 8 area

The air in an ISO class 8 area has a count of no more than 3,520,000 particles 0.5 micron or larger per cubic meter. This area is equivalent to a class 100,000 area under Federal Standard 209E, where the air has a count of no more than 100,000 particles 0.5 micron or larger per cubic foot of air. The antearea should have ISO class 8 air or better.

5-5. Sterile Product Preparation Area

The following are examples of PECs that provide the ISO class 5 area for compounding of CSPs.

Horizontal Laminar Flow Workbench

The horizontal laminar flow workbench (HLFW) works by drawing air in through a prefilter. The prefiltered air is pressurized in the plenum for consistent distribution of air to the high-efficiency particulate air (HEPA) filter (Figure 5-1).

The prefilter protects the HEPA filter from prematurely clogging. Prefilters should be checked regularly and changed as needed. A record of these checks and changes of the prefilter must be kept.

The plenum of the hood is the space between the prefilter and the HEPA filter. Air is pressurized here and distributed over the HEPA filter.

Laminar flow is the air in a confined space moving with uniform velocity along parallel lines. The term *unidirectional flow* has taken the place of laminar flow in more recent publications. Unidirectional flow is airflow moving in a single direction in a robust and uniform manner and at sufficient speed to sweep particles away from the critical processing area. Inside the HLFW is an ISO class 5 area (class 100 area).

Vertical Laminar Flow Workbench

The vertical laminar flow workbench (VLFW) works like an HLFW in that the air is drawn in through the prefilter and is pressurized in the plenum for distribution over the HEPA filter. However, the air is blown down from the top of the workstation onto the work surface, not across it (Figure 5-2).

Working in vertical laminar flow requires different techniques than does working in horizontal laminar flow. In vertical laminar flow, an object or the hands of the operator must not be above an object in the hood. In horizontal laminar flow, an object or the hands of the operator must not be in back of another object. The hands of the operator must never come between the HEPA filter and the object.

A biological safety cabinet, CAI, and CACI also use vertical unidirectional airflow to provide an ISO class 5 environment and are other examples of PECs.

Figure 5-1. Horizontal Laminar Flow Workbench

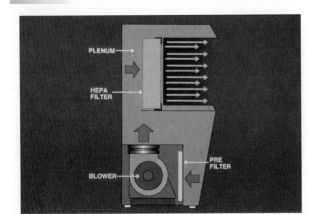

Illustration courtesy of the University of Tennessee Parenteral Medications Lab.

Figure 5-2. Vertical Laminar Flow Workbench

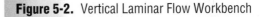
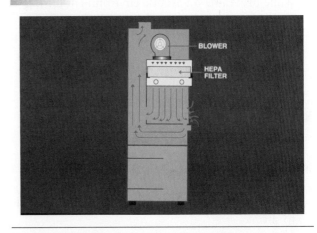

Illustration courtesy of the University of Tennessee Parenteral Medications Lab.

The HEPA Filter

The HEPA filter consists of a bank of filter media separated by corrugated pleats of aluminum. These pleats act as baffles to direct the air into laminar sheets. The HEPA filter is 99.97% efficient at removing particles 0.3 micron in size. Particles that are smaller or larger than 0.3 micron will be removed more efficiently.

Certification of the HEPA filter

The velocity of air from the HEPA filter is checked with a velometer or hot wire anemometer. ISO 14644 recommends that the average air velocity should be greater than 0.2 m/second.

Integrity of the HEPA filter: The dioctyl phthalate (DOP) test

The integrity of the HEPA filter is checked by introducing a high concentration of aerosolized Emery 3004 (a synthetic hydrocarbon) upstream of the filter on a continuous basis, while monitoring the penetration on the downstream side of the HEPA filter.

The aerosol has an average particle size of 0.3 micron. An aerosol photometer is used to check for leaks by passing the wand slowly over the filter and the gasket. None of the surfaces shall yield greater than 0.01% of the upstream smoke concentration. Any value greater than 0.01% indicates that a serious leak is present and must be sealed. All repaired areas must be retested for compliance. At one time, DOP was used to generate the aerosol. However, because DOP is a carcinogen, Emery 3004 is now used. An electronic particle counter cannot be used to certify the integrity of the HEPA filter. The particle counter is used to determine room classification.

Buffer Area (Controlled Area)

The PEC provides an ISO class 5 (class 100) area. It must be located in a controlled environment, away from excess traffic, doors, air vents, or anything that could produce air currents greater than the velocity of the airflow from the HEPA filter. Air currents greater than the velocity of the airflow from the HEPA filter may introduce contaminants into the hood. It is very easy to overcome air flowing at 90 feet per minute.

The buffer area shall be enclosed from other pharmacy operations. Floors, walls, ceiling, shelving, counters, and cabinets of the controlled area must be of nonshedding, smooth, and nonporous material to allow for easy cleaning and disinfecting. All surfaces shall be resistant to sanitizing agents. Cracks, crevices, and seams shall be avoided, as should ledges or other places that could collect dust. The floor of the buffer area shall be smooth and seamless with coved edges up the walls.

The walls of the buffer area can be sealed panels caulked with silicone or, if drywall is used, painted with epoxy paint, which is nonshedding. The corners of the ceiling and the walls shall be sealed to avoid cracks. A solid ceiling may be painted with epoxy paint, or nonshedding washable ceiling tiles that are caulked into place may be used.

Light fixtures shall be mounted flush with the ceiling and sealed. Anything that penetrates the ceiling or walls shall be sealed.

Air entering the room shall be fresh, HEPA filtered, and air conditioned. The room must be maintained in positive pressure (0.02–0.05 inch of water column) in relation to the adjoining rooms or corridors. If the buffer area is used for compounding of cytotoxic drugs, 0.01 inch of water column negative pressure is required. At least 30 air changes per hour shall occur, with the PECs allowed to provide up to 15 of the 30 required air changes per hour.

People entering the buffer area shall be properly scrubbed and gowned. Access to the buffer area shall be restricted to qualified personnel only.

Controlling the traffic in the buffer area is a critical factor in keeping the area clean. Only items required for compounding shall be brought into the buffer area. These items must be cleaned and sanitized before being taken into the buffer area. Items may be stored in the buffer area for a limited time. However, the number of items stored in the buffer area shall be kept to a minimum. All equipment used in the buffer area should remain in the room except during calibration or repair.

Because they can harbor many organisms, refrigerators and freezers should be located out of the buffer area. Computers and printers should be located outside of the buffer area because they generate many particles. However, if they are required to be in the buffer area, monitor the environment and evaluate their effect on the environment. Cardboard boxes shall not be stored in the buffer area. The items shall be removed from the boxes on the dirty side of the antearea and sanitized and transferred to the clean side of the antearea or to the buffer area for storage.

Vials stored in laminated cardboard may be stored in the buffer area. Sinks or floor drains shall not be in the buffer area because potable water contains many organisms and endotoxins.

Preparation of Operators

An operator must be trained and evaluated to be capable of properly scrubbing and garbing before entering the buffer area. This requirement is critical to the maintenance of asepsis. The greatest source of contamination in a clean room is the people in the area. A seated or standing person without movement releases an average of 100,000 particles greater than 0.3 micron in diameter per minute. A person standing with full body movement releases an average of 2,000,000 particles per minute greater than 0.3 micron in diameter, and if moving at a slow walk, he or she releases an average of 5,000,000 particles. The garb is designed to help contain the particles that are being shed.

Before entering the antearea, an operator must remove all cosmetics and all hand, wrist, and other visible jewelry or piercings. Artificial nails or extenders are prohibited while working in the sterile compounding environment, and natural nails must be kept neat and trimmed. Garb is donned in an order proceeding from that considered dirtiest to that considered cleanest. Shoe covers, head and facial hair covers, and facemask or eye shields are donned before performing hand hygiene. Hands and forearms are then washed for 30 seconds with soap and water in the antearea, and hands and forearms are dried using a lint-free disposable towel or an electric hand dryer. While still in the antearea, an operator must don a nonshedding gown that zips or buttons up to the neck, falls below the knees, and has sleeves that fit snugly around the wrists. After entering the buffer area, an operator must use a waterless alcohol-based surgical hand scrub with persistent activity to again cleanse the hands before putting on sterile gloves. Sterile contact agar plates must be used to sample the gloved fingertips of compounding personnel after garbing to assess garbing competency. For successful completion of this competency, no colony-forming units can be found on any of the agar plate samples. Three consecutive, successful garbing and gloving exercises must be completed before sterile compounding is allowed. Routine application of sterile 70% isopropyl alcohol (IPA) must occur throughout the compounding process and whenever nonsterile surfaces are touched. After this initial evaluation, the entire process is repeated

at least once a year for low- and medium-risk compounding and semiannually for high-risk compounding during any media-fill test procedure. The colony-forming unit action level for gloved hands will be based on the total number of colony-forming units on both gloves, not per hand.

Validation of the Operator

A *media fill* or *media transfer* is when a growth promotion media is used instead of the drug product, and all the normal compounding manipulations are done. It is critical that the process mimics the actual compounding process as closely as possible and represents worst-case conditions. Usually, the medium used is soybean-casein digest, which is also known as trypticase soy broth (TSB). This medium will support the growth of organisms that are likely to be transmitted to CSPs from the compounding personnel and environment. A media fill is used to check the quality of the compounding personnel's aseptic technique. It is also used to verify that the compounding process and the compounding environment are capable of producing sterile preparations.

Initially, before an operator can compound low- or medium-risk sterile injectable products, he or she must successfully complete one media fill using sterile fluid culture media such as 3% soybean-casein digest medium. Media fill units must be incubated at 20–25°C for a minimum of 14 days or at 20–25°C for a minimum of 7 days and then at 30–35°C for a minimum of 7 days. A successful media fill is indicated by no growth in any of the media fill units. The media fill shall closely simulate the most challenging or stressful conditions encountered during the compounding of low- and medium-risk preparations. The compounding personnel shall perform a revalidation at a minimum of once a year by successfully completing one media fill. The media fills shall be designed to mimic the most challenging techniques the operator will use during a normal day. Validation for high-risk compounding focuses on ensuring that both the process and the compounding personnel are capable of producing a sterile preparation with all its purported quality attributes. Revalidation must be done on at least a semiannual basis. An example of a high-risk operation is the compounding of a sterile preparation from nonsterile drug powder. To mimic this operation, the compounder must use commercially available soybean-casein digest medium made up to a 3% concentration and perform normal processing steps, including filter sterilization. All media fills must occur in an ISO class 5 environment and must be completed without interruption.

5-6. Working in the Laminar Flow Workbench

Items not in a protective overwrap shall be wiped with a lint-free wipe soaked with sterile 70% IPA before being placed in the hood. Containers and packages must be inspected for cracks, tears, or particles as they are decontaminated and placed in the hood. Items in a protective overwrap, such as bags, must be taken from the overwrap at the edge of the hood (within the first 6 inches of the hood) and placed in the hood with the injection port facing the HEPA filter. The overwrap should not be placed in the hood, because doing so would introduce particles and organisms into the hood.

When working in the HLFW, an operator shall arrange supplies to the left or right of the direct compounding area (DCA). The critical site must be in uninterrupted unidirectional airflow at all times. The compounder must be careful not to place an object or hand between the HEPA filter and the critical site because doing so would interrupt the airflow to the critical site and potentially cause particles to be washed from the hand or object onto the critical site.

All work performed in the HLFW must be done at least 6 inches inside the hood. The unidirectional airflow is blowing toward the operator, who acts as a barrier to the airflow, causing it to pass around the body and create backflow. This turbulence can cause room air to be carried into the front of the hood.

Items placed in the HLFW disturb the unidirectional airflow. The unidirectional airflow is disturbed downstream of the item for approximately three times the diameter of the object. If the item is placed next to the sidewall of the hood, the unidirectional airflow is disturbed downstream of the item for approximately six times the diameter of the object. The area downstream from the nonsterile object is no longer bathed in unidirectional airflow and may become contaminated with particles. For these reasons, it is very important that a direct path exists between the HEPA filter and the area where the manipulations will occur.

With the VLFW, supplies in the hood should be placed so that the operator may work without placing a hand or object above the critical site. An operator can place many more items in the VLFW and still work without compromising the unidirectional airflow. Remember that within 1 inch of the work surface the air is turbulent. The unidirectional air, which is coming down from the HEPA filter, strikes the work surface and changes direction to move horizontally across the work surface. Therefore, all work in the VLFW should be done at least 1 inch above the work surface. During the compounding of sterile preparations, all movements into and out of the hood must be minimized to decrease the risk of carrying contaminants into the DCA. This can be achieved by introducing all items needed for the aseptic manipulation into the work area at one time and by waiting until the procedure is completed before removing used syringes, vials, and other supplies from the PEC.

5-7. Syringes, Needles, Ampuls, and Vials

Syringes

The basic parts of the syringe are the barrel, plunger, collar, rubber tip of the plunger, and tip of the syringe. Syringes are sterile and free of pyrogens. They are packaged either in paper or in a rigid plastic container. Syringe packages must be inspected to ensure that the wrap is intact and the syringe is still sterile. Syringes have either a Luer-Lok tip, in which the needle is screwed tightly onto the threaded tip, or a slip tip, in which the needle is held on by friction (Figure 5-3). Syringes are supplied with and without needles attached and are available in a variety of

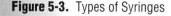

Figure 5-3. Types of Syringes

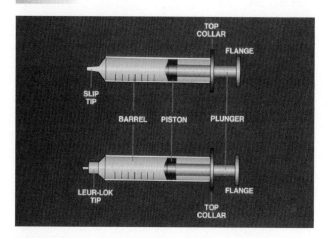

Illustration courtesy of the University of Tennessee Parenteral Medications Lab.

sizes. When removing the syringe from its package, take care not to let the syringe tip touch the surface of the hood.

Calibration marks are on the barrel of the syringe. These marks are accurate to one-half the interval marked on the syringe. The critical sites on the syringe are the tip of the syringe and the ribs of the plunger. The ribs of the plunger go back inside the syringe on injection of the fluid from the syringe and could potentially contaminate the syringe.

Needles

The basic parts of a needle include the hub, needle shaft, bevel, bevel heel, and tip of the needle (Figure 5-4).

Needles are sterile and are wrapped either in plastic with a twist-off top or in paper. This wrap must be inspected for integrity before the needle is used. The gauge of the needle refers to its outer diameter. The larger the number, the smaller the bore of the needle. The smallest is 27 gauge, and the largest is 13 gauge. The length of the needle is measured in inches, and some common lengths are 1–1.5 inches.

The critical sites on the needle are the hub of the needle, the entire needle shaft, and the tip of the needle.

Ampuls

Ampuls are single-dose containers. Once ampuls are broken, they are an open-system container; air can pass freely in and out of the ampul. Any solution taken from an ampul must be filtered with a 5 micron filter needle or filter straw, because glass particles fall into the ampul when it is broken. Before breaking the ampul, wipe the neck of the ampul with a sterile 70% IPA prep pad.

Vials

A vial is a molded glass or plastic container with a rubber closure secured in place with an aluminum seal. It may contain sterile solutions, dry-filled powders, or lyophilized drugs, or it may be an empty evacuated container. Vials may be single-dose or multiple-dose containers.

A single-dose container usually contains no preservative system to prevent the growth of micro-organisms if they are accidentally introduced into the container. A single-dose vial punctured in an environment worse than ISO class 5 air must be used within 1 hour. A single-dose vial continuously exposed to ISO class 5 air may be used up to 6 hours after initial needle puncture. When the vial is first used, it should be labeled with the date, time, and initials of the person using the vial so the beyond-use date (BUD) can be determined. A multidose vial contains preservatives, and these vials can be entered more than once. The pharmaceutical manufacturer has done studies to prove that the preservative system will remain effective and the closure will reseal after penetration by the needle. Therefore, the BUD for opened or entered multidose containers is 28 days, unless otherwise specified by the manufacturer.

5-8. Biological Safety Cabinets

A class II biological safety cabinet (BSC) should be used to prepare cytotoxic and other hazardous drugs. Four different types of class II BSCs exist. Types A1 and A2 exhaust 30% of HEPA-filtered air either into the room or to the outside through a canopy connection. Type A1 mixes the supply air in a common plenum and may have ducts and plenum under positive pressure. Type A2 has all contaminated ducts and plenum under negative pressure or surrounded by negative pressure. Type B1 exhausts 70% of total air through a dedicated exhaust duct and must be hard ducted. Type B2 exhausts 100% of total air to the outside without any recirculation and must be hard ducted also. With types B1 and B2, all the ducts and the plenum are under negative pressure and are surrounded by negative pressure.

Figure 5-4. Needle

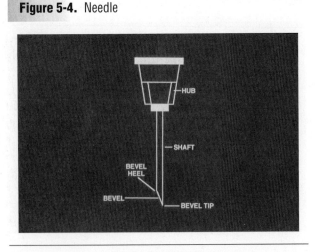

Illustration courtesy of the University of Tennessee Parenteral Medications Lab.

Preparation of Hazardous Drugs

When working with hazardous drugs, personnel must wear appropriate protective equipment, including solid-front gowns, face masks, eye protection, hair and shoe covers, and double sterile chemotherapy-type gloves. Personnel must handle all hazardous drugs with caution at all times, using appropriate chemotherapy gloves, not only during preparation, but also during receiving, distribution, stocking, inventorying, and disposal.

It is imperative that positive pressure not be allowed to build up in the vial. Proper training on the use of a chemotherapy-venting device, which uses a 0.2 micron hydrophobic filter or the negative pressure technique to prevent the build up of positive pressure within the vial, must be done before preparing hazardous drugs and on an annual basis. When a closed system transfer device (one that allows no venting or exposure of hazardous substance to the environment) is used, it shall be used within the ISO class 5 environment of a BSC or CACI.

When compounding, personnel must use syringes and IV sets with Luer-Lok fittings if possible. Use a large enough syringe so that the plunger does not separate from the barrel of the syringe when filled with solution. Syringes should be filled with no more than 75% of their total volume. When possible, attach IV sets and prime them before adding the hazardous drug. Wipe the outside of the bag or bottle to remove any inadvertent contamination. The use of nonshedding plastic-backed absorbent pads is also conducive to keeping the BSC as clean as possible.

The PEC shall be located in an ISO class 7 area physically separated from other preparation areas and maintained under negative pressure of not less than 0.01 inch water column to the surrounding area.

5-9. Overview of the Standard of Practice Related to Sterile Preparations: The United States Pharmacopeia (USP) 37/National Formulary (NF) 32

Chapter <797>, *Pharmaceutical Compounding—Sterile Preparations* in USP 32/NF 27, became the official standard for sterile pharmaceutical compounding in June 2008. Chapter <797> has three microbial risk levels of compounded sterile preparations. The risk levels are determined on the basis of the potential for the introduction of microbial, chemical, or physical contamination into the product. The chapter covers topics such as validation of sterilization and of the aseptic process, environmental control and sampling, end-product testing, bacterial endotoxins, training, and a quality assurance program.

Low-Risk Compounding

Compounding is classified as *low risk* when all of the following conditions prevail:

- Commercially available sterile products, components, and devices are used in compounding within air quality of ISO class 5 or better.
- Compounding involves few aseptic manipulations, using not more than three commercially manufactured sterile products and not more than two entries into any one sterile container.
- Closed-system transfers are used. Withdrawal from an open ampul is classified as a closed system.
- In the absence of passage of a sterility test, the storage periods for the CSPs cannot exceed the following time periods before administration:
  - Storage for not more than 48 hours at a controlled room temperature of 20–25°C
  - Storage for not more than 14 days at a cold temperature of 2–8°C
  - Storage for not more than 45 days in a solid frozen state between –25°C and –10°C.

Medium-Risk Compounding

Medium-risk CSPs are those compounded under low-risk conditions when one or more of the following conditions exist:

- Compounding involves pooling of additives for the administration to either multiple patients or to one patient on multiple occasions.
- Compounding involves complex manipulations other than a single volume transfer.
- The compounding process requires a long time period to complete dissolution or homogeneous mixing.
- In the absence of passage of a sterility test, the storage periods for the CSPs cannot exceed the following time periods before administration:
  - Exposure for not more than 30 hours at a controlled room temperature of 20–25°C

- Storage for not more than 9 days at a cold temperature of 2–8°C
- Storage for not more than 45 days in a solid frozen state between –25°C and –10°C.

High-Risk Compounding

High-risk compounds are compounded under any of the following conditions and are either contaminated or at high risk to become contaminated with infectious microorganisms:

- A sterile preparation is compounded from non-sterile ingredients.
- Sterile ingredients or components are exposed to air quality inferior to ISO class 5 for more than 1 hour, including storage in environments inferior to ISO class 5 of opened or partially used packages of manufactured sterile products with no antimicrobial preservative system.
- Nonsterile water–containing preparations are exposed for more than 6 hours before being sterilized.
- No examination of labeling and documentation from suppliers or direct determination that the chemical purity and content strength of ingredients meet their original or compendia specification occurs.
- Compounding personnel are improperly garbed and gloved.
- In the absence of passage of a sterility test, the storage periods for the CSPs cannot exceed the following time periods before administration:
  - Storage for not more than 24 hours at a controlled room temperature of 20–25°C
  - Storage for not more than 3 days at a cold temperature of 2–8°C
  - Storage for not more than 45 days in a solid frozen state between –25°C and –10°C.

5-10. Sterilization Methods

Filtration

Filtration works by a combination of sieving, adsorption, and entrapment. Care must be taken to choose the correct filter to sterilize the preparation. Membrane filters generally are compatible with most pharmaceutical solutions, but interactions do occur—often because of sorption or leaching. *Sorption* is the binding of drug or other formulation components to the filter, which can occur with peptide or protein formulations. There are filters that have little or no affinity for peptides or proteins. *Leaching* is the extracting of components of the filter into the solution. Surfactants are often added to the filter to make it hydrophilic, and they may leach into the product. Large-molecular-weight peptides may be affected by filtration. Their passage through a filter with a small pore size may cause shear stress and alter the three dimensional structure of the peptide. Solvents in the parenteral formulation may also affect filters. All filter manufacturers have compatibility data on their membrane type and can be a great source of information when choosing a membrane.

Filter choice

Choose the appropriate size and configuration of filtration device to accommodate the volume being filtered and permit complete filtration without clogging of the membrane. A 25 mm syringe disk filter should filter no more than 100 mL of solution. If the solution being filtered has a heavy particulate load, a 5 micron filter should be used before the 0.2 micron filter to decrease the particulate load to the 0.2 micron filter. The filter membrane and housing must be physically and chemically compatible with the product to be filtered and capable of withstanding the temperature, pressures, and hydrostatic stress imposed on the system.

A pharmacy may rely on the certificate of quality provided by the vendor. Certification shall include microbial retention testing with *Brevundimonas diminuta* at a minimum concentration of 10^7 organisms per cm^2, as well as testing for membrane and housing integrity, nonpyrogenicity, and extractables.

Hydrophobic and hydrophilic filters

Hydrophilic membranes wet spontaneously with water. They are used for filtration of aqueous solutions and aqueous solutions containing water-miscible solvents. *Hydrophobic filters* do not wet spontaneously with water. They are used for filtering gases and solvents.

Filter integrity

A sterilizing filter assembly shall be tested for integrity after filtration has occurred. The *bubble point* is a simple, nondestructive check of the integrity of the filtration assembly, including the filter membrane. The basis for the test is that liquid is held in the capillary structure of the membrane by surface tension.

The minimum pressure required to force the liquid out of the capillary space is a measure of the largest pores in the membrane.

A bubble point test is performed by wetting the filter with water, increasing the pressure of air upstream of the filter, and watching for air bubbles downstream to indicate passage of air through the filter capillaries. The typical water bubble point pressure of a sterilizing filter with a pore size rating of 0.2 micron is greater than 50 pounds per square inch gauge (psig). As pore size decreases, the bubble point increases. Remember that the bubble point given on the certificate of quality from the filter manufacturer is usually the water bubble point. Many drug formulations have a lower surface tension than water and will have a lower bubble point.

After the solution is filtered and before the integrity of the filter membrane is checked, the filter should be flushed with water to wash as much of the product off the membrane as possible. The integrity test may then be performed. Bubble points are also often given for 70% IPA and water. Use the alcohol test for a hydrophobic filter.

Heat Sterilization

Moist-heat sterilization (autoclave)

Moist-heat sterilization is one of the most widely used methods of sterilization. Saturation of steam at high pressure is the foundation for the effectiveness of moist-heat sterilization. When steam makes contact with a cooler object, it condenses and loses latent heat to the object. The amount of energy released is ~524 kcal/g at 121°C. Most sterilization cycles are at 121°C at 15 psig for 20–60 minutes. Moist-heat sterilization is faster and does not require as high a temperature as dry-heat sterilization. Steam must make contact with the object to be sterilized. Oils cannot be sterilized by steam nor can an empty dry vial. Biological indicators of *Geobacillus stearothermophilus* and temperature-sensing devices shall be used to verify the effectiveness of the steam sterilization cycle.

Dry-heat sterilization

Dry-heat sterilization is usually done as a batch process in an oven designed for sterilization. It provides heated filtered air that is evenly distributed throughout the chamber by a blower. The oven is equipped with a system to control the temperature and exposure period. Dry-heat sterilization requires higher temperatures and longer exposure times than does moist-heat sterilization. Typical sterilization cycles are 120–180 minutes at 160°C or 90–120 minutes at 170°C. Biological indicators of *Bacillus subtilis* and temperature-sensing devices shall be used to verify the effectiveness of the dry-heat sterilization cycle.

Depyrogenation by dry heat

Dry heat can also be used for depyrogenation of glass and stainless steel equipment and of vials. The pyrogens are destroyed when the equipment is kept at 250°C for 30 minutes. The effectiveness of the dry-heat depyrogenation cycle shall be verified by using endotoxin challenge vials to determine whether the cycle is adequate to achieve a 3-log reduction in endotoxins.

Beyond-Use Date

Each compounded sterile preparation must have a label that specifies the correct names and amount of ingredients, the total volume, the storage requirements, route of administration, and BUD. The BUD is the date after which a compounded preparation is not to be used and is determined from the date the preparation is compounded. In the absence of passing the sterility test, the CSPs must comply with the microbial BUD. If the lot of CSP has met the requirements of the sterility test, then the BUD may be based on chemical and physical stability. When assigning a BUD, compounding personnel should consult and apply drug-specific and general stability documentation and literature where available. They should consider the nature of the drug, its degradation mechanism, the container in which it is packaged, the expected storage conditions, and the intended duration of therapy.

5-11. Stability

Stability refers to physical, chemical, and microbial stability.

Instability usually refers to chemical reactions that are incessant and irreversible and result in distinctly different chemical entities. These new chemical entities can be therapeutically inactive and possibly exhibit greater toxicity.

Incompatibility usually refers to physicochemical phenomena such as concentration-dependent precipitation and acid–base reactions that occur when one drug is mixed with others to produce a product unsuitable for administration to the patient. An incompatibility could cause the patient not to receive the full therapeutic effect, or it could cause toxic decomposition products to form. A precipitated incompatibility may irritate the vein or cause occlusion of vessels.

There are three categories of incompatibilities: *therapeutic incompatibility*, *physical incompatibility*, and *chemical incompatibility*.

Therapeutic Incompatibility

Therapeutic incompatibility occurs when two or more drugs administered at the same time result in undesirable antagonistic or synergistic pharmacologic action.

Physical Incompatibility

Physical incompatibility is the combination of two or more drugs in solution, resulting in a change in the appearance of the solution, a change in color, the formation of turbidity or a precipitate, or the evolution of a gas. Physical incompatibilities are related to solubility changes or container interactions rather than to molecular change to the drug entity itself.

Six major areas of concern about physical incompatibility

Compatibility or incompatibility of two or more drugs mixed in the same syringe

For example, preoperative medications—a combination of a narcotic, an analgesic, an antiemetic, and an anticholinergic—are mixed in the same syringe to save the patient from multiple intramuscular injections.

Compatibility of two or more drugs given through the same IV administration line

This concern is common in intensive care units, where patients are often on a number of IV medications and could also be fluid restricted. For example, dopamine HCl 800 mg in 500 mL D_5W (5% dextrose in water) is prescribed. The nurse wants to push 2 amps of sodium bicarbonate through the IV line. The pH of dopamine is 3–4.5, and that of $NaHCO_3$ is approximately 8. If this push is done, a color change occurs because of decomposition of the product. The pH of the bicarbonate is too high for dopamine stability.

Compatibility of two or more drugs placed in the same bottle or bag of IV fluid

KCl, the most common additive, is a neutral salt composed of monovalent ions that are not likely to produce compatibility problems. Therefore, if a drug is compatible in a neutral salt, it is probably compatible in KCl.

Parenteral nutrition solutions can be especially difficult. The number of components, the long duration of contact time, and exposure to ambient temperature and light enhance the potential for an adverse compatibility interaction to occur. The interaction of Ca and PO_4 to form $CaPO_4$, which appears as fine white particles that create a milky solution, is a problem.

Some ways to decrease the risk of injury follow:

- Calculate the solubility of the added calcium from the volume at the time when calcium is added. Flush the line in between the addition of any potentially incompatible components.
- Add the calcium before the lipid emulsion. Therefore, if a precipitate forms, the lipid will not obscure its presence.
- Periodically agitate the admixture, and check for precipitates. Train patients and caregivers to visually inspect for signs of precipitation and to stop the infusion if precipitation is noted.

The following factors enhance formation of precipitate of calcium and phosphate:

- High concentrations of calcium and phosphate
- Increases in solution pH
- Decreases in amino acid concentrations
- Increases in temperature
- Addition of calcium before phosphate
- Lengthy time delay or slow infusion rates
- Use of the chloride salt of calcium

Do not exceed 15 mEq of Ca with up to 15 mL PO_4 per 1,000 mL of solution.

Compatibility of the additive with the composition of the IV container itself

Nitroglycerin readily migrates into many plastics, especially polyvinylchloride (PVC). Insulin adsorbs to IV tubing, filters, and both glass and plastic containers.

Compatibility of the additive with the additional equipment used to prepare or administer the IV admixture

Cisplatin interacts with aluminum by forming a black precipitate when coming in contact with it.

Stability of the drug after admixture

Ampicillin sodium is stable for 72 hours when refrigerated and 24 hours at room temperature in normal saline. However, if it is added to D_5W, it is stable for only 4 hours when refrigerated and 2 hours at room temperature.

Other potential sources of physical incompatibilities

Concentration

A drug will remain in aqueous solution as long as its concentration is less than its saturation solubility.

Cosolvent system

Drugs that are poorly water soluble are often formulated using water-miscible cosolvents. Examples of water-miscible cosolvents include ethanol, propylene glycol, and polyethylene glycol. Dilution of drugs that are in a cosolvent system often causes precipitation of the drug. A good example is diazepam injection. Dilution of the drug results in precipitation in some concentrations, but sufficient dilution to a point below diazepam's saturation solubility results in a physically stable admixture.

pH

The greatest single factor in causing an incompatibility is a change in acid–base environment. Solubility of drugs that are weak acids or bases is a direct function of solution pH. The drug's dissociation constant and pH control the portion of drug in its ionized form and the solubility of the un-ionized form. A drug that is a weak acid may be formulated at a pH sufficient to yield the desired solubility. Sodium salts of barbiturates, phenytoin, and methotrexate are formulated at high pH values to achieve adequate solubility.

Sodium salts of weak acids precipitate as free acids when added to IV fluids having an acidic pH. If the pH of these drugs is lowered, the drug's solubility at the final pH may be exceeded, resulting in possible precipitation. Drugs that are salts of weak bases may precipitate in an alkaline solution.

Ionic interactions

Large organic anions and cations may also form precipitates, such as the precipitation that occurs when heparin (anionic) and aminoglycoside antibiotics (cationic) are mixed. These heparin salts of the cationic drug are relatively insoluble in water.

Sorption phenomena

The intact drug is lost from the solution by adsorption to the surface or absorption into the matrix of container material, administration set, or filter.

Adsorption to the surface can result from interactions of functional groups within the drug's molecule to binding sites on the surfaces.

Absorption of lipid-soluble drugs into the matrix of plastic containers and administration sets, especially those made from PVC, does occur. The substantial amount of phthalate plasticizer used to make the PVC bag pliable and flexible allows the lipid-soluble drugs to diffuse from the solution into the plasticizer in the plastic matrix. Plastics such as polyethylene and polypropylene, which contain little or no phthalate plasticizer, do not readily absorb lipid-soluble drugs into the polymer core. Leaching of the phthalate plasticizer into the solution may also occur, especially if surface-active agents or a large amount of organic cosolvent is present in the formulation.

Chemical Incompatibility

Chemical incompatibilities are interactions resulting in molecular changes or rearrangements to different chemical entities. Most chemical interactions are not observable by the unaided eye.

Chemical degradation pathways

Hydrolysis is a common mode of chemical decomposition. Water attacks labile bonds in dissolved drug molecules. Functional groups labile to hydrolysis are carboxylic acid and phosphate esters, amides, lactams, and imines.

Oxidation is an electron loss that causes a positive increase in valence. Many drugs are in the reduced form, and oxygen creates stability problems. Steroids, epinephrine, and tricyclic compounds are sensitive to oxygen. For control of the stability problem, oxygen can be excluded, pH can be adjusted, and chelating agents or antioxidants can be added.

Reduction is when an electron is gained, causing a decrease in valence and the addition of halogen or hydrogen to the double bond. β-lactam antibiotics can produce reducing aldehydes on hydrolysis.

Photolysis is the catalysis by light of degradation reactions such as oxidation or hydrolysis. Examples of drugs that are light sensitive are amphotericin B, furosemide, and sodium nitroprusside. The reaction rate depends on the intensity and wavelength of light. Sodium nitroprusside in D_5W has a faint brownish cast, but exposure to light causes deterioration, which is evident by a change in color to blue caused by the reduction of the ferric to ferrous ion.

Extreme pH can be a catalysis of drug degradation. Drug reaction rates are generally less at intermediate pH values than at high or low ranges. A buffer system is often used to ensure the maintenance of the proper pH.

Effects of temperature may be evident. Usually, but not always, an elevation in temperature may increase reaction rates.

An increase in drug concentration will usually increase the degradation rate exponentially. However, this rule does not always apply. Some drugs appear to have a lower rate of decomposition at a high concentration, such as the reduced hydrolysis of nafcillin in the presence of aminophylline. Greater buffer concentration at higher nafcillin concentrations protects the drug from aminophylline's high pH and slows the hydrolysis.

Expiration dates and removal of the IV bag overwrap are important. The overwrap protects against evaporation of the solution, desiccation of the container, drug oxidation, and photochemical inactivation of the drug. Substantial moisture loss may occur, increasing drug concentration. With ready-to-use dopamine or dobutamine injections, removal of the overwrap can allow oxygen to enter the container, thereby reducing drug stability. After removal of the overwrap, the expiration date should be changed at once.

5-12. Sterile Products Compounded from Nonsterile Drugs

When a sterile preparation is compounded from a nonsterile component, several concerns arise: how to sterilize the drug, how to sterilize the container and closure, and how to ensure that the drug and components are sterile. Every sterilization process must be verified, whether it is terminal sterilization of the CSP in the final container or aseptic processing of the CSP. Sterility testing must be done on all high-risk compounded sterile preparations if they are prepared in groups of more than 25 single-dose packages or in multidose vials for administration to multiple patients. Such testing must also be done if prior to sterilization the preparations are exposed longer than 12 hours to temperatures of 2–8°C or longer than 6 hours to temperatures warmer than 8°C. If the high-risk CSPs are dispensed before the results of the sterility test are known, a method must be in place requiring daily observation of the test specimens and immediate recall of the CSP if there is evidence of microbial growth in the test sample.

Sterility Testing

There are two methods of sterility testing: *direct inoculation* and *membrane filtration*. The USP states that, when possible, membrane filtration should be performed and that two culture media are required: fluid thioglycollate medium (FTM) and TSB, which is also known as soybean-casein digest medium.

Media suitability test

Before beginning the test, one must confirm that the medium being used is sterile and will support the growth of microorganisms.

Sterility
Confirm the sterility of each sterilized batch of medium by (1) incubating a portion of the batch at the specified incubation temperature (TSB, 20–25°C; FTM, 30–35°C) for 14 days or (2) incubating uninoculated containers as negative controls during a sterility test procedure. When purchasing a new batch of sterile media from a vendor, incubate a portion for several days to ensure that it did not become contaminated during shipment.

Growth promotion test
Each lot of ready-prepared medium and each batch of dehydrated medium bearing the manufacturer's lot number must be tested for its growth-promoting qualities. Separately inoculate, in duplicate, containers of each medium with fewer than 100 viable microorganisms of each of the strains listed in the next paragraph. If visual evidence of growth appears in all inoculated media containers within 3 days of incubation in the case of bacteria and 5 days of incubation in the case of fungi, the test media is satisfactory. The test may be conducted simultaneously with testing of the media for sterility.

The organisms to be used for the growth promotion test of FTM are *Staphylococcus aureus* (*Bacillus subtilis* may be used instead), *Pseudomonas aeruginosa* (*Micrococcus luteus* may be used instead), and *Clostridium sporogenes* (*Bacteroides vulgatus* may be used instead). The test organisms for soybean-casein digest media are *B. subtilis*, *Candida albicans*, and *Aspergillus brasiliensis* (*A. niger*). Soybean-casein digest media are incubated at 20–25°C, and FTM are incubated at 30–35°C, both under aerobic conditions for a minimum of 14 days.

Validation test: Bacteriostasis and fungistasis test
The bacteriostasis and fungistasis test must be done on each product to determine if the product itself

will inhibit the growth of microorganisms. This test needs to be done only once for each product tested. The organisms used are the same as those used for growth promotion. The test uses two sets of containers. One set is inoculated with the drug product and microorganisms, and the other set is inoculated with just the microorganisms. Both sets will be incubated at the appropriate temperature for no more than 5 days. The same amount of growth should be seen in both sets. If the drug is inhibiting the growth of the microorganisms, the conditions of the test must be modified so the drug will not inhibit growth. The modifications made will now become the method for performing the sterility test on the drug preparation.

Number of articles to test

The minimum number of articles to be tested in relation to the number of articles in the batch is as follows:

- For up to 100 articles, test 10% or 4 articles, whichever is greater.
- For more than 100 but not more than 500 articles, test 10 articles.

Interpretation of results

No growth

At days 3, 5, 7, 10, and 14, examine the media visually for growth. If no microbial growth is seen, the article complies with the test for sterility. Lack of growth of the media does not prove that all units in the lot are sterile.

Observed growth

When microbial growth is observed and confirmed microscopically, the article does not meet the requirements of the test for sterility. If there is no doubt that the microbial growth can be ascribed to faulty aseptic techniques or materials used in conducting the testing procedure, the test is invalid and must be repeated.

An investigation must occur, and the organism must be identified down to the species. All records must be reviewed, including all employee training procedures and records, aseptic gowning practices, equipment maintenance records, component sterilization data, and environmental monitoring data.

Visual inspection

Every unit compounded in the pharmacy should be subjected to a physical inspection against a white background and a black background. Any container whose contents show evidence of contamination with visible foreign material must be rejected.

Pyrogens

A pyrogen is a substance that produces fever. An endotoxin is a type of pyrogen.

Gram-negative bacteria produce more potent endotoxins than do Gram-positive bacteria and fungi. The lipopolysaccharide (LPS) portion of the cell wall causes the pyrogenic response. The LPS can be sloughed off, and the bacteria do not have to be living for the LPS to be pyrogenic.

Some of the effects caused by pyrogens in the body are an increase in body temperature, chills, cutaneous vasoconstriction, a decrease in respiration, an increase in arterial blood pressure, nausea and malaise, and severe diarrhea.

The official endotoxin limits are 5 endotoxin units (EU)/kg per hour or 350 EU/total body per hour for drugs and biologicals. Drugs for intrathecal use have a much lower endotoxin limit of 0.2 EU/kg.

Water is the primary source of endotoxins because *Pseudomonas,* a Gram-negative bacterium, grows readily in water. Other sources of endotoxins or pyrogens are raw material, equipment, processing, and human contamination. It is very important to use good-quality raw materials and request a certificate of analysis with each lot of material when compounding. Endotoxins can be destroyed by dry heat. Three to five hours at 200°C will depyrogenate glass vials and beakers. The endotoxin concentration can be reduced by rinsing with sterile water for injection. When a sterile preparation is compounded from a nonsterile product, any equipment that can withstand the heat of 200°C should be depyrogenated. An article that is depyrogenated is also sterile. Endotoxins are not completely removed by filtration, and steam sterilization reduces endotoxin levels by only a small amount.

Pyrogen test (rabbit test)

The pyrogen test is designed to limit, to an acceptable level, the patient's risk of febrile reaction in the administration—by injection—of the product concerned. The test involves measuring the rise in temperature of rabbits following the IV injection of a test solution, and it is designed for products that can be tolerated by the test rabbit in a dose—not to exceed 10 mL/kg—injected intravenously within a period of no more than 10 minutes.

The rabbit test has several limitations. It is an in vivo method, it is an expensive and time-consuming test, and it is not a very sensitive test. Drugs that have pyretic side effects or that are antipyretics cannot be tested using the rabbit test. The test is not quantitative, and the pyrogenic response is dose dependent, not concentration dependent.

Bacterial endotoxin test (limulus amebocyte lysate test)

The bacterial endotoxin test (BET) provides a method for estimating the concentration of bacterial endotoxins that may be present in, or on the sample of, the article to which the test is applied using limulus amebocyte lysate (LAL) reagent. Because the blood cells of the horseshoe crab are sensitive to endotoxin and form a gel in its presence, LAL reagent is made from the lysate of amebocytes from the horseshoe crab.

There are two types of techniques for this test: the *gel-clot technique,* which is based on the formation of the gel, and the *photometric technique,* which is based on either the development of turbidity or the development of color in the test sample.

The routine gel-clot test requires 0.1 mL of test sample to be mixed with 0.1 mL of LAL reagent. This mixture is incubated for 1 hour at 37°C. A positive reaction is confirmed by formation of a firm gel that remains intact when the tube is slowly inverted 180 degrees.

The BET is 5–50 times more sensitive, more simple and rapid, and less expensive than the pyrogen test. However, the clotting enzyme is heat sensitive, pH sensitive, and chemically related to trypsin. It is dependable for detection of only pyrogens originating from Gram-negative bacteria. Also, some drugs can inhibit the reaction, and other drugs can enhance the reaction. The BET does not determine the fever-producing potential of the bacterial endotoxins.

The photometric technique requires the establishment of a standard regression curve. The endotoxin content of the test material is determined by interpolation from the curve. The test can be either an endpoint determination, in which the reading is made immediately at the end of the incubation period, or a kinetic test, in which the absorbance is measured throughout the reaction period.

All high-risk CSPs (except those for inhalation and ophthalmic use) that are prepared in groups of 25 or more individual single-dose units or in multi-dose vials for administration to multiple patients, or that are exposed longer than 12 hours to temperatures of 2–8°C and longer than 6 hours to temperatures warmer than 8°C before sterilization, must comply with the BET.

5-13. Questions

1. Which of the following tests does *not* have to be completed on a high-risk compounded sterile preparation that will be administered by intravascular injection and is prepared in a lot size of 30 single-dose vials before release to a patient?

    A. Bacterial endotoxin test
    B. Visual inspection
    C. Sterility test
    D. Verification of the sterilizing filter integrity
    E. LAL test

2. Which of the following is correct concerning certification of a laminar flow workbench?

    A. The particles introduced into the plenum of the hood must be approximately 0.5 micron.
    B. Airflow from the HEPA filter must be 120 ft/min.
    C. A leak greater than 0.01% of the upstream smoke concentration through the filter is considered a serious leak.
    D. A total particle counter can be used to check the integrity of the HEPA filter.
    E. If a HEPA filter leaks, it cannot be patched; it must be replaced.

3. The bacterial endotoxin test is used to determine

    A. the amount of pyrogens.
    B. the level of pyrogens from Gram-negative bacteria.
    C. the fever-producing potential of bacterial endotoxins from Gram-negative bacteria.
    D. the level of bacterial endotoxin from Gram-positive bacteria.
    E. the amount of live bacteria present in the drug solution.

4. Which of the following is correct concerning USP media transfers?

    A. An operator must successfully complete one media fill before compounding any CSPs.
    B. An operator who passes a written exam may compound sterile preparations until the chief pharmacist finds time to watch his or her aseptic technique.

C. An operator who has successfully completed a media fill must requalify semiannually if he or she is preparing low-risk CSPs.
D. When an operator successfully completes one media fill for high-risk compounding, he or she needs to revalidate quarterly by completing one media fill.
E. Fluid thioglycollate media are used for media transfers.

5. For a transfer of product into the controlled area,

   A. bottles, bags, and syringes must be removed from brown cardboard boxes before being brought into the buffer area.
   B. vials stored in laminated cardboard may not be brought into the controlled area.
   C. stainless steel carts may be used to transfer items into the controlled area directly from the storage area.
   D. large-volume parenteral bags of IV solution must be removed from their protective overwrap before being brought into the controlled area.
   E. the refrigerator should be placed next to the laminar flow hood for easy access.

6. Which of the following is correct concerning a vertical laminar flow hood?

   A. It is always a biological safety cabinet.
   B. In vertical laminar flow, the hands of the operator must not be behind an object.
   C. A vertical laminar flow hood has turbulent airflow within 1 inch of the work surface.
   D. A vertical laminar flow hood has the laminar airflow blowing at the operator.
   E. The operator works in a vertical flow hood and a horizontal flow hood in the same manner.

7. Certain factors may increase the risk of microbial contamination of a CSP. Which of the following would *not* be a risk factor?

   A. Very complex compounding steps
   B. Lengthy exposure of a critical site during compounding
   C. Use of appropriate aseptic technique
   D. Batch compounding without preservatives for multiple patients
   E. Preparation of a CSP from nonsterile powders

8. Which of the following is correct concerning the USP risk levels of compounded sterile preparations?

   A. Preparations intended for administration over 3 days would be classified as low risk.
   B. A high-risk sterile preparation that has met the requirements of the sterility test can be stored for not more than 24 hours at a controlled room temperature.
   C. The storage time for a medium-risk preparation under refrigeration is no longer than 9 days.
   D. A CSP that will be administered to multiple patients or to a single patient multiple times is classified as a high-risk CSP.
   E. After meeting the requirements of the sterility test, a sterile preparation can be stored indefinitely.

9. Which of the following is correct?

   A. For work done in a horizontal laminar flow workbench, arrange items in the hood so that your hand is never between the HEPA filter and an object.
   B. For work done in a horizontal laminar flow workbench, vials that are not being used should be stacked up along the side of the hood to increase workspace in the hood.
   C. Before each shift, 70% isopropyl alcohol is used to sterilize the laminar flow workbench.
   D. An object placed in the horizontal laminar flow workbench disturbs the airflow downstream of the object equal to two times the diameter of the object.
   E. Syringes and IV bags are placed in the hood in their protective overwrap.

10. Which of the following is correct concerning the necessity that operators in the buffer area be properly gowned?

   A. Operators don gowns because they shed particles, and the nonshedding gowns keep them sterile.
   B. Sterile gloves are used to avoid contamination of the CSP in case the operator accidentally touches a critical site during compounding of the preparation.
   C. Frequent sanitization with sterile 70% isopropyl alcohol is essential to keep the operators' hands sterile during the compounding process.
   D. Nonshedding garb and sterile gloves help contain the particles shed from the operators.

E. Operators must don gowns before working at the laminar flow workbench but not before entering the buffer area.

11. Which of the following is correct concerning placement of items and work performed in the laminar flow workstation?

A. Items should be placed in a horizontal flow hood to the right or left of the work area.
B. Items in a vertical laminar flow hood should be placed so that an operator's hand never goes over the top of a critical site while the operator is working in the hood.
C. An object placed in a horizontal laminar flow hood disturbs the airflow downstream of the object equal to three times the diameter of the object.
D. When working in a horizontal laminar flow workstation, an operator must perform all work at least 6 inches inside the hood.
E. All of the above are correct.

12. Which parts of the syringe are considered critical sites?

A. Ribs only
B. Collar only
C. Ribs and tip only
D. Collar and tip only
E. Ribs, collar, and tip

13. Which parts of the needle are considered critical sites?

A. The hub only
B. The needle shaft only
C. The hub and the bevel and bevel tip only
D. The needle shaft and the bevel and bevel tip only
E. The hub, the needle shaft, and the bevel and bevel tip

14. Which of the following are correct concerning ampuls?

A. Ampuls can be left in the hood and used for several days once opened.
B. Ampuls are single-dose containers and can be left in the hood and used for several days once opened.
C. Ampuls are single-dose containers and must have the neck wiped with a sterile alcohol pad before being broken
D. None of the above

15. Which of the following is correct?

A. Filter integrity testing of the filter membrane is done to determine at what pressure the filter will break.
B. The manufacturer of the filter membrane determines the bubble point of the membrane; this value is always the same, no matter what solution has been filtered.
C. As the pore size of the filter membrane decreases, the pressure at which the air can be pushed from the largest pore increases.
D. The bubble point test is a destructive test.
E. It is not necessary to perform the bubble point test if a certificate of quality from the filter manufacturer is provided.

16. Which of the following factors should be considered when choosing a sterilizing filter?

A. The volume of solution to be filtered
B. The compatibility of the membrane with the solution to be filtered
C. Whether the solution to be filtered is hydrophobic or hydrophilic
D. The compatibility of the filter housing with the product to be filtered
E. All of the above

17. Which of the following is correct concerning the USP sterility test?

A. The validation test must be done on each CSP to determine if the article to be tested adversely affects the reliability of the test.
B. The growth promotion test does not require that the test organisms listed in the USP be used.
C. After inoculation, the media must be incubated for 14 days or fewer at the appropriate temperature.
D. No growth on the sterility test proves that the aseptically produced product is sterile.
E. Trypticase soy broth is incubated at 30–35°C, and fluid thioglycollate is incubated at 20–25°C.

18. Which of the following is correct?

A. Gram-negative bacteria must be alive to cause a pyrogenic response.

B. The lipopolysaccharide portion of the cell wall of Gram-negative bacteria causes the pyrogenic response.

C. Endotoxin can be removed by a 0.2 micron filter.

D. Steam sterilization will depyrogenate an object just as well as the hot air oven.

E. An article that is depyrogenated is not necessarily sterile.

19. Which of the following is correct?

   A. The rabbit test and the LAL test are the same test.

   B. LAL reagent will determine the fever-producing potential of the pyrogens.

   C. There are two types of techniques for the BET: the gel-clot technique and the photometric technique.

   D. The CSP being tested has no effect on the test.

   E. All CSPs may be tested using the rabbit test.

20. Which of the following is correct?

   A. The rabbit test is the most sensitive because it can detect pyrogens from all sources.

   B. The rabbit test is an in vitro test.

   C. Some drugs may inhibit the formation of a gel in the BET.

   D. No drug will enhance the formation of the gel in the BET.

   E. The pyrogen test is a quantitative test.

21. The plenum in a laminar flow workbench is the area

   A. where the air is prefiltered.

   B. where air is pressurized for distribution over the HEPA filter.

   C. where compounding takes place.

   D. that serves no purpose.

   E. directly above the HEPA filter in a horizontal laminar flow hood.

22. Calcium and phosphate can interact to form a precipitate in parenteral nutrition solutions. Of the following situations, which would *not* enhance calcium and phosphate precipitate formation?

   A. High concentration of calcium and phosphate

   B. Increase in solution pH

   C. Decrease in temperature

   D. Use of the chloride salt of calcium

   E. A slow infusion rate

23. Which of the following is *not* a potential source of physical or chemical incompatibility?

   A. Dilution of a drug in a cosolvent system into an aqueous system

   B. Addition of a drug solution with a high pH into a solution with a low pH

   C. Adsorption of a lipid-soluble drug into the matrix of a polypropylene container

   D. A photosensitive drug such as sodium nitroprusside in 5% dextrose in water exposed to light

   E. Leaching of phthalate plasticizer into the solution from a polyvinyl chloride container

5-14. Answers

1. **C.** The bacterial endotoxin test (LAL test), visual inspection test, and bubble point test should all be completed before the CSP is dispensed. Because the sterility test takes 14 days, the preparation may be dispensed before the results are known. However, a system to recall the CSP must be in place if it does not meet the test's requirement.

2. **C.** Any leak greater than 0.01% of upstream smoke concentration is a serious leak. The smoke particles are 0.3 micron. The airflow from the HEPA filter should be 90 ft/min, plus or minus 20%. A total particle counter is used to classify the environment, not to certify the integrity of the HEPA filter. The HEPA filter can be patched.

3. **B.** The BET determines the level of bacterial endotoxin from Gram-negative bacteria only. The BET cannot determine fever-producing potential of the endotoxins. The Gram-negative bacteria do not have to be alive for the endotoxin to produce an effect.

4. **A.** The operator must successfully complete one media fill before compounding a sterile preparation. Once validated for low- or medium-risk compounding, the operator must revalidate annually. For high-risk compounding, the operator must revalidate semiannually. Passing only a written exam does not allow the operator to

compound a CSP. Trypticase soy broth is the medium most often used in media fills.

5.   **A.** Cardboard must be kept out of the buffer area. Vials stored in laminated cardboard may be stored in the buffer area. No items should be brought into the buffer area without being sanitized. Large-volume parenteral bags should be removed from their overwrap just before being used. The refrigerator should not be in the buffer room because it is a source of contamination.

6.   **C.** There are several types of vertical laminar flow hoods, of which the biological safety cabinet is one. The operator must never work over the top of items in the hood, and all work should be done at least 1 inch above the work surface.

7.   **C.** Use of good aseptic technique is one way to ensure a good preparation.

8.   **C.** A medium-risk CSP may not be stored longer than 9 days at cold temperature. USP <797> does not address administration at all; it applies only up to the time of administration. Once a CSP has met the requirement of the sterility test, the storage periods specified under the risk levels no longer apply. However, the beyond-use date based on chemical stability always applies. A CSP that will be administered to multiple patients or to a single patient multiple times is a medium-risk CSP.

9.   **A.** In an HLFW, never put your hand behind an object, and in a VLFW, never put your hand above an object. In an HLFW, a vial disturbs the laminar airflow equal to three times the diameter of the object. If the vial is next to the side wall, the airflow is disturbed equal to six times the diameter of the object. Syringes and IV bags should be taken from their overwrap at the edge of the hood.

10.   **D.** Operators in the buffer area should wear clean, nonshedding gowns and gloves to help contain the particles that they shed. The sterile gloves are no longer sterile once they are out of the package. Proper aseptic technique must always be used.

11.   **E.** All of the statements are correct concerning placement of items and work performed in the laminar flow workstation.

12.   **C.** The ribs of the plunger and the tip of the syringe are critical sites of the syringe.

13.   **E.** The hub, the needle shaft, and the bevel and bevel tip of the needle are all critical sites.

14.   **C.** Once an ampul is opened, it must be used immediately.

15.   **C.** The bubble point test is not a destructive test, and the value depends on the solution being filtered. When a CSP is filter sterilized, the bubble point test must be done before the preparation may be dispensed.

16.   **E.** All of the factors should be considered.

17.   **A.** The validation (bacteriostasis and fungistasis test) must be completed one time for each CSP. The growth promotion organisms listed in the USP are used for the validation test and for the growth promotion test.

18.   **B.** Endotoxin will pass through a 0.2 micron filter. Steam sterilization will not depyrogenate an article. Bacteria do not have to be alive to be pyrogenic.

19.   **C.** The pyrogen test, also known as the rabbit test, determines the fever-producing potential of the pyrogens. The BET is also known as the LAL test. The drug product can inhibit or enhance the gel formation in the BET.

20.   **C.** The pyrogen (rabbit) test is an in vivo test and is not as sensitive as the BET. It is not a quantitative test.

21.   **B.** The plenum is the area behind the HEPA filter in an HLFW that allows air to be pressurized for even distribution over the filter.

22.   **C.** An increase in temperature could enhance precipitate formation.

23.   **C.** Absorption of a lipid-soluble drug into the matrix of polyvinylchloride containers does occur. Polypropylene and polyethylene contain little or no phthalate plasticizer.

5-15. References

Akers MJ, Larrimore D, Guazzo D. *Parenteral Quality Control: Sterility, Pyrogen, Particulate and Package Integrity Testing*. 3rd ed. New York, NY: Marcel Dekker; 2003.

American Society of Health-System Pharmacists. ASHP guidelines on compounding sterile preparations. *Am J Health-Syst Pharm* 2014;71(2):145–66

American Society of Health-System Pharmacists. ASHP guidelines on handling hazardous drugs. *Am J Health-Syst Pharm*. 2006;63:1172–93.

Buchanan C, McKinnon B, Scheckelhoff D, Schneider P. *Principles of Sterile Product Preparation.* Bethesda, MD: American Society of Health-System Pharmacists; 2002:50.

General Services Administration. Federal standard 209e: Clean room and work station requirements, controlled environments. Washington, DC: U.S. Government Printing Office; 1992.

McKinnon B, Avis K. Membrane filtration of pharmaceutical solutions. *Am J Hosp Pharm.* 1993;50:1021–36.

Trissel LA. *Handbook on Injectable Drugs.* 15th ed. Bethesda, MD: American Society of Health-System Pharmacists; 2009.

United States Pharmacopeial Convention. Bacterial endotoxin test. In: *United States Pharmacopeia 37/National Formulary 32.* Rockville, MD: United States Pharmacopeial Convention; 2014:92–96.

United States Pharmacopeial Convention. Pharmaceutical compounding: Sterile preparations. In: *United States Pharmacopeia 37/National Formulary 32.* Rockville, MD: United States Pharmacopeial Convention; 2014:410–53.

United States Pharmacopeial Convention. Pyrogen test. In: *United States Pharmacopeia 37/National Formulary 32.* Rockville, MD: United States Pharmacopeial Convention; 2014:135–37.

United States Pharmacopeial Convention. Sterility tests. In: *United States Pharmacopeia 37/National Formulary 32.* Rockville, MD: United States Pharmacopeial Convention; 2014:71–77.

Nuclear Pharmacy

6

Vivian S. Loveless
Fred P. Gattas

6-1. Key Points

- Radiopharmaceuticals are mainly used for diagnostic purposes, but can also be used for palliative and therapeutic indications.
- Technetium Tc-99m is eluted from a molybdenum Mo-99/Tc-99m generator at the pharmacy and can be used as a compounded ingredient or directly injected as a radiopharmaceutical.
- Cardiac imaging is performed to help visualize perfusion, calculate the ejection fraction and ventricular wall motion, and help diagnose myocardial infarction.
- Cerebral imaging is performed to help detect perfusion in stroke patients, diagnose brain death, and help identify Parkinsonian syndrome. It can also be used to visualize cerebral spinal flow patterns and help diagnose cognitive impairment by estimating the density of beta-amyloid neuritic plaque.
- Radiolabeled white blood cells or gallium citrate Ga-67 may be intravenously injected to help detect sites of infection.
- Radiopharmaceuticals are used to help identify tumors that are metabolically active or have a high density of somatostatin receptors. They can identify prostate cancer cells and image pheochromocytomas or neuroblastomas.
- Radiopharmaceuticals can also help remove residual tumor tissue in the brain and are also used therapeutically to treat non-Hodgkin lymphoma.
- Pulmonary imaging is performed for two purposes: ventilation and perfusion.
- Tc-99m albumin aggregated (Tc-99m MAA) is the radiopharmaceutical for pulmonary perfusion studies.
- Xenon (Xe)-133 gas and Tc-99m pentetate (Tc-99m DTPA) aerosol can be used for ventilation studies.
- Renal scintigraphy can be divided into the following categories: perfusion imaging, function studies, evaluation for renal artery stenosis, and cortical imaging.
- The three radiopharmaceuticals used in renal studies are Tc-99m DTPA, Tc-99m mertiatide (Tc-99m MAG3), and Tc-99m succimer (DMSA).
- Nonradioactive interventional pharmaceuticals can be used to enhance the diagnostic accuracy of these studies.
- Tc-99m sulfur colloid is indicated for reticuloendothelial system (RES) scintigraphy.
- Tc-99m disofenin or Tc-99m mebrofenin are both indicated for hepatobiliary imaging, and nonradioactive interventional agents can be used with these radiopharmaceuticals.
- Gastric emptying and motility studies can be performed with Tc-99m sulfur colloid incorporated into various foods.
- Gastroesophageal reflux studies can be performed with Tc-99m sulfur colloid or In-111 pentetate (In-111 DTPA) compounded into liquids.
- Diagnostic skeletal imaging studies can be performed with either a Tc-99m-labeled diphosphonate compound or F-18 sodium fluoride.
- Palliative therapeutic radiopharmaceuticals for the treatment of bone pain from metastatic lesions include strontium-89 chloride and samarium Sm-153 lexidronam (Sm-153 EDTMP).

- Tc-99m sodium pertechnetate, I-123 sodium iodide, or I-131 sodium iodide can be used for diagnostic studies of the thyroid gland.
- I-123 sodium iodide and I-131 sodium iodide are used in whole body imaging for the detection of metastatic sites from thyroid cancer.
- I-131 sodium iodide can be used as a therapeutic radiopharmaceutical for the treatment of hyperthyroidism or the ablation of metastatic sites originating from thyroid carcinoma.

6-2. Study Guide Checklist

The following topics may guide your study of this subject area:

- The difference between diagnostic and therapeutic medications
- Mechanism of action for the medications
- Knowledge of which radiopharmaceuticals are compounded and which are procured from manufacturers
- Food, drug, and disease state interactions that can alter study results

- When performing a pair of nuclear imaging studies, which one should be performed first
- Specific dosing for pediatric patients

6-3. Introduction

Nuclear pharmacy is the practice of using radionuclides as a component of a diagnostic, palliative, or therapeutic drug. The difference largely involves the decay scheme of the radioactive nuclides. Radionuclides decay by different schemes, and each emission involves a signature energy measured in electron volts (eV). Radionuclides can decay and emit gamma and x-ray photons that can be used for imaging. Some radionuclides emit alpha or beta particles that have mass and cause cellular damage, and some have both gamma and alpha or gamma and beta emission. Some radionuclides emit positrons that are useful in imaging, such as in positron emission tomography (PET) (see Table 6-1).

All radionuclides have a physical half-life that follows first-order kinetics: $A_1 = A_0e^{-\lambda t}$, where A_1 = activity after a certain time in the future, A_0 = initial activity, $\lambda = 0.693$/half-life time, and t = time of decay.

Table 6-1. Properties of Radionuclides

Radionuclide	Primary production	Physical half-life	Emission type	Primary energy (MeV)
F-18	Cyclotron	110 minutes	Positron	2 × 0.511 gamma
Ga-67	Cyclotron	77.9 hours	Gamma	0.093
I-123	Cyclotron	13.22 hours	Gamma	0.159
I-131	Reactor	8.02 days	Gamma	0.364
			Beta	0.191
In-111	Cyclotron	2.8 days	Gamma	0.173 and 0.247
Ra-223	Generator	11.4 days	Alpha	5–7.5
Rb-82	Generator	76 seconds	Positron	2 × 0.511 gamma
Sm-153	Cyclotron	46.5 hours	Gamma	0.103
			Beta	0.704
Strontium-89	Reactor	50.53 days	Beta	0.585
Tc-99m	Generator	6.02 hours	Gamma	0.14
Tl-201	Cyclotron	73 hours	Gamma, x-rays	0.08
Xe-133	Reactor	5.3 days	Gamma	0.081
Y-90	Reactor	2.7 days	Beta	0.934

Note that both times must be expressed in the same units. Activities of radiation for administration in the United States are expressed in curie (Ci) units.

Some radionuclides and the ligands to which they are sometimes tagged are produced by a commercial manufacturer in a cyclotron (i.e., thallous chloride Tl-201 and indium In-111 oxine). Some radionuclides are produced by a commercial manufacturer in a nuclear reactor (i.e., I-131). Some radionuclides are produced by a commercially available generator on site (i.e., technetium Tc-99m and rubidium Rb-82).

Commercially available nonradioactive ligands (kits) approved by the U.S. Food and Drug Administration (FDA) are available for inventory storage from various manufacturers, and the compounder can label the ligands with a radionuclide. The radionuclide allows detection or the therapy of the localization site of the radioactive ligand complex. Most labeling uses Tc-99m, In-111, fluorine F-18, or yttrium Y-90 as the radionuclide, with Tc-99m being in the vast majority. Most ligand kits require stannous chloride to reduce the Tc-99m from the +7 valence state to a lower one for radiolabeling. Radiochemical purity tests must be performed for all radiolabeled kits to ensure purity is within United States Pharmacopeia (USP) specifications.

F-18, In-111, and Y-90 are supplied from FDA-approved manufacturers. Tc-99m is supplied from eluting a molybdenum Mo-99/Tc-99m generator. The generator expires 2 weeks postcalibration and is available in a variety of activities.

Tc-99m Sodium Pertechnetate (Na^{99m}TcO$_4$)

Radiopharmaceutical Na^{99m}TcO$_4$ is produced from a Mo-99/Tc-99m generator. The generator has Mo-99 in various activities loaded onto an alumina column by the manufacturer. Tc-99m is produced via Mo-99 decay. When the generator is received, a 0.9% saline charge is placed on one port of the generator, and a shielded, sterile, evacuated vial is placed on the other port; the tubing is connected through the Mo-99 column. The evacuated vial pulls the normal saline through the column, the pertechnetate ion is displaced from the column by the chloride (Cl$^-$) ion, and the evacuated vial fills with Na^{99m}TcO$_4$ solution that is isotonic in nature. That solution is used either to label a variety of different ligands or to be directly injected as a radiopharmaceutical. Radiochemical purity, chemical purity, and radionuclidic purity tests should be performed to ensure the product is within USP specifications (see Table 6-2).

Table 6-2. Tc-99m Pertechnetate USP Purity Specifications

Purity	Specification
Radiochemical purity	95%
Radionuclidic purity	0.15 μCi of Mo-99/1 mCi of Tc-99m at administration
Chemical purity	10 mcg of Al/mL

USP, United States Pharmacopeia.

6-4. Cardiac Imaging

Cardiac imaging can be performed with planar imaging, single photon emission computed tomography (SPECT), or PET. These cardiac studies provide information on perfusion, function, viability, and metabolic activity. A variety of radiopharmaceuticals are used, and these studies may be performed at rest or during stress. Stress studies can be performed through exercise, pharmacologic intervention, or both.

Pharmacologic stress agents include the following:

- Dipyridamole
- Adenosine (Adenoscan)
- Regadenoson (Lexiscan)
- Dobutamine

Thallous Chloride Tl-201

Thallous chloride Tl-201 is a monovalent cation and an analog of potassium that accumulates in viable myocardium through the Na$^+$/K$^+$ ATPase pump. It is useful in the diagnosis of coronary artery disease for assessing myocardial perfusion. By performing rest and stress studies, diagnosticians can distinguish reversible ischemia from irreversible ischemia or infarct. The intravenous (IV) radiopharmaceutical dosage ranges from 2 to 4 mCi. Tl-201 must be administered before a Tc-99m heart agent if performing dual isotope imaging.

Fludeoxyglucose F-18 (F-18 FDG)

F-18 is a positron emitter, and F-18 FDG is a metabolic indicator of glucose uptake in cells. Both glucose and F-18 FDG undergo active transport into cells by using glucose transporters, but F-18 FDG becomes trapped inside the cell once it is phosphorylated. Because this agent demonstrates metabolic activity, it is useful in determining viability of the myocardial tissue. It is used in combination with a myocardial perfusion radiopharmaceutical study to determine whether a patient will benefit from revascularization of coronary arteries. The IV dosage ranges from 5 to 15 mCi. Because F-18 is a cyclotron product with a 110-minute physical half-life, proximity to the site of production can be a limitation in acquiring this radiopharmaceutical.

Tc-99m Sestamibi (Tc-99m MIBI, Cardiolite)

Tc-99m sestamibi is a monovalent cationic complex, but unlike Tl-201, it is not a potassium analog. It is a lipophilic complex that undergoes passive diffusion into the myocardium and becomes attached to myocyte mitochondria. It is thought to be an indicator of both viability and perfusion. It is indicated for the identification of reversible myocardial ischemia and infarction and for the assessment of myocardial function. The recommended IV dosage range for this agent is 10 to 30 mCi, and a separate injection is required for both the rest and the stress studies.

Tc-99m Tetrofosmin (Myoview)

This radiotracer is a lipophilic, monovalent cationic complex that does not involve the Na$^+$/K$^+$ ATPase pump for localization into the myocardium. It provides information on both myocardial perfusion and left ventricular function. Tc-99m tetrofosmin scintigraphic imaging is performed both at rest and under stress, and this procedure identifies regions of reversible myocardial ischemia whether or not myocardial infarct is present. The recommended IV dosage range for this tracer is 5 to 33 mCi, and a separate injection is required for both the rest and the stress studies.

Rb-82 Chloride

Rb-82 chloride is a PET radiopharmaceutical produced in a commercially available strontium (Sr)-82/Rb-82 generator. Sr-82 is the parent radionuclide, and it decays to Rb-82. The generator is eluted with normal saline, and the Rb-82 chloride is administered directly to the patient from the generator via an IV infusion system. Rb-82 is a potassium analog, and it is transported inside the myocyte by the Na$^+$/K$^+$ ATPase pump; thus, uptake is greater in viable myocardium, whereas there is an absence of radioactivity in nonviable tissue. This radiopharmaceutical in combination with PET is used for the assessment of regional myocardial perfusion in patients known to have or suspected of having coronary artery disease,

and it can be used in rest or with pharmacologic stress studies. Two separate doses are required for rest and stress myocardial perfusion imaging, and 30–60 mCi is the range for a single dose of Rb-82 chloride.

UltraTag RBC (Tc-99m-Labeled Red Blood Cells)

Whole blood in 1–3 mL amounts is added to the reaction vial containing stannous ion. The stannous ion is distributed into the red blood cells via passive diffusion, and other components are added to inactivate extracellular tin. Then, 10–100 mCi of Tc-99m Na^{99m}TcO$_4$ is added. Once the Tc-99m enters the red blood cells, it is reduced by the tin and prevented from diffusing out of the cell. Labeling yields average about 95%. Then, 10–20 mCi of whole blood containing the radioactive red blood cells is reinjected back into the patient to visualize blood pool imaging, including cardiac first pass and gated equilibrium imaging. Evaluation of ventricular function is performed by having the patient attached to an electrocardiogram (ECG) synchronizer and timing the camera images to the R wave. Determination of left ventricle ejection function of the heart in addition to the wall motion during contraction can be accomplished with this study.

Tc-99m Pyrophosphate (Tc-99m PYP)

In addition to labeling the red blood cells in vitro, in vivo radiolabeling can be performed with Tc-99m PYP. A PYP vial is reconstituted with normal saline, and 15 mcg of stannous per kilogram of body weight is injected into the patient. After 15–30 minutes, the Tc-99m is injected and the red blood cell–labeling occurs. Labeling yields range from 60% to 80%.

A modified in vivo method can also be performed to increase labeling efficiency to approximately 90% by pulling 3–5 mL of the "tinned" blood into a syringe and adding Tc-99m Na^{99m}TcO$_4$ via a three-way stop cock.

Myocardial Infarct Imaging with Tc-99m PYP

To help diagnose a myocardial infarction, one can inject 24–48 hours postinfarct, 20 mCi of Tc-99m PYP into a patient. After cell death from a myocardial infarction, calcium is released from the cardiac mitochondria with the resulting calcium phosphate complexes allowing Tc-99m PYP binding. Note that at least minimal blood flow to the affected necrotic tissue is necessary to deliver the drug. Imaging can take place from 1 to 4 hours after administration.

6-5. Central Nervous System Imaging

Brain imaging or scintigraphy is performed to assess regional cerebral perfusion in suspected stroke patients, to assist in the clinical diagnosis of brain death, to determine an alteration in the blood–brain barrier (BBB), or to visualize striatal dopamine transporter in adult patients suspected of having Parkinsonian syndromes. Cisternography can be used to evaluate the flow pattern of the cerebrospinal fluid, and PET can be used to image beta-amyloid neuritic plaques in patients exhibiting cognitive impairment.

Cerebral Perfusion in Suspected Stroke Patients

Tc-99m exametazime (Ceretec)

One of the indications for Tc-99m exametazime is for cerebral scintigraphy as an adjunct in the identification of altered regional cerebral perfusion in stroke patients. The active moiety is the lipophilic Tc-99m complex, which is capable of crossing the BBB. The maximum brain uptake is 3.5–7%, and this occurs within 1 minute post-IV administration. The recommended average adult (70 kg) dosage is 10–20 mCi of Tc-99m exametazime. When methylene blue is used as a stabilizer, the preparation will be blue in color. A filter is attached to the syringe, and the preparation is filtered during the injection. When used to differentiate between ischemic and infarct areas, acetazolamide acts as an interventional agent to assess hemodynamic reserve.

Tc-99m bicisate (Neurolite)

This agent is indicated for use with SPECT as an adjunct to magnetic resonance imaging or conventional computed tomography (CT) in determining the site of stroke in patients previously diagnosed with a stroke. Tc-99m bicisate crosses an intact BBB via passive diffusion as a result of its lipophilic characteristic. In normal volunteers, cellular uptake in the brain at 5 minutes was reported to be 4.8–6.5%. The recommended IV radiopharmaceutical dosage for a patient weighing 70 kg is 10–30 mCi.

Clinical Diagnosis of Brain Death

Tc-99m pentetate (Tc-99m DTPA)

Because this chelate cannot cross an intact BBB, it is characterized as a nondiffusible radiopharmaceutical. An off-label use is the assessment of dynamic blood flow in the brain to assist in evaluation of a patient suspected of being brain dead. Brain death correlates with an absence of cerebral perfusion upon IV administration of 15–20 mCi of the radiopharmaceutical.

Tc-99m exametazime (Ceretec)

The use of this tracer to assist in determining brain death is an off-label use. In contrast to Tc-99m DTPA, interpretation of brain death with Tc-99m exametazime relies more on the evaluation of parenchymal brain uptake on delayed imaging; however, dynamic blood flow in the brain can also be identified with this radiopharmaceutical. The presence of radioactivity in the brain with time indicates brain perfusion. The IV dosage of this tracer is 10–30 mCi.

Tc-99m bicisate (Neurolite)

Just as Tc-99m exametazime is a diffusible brain-imaging agent, so is Tc-99m bicisate. An off-label use of this radiopharmaceutical is for assisting in the determination of brain death. Brain imaging with this tracer provides both dynamic blood and parenchymal uptake information. The conservation of brain perfusion is indicated by accumulation of radioactivity in the brain. The IV dosage of this radiopharmaceutical is 10–30 mCi.

Suspected Parkinsonian Syndromes

I-123 ioflupane (DaTscan)

Not only is this a radiopharmaceutical, but it is also a controlled drug (C-II). With SPECT imaging, I-123 ioflupane is used for striatal dopamine transporter visualization to aid in the assessment of adult patients with suspected Parkinsonian syndromes. It is helpful in distinguishing essential tremor from tremor resulting from Parkinsonian syndromes, and this tracer is considered an adjunct to other diagnostic modalities. A thyroid-blocking agent should be administered to the patient at a minimum of 1 hour prior to radiopharmaceutical administration. The IV dosage of I-123 ioflupane is 3–5 mCi.

Cisternography

In-111 pentetate (In-111 DTPA)

In-111 DTPA is the only radiopharmaceutical with FDA approval for cisternography studies. After intrathecal administration, the radiopharmaceutical follows the path of the cerebrospinal fluid and can be used to identify abnormal flow patterns, including cerebrospinal fluid rhinorrhea and otorrhea. In a normal patient, approximately 65% of the administered radiopharmaceutical is excreted via the kidneys within 24 hours. In the average 70 kg patient, the maximum radiopharmaceutical dosage is 0.5 mCi.

PET

Florbetapir F-18 (Amyvid)

Florbetapir F-18 injection received FDA approval in April 2012 for PET brain imaging to estimate the density of beta-amyloid neuritic plaque in patients being evaluated for Alzheimer's disease and other causes of cognitive impairment. PET with florbetapir F-18 is considered an adjunctive diagnostic procedure to other diagnostic modalities, and a positive study with this radiopharmaceutical does not establish a diagnosis of a cognitive disorder. The recommended dosage of this PET radiopharmaceutical is 10 mCi in 10 mL of volume or less.

6-6. Infection and Inflammatory Imaging

Infection and inflammatory-site imaging are performed with either gallium citrate (Ga-67) or autologous radiolabeled leukocytes. The clearance of the radiopharmaceuticals from nontarget areas determines when imaging or scintigraphy commences.

In-111 Oxyquinoline (In-111 oxine)

This diagnostic radiopharmaceutical is used to radiolabel autologous white blood cells as an adjunct in localizing sites of infection. After blood is withdrawn from a patient, the white blood cells are separated and then radiolabeled with In-111 oxine via passive diffusion. The radiolabeled leukocytes are then intravenously administered to the patient. The rationale for this procedure is that leukocytes are attracted to sites of infection and inflammation; thus, radiolabeled leukocytes in combination with scintigraphy can be useful adjuncts in identifying these sites. An adequate number of leukocytes is critical for study sensitivity; thus, patients who are leukopenic are not good candidates. The recommended dosage is 0.2–0.5 mCi of In-111 oxine–labeled autologous leukocytes. The labeled cells should be reinjected into the patient no later than 5 hours after the initial blood harvesting.

Tc-99m Exametazime (Tc-99m Ceretec)

In addition to cerebral imaging, Tc-99m exametazime is indicated for leukocyte-labeled scintigraphy as an adjunct in the localization of intra-abdominal infection and inflammatory bowel disease. White blood cell separation is the same as for In-111 oxine–labeled cells, and the normal dosage is 7–25 mCi. Optimal imaging is 2–4 hours postadministration.

Gallium Citrate (Ga-67)

Gallium citrate is beneficial in aiding in the detection of an infectious site in patients with fever of unknown origin, in assisting with the diagnosis of opportunistic infections, and in identifying some inflammatory sites. Because one cannot distinguish between tumor uptake and inflammatory sites, additional diagnostic procedures must be used to delineate the underlying disease states. The dosage ranges from 2 to 5 mCi.

6-7. Oncology

Both diagnostic and therapeutic radiopharmaceuticals are available for use in oncology. The diagnostic radiopharmaceuticals include traditional tracers, a radiolabeled peptide, a monoclonal antibody, and a PET agent. The therapeutic radiopharmaceutical is a radiolabeled monoclonal antibodies.

Fludeoxyglucose F-18 (F-18 FDG)

Fludeoxyglucose is a glucose analog in which F-18 has replaced a hydroxyl group. After the radiolabeled fludeoxyglucose is transported into a cell by facilitated diffusion, it becomes trapped inside the cell after being phosphorylated. Metabolically active cells take up this PET radiopharmaceutical according to their glucose utilization rate, so the more metabolically active (as in cancer), the greater the degree of uptake. Imaging of various neoplasms is performed with a PET scanner. The dosage range for an adult is 10–20 mCi, and the pediatric dosage range is 0.14–0.2 mCi/kg.

In-111 Pentetreotide (OctreoScan)

This tracer is a pentetate conjugate of octreotide, which is radiolabeled with In-111, and it attaches to somatostatin receptors throughout the body. Tumors having a high density of somatostatin receptors will take up this radiolabeled peptide and be demonstrated with scintigraphy. The FDA has approved this radiopharmaceutical for the scintigraphic localization of primary and metastatic neuroendocrine tumors having somatostatin receptors.

The patient should be well hydrated prior to and after radiopharmaceutical administration; bowel cleansing with a mild laxative is suggested the night before injection of the tracer and continuing for 48 hours. If a patient has an insulinoma, bowel cleansing should be conducted only if the patient's endocrinologist approves. The recommended adult radiopharmaceutical dosage for use in planar imaging is 3 mCi, while the dosage for SPECT imaging is 6 mCi. The sensitivity of the imaging study may be compromised in patients on therapeutic octreotide acetate.

In-111 Capromab Pendetide (ProstaScint)

In-111 capromab pendetide is a diagnostic radiolabeled murine monoclonal antibody that recognizes an antigen present on prostate epithelium. This particular antigen is found on many primary and metastatic prostate cancer cells. In-111 capromab pendetide is indicated for patients having newly diagnosed biopsy-proven prostate cancer who are considered to have localized cancer, as demonstrated by standard diagnostic studies, but are at high risk of pelvic lymphnode metastases. Also, this diagnostic radiopharmaceutical is indicated in postprostatectomy patients who have a rising prostate-specific antigen level, a negative or equivocal standard metastatic evaluation, and a high clinical suspicion of occult metastatic lesions. Clinical trials with this radiotracer reported an 8% incidence of human anti-mouse antibody levels after a single administration, and this should be considered when performing repeat studies or some immunoassays. The recommended dosage is 5 mCi of In-111 radiolabeled to 0.5 mg of capromab pendetide, and the dose should be filtered before administration with a 5 micron filter.

I-123 Iobenguane (I-123 MIBG, AdreView)

I-123 iobenguane is a diagnostic imaging radiopharmaceutical that is used as an adjunct in the identification of primary or metastatic pheochromocytomas or neuroblastomas. Structurally, iobenguane is similar to norepinephrine and guanethidine and follows the same cellular uptake and pathways as norepinephrine. This radiopharmaceutical is subject to interactions with drugs that reduce norepinephrine uptake, and those drugs should be discontinued for a minimum of five biological half-lives if tolerated by the patient. Any norepinephrine uptake inhibition cannot be over-

come by increasing the dosage of I-123 iobenguane. A thyroid-blocking agent is recommended prior to administration of this radiopharmaceutical. The recommended adult dosage is 10 mCi, and the pediatric dosage is based on body weight. This preparation contains benzyl alcohol in a concentration of 10.3 mg/mL; thus, the risks of benzyl alcohol should be considered.

Gallium Citrate Ga-67

Gallium citrate is a diagnostic radiopharmaceutical that has indications in both oncology and infectious and inflammatory diseases. After Ga-67 citrate is intravenously injected, the Ga-67 disassociates from the citrate and becomes bound to plasma transferrin. The exact mechanism of localization of this tracer is not known even though it has been studied at great length. Its oncological indications include identifying the presence and extent of Hodgkin disease, lymphoma, and bronchogenic carcinoma. The dosage range is 3–10 mCi, depending on the disease state and whether planar or SPECT imaging is used.

I-125 Lotrex

It is used to deliver intracavitary radiation therapy in patients with malignant brain tumors following tumor resection surgery. A balloon is surgically placed in the cavity of the removed tumor and filled with the radiopharmaceutical. The radiopharmaceutical, but not the balloon, is removed after the intended radiation treatment is completed. The patient stays in the hospital the entire time the balloon is filled.

Y-90 Ibritumomab Tiuxetan (Y-90 Zevalin)

Y-90 ibritumomab tiuxetan is a CD20-directed radiotherapeutic antibody for patients with relapsed or refractory, low-grade or follicular B-cell non-Hodgkin lymphoma (NHL) or patients with previously untreated follicular NHL who achieved a partial or complete response to first-line chemotherapy. The CD20 antigen is expressed on pre-B-lymphocytes and mature B-lymphocytes and on > 90% of B-cell NHLs.

Ra-223 Dichloride (Xofigo)

It is an alpha particle–emitting radioactive therapeutic agent indicated for the treatment of patients with castration-resistant prostate cancer, symptomatic bone metastases, and no known visceral metastatic disease. The dose regimen is 1.35 mCi/kg patient body weight, administered at 4 week intervals for a total of six injections. The active moiety of Ra-223 dichloride is the alpha particle–emitting radionuclide radium 223, which mimics calcium and forms complexes with the bone mineral hydroxyapatite at areas of increased bone turnover, such as bone metastases. The high linear energy transfer of alpha emitters (80 keV/micrometer) leads to a high frequency of double-strand DNA (deoxyribonucleic acid) breaks in adjacent cells, resulting in an antitumor effect on bone metastases. The alpha particle range from Ra-223 dichloride is less than 100 micrometers (less than 10 cell diameters), which limits damage to the surrounding normal tissue.

6-8. Pulmonary Imaging

Pulmonary imaging is performed for two purposes, ventilation and perfusion, which are often ordered as a V/Q or V/P scan. Ventilation and perfusion studies will match in some disease states and will not match in others. The results of both imaging procedures help identify different diagnoses.

Ventilation

Xenon (Xe)-133 gas

Xe-133 gas is indicated for the diagnostic evaluation of pulmonary function. A side beta emission causes a higher-than-ideal radiation exposure for imaging and may be avoided in pediatrics for this reason. The radiopharmaceutical is administered via inhalation from a closed respirator system with dosage ranges listed in Table 6-3. The patient is asked to inhale and hold his or her breath for a static image and then breathes in fresh air and exhales Xe-133 gas into a collecting bag or trapping machine while images are acquired to determine the washout period. Obstruction in airways will be detected as radioactive after the washout. The advantage of Xe-133 gas is that it is more physiologic than aerosolized Tc-99m DTPA and affords the ability to perform not only a wash-in phase but also a washout phase. Xe-133 is produced by a cyclotron and is manufactured in 10 mCi and 20 mCi vials every week. It typically expires 1 week past calibration date and may be dispensed as early as 1 week precalibration date. The ventilation study is routinely performed before the perfusion study.

Tc-99m pentetate (Tc-99m DTPA)

The kit for the preparation of Tc-99m pentetate injection is used off label as a standard of practice for pulmonary ventilation studies. The radiopharmaceutical is administered via a commercially available nebulizer in 2–3 mL in the dosage ranges listed in Table 6-3. The patient inhales the aerosol and exhales for 5–10 minutes. The higher-than-Xe-133 gas activity is attributable to the fact that less than 5% of the nebulized activity is retained in the lungs. The advantage over Xe-133 gas is the preferable imaging decay characteristics of Tc-99m as well as the ability to image in multiple angles compared with usually just the posterior angle; however, only wash-in images can be obtained. The ventilation study is routinely performed before the perfusion study.

Table 6-3. Radiopharmaceuticals for Pulmonary Imaging

Drug	Xe-133	Tc-99m pentetate	Tc-99m MAA
Normal activity range	5–20 mCi	30–50 mCi	1–5 mCi
			200,000–1,200,000 particles
Pediatric	0.3 mCi/kg		0.025–0.05 mCi/kg
	No less than 3 mCi total		No less than 0.4 mCi except for newborns, which is 0.2–0.5 mCi total
			10,000–50,000 particles for newborns
			50,000–100,000 particles for 1-year-olds
			200,000–300,000 for 5-year-olds
			200,000–700,000 for 15-year-olds
Pulmonary hypertension			60,000 particles
Pregnancy			60,000 particles

Perfusion

Tc-99m albumin aggregated (Tc-99m MAA)

The kit for the preparation of Tc-99m albumin-aggregated injection is indicated as a lung-imaging agent that may be used as an adjunct in the evaluation of pulmonary perfusion in adult and pediatric patients. Primarily, it is used in the detection of a pulmonary embolism. The radiopharmaceutical is administered intravenously in dosage ranges listed in Table 6-3. An average of 200,000–700,000 macro aggregated albumin particles (10–150 micrometers in diameter) tagged to Tc-99m are injected and occlude pulmonary capillaries in a uniform distribution, assuming the patient is supine when injected. Any areas of decreased activity indicate a decrease in blood flow or blocking of that capillary. Decreasing activity and particle numbers should be considered with pediatric and pregnant patients as well as those with a left-to-right cardiac shunt and with pulmonary hypertension. Severe pulmonary hypertension is a contraindication.

6-9. Renal Imaging

Renal function refers to the glomerular filtration and the tubular secretion in the nephron. In a healthy patient, 20% of the renal plasma flow undergoes filtration and 80% undergoes tubular secretion. Renal scintigraphy can be divided into a few main studies: perfusion, diuresis, angiotensin-converting enzyme (ACE) inhibition, and cortical. Three different drugs play an important and particular role in each of these (see Table 6-4).

Perfusion and Diuresis Studies

Renograms are separated into three different areas: arrival of the radiopharmaceutical, renal accumulation of the radiopharmaceutical, and excretion of the radiopharmaceutical into the urine. The patient should be well hydrated before the study and must void before administration and initiation of the study. Imaging takes place immediately after administration. Functional information is obtained with these studies.

If obstruction needs to be ruled out, a loop diuretic is used to see if washout of activity occurs. If none occurs, an obstruction is suspected.

Tc-99m mertiatide (Tc-99m MAG3)

About 40–50% of the injected drug is extracted by the tubules with each pass through the kidneys, and this drug is extracted 100% by the tubules. The high extraction efficiency makes it ideal for patients with and without renal insufficiency.

Tc-99m pentetate (Tc-99m DTPA)

For this pure glomerular filtration agent, the extraction percentage with each pass through the kidneys of this drug is 10–20% in patients with normal renal function.

ACE Inhibitor Studies

With renal artery stenosis, glomerular filtration rate is maintained because of the pressure exerted by the constricted efferent arteriole but maintains normal Tc-99m DTPA extraction. An hour after the baseline study, an ACE inhibitor is administered, followed by another injection of the radiopharmaceutical. Decreased urine flow caused by administration of ACE inhibitor produces a delayed washout of Tc-99m MAG3, resulting in cortical retention. Whereas when Tc-99m DTPA is the radiopharmaceutical, the ACE inhibitor reduces extraction of the radiopharmaceutical. Care must be taken to know which drug is used in the study to properly interpret the results. Captopril 25 mg or 50 mg is typically administered with the radiopharmaceutical injected 1 hour afterward. Enalaprilat (Vasotec) 0.04 mg/kg

Table 6-4. Radiopharmaceuticals for Renal Imaging

Radiopharmaceutical	Adult dosage	Pediatric dosage	Dosage with ACE inhibitor study	Mechanism of uptake
Tc-99m mertiatide	5–10 mCi	0.7–1.4 mCi/kg, minimum of 1 mCi	2 mCi, then 8 mCi	Tubular secretion
Tc-99m DTPA	15 mCi	0.2 mCi/kg, minimum of 2 mCi		Glomerular filtration
Tc-99m succimer	2–6 mCi	0.04–0.05 mCi/kg, minimum of 0.6 mCi		Cortical Binding

(2.5 mg maximum) can also be used with the radiopharmaceutical injected 15 minutes afterward.

Cortical Studies

Imaging is used to help detect renal infection or scarring, mostly in the diagnoses of acute pyelonephritis. This imaging is primarily performed in pediatric patients.

Tc-99m succimer (DMSA)

Approximately 40–50% of the injected dose is bound in the cortex, and imaging is acquired 1.5–3 hours after administration to ensure maximal uptake and background clearance. Delayed imaging can be performed for up to 24 hours.

6-10. Reticuloendothelial, Hepatobiliary, and Gastrointestinal Systems

The reticuloendothelial system (RES) includes the imaging of the liver Kupffer cells, spleen, and bone marrow. The hepatobiliary system includes the liver, gall bladder, and bile ducts. The gastrointestinal system includes the mouth, esophagus, stomach, and small and large intestines.

RES Imaging

RES imaging is based on the use of radiocolloids (Tc-99m sulfur colloid) to take advantage of the Kupffer cells for liver imaging. Distribution of the drug is based on blood flow, presence of any disease states, and the particle size and numbers administered. The anatomy of the RES can be imaged as early as 10 minutes after administration, and function can be determined as well. For instance, liver disease and tumors will decrease or restrict blood flow to certain areas, creating photopenic areas on a scintigraphic image. When cells are damaged by disease or other means, such as radiation or other trauma, Tc-99m sulfur colloid is not taken up and the drug is shunted to other areas. Accumulation in a healthy patient is 80–85% in the liver, 5–10% in the spleen, and the rest in the bone marrow via adventitial cells; the smaller particles preferentially are accumulated in the bone marrow and larger particles preferentially in the liver. A greater number of particles facilitates with bone marrow imaging.

Tc-99m sulfur colloid

Imaging can begin within 20 minutes of administration. Particles range in size from 1.5 micrometers to less, depending on compounding parameters. The drug can be filtered through a 0.1 or 0.22 micrometer filter to reduce particle sizes and help enhance bone marrow imaging.

Technetium sulfur colloid contains only inorganic sulfur and is completely void of any sulfhydryl or disulfide groups, and as such is not contraindicated in patients with a known allergy to sulfa drugs.

Hepatobiliary System

Also known as HIDA scans, these radiopharmaceuticals have the same hepatocyte uptake, transport, and excretion pathways as bilirubin, which means they are extracted by the hepatocyte, secreted into the bile canaliculi, and cleared through the biliary tract into the bowel. As such, the bilirubin level in a patient can interfere with the study, and larger dosages of radioactivity must be administered to compensate (Table 6-5). Clinical diagnoses that can be evaluated with this procedure are listed in Box 6-1.

Tc-99m mebrofenin (Choletec)

This kit contains methylparaben and propylparaben, giving it a beyond-use date of 18 hours. It is less sensitive to bilirubin interaction than is disofenin.

Tc-99m disofenin (Hepatolite)

The compounded kit has a beyond-use date of 6 hours and is more sensitive to bilirubin interaction than is mebrofenin.

Sincalide (Kinevac)

Sincalide is a nonradioactive cholecystopancreatic-gastrointestinal hormone peptide for parenteral administration that constricts the gall bladder. It can be used to establish whether a complete or near-complete obstruction of the common bile duct exists, to obtain the gall bladder ejection fraction, or to increase diagnostic ability to detect acute cholecystitis with a prolonged fasting patient.

Morphine

Morphine can be used to help evaluate cystic duct obstruction by constricting the sphincter of Oddi and restricting the radiopharmaceutical from entering the

Table 6-5. Radiopharmaceuticals for Hepatobiliary Imaging

Pharmaceutical	Liver/spleen, adults	Liver/spleen, children	Liver/spleen, newborns	Bone marrow, adults	Bone marrow, pediatric	Hepatobiliary	Hepatobiliary with elevated bilirubin
Sulfur colloid	1–8 mCi	0.015–0.075 mCi/kg	0.2–0.5 mCi	3–12 mCi	0.03–0.15 mCi/kg		
Mebrofenin						2–5 mCi	3–10 mCi
Disofenin						1–5 mCi	3–8 mCi
Sincalide						0.2 mcg/kg	
Morphine						0.04–0.1 mg/kg over 2–3 min	
Phenobarbital						(5 mg/kg/day, for 5 days)	

duodenum and forcing the flow into the gallbladder if the cystic duct is patent.

Phenobarbital

Pretreatment (5 days) with phenobarbital can be used to detect biliary atresia and to differentiate it from other causes of neonatal jaundice. It maximizes sensitivity by activating the liver excretory enzymes, and the lack of any biliary clearance into the bowel within 24 hours indicates a true positive test.

Gastrointestinal System

Solid gastric emptying and motility studies are performed using Tc-99m sulfur colloid compounded into liquid egg whites, whole eggs, and other various foods. The patient should be fasting for 4 hours before the procedure and should be off any medications that are prokinetic or delay gastric emptying (see Table 6-6 and Box 6-2). Transit times should be compared to local institutional baselines from the same delivery meal. Testing for gastroesophageal reflux disease is also available using Tc-99m sulfur colloid or In-111 DTPA compounded into a liquid solution such as milk (Table 6-7). This can also be used to test for the liquid phase of gastric emptying.

6-11. Skeletal System Imaging, Pain Palliation, and Therapy

Nuclear medicine procedures involving the skeletal system can be used for diagnostic or therapeutic purposes. Diagnostic skeletal agents are used in the adult and pediatric populations for imaging areas of altered osteogenesis. Therapeutic radiopharmaceuticals for

Box 6-1. Clinical Indications for Hepatobiliary Imaging

Acute cholecystitis
Chronic cholecystitis
Common duct obstruction
Choledochal cyst
Biliary atresia
Postoperative biliary tract
Liver transplants
Trauma
Primary benign and malignant tumors
Enterogastric bile reflux

Table 6-6. Normal Limits for Gastric Retention

Time point (hours)	Lower limit (%)[a]	Upper limit (%)[b]
0.5	70	
1	30	90
2		60
3		30
4		10

a. A lower value suggests abnormally rapid emptying.
b. A greater value suggests abnormally delayed gastric emptying.

Box 6-2. Drugs That Could Affect a Gastric Emptying Study

Aluminum-containing antacids
Antispasmodic agents
Atropine
Benzodiazepine
Calcium channel blockers
Domperidone
Erythromycin
Histamine-2 blockers
Metoclopramide
Nifedipine
Nonsteroidal anti-inflammatory drugs
Octreotide
Opiates
Phentolamine
Progesterone
Tegaserod
Theophylline

the skeletal system are indicated for the palliative treatment of painful, osteoblastic metastatic bone lesions that have been confirmed prior to treatment.

Tc-99m Medronate (Tc-99m MDP)

This diagnostic agent is a radioactive diphosphonate complex that localizes in the hydroxyapatite crystals of bone as a function of blood flow and osteoblastic activity. Tc-99m MDP bone scintigraphy can identify both benign and metastatic lesions, but this procedure cannot distinguish between the two. Three-phase bone imaging can be used to differentiate between shin splints and stress fractures, and it can also be used to distinguish between osteomyelitis and cellulitis. To obtain an optimal study, the patient should be well hydrated if the patient's condition permits, and the patient should void frequently postinjection to decrease background activity and reduce the radiation dose to the urinary bladder wall. Imaging can begin 1–4 hours postinjection of 10–20 mCi (70 kg adult patient). Anaphylactic and anaphylactoid reactions have been reported with the use of this radiopharmaceutical.

Table 6-7. Gastric-Emptying Radiopharmaceuticals

Radiopharmaceutical	Dosage (mCi)
Tc-99m sulfur colloid	0.3–1
In-111 DTPA	0.25–1

F-18 Sodium Fluoride

F-18 sodium fluoride is a PET radiopharmaceutical. It was introduced in the early 1960s, but availability and imaging equipment issues prevented its widespread use. When the Tc-99m bone-imaging complexes were introduced, F-18 sodium fluoride was abandoned. It has recently been reintroduced as a bone-imaging agent because of its excellent biologic characteristics, current availability from commercial vendors, and improved PET scanners. It can be used in the assessment of benign and malignant skeletal disease, and it is useful in adult and pediatric patients. The recommended dosage range for adult patients is 5–10 mCi. The pediatric patient's dosage is based on 0.06 mCi/kg, with a minimum dose of 0.5 mCi and a maximum dose of 5 mCi.

Strontium-89 Chloride (Metastron)

This radiopharmaceutical is used as a palliative therapeutic agent to reduce bone pain from metastatic lesions with the goal of reducing the amount of opioid analgesics required. Strontium-89 chloride localizes in bone mineral, with more uptake seen in areas of active osteogenesis as compared to normal bone. The palliative effect of this radiopharmaceutical is due to strontium-89 chloride being a beta emitter, resulting in irradiation of the bone in which it is localized. It is retained for a longer period in metastatic bone lesions as compared to normal bone. Because this agent is toxic to bone marrow, it should be used cautiously in patients with leukocyte counts less than 2,400 and platelet levels less than 60,000. Because strontium-89 chloride is a calcium analog, it should be administered slowly over 1–2 minutes to prevent a flushing sensation. The dosage of radioactivity is 4 mCi, or it can be based on 0.04–0.06 mCi/kg of body weight. Hematologic monitoring should be conducted at least every other week after injection until bone marrow function has recovered.

Samarium (Sm)-153 Lexidronam (Sm-153 EDTMP, Quadramet)

Sm-153 lexidronam is a beta and gamma emitter; its palliative therapeutic effect is due to the beta emission, but the gamma emission allows it to be imaged for biodistribution knowledge. Localization of the product in areas of active osteoblastic activity is the result of the lexidronam complex, which is a tetraphosphonate chelator. As with strontium-89 chloride, this radiopharmaceutical accumulates in areas of osteoblastic lesions more than in normal bone. As bone pain is reduced, the amount of opioid analgesics can be decreased. Because of the bone marrow toxicity occurring with this radiopharmaceutical, it should be administered only to patients having adequate hematologic status and bone marrow reserve. There is a risk of bone marrow suppression, thus necessitating weekly monitoring of blood counts, beginning 2 weeks after Sm-153 EDTMP injection and continuing for a minimum of 8 weeks or until return of bone marrow function. The dosage of Sm-153 EDTMP is 1 mCi/kg by IV injection over a time period of 1 minute.

Tc-99m Oxidronate (Tc-99m HDP)

This tracer is a diagnostic bone-imaging agent used in both adult and pediatric patient populations to identify areas of altered osteogenesis and areas of actively metabolizing bone. Oxidronate is a diphosphonate complex that is responsible for localization of the radiopharmaceutical in the hydroxyapatite crystals in the bone. Adverse reactions are uncommon, but the following have been linked to this agent: nausea, vomiting, and hypersensitivity reactions. To optimize imaging quality, the patient should be well hydrated if the patient's condition permits. The recommended radiopharmaceutical dosage range for an adult patient is 10–20 mCi, and the dosage range for a pediatric patient is 0.20 mCi/kg to 0.35 mCi/kg. A minimum pediatric dosage of 1 mCi is recommended for a diagnostic imaging study.

6-12. Thyroid Imaging and Therapy

Nuclear medicine procedures related to the thyroid are based on the association of iodine uptake in relation to the status of the thyroid glands. The body cannot distinguish between iodine found in nature and radioactive isotopes of iodine that can be used for diagnosis and therapy. The percentage uptake of iodine in addition to T_4 and thyroid-stimulating hormone levels is used to help identify various thyroid diseases and cancers (Tables 6-8 and 6-9). I-131 sodium iodide can be administered to treat the disease directly or to help address any tissue remaining from surgical removal of a thyroid carcinoma.

Imaging

I-131 sodium iodide

I-131 sodium iodide is indicated for use in performing the radioactive iodide uptake test to evaluate thyroid

Table 6-8. Radiopharmaceuticals for Thyroid Imaging

Radiopharmaceutical	Normal imaging dosage amount (mCi)	Normal whole-body imaging amount (mCi)
I-131	0.015	5–10
I-123	0.1–0.4	1–10
Tc-99m	10	

function. The beta decay causes an unnecessary radiation exposure burden to the patient, and the high-energy gamma emission is also less than desirable. An anatomical image of the thyroid is usually taken 24 hours after administration, and uptake counts are taken at 6 hours and 24 hours postadministration.

Table 6-9. Factors Affecting Thyroidal Uptake of Radioiodine

Uptake

Decreased uptake

Thyroxine

Triiodothyronine

Lugol's solution

Saturated solution of potassium iodide

Some mineral supplements, cough medicines, and vitamin preparations

Iodine food supplements

Iodinated drugs

Iodinated skin ointments

Congestive heart failure

Renal failure

Adrenocorticotropic hormone, adrenal steroids

Penicillin

Goitrogenic foods

Antithyroid drugs

Prior radiation to neck

Increased uptake

Pregnancy

Rebound after therapy

Recovery from subacute thyroiditis

Lithium

Normal uptake percentages vary from 7% to 20% for 6 hours and from 10% to 35% for 24-hour counts. Whole-body imaging may be used to detect thyroid cancer that has metastasized.

I-123 sodium iodide

I-123 sodium iodide is indicated the same as I-131 sodium iodide diagnostic capsules, and uptake and imaging protocols are the same as I-131 sodium iodide diagnostic capsules.

Tc-99m sodium pertechnetate

The physical attributes of $Na^{99m}TcO_4$ are similar to those of iodide, allowing this drug to also be used for thyroid imaging because it is taken up similarly to iodide; however, it is not organified. Tc-99m sodium pertechnetate can be administered intravenously or given as an oral solution. Anatomical images can be taken 10–30 minutes after IV administration and 1 hour after oral administration. Uptake values cannot be performed with this drug.

Therapy

I-131 sodium iodide

Because of the damaging nature of the beta particles from I-131 sodium iodide decay and the specificity to which iodine accumulates in the thyroid (especially one that is hyperfunctioning), I-131 sodium iodide is a common therapeutic option for almost all thyroid cancers except medullary (because the latter does not accumulate radioiodine). Thyroid cancer is treated with surgery, and then I-131 sodium iodide is used for ablation of remaining tissue. Dosages vary considerably on the basis of the physician's decisions about how much radiation with which to ablate any remaining thyroid tissue after thyroidectomy and whether a functioning primary or metastatic carcinoma exists. Typical dosages for hyperthyroidism loosely range from 25 to 30 mCi, and metastatic therapies can loosely range from 100 to 200 mCi.

6-13. Questions

1. Which of the following radiopharmaceuticals is indicated to image beta-amyloid neuritic plaques in patients exhibiting cognitive impairment?

   A. Tc-99m DTPA
   B. Tc-99m bicisate
   C. In-111 DTPA
   D. Florbetapir F-18

2. Which of the following radiopharmaceuticals is a controlled substance?

   A. I-123 ioflupane
   B. Florbetapir F-18
   C. Thallous chloride Tl-201
   D. Tc-99m exametazime

3. Which of the following radiopharmaceuticals accumulates in viable myocardium via the Na^+/K^+ ATPase pump?

   A. F-18 FDG
   B. Tc-99m tetrofosmin
   C. Rb-82 chloride
   D. Tc-99m sestamibi

4. Which of the following radiopharmaceuticals is a monovalent cation and a potassium analog?

   A. F-18 FDG
   B. Tc-99m tetrofosmin
   C. Tc-99m sestamibi
   D. Thallous chloride Tl-201

5. Which of the following PET radiopharmaceuticals is commercially available from a generator?

   A. F-18 FDG
   B. I-23 ioflupane
   C. Florbetapir F-18
   D. Rb-82 chloride

6. Which of the following is a myocardial radiopharmaceutical that provides information on both perfusion and left ventricular function?

   A. Rb-82 chloride
   B. Tc-99m tetrofosmin
   C. F-18 FDG
   D. Thallous chloride Tl-201

7. An example of a diagnostic skeletal agent is

   A. Tc-99m bicisate.
   B. Tc-99m MDP.
   C. Sr-82 chloride.
   D. Florbetapir F-18.

8. What patient preparation is recommended for skeletal imaging if the patient's condition permits?

   A. Bowel cleansing
   B. Hydration
   C. Thyroid blockade
   D. Sincalide administration

9. Which of the following correctly characterizes Tc-99m HDP?

   A. Localizes in areas of high bone metabolic activity
   B. Limited to use in adult patients with metastatic skeletal lesions
   C. Frequent adverse reactions
   D. Lipophilic cationic complex

10. Which of the following radiopharmaceuticals exerts it palliative effect through its beta particle emission?

    A. Tc-99m MDP
    B. In-111 oxyquinoline
    C. I-123 iobenguane
    D. Sm-153 EDTMP

11. Which of the following radiopharmaceuticals is indicated for radiolabeling leukocytes?

    A. Tc-99m DTPA
    B. F-18 FDG
    C. In-111 oxine
    D. I-123 iobenguane

12. An example of a radiolabeled peptide that is used in localizing primary and metastatic neuroendocrine tumors is

    A. In-111 pentetreotide.
    B. I-123 iobenguane.
    C. In-111 capromab pendetide.
    D. I-123 ioflupane.

13. Which of the following PET radiopharmaceuticals is used for assessing malignant and benign skeletal disease?

    A. F-18 FDG
    B. Florbetapir F-18
    C. Rb-82 chloride
    D. F-18 sodium fluoride

14. Which of the following radiopharmaceuticals is a calcium analog?

    A. Thallous chloride Tl-201
    B. Rb-82 chloride
    C. Florbetapir F-18
    D. Strontium-89 chloride

15. What is the recommended minimum leukocyte count prior to a patient receiving strontium-89 chloride?

    A. 2,400
    B. 6,200
    C. 8,800
    D. 10,000

16. Which of the following radiopharmaceuticals has indications for both cardiology and oncology?

    A. I-123 iobenguane
    B. I-123 ioflupane
    C. In-111 capromab pendetide
    D. F-18 FDG

17. Which of the following statements describes the use of In-111 oxine?

    A. Autologous white blood cells are used.
    B. It is ideal for leukopenic patients with a fever.
    C. Radiolabeling occurs in vivo.
    D. It provides palliative therapeutic benefit.

18. Which of the following correctly characterizes I-123 MIBG?

    A. Has similar structure to somatostatin
    B. Follows cellular pathway of norepinephrine
    C. Is therapeutic agent for treatment of thyroid disease
    D. Interacts with drugs that affect glucose uptake

19. Following an intravenous injection of Ga-67 citrate, Ga-67 disassociates from citrate and becomes immediately bound to

    A. erythrocytes.
    B. leukocytes.
    C. platelets.
    D. transferrin.

20. Which of the following radiopharmaceuticals is useful in assisting with the diagnosis of opportunistic infections?

    A. Thallous chloride Tl-201
    B. I-123 iobenguane
    C. In-111 pentetreotide
    D. Ga-67 citrate

21. Which of the following statements is true concerning In-111 pentetreotide?

    A. It is an analog of guanethidine.
    B. It is primarily a therapeutic radiopharmaceutical.
    C. One day pretreatment with octreotide is recommended.
    D. Its planar imaging dosage is different from its SPECT dosage.

22. Which of the following is true regarding Sm-153 lexidronam?

    A. Localizes in areas of osteoblastic activity
    B. Localizes in medullary thyroid cancer
    C. Is a calcium analog
    D. Is given orally

23. Which of the following radiopharmaceuticals is used as an adjunct in determining the site of stroke in patients previously diagnosed with stroke?

    A. In-111 DTPA
    B. Tc-99m sestamibi
    C. Tc-99m bicisate
    D. I-123 ioflupane

24. Which of the following radiopharmaceuticals is indicated in cisternography studies?

    A. In-111 DTPA
    B. Tc-99m sestamibi
    C. Tc-99m bicisate
    D. I-123 ioflupane

25. Which of the following describes Tc-99m sestamibi?

    A. It is an anionic complex.
    B. It localizes in myocytes via passive diffusion.
    C. It is transported into cells via glucose transporters.
    D. It is a potassium analog.

6-14. Answers

1. **D.** Florbetapir F-18 is the only one with this indication. Tc-99m DTPA is used to evaluate patients for brain death, and Tc-99m bicisate is used in evaluation of stroke patients and in the evaluation of brain death. In-111 DTPA is indicated for cisternography studies.

2. **A.** All are radiopharmaceuticals, but I-123 ioflupane is the only one that is a controlled drug.

3. **C.** F-18 FDG is transported via glucose transporters whereas Tc-99m tetrofosmin and Tc-99m sestamibi enter the cell via passive diffusion.

4. **D.** F-18 FDG is a glucose analog. Tc-99m tetrofosmin and Tc-99m sestamibi are monovalent cations but not potassium analogs. Thallous chloride Tl-201 is a monovalent cation and a potassium analog.

5. **D.** F-18 and I-123 are not available from a generator.

6. **B.** F-18 FDG is an indicator of metabolism, and Rb-82 chloride and thallous chloride Tl-201 provide information on myocardial perfusion. Tc-99m tetrofosmin provides information on both myocardial perfusion and left ventricular function.

7. **B.** Tc-99m bicisate and florbetapir F-18 are for central nervous system imaging, and Sr-82 chloride is a palliative therapeutic agent.

8. **B.** Bowel cleansing, thyroid blockade, and sincalide administration provide no benefit in skeletal imaging.

9. **A.** Tc-99m HDP can be used in the pediatric population, and adverse reactions are uncommon. It is a diphosphonate complex but not a lipophilic complex.

10. **D.** Sm-153 EDTMP is the only radionuclide listed that produces beta particles, so it is the only one that can be used in therapy.

11. **C.** Tc-99m DTPA is used in brain and renal studies, F-18 FDG is used as a metabolic indicator, and I-123 iobenguane is used in the detection of pheochromocytomas and neuroblastomas.

12. **A.** In-123 iobenguane is used in the detection of pheochromocytomas and neuroblastomas,

but it is not a peptide. In-111 capromab pendetide is a monoclonal antibody used in patients with prostate cancer. I-123 ioflupane is used in the evaluation of patients with Parkinsonian syndromes.

13. **D.** F-18 FDG is used in the assessment of other oncology pathologies as well as cardiac disease, and florbetapir F-18 is used in estimating density of beta-amyloid plaques in patients being evaluated for cognitive impairment. Rb-82 chloride is used in cardiac studies.

14. **D.** Tl-201 chloride and Rb-82 chloride are potassium analogs, and florbetapir F-18 is not a calcium analog.

15. **A.** Any level over 2,400 is above the minimum level of leukocytes recommended before a patient receives strontium-89 chloride.

16. **D.** I-123 iobenguane and In-111 capromab pendetide have oncology indications but not cardiology indications. I-123 ioflupane does not have either a cardiology or an oncology indication.

17. **A.** In-111 oxine is not useful for leukopenic patients, and radiolabeling occurs in vitro. It is a diagnostic agent rather than a therapeutic radiopharmaceutical.

18. **B.** It is structurally similar to norepinephrine and guanethidine and interacts with drugs that reduce norepinephrine uptake. It is a diagnostic agent.

19. **D.** Ga-67 immediately binds to plasma transferrin, and it is not dependent on white blood cells, erythrocytes, or platelets for localization.

20. **D.** Tl-201 chloride is indicated for cardiology, not infectious diseases. I-123 iobenguane and In-111 pentetreotide are both for oncology indications, not infectious diseases. Ga-67 citrate is useful for diagnosis of opportunistic infections, and it has application in oncology as well.

21. **D.** It is a diagnostic radiopharmaceutical and an analog of somatostatin. If possible, octreotide administration should be suspended before administration of this radiopharmaceutical. Dosage for SPECT imaging is twice as great as for planar imaging.

22. **A.** It localizes in areas of osteoblastic metastatic bone disease, and it is administered intravenously.

23. **C.** In-111 DTPA is used for cisternography studies, and Tc-99m sestamibi does not have an indication for the central nervous system. I-123 ioflupane is used in the assessment of patients suspected of having Parkinsonian syndromes.

24. **A.** Tc-99m sestamibi does not have an indication for central nervous system diseases or disorders. Tc-99m bicisate is used in stroke patients and patients suspected of being brain dead, and I-123 ioflupane is used in the assessment of patients suspected of having Parkinsonian syndromes.

25. **B.** It is a monovalent cation but not a potassium analog. Glucose transporters are not involved in the localization of this agent.

6-15. References

AdreView [package insert]. Arlington Heights, IL: GE Healthcare; revised September 2008.

Amyvid (Florbetapir F 18 Injection) [package insert]. Indianapolis, IN: Lilly USA, LLC; revised April 2012.

Cardiogen-82 [package insert]. Princeton, NJ: Bracco Diagnostics Inc.; revised February 2012.

Cardiolite [package insert]. N. Billerica, MA: Lantheus Medical Imaging; July 2010.

Ceretec [package insert]. Arlington Heights, IL: GE Healthcare; revised February 2013.

DaTscan [package insert]. Arlington Heights, IL: GE Healthcare; revised April 2011.

Delbeke D, Coleman RE, Guiberteau MJ, et al. Procedure guideline for tumor imaging with ^{18}F-FDG PET/CT 1.0. Society of Nuclear Medicine and Molecular Imaging Practice Guidelines, approved February 11, 2006. http://snm.org/guidelines.

Gallium Citrate Ga-67 Injection [package insert]. St. Louis, MO: Mallinckrodt Inc.; revised April 2012.

Indium DTPA In 111 [package insert]. Arlington Heights, IL: GE Healthcare; revised February 2006.

Indium In 111 Oxyquinoline Solution [package insert]. Arlington Heights, IL: GE Healthcare; revised February 2006.

Iotrex I-125 [package insert]. Richland, WA: IsoRay Medical, Inc.

KINEVAC Sincalide for Injection [package insert]. Princeton, NJ: Bracco Diagnostics Inc.; revised May 2011.

Kit for the preparation of Technetium Tc-99m Mebrofenin [package insert]. Princeton, NJ: Bracco Diagnostics Inc.; revised March 2007.

Kit for the Preparation of Technetium Tc-99m Mertiatide [package insert]. St. Louis, MO: Mallinckrodt Inc.; revised December 2011.

Kit for the Preparation of Technetium Tc-99m Pentetate Injection [package insert]. Kirkland, Quebec, Canada: Jubilant DraxImage Inc.; revised June 2011.

Kit for the Preparation of Technetium Tc-99m Sulfur Colloid Injection [package insert]. Bedford, MA: Pharmalucence, Inc.; revised July 2011.

Kit for the Preparation of Technetium Tc-99m Succimer Injection [package insert]. Arlington Heights, IL: GE Healthcare; revised February 2006.

Kowalsky RJ, Falen SW, eds. *Radiopharmaceuticals in Nuclear Pharmacy and Nuclear Medicine*. 3rd ed. Washington, DC: American Pharmacists Association; 2011.

MAA Kit for the Preparation of Technetium Tc-99m Albumin Aggregated Injection [package insert]. Kirkland, Quebec, Canada: Jubilant DraxImage Inc.; 2011.

MDP Multidose [package insert]. Arlington, Heights, IL: GE Healthcare; revised September 2007.

Metastron [package insert]. Arlington Heights, IL: GE Healthcare; revised February 2006.

Myoview [package insert]. Arlington Heights, IL: GE Healthcare; revised May 2011.

Neurolite [package insert]. N. Billerica, MA: Lantheus Medical Imaging; June 2008.

OctreoScan [package insert]. St. Louis, MO: Mallinckrodt Inc.; revised October 25, 2006.

ProstaScint [package insert]. Langhorne, PA: EUSA Pharma (USA), Inc.; revised December 2010.

Quadramet [package insert]. N. Billerica, MA: Lantheus Medical Imaging; 2009.

Saha G. *Fundamentals of Nuclear Pharmacy*. 6th ed. New York, NY: Springer; 2010.

Smith BT, Weatherman KD, eds. *Diagnostic Imaging for Pharmacists*. Washington, DC: American Pharmacists Association; 2012.

Sodium Iodide I-123 Capsules [package insert]. St. Louis, MO: Mallinckrodt Inc.; revised October 12, 2006.

Sodium Iodide I-131 Capsule USP Diagnostic Oral [package insert]. Kirkland, Quebec, Canada: Jubilant DraxImage Inc.; January 2011.

Taylor A, Schuster D, Alazraki N. *A Clinician's Guide to Nuclear Medicine*. 2nd ed. Reston, VA: Society of Nuclear Medicine; 2006.

TechneScan HDP [package insert]. St. Louis, MO: Mallinckrodt Inc.; revised December 2011.

TechneScan PYP [package insert]. St. Louis, MO: Mallinckrodt Inc.; revised February 2012.

Thallous Chloride Tl 201 Injection [package insert]. Arlington Heights, IL: GE Healthcare; revised April 2006.

Thrall J, Ziessman H. *Nuclear Medicine: The Requisites*. 4th ed. St. Louis, MO: Mosby; 2013.

UltraTag RBC Kit for the preparation of Technetium Tc-99m-Labeled Red Blood Cells [package insert]. St. Louis, MO: Mallinckrodt Inc.; revised December 2012.

Ultra-TechneKow DTE (Technetium Tc-99m Generator) [package insert]. St. Louis, MO: Mallinckrodt Inc.; revised February 2014.

Xenon Xe 133 Gas [package insert]. N. Billerica, MA: Lantheus Medical Imaging; revised August 2011.

Xofigo (radium Ra 223 dichloride) Injection [package insert]. Wayne, NJ: Bayer HealthCare Pharmaceuticals Inc.; revised May 2013.

Zevalin (ibritumomab tiuxetan) [package insert]. Irvine, CA: Spectrum Pharmaceuticals, Inc.; revised November 2011.

Pharmacokinetics, Drug Metabolism, and Drug Disposition

Bernd Meibohm
Charles R. Yates

7-1. Key Points

- The clearance CL can be determined from the relationship

$$CL = \frac{DR}{C_{ss,av}} \text{ or } CL = \frac{D}{AUC}$$

- The volume of distribution can be determined from the relationship

$$V = \frac{CL}{K}$$

- The average steady-state concentration $C_{ss,av}$ during multiple dosing is determined only by the dose D, the dosing interval τ (or both together as dosing rate $DR = D/\tau$), and the clearance CL:

$$C_{ss,av} = \frac{D}{\tau \times CL}$$

- The area under the curve resulting from administration of a single dose AUC_{single} is equal to the area under the curve during one dosing interval at steady-state AUC_{ss}, provided that the same dose is given per dosing interval τ:

$$C_{ss,av} = \frac{AUC_{ss}}{\tau} = \frac{D}{\tau \times CL} = \frac{AUC_{single}}{\tau}$$

- The volume of distribution at steady state is by definition the sum of the pharmacokinetic volumes of distribution for the different pharmacokinetic compartments. It is the theoretical

$$V_{ss} = V_p + \frac{f_u}{f_{ut}} \times V_t$$

where V_p is the volume of plasma (3 L), V_t is the volume of tissue water (total body water minus plasma volume: $42 - 3 = 39$ L based on a "standard" person), and f_u and f_{ut} are the fraction unbound for the drug in plasma and in plasma and tissue, respectively.

- *Clearance* is defined as the irreversible removal of a drug from the body by an organ of elimination. CL by the eliminating organ (CL_{organ}) is defined as the product of blood flow to the organ (Q) and the extraction ratio of that organ (ER). The fraction of drug escaping first-pass metabolism (F^*) can be described in terms of the hepatic ER ($F^* = 1 - ER$).

- The venous equilibrium model relates hepatic ER to hepatic blood flow Q, unbound drug fraction f_{up}, and intrinsic clearance CL_{int}:

$$CL_H = \frac{Q \times f_{up} \times CL_{int}}{Q + f_{up} \times CL_{int}}$$

- The venous equilibrium model can be simplified for drugs with low ER (<0.3) and high ER (>0.7). For low-ER drugs, $CL_H \approx f_{up} \times CL_{int}$. For high-$ER$ drugs, $CL_H \approx Q$.

- Bioavailability is the fraction (or percentage) of a dose administered nonintravenously (or extravascularly) that is systemically available as compared to an intravenous dose. The overall oral bioavailability (F) of a drug is dependent on the fraction absorbed (f_a), the fraction escaping metabolism in the intestinal wall (f_g), and the fraction escaping hepatic first-pass metabolism (F^*).

Drugs may undergo three processes in the kidney. Two act to remove a drug from the body: filtration and secretion. The other acts to return a drug to the body: reabsorption. The net process a drug undergoes can be determined by calculating the excretion ratio (E_{ratio}) using total renal clearance (CL_R) and filtration clearance (CL_F):

$$E_{ratio} = \frac{CL_R}{CL_F} = \frac{CL_R}{f_{up} \times 125 \text{ mL/min}}$$

where the CL_F is the product of glomerular filtration rate (125 mL/min for a "standard" person) and the fraction of a drug that is not bound to plasma proteins (unbound fraction f_{up}).

7-2. Study Guide Checklist

The following topics may guide your study of this subject area:

- Principles of first-order elimination kinetics
- Factors that affect a drug's bioavailability after extravascular administration
- Considerations for drug selection when trying to minimize the potential for drug–drug or drug–disease interactions
- Differences between high-extraction and low-extraction drugs when interpreting clinical significance of changes in protein binding and intrinsic clearance

7-3. Introduction

Pharmacokinetics is the science of a drug's fate in the body. A drug's therapeutic potential is intimately linked to its pharmacokinetic profile. For example, a drug's pharmacologic response may be severely diminished by poor absorption, rapid elimination from the body, or both. The most important factors contributing to drug disposition include absorption, distribution, metabolism, and excretion.

Absorption

The rate and extent of drug absorption is referred to as *bioavailability*. The fraction of drug absorbed (f_a), an important determinant of the extent of bioavailability (represented by F), is affected not only by the drug's physicochemical properties but also by physi-ologic barriers at the site of absorption. For example, intestinal expression of the drug efflux transporter P-glycoprotein is known to limit oral drugs.

Distribution

Many drugs circulate in the body bound to plasma proteins (e.g., human serum albumin). The fraction of drug not bound to plasma protein (f_{up}) is responsible for the pharmacologic effect. A drug may also bind significantly to tissue proteins (f_{ut}). Drugs with a large f_{up}-to-f_{ut} ratio have a large volume of distribution, whereas drugs with a small f_{up}-to-f_{ut} ratio are largely confined to the vascular space. Volume of distribution is directly related to *half-life* ($t_{1/2}$), the time required to eliminate half the drug from the body.

Metabolism

Approximately 50% of drugs undergo some form of hepatic metabolism. The cytochrome P450 (CYP450) family of drug-metabolizing enzymes is primarily responsible for drug inactivation in the liver. For a specific drug, however, other hepatic or nonhepatic enzymes may play a major role in their metabolism as well. Hepatic clearance depends on liver blood flow and the extraction ratio (ER). Hepatic ER can be used to estimate the fraction of drug escaping first-pass metabolism (F^*), which is an important determinant of oral bioavailability. Intestinal inactivation of drugs by CYP450 enzymes in the gut is responsible for reduced F of a number of drugs.

Excretion

The primary purpose of hepatic metabolism is to increase a drug's water solubility to facilitate its excretion through renal as well as nonrenal pathways. The kidneys also serve as the primary eliminating organ for drugs that do not undergo hepatic metabolism. Renal clearance comprises three main physiologic processes: glomerular filtration, reabsorption, and secretion. *Filtration clearance* is the product of f_{up} and glomerular filtration rate (a physiologic parameter that diminishes with age). Renal reabsorption is a predominantly passive process dependent on physicochemical drug properties and on urine drug concentration and pH, whereas secretion is an active process facilitated by various transport mechanisms. The net of filtration, reabsorption, and secretion determines a drug's total renal clearance.

Interindividual differences in drug pharmacokinetics can at least partially explain variability in drug response. Thus, a thorough understanding of the physiologic processes affecting drug disposition is essential to drug individualization and optimization.

7-4. Absorption and Disposition

Drug Input

Drugs are administered to the body by one of two routes, intravascular or extravascular. For intravascular administration, drugs are usually administered in intravenous (IV) infusion (continuous, short term, or bolus). The concentration (C) is given by the following expressions.

IV bolus

$$C = \frac{Dose}{V} \times e^{-K \times t}$$

$\dfrac{dC}{dt}$ (rate of change in plasma concentration)

$\quad$ = (rate of drug elimination, or output rate)
$\quad K$ = elimination rate constant = CL/V
$\quad CL$ = clearance = Dose/AUC
$\quad V$ = Volume

IV infusion

For drugs that are administered extravascularly (by mouth, intramuscularly, or subcutaneously) and act systemically, absorption must occur. See section 7-6.

First-order absorption

$$C = \frac{k_a \times F \times Dose}{V \times (k_a - K)} \times \left(e^{-K \times t} - e^{-k_a \times t}\right)$$

where k_a = first-order rate constant for drug absorption; absorption half-life = $0.693/k_a$; K = first-order rate constant for drug elimination (CL/V); CL = $F \times$ Dose/AUC, oral clearance = CL/F = Dose/AUC; and F = bioavailability, or fraction of drug absorbed. F refers to the rate *and* extent of absorption.

7-5. Constant Rate Regimens

For many drugs to be therapeutically effective, drug concentrations of a certain level have to be maintained at the site of action for a prolonged period (e.g., β-lactam antibiotics, antiarrhythmics), whereas

for others, alternating plasma concentrations are more preferable (e.g., aminoglycoside antibiotics such as gentamicin).

Two basic approaches to administering the drug can be applied to continuously maintain drug concentrations in a certain therapeutic range over a prolonged period:

- Drug administration at a constant input rate
- Sequential administration of discrete single doses (multiple dosing)

Drug Administration as Constant Rate Regimens

At any time during the infusion, the rate of change in drug concentration is the difference between the input rate (infusion rate R_0/volume of distribution V) and the output rate (elimination rate constant $K \times$ concentration C):

$$\text{Rate of change} = \text{input rate} - \text{output rate}$$

In concentrations:

$$\frac{dC}{dt} = \frac{R_0}{V} - K \times C$$

In amounts:

$$V \times \frac{dC}{dt} = R_0 - CL \times C$$

$\quad R_0$ = infusion rate (in amount/time, e.g., mg/h)
$\quad V$ = volume of distribution
$\quad CL$ = clearance
$\quad K$ = first-order rate constant for drug elimination (CL/V)

$$\frac{dC}{dt} = 0, \quad \frac{R_0}{V} = K \times C_{ss}, \text{ or } R_0 = CL \times C_{ss}$$

Hence, the steady-state concentration C_{ss} is determined only by the infusion rate R_0 and the clearance CL.

Drug concentration at steady state:

$$C_{ss} = \frac{R_0}{CL}$$

Drug concentration before steady state:

$$C = \frac{R_0}{CL} \times \left(1 - e^{-K \times t}\right)$$

Time to Reach Steady State

For therapeutic purposes, knowing how long after initiation of an infusion reaching the targeted steady-state concentration C_{ss} will take is often critical.

Concentration during an infusion before steady state:

$$C = \frac{R_0}{CL} \times \left(1 - e^{-K \times t}\right)$$

Concentration during an infusion at steady state:

$$C_{ss} = \frac{R_0}{CL}$$

The fraction of steady-state f is then

$$f = \frac{C}{C_{ss}} = \left(1 - e^{-K \times t}\right)$$

After a duration of infusion of

1.0 $t_{1/2} \rightarrow 50\%$ of steady state is reached
2.0 $t_{1/2} \rightarrow 75\%$ of steady state is reached
3.0 $t_{1/2} \rightarrow 87.5\%$ of steady state is reached
3.3 $t_{1/2} \rightarrow 90\%$ of steady state is reached
4.0 $t_{1/2} \rightarrow 93.8\%$ of steady state is reached
5.0 $t_{1/2} \rightarrow 96.9\%$ of steady state is reached

The following conclusions can be drawn:

- The approach to the steady-state concentration C_{ss} is exponential in nature and is controlled by the elimination process (elimination rate constant K), *not* the infusion rate R_0.
- Only the value of the steady-state concentration C_{ss} is controlled by the infusion rate R_0 (and of course by the clearance CL).
- If one assumes for clinical purposes that a concentration of > 95% of steady state is therapeutically equivalent to the final steady-state concentration C_{ss}, approximately five elimination half-lives $t_{1/2}$ are necessary to reach steady state after initiation of an infusion.

Concentration-Time Profiles Postinfusion

The plasma concentration postinfusion cannot be distinguished from giving an IV bolus dose. Because the drug input has been discontinued, the rate of change in drug concentration is determined only by the output rate. If the drug follows one-compartment characteristics, then the plasma concentration profile can be described by

$$C = C' \times e^{-K \times t_{pi}}$$

where C' is concentration at the end of the infusion and t_{pi} is time postinfusion (i.e., time after the infusion has stopped).

Thus, a general expression can be used to calculate the plasma concentration during and after a constant rate infusion:

$$C = \frac{R_0}{CL} \times \left(1 - e^{-K \times t}\right) \times e^{-K \times t_{pi}}$$

where t is the elapsed time after the beginning of the infusion and t_{pi} is the postinfusion time—that is, the difference between the duration of the infusion (infusion time T_{inf}) and t: $t_{pi} = t - T_{inf}$. For describing concentrations during the infusion, t_{pi} is set to zero. For describing concentrations postinfusion, t is set to T_{inf}.

Four different cases can be distinguished:

1. During the infusion, but before steady state is reached:

$$t = t, \ t_{pi} = 0 \Rightarrow C = \frac{R_0}{CL} \times \left(1 - e^{-K \times t}\right)$$

2. During the infusion at steady state:

$$t \rightarrow \infty, \ t_{pi} = 0 \Rightarrow C = \frac{R_0}{CL}$$

3. After cessation of the infusion before steady state:

$$t = T_{inf}, \ t_{pi} = t - T_{inf}$$

$$\Rightarrow C = \frac{R_0}{CL} \times \left(1 - e^{-K \times T_{inf}}\right) \times e^{-K \times (t - T_{inf})}$$

4. After cessation of the infusion at steady state:

$$t \rightarrow \infty, \ t_{pi} = t - T_{inf} \Rightarrow C = \frac{R_0}{CL} \times e^{-K \times (t - T_{inf})}$$

Determination of Pharmacokinetic Parameters

The elimination rate constant K and the elimination half-life $t_{1/2}$ can be determined from

- The terminal slope after the infusion has been stopped
- The time to reach half of C_{ss}

■ The slope of the relationship of $\ln(C_{ss} - C)$ versus t, based on

$$C = C_{ss} \times \left(1 - e^{-K \times t}\right)$$

and the resulting $\ln(C_{ss} - C) = \ln C_{ss} - K \times t$

The clearance CL from the relationship can be determined from

$$CL = \frac{R_0}{C_{ss}}$$

The volume of distribution from the relationship can be determined from

$$V = \frac{CL}{K}$$

Loading Dose and Maintenance Dose

The loading dose LD is supposed to immediately ($t = 0$) reach the desired target concentration C_{target}. It is administered as an IV bolus injection or, more frequently, as a short-term infusion. Following is an expression of target concentration calculated for a drug with one-compartment characteristics:

$$C_{target} = \frac{LD}{V} \rightarrow LD = C_{target} \times V$$

The maintenance dose MD is intended to sustain C_{target}. It is administered as a constant rate infusion. The maintenance dose is the infusion rate necessary to sustain the target concentration:

$$C_{target} = \frac{MD}{CL} \rightarrow MD = R_0 = C_{target} \times CL$$

7-6. Multiple Dosing

Continuous drug concentrations for a prolonged therapy can be maintained either by administering the drug at a constant input rate or by sequentially administering discrete single doses of the drug. The latter is the approach more frequently used and can be applied for extravascular as well as intravascular routes of administration.

Multiple-dose regimens are defined by two components, the dose D that is administered at each dos-ing occasion, and the dosing interval τ, which is the time between the administrations of two subsequent doses. Dose and dosing interval can be summarized in the dosing rate DR:

$$DR = \frac{D}{\tau}$$

Concentration-Time Profiles during Multiple Dosing

The multiple-dose function MDF can be used for calculating drug concentrations before steady state has been reached during a multiple-dose regimen:

$$MDF = \frac{1 - e^{n \times K \times \tau}}{1 - e^{-K \times \tau}}$$

where K is the respective rate constant of the drug, τ is the dosing interval, and n is the number of the dose.

Once steady state has been reached, n approaches infinity, and MDF simplifies to the accumulation factor AF:

$$AF = \frac{1}{1 - e^{-K \times \tau}}$$

Multiple-Dosing Regimens: Instantaneous Input (IV Bolus)

For an IV bolus multiple-dose regimen, the concentrations during the first dosing interval, the nth dosing interval, and at steady state are described by the relationships shown in Table 7-1.

The peak and trough concentrations at steady state can thus be expressed as the peak and trough after the first dose multiplied by the accumulation factor AF:

$$C_{ss,max} = \frac{C_{1,max}}{1 - e^{-K \times \tau}}$$

$$C_{ss,min} = \frac{C_{1,min}}{1 - e^{-K \times \tau}} = \frac{C_{1,max} \times e^{-K \times \tau}}{1 - e^{-K \times \tau}}$$

Average steady-state concentration

By definition, the average drug input rate is equal to the average drug output rate at steady state. Whereas the *average input rate* is the drug amount entering the

Table 7-1. IV Bolus Multiple-Dose Regimen

Dose number	Equation	Maximum or peak concentration	Minimum or trough concentration at the end of the dosing interval
1	$C = \dfrac{D}{V} \times e^{-K \times t}$	$C_{1,\max} = \dfrac{D}{V}$	$C_{1,\min} = \dfrac{D}{V} \times e^{-K \times \tau}$
n	$C = \dfrac{D}{V} \times e^{-K \times t} \times \dfrac{1 - e^{-n \times K \times \tau}}{1 - e^{-K \times \tau}}$	$C_{n,\max} = \dfrac{D}{V} \times \dfrac{1 - e^{-n \times K \times \tau}}{1 - e^{-K \times \tau}}$	$C_{n,\min} = \dfrac{D}{V} \times e^{-K \times \tau} \times \dfrac{1 - e^{-n \times K \times \tau}}{1 - e^{-K \times \tau}}$
Steady state	$C = \dfrac{D}{V} \times \dfrac{e^{-K \times t}}{1 - e^{-K \times \tau}}$	$C_{ss,\max} = \dfrac{D}{V} \times \dfrac{1}{1 - e^{-K \times \tau}}$	$C_{ss,\min} = \dfrac{D}{V} \times \dfrac{e^{-K \times \tau}}{1 - e^{-K \times \tau}}$

systemic circulation per dosing interval, the *average output rate* is equal to the product of clearance *CL* and the average plasma concentration within one dosing interval $C_{ss,av}$:

$$\frac{D}{\tau} = CL \times C_{ss,av}$$

Thus, the average steady-state concentration $C_{ss,av}$ during multiple dosing is determined only by the dose *D*, the dosing interval τ (or both together as dosing rate $DR = D/\tau$), and the clearance *CL*:

$$C_{ss,av} = \frac{D}{\tau \times CL}$$

The area under the curve resulting from administration of a single dose AUC_{single} is equal to the area under the curve during one dosing interval at steady state AUC_{ss} if the same dose is given per dosing interval τ:

$$C_{ss,av} = \frac{AUC_{ss}}{\tau} = \frac{D}{\tau \times CL} = \frac{AUC_{single}}{\tau}$$

Thus,

$$AUC_{single} = AUC_{ss}$$

Extent of accumulation

The extent of accumulation during multiple dosing at steady state is determined by the dosing interval τ and the half-life of the drug $t_{1/2}$ (or the elimination rate constant *K*):

$$AF = \frac{1}{1 - e^{-K \times \tau}}$$

Thus, the extent of accumulation is dependent not only on the pharmacokinetic properties of a drug but also on the multiple-dosing regimen chosen.

Fluctuation

The degree of fluctuation between peak and trough concentrations during one dosing interval—that is, $C_{ss,\max}$ and $C_{ss,\min}$—is determined by the relationship between elimination half-life $t_{1/2}$ and dosing interval τ:

$$Fluctuation = \frac{C_{ss,\max} - C_{ss,\min}}{C_{ss,\min}}$$

Multiple-Dosing Regimens: First-Order Input (Oral Dosing)

The average steady-state concentration $C_{ss,av}$ is now determined by the bioavailable fraction *F* of the dose *D* administered per dosing interval τ and the clearance *CL*:

$$C_{ss,av} = \frac{F \times D}{\tau \times CL}$$

The concentration-time profile after a single oral dose is given by

$$C = \frac{F \times D \times k_a}{V \times (k_a - K)} \times \left(e^{-K \times t} - e^{-k_a \times t} \right)$$

Hence, the concentration at any time within a dosing interval during multiple dosing at steady state is determined by

$$C = \frac{F \times D \times k_a}{V \times (k_a - K)} \times \left(\frac{e^{-K \times t}}{1 - e^{-K \times \tau}} - \frac{e^{-k_a \times t}}{1 - e^{-k_a \times \tau}} \right)$$

Thus, the trough concentration is readily available, if one assumes that the absorption is completed:

$$C_{ss,min} = \frac{F \times D \times k_a}{V \times (k_a - K)} \times \left(\frac{e^{-K \times \tau}}{1 - e^{-K \times \tau}} \right)$$

The peak concentration is assessable via the time-to-peak t_{max}, which is dependent on the rate of absorption and has to be determined through

$$t_{max} = \frac{\ln \left(\frac{k_a \times (1 - e^{-k_e \times \tau})}{K \times (1 - e^{-K \times \tau})} \right)}{(k_a - K)}$$

7-7. Volumes of Distribution and Protein Binding

Drug distribution means the reversible transfer of drug from one location to another within the body. After the drug has entered the vascular system, it becomes distributed throughout the various tissues and body fluids. However, most drugs do not distribute uniformly and in a similar manner throughout the body, as reflected by the difference in their volumes of distribution. Thus, the following material focuses on the factors and processes determining the rate and extent of distribution and the resulting consequences for pharmacotherapy.

Following are factors affecting distribution:

- Binding to blood or tissue elements
- Blood flow (i.e., the delivery of drug to the tissues)
- Ability to cross biomembranes
- Physicochemical properties of the drug (lipophilicity, extent of ionization) that determine partitioning into tissues

Protein Binding

The fraction unbound in plasma varies widely among drugs. Drugs are classified as follows:

- Highly protein bound:

$$f_u \leq 0.1 (\leq 10\% \text{ unbound}, \geq 90\% \text{ bound})$$

- Moderately protein bound:

$$f_u = 0.1 - 0.4 (10 - 40\% \text{ unbound}, 60 - 90\% \text{ bound})$$

- Low protein bound:

$$f_u \geq 0.4 (\geq 40\% \text{ unbound}, \leq 60\% \text{ bound})$$

Factors Determining the Degree of Protein Binding

The reversible binding of a drug to proteins obeys the law of mass action,

$$[\text{Drug}] + [\text{Protein}] \underset{k_1}{\overset{k_2}{\rightleftharpoons}} [\text{Drug-Protein-Complex}]$$

where the expressions in brackets represent the molar concentrations of the components, and k_1 and k_2 are rate constants for the forward and reverse reactions, respectively. The equilibrium association constant K_a is defined as k_1/k_2.

This reaction results in the following relationship for the fraction unbound:

$$f_u = \frac{1}{1 + \frac{N}{(1/K_a) + C_u}}$$

where N is the number of available binding sites and C_u is the unbound concentration.

Binding Proteins

Human plasma contains more than 60 proteins. Of these, three proteins account for the binding of most drugs. Albumin, which comprises approximately 60% of total plasma protein, fully accounts for the plasma binding of most anionic drugs and many endogenous anions (high-capacity, low-affinity binding site). Many cationic and neutral drugs bind appreciably to α_1-acid glycoprotein (high-affinity, low-capacity binding site) or lipoproteins in addition to albumin. Other proteins, such as transcortin, thyroid-binding globulin, and certain antibodies have specific affinities for a small number of drugs.

Volumes of Distribution

Volume of distribution at steady-state V_{ss}

The volume of distribution at steady state is by definition the sum of the pharmacokinetic volumes of distribution for the different pharmacokinetic compartments. It is the theoretical

$$V_{ss} = V_p + \frac{f_u}{f_{u,t}} \times V_t$$

where V_p is the volume of plasma (3 L); V_t is the volume of tissue water (total body water minus plasma volume: $42 - 3 = 39$ L based on a "standard" person);

and f_u and f_{ut} are the fraction unbound for the drug in plasma and in tissue, respectively.

Besides physicochemical properties of the drug, the relationship for V_{ss} shows that the extent of distribution is largely determined by the differences in protein binding in plasma and tissue, respectively:

$$V_{ss} = 3L + \frac{f_u}{f_{ut}} \times 39L$$

Unbound steady-state concentrations

The average steady-state concentration during a multiple-dose regimen or during a constant rate infusion is determined by

$$C_{ss} = \frac{Dose\ rate}{CL} = \frac{Dose\ rate}{f_u \times CL_u}$$

The free steady-state concentration $C_{ss,u}$ is given by

$$C_{ss,u} = f_u \times C_{ss}$$

Thus, the unbound steady-state concentration $C_{ss,u}$ is determined by

$$\frac{C_{ss,u}}{f_u} = \frac{Dose\ rate}{f_u \times CL_u} \Rightarrow C_{ss,u} = \frac{Dose\ rate}{CL_u}$$

7-8. Bioavailability and Bioequivalence

The Food and Drug Administration (FDA) (21 Code of Federal Regulations 320) defines *bioavailability* as "the rate and extent to which the active ingredient or active moiety is absorbed from a drug product and becomes available at the site of action." Because, in practice, drug concentrations can rarely be determined at the site of action (e.g., at a receptor site), bioavailability is more commonly defined as "the rate and extent that the active drug is absorbed from a dosage form and becomes available in the systemic circulation."

Following are factors affecting bioavailability:

- Drug product formulation
- Properties of the drug (salt form, crystalline structure, formation of solvates, and solubility)
- Composition of the finished dosage form (presence or absence of excipients and special coatings)
- Manufacturing variables (tablet compression force, processing variables, particle size of drug or excipients, and environmental conditions)

- Rate and site of dissolution in the gastrointestinal tract
- Physiology

With respect to physiology, the following factors affect bioavailability:

- Contents of the gastrointestinal tract (fluid volume and pH, diet, presence or absence of food, bacterial activity, and presence of other drugs)
- Rate of gastrointestinal tract transit (influenced by disease, physical activity, drugs, emotional status of subject, and composition of the gastrointestinal tract contents)
- Presystemic drug metabolism or degradation (influenced by local blood flow; condition of the gastrointestinal tract membranes; and drug transport, metabolism, or degradation in the gastrointestinal tract or during the first pass of the drug through the liver)

Absolute Bioavailability

Absolute bioavailability is the fraction (or percentage) of a dose administered nonintravenously (or extravascularly) that is systemically available as compared to an intravenous dose. If given orally, absolute bioavailability (*F*) is

$$F = \frac{AUC_{PO}}{AUC_{IV}} \times \frac{D_{IV}}{D_{PO}}$$

Relative Bioavailability

Relative bioavailability refers to a comparison of two or more dosage forms in terms of their relative rate and extent of absorption:

$$F = \frac{AUC_{test\ formulation}}{AUC_{reference}} \times \frac{D_{reference}}{D_{test\ formulation}}$$

Bioequivalence

Two dosage forms that do not differ significantly in their rate and extent of absorption are termed *bioequivalent*. In general, bioequivalence evaluations involve comparisons of dosage forms that are

- *Pharmaceutical equivalents:* Drug products that contain identical amounts of the identical active drug ingredient (i.e., the same salt or ester of the same therapeutic moiety, in identical dosage forms)
- *Pharmaceutical alternatives:* Drug products that contain the identical therapeutic moiety, or its precursor, but not necessarily in the same amount or dosage form or as the same salt or ester

Biopharmaceutics Classification System

With minor exceptions, the FDA requires that bioavailability and bioequivalence of a drug product be demonstrated through in vivo studies. However, the Biopharmaceutics Classification System (BCS) can be used to justify the waiver of the requirement for in vivo studies for rapidly dissolving drug products containing active moieties or active ingredients that are highly soluble and highly permeable (Class 1 drugs).

The BCS divides drugs into classes on the basis of their solubility and permeability:

- Class 1: high solubility and high permeability
- Class 2: low solubility and high permeability
- Class 3: high solubility and low permeability
- Class 4: low solubility and low permeability

7-9. Elimination and Clearance Concepts

Clearance is defined as the irreversible removal of a drug from the body by an organ of elimination. Because the units of CL are flow (e.g., mL/minute or L/h), CL is often defined as the volume of blood irreversibly cleared of a drug per unit of time.

CL by the eliminating organ (CL_{organ}) is defined as the product of blood flow (Q) to the organ and the ER of that organ:

$$CL_{organ} = Q \times ER$$

Individual organ clearances are additive. For the majority of drugs used clinically, the liver is the major—and sometimes only—site of metabolism; the kidneys are the major site of excretion for drugs and metabolites. Thus, the equation for total clearance can be written to include renal clearance (CL_R) and hepatic clearance (CL_H):

$$CL = CL_R + CL_H$$

The fraction of drug excreted unchanged by the kidneys (f_e) indicates what fraction of the drug administered will be excreted into the urine:

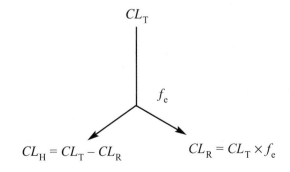

7-10. Renal Clearance

Drugs may undergo three processes in the kidney. Two act to remove a drug from the body: *filtration* and *secretion*. The other acts to return a drug to the body: *reabsorption*. Thus, one may express renal clearance of a drug as follows:

$$CL_R = \left[CL_{filtration} + CL_{secretion} \right] \times \left(1 - f_{reabsorbed} \right)$$

Calculating Filtration Clearance of Creatinine

Normal serum concentrations of creatinine are 0.8–1.3 mg/dL for men and 0.6–1 mg/dL for women.

Creatinine is a useful marker of renal function because it is an endogenous by-product of muscle breakdown. The kidney eliminates creatinine at a rate approximately equal to the glomerular filtration rate (GFR). A number of formulas have been developed that allow creatinine clearance (CL_{cr}) to be estimated from serum creatinine concentrations. The most widely used clinically is the Cockroft–Gault equation:

$$CL_{cr} = \frac{(140 - age) \times IBW}{S_{cr} \times 72}$$

$$\left(\text{multiply by } 0.85 \text{ if patient is female} \right)$$

where S_{cr} is the serum creatinine concentration in mg/dL, and IBW is the ideal body weight.

$$IBW_{males}(kg) = 50 + (2.3 \times \text{height in inches} > 5 \, ft)$$

$$IBW_{females}(kg) = 45.5 + (2.3 \times \text{height in inches} > 5 \, ft)$$

Secretion Clearance

A drug in blood may also be secreted into the kidney tubule. This process occurs against a concentration gradient (concentration of a drug in the kidney tubule is very high because of water reabsorption) and therefore is an active process.

Cellular processes (e.g., presence of active transporters) exist to facilitate tubular secretion. The two most well characterized of these processes include transporters responsible for the secretion of basic (anionic) and acidic (anionic) drugs.

Reabsorption

Passive reabsorption of many drugs also occurs in the kidneys. Because reabsorption is a passive process (i.e., diffusion), reabsorption will depend on the physicochemical properties of the drug (e.g., molecular weight, polarity, and acid disassociation content pK_a).

Weak bases: $B + H^+ \Leftrightarrow BH^+$
Low urine pH = more ionized, less reabsorption
High urine pH = less ionized, more reabsorption

Thus, only weak bases with pK_a between 6 and 12 show changes in the extent of reabsorption (and thus CL_R) with changes in urine pH.

Weak acids: $HA \Leftrightarrow A^- + H^+$
Low urine pH = less ionized, more reabsorption
High urine pH = more ionized, less reabsorption

Thus, only weak acids with pK_a in the range of 3 to 7.5 show changes in the extent of reabsorption (and thus CL_R) with changes in urine pH.

All drugs that are not bound to plasma proteins are filtered; therefore, filtration clearance is

$$CL_{\text{filtration}} = f_{\text{up}} \times GFR = 125\,\text{mL/minute}$$

Some drugs are secreted or reabsorbed, or both. One can determine the net process a drug undergoes by calculating the excretion ratio (E_{ratio}):

$$E_{\text{ratio}} = \frac{CL_R}{CL_{\text{filtration}}} = \frac{CL_R}{f_{\text{up}} \times 125\,\text{mL/minute}}$$

7-11. Hepatic Clearance

The fraction of drug escaping first-pass metabolism (F^*) can be described in terms of the hepatic extraction ratio:

$$F^* = 1 - ER$$

The overall oral bioavailability (F) of a drug is dependent on the fraction absorbed (f_a), the fraction escaping metabolism in the intestinal wall (f_g), and the fraction escaping hepatic first-pass metabolism (F^*).

$$F = f_a \times f_g \times F^*$$

Venous Equilibrium Model for Hepatic Clearance

The venous equilibrium model relates hepatic extraction ratio ER to its determinants as follows:

$$ER = \frac{f_{\text{up}} \times CL_{\text{int}}}{Q + f_{\text{up}} \times CL_{\text{int}}}$$

and (remembering that $CL_H = Q_H \times ER_H$)

$$CL_H = \frac{Q \times f_{\text{up}} \times CL_{\text{int}}}{Q + f_{\text{up}} \times CL_{\text{int}}}$$

The fraction of drug escaping hepatic first-pass metabolism using the venous equilibrium model is

$$F^* = \frac{Q}{Q + f_{\text{up}} \times CL_{\text{int}}}$$

Drugs undergoing hepatic metabolism can be divided into three broad categories:

1. Low-extraction drugs: $ER < 0.3$ and thus $F^* > 0.7$
2. Intermediate-extraction drugs: $0.3 < ER < 0.7$ and thus $0.3 < F^* < 0.7$
3. High-extraction drugs: $ER > 0.7$ and thus $F^* < 0.3$

Determinants of Hepatic Clearance

Thus, the determinants of hepatic extraction ratio, hepatic clearance, and the fraction escaping hepatic first-pass metabolism are liver blood flow (Q), protein binding (f_{up}), and CL_{int}.

For some drugs, hepatic clearance is limited or restricted to the unbound or free drug ($ER < f_{\text{up}}$). This is known as *restrictive clearance*. Because clearance is limited to unbound drug, changes in protein binding will alter the concentration of the drug that is available for elimination.

Some drugs defy this principle so that the hepatic extraction ratio is greater than the fraction of drug unbound in plasma ($ER > f_{\text{up}}$). When this occurs, it suggests that drug clearance is not restricted to unbound drug. Drugs behaving in this manner are said to undergo *nonrestrictive clearance*. Because nonrestrictive clearance is not limited to the fraction unbound in plasma, changes in protein binding will *not* alter the concentration of drug that is available for elimination (i.e., all of a drug is available for elimination regardless of whether it is bound or unbound).

Intrinsic clearance (CL_{int}) is defined as the intrinsic ability of the hepatic enzymes to eliminate a drug when blood flow or protein binding causes no limitations. CL_{int} is a measure of the capacity and affinity of drug-metabolizing enzymes (e.g., CYP450s) for the drug. The determinants of CL_{int}

can be explained using the Michaelis–Menten equation:

$$\upsilon = \frac{V_{\max} \times C_{\mathrm{u}}}{K_{\mathrm{m}} + C_{\mathrm{u}}} \text{ and } CL_{\mathrm{u}} = \frac{V_{\max}}{K_{\mathrm{m}} + C_{\mathrm{u}}}$$

where υ is the rate of drug metabolism (amount/time), $V_{\max}$ is the maximal rate of metabolism for a given metabolic pathway (amount/time), K_{m} is the concentration of the drug at which the rate of metabolism is half-maximal (amount/volume), and C_{u} is the unbound drug concentration (amount/volume).

Physiologically, $V_{\max}$ describes the quantity (capacity) of a drug-metabolizing enzyme to metabolize a drug. K_{m} describes the interaction between the drug-metabolizing enzyme and the drug.

Factors that affect CL_{int} are

- *Enzyme induction:* Enzyme induction refers to an increased number (capacity) of drug-metabolizing enzymes, which results in an increase in clearance. An increased number (capacity) of drug-metabolizing enzymes results in an increase in $V_{\max}$ and CL_{int}.
- *Enzyme inhibitors:* Competitive inhibition of the drug-metabolizing enzyme by another drug increases the apparent K_{m} (i.e., a higher concentration of drug will be required to achieve a half-maximal rate of metabolism). Increase in apparent K_{m} results in decrease in CL_{int}.

An extensive list of potential P450 inducers and inhibitors can be found at www.drug-interactions.com.

7-12. Drug, Disease, and Dietary Influences on Absorption, Distribution, Metabolism, and Excretion

Pharmacokinetics is the science of a drug's fate in the body. Typical reported pharmacokinetic parameters are determined in healthy individuals. However, drugs are prescribed to individuals with one or more altered physiological or pathological conditions. *Clinical pharmacokinetics* focuses on tailoring therapeutic dosing regimens to individuals on the basis of these altered physiological and pathological states. Thus, it is important to consider patient-specific factors that potentially contribute to drug interactions: drug–drug, drug–disease, and drug–dietary factors.

Drug interactions alter the effects of a drug by reaction with another drug or drugs, with foods or beverages, or with a preexisting medical condition. Drug interactions can be broadly classified as

- Drug–drug
- Drug–disease
- Drug–diet

Drug–Drug Interactions

- Induction of CYP450 enzymes
  - An increased number ($V_{\max}$) of drug-metabolizing enzymes leads to increased clearance.
  - Example: Rifampin increases clearance of warfarin.
- Inhibition of cytochrome P450 enzymes
  - Competitive inhibition of the drug-metabolizing enzyme by another drug leads to increase in apparent K_{m}, which leads to decreased clearance.
  - Example: Cimetidine decreases the clearance of warfarin.
- Inhibition of drug efflux transporter P-glycoprotein
  - Competitive inhibition of P-glycoprotein occurs.
- Decreased renal clearance for drugs undergoing net secretion
  - Example: Quinidine inhibits the renal secretion of digoxin.
- Increased f_{a} and F
  - Example: Ketoconazole increases the oral absorption of cyclosporine.
- Protein-binding displacement
  - A drug or drugs is displaced from major binding proteins.
- Increased f_{up}
- Increased volume of distribution
- Increased clearance for restrictively cleared drugs
  - Example: Aspirin displaces warfarin from albumin, leading to an increased distribution and clearance for warfarin.

Drug–Disease Interactions

Cardiovascular disease

Reduced cardiac output associated with congestive heart failure leads to reduced perfusion of key eliminating organs such as the liver and kidney. The following pharmacokinetic effects have been reported:

- Decreased absorption rate (e.g., digoxin, hydrochlorothiazide, procainamide, and quinidine)
- Prolonged hepatic clearance for high extraction ($E > 0.7$) drugs (e.g., lidocaine and theophylline)
- Reduced volume of distribution (e.g., digoxin)

Renal disease

Creatinine clearance is commonly used to assess renal function, and the CL_R of many drugs is known to vary in proportion to CL_{cr}. Thus, renal impairment can be inferred from changes in CL_{cr}.

CL_{cr} is most often estimated by measuring serum creatinine concentration, using the Cockroft–Gault equation, as discussed previously.

Serum creatinine concentrations remain relatively constant (about 1 mg/dL) in adults over age 20. However, patients with compromised renal function may exhibit higher concentrations.

Renal function (RF) in a patient may be estimated by comparing the patient's creatinine clearance to what CL_{cr} would be in a normal individual (i.e., $f_{up} \times GFR$ or 125 mL/minute).

$$ RF = \frac{CL_{cr}^{patient}}{CL_{cr}^{normal}} = \frac{CL_{cr}^{patient}}{125 \text{ mL/minute}} $$

Use of this equation to estimate RF assumes the intact nephron hypothesis (i.e., that renal disease results in the dysfunction of a certain fraction of nephrons but allows the remaining nephrons to remain intact).

To individualize drug treatment in patients with renal impairment, one needs to know the drug clearance *in a patient*. This knowledge will allow one to calculate the dose rate of the drug that will maintain an individualized C_{target}. Clearance in a patient with renal impairment will be designated CL^*. Three parameters are needed to calculate CL^*:

- CL of the drug and f_e in normal subjects. These values can be found in textbooks, primary literature, or package inserts.
- RF in a patient is usually estimated using a recent serum creatinine concentration and the equations presented above.

One can then calculate clearance in your patient with renal impairment using the following equation:

$$ CL^* = CL \times \left[1 - f_e \times \left(1 - RF \right) \right] $$

CL^* represents *total* clearance in the renally impaired individual.

Liver disease

Hepatic disease results in numerous pathophysiologic changes in the liver that may influence drug pharmacokinetics, including the following:

- Reduction in liver blood flow
  - Decreased clearance for high-extraction drugs

- Reduction in number and activity of hepatocytes
  - Decreased first-pass metabolism for high-extraction drugs
  - Decreased clearance for low-extraction drugs
- Impaired production of human serum albumin
  - Increased distribution of drugs

Drug–Diet Interactions

- Drug–food interactions
  - Type I: Ex vivo bioinactivation
  - Type II: Interactions affecting oral absorption
  - Type III: Interactions affecting systemic disposition
  - Type IV: Interactions affecting either renal or hepatic clearance
- Ex vivo bioinactivation
  - It typically occurs in the delivery device before drugs enter body.
  - Interaction occurs between the drug and the nutritional element or formulation through biochemical or physical reactions.
  - Interaction examples include hydrolysis, oxidation, neutralization, precipitation, and complexation.
  - High ethanol content may precipitate inorganic salts present in enteral feeding formulas.
  - Syrups are acidic solvents and may cause precipitation of inorganic salts.
- Interactions affecting absorption
  - This type of interaction affects drugs and nutrients delivered by mouth only.
  - It may result in either an increase or a decrease in oral bioavailability.
  - The interacting agent may alter function of either the metabolizing enzyme (e.g., CYP3A4) or the active transport protein (e.g., P-glycoprotein).
  - Meal intake alters oral absorption through mechanisms involving altered (1) gastric pH, (2) gastrointestinal transit time, and (3) dissolution of solid dosage forms.
  - Grapefruit juice inactivates gut CYP3A4, enhancing oral absorption of CYP3A4 substrates (e.g., cyclosporine, midazolam, and nifedipine).
- Interactions affecting systemic disposition
  - These interactions occur after drug or nutrient has entered the systemic circulation.
  - They involve alteration in tissue disposition or response.
  - Example: Foods high in vitamin K (e.g., broccoli) can alter systemic clotting factors, reducing effectiveness of warfarin.

- Interactions affecting either renal or hepatic clearance
  - These interactions arise from modification of drug elimination mechanisms in the liver, kidney, or both.
  - Acute ethanol ingestion may potentiate central nervous system effects of benzodiazepines (e.g., alprazolam).

7-13. The Pharmacokinetic–Pharmacodynamic Interface

Pharmacokinetics (PK) establishes the relationship between dose and concentration. *Pharmacodynamics* (PD) establishes the relationship between concentration and effect. When individualizing pharmacotherapy, one must account for both PK and PD variability. For a number of drugs, the PK variability is much larger than the PD variability. Thus, concentration-based therapeutic drug monitoring is useful for a number of drugs (e.g., theophylline). However, for some drugs, PD variability exceeds PK variability.

Linking the PK and PD allows a more thorough understanding of the effect of dosage adjustments on pharmacologic response.

The simple E_{max} model represents the most widely used model to describe the relationship between drug concentration and effect:

$$Intensity\ of\ effect = E = \frac{E_{max} \times C}{EC_{50} + C}$$

where E_{max} is the maximum effect possible (intrinsic activity) and EC_{50} is the concentration achieving 50% maximal effect (potency).

Figure 7-1 illustrates the three concentration-dependent phases as follows:

- Linear phase (1)
  - Drug concentration is much smaller than EC_{50} ($C << EC_{50}$).
  - A linear relationship exists between concentration C and effect E:

$$E = \frac{E_{max} \times C}{EC_{50}}$$

- Constant phase (3)
  - Drug concentration is much larger than EC_{50} ($C >> EC_{50}$).
  - Effect E is independent of concentration:

$$E = E_{max}$$

Figure 7-1. The Three Concentration-Dependent Phases

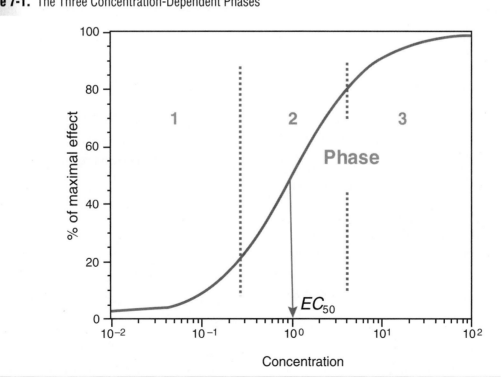

- Log-linear phase (2)
  - A log-linear relationship exists between C and E when E is between 20% and 80% of E_{max}. $E_{max}/4$ is the slope describing this relationship:

$$E = \frac{E_{max}}{4} \times \ln C + \frac{E_{max}}{4} \times \left(\ln EC_{50} + 2 \right)$$

7-14. Hysteresis

Response is linked to concentration and time. In other words, a given concentration may have a different effect depending on time. Therefore, the concentration–effect relationship is described by a *hysteresis loop*, which may be either clockwise or counterclockwise.

- Counterclockwise hysteresis
  - Distributional delay to effect site
  - Indirect response mechanism
  - Active metabolite (agonism)
  - Sensitization
- Clockwise hysteresis
  - Functional tolerance
  - Active metabolite (antagonism)

7-15. Clinical Examples

Clinical Example 1

A patient (55 years old, weighing 73 kg) was started on a multiple-dose regimen with gentamicin 80 mg every 8 hours given as IV short-term infusion over 30 minutes. Because his infection is serious, it is decided to target for a peak concentration of 10 mg/L and a trough concentration of 1 mg/L. Three blood samples were drawn 30 minutes prior to the third dose and 30 minutes and 7 hours after the end of the infusion of the third dose, respectively. The measured plasma concentrations are 1.73, 5.96, and 1.80 mg/L, respectively.

Optimize the gentamicin dosing regimen on the basis of the individual pharmacokinetic parameters of the patient to achieve the therapeutically targeted concentrations.

- *Step 1:* Calculate the elimination rate constant K:

$$K = \frac{\ln\left(\dfrac{C_{max}^*}{C_{min}^*}\right)}{\Delta t} = \frac{\ln\left(\dfrac{5.96}{1.80}\right)}{(8-1-0.5)\,h} = 0.184 \ h^{-1}$$

- *Step 2:* Calculate volume of distribution V:

$$C_{max} = \frac{C_{max}^*}{e^{-K \times t^*}} = \frac{5.96 \ \text{mg/L}}{e^{-0.184 \ h^{-1} \times 0.5 \ h}} = 6.53 \ \text{mg/L}$$

$$C_{min} = C_{min}^* \times e^{-K \times t^*}$$
$$= 1.73 \ \text{mg/L} \times e^{-0.184 \ h^{-1} \times 0.5 \ h} = 1.58 \ \text{mg/L}$$

$$V = \frac{R_0}{K} \times \frac{1 - e^{-K \times T_{inf}}}{C_{max} - C_{min} \times e^{-K \times T_{inf}}}$$

$$= \frac{80 \ \text{mg}}{0.184 \ h^{-1} \times 0.5 \ h}$$

$$\times \frac{1 - e^{-0.184 \ h^{-1} \times 0.5 \ h}}{6.53 \ \text{mg/L} - 1.58 \times e^{-0.184 \ h^{-1} \times 0.5 \ h}}$$

$$= 15 \ \text{L}$$

- *Step 3:* Calculate recommended dosing interval τ:

$$\tau = \frac{\ln\left(\dfrac{C_{ss,max(desired)}}{C_{ss,min(desired)}}\right)}{K} + T_{inf} = \frac{\ln\left(\dfrac{10}{1}\right)}{0.184 \ h^{-1}} + 0.5 \ h$$

$$= 13 \ h$$

The practically reasonable, recommended dosing interval is 12 hours.

- *Step 4:* Calculate recommended dose D:

$$D = C_{ss,max(desired)} \times K \times V \times T_{inf} \times \frac{1 - e^{-K \times \tau}}{1 - e^{-K \times T_{inf}}}$$

$$D = 10 \ \text{mg/L} \times 0.184 \ h^{-1} \times 15 \ \text{L} \times 0.5 \ h$$

$$\times \frac{1 - e^{-0.184 \ h^{-1} \times 12 \ h}}{1 - e^{-0.184 \ h^{-1} \times 0.5 \ h}} = 139.7 \ \text{mg}$$

The recommended dosing regimen is 140 mg every 12 hours.

- *Step 5:* Check expected peak $C_{ss,max}$ and trough $C_{ss,min}$:

$$C_{ss,max} \frac{R_0}{K \times V} \times \frac{1 - e^{-K \times T_{inf}}}{1 - e^{-K \times \tau}} = \frac{140 \ \text{mg}}{0.184 \ h^{-1} \times 15 \ \text{L} \times 0.5 \ h}$$

$$\times \frac{1 - e^{-0.184 \ h^{-1} \times 0.5 \ h}}{1 - e^{-0.184 \ h^{-1} \times 12 \ h}} = 10 \ \text{mg/L}$$

$$C_{ss,min} = C_{ss,max} \times e^{-K \times (\tau - T_{inf})}$$

$$= 10 \ \text{mg/L} \times e^{-0.184 \ h^{-1} \times (12 \ h - 0.5 \ h)} = 1.21 \ \text{mg/L}$$

Clinical Example 2

A 70-year-old white male weighing 95 lb is 5 feet tall and has a serum creatinine of 1.1 mg/dL. He is admitted to the hospital complaining of shortness of breath; he denies chest pain. Digoxin is prescribed for him. You are asked to design a dosage regimen using tablets for him to achieve and maintain a $C_{target,ss}$ of 1 ng/mL. The PK parameters for digoxin are as follows: CL = 2.7 mL/minute/kg (total body weight, or TBW); f_e = 0.68; V_{ss} = 6.7 L/kg (IBW); F of tablet = 0.75.

- **Step 1:** Estimate CL, CL_{cr}, RF, and CL^* of digoxin in this patient.

    IBW = 45.5 kg; TBW = 43 kg. Therefore, use TBW for all calculations.
    CL for a normal 43 kg patient = 116 mL/minute.
    CL_{cr} and RF are

$$CL_{cr} = \frac{(140-70) \times 43}{1.1 \times 72} = 38 \text{ mL/minute}$$

$$RF = \frac{38 \text{ mL/minute}}{125 \text{ mL/minute}} = 0.304$$

- **Step 2:** Estimate CL^* of digoxin in this patient with renal impairment:

$$CL^* = 116 \text{ mL/minute} \times \left[1 - 0.68(1 - 0.304)\right]$$
$$= 61.1 \text{ mL/minute}$$

- **Step 3:** Calculate Dose Rate*:

$$\text{Dose Rate}^* = \frac{1 \text{ ng/mL} \times 61.1 \text{ mL/minute}}{0.75}$$
$$= 81.5 \text{ ng/minute}$$

- **Step 4:** Determine dosing interval τ^* by estimating the half-life of digoxin:

$$\tau^*_{1/2} = \frac{0.693 \times V_{ss}}{CL^*}$$

V_{ss} (V_d) for digoxin from PK tables is 6.7 L/kg, or 289 L in this patient. Thus,

$$\tau^*_{1/2} = \frac{0.693 \times 289 \text{ L}}{0.061 \text{ L/minute}} = 3{,}283 \text{ minutes} \cong 55 \text{ hours}$$

Digoxin is normally administered every 24 hours (τ = 24 h); it could be administered 0.25 mg every 48 hours (τ = 48 h). Here, however, changing the dosing interval is not recommended, because 24 hours is very convenient, and the resultant peak:trough ratio would be lower with τ = 24 h as compared with τ = 48 h.

Clinical Example 3

A. M. is a 61-year-old white male, 6 feet tall, weighing 195 lb. He has a diagnosis of pneumonia. His serum creatinine is 2.3 mg/dL. Design a dosage regimen of gentamicin to achieve C_{peak} and C_{trough} values of 8 mg/L and 1 mg/L, respectively. V_d = 0.2 L/kg IBW.

- **Step 1:** The CL of gentamicin is 85 mL/minute and the f_e = 1.0. Calculate the degree of renal impairment:

$$CL = CL_{cr} = \frac{(140-61) \times 77.6}{2.3(72)} = 37 \text{ mL/minute}$$

$$RF = \frac{37 \text{ mL/minute}}{125 \text{ mL/minute}} = 0.296$$

- **Step 2:** Calculate the CL^* of gentamicin in this patient:

$$CL^* = 85 \text{ mL/minute} \times \left[1 - 1 \times (1 - 0.296)\right]$$
$$= 25.2 \text{ mL/minute} = 1.5 \text{ L/h}$$

- **Step 3:** Calculate the elimination rate constant in this patient:

$$k = \frac{CL}{V_{ss}} = \frac{1.5 \text{ L/h}}{0.2 \text{ L/kg} \times 77.6 \text{ kg}} = 0.097 \text{ h}^{-1}$$

- **Step 4:** Calculate the infusion rate and dosing interval:

$$\tau = \frac{\ln\left(\dfrac{C_{ss,max(desired)}}{C_{ss,min(desired)}}\right)}{K} + T_{inf} = \frac{\ln\left(\dfrac{8 \text{ mg/L}}{1 \text{ mg/L}}\right)}{0.097 \text{ h}^{-1}} + 0.5 \text{ h}$$
$$= 22 \text{ hours} \cong 24 \text{ hours}$$

$$D = C_{ss,max} \times K \times V \times T_{inf} \times \frac{1 - e^{-K \times \tau}}{1 - e^{-K \times T_{inf}}}$$

$$= 8 \text{ mg/L} \times 0.097 \text{ h}^{-1} \times (0.2 \times 77.6) \times 0.5$$

$$\times \frac{1 - e^{-0.097 \text{ h}^{-1} \times 24}}{1 - e^{-0.097 \text{ h}^{-1} \times 0.5}}$$

$$= 115 \text{ mg} \cong 120 \text{ mg}$$

Clinical Example 4

Patient D. M. is a 50-year-old white male (weighing 74.1 kg) who is being treated for seizure control with phenytoin ($V_d = 0.6$ L/kg), 300 mg/day, using the capsule formulation. He has been taking phenytoin for 2 weeks. He experienced a seizure on day 14 of treatment. His blood level was 5.2 mg/L. His dose rate was increased to 400 mg/day of the capsule formulation. Three weeks later his blood level was 11.8 mg/L.

- Phenytoin capsules and parenteral solution = sodium phenytoin
- Phenytoin tablets and suspension = phenytoin acid
- 100 mg phenytoin sodium = 92 mg phenytoin acid
- **Step 1:** The V_{max} (mg/day) for phenytoin in patient D. M. is

  a. 491
  b. 499
  c. 542
  d. 590
  e. 614

Because D. M. is using capsules, you need to multiply the original dose rate by 0.92.

Dose rate (mg/day)	C_{ss} (mg/L)	Dose rate/C_{ss} (L/day)
300 × 0.92 = 276	5.2	53.08
400 × 0.92 = 368	11.8	31.19

$$DR = V_{max} - \left(\frac{DR}{C_{ss}}\right) \times K_m$$

$$Y = \text{intercept} + X \times (-\text{slope})$$

Plot DR vs DR/C_{ss}

Y-intercept = V_{max} = 499 mg/day phenytoin
slope = $-K_m$ = -4.2 mg/L; therefore K_m = 4.2 mg/L

- **Step 2:** What dosage regimen would you recommend to achieve an average steady-state phenytoin concentration of 15 mg/L in patient D. M. using the capsule formulation?

  a. 100 mg q6h
  b. 100 mg q8h
  c. 200 mg q6h
  d. 200 mg q8h

$$DR = CL \times C_{ss,target} = \frac{V_{max} \times C_{ss,target}}{K_m + C_{ss,target}}$$

$$= \frac{499 \text{ mg/day} \times 15 \text{ mg/L}}{4.2 \text{ mg/L} + 15 \text{ mg/L}} = 390 \text{ mg/day phenytoin}$$

390 mg/day phenytoin = 424 mg/day sodium phenytoin

Recommend 400 mg Dilantin Kapseals in three or four divided doses (e.g., 100 mg q6h).

- **Step 3:** Estimate the time required to achieve steady-state levels of phenytoin in patient D. M. at the dosage regimen if it were changed to 100 mg capsule q6h.

  a. 1 day
  b. 5 days
  c. 9 days
  d. 13 days
  e. 17 days

$$t_{90} = \frac{K_m \times V_{ss}}{(V_{max} - DR)^2} \times (2.3 \times V_{max} - 0.9 \times DR)$$

$$t_{90} = \frac{4.2 \text{ mg phenytoin/L} \times 0.6 \text{ L/kg} \times 74.1 \text{ kg}}{(499 \text{ mg phenytoin} - 368 \text{ mg phenytoin/day})^2}$$

$$\times (2.3 \times 499 \text{ mg phenytoin/day}) - 0.9$$

$$\times 368 \text{ mg phenytoin/day}$$

$$t_{90} = 8.9 \text{ days}$$

About 9 days are needed to reach 90% of new steady-state plasma concentration.

- **Step 4:** Calculate the loading dose of phenytoin in this patient that would be needed to achieve a phenytoin blood level of 12 mg/L. (Assume that blood levels of phenytoin = 0 at time of administration of the loading dose.)

  a. 491 mg
  b. 535 mg
  c. 580 mg
  d. 603 mg

$$LD = C_{ss,target} \times V_{ss} = 12 \text{ mg/L phenytoin} \times 0.6 \text{ L/kg}$$

$$\times 74.1 \text{ kg} = 534 \text{ mg phenytoin}$$

$$= 580 \text{ mg phenytoin sodium (parenteral)}$$

Clinical Example 5

To treat her asthma exacerbation, L. Y., a 68-year-old woman who weighs 55 kg, has received a continuous infusion of aminophylline (infusion rate 0.45 mg/kg/h) for 5 days. This morning, she suffers from theophylline toxicity indicated by tachycardia, headache, and dizziness. A blood sample is drawn, and the theophylline plasma concentration is 24.3 mg/L. The therapeutic range is 10–20 mg/L; the population average of the volume of distribution is 0.5 L/kg.

■ **Step 1:** What is the theophylline clearance in this patient under the assumption that steady state had already been reached at the time the blood sample was obtained?

a. 0.81 L/h
b. 0.95 L/h
c. 1.35 L/h
d. 2.15 L/h
e. 2.80 L/h

$$CL = \frac{R_0}{C_{ss}} = \frac{0.45 \text{ mg/kg/h} \times 0.8 \times 55 \text{ kg}}{24.3 \text{ mg/L}} = 0.81 \text{ L/h}$$

■ **Step 2:** To what aminophylline infusion rate should the infusion be reduced to achieve a steady-state concentration in the middle of the therapeutic range, that is, 15 mg/L?

a. 0.17 mg/kg/h
b. 0.18 mg/kg/h
c. 0.20 mg/kg/h
d. 0.22 mg/kg/h
e. 0.28 mg/kg/h

$$MD = C_{target} \times CL = 15 \text{ mg/L} \times 0.81 \text{ L/h}$$
$$= 12.15 \text{ mg/h theophylline}$$
$$= 15.2 \text{ mg/h aminophylline}$$

Because the patient weighs 55 kg, $MD = 0.28$ mg/kg/h.

■ **Step 3:** How long does it take approximately to achieve the new steady state after the infusion rate has been changed?

a. 26 hours
b. 68 hours
c. 118 hours
d. 156 hours
e. 192 hours

Estimated $V = 55$ kg $\times 0.5$ L/kg $= 27.5$ L

$$t_{1/2} = \frac{\ln 2}{K} = \frac{\ln 2 \times V}{CL} = \frac{0.693 \times 27.5 \text{ L}}{0.81 \text{ L/h}} = 23.5 \text{ h}$$

Time to new steady state approximately $5 \, t_{1/2} \approx 118$ hours

■ **Step 4:** The pharmacist suggests that the new target concentration can be achieved faster

if the first infusion with the higher infusion rate is completely stopped and the second infusion with the lower infusion rate is not initiated until the plasma concentration has decreased to 15 mg/L, the target concentration. Calculate the time the therapy has to pause (i.e., the time one waits after cessation of the first infusion before the second infusion is started).

a. 14.7 hours
b. 16.4 hours
c. 20.7 hours
d. 36.1 hours
e. 55.1 hours

$$C_{target} = C_{ss,old} \times e^{-K \times t_{pause}}$$

$$t_{pause} = \frac{\ln\left(\dfrac{C_{target}}{C_{ss,old}}\right)}{-K} = \frac{\ln\left(\dfrac{15 \text{ mg/L}}{24.3 \text{ mg/L}}\right) \times 27.5 \text{ L}}{-0.81 \text{ L/h}} = 16.4 \text{ h}$$

7-16. Questions

1. A pediatric patient receives an immuno-suppressive therapy with oral cyclosporine solution. His concentration-adjusted dosing regimen is 85 mg every 12 hours. Because of a recent change in his insurance coverage, he needs to be switched from the drug product he is currently using to a generic solution dosage form of cyclosporine that is covered by his insurance. The bioavailability of the dosage form he previously used is 43%; the bioavailability of the generic dosage form is 28%. What is the appropriate dosage regimen for the generic dosage form to maintain the same systemic exposure as obtained from the previously used dosage form?

A. 25 mg every 12 hours
B. 55 mg every 12 hours
C. 184 mg every 12 hours
D. 130 mg every 12 hours
E. 305 mg every 12 hours

2. A drug is administered via continuous infusion at a rate of 60 mg/h, resulting in a steady-state plasma concentration of 5 mcg/mL. If the plasma concentration is

intended to be doubled to 10 mcg/mL, the infusion rate must be

A. left the same.
B. increased by 30 mg/h.
C. increased by 60 mg/h.
D. increased by 120 mg/h.
E. decreased by 30 mg/h.

3. Valtrex (valacyclovir) is a pro-drug for the antiviral acyclovir. It is enzymatically converted to acyclovir in the intestine and the liver. Probenecid and cimetidine increase the mean acyclovir *AUC* by 48 and 27%. Neither cimetidine nor probenecid affects the absorption of valacyclovir. Assume a glomerular filtration rate of 125 mL/minute. The pharmacokinetic parameters for acyclovir after valacyclovir administration are

    Clearance: 255 mL/minute

    $f_e = 0.90$

    Plasma protein binding: 15%

    According to the above information, which of the following statements is accurate regarding acyclovir pharmacokinetics after oral administration of valacyclovir?

    A. Tagamet (cimetidine) and probenecid increase the acyclovir fraction absorbed (f_a).
    B. Acyclovir clearance would be increased by increasing urine pH.
    C. Changes in acyclovir *AUC* after co-administration of probenecid and cimetidine likely result from inhibition of acyclovir renal secretion.
    D. Cimetidine and probenecid alter acyclovir protein binding

4. Lidocaine will be given as a constant rate infusion for the treatment of ventricular arrhythmia. A plasma concentration of 3 mcg/mL was decided on as the therapeutic target concentration. The concentration of the infusion solution is 20 mg/mL lidocaine. The average volume of distribution of lidocaine is 90 L; the elimination half-life is 1.1 hours. What infusion rate (in mL/minute) has to be set on the infusion pump to achieve the desired target concentration?

    A. 5 mL/h
    B. 8.5 mL/h
    C. 14 mL/h
    D. 23.5 mL/h
    E. 194 mL/h

5. After termination of an intravenous constant rate infusion, the plasma concentration of a drug declines monoexponentially ($C = C_0 \times e^{-k \times t}$). Concentrations measured at 2 hours and 12 hours after the end of the infusion are 12.9 mcg/mL and 6 mcg/mL, respectively. Calculate the initial concentration at the end of the infusion, and predict the concentration 24 hours after termination of the infusion.

    A. 13.5 and 2.9 mcg/mL
    B. 16.5 and 3.8 mcg/mL
    C. 16.5 and 1.3 mcg/mL
    D. 15 and 2.4 mcg/mL
    E. 15 and 1.3 mcg/mL

6. Margaret Q. (100 kg, 26 years old) presents to the emergency room with acute symptoms of asthma. She recently started smoking again and has been taking oral theophylline for several years. The immediate determination of her theophylline plasma concentration results in a level of 4 mg/L.

    Theophylline population pharmacokinetic parameters: *CL* 0.04 L/h/kg; *V* 0.5 L/kg
    Therapeutic range: 10–20 mg/L

    What is the appropriate intravenous loading dose of aminophylline for Margaret to achieve a target concentration of 12 mg/L?

    A. 300 mg
    B. 400 mg
    C. 500 mg
    D. 600 mg
    E. 750 mg

7. For a drug product in clinical drug development, an oral dosing regimen needs to be established for a phase III study that maintains an average steady-state concentration of 50 ng/mL. In single-dose studies, an oral dose of 80 mg resulted in an *AUC* of 962 ng · h/mL and an elimination half-life of 10.3 hours. What dosing regimen should be used?

    A. 35 mg every 12 hours
    B. 50 mg every 12 hours
    C. 72 mg every 12 hours
    D. 95 mg every 12 hours
    E. 125 mg every 12 hours

8. Mary D. (68 kg, 47 years old) has recently received her first 0.25 mg dose of digoxin. Plasma digoxin concentrations 12 and 24 hours

following oral administration of this dose are 0.72 and 0.33 mcg/L, respectively. The therapeutic plasma concentration range is 0.8–2 mcg/L. Predict Mary's digoxin trough concentration at steady state, assuming that oral digoxin therapy is continued at a dose rate of 0.25 mg once daily.

A. 0.62 mcg/L
B. 0.93 mcg/L
C. 1.32 mcg/L
D. 1.57 mcg/L
E. 1.95 mcg/L

9. The population average values for the clearance and volume of distribution of nifedipine have been reported as 0.41 L/h/kg and 1.2 L/kg, respectively. What would be the maximum dosing interval you can use for a multiple-dose regimen with an immediate-release oral dosage form of nifedipine if peak-to-trough fluctuation should not exceed 100%?

A. 2 hours
B. 4 hours
C. 6 hours
D. 8 hours
E. 12 hours

10. Beth R. (58 kg, 63 years old) is suffering from symptomatic ventricular arrhythmia. She will be started on an oral multiple-dose regimen with the antiarrhythmic mexiletine. The population average values of mexiletine for clearance and volume of distribution are $CL = 0.5$ L/h/kg and $V = 6$ L/kg, respectively. Although a therapeutic range of 0.5–2 mg/L has been described, avoiding large peak-to-trough fluctuations is recommended. The available oral dosage forms are 150, 200, and 250 mg capsules with an oral bioavailability of $F = 0.9$. Design an appropriate and practically reasonable oral dosing regimen that keeps the plasma concentrations at an average concentration of approximately 1 mg/L, with a peak-to-trough fluctuation $\leq 100\%$ (e.g., with concentrations within the limits of 0.75 and 1.5 mg/L).

A. 150 mg q6h
B. 200 mg q6h
C. 200 mg q8h
D. 250 mg q8h
E. 375 mg q12h

11. Edgar W. (58 kg, 20 years old) is receiving 80 mg of gentamicin as IV infusion over a 30-minute period q8h. Two plasma samples are obtained to monitor serum gentamicin concentrations as follows: one sample 30 minutes after the end of the short-term infusion and one sample 30 minutes before the administration of the next dose. The serum gentamicin concentrations at these times are 4.9 and 1.7 mg/L, respectively. Assume steady state. Develop a practically reasonable dosing regimen that will produce peak and trough concentrations of approximately 8 and 1 mg/L, respectively.

A. 120 mg q8h
B. 160 mg q8h
C. 140 mg q12h
D. 180 mg q12h
E. 280 mg q24h

12. A patient who is receiving chronic phenytoin therapy is hospitalized for an elective surgical procedure. Admission labs note that the patient has a phenytoin concentration of 8 mcg/mL (therapeutic range: 10–20 mcg/mL) and an albumin concentration of 3 g/dL. Phenytoin: $F = 0.2$–0.9, CL-variable, < 1% excreted unchanged in the urine, 88–93% bound to plasma proteins (primarily albumin). Given this information and the therapeutic range of phenytoin, you would recommend that the physician

A. decrease the dose of phenytoin, because high-extraction drugs (e.g., phenytoin) exhibit increased unbound concentrations with increases in fraction unbound in the plasma.
B. increase the dose rate of phenytoin, because low-extraction drugs (e.g., phenytoin) exhibit increased CL with increases in fraction unbound in the plasma.
C. not change the dose rate of phenytoin because low-extraction drugs (e.g., phenytoin) do not exhibit changes in unbound concentrations with increases in fraction unbound in the plasma.
D. not change the dose rate of phenytoin because low-extraction drugs (e.g., phenytoin) exhibit equal and offsetting changes in CL and F with increases in fraction unbound in plasma.

13. Which of the following conditions indicate the possibility of renal clearance of a weakly acidic drug being sensitive to changes in urine pH?

    A. The drug is secreted and not reabsorbed.
    B. The drug has a pK_a value of 5.
    C. The drug has a small volume of distribution.
    D. All of the drug is excreted unchanged by the kidneys (i.e., $f_e = 1$).

14. A young man (73 kg, 28 years old, creatinine clearance 124 mL/minute) receives a single 200 mg oral dose of an antibiotic. The following pharmacokinetic parameters of the antibiotic are reported in the literature:

    $F = 90\%$
    $V_d = 0.31$ L/kg
    $t_{1/2} = 2.1$ h
    $f_{up} = 0.77$
    67% of the antibiotic's absorbed dose is excreted unchanged in the urine.

    Determine the renal clearance of the antibiotic. What is the probable mechanism for renal clearance of this drug?

    A. 84 mL/minute, glomerular filtration and tubular reabsorption
    B. 98 mL/minute, glomerular filtration and tubular reabsorption
    C. 112 mL/minute, glomerular filtration
    D. 167 mL/minute, glomerular filtration and tubular reabsorption
    E. 236 mL/minute, glomerular filtration and tubular secretion

15. The pharmacokinetic parameters for captopril in healthy adults are

    Clearance: 800 mL/minute
    $f_e = 0.5$
    V_{ss}: 0.81 L/kg
    Plasma protein binding: 75%

15a. Captopril is a weakly basic drug that is used in the treatment of hypertension. Assume a glomerular filtration rate of 125 mL/minute. What is (are) the mechanism(s) for renal clearance of captopril?

    A. Filtration only
    B. Reabsorption only
    C. Secretion only
    D. Filtration and net secretion
    E. Filtration and net reabsorption

15b. When cimetidine (a highly lipid soluble weak base that is highly secreted in the renal proximal tubules) and captopril are coadministered, the renal clearance of captopril is reduced to approximately 125 mL/minute. What is the most likely mechanism to account for this reduction in renal clearance?

    A. Cimetidine reduces the filtration clearance of captopril.
    B. Cimetidine enhances the reabsorption of captopril.
    C. Cimetidine increases the unbound fraction of captopril.
    D. Cimetidine blocks the renal secretion of captopril.

16. One of the most severe drug interactions is that between digoxin and quinidine. Administration of quinidine to patients taking digoxin results in a two- to threefold increase in digoxin C_{ss} and AUC after oral and intravenous administration of digoxin. Digoxin and quinidine are substrates for the multidrug resistance transporter, P-glycoprotein. According to the following pharmacokinetic data for digoxin, what is the most likely mechanism to explain this drug–drug interaction?

    CL: 125 mL/minute
    V_{ss}: 1.2 L/kg (IBW)
    f_e: > 0.99
    f_{up}: 0.25

    A. Quinidine reduces the digoxin fraction escaping first-pass metabolism.
    B. Quinidine inhibits renal secretion of digoxin by blocking P-glycoprotein.
    C. Quinidine decreases digoxin fraction reabsorbed in the kidney tubule.
    D. Quinidine reduces the fraction of digoxin absorbed.

17. The drug transporter P-glycoprotein is involved in numerous processes in drug disposition. P-glycoprotein activity is directly responsible for the following processes:

    I. Glomerular filtration
    II. Transport of drug from hepatocytes into the bile
    III. Transport of drug from the small intestine into the systemic circulation (i.e., bloodstream)

IV. Degradation of drug in the lumen of the duodenum

V. Maintenance of the integrity of the blood–brain barrier by transport of drug out of the brain

A. V only
B. II and V only
C. II and III only
D. I, II, and V only
E. All of the above

18. Inhibition of platelet aggregation by clopidogrel is due to an active metabolite formed by CYP2C19. Studies have shown that the proton pump inhibitor (PPI) omeprazole, a moderate CYP2C19 inhibitor, reduces clopidogrel's antiplatelet activity when given concomitantly or if given 12 hours apart. Consequently, the package insert for Plavix (clopidogrel) warns against concomitant use of Plavix and strong or moderate CYP2C19 inhibitors.

Which of the following dose regimens would you recommend for this patient?

A. The use of PPIs should be avoided in patients taking clopidogrel.
B. The PPI pantoprazole, a weak CYP2C19 inhibitor, should be considered as an acid-reducing agent in patients taking clopidogrel.
C. Concomitant use of CYP2C19 inducers would not be expected to affect the antiplatelet activity of clopidrogrel.
D. Individuals who lack the ability to metabolize clopidrogel because of a genetic polymorphism in CYP2C19 would experience increased antiplatelet activity when taking clopidrogrel.

19. J. D. is a 47-year-old white male who has been prescribed codeine for lower back pain. The pharmacist dispensing the medication remembers reading a study in which patients who took codeine with grapefruit juice experienced an enhanced analgesic effect. The study found that grapefruit juice enhanced oral bioavailability (*F*) of codeine. Interestingly, there was no effect on codeine hepatic clearance or volume of distribution. Thus, the pharmacist counseled the patient not to take his codeine with grapefruit juice. Based on the pharmacokinetic data for codeine (listed below), what is the most likely explanation

for the enhanced oral bioavailability of codeine?

CL: 1,350 mL/minute
f_e: 0.10
V_{ss}: 3.3 L/kg
Plasma protein binding: 35%

A. Grapefruit juice increases the absorption (f_a) of codeine.
B. Grapefruit juice decreases the fraction escaping first-pass metabolism (*F**).
C. Grapefruit juice increases renal secretion of codeine.
D. Grapefruit juice increases the fraction escaping first-pass metabolism (*F**).

20. The pharmacokinetic parameters for codeine in healthy adults are as follows:

Oral *F*: 50%
$f_e < 0.01$
V_{ss}: 2.6 L/kg
Plasma protein binding: 7%

Codeine is well absorbed ($f_a = 1$, $f_g = 0.8$). You may assume that hepatic blood flow in a 70 kg adult is 1,350 mL/minute. The hepatic clearance of codeine is

A. 851 mL/minute.
B. 1,350 mL/minute.
C. 500 mL/minute.
D. 675 mL/minute.

7-17. Answers

1. **D.** The systemic exposure or average steady-state concentration for an oral dosing regimen is given by

$$C_{ss,av} = \frac{F \times DR}{CL}$$

where *DR* is the dose rate and *F* the oral bioavailability of the respective dosing regimens. If $C_{ss,av}$ should be maintained constant, if follows that

$$C_{ss,av} = \frac{F_1 \times DR_1}{CL} = \frac{F_2 \times DR_2}{CL}$$

or $F_1 \times DR_1 = F_2 \times DR_2$

where the subscript denotes the different dosing regimens. Thus DR_2, the dose rate for the generic dosage form, can be calculated as

$$DR_2 = \frac{F_1 \times DR_1}{F_2} = \frac{43\% \times 85\ \text{mg}/12\ \text{h}}{28\%}$$

$$= 130.5\ \text{mg}/12\ \text{h}$$

2. **C.** Steady-state plasma concentration of a constant-rate infusion is directly proportional to the infusion rate R_0 through

$$C_{ss} = \frac{R_0}{CL}$$

Thus, R_0 has to be doubled from 60 mg/h to 120 mg/h to increase C_{ss} from 5 to 10 mcg/mL, that is, an increase of infusion rate by 60 mg/h.

3. **C.** Changes in acyclovir *AUC* after co-administration of probenecid and cimetidine likely result from inhibition of acyclovir renal secretion.

The predominant renal clearance mechanism can be estimated by determining the E_{ratio}:

$$E_{ratio} = \frac{CL_R}{f_{up} \times GFR} = \frac{83.3\ \text{mL/minute}}{0.77 \times 124\ \text{mL/minute}}$$

$$= 0.87$$

$$CL_R = CL_T \times f_e$$

$$CL_R = 255\ \text{mL/minute} \times 0.9 = 229.5\ \text{mL/minute}$$

$$E_{ratio} = \frac{CL_R}{f_{up} \times GFR} = \frac{229.5\ \text{mL/minute}}{0.85 \times 125\ \text{mL/minute}}$$

$$= 2.2 = \text{filtration and net secretion}$$

The $E_{ratio} > 1$ indicates that glomerular filtration and net secretion are the probable renal clearance mechanisms. Thus, alterations in protein binding or urine pH will have little effect on the clearance and *AUC* of acyclovir.

4. **B.** The infusion rate R_0 or maintenance dose *MD* needed to achieve and maintain a steady-state concentration of 3 mcg/mL is given by

$$MD = R_0 = C_{ss} \times CL = C_{ss} \times V \times \frac{0.693}{t_{1/2}}$$

$$= 3\ \text{mcg/mL} \times 90\ \text{L} \times \frac{0.693}{1.1\ \text{h}} = 170\ \text{mg/h}$$

The infusion pump setting can then be calculated as

$$\text{Infusion volume/time} = \frac{170\ \text{mg/h}}{20\ \text{mg/mL}} = 8.5\ \text{mL/h}$$

5. **D.** The first step is to calculate the elimination rate constant k from the measured plasma concentrations:

$$k = \frac{\ln\left(\frac{C_{12\,h}}{C_{2\,h}}\right)}{12\ \text{h} - 2\ \text{h}} = \frac{\ln\left(\frac{12.9\ \text{mcg/mL}}{6\ \text{mcg/mL}}\right)}{12\ \text{h} - 2\ \text{h}} = 0.077\ \text{h}^{-1}$$

The initial concentration C_0 at the end of the infusion can then be back-extrapolated by solving the following relationship for C_0:

$$C = C_0 \times e^{-k \times t}$$

$$C_0 = \frac{12.9\ \text{mcg/mL}}{e^{-0.077\ \text{h}^{-1} \times 2\ \text{h}}} = 15\ \text{mcg/mL}$$

The concentration 24 hours after termination of the infusion can be predicted by

$$C_{24\,h} = 15\ \text{mcg/mL} \times e^{-0.077\ \text{h}^{-1} \times 24\ \text{h}} = 2.4\ \text{mcg/mL}$$

6. **C.** The loading dose can be determined on the basis of the target concentration to be achieved and the volume of distribution. The predose level of 4 mg/L needs to be subtracted from the target concentration, because the loading dose has to account for only the concentration difference. The calculated theophylline dose needs to be converted to aminophylline:

$$LD = \left(C_{target} - C_{predose}\right) \times V_d$$

$$= (12 - 4)\ \text{mg/L} \times 0.5\ \text{L/kg}$$

$$\times 100\ \text{kg} = 400\ \text{mg theophylline}$$

A loading dose of 400 mg theophylline is equivalent to 500 mg aminophylline.

7. **B.** The maintenance dose *MD* required to achieve an average steady-state concentration of 50 ng/mL for an oral dosing regimen is given by

$$MD = C_{ss,av} \times CL/F$$

The oral clearance CL/F can be determined from the relationship between dose and area under the plasma concentration-time curve AUC:

$$CL/F = \frac{D}{AUC}$$

Thus, the required MD can be calculated as

$$MD = C_{ss,av} \times \frac{D}{AUC} = 50 \text{ ng/mL} \times \frac{80 \text{ mg}}{962 \text{ ng*h/mL}}$$

$$= 4.16 \text{ mg/h}$$

This corresponds to a dosing regimen of 50 mg (4.16 mg/h × 12 h) given every 12 hours.

8. **D.** Because trough concentrations after the first dose are known (0.33 mcg/L), trough concentrations during multiple dose at steady state can be predicted by multiplying the trough after the first dose with the accumulation factor

$$C_{ss,min} = C_{ss,1} \times \frac{1}{e^{-k \times \tau}}$$

The dosing interval τ is 24 hours; k can be calculated from

$$k = \frac{\ln\left(\dfrac{C_1}{C_2}\right)}{\Delta t} = \frac{\ln\left(\dfrac{0.72}{0.33}\right)}{(24-12)\text{h}} = 0.065 \text{ h}^{-1}$$

Thus,

$$C_{ss,min} = 0.33 \text{ mcg/L} \times \frac{1}{e^{-0.065 \text{ h}^{-1} \times 24 \text{ h}}} = 1.57 \text{ mcg/L}$$

9. **A.** For immediate-release formulations, upper limits for peak concentrations ($C_{ss,max}$) and lower limits for trough concentrations ($C_{ss,min}$) can be estimated by assuming immediate drug absorption. If fluctuation is equal to 100%, $C_{ss,min}$ is exactly one-half of $C_{ss,max}$. This is the case when the dosing interval τ is equal to the elimination half-life $t_{1/2}$ of the drug. A population average half-life for nifedipine can be calculated as

$$k = \frac{CL}{V} = \frac{0.41 \text{ L/h/kg}}{1.2 \text{ L/kg}} = 0.34 \text{ h}^{-1}$$

$$t_{1/2} = \frac{0.693}{0.34 \text{ h}^{-1}} = \frac{0.41 \text{ L/h/kg}}{1.2 \text{ L/kg}} = 2.03 \text{ h}$$

Thus, τ has to be smaller than 2.03 hours to avoid peak-to-trough fluctuation exceeding 100%.

10. **D.** Calculate necessary dose rate DR to maintain $C_{ss,av} = 1$ mg/L:

$$DR_{necessary} = \frac{D}{\tau} = \frac{C_{ss,av} \times CL}{F}$$

$$= \frac{1 \text{ mg/L} \times 0.5 \text{ L/h/kg} \times 58 \text{ kg}}{0.9}$$

$$= 32.22 \text{ mg/h}$$

$$= 773.3 \text{ mg/day}$$

Determine the maximum dosing interval:

$$\tau_{max} = \frac{\ln\left(\dfrac{C_{ss,max}}{C_{ss,min}}\right)}{K} = \frac{\ln\left(\dfrac{C_{ss,max}}{C_{ss,min}}\right) \times V}{CL}$$

$$= \frac{\ln\left(\dfrac{1.5}{0.75}\right) \times 6 \text{ L/kg}}{0.5 \text{ L/h/kg}} = 8.3 \text{ h}$$

Practical dosing interval: 8 hours

$$D = DR_{necessary} \times \tau = 32.22 \text{ mg/h} \times 8 \text{ h}$$

$$= 257.8 \text{ mg}$$

Recommended dosing regimen: 250 mg every 8 hours

11. **C.** Calculate the elimination rate constant k:

$$k = \frac{\ln\left(\dfrac{C_1}{C_2}\right)}{\Delta t} = \frac{\ln\left(\dfrac{4.9}{1.7}\right)}{6.5 \text{ h}} = 0.163 \text{ h}^{-1}$$

Calculate the volume of distribution assuming steady state:

$$C_{ss,max} = \frac{C_{measured \ peak}}{e^{-k \times t}} = \frac{4.9 \text{ mg/L}}{e^{-0.163 \text{ h}^{-1} \times 0.5 \text{ h}}} = 5.32 \text{ mg/L}$$

$$C_{ss,min} = C_{measured\ trough} \times e^{-k \times t}$$

$$= 1.7\ \text{mg/L} \times e^{-0.163\ \text{h}^{-1} \times 0.5}$$

$$= 1.57\ \text{mg/h}$$

$$V = \frac{R_0}{k} \times \frac{1 - e^{-k \times T_{inf}}}{C_{max} - C_{min} \times e^{-k \times T_{inf}}}$$

$$= \frac{80\ \text{mg}}{0.163\ \text{h}^{-1} \times 0.5\ \text{h}}$$

$$\times \frac{1 - e^{-1.163\ \text{h}^{-1} \times 0.5\ \text{h}}}{5.32\ \text{mg/h} - 1.57\ \text{mg/h} \times e^{-0.163\ \text{h}^{-1} \times 0.5\ \text{h}}}$$

$$= 19.8\ \text{L}$$

Calculate the recommended dosing interval:

$$\tau = \frac{\ln\left(\dfrac{C_{ss,max(desired)}}{C_{ss,min(desired)}}\right)}{k} + T_{inf}$$

$$= \frac{\ln\left(\dfrac{8}{1}\right)}{0.163\ \text{h}^{-1}} + 0.5\ \text{h} = 13.3\ \text{h}$$

Recommended dosing interval: 12 hours
Calculate the recommended dose:

$$D = C_{ss,max(desired)} \times K \times V \times T_{inf} \times \frac{1 - e^{-K \times \tau}}{1 - e^{-K \times T_{inf}}}$$

$$= 8\ \text{mg/L}$$

$$\times 0.163\ \text{h}^{-1} \times 19.8\ \text{L} \times 0.5\ \text{h}$$

$$\times \frac{1 - e^{-0.163\ \text{h}^{-1} \times 12\ \text{h}}}{1 - e^{-0.163\ \text{h}^{-1} \times 0.5\ \text{h}}}$$

$$D = 142\ \text{mg}$$

Recommended dosing regimen: 140 mg every 12 hours

12. **C.** Phenytoin has to be a low-extraction drug because its bioavailability is as high as 90%. The large range in F is due to variability in the absorption of the drug. You know it is not high extraction because if it were, you could never get an F of 90%. Assume $ER < 0.1$, $f_{up} = 0.07$–0.12. Phenytoin is a low-extraction drug and restrictively cleared (assume all low-ER drugs are restrictively cleared for the purposes of this course). Normal albumin range: 3.5–5 gm/dL. Thus, the patient probably has increased f_{up} because of decreased albumin. F_{up} (according to the following equation) would be 0.14 (slightly elevated).

$$f_{up} = \frac{1}{1 + 2.1 \times \text{Albumin}}$$

Because phenytoin is a low-extraction drug, CL is dependent on f_{up} and CL_{int}. Increased f_{up} would lead to increased CL and decreased total plasma concentrations (thus C_p of 8, which is below therapeutic range). However, unbound concentrations would be predicted to be normal (therapeutic) even though total concentration is low. You would not recommend an increase in patient's phenytoin dose because it may result in toxic concentrations. Obtaining free phenytoin plasma concentration, if available from the hospital's lab, may be reasonable to document therapeutic concentrations.

13. **B.** Answer A is incorrect. No pH sensitivity in CL_R is expected unless the drug is reabsorbed (i.e., $E_{ratio} \ll 1$). Answer B is possible. Weakly acidic drugs with pK$_a$ values between 3 and 7.5 can be highly un-ionized in the range of urine pH (5–8) and can thus undergo significant reabsorption if the un-ionized form is non-polar. Answer C is incorrect. Clearance and volume have nothing to do with a drug's likelihood of being affected by changes in urine pH. Answer D is incorrect. The fraction excreted unchanged says nothing about the mechanisms of renal elimination. However, it is important to note that for drugs with high f_e values that are susceptible to changes in urine pH, large changes in the PK of the drug (i.e., CL_R) may be observed.

14. **A.** The antibiotic's total clearance can be determined from the reported V_d and $t_{1/2}$:

$$CL = V_d \times \frac{\ln 2}{t_{1/2}} = 0.31\ \text{L/kg} \times 73\ \text{kg} \times \frac{0.693}{2.1\ \text{h}}$$

$$= 7.47\ \text{L/h}$$

Renal clearance CL_R is then given by total clearance and the fraction excreted f_e:

$$CL_R = f_e \times CL = 0.67 \times 7.47\ \text{L/h} = 5\ \text{L/h}$$

$$= 83.3\ \text{mL/minute}$$

The predominant renal clearance mechanism can be estimated by determining the E_{ratio}:

$$E_{ratio} = \frac{CL_R}{f_{up} \times GFR} = \frac{83.3\ \text{mL/minute}}{0.77 \times 124\ \text{mL/minute}}$$

$$= 0.87$$

The $E_{\text{ratio}} < 1$ indicates that glomerular filtration and net reabsorption are the probable renal clearance mechanisms.

15a. D.

$$CL_R = CL_T \times f_e$$

$$CL_R = 800 \text{ mL/minute} \times 0.5 = 400 \text{ mL/minute}$$

$$E_{\text{ratio}} = \frac{CL_R}{f_{\text{up}} \times GFR} = \frac{400 \text{ mL/minute}}{0.25 \times 125 \text{ mL/minute}}$$

$$= 12.8 = \text{filtration and net secretion}$$

15b. D. The most likely mechanism to account for this reduction in renal clearance is that cimetidine blocks the renal secretion of captopril.

16. B.

$$CL_R = CL_T \times f_e$$

$$CL_R = 125 \text{ mL/minute} \times 1 = 125 \text{ mL/minute}$$

$$E_{\text{ratio}} = \frac{CL_R}{f_{\text{up}} \times GFR} = \frac{125 \text{ mL/minute}}{0.25 \times 125 \text{ mL/minute}}$$

$$= 4 = \text{filtration and net secretion}$$

17. B. The drug transporter P-glycoprotein is directly responsible for the transport of drug from hepatocytes into the bile and maintenance of the integrity of the blood–brain barrier by transport of drug out of the brain.

18. B. The PPI Protonix (pantoprazole), a weak CYP2C19 inhibitor, should be considered as an acid-reducing agent in patients taking Plavix (clopidogrel). The package insert warns against use of strong or moderate CYP2C19 inhibitors. Since Protonix is a weak inhibitor, its use is permissible.

19. A.

$$CL_H = 1,350 \times 0.9 = 1,215 \text{ mL/minute}$$

$$ER = \frac{1,215 \text{ mL/minute}}{1,350 \text{ mL/minute}} \approx 1$$

$$F = f_a \times f_g \times F^*$$

No effect on CL_H. No effect on F^*.

20. C.

$$F = f_a \times f_g \times F^*$$

$$F^* = \frac{F}{F_a \times f_g} = \frac{0.5}{1 \times 0.8} = 0.63$$

$$ER = 1 - F^* = 1 - 0.63 = 0.37$$

$$CL_H = Q \times ER = 1,350 \text{ mL/minute} \times 0.37$$

$$= 500 \text{ mL/minute}$$

7-18. References

Atkinson A, Daniels C, Dedrick R, et al. *Principles of Clinical Pharmacology.* San Diego, Calif.; Academic Press; 2001.

Ensom MH, Davis GA, Cropp CD, Ensom RJ. Clinical pharmacokinetics in the 21st century: Does the evidence support definitive outcomes? *Clin Pharmacokinet.* 1998;34:265–79.

Levy RH, Bauer LA. Basic pharmacokinetics. *Ther Drug Monit.* 1986;8(1):47–58.

Meibohm B, Derendorf H: Basic concepts of pharmacokinetic/pharmacodynamic (PK/PD) modelling. *Int J Clin Pharmacol Ther.* 1997;35:401–13.

Rolan, PE. Plasma protein binding displacement interactions: Why are they still regarded as clinically important? *Br J Clin Pharmacol.* 1994;37:125–8.

Rowland M, Tozer T. *Clinical Pharmacokinetics.* 3rd ed. Media, Pa.: Williams & Wilkins; 1995.

Saitoh A, Jinbayashi H, Saitoh AK, et al. Parameter estimation and dosage adjustment in the treatment with vancomycin of methicillin-resistant *Staphylococcus aureus* ocular infections. *Ophthalmologica.* 1997; 211(4):232–35.

Sawchuk RJ, Zaske DE, Cipolle RJ, et al. Kinetic model for gentamicin dosing with the use of individual patient parameters. *Clin Pharmacol Ther.* 1977;21:362–69.

Tod MM, Padoin C, Petitjean O. Individualising aminoglycoside dosage regimens after therapeutic drug monitoring: Simple or complex pharmacokinetic methods? *Clin Pharmacokinet.* 2001;40:803–14.

Wilkinson, GR, Shand, DG. Commentary: A physiological approach to hepatic drug clearance. *Clin Pharmacol Ther.* 1975;18:377–90.

Biotechnology and Pharmacogenomics

Stephanie A. Flowers
P. David Rogers

8-1. Key Points

- *Biotechnology,* as defined by Merriam-Webster's Dictionary, is "the manipulation (as through genetic engineering) of living organisms or their components to produce useful usually commercial products (as pest resistant crops, new bacterial strains, or novel pharmaceuticals)."
- The central dogma of molecular biology is that deoxyribonucleic acid (DNA) encodes ribonucleic acid (RNA), which, in turn, encodes protein.
- Recombinant DNA technology makes use of several molecular biological tools that allow for the placement of a desired DNA fragment in proximity to other DNA fragments within a DNA molecule for a specific purpose.
- Cytokines are molecules secreted by cells that orchestrate the immune response. They activate immune cells such as lymphocytes, macrophages, monocytes, and neutrophils.
- An enzyme is a protein that catalyzes a specific chemical reaction.
- Hormones are chemical substances transmitted by the bloodstream to cells distant from their physiologic source that impart specific cellular effects.
- Clotting or blood factors are chemical blood constituents that interact to cause blood coagulation.
- Vaccines are preparations of antigenic material administered to stimulate the development of antibodies for the purpose of conferring active immunity against a particular pathogen or disease.
- Subsets of β-lymphocyte clones produce identical antibodies that recognize the same antigen. These identical antibodies are said to be monoclonal. Fusing β-lymphocytes with lymphocyte tumor cells produces a hybridoma that can be cultured in large quantities for the mass production of a given monoclonal antibody.
- Gene therapy, an application of biotechnology, has great potential therapeutic benefit.
- Biotechnology has facilitated the development of novel drug delivery strategies, including liposomal technology, immunotoxins, and PEGylation.
- Pharmacogenomics is the scientific discipline of using genomewide approaches to understand the inherited basis of differences between individual responses to drugs.
- Single nucleotide polymorphisms are differences in a single nucleotide base occurring at a significant frequency (usually > 5%) within the population. They may result in no change in the encoded amino acid of a codon or a change in the encoded amino acid with no change in the function of the encoded protein. However, when the amino acid substitution attributable to a single nucleotide polymorphism (SNP) results in a phenotypic difference, it may carry clinical relevance.

8-2. Study Guide Checklist

The following topics may guide your study of this subject area:

- Familiarize yourself with marketed biological products (Table 8-1). Focus on products included in the list of "Top 100 drugs."
- Gain a general sense of the types of biological products that are currently approved by the U.S. Food and Drug Administration (FDA).
- Study recombinant technology and the production of vaccines.

Table 8-1. Approved Biological Products

Generic name	Brand name (manufacturer)	Indications
Blood factors		
Factor VII	NovoSeven (Novo Nordisk)	Hemophilia
Factor VIII	Bioclate, Recombinate, Advate (Baxter); Kogenate, Helixate (Bayer); ReFacto (Genetics Institute); Xyntha (Wyeth)	Hemophilia A
Factor IX	BeneFix (Genetics Institute)	Hemophilia B
Factor XIII	Corifact (CSL Behring)	Congenital FXIII deficiency
Cytokines		
Aldesleukin (IL-2)	Proleukin (Chiron)	Metastatic renal cell carcinoma and melanoma
Denileukin diftitox	Ontak (Ligand)	Cutaneous T-cell lymphoma
Interferon alfacon-1	Infergen (InterMune)	Hepatitis C
Interferon alfa-n1	Wellferon (GlaxoSK)	Chronic hepatitis C
Interferon alfa-2a	Roferon-A (Roche)	Hairy cell leukemia; AIDS-related Kaposi's sarcoma; chronic myelogenous leukemia
Interferon alfa-2b	Intron-A (Schering)	Hairy cell leukemia; AIDS-related Kaposi's sarcoma; chronic hepatitis B and C; condylomata acuminata; malignant melanoma
Interferon alfa-n3	Alferon-N (InterMune)	Condylomata acuminata
Interferon beta-1b	Betaseron (Berlex)	Acute relapsing–remitting multiple sclerosis
Interferon beta-1a	Avonex (Biogen); **Rebif (EMD Serono)**	Acute relapsing–remitting multiple sclerosis
Interferon gamma-1b	Actimmune (InterMune)	Chronic granulomatous disease; osteoporosis
Oprelvekin (IL-11)	Neumega (Genetics Institute)	Thrombocytopenia from chemotherapy
Peginterferon alfa-2a	Pegasys (Roche)	Hepatitis C
Peginterferon alfa-2b	PegIntron (Schering)	Hepatitis C
Enzymes		
Agalsidase beta	Fabrazyme (Genzyme)	Fabry disease
Alglucosidase alfa	Myozyme, Lumizyme (Genzyme)	Lysosomal alpha-1, 4-glucosidase deficiency
Alpha-1-proteinase inhibitor	Zemaira (Aventis), Glassia (Kamada)	Alpha-1-proteinase inhibitor deficiency
Alteplase	Activase (Genentech)	Acute myocardial infarction; pulmonary embolism; stroke
Bivalirudin	Angiomax (Medicines Co.)	Coronary angioplasty (PTCA); unstable angina
Dornase alfa	Pulmozyme (Genentech)	Respiratory complication from cystic fibrosis
Elosulfase alfa	Vimizim (Biomarin)	Morquio A syndrome (MPS IVA)
Eptifibatide	Integrilin (Millennium)	Acute coronary syndromes; angioplasties
Galsulfase	Naglazyme (Biomarin)	Mucopolysaccharidosis
Idursulfase	Elaprase (Shire Human Genetic Therapies)	Mucopolysaccharidosis
Imiglucerase	Cerezyme (Genzyme)	Type 1 Gaucher's disease
Laronidase	Aldurazyme (Biomarin)	Mucopolysaccharidosis
Lepirudin	Refludan (Berlex)	Heparin-induced thrombocytopenia
Pancrelipase	Pancreaze (Ortho-McNeil-Janssen)	Exocrine pancreatic insufficiency
Pegloticase	Krystexxa (Savient)	Treatment of severe, treatment-refractory, chronic gout

Table 8-1. Approved Biological Products *(Continued)*

Generic name	Brand name (manufacturer)	Indications
Rasburicase	Elitek (Sanofi-Synthelabo)	Elevated plasma uric acid in pediatric malignancy
Reteplase	Retavase (Centocor/J&J)	Acute myocardial infarction
Tenecteplase	TNKase (Genentech)	Acute myocardial infarction
Tirofiban	Aggrastat (Merck)	Acute coronary syndromes
Growth factors		
Becaplermin (PDGF)	Regranex (Ortho-McNeil-Janssen)	Diabetic foot ulcer
Darbepoetin alfa	**Aranesp (Amgen)**	Anemia associated with end-stage renal disease and chronic renal insufficiency
Epoetin alfa	**Epogen (Amgen); Procrit (Janssen Pharmaceuticals)**	Anemia attributable to chronic renal disease; zidovudine-induced anemia; anemia due to chemotherapy; surgery patients
Filgrastim	**Neupogen (Amgen)**	Neutropenia attributable to myelosuppressive chemotherapy; myeloid reconstitution after bone marrow transplant; severe chronic neutropenia; peripheral blood progenitor cell transplant; induction and consolidation therapy in acute myelogenous leukemia
Methoxy polyethylene glycol-epoetin beta	Mircera (Roche)	Anemia attributable to chronic renal failure
Palifermin	Kepivance (Biovitrum)	Oral mucositis; mucositis following chemotherapy
Pegfilgrastim	**Neulasta (Amgen)**	Febrile neutropenia attributable to myelo-suppressive chemotherapy
Sargramostim	Leukine (Berlex)	Myeloid reconstitution after bone marrow transplant; bone marrow transplant failure; adjunct to chemotherapy in acute myelogenous leukemia; peripheral blood progenitor cell transplant
Hormones		
Choriogonadotropin alfa	Ovidrel (Serono)	Fertility
Exenatide	Byetta (Amylin)	Diabetes mellitus type 2
Follitropin alfa	Gonal-F (Serono)	Ovulatory failure
Follitropin beta	Follistim (Organon)	Ovulatory failure
Human growth hormone	Protopin, Nutropin (Genentech)	Growth hormone deficiency in pediatric patients
	Humatrope (Eli Lilly)	Growth retardation in chronic renal disease
	Saizen, Serostim (Serono)	AIDS wasting
	Norditropin (Novo Nordisk)	Turner's syndrome
	Genotropin (Pharmacia); Bio-Tropin (Sol Source Technologies)	Growth hormone deficiency in adults
Human insulin	Humulin, **Humalog (Eli Lilly);** Novolin, **NovoLog FlexPen, Levemir (Novo Nordisk Inc.); Lantus,** Lantus SoloSTAR **(Sanofi-Aventis)**	Insulin-dependent diabetes mellitus
Ganirelix	Antagon (Organon)	Luteinizing hormone surge during fertility therapy

(continued)

Table 8-1. Approved Biological Products *(Continued)*

Generic name	Brand name (manufacturer)	Indications
Glucagon	GlucaGen (Novo Nordisk)	Hypoglycemia
Growth hormone-releasing hormone	Geref (Serono)	Growth hormone deficiency in pediatric patients
Liraglutide recombinant	**Victoza (Novo Nordisk)**	Diabetes mellitus type 2
Metreleptin	Myalept (Amylin)	Leptin deficiency in patients with congenital or acquired generalized lipodystrophy
Repository corticotropin injection	H. P. Acthar Gel (Questcor)	Acute exacerbations of multiple sclerosis in adults; infantile spasms
Tesamorelin acetate	Egrifta (Theratechnologies)	HIV-induced lipodystrophy
Testosterone cypionate	Testosterone Cypionate Injection, USP (Sun Pharma)	Primary hypogonadism; hypogonadotropic hypogonadism
Testosterone undecanoate	Aveed (Endo Pharma)	Primary hypogonadism; hypogonadotropic hypogonadism
Thyrotropin	Thyrogen (Genzyme)	Thyroid cancer
Monoclonal antibodies		
Abciximab	ReoPro (Centocor)	Prevention of blood clots following percutaneous coronary intervention; unstable angina prior to percutaneous coronary intervention
Adalimumab	**Humira (AbbVie)**	Acute rheumatoid arthritis
Alemtuzumab	Campath (Berlex)	Chronic lymphocytic leukemia
Basiliximab	Simulect (Novartis)	Acute organ transplant rejection
Belimumab	Benlysta (Human Genome Sciences)	Systemic lupus erythmatosus
Bevacizumab	**Avastin (Genentech)**	Colorectal cancer
Canakinumab	Ilaris (Novartis)	Cryopyrin-associated periodic syndrome
Certolizumab pegol	Cimzia (UCB)	Crohn's disease
Cetuximab	Erbitux (ImClone Systems)	Colorectal cancer
Daclizumab	Zenapax (Roche)	Kidney transplant; acute rejection
Denosumab	Prolia, Xgeva (Amgen)	Postmenopausal osteoporosis; skeletal-related events in patients with bone metastases from solid tumors
Eculizumab	Soliris (Alexion)	Paroxysmal nocturnal hemoglobinuria
Efalizumab	Raptiva (Genentech)	Psoriasis
Gemtuzumab (ozogamicin)	Mylotarg (Wyeth/PDL)	Acute myeloid leukemia (CD33+)
Golimumab	Simponi Aria (Janssen Biotech)	Rheumatoid arthritis; psoriatic arthritis; ankylosing spondylitis; and ulcerative colitis
Ibritumomab (tiuxetan)	Zevalin (IDEC)	B-cell non-Hodgkin's lymphoma
Infliximab	**Remicade (Janssen Biotech)**	Crohn's disease; rheumatoid arthritis
Ipilimumab	Yervoy (Bristol-Meyers Squibb)	Late-stage melanoma
Natalizumab	Tysabri (Amgen)	Crohn's disease; multiple sclerosis
Obinutuzumab	Gazyva (Genentech)	Chronic lymphocytic leukemia (CD20+)
Ofatumumab	Arzerra (Glaxo Group Ltd)	Chronic lymphocytic leukemia (CD20+)
Omalizumab	**Xolair (Genentech)**	Asthma

Table 8-1. Approved Biological Products *(Continued)*

Generic name	Brand name (manufacturer)	Indications
Palivizumab	Synagis (MedImmune)	Prevention of respiratory syncytial virus and fatal pneumonia in pediatrics
Panitumumab	Vectibix (Amgen)	Metastatic colorectal cancer
Ranibizumab	**Lucentis (Genentech)**	Exudative age-related macular degeneration
Rituximab	**Rituxan** (IDEC/**Genentech**)	Low-grade non-Hodgkin's lymphoma
Tocilizumab	Actemra (Genentech)	Moderate to severe rheumatoid arthritis
Tositumomab	Bexxar (Corixa)	CD20+ non-Hodgkin's lymphoma
Trastuzumab	**Herceptin (Genentech**/PDL**)**	Metastatic breast cancer (Her 2 Neu+)
Ustekinumab	Stelara (Centocor Ortho Biotech)	Plaque psoriasis
Vaccines		
Haemophilus b/hepatitis B	Comvax (Merck)	Prevention of *Haemophilus influenzae* and hepatitis B
Hepatitis B vaccine	Engerix-B (GlaxoSK); Recombivax HB (Merck)	Prevention of hepatitis B
Streptococcus pneumoniae	**Prevnar 13 (Wyeth)**	Prevention of *Streptococcus pneumoniae* in children
Neisseria meningitidis	Menveo (Novartis)	Prevention of *Neisseria meningitidis*
Adenovirus Type 4 and Type 7 Vaccine, Live, Oral	(Barr Labs)	Acute respiratory disease caused by Adenovirus Type 4 and Type 7
Varicella zoster virus (VZV), Live, Attenuated	**Varivax (Merck)**	Prevention of varicella in individuals 12 months of age and older.
Others		
Abatacept	**Orencia (Bristol-Meyers Squibb)**	Rheumatoid arthritis
Anakinra	Kineret (Amgen)	Rheumatoid arthritis
BCNU polymer	Gliadel (Guilford)	Recurrent glioblastoma multiforme
Daunorubicin-liposomal	DaunoXome (Gilead)	Kaposi's sarcoma
Doxorubicin-liposomal	DOXIL (Alza)	Kaposi's sarcoma; ovarian cancer
Etanercept	**Enbrel (Amgen)**	Rheumatoid arthritis; psoriatic arthritis
Fomivirsen	Vitravene (Isis)	Cytomegalovirus retinitis
Glatiramer	Copaxone (Teva)	Relapsing multiple sclerosis
Incobotulinumtoxin A	Xeomin (Merz)	Cervical dystonia; blepharospasm
Lipid-based amphotericin B	Abelcet (Elan); Amphotec (Sequus); AmBisome (Fujisawa/Gilead)	Aspergillosis; cryptococcal meningitis in HIV; systemic fungal infections
Nesiritide	Natrecor (Scios/Innovex)	Congestive heart failure
Rilonacept	Arcalyst (Regeneron)	Cryopyrin-associated periodic syndromes
Romiplostim	Nplate (Amgen)	Idiopathic thrombocytopenic purpura
Centruroides (Scorpion) Immune F(ab')$_2$ (Equine) Injection	Anascorp (Rare Disease Therapeutics)	Scorpion envenomation
Azficel-T	LaViv (Fibrocell Science)	Nasolabial fold wrinkles in adults

Boldface indicates one of top 100 drugs for 2012 by units sold at retail outlets, www.drugs.com/stats/top100/2012/units.
AIDS, acquired immune deficiency syndrome; BCNU, bis-chlorethylnitrosourea; HIV, human immunodeficiency virus; IL, interleukin; PDGF, platelet-derived growth factor; PTCA, percutaneous transluminal coronary angioplasty.

- Review the nomenclature of monoclonal antibodies.
- Familiarize yourself with the concept of pharmacogenomics and major genetic polymorphisms that determine drug response.

8-3. Introduction

Since the discovery of the DNA (deoxyribonucleic acid) double helix half a century ago, significant use of biotechnology has been made for the improvement of human health (Table 8-2). A number of biological products with therapeutic applications has accompanied these advances. With the arrival of the postgenomic era, the field of pharmacogenomics has emerged and shows great promise to revolutionize the way in which pharmacy and medicine are practiced. This chapter highlights key concepts relevant to the practicing pharmacist in the areas of biotechnology and pharmacogenomics.

Biotechnology has revolutionized the pharmaceutical industry by imparting the ability to mass produce safe and pure versions of chemicals produced naturally in the body. A multitude of disease states have been affected by therapeutic agents derived through biotechnology, including AIDS (acquired immune deficiency syndrome), anemia, cancer, congestive heart failure, cystic fibrosis, diabetes, growth hormone deficiency, hemophilia, hepatitis B and C, and multiple sclerosis, to name a few.

Biotechnology is defined by Merriam-Webster's Dictionary as "the manipulation (as through genetic engineering) of living organisms or their components to produce useful usually commercial products (as pest resistant crops, new bacterial strains, or novel pharmaceuticals)."

8-4. Key Terms

- *Antibody (immunoglobulin):* A protein produced by β-lymphocytes in response to antigen molecules determined to be nonself. Antibodies recognize and bind to antigens, resulting in their inactivation or opsonization for phagocytosis or complement-mediated destruction. A number of immunoglobulin G products have been developed for therapeutic use in various immune disorders.
- *Antigen:* A molecule that elicits an antibody-mediated immune response.
- *Bioinformatics:* The application of computer sciences and information technology to the management and analysis of biological information.
- *Biotherapy:* Any treatment involving the administration of a microorganism or other biologic material.

Table 8-2. Milestones in Biotechnology

Event	Year
Identification of DNA as a genetic material	1940
Discovery of DNA double helix by James Watson and Francis Crick	1953
Elucidation of the genetic code (64 nucleic acid triplets, or codons, encode 20 amino acids)	1961
Cloning of DNA and production of the first recombinant DNA–derived protein	1973
Introduction of monoclonal antibodies	1975
Production of the first human protein (somatostatin) from recombinant DNA technology	1977
Cloning of the human insulin gene	1978
Licensing in the United States of technology to derive human insulin from recombinant DNA	1982
Conception of the polymerase chain reaction for amplification of DNA	1983
Initiation of the Human Genome Project	1990
Discovery of the first breast cancer susceptibility gene, BRCA1	1994
Sequencing of the first bacterial genome, *Haemophilus influenza*	1995
Sequencing of the first eukaryotic genome, *Saccharomyces cerevisiae*	1996
Sequencing of the human genome	2001

- *Clotting factor (blood factor):* Chemical blood constituents that interact to cause blood coagulation.
- *Combinatorial chemistry:* A drug development strategy that uses nucleic acids and amino acids in various combinations to synthesize vast libraries of oligonucleotide or peptide compounds for high-throughput lead compound screening.
- *Cytokine:* An extracellular signaling protein that mediates communication between cells.
- *DNA (deoxyribonucleic acid):* A polynucleotide molecule consisting of covalently linked nucleic acids. DNA serves as the genetic material.
- *Enzyme:* A protein that catalyzes a chemical reaction.
- *Gene:* A region of DNA that encodes a specific RNA (ribonucleic acid) or protein responsible for a specific hereditary characteristic.
- *Gene therapy:* Therapeutic technologies that directly target human genes responsible for disease.
- *Genome:* The complete set of genetic information for a given organism.
- *Genomics:* The scientific discipline of mapping, sequencing, and analyzing genomes. It encompasses structural genomics, functional genomics, and pharmacogenomics.
- *Hormone:* A chemical substance imparting specific cellular effects that is transmitted by the bloodstream to cells distant from its physiologic source.
- *Hybridoma:* A cell line generated by the fusion of antibody-producing β-lymphocytes with lymphocyte tumor cells for the production of monoclonal antibodies.
- *Interferon:* A member of a group of cytokines that prevents viral replication and slows the growth and replication of cancer cells.
- *Interleukin:* A member of a group of cytokines involved in orchestration and regulation of the immune response.
- *Liposome:* A microscopic, sphere-like lipid droplet that functions as a therapeutic carrier.
- *Monoclonal antibody:* An antibody derived from a hybridoma cell line.
- *Pharmacogenomics:* The scientific discipline of using genomewide approaches to understand the inherited basis of differences between individuals in the response to drugs. This field is an expansion of the field of pharmacogenetics, which traditionally considered such inherited differences on a gene-by-gene basis.
- *Plasmid:* A small, circular, extrachromosomal DNA molecule capable of replication independent of that of the genome.

- *Polymerase chain reaction (PCR):* A molecular biologic technique for amplification of specific DNA molecules.
- *Protein:* A functional product of a specific gene consisting of amino acids linked together through peptide bonds in a specific sequence.
- *Proteomics:* The scientific field of the study of sequencing and analyzing the expression, modification, and function of proteins on a genomewide or global scale.
- *Recombinant DNA (rDNA) technology:* The application of DNA molecules derived by joining two DNA molecules from different sources.
- *Restriction endonuclease:* An enzyme capable of cleaving a DNA molecule in a site-specific manner.
- *Ribozymes:* RNA molecules with intrinsic enzymatic activity.
- *RNA (ribonucleic acid):* A polynucleotide molecule consisting of covalently linked ribonucleic acids. Messenger RNA (mRNA) serves as the template for protein synthesis. Transfer RNA (tRNA) serves as the adaptor molecules between amino acids and mRNA during protein synthesis. Ribosomal RNA (rRNA) serves as a component of the ribosome and participates in protein synthesis.
- *Small molecule chemistry:* The field of drug development focusing on small organic nucleotide- or peptide-based molecules derived through either combinatorial chemistry or rational drug design.
- *Single nucleotide polymorphism:* Common DNA sequence variations among individuals involving a single nucleotide substitution.
- *Vaccine:* A preparation of antigenic material administered to stimulate the development of antibodies conferring active immunity against a particular pathogen or disease.

Biological Products

Many U.S. Food and Drug Administration (FDA)–approved biological products are currently on the market, including blood factors, cytokines, enzymes, growth factors, hormones, interferons, monoclonal antibodies, and vaccines. A list of such biological products is provided in Table 8-1.

Gene Expression and Protein Synthesis

Proteins are the major macromolecular component of the cell and are responsible for conducting most of a cell's biological activity. Proteins consist of a linear polymer of amino acids linked together in a specific sequence. This specific sequence is responsible for a protein's structure and function. The initial code for the synthesis of a given protein is stored in a gene on a sequence of DNA that is part of a chromosome within the nucleus of a cell.

The central dogma of molecular biology is that DNA encodes RNA, which, in turn, encodes protein. A given amino acid within a protein is encoded by a triplet of nucleic acid base pairs within the gene encoding the protein. This triplet is called a *codon*. There are 64 codons encoding 20 different amino acids as dictated by the genetic code.

An overview of transcription, translation, and post-translational modification is shown in Figure 8-1.

Recombinant DNA Technology

Recombinant DNA technology uses several molecular biological tools to insert a desired DNA fragment with a specific purpose in proximity to other DNA fragments within a DNA molecule. Most often, a gene encoding a desired protein is isolated through screening of the genomic library or by use of the viral enzyme reverse transcriptase to generate complementary DNA (cDNA) from the mRNA transcript of the gene. Enzymes called *restriction endonucleases* allow the cleavage of DNA in the plasmid at very specific locations. The gene is then ligated into a vector, such as a plasmid, for gene cloning or for control of the expression of the encoded protein.

Figure 8-1. Gene Expression: The Synthesis of Proteins

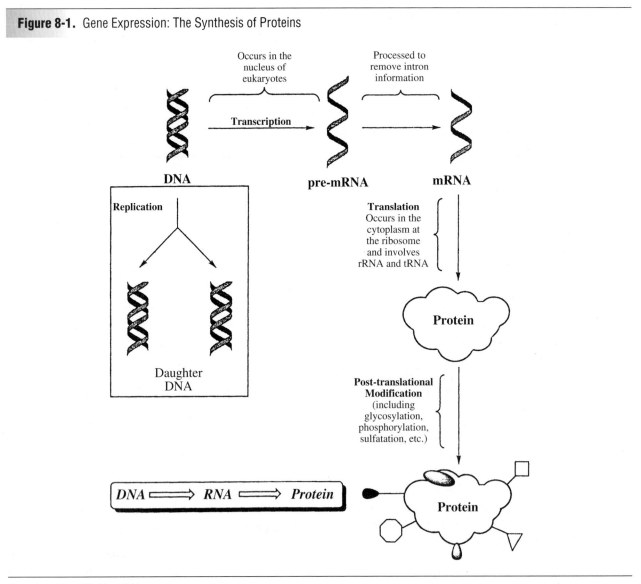

An *expression vector* is a plasmid designed to allow inducible expression of the inserted gene within a host cell (such as the bacterium *Escherichia coli* or the yeast *Saccharomyces cerevisiae*). This mechanism permits production of large quantities of the desired protein. The protein must then be isolated and purified for further use. Such techniques, used on an industrial scale, mass produce therapeutically useful biological products such as cytokines, enzymes, hormones, blood factors, and vaccines (Figure 8-2).

Cytokines (i.e., molecules secreted by cells) orchestrate the immune response and activate immune cells

Figure 8-2. Summary of Typical rDNA Production of a Protein from Either Genomic DNA or cDNA

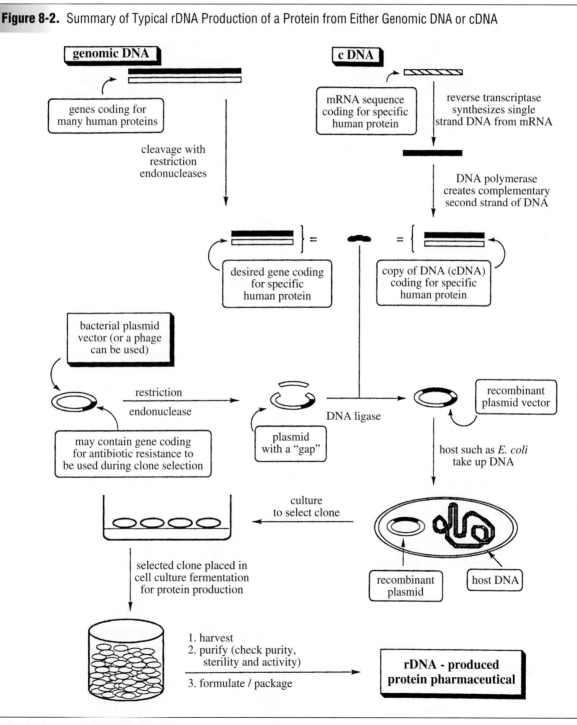

Reprinted with permission from Sindelar, 2002.

such as lymphocytes, monocytes, macrophages, and neutrophils. Therapeutically useful recombinant cytokines include interferons, interleukins, and colony-stimulating factors. Examples of these include interferon beta-1b (Betaseron), which is used to treat acute relapsing–remitting multiple sclerosis; aldesleukin (IL-2) (Proleukin), which aids in the management of metastatic renal cell carcinoma and melanoma; and oprelvekin (IL-11) (Neumega), which treats thrombocytopenia caused by chemotherapy.

An *enzyme* is a protein that catalyzes a specific chemical reaction. Numerous different enzymes with therapeutic use have been produced using rDNA technology. Alteplase (Activase), for example, treats acute myocardial infarction, pulmonary embolism, and stroke. Dornase alfa (Pulmozyme) treats respiratory complications that develop in cystic fibrosis. Eptifibatide (Integrilin) is used to treat acute coronary syndromes.

Hormones—chemical substances transmitted through the bloodstream—are designed to impart specific cellular effects to cells distant from their physiologic source. Since the introduction and success of recombinant human insulin in 1982, many other recombinant hormones have been developed, such as human growth hormone, which treats growth hormone deficiency in pediatric patients, and follitropin alfa and beta (Gonal-F and Follistim, respectively), which are used to remedy ovulatory failure.

Clotting or blood factors are chemical blood constituents that interact to cause blood coagulation. Patients suffering from hemophilia A (caused by factor VIII deficiency) and hemophilia B (caused by factor IX deficiency) have benefited greatly from rDNA technology. Factors VII, VIII, and IX are available in recombinant forms for clinical use.

Vaccines—preparations of antigenic material administered to stimulate the development of antibodies—confer active immunity against a particular pathogen or disease. Vaccine development has also benefited from advances in rDNA technology. Traditional vaccine production used killed or nonvirulent organisms, microbial toxins, or actual microbial components to elicit long-term immune protection. Safer and more specific vaccine antigens have been devised as recombinant proteins. This technology has led to the very successful recombinant hepatitis B vaccine.

Monoclonal Antibodies

Antibodies, proteins produced by the immune system's β-lymphocytes, use specific methods to recognize foreign molecules within the body. Subsets of β-lymphocyte clones produce identical antibodies that recognize the same antigen. These identical antibodies are *monoclonal*. Fusing β-lymphocytes with lymphocyte tumor cells produces a hybridoma. This fused cell type is immortal and can be cultured in large quantities for the mass production of a given monoclonal antibody.

Monoclonal antibodies that bind to and inactivate their targets can be developed and have great therapeutic utility (Figure 8-3). Nomenclature of monoclonal antibodies is highly structured. The first component of the name is product specific. The second component indicates its therapeutic use: *ci* for cardiovascular use, *li* for use in inflammation, and *tu* for use in cancer. The third component indicates the type of monoclonal antibody: *mo* for murine, *xi* for chimeric, and *zu* for humanized. The fourth component, *mab,* represents monoclonal antibody. An example of a monoclonal antibody used clinically is abciximab (ReoPro), which prevents blood clots following percutaneous transluminal coronary angioplasty (PTCA) and prevents unstable angina prior to PTCA. Another example, infliximab (Remicade), is used to treat Crohn's disease and rheumatoid arthritis.

Gene Therapy

Gene therapy is an excellent example of the therapeutic application of biotechnology. This technology holds promise for the treatment of inherited disorders, as well as acquired illnesses such as infectious diseases and cancer.

The molecular goal of gene therapy is to repair or correct a dysfunctional gene by selectively introducing rDNA into cells or tissues, thereby allowing the expression of a functional gene product.

Novel drug delivery strategies must be used to introduce exogenous DNA into the cell to treat retroviruses, lentiviruses, and adeno-associated viruses. These novel drug delivery strategies also have applications for nonviral delivery systems (e.g., liposomes or uncomplexed plasmid DNA).

Alternative approaches using ribozymes (e.g., RNA repair) may prove effective. The enzymatic activity of these RNA molecules can be used to repair defective mRNAs.

Chimeric RNA and DNA oligonucleotides make use of the cell's DNA mismatch repair apparatus to correct mutations at the genomic level. Antisense oligonucleotides for gene inactivation have proved clinically useful. Fomivirsen (Vitravene), one such agent, targets the mRNA of human cytomegalovirus (CMV). This agent is indicated for the treatment of CMV retinitis in patients with AIDS.

Figure 8-3. Production of Monoclonal Antibodies

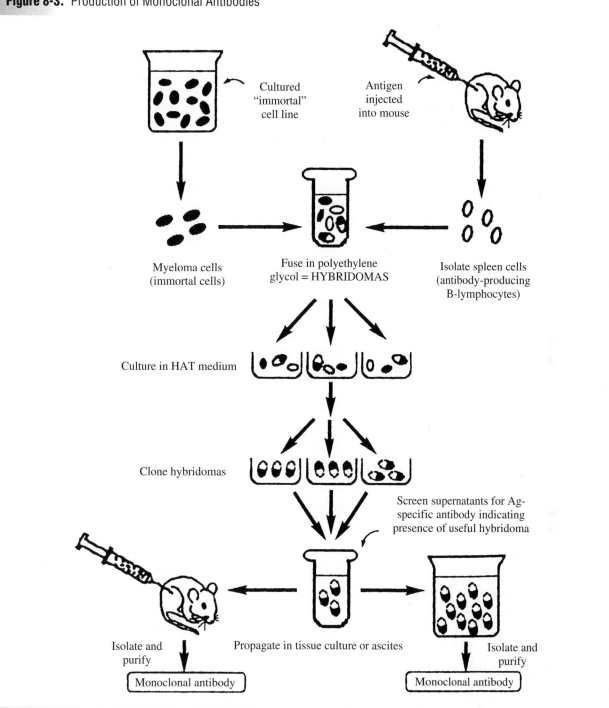

Cultured "immortal" cell line

Antigen injected into mouse

Myeloma cells (immortal cells)

Fuse in polyethylene glycol = HYBRIDOMAS

Isolate spleen cells (antibody-producing B-lymphocytes)

Culture in HAT medium

Clone hybridomas

Screen supernatants for Ag-specific antibody indicating presence of useful hybridoma

Isolate and purify

Propagate in tissue culture or ascites

Isolate and purify

Monoclonal antibody

Monoclonal antibody

Reproduced from Sindelar, 2002.

Drug Delivery

Biotechnology has facilitated the development of novel drug delivery strategies. The use of liposomes has had a positive effect on drug delivery. Drugs can be formulated into liposomes (i.e., microscopic, spherical lipid droplets). The outer membrane of the liposome fuses with the membrane of the target cell, thereby facilitating highly targeted drug delivery. Such technology has greatly improved the therapeutic index of the antifungal drug amphotericin B. Lipid-based formulations now allow greater quantities of the drug to be delivered with substantially less toxicity to the patient.

Another promising approach is the use of immunotoxins. These delivery agents combine a monoclonal antibody with a toxin such as an anticancer or antimicrobial agent, thereby allowing targeted drug delivery with minimal toxicity.

Another novel strategy is the use of PEGylation—that is, the addition of polyethylene glycol (PEG) to therapeutic proteins to minimize the deleterious immune response to an individual protein.

Pharmacogenomics

Pharmacogenomics is the scientific discipline of using genomewide approaches to understand the inherited basis of differences between individuals in the response to drugs. This field is an expansion of the field of pharmacogenetics, which traditionally considered such inherited differences on a gene-by-gene basis.

Genetic differences in drug metabolism, drug disposition, and drug targets have a large effect on efficacy and toxicity. Comprehension of the relationships between specific genetic factors and drug response can be used to predict drug response and optimize drug therapy in any given individual. Currently, more than 100 drugs contain FDA labeling regarding potentially applicable pharmacogenetic biomarkers. The Clini-cal Pharmacogenetics Implementation Consortium (CPIC), formed in 2009, produces peer-reviewed guidelines that enable the translation of genetic tests into prescribing decisions for specific drugs (www.pharmgkb.org). The top three therapeutic areas in which this type of genetic testing is being implemented are oncology, psychiatry, and cardiovascular medicine.

Of particular significance to genetic testing are single nucleotide polymorphisms (SNPs). SNPs are differences in a single nucleotide base that occur at a significant frequency (usually > 5%) within the population. An SNP may or may not promote change in the encoded amino acid of a codon, or it may change the encoded amino acid but yield no change in the function of the encoded protein. When an SNP causes amino acid substitution, a phenotypic difference that carries clinical relevance may result. Even when the SNP results in no change in the encoded amino acid, it may be associated with a phenotypic change, thereby serving as a predictive marker of that change.

Examples of significant genetic polymorphisms that can influence drug response are shown in Tables 8-3 and 8-4.

Examples of significant genetic polymorphisms in drug-metabolizing enzymes are shown in Tables 8-5 and 8-6.

Table 8-3. Genetic Polymorphisms in Drug Target Genes That Can Influence Drug Response[a]

Gene or gene product	Medication	Drug effect associated with polymorphism
Angiotensin-converting enzyme (ACE)	ACE inhibitors (e.g., enalapril)	Renoprotective effects; blood pressure reduction; reduction in left ventricular mass; endothelial function
	Fluvastatin	Lipid changes (reductions in low-density lipoprotein cholesterol and apolipoprotein B); progression or regression in coronary atherosclerosis
Arachidonate 5-lipoxygenase	Leukotriene inhibitors	Improvement of FEV_1
β_2-adrenergic receptor	β_2-agonists	Bronchodilatation; susceptibility to agonist-induced desensitization; cardiovascular effects
Bradykinin B_2 receptor	ACE inhibitors	ACE inhibitor–induced cough
Dopamine receptors (D_2, D_3, D_4)	Antipsychotics (e.g., haloperidol and clozapine)	Antipsychotic response (D_2, D_3, D_4); antipsychotic-induced tardive dyskinesia (D_3); antipsychotic-induced acute akathisia (D_3)
Estrogen receptor-α	Conjugated estrogens	Increase in bone mineral density
	Hormone replacement therapy	Increase in high-density lipoprotein cholesterol
Glycoprotein IIIa subunit of glycoprotein IIb/IIIa	Aspirin or glycoprotein IIb/IIIa inhibitors	Antiplatelet effect
Serotonin (5-hydroxytryptamine transporter	Antidepressants (e.g., clomipramine, fluoxetine, paroxetine)	5-Hydroxytryptamine neurotransmission, antidepressant response)

Reprinted with permission from Evans, McLeod, 2003.
FEV_1, forced expiratory volume in 1 second.
a. The examples shown are illustrative and are not representative of all published studies.

Table 8-4. Genetic Polymorphisms in Disease-Modifying or Treatment-Modifying Genes That Can Influence Drug Response[a]

Gene or gene product	Disease or response association	Medication	Influence of polymorphism on drug effect or toxicity
Adducin	Hypertension	Diuretics	Myocardial infarction or strokes
Apolipoprotein E	Progression of atherosclerosis; ischemic cardiovascular events	Statins (e.g., simvastatin)	Enhanced survival
	Alzheimer's disease	Tacrine	Clinical improvement
Human leukocyte antigen	Toxicity	Abacavir	Hypersensitivity reaction
Cholesterol ester transfer protein	Progression of atherosclerosis	Statins (e.g., pravastatin)	Slowing of progression of atherosclerosis
Ion channels (HERG, KvLQT1, Mink, and MiRP1)	Congenital long-QT syndrome	Erythromycin; terfenadine; cisapride; clarithromycin; and quinidine	Increased risk of drug-induced torsades de pointes
Methylguanine methyltransferase	Glioma	Carmustine	Response of glioma to carmustine
Parkin	Parkinson's disease	Levodopa	Clinical improvement and levodopa-induced dyskinesias
Prothrombin and factor V	Deep-vein thrombosis; cerebral-vein thrombosis	Oral contraceptives	Increased risk of deep-vein thrombosis and cerebral-vein thrombosis with oral contraceptives
Stromelysin-1	Atherosclerosis progression	Statins (e.g., pravastatin)	Reduction in cardiovascular events by pravastatin (death, myocardial infarction, stroke, angina, and others); reduction in risk of repeated angioplasty

Reprinted with permission from Evans, McLeod, 2003.
a. The examples shown are illustrative and are not representative of all published studies.

Table 8-5. Pharmacogenomics of Phase I Drug Metabolism[a]

Drug-metabolizing enzyme	Frequency of variant poor-metabolism phenotype	Representative drugs metabolized	Effect of polymorphism
Butyrylcholinesterase (pseudocholinesterase)	Approximately 1 in 3,500 Europeans	Succinylcholine	Enhanced drug effect
Cytochrome P-450 2D6 (CYP2D6)	6.8% of Swedes	Debrisoquin	Enhanced drug effect
	1% of Chinese	Sparteine	Enhanced drug effect
		Nortriptyline	Enhanced drug effect
		Codeine	Decreased drug effect
Cytochrome P-450 2C9 (CYP2C9)	Approximately 3% of English (those homozygous for the *2 and *3 alleles)	Warfarin	Enhanced drug effect
		Phenytoin	Enhanced drug effect
Cytochrome P-450 2C19 (CYP2C19)	2.7% of white Americans; 3.3% of Swedes; 14.6% of Chinese; 18% of Japanese	Omeprazole	Enhanced drug effect
Dihydropyrimidine dehydrogenase	Approximately 1% of population is heterozygous	Fluorouracil	Enhanced drug effect

Reprinted with permission from Weinshilboum, 2003.
a. Examples of genetically polymorphic phase I enzymes that catalyze drug metabolism are listed, including selected examples of drugs that have clinically relevant variations in their effect.

Table 8-6. Pharmacogenomics of Phase II Drug Metabolism[a]

Drug-metabolizing enzyme	Frequency of variant poor-metabolism phenotype	Representative drugs metabolized	Effect of polymorphism
N-acetyltransferase 2	52% of white Americans	Isoniazid	Enhanced drug effect
	17% of Japanese	Hydralazine	Enhanced drug effect
Uridine diphosphate-glucuronosyltransferase 1A1 (TATA box polymorphism)	10.9% of whites	Procainamide	Enhanced drug effect
	4% of Chinese	Irinotecan	Enhanced drug effect
	1% of Japanese	Bilirubin	Gilbert's syndrome
Thiopurine *S*-methyltransferase	Approximately 1 in 300 whites	Mercaptopurine	Enhanced drug effect (toxicity)
	Approximately 1 in 2,500 Asians	Azathioprine	Enhanced drug effect (toxicity)
Catechol *O*-methyltransferase	Approximately 25% of whites	Levodopa	Enhanced drug effect

Reprinted with permission from Weinshilboum, 2003.
a. Examples of genetically polymorphic phase II (conjugating) enzymes that catalyze drug metabolism are listed, including selected examples of drugs that have clinically relevant variations in their effects.

8-5. Questions

1. The process whereby the ribosome in the cytoplasm reads mRNA codons and matches them with the appropriate tRNAs (which, in turn, carry amino acids responsible for protein synthesis) is referred to as

    A. transcription.
    B. translation.
    C. transformation.
    D. transfection.
    E. transduction.

2. How many nucleotide triplets (or codons) exist for the encoding of the 20 possible amino acids specified by the genetic code?

    A. 4
    B. 12
    C. 20
    D. 61
    E. 64

3. Which of the following refers to a plasmid designed to allow for the expression of an inserted gene within a host cell for the production of the specified protein?

    A. Cloning vector
    B. Expression vector
    C. Transcription factor
    D. Translation initiation factor
    E. Transposable genetic element

4. Which of the following is an example of an rDNA-generated cytokine used for the management of acute relapsing–remitting multiple sclerosis?

    A. Interferon beta-1b (Betaseron)
    B. Aldesleukin (IL-2) (Proleukin)
    C. Eptifibatide (Integrilin)
    D. Bivalirudin (Angiomax)
    E. Abciximab (ReoPro)

5. Alteplase (Activase) is an rDNA protein of which of the following types?

    A. Hormone
    B. Enzyme
    C. Clotting factor
    D. Chemokine
    E. Cytokine

6. Which of the following biological agents is indicated for treatment of ovulatory failure?

    A. Ganirelix (Antagon)
    B. Glucagon (GlucaGen)
    C. Follitropin alfa (Gonal-F)
    D. Eptifibatide (Integrilin)
    E. Thyrotropin (Thyrogen)

7. Which of the following recombinant blood factors is available in recombinant form for clinical therapeutic use?

    A. Factor III
    B. Factor V
    C. Factor VI

D. Factor VII
E. Factor X

8. Recombinant DNA technology has led to the development of vaccines for which of the following diseases?

   A. Hepatitis B
   B. Hepatitis A
   C. *Haemophilus influenzae* type B infection
   D. Malaria
   E. AIDS

9. As dictated by the nomenclature for mono-clonal antibodies, which of the following is a chimeric monoclonal antibody therapeutically used for inflammatory disease?

   A. Abciximab
   B. Infliximab
   C. Palivizumab
   D. Rituximab
   E. Trastuzumab

10. Which of the following is best described as the repair or correction of a dysfunctional gene by selectively introducing rDNA into cells or tissues (ultimately leading to the expression of a functional gene product)?

    A. Monoclonal antibody therapy
    B. Gene therapy
    C. Antiviral therapy
    D. Cell therapy
    E. rDNA therapy

11. Fomivirsen (Vitravene) is an example of which of the following biological products?

    A. A liposomal formulation
    B. An antisense oligonucleotide
    C. An siRNA molecule
    D. An rDNA-produced protein
    E. A monoclonal antibody

12. The use of liposomal technology has favor-ably affected the therapeutic index of which of the following drugs?

    A. Cyclosporine
    B. Itraconazole
    C. Amphotericin B
    D. Cisplatin
    E. Propofol

13. Which of the following is best described as the scientific discipline of using genomewide approaches to understand the inherited basis of differences between individuals in their response to drugs?

    A. Pharmacogenomics
    B. Functional genomics
    C. Comparative genomics
    D. Pharmacodynamics
    E. Molecular genetics

14. An SNP always results in a change in which of the following?

    A. The nucleotide sequence in the genome
    B. The nucleotide sequence of a codon
    C. The encoded amino acid of the codon
    D. The encoded amino acid of the codon, with no change in function of the encoded protein
    E. The encoded amino acid of the codon, with a clinically relevant change in the function of the encoded protein

15. Which of the following is best described as "the manipulation (as through genetic engi-neering) of living organisms or their compo-nents to produce useful usually commercial products (as pest resistant crops, new bacte-rial strains, or novel pharmaceuticals)"?

    A. Biology
    B. Biotechnology
    C. Biotherapy
    D. Bioinformatics
    E. Nanotechnology

16. Which of the following is a drug discovery strat-egy that uses nucleic acids and amino acids in various combinations to synthesize vast libraries of oligonucleotide or peptide compounds for high-throughput lead compound screening?

    A. Whole cell screening
    B. Natural product screening
    C. Gene therapy
    D. Combinatorial chemistry
    E. rDNA technology

17. Which of the following is best defined as the application of computer sciences and infor-mation technology to the management and analysis of biological information?

    A. Biometrics
    B. Biotherapy
    C. Bioinformatics
    D. Biostatistics
    E. Biotechnology

18. Which of the following best outlines the central dogma of molecular biology?

    A. mRNA→DNA→Protein
    B. DNA→mRNA→Protein
    C. Protein→RNA→DNA
    D. DNA→Protein→mRNA
    E. Protein→DNA→mRNA

19. Which of the following biotechnology agents is indicated for treating anemia caused by chronic renal disease?

    A. Epoetin alfa
    B. Becaplermin
    C. Filgrastim
    D. Alemtuzumab
    E. Sargramostim

20. Which of the following products is indicated for prevention of blood clots post-PTCA?

    A. Abciximab
    B. Basiliximab
    C. Infliximab
    D. Trastuzumab
    E. Becaplermin

8-6. Answers

1. **B.** *Transcription* is the process by which RNA polymerase copies a strand of DNA into complementary RNA. *Transformation* refers to the alteration of the heritable properties of a eukaryotic cell. *Transfection* is the introduction of foreign DNA into a eukaryotic cell. *Transduction* can refer to the transfer of DNA from one bacterium to another through a bacteriophage.

2. **D.** There is degeneracy in the genetic code. Some amino acids may be encoded by as many as six codons, whereas others may be encoded by only one. Of the 64 possible codons, three are stop codons (UAA, UGA, and UAG).

3. **B.** A *cloning vector* is used to carry a fragment of DNA into a cell for cloning. A *transcription factor* is a protein that regulates transcription in eukaryotic cells. A *translation initiation factor,* as its name implies, is involved in the initiation of translation. A *transposable genetic element,* or *transposon,* is a portion of DNA that can move from one part of the genome to another.

4. **A.** Aldesleukin (IL-2) (Proleukin) is a recombinant cytokine indicated for the treatment of metastatic renal cell carcinoma and melanoma. Eptifibatide (Integrilin) is a recombinant enzyme indicated for treatment of acute coronary syndromes. Bivalirudin (Angiomax) is an enzyme indicated for use in coronary angioplasty and unstable angina. Abciximab (ReoPro) is a monoclonal antibody indicated for prevention of blood clots post-PTCA and unstable angina prior to PTCA.

5. **B.** Alteplase (Activase) is an rDNA protein of the enzyme type.

6. **C.** Ganirelix (Antagon) is a recombinant hormone indicated for the treatment of luteinizing hormone surge during fertility therapy. Glucagon (GlucaGen) is a recombinant hormone indicated for treatment of hypoglycemia. Eptifibatide (Integrilin) is a recombinant enzyme indicated for the treatment of acute coronary syndromes. Thyrotropin (Thyrogen) is a recombinant hormone indicated for the treatment of thyroid cancer.

7. **D.** The other factors listed are not clinically available in recombinant form.

8. **A.** Although promising, this technology has not yet yielded vaccines for hepatitis A, malaria, AIDS, or infections caused by *Haemophilus influenzae* type B.

9. **B.** Nomenclature of monoclonal antibodies is highly structured. The first component of the name is product specific; the second component indicates its therapeutic use (*ci* for cardiovascular use, *li* for use in inflammation, *tu* for use in cancer); the third component indicates the type of monoclonal antibody (*mo* for murine, *xi* for chimeric, *zu* for humanized); and the fourth component (*mab*) represents monoclonal antibody.

10. **B.** The repair or correction of a dysfunctional gene by selectively introducing recombinant DNA into cells or tissues, ultimately leading to the expression of a functional gene product, is called *gene therapy.*

11. **B.** Fomivirsen (Vitravene) is the first product based on this technology to come to market.

12. **C.** Formulation of this antifungal agent as a liposomal preparation (AmBisome) has significantly reduced the nephrotoxicity and other adverse effects associated with this drug.

13. **A.** The scientific discipline of using genomewide approaches to understand the inherited basis of differences between individuals in their response to drugs best describes pharmacogenomics.

14. **A.** An SNP may occur outside of an open reading frame (coding region), it may induce a mutation where no change in encoded amino acid occurs, and it may or may not cause a functional change in an encoded protein.

15. **B.** This definition by Merriam-Webster's Dictionary best describes *biotechnology*.

16. **D.** A drug discovery strategy that uses nucleic acids and amino acids in various combinations to synthesize vast libraries of oligonucleotide or peptide compounds for high-throughput lead compound screening is called *combinatorial chemistry*.

17. **C.** The application of computer sciences and information technology to the management and analysis of biological information best defines *bioinformatics*.

18. **B.** DNA is transcribed into mRNA, which is translated ultimately to protein.

19. **A.** Becaplermin is indicated for the management of diabetic foot ulcers. Filgrastim is indicated for treatment of neutropenia. Alemtuzumab is indicated for treatment of chronic lymphocytic leukemia. Sargramostim is indicated for myeloid reconstitution after bone marrow transplant; after bone marrow transplant failure, as an adjunct to chemotherapy in acute myelogenous leukemia; and in peripheral blood progenitor cell transplant.

20. **A.** Basiliximab is indicated for management of acute organ transplant rejection. Infliximab is indicated for the treatment of Crohn's disease and rheumatoid arthritis. Trastuzumab is indicated for the management of metastatic breast cancer. Becaplermin is indicated for the treatment of diabetic foot ulcers.

8-7. References

Adams VR, Karlix JL. Monoclonal antibodies. In: Koeller J, Tami J, eds. *Concepts in Immunology and Immunotherapeutics.* 3rd ed. Bethesda, MD: American Society of Health-System Pharmacists' Production Office; 1997:269–99.

Alberts B, Bray D, Lewis J, et al., eds. *Molecular Biology of the Cell.* 3rd ed. New York, NY: Garland; 1994.

Carrico JM. Human Genome Project and pharmacogenomics—implications for pharmacy. *J Am Pharm Assoc.* 2000;40:115–16.

Center for Biologics Evaluation and Research. U.S. Food and Drug Administration Web site. http://www.fda.gov/cber.

Center for Drug Evaluation and Research. U.S. Food and Drug Administration Web site. http://www.fda.gov/cder/.

Evans WE, McLeod HL. Pharmacogenomics: Drug disposition, drug targets, and side effects. *N Engl J Med.* 2003;348:538–49.

Glick BR, Pasternak JJ, eds. *Molecular Biotechnology: Principles and Applications of Recombinant DNA.* 2nd ed. Washington, DC: ASM Press; 1998.

Hollinger P, Hoogenboom H. Antibodies come back from the brink. *Nature Biotech.* 1998;16:1015–16.

Regan JW. Biotechnology and drug discovery. In: Delgado JN, Remers WA, eds. *Textbook of Organic Medicinal and Pharmaceutical Chemistry.* 10th ed. Philadelphia, PA: Lippincott-Raven; 1998:139–52.

Rogers CS, Sullenger BA, George AL Jr. Gene therapy. In: Hardman JG, Limbird LE, eds. *Goodman and Gilman's The Pharmacological Basis of Therapeutics.* 10th ed. New York, NY: McGraw-Hill; 2001:81–112.

Sindelar RD. Pharmaceutical biotechnology. In: Williams DA, Lemke TL, eds. *Foye's Principles of Medicinal Chemistry.* 5th ed. Philadelphia, PA: Lippincott Williams & Wilkins; 2002:982–1015.

Table of Pharmacogenomic Biomarkers in Drug Labels. U.S. Food and Drug Administration Website. http://www.fda.gov/drugs/scienceresearch/researchareas/pharmacogenetics/ucm083378.htm. Accessed March 6, 2014.

Vaughan TJ, Osbourn JK, Tempest PR. Human antibodies by design. *Nature Biotech.* 1998;16:535–39.

Weinshilboum R. Inheritance and drug response. *N Engl J Med.* 2003;348:529–37.

Biostatistics

9

Junling Wang

9-1. Key Points

- *Statistics* can be defined as a field of study that focuses on (1) the collection and analysis of data and (2) the drawing of inferences about a collection of data when only a part of the data is available for analysis. Statistical analysis can help researchers distinguish random variation from real differences when drawing conclusions. In the case of medical and biological data, statistics are most commonly referred to as *biostatistics*.

- In statistics, a *population* includes every member of all entities that one is interested in at a particular time.

- A *sample* is a collection of entities that are part of a population.

- A spreadsheet program can provide simple descriptive statistical analysis, but one typically uses statistical software for data analysis.

- When grouping data, an investigator counts the number of observations falling into a certain class interval. The investigator can then produce a frequency distribution that typically includes four statistical measures: frequency, cumulative frequency, relative frequency, and cumulative relative frequency.

- The mean, the median, and the mode are the three most commonly used measures of central tendency.

- Measures of dispersion reflect variability in a set of values.

- A test result can be evaluated using four measures of probability estimates: sensitivity, specificity, predictive value positive, and predictive value negative.

- For each parameter of interest, the investigator can compute two estimates: a point estimate and an interval estimate.

- The *null hypothesis* is the hypothesis to be tested, typically designated as H_0. The null hypothesis is a statement presumed to be true in the study population. The *alternative hypothesis* complements the null hypothesis. It is a statement of what may be true if the process of hypothesis testing rejects the null hypothesis. The alternative hypothesis is typically designated as H_A.

- The *p* value for a hypothesis testing is the probability of seeing a test statistic that is as extreme as or more extreme than the value of the test statistic observed.

- Regression analysis focuses on the assessment of the nature of the relationships with an ultimate objective of predicting or estimating the value of one variable given the value of another variable. Correlation analysis is related to the strength of the relationships between two variables.

- One way to evaluate the regression equation is to calculate the coefficient of determination, which describes the relative magnitude of the scatter of data points about the regression line. The coefficient of determination ranges from 0 to 1.

- The sample estimate of the correlation coefficient is designated as *r*, and the population parameter for the correlation coefficient is designated as ρ.

Much of the material in the chapter is a summary of work done by Wayne W. Daniel (Daniel WW. *A Foundation for Analysis in the Health Sciences.* 8th ed. Hoboken, NJ: Wiley; 2005) and Stephen B. Hulley (Hulley SB. *Designing Clinical Research: An Epidemiological Approach.* Baltimore, MD: Williams & Wilkins; 1988).

The value of the correlation coefficient ranges from −1 to 1.

- The chi-square test is the most frequently used test when an investigator has frequency or count data and when the variables are categorical.
- Nonparametric tests have at least two advantages compared to parametric tests. First, nonparametric tests apply when the data are merely rankings or classifications. Rankings and classifications may not represent a measurement level strong enough for parametric tests. Second, nonparametric tests tend to be more easily and quickly applied than do parametric tests.

9-2. Study Guide Checklist

The following topics may guide your study of this subject area:

- Basic concepts: data, biostatistics, sources of data, variable, quantitative variable, qualitative variable, random variable, discrete random variable, continuous random variable, population, sample, and simple random sample
- Steps of data management
- Descriptive statistics: ordered array, grouped data, measures of central tendency (mean, median, and mode), and measures of dispersion (range, variance, standard deviation, and coefficient of variation)
- Evaluation of screening tests using sensitivity, specificity, predictive value positive, and predictive value negative
- Concepts related to confidence interval: point estimate, interval estimate, reliability coefficient, precision, and margin of error
- Estimation of the confidence intervals for a population mean or proportion
- Basic concepts related to hypothesis testing: research hypothesis, statistical hypothesis, null hypothesis, alternative hypothesis, test statistic, rejection region and nonrejection region, significance level, type I and type II errors, p value, and one-sided and two-sided tests
- Hypothesis testing for a population mean or proportion
- Regression and correlation: independent and dependent variables, method of least squares, evaluation and use of the regression equation, correlation model, and precautions for using regression and correlation analyses
- Chi-square tests: observed and expected frequencies

- Nonparametric tests: advantages, disadvantages, and sign test
- Limitations of statistical analysis

9-3. Some Basic Concepts

One important part of research is to draw conclusions on the basis of limited amounts of data. Statistical analysis can facilitate the achievement of this goal. The following basic concepts are important to understanding statistics:

- *Data:* The raw material that researchers use for statistical analysis is data. In statistics, data can be defined as numbers. These numbers can be the result of measuring (e.g., height, weight, blood pressure) or counting (e.g., the number of patients discharged from a hospital on a given day). Each of these numbers is a *datum,* and all numbers taken together are *data.*
- *Biostatistics: Statistics* can be defined as a field of study that focuses on (1) the collection and analysis of data and (2) the drawing of inferences about a collection of data when only a part of the data is available for analysis. Statistical analysis can help researchers distinguish random variation from real differences when drawing conclusions. In the case of medical and biological data, statistics are most commonly referred to as *biostatistics.*
- *Sources of data:* Data for statistical analysis may be obtained from one or more of the following sources:
  - *Routinely kept records:* Organizations typically keep records of day-to-day activities. For example, hospital discharge data provide a wealth of data on the organization's patient care activities.
  - *Surveys:* If the data required to answer a research question are not available from routinely kept records, one may need to carry out a survey. For example, one may conduct a survey on patients' transportation costs.
  - *Experiments:* Often, the data required to answer a research question are available only as a result of conducting an experiment. For instance, a pharmacist may wish to determine whether pharmacy-based medication therapy management services can improve patient compliance with diabetes medications.
  - *External sources:* The data required to answer a research question may exist as published reports, research literature, data banks that

are commercially available, or databases that are in the public domain.

■ *Variable:* A *variable* is a characteristic that takes on different values for different possessors. Some examples of variables include ages of patients vaccinated in a community pharmacy and the heights of patients in a clinic. Different types of variables exist:

  • *Quantitative variable:* A *quantitative variable* is a variable whose amount can be measured (e.g., height, blood pressure, age).

  • *Qualitative variable:* A *qualitative variable* is a variable whose attributes can be measured. An example of a qualitative variable is sex, which can be female or male. A pharmacist may be interested in counting the number of female and male patrons who visit the pharmacy. These counts are also called *frequencies*.

  • *Random variable:* Whenever one measures the height, weight, or blood pressure of an individual, the result is typically called the *value of a variable*. When the values are determined by random factors and cannot be exactly predicted in advance, the variable is called a *random variable*. One example of a random variable is adult height, which cannot be exactly predicted at birth.

  • *Discrete random variable:* A *discrete random variable* is characterized by interruptions or gaps in its values. In other words, values are absent between particular values. One example of a discrete random variable is the number of admissions to a hospital in a given time period. The value of this variable cannot be, for example, 3.5 or 1.07 but rather must be a whole number such as 4 or 1.

  • *Continuous random variable:* A *continuous random variable* does not have interruptions or gaps in its values, or it can assume any value within an interval between any two of its values. Two individuals' weights may be very close together, but theoretically one can always find another person with a weight falling somewhere in between. In some situations, continuous variables may be recorded as discrete because of the limitations of available measuring instruments. Height, for instance, although a continuous variable, can be measured to the whole inch.

■ *Population:* In statistics, a *population* includes every member of all entities that one is interested in at a particular time. A population of values includes every member of all the possible values

of a random variable that one is interested in at a particular time. A population may be infinite or finite. If a population of values has an endless number of values, the population is infinite. In contrast, if a population of values has a fixed number of values, the population is finite.

■ *Sample:* A *sample* is a collection of entities that are part of a population. Suppose one's population consists of all patients who filled prescriptions through a chain pharmacy in a given month. If one measures the weights of only a part of those patients, that portion of patients becomes the sample.

■ *Simple random sample:* A *simple random sample* is a sample selected from a population such that every possible sample of the same size has the same chance of being drawn. The process of drawing a simple random sample is called *simple random sampling*.

9-4. Data Management

Although data analysis is typically conducted after the data are collected, preparation for data collection and data analysis should occur as part of research planning. The first step in planning for data management is to develop coding rules for data entry. Every variable is given a name in the data set, and these names are typically self-explanatory. For example, "sex" may be given to the variable for individuals' sex. For every variable, every possible value is then given a number so that the variable's values can be entered into the computer. For example, "1" can be given to female, and "2" can be given to male. Missing data and the response "don't know" are typically given extreme codes such as "9," "99," or "–8."

Generally, all coding decisions should be made before data collection. Often, coding instructions are printed on the data collection forms. Such precoding makes data entry more accurate and faster. Open-ended questions that require interpretation and coding judgment after data collection are more difficult to use.

After determining the coding rules, the investigator must select a data-entry program, which may be spreadsheet software, database managers' software, or statistical software. The most commonly used among these options is spreadsheet software, such as Microsoft Excel. When using spreadsheet software, one enters the data into rows (for the names of the variables) and columns (for the observations). Spreadsheet programs can themselves provide simple descriptive statistics and distributions. One can also use a spreadsheet program to sort the data to identify errors in the data set. For example, the observation taking the value "3" would be an error for the variable "gender" when "1" represents female and "2" represents male.

In modern times, most data collection, data entry, and data analysis can be conducted using microcomputers. Some projects require a complicated analytic plan and large data sets, and these projects require large mainframe computers. However, microcomputers are typically adequate for data processing and analyses for most research projects.

For a typical research project, the data can be stored on a compact disk or a thumb drive, but in general, storing data on a hard disk is a better practice. Regardless of where the data are stored, making a copy of the data at regular intervals is important to guard against data losses caused by system failure. Additionally, backing up the data set onto another storage system is recommended.

9-5. Descriptive Statistics

In terms of steps for data analysis, a deliberate approach is recommended, which involves first descriptive and then analytic analyses. The investigator should always conduct descriptive analysis as the first step by describing the distribution of each individual variable. Next, the investigator can estimate confidence intervals and conduct hypothesis testing. Using the results from these analyses, the investigator can then draw statistical conclusions. A spreadsheet program can provide simple descriptive statistical analysis, but one typically uses statistical software for data analysis. The existing statistical programs include but are not limited to SAS, SPSS, and Stata. The main descriptive statistical analysis techniques are described as follows.

The Ordered Array

A first step in organizing data is to prepare an ordered array by sorting the data in order of magnitude from the smallest to the largest. With an ordered array, the investigator can quickly determine the smallest measurement, the largest measurement, and other facts about the data.

Grouped Data

An ordered array is useful, but grouping data is required for further summarization. One can group values or observations into class intervals—a set of

contiguous, nonoverlapping intervals—so that each observation in the data set belongs to one and only one interval. A commonly used rule of thumb is that one should have between 6 and 15 class intervals. Fewer than 6 intervals would mean a loss of information in the data set because the data have been summarized too much; greater than 15 intervals could suggest that the data have not been summarized enough.

Class intervals generally should be the same width, but this rule has exceptions when it is impossible to achieve. The width of the interval may be determined by dividing the range of the data by the number of class intervals. Other helpful rules of thumb can be used when setting up class intervals. Class interval widths that are multiples of 5 or 10 tend to make the summarization more meaningful. Additionally, having the lower limit of each interval end in a 5 or 0 is common practice.

When grouping data, an investigator counts the number of observations falling into a certain class interval. The investigator can then produce a frequency distribution that typically includes four statistical measures: frequency, cumulative frequency, relative frequency, and cumulative relative frequency. *Frequency* is the number of observations falling in a particular class interval. *Cumulative frequency* is the sum of all observations within a certain interval and within all preceding intervals. *Relative frequency* is the proportion of observations within a certain class interval. *Cumulative relative frequency* is the sum of the proportion of observations within a certain class interval and within all preceding intervals. Table 9-1 shows an example of a frequency distribution.

Measures of Central Tendency

The mean, the median, and the mode are the three most commonly used measures of central tendency. The *mean* is calculated by summing all values for a variable and dividing the total by the number of values for the variable. The *median* is the value in a data set for which the number of values less than or equal to the median is equal to the number of values greater than or equal to the median. When an odd number of values exists, the median is the middle value in the ordered array. When an even number of values exists, the median is the average of the two middle values in the ordered array. The *mode* is the most frequent observation in a set of observations. If all observations are different within the data set, there is no mode. A set of values can have more than one mode.

Table 9-1. A Frequency Distribution of the Ages of 100 Individuals

Class intervals	Frequency	Cumulative frequency	Relative frequency	Cumulative relative frequency
10–19	10	10	0.1429	0.1429
20–29	15	25	0.2143	0.3571
30–39	15	40	0.2143	0.5714
40–49	10	50	0.1429	0.7143
50–59	15	65	0.2143	0.9286
60–69	5	70	0.0714	1.0000
Total	70		1.0000	

Measures of Dispersion

Measures of dispersion reflect variability in a set of values.

The range

One way to measure dispersion is to use the *range*, which is the difference between the largest value and the smallest value in the data.

Variance

The *variance* measures the scatter of the observations about their mean. When computing the variance of a sample, one subtracts the mean from each observation in the set, squares the differences obtained, sums all squared differences, and divides the total by the number of values in the set minus 1. The calculation of the variance of a sample can be given by

$$s^2 = \frac{\sum_{i=1}^{n}(x_i - \bar{x})^2}{n-1}$$

where s^2 stands for the sample variance, $\sum$ is the summation sign, and $\sum_{i=1}^{n}$ stands for the sum of all values of a variable. In addition, x_i represents the ith observation for the variable X, and $\bar{x}$ stands for the sample mean.

The denominator here is $n - 1$ because of the theoretical consideration degree of freedom. If an investigator knows $n - 1$ deviations of the values for a variable from its mean, the investigator will be able to determine the unknown nth deviation because the sum of deviations of all values from their mean equals zero.

The preceding equation for the calculation of variance is for sample variance. If the investigator needs to calculate population variance, the denominator of the calculation would be the total number of values in the population instead of the total number of values minus 1.

Standard deviation

The unit for variance is squared. If the investigator wishes to use the same concept as the variance but express it in the original unit, a measure called *standard deviation* can be used. Standard deviation equals the square root of the variance.

The coefficient of variation

The standard deviation is useful as a measure of dispersion, but its use in some situations may be misleading. For example, one may be interested in comparing the dispersion of two variables measured in different units, such as serum cholesterol level and body weight. The former may be measured in milligrams per 100 mL, and the latter may be measured in pounds. Comparing them directly may produce erroneous findings.

The coefficient of variation can be expressed as the standard deviation as a percentage of the mean, which is given by

$$\text{coefficient of variation} = \frac{s}{\bar{x}}(100)$$

where s is the standard deviation and $\bar{x}$ is the mean of the variable. Because the mean and standard deviation have the same units of measurement, the units cancel out when computing the coefficient of variation. Thus, the coefficient of variation is independent of the unit of measurement.

9-6. Evaluation of Screening Tests

In the health sciences, investigators often need to evaluate diagnostic criteria and screening tests. Clinicians frequently need to predict the absence or presence of a disease depending on whether test results are positive or negative or whether certain symptoms are present or absent. A conclusion based on the test results and symptoms is not always correct. There can be false positives and false negatives. When an individual's true status is negative, but the test result shows positive, the test result is false positive. When an individual's true status is positive, but the test result shows negative, the test result is false negative. A test result can be evaluated using four measures of probability estimates: sensitivity, specificity, predictive value positive, and predictive value negative:

- *Sensitivity:* The sensitivity of a test is the probability of the test result being positive when an individual has the disease. Using notations in Table 9-2, one can show that this probability equals $\dfrac{a}{a+b}$.

- *Specificity:* The specificity of a test is the probability of the test result being negative when an individual does not have the disease. Using the notations in Table 9-2, one can show that this probability equals $\dfrac{d}{c+d}$.

- *Predictive value positive:* The predictive value positive of a test is the probability of an individual having the disease when the test result is positive. Using the notations in Table 9-2, one can show that this probability equals $\dfrac{a}{a+c}$.

- *Predictive value negative:* The predictive value negative of a test is the probability of an indi-

vidual not having the disease when the test result is negative. Using the notations in Table 9-2, one can show that this probability equals $\dfrac{d}{b+d}$.

9-7. Estimation

In the field of health sciences, although many populations are finite, including every observation from the population, the sample is still prohibitive. Therefore, an investigator needs to estimate population parameters, such as the population mean and the population proportion, on the basis of data in the sample. For each parameter of interest, the investigator can compute two estimates: a point estimate and an interval estimate. A *point estimate* is a single value estimated to represent the corresponding population parameter. For example, the sample mean is a point estimate of the population mean. An *interval estimate* is a range of values defined by two numerical values. With a certain degree of confidence, the investigator thinks that the range of values includes the parameter of interest. The composition of a confidence interval can be described as

$$\text{estimator} \pm \left(\text{reliability coefficient}\right) \times \left(\text{standard error}\right)$$

The center of the confidence interval is the point estimate of the parameter of interest. The reliability coefficient is a value typically obtained from the standard normal distribution or *t* distribution. If the investigator needs to estimate a 95% confidence interval, for instance, the reliability coefficient indicates within how many standard errors lie 95% of the possible values of the population parameter. The value obtained by multiplying the reliability coefficient and the standard error is referred to as the *precision* of the estimate. It is also called the *margin of error*.

Confidence intervals can be calculated for the population mean, population proportion, difference in population means, difference in population proportions, and other measures. The first two are discussed here.

Confidence Interval for Population Mean

When estimating the confidence interval for a population mean, after calculating the sample mean, the investigator needs to determine the reliability coefficient. When the sample size is large (a rule of thumb is greater than 30), reliability coefficients can

---

Table 9-2. Elaboration of Individuals Cross-Classified on the Basis of Disease Status and Test Results

Disease status	Test results	
	Positive	**Negative**
Disease	a	b
No disease	c	d

Adapted from Daniel, 2005.

be obtained from the standard normal distribution. When an investigator needs to estimate 90%, 95%, and 99% confidence intervals, the corresponding reliability coefficients are 1.645, 1.96, and 2.58, respectively.

For example, in a study of patients' punctuality for their appointments, a sample of 35 patients were found to be on average 17.2 minutes late for their appointments with a standard deviation of 8 minutes. The 90% confidence interval for population mean is given by

$$17.2 \pm (1.645) \times \left(\frac{8}{\sqrt{35}} \right)$$

$$15, 19.4$$

This confidence interval can be interpreted using the following practical interpretation: the investigators are 90% confident that the interval [15, 19.4] contains the population mean.

The method followed in this example applies if the sample size is large. When the sample size is small, the reliability coefficient would be obtained from a *t* distribution.

Confidence Interval for Population Proportion

To estimate the population proportion, an investigator first needs to draw a sample of size *n* from the population and compute the sample proportion, $\hat{p}$. Then the confidence interval for the population proportion can be estimated using the same composition as given for a confidence interval. When both np and $n(1 - p)$ are greater than 5 (p is population proportion), the reliability coefficients can be estimated from the standard normal distribution. The standard error can be estimated as $\sqrt{\frac{\hat{p}(1-\hat{p})}{n}}$.

For example, among a sample of 1,000 individuals, 15% exercise at least twice a week. The 95% confidence interval for the population proportion is given by

$$0.15 \pm 1.96 \times \sqrt{\frac{0.15(1-0.15)}{1,000}}$$

$$0.128, 0.172$$

The interpretation of this confidence interval is that the investigators are 95% confident that the population proportion is in the interval between 0.128 and 0.172.

9-8. Hypothesis Testing

Both hypothesis testing and estimation examine a sample from a population with the purpose of aiding the researchers or decision makers in drawing conclusions about the population.

Basic Concepts

Null hypothesis and alternative hypothesis

When conducting research, an investigator typically has two types of hypotheses: a research hypothesis and a statistical hypothesis. A *research hypothesis* is the investigator's theories or suspicions that need to be subjected to the rigors of scientific testing. A *statistical hypothesis* is a hypothesis stated in a way that can be tested using statistical techniques. In the process of hypothesis testing, two statistical hypotheses are used: the null hypothesis and the alternative hypothesis. The *null hypothesis* is the hypothesis to be tested and is typically designated as H_0. The null hypothesis is a statement presumed to be true in the study population. As the result of hypothesis testing, the null hypothesis is either not rejected or rejected. Typically, an indication of equality ($=$, $\geq$, or $\leq$) is included in the null hypothesis. The *alternative hypothesis* complements the null hypothesis. It is a statement of what may be true if the process of hypothesis testing rejects the null hypothesis. The alternative hypothesis is typically designated as H_A. Usually, the alternative hypothesis is the same as the research hypothesis.

A word of caution regarding null hypothesis is warranted here. When hypothesis testing does not reject the null hypothesis, it does not mean proof of the null hypothesis. Hypothesis testing indicates only whether the available data support or do not support the null hypothesis.

Test statistic

The *test statistic* is a numerical value calculated from the data in the sample. The test statistic can assume many different values, and the particular sample determines the specific value that the test statistic assumes. The test statistic can be considered as the decision rule. The value of the test statistic determines whether to reject the null hypothesis.

The general formula for the test statistic is given as follows:

$$\text{test statistic} = (\text{a statistic} - \text{hypothesized parameter}) / (\text{standard error of the statistic})$$

Values that the test statistic can assume are divided into two groups that fall into two regions for hypothesis testing: the rejection region and the nonrejection region. The values in the nonrejection region are more likely to occur than the values in the rejection region if the null hypothesis is true. Therefore, the decision rule of hypothesis testing is that if the value of the test statistic is within the rejection region, then the investigator should reject the null hypothesis and vice versa.

Significance level

The critical values that separate the rejection region from the nonrejection region are determined by the level of significance, which is typically designated by α. Thus, hypothesis testing is frequently called *significance testing*. If the test statistic falls into the rejection region, then the test is said to be significant.

Type I and type II errors

Because significance level determines the critical values for separating the rejection and nonrejection regions of a test, an investigator obviously has a probability of committing errors when conducting hypothesis testing. There are two types of errors for hypothesis testing (Table 9-3). When the null hypothesis is true, but the statistical decision is to reject the null hypothesis, the investigator has committed a type I error. If the null hypothesis is not true, and the statistical decision is not to reject the null hypothesis, then the investigator has committed a type II error. The probability of a type I error is the level of the significance for the test, which is α. The probability of a type II error is typically designated as β. Another concept often used in statistics is *power,* which is the probability of not rejecting a false null hypothesis.

In a hypothesis testing, the level of significance, or α, is typically made small so that there is a small probability of rejecting a true null hypothesis. Typical levels of significance for statistical tests are 0.01, 0.05, and 0.1. However, the investigator exercises less

control over the probability of a type II error. Keep in mind that the investigator never knows the true status of the null hypothesis. Therefore, to have a lower probability of committing any errors, investigators take more comfort when a null hypothesis is rejected.

The *p* value

The *p* value for hypothesis testing is the probability of seeing a test statistic that is as extreme as or more extreme than the value of the test statistic observed. Reporting *p* value as part of the results is more informative than reporting only the statistic decision of rejecting or not rejecting the null hypothesis.

One-sided and two-sided tests

When the rejection region includes two tails of the distribution of the test statistic in testing a hypothesis, it is a two-sided test. If the rejection region includes only one tail of the distribution, then it is a one-sided test. In other words, if both sufficiently large and small values of a test statistic lead to rejection of the null hypothesis, then the investigator needs a two-sided test. If only sufficiently large or small values of a test statistic can lead to rejection of the null hypothesis, then the investigator needs a one-sided test.

Hypothesis Testing for a Population Mean

When testing a hypothesis for a population mean, an investigator uses a Z statistic or a t statistic, depending on whether the sample size is large (this may remind readers of the determination of the reliability coefficient for the confidence interval). When the sample size is small, the investigator should use the t statistic, which is given by

$$t = \frac{\bar{x} - \mu_0}{s/\sqrt{n}}$$

where $\bar{x}$ stands for the sample mean, μ_0 represents the hypothesized population mean, s stands for sample standard deviation, and n represents sample size.

Hypothesis Testing for a Population Proportion

When one tests a hypothesis for a population proportion and when the sample size is large, the test statistic is given by

$$z = \frac{\hat{p} - p_0}{\sqrt{\dfrac{p_0(1 - p_0)}{n}}}$$

Table 9-3. Type I and Type II Errors

Status of null hypothesis	Statistical decision	
	Not to reject H$_0$	**Reject H$_0$**
True	Correct decision	Type I error
False	Type II error	Correct decision

Adapted from Daniel 2005.

where $\hat{p}$ stands for the sample proportion, p_0 represents the hypothesized population proportion, and n stands for sample size.

9-9. Simple Linear Regression and Correlation Analyses

Regression and correlation analyses are used when analyzing the relationship between two numerical variables. Regression and correlation are closely related, but they serve different purposes. Regression analysis focuses on the assessment of the nature of the relationships with an ultimate objective of predicting or estimating the value of one variable given the value of another variable. Correlation analysis is related to the strength of the relationships between two variables.

The Regression Model

Independent variable and dependent variable

In a simple linear regression, two variables are of interest: the independent variable X and the dependent variable Y. Variable X is usually controlled by the investigator, and its values may be preselected by the investigator. Corresponding to each value of X are one or more values of Y. When the investigator conducts simple linear regression analysis, the objective is to estimate the linear relationship between the independent and dependent variables. The investigator needs to first draw a sample from the population and then plot a scatter diagram of the relationship between the two variables by assigning the values of the independent variables to the horizontal axis and the values of the dependent variable to the vertical axis. An example of such a diagram is the relationship between age and the forced expiratory volume (liters) among a group of children between 10 and 16 years of age (Figure 9-1). It is clear from this diagram that the older the children are, the greater the forced expiratory volume. In other words, a linear relationship may exist between the two variables.

Estimation of the linear line

The method usually followed to obtain the linear line is known as the *method of least squares*, and the line obtained is the *least squares line*. The least squares line has this characteristic: the squared vertical deviations of any data point from the least squares line are the smallest among all possible lines that describe the linear relationship between the independent and dependent variables.

The general format of the least squares line is $\hat{y} = a + bx$, where a is the sample estimate of the intercept of the line, and b is the sample estimate of the slope of the line. The population parameters for the intercept and the slope of the line are designated α and β, respectively. The estimated least squares line for the linear relationship depicted in Figure 9-1 is given by

$$\hat{y} = 0.23 + 0.14x$$

where a, the intercept of the line, has a positive sign, suggesting that the line crosses the vertical axis above the origin; and b, the slope of the line, has a

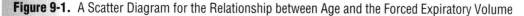

Figure 9-1. A Scatter Diagram for the Relationship between Age and the Forced Expiratory Volume

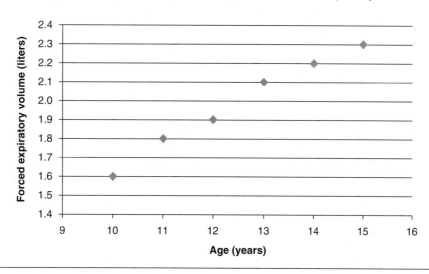

value of 0.14, suggesting that when x increases by 1 unit, y increases by 0.14 unit.

Evaluation of the regression equation

After the regression equation is estimated, the investigator must evaluate whether the estimate of the slope of the line adequately describes the relationship between the independent and dependent variables. One way to evaluate the regression equation is to calculate the coefficient of determination, which describes the relative magnitude of the scatter of data points about the regression line. The coefficient of determination ranges from 0 to 1. The closer the coefficient of determination is to 1, the closer the observations lie to the regression line. The coefficient of determination for the preceding example is 0.98.

Use of the regression equation

With an estimated linear line, the investigator can then predict the value of the dependent variable when given a value for the independent variable. For example, if $X = 11$,

$$\hat{y} = 0.23 + 0.14(11) = 1.77$$

The Correlation Model

Different from the regression model, which often pre-selects the values of the independent variables, the correlation model selects a sample of the observation units and then measures the values of the two variables X and Y for each unit of observation. In other words, the two variables X and Y have equal footing. Therefore, in the framework of correlation analysis, two linear regression models may be estimated: either of the two variables can be the dependent variable, and the other becomes the independent variable.

In a correlation model, the correlation coefficient is used to describe and measure the relationship between the variables X and Y. The sample estimate of the correlation coefficient is designated as r, and the population parameter for the correlation coefficient is designated as ρ. The value of the correlation coefficient ranges from -1 to 1. The absolute value of the correlation coefficient equals the square root of the coefficient of determination. The sign of the correlation coefficient is the same as the sign of the slope of the regression line for the variables X and Y.

If $\rho = 1$, X and Y have a perfect direct linear correlation. If $\rho = -1$, X and Y have a perfect inverse linear correlation. If $\rho = 0$, the two variables are not linearly correlated.

Some Precautions

Simple linear regression and correlation analyses are powerful tools when they are appropriately used. However, the investigator may get useless and meaningless information when these analyses are not used properly. The following few precautions should be kept in mind. First, in simple linear regression and correlation analyses, the variables X and Y are measured on the same unit of association. Therefore, discussing the association between the weights of some individuals and the heights of some other individuals would be meaningless.

Second, even when a strong linear relationship is identified from the analysis between the two variables, it should not be mistaken as evidence of cause and effect. In that situation, the relationship may be causal, but a third factor may also possibly directly or indirectly cause both the independent and the dependent variables.

Third, an investigator should guard against extrapolation. In other words, the regression equation may not be used to predict the values of the dependent variable outside the range of the values of the independent variable. The reason for this precaution is that the relationship between the variables may not be the same (e.g., nonlinear) outside the range of the values of the independent variables.

9-10. Chi-Square Tests

The chi-square test is the most commonly used test when an investigator is working with frequency or count data and when the variables are categorical. A pharmacy investigator may have a number of pharmacy patrons using different types of insurance at the pharmacy: private insurance, Medicaid, Medicare, and others. These are count data. The investigator may be interested in comparing the insurance status between his or her pharmacy and another pharmacy. Another researcher might be concerned with the rates of compliance with diabetes medications between females and males. The chi-square test is suitable for these scenarios because the variables are categorical.

Two sets of frequencies matter for a chi-square test: observed frequencies and expected frequencies. The *observed frequencies* are the number of observed individuals or other entities that fall into the various categories of the variable of interest (e.g., the health insurance status). For example, among 100 pharmacy patrons, 30 might be privately insured, 40 might have Medicare, 20 might have Medicaid, and 10 might not have any insurance. The expected frequencies are the number of individuals who fall into the various categories of the variable of interest if the null hypothesis is true. For this example, if the null hypothesis is that individuals are equally likely to have any one of the four insurance categories, 25 individuals are expected to have each of the four types of insurance.

The test statistic for the chi-square test is typically

$$X^2 = \sum \left[\frac{(O_i - E_i)^2}{E_i} \right]$$

where O_i is the observed frequency for the ith category and E_i is the expected frequency for the ith category. The quantity of X^2 measures the degrees of agreement between the observed frequencies and the expected frequencies: the poorer the agreement, the greater the quantity of X^2. Therefore, a large enough X^2 value would lead to rejection of the null hypothesis. When the null hypothesis is true, X^2 follows a chi-square distribution, which determines the critical values that separate the rejection region from the nonrejection region.

A word of caution about the chi-square test is needed. When the expected frequencies are too small, a chi-square test would not be appropriate. For example, some writers have suggested that all expected values should be greater than 5 or 10. Otherwise, an alternative test, such as Fisher's exact test, should be used.

Using the pharmacy patron insurance example,

$$X^2 = \sum \left[\frac{(O_i - E_i)^2}{E_i} \right] = \frac{(30-25)^2}{25} + \frac{(40-25)^2}{25}$$
$$+ \frac{(20-25)^2}{25} + \frac{(10-25)^2}{25} = 20$$

By consulting a chi-square distribution table, the investigator would obtain a critical value of 7.815, which is less than the X^2 value calculated for this example. Therefore, the null hypothesis is rejected. The pharmacy patrons might not be equally likely to have any one of the four types of insurance.

9-11. Nonparametric Tests

Most of the statistical tests that have been described so far are parametric statistics, with the exception of the chi-square test. For parametric tests, the investigators are interested in estimating or testing hypotheses about population parameters, such as the population mean or the population proportion. Additionally, not emphasized earlier, but required,

is that the investigator know the form of the population distribution from which the sample is drawn.

Nonparametric tests have at least the following two advantages compared to parametric tests. First, nonparametric tests apply when the data are merely rankings or classifications. Rankings and classifications may not represent a measurement level strong enough for parametric tests. Second, nonparametric tests tend to be more easily and quickly applied than are parametric tests.

Nonparametric tests also have disadvantages. When the data can be analyzed with parametric tests, using nonparametric tests is a waste of data. Additionally, when the sample size is large, conducting a nonparametric test can be too time consuming.

One type of nonparametric test is the sign test, which focuses on the median of the distribution. The only requirement for using the sign test is that the variable be continuous. The raw data used in the calculation of the test statistic for the sign test are plus and minus signs.

For example, the appearance scores among a group of girls with mental retardation are 4, 5, 8, 8, 9, 6, 10, 7, 6, and 6. Researchers are interested in determining whether the median appearance score among them is 5.

Using a sign test, researchers count the number of values greater than 5 as the number of pluses and the number of values less than 5 as the number of minuses. Values equal to 5 are dropped from further analysis as is typically done for the sign test. Therefore, this example has eight pluses and one minus. If the median for the distribution is indeed 5, one would expect to see an equal number of plus and minus signs. The probability of seeing as many pluses and minuses as in this example can be calculated on the basis of a binomial distribution. The probability turns out to be 0.039 for this test. At the level of significance of 0.05, the statistical decision is to reject the null hypothesis that the median of the distribution is 5.

9-12. Limitation of Statistical Analysis

Statistical analysis can be crucial to helping decision makers and researchers in decision-making processes. However, statistical significance should not be considered definitive, and statistical conclusions should be taken as only one piece of information needed for decision making. Other relevant information, such as safety, cost, and accessibility of a program, should also be considered. Additionally, keeping in mind the difference between statistical significance and clinical significance is important. Although statistical significance is tested objectively using hypothesis testing, clinical significance is assessed subjectively by a patient, a caregiver, or a medical professional. As an example, certain points of blood pressure reduction resulting from an intervention program might be statistically significant according to hypothesis testing. However, if patients, doctors, and caregivers do not perceive patients as having benefited, concluding that the amount of blood pressure reduction is clinically significant would be difficult.

9-13. Questions

1. Which of the following statements about statistics is true?

   A. Data used in statistical analysis have to include all entities in a population.
   B. If an investigator has a research question, she or he has to collect original data.
   C. Statistical analysis draws conclusions on the basis of data from the whole population.
   D. Statistics can help distinguish random variation from real differences when drawing conclusions.

2. Which of the following statements is *not* true for variables?

   A. A continuous random variable has interruptions or gaps in its values.
   B. Height is a quantitative variable.
   C. Blood pressure can be a random variable.
   D. Weight is a continuous variable.

3. Which of the following statements is *not* true about data management?

   A. Data analysis planning needs to start before data collection.
   B. An investigator has to use large mainframe computers for data storage.
   C. Open-ended questions are more challenging because precoding for them is difficult.
   D. Spreadsheet programs can be used for data analysis for some projects.

4. Which of the following statements is true?

   A. The response "don't know" should be left blank in the data set.
   B. Missing data should always be left blank in the data set.

   C. All coding decisions have to be made after data collection and before data entry.
   D. Coding instructions may be printed on the data collection form.

5. Which of the following is *not* a measure of central tendency?

   A. Median
   B. Mean
   C. Range
   D. Mode

6. Which of the following measures of dispersion is independent of the measurement unit?

   A. Range
   B. Variance
   C. Standard deviation
   D. Coefficient of variation

The following table shows 100 individuals cross-classified according to disease status and test results. Use data from this table for Questions 7–10.

	Disease		
Test results	**Present**	**Absent**	**Total**
Positive	30	40	70
Negative	20	10	30
Total	50	50	100

7. What is the sensitivity for the test?

   A. 30/50
   B. 10/50
   C. 30/70
   D. 10/30

8. What is the specificity for the test?

   A. 30/50
   B. 10/50
   C. 30/70
   D. 10/30

9. What is the predictive value positive for the test?

   A. 30/50
   B. 10/50
   C. 30/70
   D. 10/30

10. What is the predictive value negative for the test?

   A. 10/30
   B. 10/50

C. 30/50

D. 30/70

11. Which of the following statements is true?

A. For a population parameter, an investigator cannot produce both a point estimate and an interval estimate.

B. The lower limit of a confidence interval is also called the precision of the test.

C. The reliability coefficient is always determined from a *t* distribution.

D. The reliability coefficient for the confidence interval can be determined on the basis of the standard normal distribution only when certain conditions are met.

12. Which of the following statements is true about statistical hypotheses?

A. An alternative hypothesis is a statement presumed to be true in the study population.

B. The null hypothesis is typically the same as the research hypothesis.

C. A statistical test can either prove or reject a null hypothesis.

D. A statistical test cannot prove a null hypothesis.

13. Which of the following statements is true?

A. If the test statistic falls into the nonrejection region, the test is said to be significant.

B. The rejection region can be on only one tail of the distribution.

C. Researchers typically prefer higher levels of significance.

D. A test statistic can assume different values when different samples are drawn from the population.

14. Which of the following statements is *not* true for type I and type II errors?

A. A type I error occurs when a true null hypothesis is rejected.

B. A type I error cannot occur at the same time as a type II error.

C. A type II error occurs when a false null hypothesis is not rejected.

D. A type I error occurs when a true hypothesis is not rejected.

15. Which of the following statements is true?

A. It is appropriate to estimate a simple linear regression equation for any two variables.

B. A negative intercept of a linear regression means the higher the independent variable is, the lower the dependent variable will be.

C. A positive slope suggests that the regression line crosses the vertical axis above the origin.

D. The investigator typically has control over the values of the independent variable.

16. Which of the following statements is *not* true?

A. The coefficient of variation ranges from 0 to 1.

B. The correlation coefficient ranges from 0 to 1.

C. The sign of the correlation coefficient is the same as the slope of the regression equation.

D. The absolute value of the correlation coefficient equals the square root of the coefficient of determination.

17. Which of the following statements is true?

A. Regression analysis can determine whether two variables have a causal relationship.

B. Correlation analysis can determine whether two variables have a causal relationship.

C. If there is a linear relationship between two variables, the relationship outside the range of the values of the independent variable is not necessarily linear.

D. A linear regression model can be used to predict the value of the dependent variable for any values of the independent variable.

18. Which of the following statements is true?

A. When two variables are correlated, only one regression model can be estimated from them.

B. Investigators can preselect values for both variables for a simple linear correlation analysis.

C. Investigators can preselect values of the dependent variable for a simple linear regression analysis.

D. Investigators have some control over the independent variable for a simple linear regression analysis.

19. Which of the following statements is *not* true about the chi-square test?

A. The chi-square test is a nonparametric test.

B. The test statistic of a chi-square test follows a chi-square distribution when the null hypothesis is true.

C. The chi-square test always applies when the data are counts or frequencies.

D. The rejection and nonrejection regions of the chi-square test are determined on the basis of the chi-square distribution.

20. Which of the following statements is true?

A. Parametric tests are always preferred over nonparametric tests.

B. When a sample size is large, a nonparametric test has the advantage of being more easily and quickly applied than a parametric test.

C. The investigator needs to know the form of the population distribution to use a nonparametric test.

D. The sign test takes into consideration only the positive and negative signs of the data.

9-14. Answers

1. D. Statistical analysis can help researchers to distinguish random variation from real differences when drawing conclusions.

2. A. A continuous random variable does not have interruptions or gaps in its values, or it can assume any value within an interval between any two of its values.

3. B. In modern times, most data collection, data entry, data storage, and data analysis can be conducted using microcomputers.

4. D. Generally, all coding decisions should be made before data collection. Coding instructions are then often printed on the data collection forms.

5. C. Range is a measure of dispersion.

6. D. The coefficient of variation can be expressed as a percentage of the mean. Because the mean and standard deviation have the same units of measurement, the units cancel out when the coefficient of variation is computed.

7. A. The sensitivity of a test is the probability of the test result being positive when an individual has the disease.

8. B. The specificity of a test is the probability of the test result being negative when an individual does not have the disease.

9. C. The predictive value positive of a test is the probability of an individual having the disease when the test result is positive.

10. A. The predictive value negative of a test is the probability of an individual not having the disease when the test result is negative.

11. D. When the sample size is large (a rule of thumb is greater than 30), reliability coefficients can be obtained from the standard normal distribution.

12. D. When hypothesis testing does not reject the null hypothesis, it does not mean proof of the null hypothesis. Hypothesis testing indicates only whether the available data support or do not support the null hypothesis.

13. D. The test statistic is a numerical value calculated from the data in the sample. The test statistic can assume many different values, and the particular sample determines the specific value that the test statistic assumes.

14. D. When the null hypothesis is true, but the statistical decision is to reject the null hypothesis, the investigator has committed a type I error.

15. D. The independent variable is usually controlled by the investigator, and the investigator may preselect its values.

16. B. The value of the correlation coefficient ranges from −1 to 1.

17. C. The relationship between the variables may not be the same (e.g., nonlinear) outside the range of the values of the independent variables.

18. D. The independent variable is usually controlled by the investigator, and the investigator may preselect its values.

19. C. When the expected frequencies are too small, a chi-square test would not be appropriate.

20. D. The sign test takes into consideration only the positive and negative signs of the data. The raw data used in the calculation of the test statistic for the sign test are plus and minus signs.

9-15. References

Daniel WW. *A Foundation for Analysis in the Health Sciences*. 8th ed. Hoboken, NJ: Wiley; 2005.

Hulley SB. *Designing Clinical Research: An Epidemiological Approach*. Baltimore, MD: Williams & Wilkins; 1988.

Drug Information

Glen E. Farr

10

10-1. Key Points

- Drug information is printed, electronic, or verbal information pertaining to medications.
- Providing evidence-based drug information is at the core of the practice of pharmacy in any setting.
- Clinical decision support systems (CDSSs) are an important part of any clinical information and electronic health record system.
- Drug information resources are categorized as tertiary, secondary, and primary literature. Pharmacists should use a combination of the different types of resources and will benefit from familiarity with commonly used sources of drug information.
- With a vast amount of specialized information available, selecting the most relevant drug information resource for the specific question is important.
- Pharmacists should use evidence-based practice (EBP) or evidence-based medicine (EBM) in clinical decision making and in responses to drug information questions. However, not all "evidence-based" information is actually based on evidence and uniformly agreed upon.
- Many major compendia of drug information provide information on U.S. Food and Drug Administration (FDA)–approved and off-label (non-FDA-approved) indications.
- With more than 20,000 biomedical journals published annually, appropriate search techniques are crucial to identify relevant primary literature.

- Electronic access to drug information databases allows a single search of millions of citations through the use of keywords and linked keywords.
- Conducting a variety of searches with various combinations of search terms is important to perform the most comprehensive search possible.
- When conducting a search of the MEDLINE database through PubMed, users are advised to first use the Medical Subject Headings (MeSH) terms to ensure that all relevant information is identified through the search.
- Several databases should be consulted when researching a drug information question to ensure a thorough and comprehensive search of available information.
- Effective written and oral communication skills are fundamental components of the practice of pharmacy and the provision of drug information.
- With a vast amount of information available, the ability to judge the reliability of drug information from various sources, particularly the Internet, is essential.
- When possible, verify drug information in multiple sources.

10-2. Study Guide Checklist

The following topics may guide your study of this subject area:

- Different actions of tertiary, secondary, and primary literature sources for drug information
- Description of the concept and use of EBP as it relates to drug information
- Considerations for the evaluation of the reliability of drug information from various sources

Editor's Note: This chapter is based on the 10th edition chapter written by Anne M. Hurley.

■ Factors to consider to respond appropriately to different levels of drug information requests, for example, from prescribers versus consumers

■ Elements of clinical decision support systems to reduce adverse events and enhance decision making

■ Use of Boolean operators (*and, or,* and *not*) and MeSH terms when conducting a literature search with the database PubMed

10-3. Fundamentals of Practice of Drug Information

Drug information is printed, electronic, or verbal information pertaining to prescription and non-prescription medications and dietary supplements. The term *medication information* is also used and pertains to the use of information to affect medication therapy outcomes. Providing drug information to health professionals and the patient is at the core of all types of pharmacy practice.

Some pharmacists specialize in providing verbal and written drug information for patient education, prescriber education, and formulary development, but most pharmacists provide drug information as a part of their overall responsibilities. Before the introduction of electronic databases and access to the World Wide Web, most pharmacists used traditional literature sources for information about medications. At that time, drug information resources were categorized as tertiary, secondary, and primary literature. Those terms are still in use, but the Internet has drastically changed how to obtain and share drug information. Today's pharmacists use a combination of the different types of resources, both written and electronic, to keep up to date and to serve as a source of drug information.

Types of Drug Information Literature

Medical and pharmaceutical literature is generally categorized as primary, secondary, and tertiary. Table 10-1 provides a listing of tertiary and secondary literature examples and general drug information; the examples include compendia, textbooks, review articles, and general information identified on the Internet.

Tertiary resources

Advantages of **tertiary resources** include convenience, ease of use, and familiarity. Most tertiary references

are available in print and electronic formats. An important consideration when choosing the most appropriate reference for a particular drug information question is the type of information being sought. Because of the variety of specialized information available, selecting the most relevant drug information resource for a specific question is important.

Major compendia contain drug monographs and are commonly used by pharmacists in a variety of practice settings. Drug monographs are typically organized by general categories of drug information, including dosage and administration, mechanism of action, pharmacokinetics, adverse effects, drug interactions, and toxicology. Many major compendia of drug information, such as *AHFS Drug Information* and *Facts & Comparisons,* provide information on indications approved by the U.S. Food and Drug Administration (FDA) as well as some documented off-label (non-FDA-approved) indications. The *Physicians' Desk Reference* (PDR), however, contains only FDA-approved medication uses.

The FDA's *Orange Book: Approved Drug Products with Therapeutic Equivalence Evaluations* (or *Orange Book*) can be accessed on the FDA Web site (www.fda.gov). (Note: www.fda.com is not the official FDA Web site.) The *Orange Book* contains information regarding medication bioequivalence, using "A," "AB," and "B" classifications.

PDR Network's *Red Book* contains information regarding availability and pricing for prescription and over-the-counter (OTC) medications, as well as information regarding dosage form, size, strength, and routes of administration. This reference also includes the product's National Drug Code (NDC) numbers and Average Wholesale Price (AWP). The AWP is a benchmark that has been used for decades for pricing and reimbursement of prescription drugs for both government and private payers. Initially, the AWP was intended to represent the average price that wholesalers used to sell medications to pharmacies. However, the AWP is not a true representation of actual market prices. AWP has often been compared to the "list price" or "sticker price," meaning it is an elevated drug price that is rarely what is actually paid. AWP is not a government-regulated figure and does not include buyer volume discounts or rebates often involved in prescription drug sales.

Lists of sugar-free, lactose-free, and alcohol-free preparations can also be found in the *Red Book.* Red Book Online is also available, offering the advantage of daily updates. The *Red Book* can be accessed on the FDA Web site (www.fda.gov).

Table 10-1. Examples of Drug Information Resources by Category (Secondary and Tertiary Literature)

Category	Title
Compendia and general drug information	*AHFS Drug Information* (McEvoy 2014) (www.ahfsdruginformation.com)
	Clinical Pharmacology (www.clinicalpharmacology.com)
	Facts & Comparisons (www.factsandcomparisons.com)
	Epocrates (www.epocrates.com)
	Lexicomp *Drug Information Handbook* (Lacy, Armstrong, Goldman 2012) (http://webstore.lexi.com/Drug-Information-Handbook)
	Micromedex Healthcare Series (www.micromedex.com)
	Micromedex Medication Management (http://micromedex.com/medication-management)
	Physicians' Desk Reference (PDR Network 2014)
	UpToDate (www.uptodate.com/home)
	The Medical Letter (www.medicalletter.org)
	Pharmacist's Letter (www.pharmacistsletter.com)
	Medscape Drug Reference (http://search.medscape.com/drug-reference-search)
	The Pink Sheet (www.thepinksheet.com)
Evidence-based practice	ACP Journal Club (http://acpjc.acponline.org)
	Evidence-Based Medicine (http://ebm.bmj.com)
	Journal Watch (www.jwatch.org/)
	PNN Pharmacotherapy News Network (www.pharmacotherapynewsnetwork.com/index.html)
Product identification and pronunciation	Drugs.com (www.drugs.com/imprints.php)
	Drugs.com (www.drugs.com/search-wildcard-phonetic.html)
Nonprescription medications and alternative medicine	Introduction to dietary supplements (Tsourounis, Dennehy 2012) (www.pharmacylibrary.com/content/617437)
	Natural Medicines Comprehensive Database (www.naturaldatabase.com)
	*Natural Standard (*www.naturalstandard.com)
	PDR for Herbal Medicines (PDR Network 2009) (www.pdrbooks.com/prod/Product-Catalog_92/PDR—for-Herbal-Medicines—4th-Edition_76.aspx)
	PDR for Nonprescription Drugs (www.pdrbooks.com/prod/Product-Catalog_92/2014-PDR—for-Nonprescription-Drugs_104.aspx)
	The Review of Natural Products (DerMarderosian, Liberti, Beutler, et al. 2010) (www.factsandcomparisons.com/review-of-natural-products-bound)
	Handbook of Nonprescription Drugs: An Interactive Approach to Self-Care (www.pharmacist.com/apha-publishes-new-edition-practitioner%E2%80%99s-quick-reference-nonprescription-drugs)
Special populations	
Geriatrics	*Geriatric Dosage Handbook* (Semla, Beizer, Higbee 2012) (http://webstore.lexi.com/Geriatric-Dosage-Handbook)
Pediatrics	*NeoFax* (Young, Mangum) (http://sites.truvenhealth.com/neofax)
	Pediatric and Neonatal Dosage Handbook (Taketomo, Hodding, Kraus 2013–14) (http://webstore.lexi.com/Pediatric-Dosage-Handbook)
	The Harriet Lane Handbook (Johns Hopkins Hospital, Tschudy, Arcara 2012) (www.us.elsevierhealth.com/pediatrics/the-harriet-lane-handbook-expert-consult/9780323079426)
	Pediatric Injectable Drugs. (Phelps, Hagemann, Lee, et al. 2013)

(continued)

Table 10-1. Examples of Drug Information Resources by Category (Secondary and Tertiary Literature) *(Continued)*

Category	Title
Pregnancy and lactation	*Drugs in Pregnancy and Lactation* (Briggs, Freeman, Yaffe 2011)
	Breastfeeding: A Guide for the Medical Professional (Lawrence, Lawrence 2011)
	LactMed (http://toxnet.nlm.nih.gov/cgi-bin/sis/htmlgen?LACT)
	Micromedex Reprotox System (www.micromedexsolutions.com/micromedex2/4.29.4.1/WebHelp/ MICROMEDEX_2.htm#Document_help/Reprotox_document.htm)
Renal dysfunction	*Drug Prescribing in Renal Failure: Dosing Guidelines for Adults and Children* (Aronoff, Bennett, Berns 2007)
	GlobalRPh.com (www.globalrph.com/nephrology.htm)
Medications in bariatric surgery patients	*Pharmacist's Letter,* December 2013 (www.pharmacistsletter.com)
Specific use	
Adverse effects	*Meyler's Side Effects of Drugs* (Aronson 2006)
	Institute for Safe Medication Practices (www.ismp.org)
	Clinical Alerts (www.nlm.nih.gov/databases/alerts/)
	U.S. FDA MedWatch Program (www.fda.gov/Safety/MedWatch/)
	Vaccine Adverse Event Reporting System (http://vaers.hhs.gov/index)
Drug interactions	*Drug Interactions Analysis and Management* (Hansten, Horn 2013) (www.hanstenandhorn.com/news.htm)
Foreign medications	*Martindale: The Complete Drug Reference* (Sweetman 2011) (www.lexi.com/institutions/products/online/ database-module-descriptions/martindale/)
	The British Pharmacopoeia (www.pharmacopoeia.co.uk/)
Immunology	Center for Biologics Evaluation and Research (www.fda.gov/BiologicsBloodVaccines/default.htm)
	ImmunoFacts 2013: Vaccines and Immunologic Drugs (Grabenstein 2013)
	Epidemiology and Prevention of Vaccine-Preventable Diseases (The Pink Book) (www.cdc.gov/vaccines/pubs/ pinkbook/index.html)
Intravenous use, compatibility and stability	*Handbook on Injectable Drugs* (Trissel 2013)
	Trissel's Tables of Physical Compatibility (Trissel 1999)
	Pediatric Injectable Drugs. (Phelps Hagemann Lee et al. 2013)
	King Guide to Parenteral Admixtures (King, Catania 2006) (www.kingguide.com)
Patient information and patient counseling	Micromedex Clinical Knowledge Integration Options (Truven Health Analytics) (http://micromedex.com/ patient-connect)
	UpToDate: Patient Information (www.uptodate.com/home)
	Pharmacist's Letter (www.pharmacistsletter.com)
	MedlinePlus (www.nlm.nih.gov/medlineplus)
	Medication Teaching Manual: The Guide to Patient Drug Information (American Society for Health-System Pharmacists 2003)
Pricing, availability, etc.	*Red Book* (PDR Network 2010) (www.pdrbooks.com/prod/Product-Catalog_92/2014-PDR—for-Nonprescription-Drugs_104.aspx)
Product identification	*Ident-a-Drug Reference* (Therapeutic Research Center) (http://identadrug.therapeuticresearch.com/ home.aspx?cs=&s=ID)
	Athena Health (www.epocrates.com)

Table 10-1. Examples of Drug Information Resources by Category (Secondary and Tertiary Literature) *(Continued)*

Category	Title
Regulatory	*Orange Book: Approved Drug Products with Therapeutic Equivalence Evaluations* (U.S. Food and Drug Administration 2014) (www.accessdata.fda.gov/scripts/Cder/ob/default.cfm)
	U.S. Drug Enforcement Administration (www.usdoj.gov/dea)
	U.S. Food and Drug Administration (www.fda.gov)
	National Association of Boards of Pharmacy (www.nabp.net)
	Code of Federal Regulations (www.ecfr.gov/cgi-bin/ECFR?page=browse)
	World Health Organization (www.who.int/en)
Toxicology	Truven Health Analytics Micromedex Toxicology Management (http://micromedex.com/toxicology-management)
	TOXNET: Toxicology Data Network (U.S. National Library of Medicine) (http://toxnet.nlm.nih.gov)
	Disposition of Toxic Drugs and Chemicals in Man (Baselt 2011)
	LiverTox: Clinical and Research Information on Drug-Induced Liver Injury (http://livertox.nih.gov)
	Goldfrank's Toxicologic Emergencies. (Nelson, Lewin, Howland, et al. 2011)
Travel	*Yellow Book: CDC Health Information for International Travel 2014* (Centers for Disease Control and Prevention 2014) (wwwnc.cdc.gov/travel/page/yellowbook-home-2014)

Disadvantages of tertiary resources include publication lag time and the potential for incomplete information as a result of space limitations or inadequate searching techniques. Because of the inherent limitations of tertiary references, a search of the secondary literature is typically appropriate to ensure identification of up-to-date primary literature.

Secondary and primary resources

Secondary references index journal article citations and abstracts, allowing retrieval of primary literature. With more than 20,000 biomedical journals published annually, appropriate search techniques are crucial to identify relevant primary literature. Electronic access to secondary databases allows the search of millions of citations through a single search with the use of keywords and linked keywords (see Table 10-2).

To be thorough and comprehensive, one should use several databases when researching a drug information question. Once relevant primary literature is identified through the secondary databases, it must be evaluated to ensure quality and relevance.

Several examples of secondary drug information services are available online, including the following:

- Clinical Trials Information: www.clinicaltrials.gov
- Clinical Guidelines: www.nhlbi.nih.gov/guidelines
- National Quality Measures Clearinghouse: www.qualitymeasures.ahrq.gov

- Systemic Reviews: www.systematicreviews journal.com
- Evidence-Based Practice reviews: www.acponline .org/clinical_information/guidelines/guidelines

There are even Web sites to obtain medical care online (see DeJong, Santa, Dubley 2014). A Google or a Google Scholar search will identify most of those information sources.

Table 10-1 lists other examples of secondary resource databases. Secondary databases may be available for access directly or through a provider, such as Embase

Table 10-2. Examples of Secondary Literature Databases

Database	Source
Cumulative Index to Nursing and Allied Health Literature (CINAHL)	www.ebscohost.com/academic/ cinahl-plus-with-full-text
Embase	www.elsevier.com/online-tools/embase
Iowa Drug Information Service (IDIS)	www.uiowa.edu/~idis/idistday.htm
The Cochrane Database of Systematic Reviews	www.cochrane.org
MEDLINE	www.pubmed.gov
Ovid	www.ovid.com

(www.elsevier.com/online-tools/embase) and Ovid (www.ovid.com). MEDLINE may be accessed free through PubMed (www.pubmed.gov). Primary literature consists of clinical studies and reports. Evaluation of the primary literature is discussed in Chapter 11, "Clinical Trial Design."

10-4. Application of Drug Information Skills for Delivery of Patient Care

Pharmacists must be able not only to retrieve drug information, but also to communicate the information effectively. Effective written and oral communication skills are a fundamental component of pharmacy practice. With more complex treatment regimens, pharmacists today require more advanced problem-solving skills than previously. They must formulate answers to increasingly complex questions that necessitate a solid foundation of drug information skills. Pharmacists must remain current with pharmacy and medical literature to provide the most up-to-date drug information available. Pharmacists are expected to be the experts on medications and to use their knowledge of medications to improve drug therapy outcomes and patient care.

Drug information provided during the patient counseling session is a type of verbal drug information. When patients contact the pharmacy with questions regarding medications, pharmacists have the opportunity to communicate drug information verbally or electronically. Any verbal, printed or electronic communication of drug information to the patient must be well thought out, thorough, and complete, containing the pertinent components of medication information and tailored to the individual patient's specific needs. During the counseling session, information regarding dosage, administration, storage, drug interactions, and side effects may need to be communicated, depending on the individual patient and situation. Each pharmacist must develop proficiency in the art of providing patient-specific drug information.

Effective patient care requires that pharmacists intervene when appropriate to advocate for the patient's well-being. Pharmacists who effectively communicate evidence-based knowledge to physicians and other prescribers can positively influence a patient's quality of life and care.

Pharmacists also provide written drug information. Responding to e-mail, patient medication guides,

pamphlets, and handouts containing information about medications are all types of written drug information. Pharmacists may contribute to the production of newsletters and other types of publications for both patients and health care providers. Pharmacists may be involved in developing important documents that guide medical practice, such as therapeutic guidelines and formulary development.

Additionally, drug information skills include the ability to identify the true question being asked, followed by a systematic approach to searching for the answer or solutions and formulation of a thorough and appropriate response.

Systematic Approach to Answering a Drug Information Request

The successful application of drug information skills requires use of a systematic approach for searching drug information resources. The first step on receipt of a drug information question or request is to obtain pertinent background and demographic information from the requester. Next, the pharmacist must confirm the ultimate question to formulate an appropriate search strategy. The question should be categorized by the type of information requested, such as "drug interactions," "adverse effects," "pharmacoeconomics," or "pediatrics." Categorizing the question is useful for deciding which drug information resources will be most appropriate to use during the search. Once the question is categorized, the pharmacist should plan how to search the literature. Finally, evaluation of the retrieved literature forms the basis for the formulation of an appropriate response to the requester.

Following the categorization of the question, a systematic approach includes a search of the tertiary and secondary literature and identifies primary literature that is relevant to the question or request. Formulating a response that has been thoroughly searched and documented and appropriately answers the initial question is a skill that is essential to the provision of drug information. One must also keep the legalities and liabilities of providing drug information in mind when formulating a response to a drug information request. For example, a pharmacist may have used a source that contained an error in dosing that was later corrected, but the pharmacist may not have seen the correction. If the patient was harmed by the information provided, the greatest liability would be on the source, but the pharmacist may share some liability. This is a reason to use multiple sources in responding to a drug information question.

Clinical decision support systems

Clinical decision support systems (CDSSs) are used to support decision making in a variety of clinical domains. These systems are computer-based programs designed to provide information support for health professionals making clinical decisions typically at the point of care and integrated in pharmacy computer systems. A CDSS system has three basic components: (1) an inference engine or artificial intelligence, (2) a knowledge base, and (3) a communication mechanism. These systems have emerged as an important part of any clinical information system, particularly in the era of computerized physician order entry (CPOE) systems that allow direct entry of orders and instructions for the treatment of patients by a clinician. The orders are communicated through a computer network to the hospital staff or other various departments responsible for fulfilling an order, including pharmacy, radiology, or laboratory. Used properly, CPOE decreases delays in order completion, reduces errors related to handwriting or transcriptions, allows order entry at the point of care or off site, provides error checking for duplicate or incorrect doses or tests, and simplifies inventory and posting of charges.

Literature Searching Skills and Sources

Some basic skills for searching the literature are necessary for identifying the most up-to-date, evidence-based information as well as for formulating the most comprehensive response possible. Millions of articles may be accessed through the Internet. To retrieve articles in a comprehensive and timely manner, pharmacists must be proficient at searching the secondary literature databases, keeping in mind the importance of searching different databases to ensure a comprehensive search.

The National Library of Medicine (NLM) is the world's largest medical library and provides several bibliographic, factual, and evidence-based drug and dietary supplement information resources. PubMed is maintained by the NLM and the National Center for Biotechnology Information (NCBI) to provide access to millions of citations from the biomedical literature. PubMed is a database of biomedical journal citations and abstracts for thousands of journals published in the United States and worldwide. Access to the NLM's MEDLINE service is available worldwide through the Internet at no cost. MEDLINE is a large electronic bibliographic database, containing citations from the late 1940s to the present, accessible through PubMed.

The "LinkOut" feature of PubMed allows direct access to full articles from the journal's Web site and related Internet resources. Depending on the individual citation, a fee may be charged for access to the full text. Most medical centers and academic institutions have subscriptions to many journals, thereby allowing direct access to selected journals.

Pharmacists conducting literature searches must be able to retrieve appropriate articles that are relevant to the inquiry. Using efficient search techniques is important to avoid retrieving an overwhelmingly excessive number of irrelevant citations.

MEDLINE citations are indexed through the controlled vocabulary developed by the NLM, known as the *Medical Subject Headings* (MeSH). When conducting a search of the MEDLINE database through PubMed, the pharmacist should first use MeSH terms to ensure that all relevant information is identified through the search. Keywords may be used to conduct a search in PubMed when a search using MeSH terms does not produce relevant results or when a MeSH term is not available for the desired search term.

Boolean operators (*and*, *or*, and *not*) are often used to combine relevant search terms, helping to narrow and focus the search. The term *and* may be used to combine two or more search terms, allowing retrieval of citations containing only both concepts. The Boolean operator *or* will allow access to citations including either term and will, therefore, potentially produce a larger number of results in a literature search than *and*. The term *not* is used to limit a search and, therefore, will likely produce fewer results; however, a disadvantage of using this term is that relevant articles may be excluded.

Literature searches can be made more effective by combining appropriate MeSH terms and by imposing appropriate limits on the search, such as by type of publication or range of publication date. Because no single search strategy will always produce satisfactory results, conducting several searches with various combinations of search terms is important to achieve the most comprehensive search possible.

Patients and health care professionals commonly ask questions of pharmacists about current health news topics. In this case, the Internet may be an appropriate source to begin a search for the requested information; however, drug information provided by news sources should be cautiously interpreted and should always be verified by reputable sources of drug information.

Information pertaining to the U.S. government or FDA can be identified through the FDA Web site and the U.S. Centers for Disease Control and Prevention (CDC) Web site (www.cdc.gov). These Web sites also include clinical information and information about new drug approvals and FDA-required information in the labeling. For example, when a product package insert is needed, the company Web site or the FDA Web site is an appropriate starting place.

The American Society of Health-System Pharmacists (ASHP) Web site (www.ashp.org) provides useful information regarding drug shortages and materials for formulary development.

Several sources provide general reviews and reports that are searchable and provide an excellent resource for many questions pharmacists receive from patients and practitioners. For example, *Pharmacist's Letter* (http://pharmacistsletter.com) and *Prescriber's Letter* (http://prescribersletter.com) offer print and online access to practical information, including patient information materials for subscribers. The publishers of *Pharmacist's Letter* and *Prescriber's Letter* also produce the *Natural Medicines Comprehensive Database* (www.natural database.com), which provides information on supplements and is of great interest to both patients and health care professionals.

Another source is *Internet Drug News.com* for Pharmaceutical News & Information: Pharmaceutical News Harvest (www.coreynahman.com), a free service updated daily that focuses on recent news and pharmaceutical manufacturers activities.

For investigational drugs and pharmaceutical manufacturer's information, First Word Pharma (www.firstwordpharma.com/#axzz2tPDNXpnN) is a free source of information.

Medscape Drug Reference (http://firstwordpharma .com) is a general drug information database that may be freely accessed through the Internet. The drug information contained in this reference is considered to be broad in scope and depth and relies on authoritative sources of drug information.

Wikipedia (www.wikipedia.org) is a free online resource that is edited by its users. Although consumers may use this source for drug information, potential problems include errors in information, lack of referenced documentation, and omissions of information. Wikipedia may be a useful source for providing information supplementary to other more reliable sources, but pharmacists should be cautious of user-edited sites as a definitive source of drug information.

Many journals and textbooks are now available electronically through the Web, allowing greater ease of use and increased availability. They are usually available online sooner than they are available in print. Many of these sources also have apps for smartphones and tablets.

Many databases and Web sites of pharmacy organizations provide patient drug information handouts that can be easily and legally printed for distribution to patients. In addition, vendors of pharmacy computer systems provide patient information and decision support modules that include basic drug information. Providing patients with not only verbal counseling but also written communication of their pertinent drug information helps reinforce the importance of the information and helps ensure the quality of pharmaceutical care provided.

Once sufficient information has been identified through the search, the literature must be evaluated for accuracy and relevance. A response can then be formulated and provided to the requester in written, electronic, or verbal format, incorporating the essential drug information skills mentioned previously.

10-5. Reliability of Information

Drug information needs to be clear, concise, and complete. Drug information resources should be free from commercial influence, relevant, and appropriately referenced. Pharmacists need to have the ability to judge the reliability of sources of information. Pharmacists also should be able to counsel patients about reliable drug information sources available on the Internet.

Although many reputable Internet sources of drug information are available to the general public free of charge, some sources of information are inaccurate and unreliable. The practicing pharmacist should verify through additional searches of the secondary literature that the information obtained from the Internet is evidence based to be able to distinguish it from misleading and potentially dangerous information.

Pertinent landmark clinical trials, when appropriate, should be included. Also important is that the resource be as free as possible from bias and errors. And if an error is later discovered and reported in a subsequent issue, the pharmacist should convey this error, when feasible and possible, to those who were provided with that information.

All information should ideally be evidence based. Evidence-based practice (EBP), or evidence-based medicine (EBM), is an interdisciplinary approach to clinical practice. Its basic principles are (1) that all practical decisions made should be based on research studies and (2) that these research studies are selected and interpreted according to some specific norms characteristic for EBP. Typically, such norms disregard theoretical studies and qualitative studies and consider quantitative studies according to a narrow set of criteria of what counts as evidence. Evidence comprises research findings derived from the systematic collection of data through observation and experimentation and the formulation of questions and testing of hypotheses.

Several evidence-based abstraction services may be accessed online, including the ACP journal club (http://acpjc.acponline.org) and evidence-based medicine (http://ebm.bmj.com). Both services target internal medicine and primary care. Journal watch series (www.jwatch.org) targets general medicine, dermatology, cardiology, psychiatry, women's health, emergency medicine, infectious disease, neurology, gastroenterology, oncology and hematology, and pediatrics. PNN Pharmacotherapy line (www.pharmacotherapynews network.com/index.html) targets pharmacists with a focus on internal medicine and primary care.

Implementing EBM and EBP in practice provides a framework and the skills to strengthen confidence in pharmacotherapeutic decisions and results in better communication with colleagues involved in decision making. However, not all EBP information is actually helpful, be it evidence based or generally agreed upon. *Clinical Evidence,* a project of the *British Medical Journal,* recently examined 3,000 medical treatments that have been studied in randomized controlled trials (RCTs) (http://clinicalevidence.bmj.com/x/set/static/cms/efficacy-categorisations.html). Findings on the treatments studied by RCTs indicated that effectiveness was unknown in 50% of the treatments. For the remaining treatments, 11% were shown to be beneficial, 24% were likely to be beneficial, 7% were trade-offs between benefit and risk, 5% were unlikely to be beneficial, and 3% were ineffective or harmful.

Another example involved the 4,000 recommendations in guidelines developed by the Infectious Diseases Society of America. For these recommendations, 14% were based on RCTs, but 55% were based only on expert opinion or case studies (Mursu J, Robien K, Harnack LJ, et al. 2011). As an example of disagreement with an EBP guideline, the American Association of Clinical Endocrinologists (AACE) does not endorse the 2013 guidelines from the American Heart Association and the American College of Cardiology regarding treatment of hyperlipidemia. The AACE has questioned the scientific basis of the guidelines and said certain at-risk populations of patients would be underserved. The AACE recommends that practitioners follow the AACE 2012 Guidelines (www.aace .com/files/lipid-guidelines.pdf). Thus, evidence-based guidelines and evidence are also subject to interpretation and should be applied in the context of individual patient needs and circumstances.

With millions of Web sites available, a method of quality assurance to assess the reliability of Internet information is not currently practical or possible. However, general guidelines can be applied case by case to make decisions about the reliability of Internet health information.

Information identified on the Internet should be carefully evaluated for the credentials of the author, evidence to support claims, and logic of the information. Additionally, the date of publication should be taken into consideration, because using outdated information regarding medications can be dangerous. The source of drug information identified on the Internet needs to be evaluated. The name, location, and sponsor of the Web site should be disclosed and evaluated for bias or conflicts of interest.

Web sites supported by a pharmacy organization, a university, or a pharmaceutical manufacturer (regulated by the FDA) may generally be considered to be credible, although information on a pharmaceutical industry Web site should be interpreted with caution because of the potential for bias. In general, information found on Web sites produced by the U.S. government and educational institutions may be considered reliable.

When possible, verifying information in multiple sources is prudent. Recommendations may vary between references, and the potential exists that one reference may contain more up-to-date information than another. In addition, a potential for error always exists, and accessing multiple sources to verify drug information accuracy and completeness minimizes the potential for errors when providing drug information.

The primary literature is vast, and practitioners need to critically evaluate it before extrapolating recommendations regarding patient care. The CONSORT (Consolidated Standards of Reporting Trials) Statement is a useful reference that pharmacists are encouraged to apply as a guide when evaluating the primary literature. Chapter 11, "Clinical Trial Design," provides more detail for considerations when judging the reliability of sources of primary literature.

Pharmacists have a long history of providing drug information to patients and health care professionals. This function is a professional responsibility—and opportunity—to positively affect patient outcomes.

10-6. Questions

1. Drug information is

    A. electronic information pertaining to medications only.
    B. written information pertaining to medications only.
    C. verbal information pertaining to medications only.
    D. written, electronic, and verbal information pertaining to medications.

2. Which of the following is *not* true of drug information provided by pharmacists?

    A. It may be tailored to a specific patient.
    B. It may be developed for the benefit of a large group of patients with a common medical need.
    C. It may be written or verbal information provided to patients or health care providers.
    D. It may be only written information provided to patients or health care providers.

3. Many career options are available to pharmacists in a variety of practice settings. Which of the following is true regarding the practice of providing drug information?

    A. Pharmacists practicing in a community pharmacy do not need to have drug information skills.
    B. Only specialty pharmacists practicing in drug information centers need to have skills in drug information.
    C. With expanding technology, pharmacists do not need to know about drug information references.
    D. All pharmacists need to have skills in providing drug information.

4. Pharmacists need to be proficient in which of the following skills?

    A. Verbal communication skills only
    B. Written communication skills only
    C. Literature evaluation skills only
    D. Written and verbal communication skills and literature evaluation skills

5. Which of the following references would be the best source to identify drug information regarding whether a medication is lactose free?

    A. *AHFS Drug Information*
    B. *Orange Book*
    C. *Red Book*
    D. *Martindale: The Complete Drug Reference*

6. When counseling patients, pharmacists have the opportunity to do which of the following?

    A. Pharmacists communicate verbal drug information only.
    B. Pharmacists provide written drug information only.
    C. Pharmacists provide patients with written and verbal drug information.
    D. Pharmacists do not use drug information skills when interacting with patients.

7. When one is conducting a search for a drug information request, a systematic approach is recommended. Which of the following, in general, is the most appropriate order for searching different types of literature?

    A. Search primary literature first, followed by a search of secondary references to identify tertiary literature.
    B. Search tertiary literature first, followed by a search of secondary references to identify primary literature.
    C. Only primary literature needs to be consulted for all types of drug information questions.
    D. Only tertiary literature needs to be consulted for all types of drug information questions.

8. Which of the following are examples of secondary literature?

    A. MEDLINE and *AHFS Drug Information*
    B. Embase and *Facts & Comparisons*
    C. MEDLINE and Embase
    D. *AHFS Drug Information* and *Facts & Comparisons*

9. Which of the following are examples of tertiary literature?

    A. MEDLINE and *AHFS Drug Information*
    B. Embase and *Facts & Comparisons*
    C. MEDLINE and Embase
    D. *AHFS Drug Information* and *Facts & Comparisons*

10. Patient information is provided by which of the following drug information resources?

    A. MedlinePlus
    B. *Martindale: The Complete Drug Reference*
    C. *Red Book*
    D. *Orange Book*

11. Which of the following drug information resources contains the *Orange Book?*

    A. *AHFS Drug Information*
    B. ASHP Web site
    C. FDA Web site
    D. CDC Web site

12. A physician calls the pharmacy and provides the name of a medication from another country. Which of the following references would be the best place to search for internationally available medications?

    A. *AHFS Drug Information*
    B. *PDR*
    C. *Red Book*
    D. *Martindale: The Complete Drug Reference*

13. Which of the following drug information references provides specific information about medications' adverse effects?

    A. *Meyler's Side Effects of Drugs*
    B. *King Guide to Parenteral Admixtures*
    C. *Red Book*
    D. *Orange Book*

14. Boolean operators that are often useful when conducting a search of secondary literature include all of the following *except*

    A. and.
    B. or.
    C. MeSH.
    D. not.

15. MeSH terms are

    A. not appropriate to include in a search strategy of the secondary literature.
    B. controlled vocabulary developed by the U.S. National Library of Medicine.
    C. the same as keywords.
    D. useful for identifying drug information in tertiary references.

16. When one is conducting a literature search in secondary literature databases, which of the following are generally useful strategies for narrowing a search?

    A. Using "limits"
    B. Using the Boolean operator *or*
    C. Using only keywords
    D. Combining only two MeSH terms at a time

17. Electronic drug information resources, such as smartphones and tablets, provide which of the following advantages in terms of patient care?

    A. They increase potential errors associated with drug information.
    B. They decrease potential errors associated with drug information.
    C. They replace the role of the clinical pharmacist.
    D. They decrease the interaction between the patient and the health care provider.

18. Drug information is often retrieved from the Internet by both patients and health care providers. Which of the following is the best advice to provide to a patient seeking drug information on the Internet?

    A. It is not usually necessary to search more than one Web site when searching for drug information on the Internet.
    B. Drug news provided by the media is an evidence-based source of drug information.
    C. Regardless of the number or types of sources consulted for drug information, it is wise to verify the information with a health care provider.
    D. All information provided by pharmaceutical manufacturers is unbiased.

19. When searching for drug information on the Internet, pharmacists should do which of the following?

    A. Verify the information in only one source on the Internet.
    B. Verify the information in multiple sources.
    C. Trust all authors of information on the Internet, as long as they have a PharmD, MD, or PhD.
    D. Disregard the potential for errors or bias in the information.

20. Once relevant primary literature is identified through secondary database sources, which of the following should occur?

    A. The relevant primary literature identified is usually accurate and reliable; therefore, no further evaluation is necessary.
    B. The pharmacist is responsible for evaluating primary literature to assess accuracy and reliability of information.
    C. Recommendations should be made on the basis of the literature identified without first evaluating the information.
    D. Because all published literature has already been evaluated for accuracy and reliability before publication, the pharmacist does not need to conduct an evaluation of the literature.

10-7. Answers

1. **D.** Drug information is defined as written, electronic, and verbal information pertaining to medications.

2. **D.** Drug information includes written or verbal information provided to patients or health care providers. Drug information provided by pharmacists may be tailored to a specific patient or developed for the benefit of a large group of patients with a common medical need.

3. **D.** All pharmacists need to have skills in providing drug information, regardless of practice setting, including specialty pharmacists practicing in drug information centers as well as those practicing in a community pharmacy. With expanding technology, it is crucial that pharmacists know about available drug information references.

4. **D.** Pharmacists need to be proficient in written and verbal communication skills as well as in literature evaluation skills.

5. **C.** Of the choices provided, the *Red Book* would be the best source to identify information regarding whether a medication is lactose free.

6. **C.** Pharmacists have the opportunity to provide patients with written and verbal drug information during the counseling session.

7. **B.** The amount of primary literature is vast. Search tertiary literature first, followed by a search of secondary references to identify primary literature.

8. **C.** MEDLINE and Embase are examples of secondary literature. Other types of secondary literature include International Pharmaceutical Abstracts (IPA) and Iowa Drug Information Service (IDIS).

9. **D.** *AHFS Drug Information* and *Facts & Comparisons* are examples of tertiary literature. Other types of tertiary literature include Lexi-Comp *Drug Information Handbook* and Micromedex Healthcare Series.

10. **A.** MedlinePlus is a drug information reference containing drug information tailored to the patient.

11. **C.** The FDA Web site contains the electronic version of the *Orange Book*.

12. **D.** *Martindale: The Complete Drug Reference* contains drug information regarding internationally available medications.

13. **A.** *Meyler's Side Effects of Drugs* is a drug information resource that provides specific information about medications' adverse effects.

14. **C.** Boolean operators that are often useful when conducting a search of secondary literature include *and*, *or*, and *not*. MeSH terms help focus a search of the secondary literature.

15. **B.** MeSH terms are controlled vocabulary developed by the U.S. National Library of Medicine.

16. **A.** Using "limits" is a useful strategy for narrowing a search of the secondary literature.

17. **B.** Electronic drug information resources, such as smartphones, have been shown to decrease potential errors associated with drug information, thereby improving patient care.

18. **C.** Although patients may be encouraged to seek information on appropriate drug information sources freely available on the Internet, patients should verify the information identified on the Internet with a health care provider to ensure appropriate use of information identified.

19. **B.** When searching for drug information on the Internet, pharmacists should verify the information in multiple sources.

20. B. Once relevant primary literature is identified through secondary database sources, the pharmacist is responsible for evaluating primary literature to assess accuracy and reliability of information.

10-8. References

Akus M, Bartick M. Lactation safety recommendations and reliability compared in 10 medication resources. *Ann Pharmacother.* 2007;41(9):1352–60.

American Society for Health-System Pharmacists. *Medication Teaching Manual: The Guide to Patient Drug Information.* 8th ed. Bethesda, MD: American Society for Health-System Pharmacists: 2003.

Aronoff GR, Bennett WM, Berns JS, et al. *Drug Prescribing in Renal Failure: Dosing Guidelines for Adults and Children.* 5th ed. Philadelphia, PA: American College of Physicians; 2007.

Aronson JK. *Meyler's Side Effects of Drugs.* 15th ed. Amsterdam: Elsevier Science; 2006.

Baselt, RC. *Disposition of Toxic Drugs and Chemicals in Man.* 9th ed. Seal Beach, CA: Biomedical Publications; 2011.

Brand KA, Kraus ML. Drug information specialists. *Am J Health-Syst Pharm.* 2006;63(8):712–14.

Briggs GG, Freeman RK, Yaffe SJ. *Drugs in Pregnancy and Lactation: A Reference Guide to Fetal and Neonatal Risk.* 9th ed. Philadelphia, PA: Lippincott Williams & Wilkins; 2011.

Centers for Disease Control and Prevention. *Yellow Book: CDC Health Information for International Travel 2014.* New York, NY: Oxford University Press; 2014.

Centers for Disease Control and Prevention, Atkinson W, Wolfe S, Hamborsky J, eds. *Epidemiology and Prevention of Vaccine-Preventable Diseases.* 12th ed. Washington, DC: Public Health Foundation; 2011.

Clauson KA, Polen HH, Kamel Boulos MN, Dzenowagis JH. Scope, completeness, and accuracy of drug information on Wikipedia. *Ann Pharmacother.* 2008;42(12):1814–21.

DeJong C, Santa J, Dubley RA. Websites that offer care over the Internet: Is there an access quality tradeoff? *JAMA.* 2014;311(13):1287.

DerMarderosian A, Liberti L, Beutler JA, et al. *The Review of Natural Products.* 6th ed. St. Louis, MO: Wolters Kluwer Health; 2010.

Galt KA, Rule AM, Houghton B, et al. Personal digital assistant-based drug information sources:

Potential to improve medication safety. *J Med Lib Assoc.* 2005;93(2):229–36.

Grabenstein JD. *ImmunoFacts: Vaccines and Immunologic Drugs 2013.* Philadelphia, PA: Lippincott Williams & Wilkins; 2012.

Gruenwald J, Brendler T, Jaenicke C, et al., eds. *PDR for Herbal Medicines.* 4th ed. Montvale, NJ: Thomson Healthcare; 2007.

Hansten PD, Horn JR, eds. *Drug Interactions Analysis and Management 2013.* St. Louis, MO: Wolters Kluwer Health; 2013.

Johns Hopkins Hospital, Tschudy MM, Arcara KM, eds. *The Harriet Lane Handbook.* 19th ed. Philadelphia, PA: Elsevier Mosby; 2012.

King JC, Catania PN. *King Guide to Parenteral Admixtures.* 35th ed. Napa, CA: King Guide Publications; 2006.

Knoben, JE, Phillips, SJ. New drug information resources for pharmacists at the National Library of Medicine. *J Am Pharm Assoc.* 2014;54:49–55.

Krinsky DL, Berardi RR, Ferreri SP, et al., eds. *Handbook of Nonprescription Drugs: An Interactive Approach to Self-Care.* 17th ed. Washington, DC: American Pharmacists Association; 2012.

Lacy CF, Armstrong LL, Goldman MP, et al., eds. *Drug Information Handbook.* 21st ed. Hudson, OH: Lexicomp; 2012.

Lawrence RA, Lawrence RM. *Breastfeeding: A Guide for the Medical Professional.* 7th ed. Maryland Heights, MO: Elsevier Mosby; 2011.

McEvoy GK, ed. *AHFS Drug Information 2014.* Bethesda, MD: American Society of Health-System Pharmacists; 2014.

Moher D, Hopewell S, Schulz KF, et al. CONSORT 2010 explanation and elaboration: Updated guidelines for reporting parallel group randomised trials. *J Clin Epidemiol.* 2010;63;e1–e37.

Mursu J, Robien K, Harnack LJ, et al. Dietary supplements and mortality rate in older women: The Iowa Women's Health Study. *Arch Intern Med.* 2011:171(18);1625–33.

Nathan JP, Gim S. Responding to a drug information request. *Am J Health-Syst Pharm.* 2009:66(8); 706–11.

Nelson LS, Lewin NA, Howland MA, et al., eds. *Goldfrank's Toxicologic Emergencies.* 9th ed. New York, NY: McGraw-Hill; 2011.

Pew Research. Pew Research Internet project: Health fact sheet. Pew Research Center, Washington, DC; 2014. Accessed at http://www.pewinternet.org/Commentary/2011/November/Pew-Internet-Health.aspx.

PDR Network. *PDR for Herbal Medicines.* 5th ed. Montvale, NJ: PDR Network; 2009.

PDR Network. *PDR for Nonprescription Drugs*. 34th ed. Montvale, NJ: PDR Network; 2013.

PDR Network. *Physicians' Desk Reference*. 68th ed. Montvale, NJ: PDR Network; 2014.

PDR Network. *Red Book*. Montvale, NJ: Thomson Healthcare/Thomson PDR; 2010.

Phelps SJ, Hagemann TM, Lee KR, et al. *Pediatric Injectable Drugs*. 10th ed. Bethesda, MD: American Society of Health-System Pharmacists; 2013.

Rosenberg JM, Schilit S, Nathan JP, et al. Update on the status of 89 drug information centers in the United States. *Am J Health-Syst Pharm*. 2009; 66(19):1718–22.

Semla TP, Beizer JL, Higbee MD. *Geriatric Dosage Handbook*. 17th ed. Hudson, OH: Lexi-Comp; 2012.

Sweetman SC, ed. *Martindale: The Complete Drug Reference*. 37th ed. London: Pharmaceutical Press; 2011.

Taketomo CK, Hodding JH, Kraus DM. *Pediatric and Neonatal Dosage Handbook*. 20th ed. Hudson, OH: Lexicomp; 2013–14.

Therapeutic Research Center. Ident-a-Drug Reference. http://identadrug.therapeuticresearch.com.

Therapeutic Research Center. Natural Medicines Comprehensive Database. http://www.naturaldatabase.therapeuticresearch.com.

Trissel LA. *Trissel's Tables of Physical Compatibility*. Lake Forest, IL; MultiMatrix; 1999.

Trissel LA. *Handbook on Injectable Drugs*. 17th ed. Bethesda, MD: American Society of Health-System Pharmacists; 2013.

Tsourounis C, Dennehy C. Introduction to dietary supplements. In: Krinsky D, Berardi R, Ferreri S, et al., eds. *Handbook of Nonprescription Drugs: An Interactive Approach to Self-Care*. 17th ed. Washington, DC: American Pharmacists Association; 2012:955–66.

U.S. Food and Drug Administration. *Orange Book: Approved Drug Products with Therapeutic Equivalence Evaluations*. 34th ed. Silver Spring, MD: U.S. Food and Drug Administration; 2014.

U.S. National Library of Medicine. Fact Sheet: PubMed: Medline retrieval on the world wide web. Bethesda, MD: U.S. National Library of Medicine. http://www.nlm.nih.gov/pubs/factsheets/pubmed.html.

U.S. National Library of Medicine. TOXNET: Toxicology Data Network. Bethesda, MD: U.S. National Library of Medicine. http://toxnet.nlm.nih.gov.

Young TE, Mangum B. *NeoFax*. New York, NY: Ann Arbor, MI: Truven Health Analytics. http://sites.truvenhealth.com/neofax.

Clinical Trial Design

Bradley A. Boucher

11-1. Key Points

- Observational research may be prospective or retrospective.
- Experimental research is usually prospective.
- Experimental designs should seek to minimize bias, confounding, and random error.
- Cohort studies may be prospective, cross-sectional, or retrospective.
- Retrospective studies are able to identify an association between variables.
- Well-designed randomized controlled trials (RCTs) can establish a cause-and-effect relationship between variables.
- Evidence-based medicine requires the critical appraisal of medical literature and the adoption of scientifically rigorous, relevant information into clinical practice.

11-2. Study Guide Checklist

The following topics may guide your study of this subject area:

- Differences between observational and experimental studies
- Similarities and differences between major experimental trial design types
- Differences between parallel and crossover randomized clinical trials
- Key aspects of RCTs to consider in reviewing published studies

This chapter is based on the 9th edition chapter with the same title, written by Trevor McKibbin.

- Three major blinding categories used in randomized clinical trials
- Difference between *per protocol* and *intention-to-treat* data analysis techniques
- Four major steps for critically appraising medical literature
- Practical methods to assist practitioners in staying current with medical literature
- Definition of evidence-based medicine
- Major steps in practicing evidence-based pharmacy

11-3. Introduction

Clinical research refers to studies conducted in humans seeking to answer a question regarding health care. It includes studies evaluating medical disease prevention, diagnosis, and treatment. Data derived from well-planned and well-executed clinical research studies are extremely important in advancing patient care. Although the basic principles of clinical research design techniques and processes are not particularly difficult to comprehend, actually conducting studies is a complex enough process that entire textbooks are devoted to trial design as well as data processing and interpretation. As such, many health care practitioners lack the time and expertise to design and execute studies themselves without additional training and may even be inadequately prepared to interpret published clinical data. Regardless, understanding the basics of clinical research design is essential for all practitioners to practice evidence-based medicine. Critical appraisal of medical literature and judicious use of new knowledge will thus aid clinicians in providing the best possible care based on current data to the patients they serve.

This chapter introduces the reader to the basic concepts of clinical research; clinical trial design, including the major types of clinical trials; and many of the key aspects of randomized clinical trials. The chapter also addresses the basic principles for evaluating the primary literature and techniques for reviewing these data and implementing useful findings in clinical practice.

11-4. Fundamentals of Research Design and Methodology

There are two basic types of clinical research: observational research and experimental research. A brief description of each type follows.

- *Observational research:* In this type of research, the investigator observes what is occurring without intervening. Typically, descriptive statistics are used to summarize the study results. This includes measures of central tendency (e.g., arithmetic mean, median, mode) and measures of variability (e.g., range, standard deviation, variance). Observational research may be retrospective or prospective. Retrospective studies involve looking back from the present, whereas prospective studies begin at the present time and observe study variables of interest from the present forward. One specific type of observational research that is very important within medicine is the case report. A case report retrospectively describes a specific clinical case or limited number of cases. Case reports are not able to establish a causal relationship but may often be the first evidence of a previously unknown or unrecognized relationship.

- *Experimental research:* In this type of research, a specific intervention or exposure to a condition is evaluated in a study group and typically compared with a control group. Experimental research is usually prospective in nature but may use historical controls or controls from medical literature for the comparator group. Familiarity with the terminology of experimental clinical study designs is useful from several vantage points. One aspect is the ability to efficiently plan and conduct clinical research based on accepted methodologies by motivated investigators. Perhaps more important for most clinicians is the ability to interpret medical literature as previously noted. Upon identification of the methodology used within a published study, the clinician should be able to readily conceptualize how a study was conducted. The following list outlines each major experimental clinical study design:

- *Case series:* This type of study is similar to a case report although it reports on a group of patients with similar clinical presentations or exposure to a particular treatment or condition compared with a single case or limited number of cases. A case series may be either retrospective or prospective. The lack of a control group and randomization limits determination of a causal relationship and rigorous statistical analysis, respectively.

- *Cohort study:* A cohort study selects participants on the basis of one or more specific characteristics and compares them over time to either a different set of patients or the rest of the general population that serves as the control group. In either case, the study group of interest is exposed to the test treatment or condition at the beginning of the evaluation period, whereas the other group is not exposed. Cohort studies are essentially the same as randomized clinical trials (discussed below) except for the absence of randomization. A cohort study can be conducted prospectively, in which case participants are selected on the basis of the study characteristics of interest and then observed following exposure until the conclusion of the study. Cohort studies can also identify participants retrospectively, in which case participant records are used to identify and prospectively evaluate individuals with the selected characteristics thereafter. Yet another design is to study prospectively one group of patients possessing the study characteristics and having been exposed to the test treatment and to compare that group to a historical participant group evaluated retrospectively. A well-designed cohort study can provide convincing evidence of an association between study variables. However, the inability to randomize patients to one group or another is a major source of bias inherent in conducting cohort studies because the participant groups may not be comparable. *Bias* denotes systematic error within clinical investigations. Bias is distinct from *confounding variables*. The latter term is used to describe variables that are not systematically introduced into the study but that may affect the outcome of interest in clinical studies. Generally speaking, confounding variables cannot be controlled in clinical studies completely (e.g., use of concurrent medications during the course of a study).

- *Case-control study:* Case-control studies are similar to cohort studies in that one group of participants has a disease and is compared to a control group that does not have the disease. However, a best attempt is made to find patients within the control group who match the participants with the disease or condition based on a predefined set of characteristics such as age or sex. Another difference is that case-control studies are always retrospective.

- *Randomized controlled trial (RCT):* In this type of trial, study participants are prospectively assigned randomly to one or more treatment or control groups upon meeting the inclusion criteria for the study. A well-designed and well-executed RCT is able to provide evidence of a causal relationship between the intervention being investigated and the primary study outcome. The two most common design subtypes of RCTs are known as parallel and crossover.

- *Parallel RCT:* In this study design, participants are randomized to one of the treatment or control arms of the study. Control groups may receive standard treatments, no treatment, usual care, or placebos. *Placebos* are inactive substances that are often used in clinical drug studies. Typically, study participants receive the assigned treatment or control for the entire trial in a parallel RCT (see Figure 11-1). Outcome responses for each treatment or control group are then compared at the conclusion of the study *between* patients assigned to each study group. Conditions being evaluated can be acute or chronic, which is one of the reasons that parallel RCTs are the most common prospective RCT design.

- *Crossover RCT:* In this design, the study participants receive one or more of the treatments or controls for a predefined period during the course of the study. Participants are then switched or "crossed over" to one or more of the other treatment or control arms (see Figure 11-2). In this instance, outcome responses are compared *within* the same participants, resulting typically in less variability. Although crossover RCTs are very efficient for evaluating causal effects of one treatment over another within the same participant, a major limitation is that only stable, chronic, or episodic conditions can be studied. Examples include

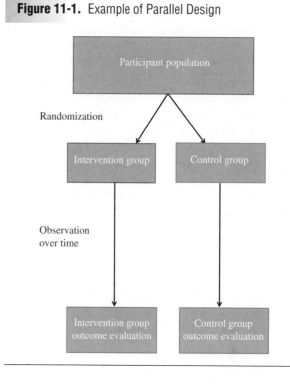

Figure 11-1. Example of Parallel Design

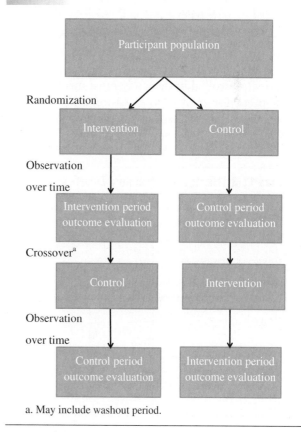

Figure 11-2. Example of Crossover Design

a. May include washout period.

glaucoma, epilepsy, migraines, and so on. Even with chronic or episodic conditions, however, a return to the same baseline state is needed to use a crossover design. This frequently requires a period of no treatment or usual treatment between study periods to avoid a carryover or residual effect as one treatment ends and the next one begins. This time period is referred to as a "washout" period.

Key Aspects of Randomized Controlled Trials

RCTs have a high weighting in the ranks of medical literature. See Figure 11-3 for a diagram illustrating general considerations regarding scientific rigor of particular study designs. Understanding the basics of RCT design will aid in interpreting the results and applying new literature to study practice. This section reviews key considerations of RCT design. Many of the principles covered here may also be applied to other types of trials.

Sampling and randomization

Sampling of a population is necessary in RCTs because enrolling every patient within a population with a particular disease state or condition in the study is not feasible. Key aspects of sampling are as follows:

- Study participants must be representative of the population to which the results of the study are to be applied.
- Patients enrolled in the study must meet all of the predetermined study inclusion criteria, and conversely, they must not have any of the characteristics listed as exclusion criteria.

Figure 11-3. Hierarchy of Literature Evidence

Trial design	Scientific validity
Systematic reviews and meta-analyses	
Randomized controlled trial	
Cohort study	
Case-control study	
Case series	
Case report	

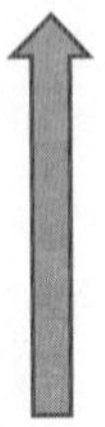

Clinicians should consider the aforementioned inclusion and exclusion criteria when applying the study results to avoid extrapolating these results to patients who may not be representative of the population being evaluated. Alternatively, one can infer that similar findings will be observed in other patients who meet these criteria within the probabilities emanating from inferential statistics used to analyze the study data. One of the basic principles of inferential statistics is that patients sampled from a particular population of interest have an equal chance of being randomized or assigned to one of the study groups or another. As such, systematic error can occur when study participants are not properly randomized into the study groups, which can lead to potentially misleading and incorrectly interpreted study results because of bias in patients being assigned to one group or another. Randomization does not ensure that study participant characteristics (e.g., sex, weight, race, and so on) are equally divided between study groups. A process known as *stratification* can be used to accomplish the latter. Stratification is a grouping that occurs before randomization, although grouping of patient characteristics can be performed retrospectively. In this latter instance, the process is often referred to as *subgroup analysis*.

Blinding

In clinical trials, *blinding* refers to the process whereby some or all of the participants are unaware of the treatment being received by the study participants. Blinding is a very important strategy for decreasing bias within any clinical trial. The underlying purpose of blinding is that study volunteers or patients may knowingly or unknowingly alter the study outcome data if they know which treatment or treatments they are receiving. Similarly, study investigators may bias data collection based on the perceived benefits of the treatment or lack of benefits they are observing if they are aware of the treatment the volunteers or patients are receiving or not receiving, respectively. Nevertheless, certain clinical studies may not be suitable for blinding because of safety or ethical concerns (e.g., administration of investigational treatments through compassionate use protocols, severely ill patients, and so on). Regardless of blinding type, the processes must be in place to break the blind if needed for safety reasons. When no blinding is used, studies are referred to as *open-label* trials. Generally accepted blinding definitions are as follows:

- *Single blind:* Patients are unaware of which treatment they are receiving.

- *Double blind:* Neither the study patients nor the investigators are aware of the treatments. This is the traditional gold standard within clinical research focused on treatment efficacy because this design has the greatest potential for minimizing bias from the study participants and investigators.
- *Triple blind:* All persons coming in contact with the study procedures or data (e.g., during the data analysis phase) are unaware of the study treatments in addition to the study participants and investigators.

Maintaining study blinding can be very challenging or virtually impossible irrespective of careful study planning and design. Such challenges can be overcome to some extent by using a group of blinded investigators—independent of those unblinded investigators or personnel directly interacting with the study participants—to gather the safety and efficacy data. Regardless of the blinding strategies used, investigators should provide details, to the greatest extent possible, on their maintenance of blinding for any trials published in medical literature.

Sample size

Selection of sample size is an extremely important issue in designing randomized clinical trials. Inadequate numbers of study participants will decrease the statistical power of any clinical trial. In this instance, patient numbers may be insufficient to report a statistically significant difference between the study treatments, although in actuality a difference does exist. Thus, *statistical power* is the probability of avoiding a false negative study result. Conversely, recruitment of an excessive number of study participants may be very inefficient despite being more than adequately powered statistically. Specifically, patient recruitment may take much longer than is necessary as well as substantially increase the study budget, thereby making the study unfeasible to conduct. Generally, the greater the expected difference between the study treatments, the fewer the number of study participants that will be needed to demonstrate a statistically significant difference between the groups. Furthermore, fewer study participants will be needed when less variability exists in the study outcomes being measured from one participant to another. Statistical power can be calculated by investigators and biostatisticians on the basis of estimates of the expected differences and variability between the study groups and should be included in any published report of the study results.

Controls

In the context of RCTs, controls are the comparator to the treatment of interest. In a crossover study design, patients serve as their own control. As previously noted, control groups may receive standard treatments, no treatment, usual care, or placebos in both RCT crossover and parallel designs. Ideally, the placebo should have dosage form properties (e.g., color, shape, taste, and so on) that are identical to the active treatment dosage forms to avoid compromising study blinding. The potential for a "placebo effect" should always be considered. This occurs when the placebo has an effect on the study outcome despite receipt of an inactive substance. Use of placebos may not be suitable for all RCTs because of ethical considerations. In these instances, an active or usual treatment would be used as the control.

Follow-up

Any RCT must follow the study participants over a sufficient period of time to demonstrate adequate safety or efficacy data or both. The length of follow-up is determined by the following:

- The period of time intended for patients to receive the study intervention
- Long-term safety concerns
- The study objectives and outcome measures (e.g., pain scale, overall survival, and so on)

During the treatment and follow-up study periods, not all participants may remain in the study. More specifically, participants may drop out of the trial. This can occur for a number of reasons, and investigators must plan how to handle the partial data in addition to the study sample size determination as previously noted. The two major analysis approaches are as follows:

- *Intention to treat:* This method includes all patients as a member of their respective study group, regardless of completion of the protocol since they began the study and were randomized. Data up to the point of withdrawal are used in the analysis.
- *Per protocol:* This method excludes data from participants with significant deviations from the protocol. If incomplete data are excluded from study outliers, this exclusion may increase precision and homogeneity of the study results. If incomplete data are related to adverse events or lack of response, this may bias results in a positive manner. For example, if many of the

patients with adverse events withdraw from the study and are not included in the data analysis, then the treatment may appear to be safer than is actually the case. As such, dropout patient characteristics and reasons for study withdrawal should be included with reporting of the other study results.

Importantly, the two analytical techniques are not mutually exclusive. Often investigators will report results from both techniques that allow the reader of the report to compare potential differences directly. The following are additional sources for guidance in designing clinical research studies:

- Spilker B. *Guide to Clinical Trials.* New York, NY: Lippincott Williams and Wilkins; 1991.
- Freidman LM, Furberg CD, DeMets DL. *Fundamentals of Clinical Trials.* 3rd ed. New York, NY: Springer; 1998.

11-5. Principles of Evaluation for Medical Literature

Critical appraisal is an objective systematic review of medical literature. The critical appraisal of original research articles can be time consuming; however, the skills required are not difficult to develop and are highly important to pharmacy practitioners. Critical appraisal of the literature can be broken down into four steps:

- Search the literature for relevant evidence.
- Determine the applicability of the study.
- Evaluate basic study design.
- Critically evaluate the validity of the study results.

The following series of questions will aid in evaluating the design of a clinical trial and validity of the results. These questions were adapted from Guyatt, Sackett, and Cook (1994) and assembled by Hill and Spittlehouse (2001):

- Did the trial address a focused research question in terms of the following?
  - Population studied
  - Intervention given
  - Outcomes considered
- Did the authors use the correct type of study design?
- Was the assignment of participants randomized?
- Were all of the participants who entered the trial appropriately accounted for as well as those not enrolled in the study?

- Were participants and study personnel blinded? If not, were appropriate efforts made to blind the study treatments, or is there appropriate justification for not blinding?
- Did the groups have similar baseline characteristics at the start of the study?
- Aside from the experimental interventions, were the groups treated equally?
- How large was the treatment effect?
- How precise was the estimate of the treatment effect?
- Can the study results be applied to the local population?
- Were all clinically important outcomes considered?
- Are the benefits worth the harm and costs?

The following are additional sources for guidance in assessing medical literature and the practice of evidence-based medicine:

- Guyatt G, Drummond R, Meade MO, Cook DJ, eds. *Users' Guides to the Medical Literature: A Manual for Evidenced-Based Clinical Practice.* 2nd ed. Columbus, OH: McGraw-Hill; 2008. Available at: http://www.jamaevidence.com/resource/520.
- Greenhalgh T. *How to Read a Paper: The Basics of Evidence-Based Medicine.* London: BMJ Books; 2001.

11-6. Practical Implications of Primary Literature

Diligently reviewing and applying appropriate primary literature can aid in improving the care of patients. However, medical knowledge is not stagnant, and new investigations are continually refining and improving the treatment of patients. Thus, treatment based on old literature may no longer meet current standards of care, and clinicians need to review the literature regularly. The amount of new literature being published daily can easily overwhelm practitioners; hence, review articles, systematic reviews, and clinical practice guidelines play an important role in keeping practitioners up to date. The following steps can help practitioners deal with the fast pace of medical literature:

- Identify three to five key journals that are relevant to your practice, and review them regularly for pertinent literature (monthly or bimonthly basis).
- Regularly attend continuing education courses, and keep up with continuing education resources and requirements.

■ Familiarize yourself with practice guidelines applicable to your area of practice (see www.guideline.gov).

■ Join or establish a group of practitioners in regular journal clubs.

11-7. Principles of Research Design and Analysis in Practicing Evidence-Based Pharmacy

According to Rosenberg and Donald (1995), "Evidence-based medicine is the process of systematically finding, appraising, and using contemporaneous research findings as the basis for clinical decisions." They propose four steps to the practice of evidence-based medicine. These steps apply broadly to the interdisciplinary practice of medicine, including the practice of pharmacy:

■ Formulate a clear clinical question from a patient's problem.

■ Search the literature for relevant clinical articles.

■ Evaluate and critically appraise the evidence for validity usefulness.

■ Implement useful findings in clinical practice.

Applying current evidence to clinical practice necessitates critical appraisal of the literature. Incorporating the following into routine practice will aid the reader of medical literature in reaching sound clinical decisions:

■ Regularly review and keep up to date with relevant medical literature.

■ Familiarize yourself with clinical practice guidelines that apply to your area of practice.

■ Critically appraise literature to determine validity of study results and applicability to practice.

11-8. Questions

1. Which of the following is *not* a descriptive statistic commonly used in characterizing data from observational studies?

   A. Arithmetic mean
   B. Normality
   C. Mode
   D. Range

2. Which of the following clinical study design characteristics is consistent with a case report?

   A. Observational
   B. Prospective
   C. Randomized
   D. Controlled

3. Clinical research generally seeks to answer questions in all of the following health care areas *except*

   A. disease prevention.
   B. diagnosis.
   C. treatment.
   D. reimbursement.

4. Which of the following statements is *true* regarding observational research design characteristics?

   A. Participants are blinded.
   B. They can be retrospective or prospective.
   C. Randomization of participants is preferred.
   D. They establish a causal relationship between variables of interest.

5. Which of the following research design types is *not* considered experimental research?

   A. Cohort study
   B. Randomized clinical trial
   C. Case-control study
   D. Retrospective epidemiologic study

6. Cohort studies are the same as randomized clinical trials except for which of the following study design characteristics?

   A. Evaluation of causal relationship between study variables
   B. Randomization of study participants
   C. Exposure to a test treatment or condition
   D. Option for use of historical control groups

7. Which of the following randomized clinical trial designs evaluate intrasubject effects between two or more study treatments?

   A. Crossover
   B. Parallel
   C. Sequential
   D. Latin square

8. Which of the following disease states is not suitable for a crossover study design?

   A. Glaucoma
   B. Migraine headaches

C. Epilepsy
D. Pneumonia

9. Blinding of subjects is an important process within clinical trials to minimize which of the following?

A. Confounding variables
B. Systematic error
C. Bias
D. Variability

10. Randomization is a key process within clinical trials to ensure which of the following?

A. Validity of inferential statistics
B. Avoidance of placebo effect
C. Avoidance of carryover effect
D. Normal distribution of study outcome

11. Which group or groups of individuals is unaware of the subject treatment in a double-blind study?

A. Subjects only
B. Subjects and investigators
C. Investigators and data analysis personnel
D. Data analysis personnel and subjects

12. Which of the following is *not* a characteristic of stratification?

A. Conducted after randomization
B. Ensures equal distribution of subject characteristics between groups
C. Requires larger number of subjects
D. Can be used in parallel or crossover studies

13. Which of the following is *true* regarding sample size in randomized clinical trials?

A. Increased sample size reduces statistical power.
B. Increased sample size is needed for a crossover design versus a parallel design.
C. Decreased sample size is needed where the expected difference in outcome between groups is large.
D. Decreased sample size is needed where large variability exists in the study outcome being measured.

14. All of the following groups can serve as a control in a randomized clinical trial *except*

A. standard treatment.
B. placebo.

C. historical.
D. usual care.

15. Which of the following is *not* an acceptable technique for managing data from those patients who withdraw from a study prior to completing the study protocol?

A. Analyzing the data using an intention-to-treat method
B. Analyzing the data using a per protocol method with categorization of withdrawal subject characteristics including reason for withdrawal
C. Analyzing the data using both intention-to-treat and per protocol methods
D. Analyzing the data from those subjects completing the protocol following purging of withdrawal subject information from the study database

16. All of the following are steps in the critical appraisal of the literature relative to a published study *except*

A. evaluating the validity of the study results.
B. searching for other studies published by the authors.
C. determining applicability of the study.
D. evaluating the basic study design.

17. Which of the following questions is *not* an aid in evaluating a clinical trial?

A. Were all confounding variables avoided in the study?
B. Did the study groups have similar baseline characteristics?
C. How large was the treatment effect?
D. Are the benefits worth the harm and costs?

18. All of the following are essential vehicles for practitioners in keeping up to date with new literature *except*

A. review articles.
B. clinical practice guidelines.
C. attendance at continuing education courses.
D. case reports.

19. Which of the following is *not* a critical step in practicing evidenced-based medicine?

A. Search the literature for relevant clinical articles.
B. Regularly converse with colleagues on their approach to a clinical problem.

C. Evaluate and critically appraise the clinical studies for validity and usefulness.

D. Formulate a clear clinical question relative to a particular patient problem.

20. All of the following are potential confounding variables *except*

A. a subject's concurrent medications.

B. medical complications that occur during study period.

C. study dropouts.

D. exclusion of patients with severe forms of the disease being studied.

21. Which of the following is *not* used to calculate a sample size?

A. Desired statistical power

B. Estimated effect size

C. Probability of the results affecting clinical practice

D. Variability and experimental error

22. In a randomized controlled trial that follows a parallel design, which of the following is *true*?

A. Patients serve as their own control.

B. All patients end up receiving all of the interventions in random different orders, depending on group assignment.

C. Only patients who complete the entire protocol are included in the final analysis.

D. Patients are assigned to groups that receive a particular treatment over time; the only planned difference in the groups is the intervention.

23. The intention-to-treat analysis includes data from which patients?

A. All patients regardless of whether they completed the protocol

B. Only patients who complete a specified protocol

C. Only patients who complete the protocol with favorable outcomes

D. None of the patients who did not complete the entire trial

24. The duration of follow-up for a randomized clinical trial is determined by all of the following *except*

A. outcome to be measured.

B. long-term safety concerns.

C. duration of time required to see an effect.

D. study budget.

25. Which of the following is an acceptable reason for excluding a patient from an intention-to-treat analysis of study data?

A. Adverse events

B. Lack of response

C. Failure to meet inclusion criteria

D. Noncompliance with study medication

11-9. Answers

1. **B.** Arithmetic mean, mode, and range are descriptive statistics. Normality is used in inferential statistics and is the exception.

2. **A.** Case reports are always observational. Prospective designs, randomization, and controls are all study design characteristics commonly used with randomized clinical trials and are not associated with case reports.

3. **D.** Clinical research generally seeks to answer questions related to disease prevention, diagnosis, and treatment. Reimbursement is a payment issue not normally addressed in clinical trials.

4. **B.** Observational studies can be retrospective or prospective. Observational studies lack randomization, are unblinded, and are unable to establish a causal relationship between variables of interest.

5. **D.** Experimental research designs include cohort studies, randomized clinical trials, and case-control studies. Retrospective epidemiologic studies are observational and are the exception.

6. **B.** Cohort studies do not randomize study participants. Cohort studies do share commonality with randomized clinical trials in that they evaluate causal relationships between study variables, involve exposure to a test treatment or condition, and may occasionally use historical control groups.

7. **A.** Intrasubject effects are analyzed in crossover study designs. Parallel, sequential, and Latin square designs analyze intersubject effects.

8. **D.** Crossover study designs can be used only for stable, chronic, or episodic conditions. Glaucoma, migraine headaches, and epilepsy meet

this criterion. Pneumonia does not meet this criterion, and therefore, is generally not suitable for a crossover design.

9. **C.** Blinding of subjects is an important process within clinical trials to minimize bias. It does not minimize confounding variables, systematic error, or variability.

10. **A.** Randomization is a key process within clinical trials to ensure the validity of inferential statistics used in analyzing the study results. It does not avoid the placebo effect or the carryover effect or ensure a normal distribution of the study outcome.

11. **B.** Subjects and investigators are unaware of the subject treatment in a double-blind study. In a single-blind study, only the subjects are unaware of the subject treatment, whereas a triple-blind study refers to blinding of all persons who come in contact with the study procedures or data.

12. **A.** Stratification ensures equal distribution of selected subject characteristics between groups. It requires a larger number of patients and can be used in both parallel and crossover study designs. Stratification is performed before randomization.

13. **C.** Decreased sample size is needed where the expected difference in outcome between groups is large. Increased sample size increases statistical power and is needed where there is large variability in the study outcome being measured. Decreased sample size is needed for a crossover study design because patients are serving as their own controls.

14. **C.** Randomized clinical trials can use standard treatment, usual care, and placebo as controls. Historical controls cannot be used in a randomized clinical trial and are the exception.

15. **D.** Patients who withdraw from a study prior to completing the study protocol can be managed by analyzing data using an intention-to-treat method and both intention-to-treat and per protocol methods and by categorizing patients according to reason for withdrawal using a per protocol method. Purging data from the study database upon withdrawal from the study and including only subjects completing the protocol is inappropriate and is the exception.

16. **B.** General steps in the critical appraisal of the literature relative to a published study include evaluating the validity of the study results, determining applicability of the study, and evaluating the basic study design. Searching for other studies published by the authors is not generally a step in appraising the literature and is the exception.

17. **A.** Asking if the groups have similar baseline characteristics, how large was the treatment effect, and if the benefits of the treatment are worth the harm and costs are aids in evaluating a clinical trial. Determining if all confounding variables were avoided in a study is not an aid in evaluating a clinical trial.

18. **D.** Important vehicles for practitioners relative to keeping up to date with new literature include review articles, clinical practice guidelines, and attendance at continuing education. Case reports are generally not an important method for keeping up to date with new literature.

19. **B.** Critical steps in practicing evidenced-based medicine include searching the literature for relevant clinical articles, evaluating and critically appraising the clinical studies for validity and usefulness, and formulating a clear clinical question relative to a particular patient problem. Regularly conversing with colleagues on their approach to a clinical problem is not a part of practicing evidence-based medicine.

20. **D.** Potential confounding variables include a subject's concurrent medications, medical complications that occur during the study period, and study dropouts. Exclusion of patients with severe forms of the disease being studied is not a confounding variable because it can be controlled.

21. **C.** The desired statistical power, estimated effect size, and variability and experimental error are all used to calculate a sample size. The probability of the results affecting clinical practice is not generally used in calculating sample size.

22. **D.** In a randomized controlled trial that follows a parallel design, patients are assigned to groups that receive a particular treatment over time; the only planned difference in the groups is the intervention. Patients do not serve as their own control; they generally receive only one study treatment depending on group

assignment; and all patients are accounted for in the final analysis, including patients who do not complete the study protocol.

23. **A.** The intention-to-treat analysis includes data from all patients regardless of whether they completed the protocol.

24. **D.** The duration of follow-up for a randomized clinical trial is determined by the outcome to be measured, long-term safety concerns, and the duration of time required to observe an effect. Study budget is not a scientific factor in determining the duration of follow-up.

25. **C.** Failure to meet the study inclusion criteria is an acceptable reason for excluding a patient from an intention-to-treat analysis of study data. Adverse events, lack of response, and noncompliance with the study treatment are unacceptable reasons for excluding patients.

11-10. References

Aparasu RR, Bently JP. *Principles of Research Design and Drug Literature Evaluation.* Burlington, MA: Jones & Bartlett Learning; 2015.

Dawson B, Trapp RG. *Basic and Clinical Biostatistics.* 4th ed. New York, NY: Lange Medical Books/McGraw-Hill; 2004.

Gluud LL. Bias in clinical intervention research. *Am J Epidemiol.* 2006;163(6):493–501.

Guyatt GH, Sackett DL, Cook DJ. Users' guides to the medical literature II: How to use an article about a therapy or prevention. *JAMA.* 1994;271(1): 59–63.

Hill A, Spittlehouse C. What is critical appraisal? *Bandolier.* 2001;3(2):1–8.

Rosenberg W, Donald A. Evidence-based medicine: An approach to clinical problem solving. *BMJ.* 1995;310(6987):1122–6.

Hypertension

Benjamin N. Gross

12-1. Key Points

- *Hypertension* is defined as a systolic blood pressure (BP) exceeding 140 mm Hg, a diastolic blood pressure exceeding 90 mm Hg, or any condition in a patient that requires antihypertensive therapy.
- The Joint National Committee on Detection, Evaluation, and Treatment of High Blood Pressure (JNC-VIII) no longer addresses definitions of hypertension and prehypertension, as was the case in the JNC-VII guidelines.
- Secondary causes of hypertension include renovascular disease, primary aldosteronism, Cushing's syndrome, pheochromocytoma, aortic coarctation, and drugs (steroids and estrogens, alcohol, cocaine, cyclosporine and tacrolimus, sympathomimetics, erythropoietin, licorice, monoamine oxidase [MAO] inhibitors, tricyclic antidepressants, and nonsteroidal anti-inflammatory drugs [NSAIDs]).
- Recommended lifestyle modifications to improve both BP and overall cardiovascular health include losing weight; limiting alcohol intake; increasing aerobic physical activity; reducing sodium intake; maintaining adequate dietary intake of potassium, magnesium, and calcium; stopping smoking; and reducing dietary cholesterol and saturated fat intake.
- JNC-VIII recommends similar treatment goals defined for all hypertensive populations except for those individuals ≥ 60 years.
- Thiazide diuretics, angiotensin converting enzyme inhibitors (ACEIs), angiotensin II receptor blockers (ARBs), or calcium channel blockers (CCBs) are considered by JNC-VIII to be the initial agent for treatment of hypertension for non–African American patients.
- JNC-VIII considers thiazide diuretics and CCBs equivalent choices as initial therapy for hypertension in African American patients.
- JNC-VIII recommends ACEIs or ARBs alone or in combination with other drug classes in all chronic kidney disease (CKD) patients regardless of race and diabetes status.
- Vasodilators, α_1-receptor antagonists, α_2-receptor agonists, and postganglionic adrenergic neuron blockers should be avoided as initial agents for hypertension.
- The classification and treatment of hypertensive urgencies and emergencies is determined by the presence or absence of acute target organ damage and not by BP.
- All causes for inadequate response should be addressed before additional agents are added to a patient's antihypertensive regimen (i.e., pseudoresistance, nonadherence, volume overload, drug-related causes, associated conditions, and secondary causes of hypertension).

12-2. Study Guide Checklist

The following topics may guide your study of this subject area:

- Proper BP measurement technique
- Risk factors for hypertension
- Secondary causes of hypertension with emphasis on drug-induced causes

- General sense of lifestyle practices in management of hypertension with particular focus on the Dietary Approaches to Stop Hypertension (DASH) diet
- General sense of changes from previous hypertension guidelines regarding classification of hypertension
- Considerations for selection of antihypertensive drugs based on a patient's condition and prior drug experience
- Actions of various categories of antihypertensive drugs
- Trade names and available dosage forms, particularly of the "Top 100 Drugs"
- Frequency of dosing regimen
- Major adverse drug reactions of antihypertensive drugs
- Significant drug interactions of antihypertensive drugs
- Any unique patient counseling points for specific antihypertensive drugs
- Indications for drugs to treat hypertensive emergencies and urgencies

12-3. Disease Overview

- *Hypertension* is defined as a systolic blood pressure (SBP) > 140 mm Hg, a diastolic blood pressure (DBP) > 90 mm Hg, or a condition in any patient requiring antihypertensive therapy.
- In the United States, 77.9 million (1 of every 3) adults are affected by hypertension.
- Incidence increases with age.
- Onset most commonly occurs in the third to fifth decades of life, and the lifetime risk of hypertension is 90% for those surviving to age 80.
- Prevalence differs by ethnic group, socioeconomic group, and geographic region. The highest prevalence is seen in non-Hispanic African Americans (42%), compared with non-Hispanic Caucasians (28%) and Mexican Americans (26%).

Classification

The Eighth Report of the Joint National Committee on Detection, Evaluation, and Treatment of High Blood Pressure (JNC-VIII) no longer addresses the definitions of hypertension and prehypertension, as was the case in the JNC-VII guidelines. JNC-VIII defines thresholds for pharmacologic treatment.

Clinical Presentation and Complications

Cardiovascular effects

- Left ventricular hypertrophy
- Congestive heart failure (CHF)
- Peripheral arterial disease
- Angina pectoris
- Myocardial infarction
- Sudden death

Renal effects

- Nephropathy
- Renal failure
- Requirements for dialysis

Cerebrovascular effects

- Transient ischemic attacks
- Stroke

Ophthalmologic effects

- Retinal hemorrhage
- Retinopathy
- Blindness

Pathophysiology and Etiology

- Blood pressure = (stroke volume × heart rate) × peripheral resistance (Figure 12-1)

Sympathetic nervous system activation

Central activation
- Presynaptic α_2 stimulation is a negative feedback mechanism, leading to decreased norepinephrine release.
- Presynaptic β stimulation leads to increased norepinephrine release.

Peripheral activation
- β_1 stimulation leads to increased heart rate and contractility, causing increased cardiac output.
- β_2 stimulation leads to arterial vasodilation.
- β stimulation also causes increased renin release, causing increased angiotensin II production.
- α_1 stimulation leads to arterial and venous vasoconstriction.

Renin–angiotensin–aldosterone system

- Decreased renal perfusion pressure causes increases in renin levels.
- Renin reacts with angiotensinogen to produce angiotensin I (AT-I).

Figure 12-1. Sympathetic Nervous System Activation

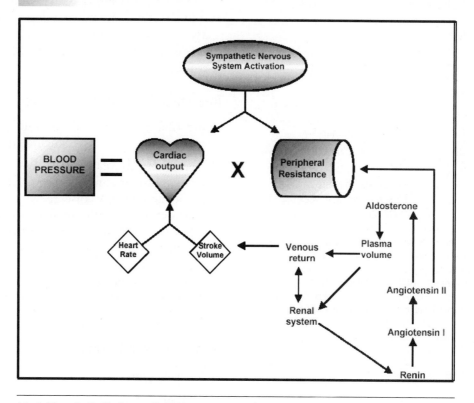

Adapted from Carter BL, Saseen JL, 2002.

- Angiotensin-converting enzyme (ACE) causes AT-I to become angiotensin II (AT-II).
- AT-II is a potent vasoconstrictor and stimulates aldosterone release, which increases sodium and fluid retention.

Water and sodium retention

- Acute: Increased fluid volume causes increased cardiac output, which causes increased blood pressure (BP).
- Chronic: Excess intracellular sodium causes vascular hypertrophy, which increases vascular resistance and response to vasoconstriction and, in turn, increases BP.

Etiology

Primary (essential) hypertension
- Unknown cause
- Found in 85–95% of all hypertension cases

Secondary hypertension
- ***Renovascular disease:*** This condition is suggested by increased blood urea nitrogen (BUN) and creatinine and by abdominal bruits.
- ***Primary aldosteronism:*** This condition is suggested by unprovoked hypokalemia.
- ***Cushing's syndrome:*** This condition is suggested by unprovoked hypokalemia and truncal obesity with purple striae.
- ***Pheochromocytoma:*** This condition is suggested by increased urinary catecholamine excretion (i.e., vanillylmandelic acid and metanephrine) accompanied by headache, palpitations, and perspiration.
- ***Aortic coarctation:*** This condition is suggested by delayed or absent femoral pulses and decreased BP in the lower extremities.
- ***Drug-induced hypertension:*** The following drugs may induce hypertension:
  - Steroids and estrogens (including oral contraceptives)
  - Alcohol
  - Cocaine
  - Cyclosporine and tacrolimus
  - Sympathomimetics
  - Erythropoietin
  - Licorice (in chewing tobacco)
  - Monoamine oxidase (MAO) inhibitors
  - Tricyclic antidepressants
  - Nonsteroidal anti-inflammatory drugs (NSAIDs)

Table 12-1. Recommendations for Follow-up Based on Initial BP Measurements for Adults

Initial BP (mm Hg)[a]

Systolic	Diastolic	Recommended follow-up[b]
< 130	< 85	Recheck in 2 years.
130–139	85–89	Recheck in 1 year.[c]
140–159	90–99	Confirm within 2 months.[c]
160–179	100–109	Evaluate or refer to source of care within 1 month.
~180	~110	Evaluate or refer to source of care immediately or within 1 week depending on clinical situation.

Adapted from JNC-7 Express, National Heart, Lung, and Blood Institute.
a. If systolic and diastolic readings are different, follow recommendations for shorter time to follow-up (e.g., a person with a reading of 160/86 mm Hg should be evaluated or referred to source of care within 1 month).
b. Modify the scheduling of follow-up according to reliable information about past BP measurements, other cardiovascular risk factors, or target organ disease.
c. Provide advice about lifestyle modifications.

Diagnostic Criteria

Diagnosis and treatment begin with proper BP measurement, assessment, and follow-up planning (Table 12-1). The patient should avoid ingesting caffeine and smoking for 30 minutes prior to BP measurement and should be resting for 5 minutes prior to BP measurement. BP is measured as follows:

- Position arm (brachial artery) at heart level.
- Uncover arm; do not put cuff over clothes.
- Determine proper size cuff.

Upper arm circumference	Cuff size required
16–22.5 cm	Pediatric cuff
22.6–30 cm	Regular adult cuff
30.1–37.5 cm	Large adult cuff
37.6–43.7 cm	Thigh cuff

- Position cuff 1 inch above antecubital crease.
- Ask patient about previous readings.
- Place stethoscope over brachial artery (medial to the center).
- Inflate cuff rapidly to approximately 30 mm Hg above previous readings.
- Deflate cuff slowly.
- Remember to deflate cuff completely when done.
- Wait 1–2 minutes before repeating.
- Take pressure in both arms.

- If orthostatic hypotension is suspected, take BP while patient is sitting, standing, and supine.
- If two readings are taken at least 2 minutes apart, average the readings.
- If readings differ by > 5 mm Hg, take additional readings.

Treatment Principles and Goals

Figure 12-2 and Table 12-2 outline some important treatment principles. Goals include the following:

- To reduce end-organ damage
- To minimize or control other risk factors for cardiovascular (CV) disease
- To maintain BP, with minimal side effects, at or below the level appropriate for the patient's risk:
  - 140/90 mm Hg for those individuals age < 60 years, with diabetes and with chronic kidney disease
  - 150/90 mm Hg for those individuals age ≥ 60 years

Monitoring and Evaluation

Initial evaluation

The initial evaluation of a patient with hypertension has the following goals:

- To identify known causes of high blood pressure
- To assess the presence or absence of target organ damage and CV disease, the extent of disease, and the patient's response to therapies (Box 12-1)
- To identify other CV risk factors or concomitant disorders that may affect prognosis and guide therapy (Box 12-1)

The patient's history should be considered in the initial evaluation:

- Duration and levels of elevated BP
- History or symptoms of coronary heart disease (CHD), heart failure, cerebrovascular disease, pulmonary vascular disease, diabetes mellitus, renal disease, or dyslipidemia
- Family history of hypertension, premature CHD, stroke, diabetes, dyslipidemia, or renal disease
- Symptoms suggesting the cause of hypertension
- Recent weight changes, physical activity levels, or smoking or other tobacco use
- Dietary assessment of intake of sodium, alcohol, saturated fat, and caffeine
- Complete medication history, including prescription, over-the-counter, and herbal or natu-

Figure 12-2. Algorithm for the Treatment of Hypertension

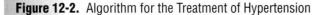

Figure. 2014 Hypertension Guideline Management Algorithm

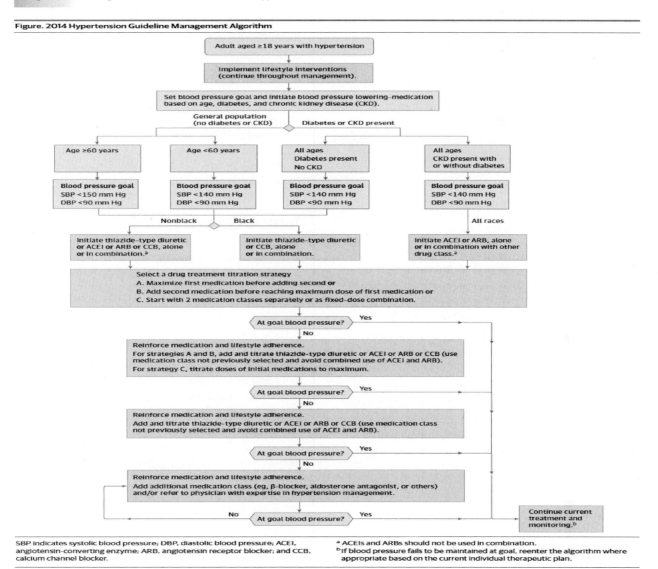

SBP indicates systolic blood pressure; DBP, diastolic blood pressure; ACEI, angiotensin-converting enzyme; ARB, angiotensin receptor blocker; and CCB, calcium channel blocker.

[a] ACEIs and ARBs should not be used in combination.
[b] If blood pressure fails to be maintained at goal, reenter the algorithm where appropriate based on the current individual therapeutic plan.

JNC-VIII, 2013.

ral products that may increase BP or decrease effectiveness of antihypertensive agents
- Results and adverse effects of previous anti-hypertensive therapy
- Psychosocial and environmental factors that may influence hypertension control

An examination should also be done:

- Two or more blood pressure measurements separated by at least 2 minutes
- Measurement of height, weight, and waist circumference
- Funduscopic exam for hypertensive retinopathy
- Exam of neck for carotid bruits, distended veins, or enlarged thyroid gland
- Exam of heart for abnormalities in rate and rhythm, increased size, precordial heave, clicks, murmurs, and third and fourth heart sounds
- Exam of lungs for rales and evidence of bronchospasm
- Exam of abdomen for bruits, enlarged kidneys, masses, and abnormal aortic pulsation
- Exam of extremities for decreased or absent peripheral arterial pulsations, bruits, and edema
- Neurologic assessment

Routine laboratory tests are necessary:

- Urinalysis
- Complete blood cell count (CBC)

Table 12-2. Identifiable Causes, Diagnostic Tests, and Clinical Findings for Secondary Hypertension

Cause or diagnosis	Diagnostic test (clinical finding)
Chronic kidney disease	Estimated GFR (abdominal or flank mass for polycystic kidney disease)
Coarctation of the aorta	CT angiography (delayed or absent femoral pulse)
Cushing's syndrome and other glucocorticoid excess states, including chronic steroid therapy	History; dexamethasone suppression test (truncal obesity, moon facies, buffalo hump, abdominal striae, and hirsutism)
Drug-induced or drug-related condition	History; drug screening
Pheochromocytoma	24-hour urinary metanephrine and normetanephrine (headache, palpitations, and sweating)
Primary aldosteronism and other mineralocorticoid excess states	24-hour urinary aldosterone level or specific measurements of other mineralocorticoids (hypokalemia)
Renovascular hypertension	Doppler flow study; magnetic resonance angiography (abdominal bruit)
Sleep apnea	Sleep study with oxygen saturation (obesity, snoring, and fatigue during wake time)
Thyroid or parathyroid disease	Thyroid-stimulating hormone; serum parathyroid hormone (goiter; hypercalcemia)

CT, computed tomography; GFR, glomerular filtration rate.

- Blood chemistries (sodium, potassium, creatinine, BUN, and glucose)
- Fasting lipid profile: total cholesterol, triglycerides, HDL (high-density lipoprotein), and LDL (low-density lipoprotein)
- Electrocardiogram (ECG)

The following laboratory tests are optional:

- Creatinine clearance
- Microalbuminuria
- 24-hour urinary protein
- Blood calcium
- Uric acid
- Glycosylated hemoglobin
- Thyroid-stimulating hormone
- Limited echocardiography
- Ankle-brachial index
- Plasma renin activity and urinary sodium determination

Box 12-1. Cardiovascular Risk Factors

Major Risk Factors

- Hypertension[a]
- Cigarette smoking
- Obesity[a] (body mass index $\geq$ 30 kg/m^2)
- Physical inactivity
- Dyslipidemia[a]
- Diabetes mellitus[a]
- Microalbuminuria or estimated GFR < 60 mL/min
- Age (> 55 for men, > 65 for women)
- Family history of premature cardiovascular disease (men under age 55, women under age 65)

Target Organ Damage

Heart
- Left ventricular hypertrophy
- Angina or prior myocardial infarction
- Prior coronary revascularization
- Heart failure

Brain
- Stroke or transient ischemic attack

Kidney
- Chronic kidney disease
- End stage renal disease

Vascular System
- Peripheral arterial disease

Eyes
- Retinopathy

Adapted from JNC-7 Express, National Heart, Lung, and Blood Institute. GFR, glomerular filtration rate.
a. Components of the metabolic syndrome.

Follow-up evaluation

Follow-up evaluation includes any of the previous exams completed during the initial evaluation that are required to monitor both response to and possible adverse effects from prescribed antihypertensive therapies, in addition to the assessment of any new symptoms of target organ damage and the assessment of patient adherence to therapy (Box 12-2).

12-4. Nondrug Therapy

Lifestyle modifications are recommended to improve both BP and overall cardiovascular health (Table 12-3).

- Be aware of signs of patient nonadherence to antihypertensive therapy.
- Establish the goal of therapy: to reduce blood pressure to nonhypertensive levels with minimal or no adverse effects.
- Educate patients about the disease, and involve them and their families in its treatment. Have them measure blood pressure at home.
- Maintain contact with patients; consider telecommunication.
- Keep care inexpensive and simple.
- Encourage lifestyle modifications.
- Integrate pill taking into routine activities of daily living.
- Prescribe medications according to pharmacologic principles, favoring long-acting formulations.
- Be willing to stop unsuccessful therapy and try a different approach.
- Anticipate adverse effects. Adjust therapy to prevent, minimize, or ameliorate side effects.
- Continue to add effective and tolerated drugs, stepwise, in sufficient doses to achieve the goal of therapy.
- Encourage a positive attitude about achieving therapeutic goals.
- Consider using nurse case management.

Adapted from JNC-7 Express, National Heart, Lung, and Blood Institute.

Research has shown that diets rich in fruits, vegetables, and low-fat dairy foods, and with reduced saturated and total fats, significantly lower blood pressure (Tables 12-4 and 12-5).

12-5. Drug Therapy

All patient factors (severity of BP elevation, presence of target organ damage, and presence of CV disease or other risk factors) must be considered when initiating therapy.

Initial Therapy

- For candidates for therapy, see Figure 12-2.
- Use of lifestyle modifications (Table 12-3) should continue to be stressed to patients after the decision to initiate drug therapy has been made to further decrease the risk of complications from cardiovascular disease.
- JNC-VIII recommends the use of thiazide diuretics, as initial therapy in non–African American patients alone or in combination with other agents.
- JNC-VIII recommends CCBs and thiazide diuretics in African American patients alone or in combination.
- JNC-VIII recommends ACEIs or ARBs alone or in combination with other drug types in CHD regardless of race or diabetes status.

Table 12-3. Lifestyle Modifications to Manage Hypertension

Modification	Recommendation	Approximate SBP reduction (Range)
Weight reduction	Maintain normal body weight (body mass index 18.5–24.9 kg/m²).	5–20 mm Hg/ 10 kg weight loss
Adopt DASH eating plan	Consume a diet rich in fruits, vegetables, and low-fat dairy products with a reduced content of saturated and total fat.	8–14 mm Hg
Dietary sodium reduction	Reduce dietary sodium intake to no more than 100 mmol per day (2.4 g sodium or 6 g sodium chloride).	2–8 mm Hg
Physical activity	Engage in regular aerobic physical activity such as brisk walking (at least 30 minutes per day, most days of the week).	4–9 mm Hg
Moderation of alcohol consumption	Limit consumption to no more than 2 drinks (1 oz or 30 mL ethanol; e.g., 24 oz beer, 10 oz wine, or 3 oz 80-proof whiskey) per day in most men and to no more than 1 drink per day in women and lighter weight persons.	2–4 mm Hg[30]

Adapted from JNC-7 Express, National Heart, Lung, and Blood Institute.
DASH, Dietary Approaches to Stop Hypertension. For overall cardiovascular risk reduction, stop smoking. The effects of implementing these modifications are dose and time dependent and could be greater for some individuals.

Table 12-4. Dietary Suggestions for Hypertensive Patients

Food group	Daily servings	Serving sizes	Examples and notes	Significance of each food group to the DASH diet pattern
Grains and grain products	7–8	1 slice bread; ½ c dry cereal; ½ c cooked rice, pasta, or cereal	Whole wheat bread, English muffins, pita bread, bagel, cereals, grits, and oatmeal	Major sources of energy and fiber
Vegetables	4–5	1 c raw leafy vegetable; ½ c cooked vegetable; 6 oz vegetable juice	Tomatoes, potatoes, carrots, peas, squash, broccoli, turnip greens, collards, kale, spinach, artichokes, beans, and sweet potatoes	Rich sources of potassium, magnesium, and fiber
Fruits	4–5	6 oz fruit juice; 1 medium fruit; ¼ c dried fruit; ¼ c fresh, frozen, or canned fruit	Apricots, bananas, dates, grapes, oranges, orange juice, grapefruit, grapefruit juice, mangoes, melons, peaches, pineapple, prunes, raisins, strawberries, and tangerines	Important sources of potassium, magnesium, and fiber
Low-fat or nonfat dairy foods	2–3	8 oz milk; 1 c yogurt; 1.5 oz cheese	Skim or 1% milk, skim or low-fat buttermilk, nonfat or low-fat yogurt, part-skim mozzarella cheese, and nonfat cheese	Major sources of calcium and protein
Meats, poultry, and fish	2 or fewer	3 oz cooked meat, poultry, or fish	Select only lean cuts; trim away visible fat; broil, roast, or boil instead of frying; and remove skin from poultry	Rich sources of protein and magnesium
Nuts, seeds, and legumes	4–5 per week	1.5 oz or ⅓ c nuts; ½ oz or 2 T seeds; ½ c cooked legumes	Almonds, filberts, mixed nuts, peanuts, walnuts, sunflower seeds, kidney beans, and lentils	Rich sources of energy, magnesium, potassium, protein, and fiber

Adapted from JNC-7 Express, National Heart, Lung, and Blood Institute.
DASH, Dietary Approaches to Stop Hypertension.

Table 12-5. The DASH Diet Sample Menu Based on 2,000 Calories per Day

Food	Amount	Servings provided
Breakfast		
Orange juice	6 oz	1 fruit
1% low-fat milk	8 oz (1 c)	1 dairy
Cornflakes (with 1 t sugar)	1 c	2 grains
Banana	1 medium	1 fruit
Whole wheat bread (with 1 T jelly)	1 slice	1 grain
Soft margarine	1 t	1 fat
Lunch		
Chicken salad	¾ c	1 poultry
Pita bread	½ large	1 grain
Raw vegetable medley		
Carrot and celery sticks	3–4 sticks each	1 vegetable
Radishes	2	1 vegetable
Loose-leaf lettuce	2 leaves	1 vegetable

Table 12-5. The DASH Diet Sample Menu Based on 2,000 Calories per Day *(Continued)*

Food	Amount	Servings provided
Lunch		
Part-skim mozzarella cheese	1.5 slices (1.5 oz)	1 dairy
1% low-fat milk	8 oz (1 c)	1 dairy
Fruit cocktail in light syrup	½ c	1 fruit
Dinner		
Herbed, baked cod	3 oz	1 fish
Scallion rice	1 c	2 grains
Steamed broccoli	½ c	1 vegetable
Stewed tomatoes	½ c	1 vegetable
Spinach salad:		
Raw spinach	½ c	1 vegetable
Cherry tomatoes	2	1 vegetable
Cucumber	2 slices	1 vegetable
Light Italian salad dressing	1 T	½ fat
Whole wheat dinner roll	1 small	1 grain
Soft margarine	1 t	1 fat
Melon balls	½ c	1 fruit
Snacks		
Dried apricots	1 oz (¼ c)	1 fruit
Mini pretzels	1 oz (¾ c)	1 grain
Mixed nuts	1.5 oz (⅓ c)	1 nuts
Diet ginger ale	12 oz	0

Total number of servings in 2,000-calorie per day menu

Food group	Servings
Grains	8
Vegetables	4
Fruits	5
Dairy foods	3
Meats, poultry, and fish	2
Nuts, seeds, and legumes	1
Fats and oils	2.5

Tips on eating the DASH way

- Start small. Make gradual changes in your eating habits.
- Center your meal around carbohydrates, such as pasta, rice, beans, or vegetables.
- Treat meat as one part of the whole meal, instead of the focus.
- Use fruits or low-fat, low-calorie foods such as sugar-free gelatin for desserts and snacks.

Remember: If you use the DASH diet to help prevent or control high blood pressure, make it part of a lifestyle that includes choosing foods lower in salt and sodium; keeping a healthy weight; being physically active; and if you drink alcohol, doing so in moderation.

Adapted from JNC-7 Express, National Heart, Lung, and Blood Institute.
DASH, Dietary Approaches to Stop Hypertension.

Table 12-6. Strategies to Dose Antihypertensive Drugs

Strategy	Description	Details
A	Begin one drug, titrate to maximum dose, and then add a second drug.	If goal BP is not achieved with the initial drug, titrate the dose of the initial drug up to the maximum recommended dose to achieve goal BP.
		If goal BP is not achieved with the use of one drug despite titration to the maximum recommended dose, add a second drug from the list (thiazide-type diuretic, CCB, ACEI, or ARB) and titrate up to the maximum recommended dose of the second drug to achieve goal BP.
		If goal BP is not achieved with 2 drugs, select a third drug from the list (thiazide-type diuretic, CCB, ACEI, or ARB), avoiding the combined use of ACEI and ARB. Titrate the third drug up to the maximum recommended dose to achieve goal BP.
B	Begin one drug, and add a second drug before achieving maximum dose of the initial drug.	Begin one drug, and add a second drug before achieving the maximum recommended dose of the initial drug, then titrate both drugs up to the maximum recommended doses of both to achieve goal BP.
		If goal BP is not achieved with 2 drugs, select a third drug from the list (thiazide-type diuretic, CCB, ACEI, or ARB), avoiding the combined use of ACEI and ARB. Titrate the third drug up to the maximum.
C	Begin with 2 drugs at the same time, either as 2 separate pills or as a single pill combination.	Initiate therapy with 2 drugs simultaneously, either as 2 separate drugs or as a single pill combination.
		Some committee members recommend beginning therapy with ≥ 2 drugs when SBP is > 160 mm Hg, DBP is > 100 mm Hg, or both, or if SBP is > 20 mm Hg above goal, DBP is > 10 mm Hg above goal, or both.
		If goal BP is not achieved with 2 drugs, select a third drug from the list (thiazide-type diuretic, CCB, ACEI, or ARB), avoiding the combined use of ACEI and ARB. Titrate the third drug up to the maximum recommended dose.

- JNC-VIII recommends three strategies to dose antihypertensive drugs (Table 12-6). For each strategy, begin with one drug, titrate to maximum dose, and then add a second drug from a second class.
- For patients who are 20/10 mm Hg greater than their goal BP, 2-drug combination therapy should be strongly considered.
- All causes for an inadequate response should be addressed before additional agents are added to a patient's antihypertensive regimen (Box 12-3).
- Vasodilators, α_1-receptor antagonists, α_2-receptor agonists, and postganglionic adrenergic neuron blockers should be avoided as initial agents for hypertension.

Diuretics

Thiazide and thiazide-like diuretics

See Table 12-7 for a list of thiazide and thiazide-like diuretics, their usual dosage range, and adverse effects associated with these medications.

Mechanism of action
- Direct arteriole dilation occurs.
- Reduction of total fluid volume occurs through the inhibition of sodium reabsorption in the distal tubules, which causes increased excretion of sodium, water, potassium, and hydrogen.
- The effectiveness of other antihypertensive agents is increased by preventing reexpansion of plasma volume.
- A significant decrease in efficacy occurs in renal failure: serum creatinine > 2 mg/dL or glomerular filtration rate (GFR) < 30 mL/min.
- Diuretics are also available in combination with other drugs (Table 12-8).

Patient instructions and counseling
- Medication may be taken with food or milk.
- Take early in the day to avoid nocturia.
- Medication may increase sensitivity to sunlight. Consider using sunscreen with SPF (sun protection factor) > 15.
- Medication may increase blood glucose in diabetics.

Box 12-3. Causes of Inadequate Responsiveness to Therapy

Pseudoresistance

- "White-coat hypertension" or office elevations
- Pseudohypertension in older patients
- Use of regular adult cuff on a very obese arm

Nonadherence to therapy

Volume overload
- Excess salt intake
- Progressive renal damage (nephrosclerosis)
- Fluid retention from reduction of blood pressure
- Inadequate diuretic therapy

Drug-related causes
- Doses too low
- Wrong type of diuretic
- Inappropriate combinations
- Rapid inactivation (e.g., hydralazine)
- Drug actions and interactions
- Sympathomimetics
- Nasal decongestants
- Appetite suppressants
- Cocaine and other illicit drugs
- Caffeine
- Oral contraceptives
- Adrenal steroids
- Licorice (as may be found in chewing tobacco)
- Cyclosporine or tacrolimus
- Erythropoietin
- Antidepressants
- Nonsteroidal anti-inflammatory drugs

Associated conditions
- Smoking
- Increasing obesity
- Sleep apnea
- Insulin resistance or hyperinsulinemia
- Ethanol intake of more than 1 oz (30 mL) per day
- Anxiety-induced hyperventilation or panic attacks
- Chronic pain
- Intense vasoconstriction (arteritis)
- Organic brain syndrome (e.g., memory deficit)

Identifiable causes of hypertension

Adapted from JNC-7 Express, National Heart, Lung, and Blood Institute.

- Report problems with muscle cramps, which may indicate decreased potassium level.

Drug–drug and drug–disease interactions
- Steroids cause salt retention and antagonize thiazide action.

- NSAIDs blunt thiazide response.
- Class IA or III antiarrhythmics (that prolong the QT interval) may cause torsades de pointes with diuretic-induced hypokalemia.
- Probenecid and lithium block thiazide effects by interfering with thiazide excretion into the urine.
- Thiazides decrease lithium renal clearance and increase the risk of lithium toxicity.

Parameters to monitor
- BP
- Weight
- Serum electrolytes and uric acid
- BUN and creatinine
- Cholesterol levels

Loop diuretics

See Table 12-7 for a list of loop diuretics, their usual dosage range, and adverse effects associated with these medications.

Mechanism of action
- Reduction of total fluid volume occurs through the inhibition of sodium and chloride reabsorption in the ascending loop of Henle, which causes increased excretion of water, sodium, chloride, magnesium, and calcium.
- Loop diuretics are more effective than thiazides in patients with renal failure: serum creatinine > 2 mg/dL or GFR < 30 mL/min.

Patient instructions and counseling
- Medication may be taken with food or milk.
- Take early in the day to avoid nocturia.
- Medication may increase sensitivity to sunlight. Consider using sunscreen with SPF > 15.
- Medication may increase blood glucose in diabetics.
- Report problems with muscle cramps, which may indicate decreased potassium level.
- Rise slowly from a lying or sitting position.

Drug–drug and drug–disease interactions
- Aminoglycosides can precipitate ototoxicity when combined with loop diuretics.
- NSAIDs blunt diuretic response.

Table 12-7. Thiazide Diuretics, Thiazide-Like Diuretics, Loop Diuretics, Potassium-Sparing Agents, and Aldosterone-Receptor Blockers

Drug	Trade name	Usual dosage range, total mg/day (frequency per day)	Adverse events and comments[a]
Thiazide diuretics			
Bendroflumethiazide	Naturetin	2.5–5 (1)	**Short-term:** increased cholesterol and glucose
Benzthiazide	Aquatag, Exna	12.5–50 (1)	**Biochemical:** decreased potassium, sodium, and magnesium; increased uric acid and calcium
Chlorothiazide	Diuril	125–500 (1)	
Chlorthalidone	Hygroton, Hylidone	12.5–25 (1)	**Rare:** blood dyscrasias, photosensitivity, pancreatitis, hyponatremia, and sulfonamide-type immune reactions
Hydrochlorothiazide	Hydrodiuril, Microzide	12.5–50 (1)	**Other:** impotence, fatigue, headache, rash, and vertigo
Hydroflumethiazide	Saluron, Diucardin	25–50 (1)	
Methyclothiazide	Aquatensen, Enduron	5 (1)	
Polythiazide	Renese	2.5–5 (1)	
Trichlormethiazide	Metahydrin, Naqua	2–4 (1)	
Thiazide-like diuretics			
Indapamide	Lozol	2.5–5 (1)	
Metolazone	Mykrox	2.5–10 (1)	(Less or no hypercholesterolemia compared to other thiazides; decreased microalbuminuria in diabetes)
Metolazone	Zaroxolyn	2.5–5 (1)	(Less or no hypercholesterolemia compared to other thiazides; decreased microalbuminuria in diabetes)
Loop diuretics			
Bumetanide	Bumex	0.5–2 (2)	Ototoxicity at high doses
Furosemide	Lasix	20–80 (2)	(Short duration and no hypercalcemia)
Torsemide	Demadex	2.5–10 (1)	(Short duration and no hypercalcemia)
Potassium-sparing agents[b]			
Amiloride	Midamor	5–10 (1–2)	Hyperkalemia
Triamterene	Dyrenium	50–100 (1–2)	(Avoid with history of kidney stones or hepatic disease)
Aldosterone-receptor blockers			
Eplerenone	Inspra	50–100 (1–2)	
Spironolactone	Aldactone	25–50 (1–2)	

Adapted from JNC-7 Express, National Heart, Lung, and Blood Institute.
a. Adverse events, or side effects, listed are for the class of drugs, except where noted for individual drugs (in parentheses).
b. See Table 12-8 for combination products.

- Class IA or III antiarrhythmics (that prolong the QT interval) may cause torsades de pointes with diuretic-induced hypokalemia.
- Probenecid blocks loop diuretic effects by interfering with excretion into the urine.

Parameters to monitor
- Weight
- Serum electrolytes
- BUN and creatinine
- Uric acid
- Hearing (in high doses)

Potassium-sparing diuretics

See Table 12-7 for a list of potassium-sparing diuretics, their usual dosage range, and adverse effects associated with these medications.

Table 12-8. Combination Drugs for Hypertension

Fixed-dose combination (mg)[a]	Trade name
ACEIs and CCBs	
Amlodipine/benazepril hydrochloride (2.5/10, 5/10, 5/20, 10/20)	Lotrel
Trandolapril/verapamil (2/180, 1/240, 2/240, 4/240)	Tarka
ACEIs and diuretics	
Benazepril/hydrochlorothiazide (5/6.25, 10/12.5, 20/12.5, 20/25)	Lotensin HCT
Captopril/hydrochlorothiazide (25/15, 25/25, 50/15, 50/25)	Capozide
Enalapril maleate/hydrochlorothiazide (5/12.5, 10/25)	Vaseretic
Lisinopril/hydrochlorothiazide (10/12.5, 20/12.5, 20/25)	Prinzide
Moexipril HCl/hydrochlorothiazide (7.5/12.5, 15/25)	Uniretic
Fosinopril HCl/hydrochlorothiazide (10/12.5, 20/12.5)	Monopril HCT
Quinapril HCl/hydrochlorothiazide (10/12.5, 20/12.5, 20/25)	Accuretic
ARBs and CCBs	
Amlodipine/valsartan (5/160, 5/320, 10/160, 10/320)	Exforge
Amlodipine/olmesartan (5/20, 5/40, 10/20, 10/40)	Azor
Amlodipine/telmisartan (5/40, 5/80, 10/40, 10/80)	Twynsta
ARBs and diuretics	
Candesartan cilexetil/hydrochlorothiazide (16/12.5, 32/12.5)	Atacand HCT
Olmesartan medoxomil/hydrochlorothiazide (20/12.5, 40/12.5, 40/25)	Benicar HCT
Eprosartan mesylate/hydrochlorothiazide (600/12.5, 600/25)	Teveten/HCT
Irbesartan/hydrochlorothiazide (150/12.5, 300/12.5)	Avalide
Losartan potassium/hydrochlorothiazide (50/12.5, 100/25)	Hyzaar
Telmisartan/hydrochlorothiazide (40/12.5, 80/12.5)	Micardis/HCT
Valsartan/hydrochlorothiazide (80/12.5, 160/12.5)	**Diovan/HCT**
Azilsartan medoxomil/chlorthalidone (40/12.5, 40/25)	Edarbyclor
ARBs, CCBs, and diuretics	
Amlodipine/valsartan/hydrochlorothiazide (5/160/12.5, 5/160/25, 10/160/12.5, 10/160/25, 10/320/25)	Exforge HCT
Olmesartan/amlodipine/hydrochlorothiazide (20/5/12.5, 40/5/12.5, 40/5/25, 40/10/12.5, 40/10/25)	Tribenzor
β-blockers and diuretics	
Atenolol/chlorthalidone (50/25, 100/25)	Tenoretic
Bisoprolol fumarate/hydrochlorothiazide (2.5/6.25, 5/6.25, 10/6.25)	Ziac
Propranolol LA/hydrochlorothiazide (50/25, 80/25)	Inderide
Metoprolol tartrate/hydrochlorothiazide (50/25, 100/25)	Lopressor HCT
Nadolol/bendroflumethiazide (40/5, 80/5)	Corzide
Metoprolol succinate/hydrochlorothiazide (25/12.5, 50/12.5, 100/12.5)	Dutoprol
Centrally acting drugs and diuretics	
Methyldopa/hydrochlorothiazide (250/15, 250/25, 500/30, 500/50)	Aldoril

(continued)

Table 12-8. Combination Drugs for Hypertension *(Continued)*

Fixed-dose combination (mg)[a]	Trade name
RI and diuretic	
Aliskiren/hydrochlorothiazide (150/12.5, 150/25, 300/12.5, 300/25)	Tekturna HCT
RI and ARB	
Aliskiren/valsartan (150/160, 300/320)	Valturna
RI and CCB	
Aliskiren/amlodipine (150/5, 300/5, 150/10, 300/10)	Tekamlo
RI, CCB, and diuretic	
Aliskiren/amlodipine/hydrochlorothiazide (150/5/12.5, 300/5/12.5, 300/5/25, 300/10/12.5, 300/10/25)	Amturnide
Other combinations	
Amiloride HCl/hydrochlorothiazide (5/50)	Moduretic
Spironolactone/hydrochlorothiazide (25/25, 50/50)	Aldactazide
Triamterene/hydrochlorothiazide (37.5/25, 50/25, 75/50)	Dyazide, Maxzide

Adapted from JNC-7 Express, National Heart, Lung, and Blood Institute.
BB, β-blocker; RI, renin inhibitor.
a. Some drug combinations are available in multiple fixed doses. Each drug dose is reported in milligrams.

Mechanism of action
- Potassium-sparring diuretics interfere with potassium and sodium exchange in the distal tubule, decrease calcium excretion, and increase magnesium loss.

Patient instructions and counseling
- Take early in the day to avoid nocturia.
- Take after meals.
- Avoid excessive ingestion of foods high in potassium and use of salt substitutes.
- Medication may increase blood glucose in diabetics.
- Report problems with muscle cramps, which may indicate decreased potassium levels.
- Sexual dysfunction is possible.

Drug–drug and drug–disease interactions
- ACEIs may increase the risk of hyperkalemia.
- Indomethacin can cause a decrease in renal function when combined with triamterene.
- Cimetidine increases bioavailability and decreases clearance of triamterene.

Parameters to monitor
- Weight
- Serum electrolytes (especially potassium)
- BUN and creatinine

Adrenergic Inhibitors

Postganglionic adrenergic neuron blockers

This medication class is best avoided unless necessary to treat refractory hypertension that is unresponsive to all other agents, because the medications are poorly tolerated. See Table 12-9 for a list of postganglionic adrenergic neuron blockers, their usual dosage range, and adverse effects associated with these medications.

Mechanism of action
Postganglionic adrenergic neuron blockers cause presynaptic inhibition of the release of the neurotransmitter from peripheral neurons by agonistic activity on the α_2 receptor and depletion of the neurotransmitter through competitive uptake into the neurosecretory vesicles.

Patient instructions and counseling
- Report symptoms of dizziness or hypotension.
- Do not take over-the-counter (OTC) cold products without first asking the doctor or pharmacist.
- Rise slowly from a lying or sitting position.
- Report new fluid retention.
- Sexual dysfunction is possible.

Table 12-9. Postganglionic Adrenergic Neuron Blockers

Drug	Trade name	Usual dosage range, total mg/day (frequency per day)	Adverse events and comments
Guanadrel	Hylorel	10–75 (2)	Postural hypotension and diarrhea
Guanethidine monosulfate	Ismelin	10–150 (1)	Postural hypotension and diarrhea
Reserpine[a]	Serpasil	0.05–0.25 (1)	Nasal congestion, sedation, depression, activation of peptic ulcer, dizziness, lethargy, memory impairment, sleep disturbances, and weight gain

Adapted from JNC-7 Express, National Heart, Lung, and Blood Institute.
a. Reserpine also acts centrally.

Drug–drug and drug–disease interactions
- OTC sympathomimetics may potentiate an acute hypertensive effect.
- Tricyclic antidepressants and chlorpromazine antagonize the therapeutic effects of guanethidine.
- Pheochromocytoma is a contraindication to this class of medications.
- This medication class should be avoided in patients with CHF, angina, and cerebrovascular disease.

Parameters to monitor
- History of depression (reserpine)
- Sleep disturbances, drowsiness, and lethargy (reserpine)
- Symptoms of peptic ulcer (reserpine)

Centrally active α₂-agonists

See Table 12-10 for a list of centrally active α_2-agonists, their usual dosage range, and adverse effects associated with these medications.

Mechanism of action
These medications cause decreased sympathetic outflow to the cardiovascular system by agonistic activity on central α_2 receptors.

Table 12-10. Centrally Active α_2-Agonists

Drug	Trade name	Usual dosage range, total mg/day (frequency per day)	Adverse events and comments[a]
Clonidine HCl[b]	Catapres	0.1–0.8 (2)	Sedation, dry mouth, bradycardia, withdrawal hypertension, orthostatic hypotension, depression, impotence, and sleep disturbances
Guanabenz acetate	Wytensin	8–32 (2)	(More withdrawal)
Guanfacine HCl	Tenex	1–3 (1)	(Less withdrawal)
Methyldopa	Aldomet	250–1,000 (2)	(Hepatic and autoimmune disorders)

Adapted from JNC-7 Express, National Heart, Lung, and Blood Institute.
a. Adverse events, or side effects, listed are for the class of drugs, except where noted for individual drugs (in parentheses).
b. Clonidine HCl is also available as a once-weekly transdermal patch.

Patient instructions and counseling
- Report symptoms of dizziness or hypotension.
- Exercise sedation precautions.
- Fever and flu-like symptoms may represent hepatic dysfunction (methyldopa).
- Report new fluid retention.
- Sexual dysfunction is possible.

Drug–drug and drug–disease interactions
- Use cautiously with other sedating medications.
- Use cautiously in patients with angina, recent myocardial infarction (MI), cerebrovascular accident (CVA), and hepatic or renal disease (guanabenz and guanfacine).

Parameters to monitor
- CBC—positive Coombs test in 25% of those tested; less than 1% develop hemolytic anemia (methyldopa)
- Sleep disturbances, drowsiness, or dry mouth
- Symptoms of depression
- Impotence
- Pulse
- Rebound hypertension

Table 12-11. Peripherally Acting α_1-Adrenergic Blockers

Drug	Trade name	Usual dosage range, total mg/day (frequency per day)	Adverse events and comments
Doxazosin mesylate	Cardura	1–16 (1)	Postural hypotension, syncopal episode with first dose, diarrhea, weight gain, peripheral edema, dry mouth, urinary urgency, constipation, priapism, nausea, dizziness, headache, palpitations, and sweating; no effects on glucose or cholesterol
Prazosin HCl	Minipress	2–20 (2–3)	
Terazosin HCl	Hytrin	1–20 (1–2)	

Reprinted with permission from JNC-VII.

Peripherally acting α_1-adrenergic blockers

See Table 12-11 for a list of peripherally acting α_1-adrenergic blockers, their usual dosage range, and adverse effects associated with these medications.

Mechanism of action
- Peripheral α_1 postsynaptic receptors are blocked, which causes vasodilation of both arteries and veins (indirect vasodilators).
- These agents cause less reflex tachycardia than do direct vasodilators (hydralazine and minoxidil).

Patient instructions and counseling
- Take first dose of no more than 1 mg of any agent, and take at bedtime.
- Rise slowly from a lying or sitting position.
- Medication may cause dizziness.
- Priapism is possible.

Drug–drug and drug–disease interactions
- NSAIDs decrease antihypertensive effects of α_1-blockers.
- Increased antihypertensive effects occur with diuretics and β-blockers.

Parameters to monitor
- BP and pulse
- Peripheral edema

β-blockers

See Table 12-12 for a list of β-blockers, their usual dosage range, and adverse effects associated with these medications.

Mechanism of action
These medications competitively block response to β-adrenergic stimulation:

- Block secretion of renin
- Decrease cardiac contractility, thereby decreasing cardiac output
- Decrease central sympathetic output
- Decrease heart rate, thereby decreasing cardiac output

Patient instructions and counseling
- Report symptoms of dizziness or hypotension.
- Exercise sedation precautions (with lipid-soluble compounds).
- Abrupt withdrawal of the drug should be avoided.
- Sexual dysfunction is possible.

Drug–drug and drug–disease interactions
- Use with caution in patients with diabetes.
- Use with caution in patients with Raynaud's phenomenon or peripheral vascular disease.
- β-blockers may decrease the effectiveness of sulfonylureas.
- Nondihydropyridines may increase the effect and toxicity of β-blockers.

Parameters to monitor
- ECG
- Rebound hypertension
- Cholesterol levels
- Pulse (apical and radial)
- Glucose levels

Direct Vasodilators

This medication class (second-line agents) is best avoided unless necessary to treat refractory hypertension that is unresponsive to all other agents.

These agents should *not* be used alone secondary to increases in plasma renin activity, cardiac output, and heart rate and should therefore be used only when β-blockers and diuretics are part of the antihypertensive regimen.

Table 12-12. β-Blockers and Combination α- and β-Blockers

Drug	Trade name	Lipid solubility/ primary (secondary) routes of elimination	Usual dosage range, total mg/day (frequency per day)	Adverse events and comments[a]
β-blockers				
Acebutolol[b,c]	Sectral	Low/H (R)	200–800 (1)	Bronchospasm, bradycardia, and heart failure; may mask insulin-induced hypoglycemia; *less serious:* impaired peripheral circulation, insomnia, fatigue, decreased exercise tolerance, and hyper-triglyceridemia, except agents with intrinsic sympathomimetic activity
Atenolol[b]	Tenormin	Low/R (H)	25–100 (1)	
Betaxolol[b]	Kerlone	Low/H (R)	5–20 (1)	
Bisoprolol fumarate[b]	Zebeta	Low/R (H)	2.5–10 (1)	
Carteolol HCl[c]	Cartrol	Low/R	2.5–10 (1)	
Metoprolol tartrate[b]	Lopressor	Moderate/H (R)	50–100 (2)	
Metoprolol succinate[b]	Toprol-XL	Moderate/H (R)	50–100 (1)	
Nadolol	Corgard	Low/R	40–120 (1)	
Nebivolol[b]	Bystolic	High/H (R)	5–20 (1)	
Penbutolol sulfate[c]	Levatol	High/H (R)	10–20 (1)	
Pindolol[c]	Visken	Moderate/H (R)	10–60 (2)	
Propranolol HCl	Inderal	High/H	40–160 (2)	
Timolol maleate	Inderal LA	High/H	60–180 (1)	
	Blocadren	Low–moderate/H (R)	20–40 (2)	
Combined α- and β-blockers				
Carvedilol	Coreg	Moderate/bile into feces	12.5–50 (2)	Postural hypotension, bronchospasm
Carvedilol	Coreg CR	Moderate/bile into feces	10–80 (1)	Postural hypotension, bronchospasm
Labetalol	Normodyne, Trandate	Moderate/R (H)	200–800 (2)	

Adapted from JNC-VII.
H, hepatic; R, renal.
a. Adverse events, or side effects, listed are for the class of drugs.
b. Cardioselective.
c. Intrinsic sympathomimetic activity.

See Table 12-13 for a list of direct vasodilators, their usual dosage range, and adverse effects associated with these medications.

Mechanism of action

These agents cause direct relaxation of peripheral arterial smooth muscle and thereby significantly decrease peripheral resistance.

Patient instructions and counseling

- Report symptoms of dizziness or hypotension.
- Hirsutism is possible (minoxidil).
- Report any new symptoms of fatigue, malaise, low-grade fever, and joint aches.
- Report rapid weight gain (> 5 pounds), unusual swelling, and pulse increases of > 20 beats per minute above normal.
- Rise slowly from a lying or sitting position.

Table 12-13. Direct Vasodilators

Drug	Trade name	Usual dosage range, total mg/day (frequency per day)	Adverse events and comments[a]
			Headaches, fluid retention, tachycardia, peripheral neuropathy, and postural hypotension
Hydralazine HCl	Apresoline	25–100 (2)	(Lupus syndrome)
Minoxidil	Loniten	2.5–80 (1–2)	(Hirsutism)

Adapted from JNC-7 Express, National Heart, Lung, and Blood Institute.
a. Adverse events, or side effects, listed are for the class of drugs, except where noted for individual drugs (in parentheses).

Drug–drug and drug–disease interactions

- Use with caution in patients with pulmonary hypertension.
- Use with caution in patients with significant renal failure or CHF.
- Use with caution in patients with coronary artery disease or a recent MI.

Parameters to monitor

- Weight (fluid status)
- BP and pulse
- CBC with antinuclear antibody test (hydralazine)

Calcium Antagonists

Low-renin hypertensive, African American, and elderly patients respond well to this class of medications. See Table 12-14 for a list of calcium antagonists, their usual dosage range, and adverse effects associated with these medications.

Mechanism of action

- Calcium antagonists inhibit the influx of calcium ions through slow channels in vascular smooth muscle and cause relaxation of both coronary and peripheral arteries.

- These agents cause sinoatrial (SA) and atrioventricular (AV) nodal depression and a decrease in myocardial contractility (nondihydropyridines).

Patient instructions and counseling

- Report symptoms of dizziness or hypotension.
- Constipation is possible (verapamil).
- Report any new symptoms of shortness of breath, fatigue, or increased swelling of the extremities.
- Rise slowly from a lying or sitting position.

Drug–drug and drug–disease interactions

- Use with caution in patients on β-blockers (nondihydropyridines), which may increase CHF and bradycardia. This combination can also cause conduction abnormalities to the AV node.
- Use with extreme caution in patients with conduction disturbances in the SA or AV node.
- Grapefruit juice may increase the levels of some dihydropyridines.

Parameters to monitor

- ECG
- Peripheral edema

Table 12-14. Calcium Antagonists

Drug	Trade name	Usual dosage range, total mg/day (frequency per day)	Adverse events and comments[a]
Nondihydropyridines			
Diltiazem HCl	Cardizem SR, Cardizem CD, Dilacor XR, Tiazac	180–420 (1) 120–360 (1)	Conduction defects, worsening of systolic dysfunction, and gingival hyperplasia
Verapamil immediate-release	Calan, Isoptin	80–320 (2)	(Nausea and headache)
Verapamil long-acting	Calan SR, Isoptin SR	120–360 (1–2)	(Constipation)
Verapamil COER	Covera HS, Verelan PM	120–360 (1)	
Dihydropyridines			
Amlodipine besylate	Norvasc	2.5–10 (1)	Edema of the ankle, flushing, headache, and gingival hyperplasia
Felodipine	Plendil	2.5–20 (1)	
Isradipine	DynaCirc	2.5–10 (2)	
	DynaCirc CR	5–20 (1)	
Nicardipine	Cardene SR	60–120 (1)	
Nifedipine	Procardia XL, Adalat CC	30–60 (1)	
Nisoldipine	Sular	10–40 (1)	

Adapted from JNC-7 Express, National Heart, Lung, and Blood Institute.

a. Adverse events, or side effects, listed are for the class of drugs, except where noted for individual drugs (in parentheses).

- BP and pulse
- Bowel habits
- Symptoms of conduction disturbances

Angiotensin-Converting Enzyme Inhibitors and Angiotensin II Receptor Blockers

Ethnic differences exist in the response to these classes of medications. These agents are relatively ineffective as monotherapy in African American patients. However, the addition of diuretic therapy has been shown to sensitize African American patients to these agents to obtain similar responses as in non–African American patients.

See Table 12-15 for a list of ACEIs and ARBs, their usual dosage range, and adverse effects associated with these medications.

Mechanism of action

ACEIs

- ACEIs inhibit the conversion of angiotensin I to angiotensin II (a potent vasoconstrictor; see Figure 12-1).
- These agents indirectly inhibit fluid volume increases by inhibiting angiotensin II–stimulated release of aldosterone.

ARBs

- ARBs inhibit the binding of angiotensin II to the angiotensin II receptor, thereby inhibiting the vasoconstrictive properties of angiotensin II as well as its ability to stimulate the release of aldosterone.
- These agents are currently considered as alternative therapy in patients not able to tolerate ACEIs because of cough.

Table 12-15. Angiotensin-Converting Enzyme Inhibitors and Angiotensin II Receptor Blockers

Drug	Trade name	Usual dose range, total mg/day (frequency per day)	Adverse events and comments
ACEIs			
Benazepril HCl	Lotensin	10–40 (1–2)	**Common:** cough
Captopril	Capoten	25–100 (2–3)	**Rare:** angioedema, hyperkalemia, rash, loss of taste, and leucopenia
Enalapril maleate	Vasotec	2.5–40 (1–2)	**Other:** vertigo, headache, fatigue, first-dose hypotension, minor GI disturbances, acute renal insufficiency in patients with predisposing factors such as renal stenosis and coadministration with thiazide diuretics, and proteinuria (especially in patients with history of renal disease)
Fosinopril sodium	Monopril	10–40 (1–2)	
Lisinopril	Prinivil, Zestril	10–40 (1)	
Moexipril	Univasc	7.5–30 (1)	
Perindopril	Aceon	4–8 (1–2)	
Quinapril HCl	Accupril	10–40 (1–2)	
Ramipril	Altace	1.25–20 (1)	
Trandolapril	Mavik	1–4 (1)	
ARBs			
Azilsartan	Edarbi	40–80 (1)	Angioedema and hyperkalemia
Candesartan	Atacand	8–32 (1)	
Eprosartan	Teveten	400–800 (1–2)	
Irbesartan	Avapro	150–300 (1)	
Losartan	Cozaar	25–100 (1–2)	
Olmesartan	**Benicar**	20 (1)	
Telmisartan	Micardis	40–80 (1)	
Valsartan	**Diovan**	80–320 (1)	

Adapted from JNC-VII.
Boldface indicates one of top 100 drugs for 2012 by units sold at retail outlets, www.drugs.com/stats/top100/2012/units.
GI, gastrointestinal.

Patient instructions and counseling

- Report symptoms of dizziness or hypotension.
- Symptoms of swelling of the lips, mouth, or face should be considered an emergency. Report immediately to a doctor's office or an emergency department.
- Report new rashes (especially with captopril).
- Do not use salt substitutes containing potassium, and do not take OTC potassium supplements.
- Rise slowly from a lying or sitting position.

Drug–drug and drug–disease interactions

- NSAIDs will decrease the effectiveness of ACEIs and ARBs.
- Potassium-sparing diuretics, potassium supplements, and salt substitutes will increase the risk of hyperkalemia when used in combination with ACEIs and ARBs.
- ACEIs and ARBs should be avoided in patients with bilateral renal artery stenosis or stenosis in a single kidney.
- ACEIs and ARBs should be avoided in pregnant patients.

Parameters to monitor

- Serum electrolytes (especially creatinine and potassium)
- Symptoms of angioedema
- BP
- Symptoms of hypotension
- CBC (especially with captopril and enalapril) for neutropenia, which is more common in patients with preexisting renal impairment
- Cough
- Urinary proteins

Direct Renin Inhibitors

See Table 12-16 for a list of direct renin inhibitors, their usual dosage range, and adverse effects associated with these medications.

Mechanism of action

Direct renin inhibitors competitively inhibit human renin, which decreases plasma renin activity and

Table 12-16. Direct Renin Inhibitors

Drug	Trade name	Usual dose range, total mg/day (frequency per day)	Adverse events and comments
Aliskiren	Tekturna	150–300 mg (1)	**Common:** diarrhea **Rare:** elevated uric acid, gout, renal stone, angioedema, and rash **Other:** headache, nasopharyngitis, dizziness, fatigue, upper respiratory tract infection, back pain, and cough

Tekturna [package insert]. East Hanover, NJ: Novartis Pharmaceuticals; revised March 2012.

inhibits the conversion of angiotensinogen to angiotensin I.

Patient instructions and counseling

- Medicine can be taken with or without food.
- Establish a routine pattern for taking aliskiren with regard to meals. High-fat meals decrease absorption significantly.
- Store the medicine in a closed container at room temperature, away from heat, moisture, and direct light.
- Report symptoms of dizziness or hypotension.
- Diarrhea is possible.
- Symptoms of swelling of the lips, mouth, or face should be considered an emergency. Report immediately to a doctor's office or an emergency department.

Drug–drug and drug–disease interactions

- Concomitant use of aliskiren with cyclosporine is not recommended.
- Potassium-sparing diuretics, potassium supplements, and salt substitutes will increase the risk of hyperkalemia when used in combination with aliskiren.

- Blood concentrations of furosemide are significantly reduced when given with aliskiren.
- Ketoconazole significantly increases aliskiren plasma levels.
- Aliskiren should be avoided in pregnant patients.
- According to recent trial data, the combination of ACEI or ARB with aliskiren should be avoided.

Parameters to monitor

- Symptoms of angioedema
- BP
- Symptoms of hypotension
- Serum electrolytes (especially creatinine and potassium)

12-6. Hypertensive Urgencies and Emergencies

The classification of hypertensive urgencies and emergencies is determined by the presence or absence of acute target organ damage, not by BP, and determines the appropriate treatment approach.

The relative rise and rate of increase in BP is more important than the actual BP.

Hypertensive Emergencies

Acute elevations of BP (> 180 mm Hg systolic or > 120 mm Hg diastolic) with the presence of acute or ongoing target organ damage constitute a hypertensive emergency (Box 12-4). This situation requires immediate lowering of BP to prevent or minimize target organ damage.

Table 12-17 shows details of parenteral drugs used for treatment of hypertensive emergencies. Such emergencies should be treated as follows:

- As an initial goal, reduce mean arterial pressure (MAP) by no more than 25% within minutes to hours. Reach BP of 160/100 mm Hg within 2–6 hours.
- Measure BP every 5–10 minutes until goal MAP is reached and life-threatening target organ damage resolves.
- Maintain goal BP for 1–2 days, and further reduce BP toward normal over several weeks.
- Excessive falls in BP may precipitate renal, cerebral, or coronary ischemia.

Box 12-4. Clinical Findings of Target Organ Damage

Target Organ Damage

Hypertensive encephalopathy
Intracranial hemorrhage
Unstable angina
Acute myocardial infarction
Acute left ventricular failure with pulmonary edema
Dissecting aortic aneurysm
Eclampsia

Clinical Findings

Funduscopic: papilledema, hemorrhage, exudates
Neurologic: somnolence, confusion, seizures, coma, visual deficits or blindness
Cardiac: S4 gallop, ischemic changes on ECG, chest x-ray consistent with pulmonary edema, chest pain
Renal: oliguria, progressive azotemia, hematuria, proteinuria
Other: dyspnea

Reprinted with permission from JNC-VII.

- Intravenous agents are preferred because of the ability to titrate dosages on the basis of BP response; however, specific agents should be chosen on the basis of patient findings (Table 12-18).

Hypertensive Urgencies

Hypertensive urgencies are accelerated, malignant, or perioperative elevations in BP in the absence of new or progressive target organ damage; therefore, immediate lowering of BP is not required.

Table 12-19 shows the agents used to treat hypertensive urgencies. Such situations require the following considerations:

- There is no agent of choice; medications should be selected on the basis of patient characteristics.
- Oral therapy is preferred.
- Onset of action should occur in 15–30 minutes, and peak effects should be seen in 2–3 hours.
- Check BP every 15–30 minutes to ensure response.
- Use of immediate-release nifedipine is inappropriate to lower BP in patients with hypertensive urgencies.

Table 12-17. Parenteral Drugs for Treatment of Hypertensive Emergencies

Drug	Dose	Onset of action	Duration of action	Adverse effects[a]	Special indications
Vasodilators					
Sodium nitroprusside	0.25–10 mcg/kg/min IV infusion[b] (maximal dose for 10 min only)	Immediate	1–2 min	Nausea, vomiting, muscle twitching, sweating, and thiocyanate and cyanide intoxication	Most hypertensive emergencies; caution with high intracranial pressure or azotemia
Nicardipine hydrochloride	5–15 mg/h IV	5–10 min	1–4 h	Tachycardia, headache, flushing, and local phlebitis	Most hypertensive emergencies, except acute heart failure; caution with coronary ischemia
Fenoldopam mesylate	0.1–0.3 mcg/kg/min IV infusion	< 5 min	30 min	Tachycardia, headache, nausea, and flushing	
Nitroglycerin	5–100 mcg/min IV infusion[b]	2–5 min	3–5 min	Headache, vomiting, methemoglobinemia, and tolerance with prolonged use	Coronary ischemia
Enalaprilat	1.25–5 mg every 6 h IV	15–30 min	6 h	Precipitous fall in pressure in high-renin states; response variable	Acute left ventricular failure; avoid in acute myocardial infarction
Hydralazine hydrochloride	10–20 mg IV; 10–50 mg IM	10–20 min; 20–30 min	3–8 h	Tachycardia, flushing, headache, vomiting, and aggravation of angina	Eclampsia
Diazoxide	50–100 mg IV bolus repeated, or 15–30 mg/min IV infusion	2–4 min	6–12 h	Nausea, flushing, tachycardia, and chest pain	Now obsolete; when no intensive monitoring available
Adrenergic inhibitors					
Labetalol hydrochloride	20–80 mg IV bolus every 10 min; 0.5–2 mg/min IV infusion	5–10 min	3–6 h	Vomiting, scalp tingling, burning in throat, dizziness, nausea, heart block, and orthostatic hypotension	Most hypertensive emergencies, except acute heart failure
Esmolol hydrochloride	250–500 mcg/kg/min for 1 min, then 50–100 mcg/kg/min for 4 min; may repeat sequence	1–2 min	10–20 min	Hypotension and nausea	Aortic dissection, perioperative
Phentolamine	5–15 mg IV	1–2 min	3–10 min	Tachycardia, flushing, and headache	Catecholamine excess

Reprinted with permission from JNC-VII.
IM, intramuscular; IV, intravenous.
a. Hypotension may occur with all agents.
b. Requires special delivery system.

Table 12-18. Selected Agents for Specific Hypertensive Emergencies

Emergency	Recommended therapy	Comments
Encephalopathy	Labetalol, nicardipine, and nitroprusside	Avoid methyldopa (sedation), diazoxide (reduces cerebral blood flow), reserpine (sedation), and hydralazine (increases intracranial pressure).
Myocardial infarction (MI) or unstable angina	Nitroglycerin and esmolol	Reduce BP until pain is relieved, and use in conjunction with conventional therapy for MI/angina.
Congestive heart failure	Nitroprusside, nitroglycerin, and enalaprilat	Avoid diazoxide and hydralazine (increase oxygen demand), dihydropyridines (may worsen angina), and nitroprusside (coronary steal). Avoid labetalol, esmolol, and other β-blockers (reduce cardiac output).
Subarachnoid hemorrhage, intracerebral hemorrhage, and stroke	Nitroprusside	BP reduction is controversial because it may cause hypoperfusion; generally recommended for severe hypertension (systolic blood pressure > 220 mm Hg or diastolic blood pressure > 120 mm Hg).
Dissecting aortic aneurysm	Trimethaphan, esmolol, and nitroprusside	Avoid diazoxide and hydralazine (increase shear force).
Pheochromocytoma and cocaine overdose	Phentolamine and labetalol	Anecdotal reports suggest increased BP with labetalol; unopposed β blockade may worsen crisis.
Renal insufficiency	Nitroprusside, calcium channel blocker, and labetalol	Monitor cyanide and thiocyanate levels.
Postoperative hypertension	Nitroprusside, nicardipine, and labetalol	Blood pressure levels of > 180/110 mm Hg should be controlled before surgery. Contributing factors to postoperative hypertension may include pain and increased intravascular volume, which may require parenteral loop diuretics.

Table 12-19. Agents Used to Treat Hypertensive Urgencies

Drug	Dose	Onset	Duration	Adverse effects
Captopril	25 mg, repeat in 1–2 hours as needed	5–15 min	4–6 h	Hypotension, acute renal failure, and angioedema
Clonidine	0.1–0.2 mg, repeat in 1–2 hours as needed (up to 0.6 mg)	5–15 min	6–12 h	Hypotension, drowsiness, sedation, and dry mouth
Labetalol	100–400 mg, repeat in 2–3 hours as needed	15–30 min	4–6 h	Hypotension, heart block, and bronchoconstriction

12-7. Questions

1. According to the JNC-VIII, which of the following agents are suitable as initial therapy for the treatment of uncomplicated hypertension?

   A. Hydrochlorothiazide, chlorthalidone, amlodipine
   B. Chlorthalidone, atenolol, amlodipine
   C. Amlodipine, hydrochlorothiazide, atenolol
   D. Hydralazine, chlorthalidone, atenolol
   E. Atenolol, amlodipine, chlorthalidone

2. Hyperkalemia is a possible adverse effect of which of the following medications?

   A. Trandolapril, captopril, felodipine
   B. Felodipine, trandolapril, doxazosin
   C. Doxazosin, captopril, amiloride
   D. Amiloride, trandolapril, captopril
   E. Captopril, felodipine, doxazosin

3. A 48-year-old patient presents with a new diagnosis of chronic kidney disease. Which agent would be an appropriate choice as initial therapy in this patient based on JNC-VIII?

    A. Clonidine
    B. Guanethidine
    C. Diltiazem
    D. Perindopril
    E. Nisoldipine

4. A 62-year-old patient with a history of hypertension and gout presents to begin pharmacotherapy for hypertension. Which agent is the most appropriate choice as initial therapy based on JNC-VIII?

    A. Chlorothiazide
    B. Torsemide
    C. Tenormin
    D. Chlorthalidone
    E. Losartan

5. All of the following medications can cause bradycardia *except*

    A. terazosin.
    B. verapamil.
    C. diltiazem.
    D. Ziac.
    E. clonidine.

6. A patient requires a cardioselective β-blocker in his or her outpatient medication regimen after recent discharge from the hospital with a new myocardial infarction. You suggest he or she take

    A. labetalol.
    B. esmolol.
    C. propranolol.
    D. atenolol.
    E. carvedilol.

Use the following case study to answer Questions 7–9:

A patient presents to your ambulatory clinic with a blood pressure of 210/125 mm Hg. Past medical history is significant for type 2 diabetes, congestive heart failure, and renal insufficiency.

7. Which of the following would cause the patient to be classified as a hypertensive emergency?

    A. Blood glucose levels > 300 mg/dL, which increase the patient's risk for acute renal failure

    B. Serum creatinine of 3 mg/dL
    C. Nausea, vomiting, and diarrhea for 3 days
    D. S₄ gallop and a chest x-ray consistent with pulmonary edema
    E. Polyuria combined with polydipsia

8. What are the treatment goals for the patient with hypertensive emergency?

    A. Systolic pressure should be reduced to 120 mm Hg within the first hour of treatment to reduce the risk of further end organ damage.
    B. Diastolic pressure should be reduced to 80 mm Hg within the first hour of treatment to reduce the risk of further end organ damage.
    C. Blood pressure should be reduced to 160/100 mm Hg in the first 2–6 hours of therapy.
    D. Mean arterial pressure should be reduced by at least 50% within the first minutes to hours of therapy.
    E. Blood pressure should be reduced to no lower than 180/110 mm Hg in the first hour, because excessive falls in blood pressure may precipitate coronary ischemia.

9. What would be the recommended treatment for the patient with hypertensive emergency?

    A. Clonidine orally, 0.1–0.2 mg; repeat in 1–2 hours as needed (up to 0.6 mg)
    B. Labetalol orally, 100–400 mg; repeat in 2–3 hours as needed
    C. Nifedipine sublingually, 10 mg; repeat in 0.5–1 hour as needed (up to 60 mg)
    D. Labetalol intravenously, 20–80 mg bolus, followed by 0.5–2 mg/min infusion
    E. Enalaprilat intravenously, 1.25–5 mg every 6 hours

10. Which of the following antihypertensive agents can cause first-dose syncope, palpitations, peripheral edema, and priapism?

    A. Hydralazine
    B. Nitroprusside
    C. Prazosin
    D. Verapamil
    E. Moexipril

11. Which of the following antihypertensive agents is most likely to cause lupus syndrome, postural hypotension, and peripheral neuropathy?

   A. Atenolol
   B. Hydralazine
   C. Guanfacine
   D. Mibefradil
   E. Nitroprusside

12. Which of the following medications is *not* associated with drug-induced hypertension?

   A. Prednisone
   B. Indomethacin
   C. Rosiglitazone
   D. Cocaine
   E. Cyclosporine

13. What is the best recommendation for anti-hypertensive medication in a patient who has atrial fibrillation, coronary artery disease with angina, and hyperthyroidism?

   A. Minoxidil
   B. Betaxolol

   C. Telmisartan
   D. Nicardipine
   E. Amiloride

14. What antihypertensive agent should *not* be used in a patient with essential hypertension and a history of depression with suicidal ideation?

   A. Captopril
   B. Prazosin
   C. Metolazone
   D. Reserpine
   E. Amlodipine

15. All of the following are secondary causes of hypertension *except*

   A. renovascular disease.
   B. pheochromocytoma.
   C. systemic lupus erythematosus.
   D. primary aldosteronism.
   E. aortic coarctation.

Use Patient Profile 12-1 to answer Questions 16–20.

Patient Profile 12-1
Date: 4/20/14

Patient: male, age 70 years

Height: 5'11″

Race: African American

Known diseases: DM (15 years), HTN (20 years), obstructive sleep apnea (5 years), osteoarthritis

OTC use: Aleve, Actron

Date of birth: 4/14/44

Weight: 248 lb

Allergies: NKDA

Pharmacist notes and other patient information: + tobacco—1.5 ppd, 4–5 cups of coffee/day, ETOH—2 drinks/week

Date	Rx No.	Drug and Strength	Route	Quantity	Regimen	Refills	Pharmacist	Prescriber
1/15/09	001	Glipizide 5 mg	po	30	1 daily	5	BCE	NTE
1/15/09	002	Lisinopril 5 mg	po	30	1 daily	5	BCE	NTE
1/15/09	003	Hydrodiuril 12.5 mg	po	30	1 daily	5	BBC	NPR
1/20/09	004	Ibuprofen 800 mg	po	90	1 tid	5	REM	FTD
2/11/09	001-RF	Glipizide 5 mg	po	30	1 daily	4	BCE	NTE
2/11/09	003-RF	Hydrodiuril 12.5 mg	po	30	1 daily	4	BBC	NPR
2/11/09	004-RF	Ibuprofen 800 mg	po	90	1 tid	4	REM	FTD
3/13/09	001-RF	Glipizide 5 mg	po	30	1 daily	3	BCE	NTE
3/13/09	002-RF	Lisinopril 5 mg	po	30	1 daily	4	BCE	NTE
3/13/09	004-RF	Ibuprofen 800 mg	po	90	1 tid	3	REM	FTD

16. Possible complications that the patient is at risk of developing secondary to uncontrolled hypertension include which of the following?

    A. Hyperaldosteronism, urinary tract infection
    B. Myocardial infarction, blindness
    C. Blindness, hyperaldosteronism
    D. Urinary tract infection, blindness
    E. Chronic obstructive pulmonary disease, pneumonia

17. Education regarding lifestyle modification issues in this patient should include all of the following *except*

    A. limit alcohol intake to no more than two drinks per day.
    B. reduce daily intake of dietary magnesium, calcium, and sodium.
    C. increase aerobic physical activity, decrease weight, and limit dietary saturated fat and cholesterol.
    D. consume a diet consistent with the DASH diet.
    E. stop smoking.

18. Possible reasons for the patient's blood pressure being uncontrolled include which of the following?

    A. Use of NSAIDs, which cause decreased effectiveness of ACEI therapy, and drug interaction between glipizide and lisinopril
    B. Use of NSAIDs, which cause decreased effectiveness of ACEI therapy, and possible problems with adherence to antihypertensive therapy
    C. Lack of blood pressure response to ACEI therapy, which should not be used in combination with diuretics in an African American patient, and possible problems with adherence to antihypertensive therapy
    D. Lack of blood pressure response to ACEI therapy, which should not be used in combination with diuretics in an African American patient, and drug interaction between glipizide and lisinopril
    E. Patients with osteoarthritis tend to have hypertension that is difficult to control.

19. The appropriate initial antihypertensive agent in this patient could be

    A. benazepril.
    B. terazosin.
    C. minoxidil.
    D. metoprolol.
    E. clonidine.

20. If the patient is not able to tolerate lisinopril because of adverse effects such as cough, an appropriate alternative agent would be

    A. telmisartan.
    B. labetalol.
    C. guanabenz.
    D. reserpine.
    E. prazosin.

12-8. Answers

1. **A.** Appropriate choices for initial agents in the treatment of uncomplicated hypertension include diuretics, ACEIs, ARBs, and CCBs. Hydralazine is a direct vasodilator, which would never be considered a first-line agent in the treatment of hypertension. Atenolol is a beta blocker and is no longer considered first-line therapy according to JNC-VIII guidelines.

2. **D.** Hyperkalemia is a possible side effect with ACEIs, angiotensin II receptor antagonists, and potassium-sparing diuretics. Doxazosin is a peripherally acting α_1-blocker, which does not cause hyperkalemia. Felodipine is a calcium channel antagonist and is not linked to causing hyperkalemia.

3. **D.** For patients who have hypertension and chronic kidney disease, JNC-VIII recommends the use of ACEIs, diuretics, ARBs, and CCBs. The only listed ACEI is perindopril.

4. **E.** For patients who have hypertension and gout, JNC-VIII would recommend not using diuretic therapy, which increases the risk of gouty attacks. The only medication listed that is not a diuretic is atenolol (Tenormin), which is a β-blocker, and losartan, which is an angiotensin II receptor blocker. β-blockers are not considered first line, so the appropriate choice would be losartan.

5. **A.** Verapamil and diltiazem are nondihydropyridine calcium channel blockers, Ziac (bisoprolol and hydrochlorothiazide) is a β-blocker, and clonidine is a centrally acting α_2-agonist. They all have negative inotropic effects on the myocardium. Terazosin is a peripherally acting α_1-blocker, which does not cause bradycardia.

6. **D.** Labetalol, propranolol, and carvedilol are all nonselective β-blockers. Esmolol is a cardioselective agent available only in injectable form and, therefore, would not be for outpatient use. Atenolol is a cardioselective β-blocker that is available as an oral tablet and, therefore, can be used for outpatient dosing.

7. **D.** The classification of hypertensive urgencies and emergencies is determined by the presence or absence of acute target organ damage and not by the actual blood pressure measurement. Presence of an S_4 gallop and a chest x-ray consistent with pulmonary edema suggest acute left ventricular failure with pulmonary edema, which represents defined target organ damage and, in turn, means the patient should be classified as a hypertensive emergency.

8. **C.** According to JNC-VII, the initial goal of blood pressure lowering in patients with hypertensive emergencies is a drop in mean arterial pressure of no more than 25% within minutes to hours and to 160/100 mm Hg within 2–6 hours.

9. **E.** In a patient with CHF and hypertensive emergency, recommended treatments include nitroglycerin, nitroprusside, and enalaprilat (Table 12-17). Clonidine and labetalol (po) are incorrect choices because the patient requires IV therapy. Nifedipine SL is not indicated for immediate reduction of blood pressure. Labetalol IV is not an appropriate choice in this patient with CHF because it could decrease cardiac output.

10. **C.** Possible side effects of peripherally acting α_1-blockers (prazosin) include first-dose syncope, palpitations, peripheral edema, and priapism (Table 12-11).

11. **B.** Possible side effects of direct vasodilators (hydralazine) include postural hypotension and peripheral neuropathy. However, lupus syndrome is unique to hydralazine and does not occur with minoxidil (Table 12-13).

12. **C.** All agents listed are possible causes of drug-induced hypertension through multiple mechanisms except rosiglitazone (Box 12-3).

13. **B.** The diagnoses of atrial fibrillation, coronary artery disease with angina, and hyperthyroidism are all considered comorbid conditions with hypertension in which the use of β-blockers may have favorable effects.

14. **D.** Because of its possible increased risk of depression, reserpine should not be used for patients for whom the risk for depression or suicide already exists.

15. **C.** All listed diseases are possible causes of secondary hypertension through various mechanisms, except systemic lupus erythematosus.

16. **B.** Uncontrolled hypertension causes multiple organ system problems, including cardiovascular (CHF, MI, and peripheral arterial disease); ophthalmologic (retinopathy and blindness); cerebrovascular (transient ischemic attack and CVA); and renovascular (nephropathy, renal failure, and dialysis) issues. Therefore, this patient is at risk for MI and blindness, not for hyperaldosteronism or urinary tract infections.

17. **B.** Lifestyle modification issues to be considered in hypertensive patients include weight loss; limit of alcohol intake; increased aerobic activity; reduced sodium intake; maintenance of adequate dietary potassium, calcium, and magnesium intake; and smoking cessation.

18. **B.** Possible causes for inadequate responsiveness to therapy are listed in Box 12-3.

19. **A.** In patients with hypertension and comorbid conditions of CHF and diabetes, the initial agent should be an ACEI.

20. **A.** In patients who cannot tolerate ACEI therapy secondary to the adverse effect of cough, angiotensin II receptor antagonists are considered good alternative agents.

12-9. References

JNC-VIII (The Eighth Report of the Joint National Committee on Prevention, Detection, Evaluation and Treatment of High Blood Pressure). *JAMA.* 2013;311:507–20.

JNC-7 Express (Joint National Committee on Prevention, Detection, Evaluation, and Treatment of High Blood Pressure [JNC-7] Express). May 2003. NIH: National Heart, Lung, and Blood Institute Web site. NIH Publication 03-5233. http://www.nhlbi.nih.gov/guidelines/hypertension/jncintro.htm.

Saseen JL, Maclaughlin EJ. Hypertension. In: DiPiro JT, Talbert RL, Yee GC, et al., eds. *Pharmacotherapy: A Pathophysiologic Approach.* 8th ed. New York, NY: McGraw-Hill; 2011:101–22.

Tekturna [package insert]. East Hanover, NJ: Novartis Pharmaceuticals; revised March 2012.

Heart Failure

Robert B. Parker

13-1. Key Points

■ Heart failure is a clinical syndrome caused by the heart's inability to pump sufficient blood to meet the body's needs.

■ Although heart failure has many causes, the most common are coronary artery disease and hypertension.

■ Several compensatory mechanisms are activated to help maintain adequate cardiac output; activation of those systems is responsible for heart failure symptoms and contributes to disease progression. Medications that improve patient outcomes antagonize those compensatory mechanisms.

■ Drugs that can precipitate or worsen heart failure should be avoided (e.g., NSAIDs, verapamil, and diltiazem).

■ All patients with stage C (symptomatic) heart failure with reduced ejection fraction (HFrEF) should be treated with angiotensin-converting enzyme inhibitors (ACEIs) or angiotensin II receptor blockers (ARBs) and β-blockers.

■ The goal of treatment with diuretics is to eliminate signs of fluid retention, thus minimizing symptoms.

■ ACEIs are an integral part of heart failure pharmacotherapy. They improve survival and slow disease progression. ARBs are the preferred alternative for patients who are intolerant to ACEIs.

■ β-blockers are recommended for all patients with systolic dysfunction and mild to moderate symptoms. β-blockers improve survival, decrease hospitalizations, and slow disease progression. Bisoprolol, carvedilol, and extended-release metoprolol succinate are agents with proven benefits. They should be started at low doses with slow upward titration to the target dose.

■ Digoxin does not improve survival in patients with heart failure but does provide symptomatic benefits. The goal plasma concentration is 0.5–1 ng/mL.

■ Spironolactone and eplerenone improve survival in patients with HFrEF when added to standard therapies such as ACEIs or ARBs and β-blockers.

■ Patients with acute decompensated heart failure (ADHF) often require hospitalization and aggressive therapy with intravenous (IV) diuretics, vasodilators, and positive inotropic drugs.

13-2. Study Guide Checklist

The following topics may guide your study of this subject area:

■ Risk factors for developing heart failure, including drugs that can precipitate or worsen the disorder

■ Clinical presentation of heart failure

■ Drugs that improve survival affect the pathophysiology of heart failure

■ Selection of appropriate pharmacotherapy based on treatment guidelines and patient characteristics

■ Mechanisms of action of classes of drugs used to treat heart failure

■ Major adverse drug reactions to drugs used to treat heart failure

■ Significant drug interactions involving medications used to treat heart failure

■ Trade names and generic names of medications used to treat heart failure

■ Patient counseling points for drugs used to treat heart failure

13-3. Overview

Heart failure is a clinical syndrome resulting from any disorder that impairs the ventricle's ability to fill with or eject blood, which leads to the heart being unable to pump blood at a sufficient rate to meet the metabolic demands of the body. Heart failure can result from abnormalities in systolic as well as diastolic dysfunction. Both abnormalities are present in many patients. Patients with heart failure symptoms and left ventricular ejection fraction (LVEF) ≤ 40% are classified as having heart failure with reduced ejection fraction (HFrEF), whereas those with LVEF ≥ 50% have heart failure with preserved ejection fraction (HFpEF). Approximately 50% of patients with heart failure have HFpEF. Most clinical trials evaluating drug therapy have focused on the population with HFrEF.

■ Over 5 million people in the United States have heart failure; approximately 825,000 new cases are diagnosed each year.

■ Approximately 300,000 patients die from heart failure each year. At the time of heart failure diagnosis, the 5-year mortality rate is approximately 50%.

■ A majority of patients with heart failure are elderly.

■ Each year, there are more than 1 million hospital discharges for heart failure, and it is the most common hospital discharge diagnosis for Medicare patients. More Medicare dollars are spent for diagnosis and treatment of heart failure than for any other disorder.

■ Current estimates indicate that annual expenditures for heart failure exceed $37 billion.

Classification

The New York Heart Association (NYHA) Functional Classification for heart failure has been widely used for many years. The classification scheme primarily reflects the severity of heart failure symptoms based on a subjective assessment by the provider. A patient's functional class can change frequently over a short period because of changes in medications, diet, or intercurrent illnesses. The classification scheme, as follows, does not recognize preventive measures nor does it recognize the progressive nature of heart failure:

■ *Functional class I* includes patients with cardiac disease but without limitations of physical activity. Ordinary physical activity does not cause undue fatigue, dyspnea, or palpitations.

■ *Functional class II* includes patients with cardiac disease that results in slight limitations of physical activity. Ordinary physical activity results in fatigue, palpitations, dyspnea, or angina.

■ *Functional class III* includes patients with cardiac disease that results in marked limitation of physical activity. Although patients are comfortable at rest, less than ordinary activity will lead to symptoms.

■ *Functional class IV* includes patients with cardiac disease that results in an inability to carry on physical activity without discomfort. Symptoms of heart failure are present even at rest. With any physical activity, increased discomfort is experienced.

The guidelines for evaluation and management of heart failure from the American College of Cardiology (ACC) and the American Heart Association (AHA) recommend an additional classification scheme that emphasizes both the evolution and the progression of the disease. This scheme more objectively identifies patients within the course of the disease and links to treatments that are appropriate for each stage. Patients in stages A and B do not have heart failure but do have risk factors that predispose them to the development of heart failure:

■ *Stage A* includes patients at high risk of developing heart failure because of the presence of conditions that are strongly associated with heart failure. Patients in stage A have no known cardiac abnormalities and no heart failure signs or symptoms. Examples include patients with hypertension, coronary artery disease, diabetes, obesity, or metabolic syndrome.

■ *Stage B* includes patients who have structural heart disease strongly associated with the development of heart failure but who have never shown signs or symptoms of heart failure. Examples include patients with previous myocardial infarction, left ventricular hypertrophy, or impaired left ventricular systolic function.

■ *Stage C* includes patients who have current or prior symptoms of heart failure associated with underlying structural heart disease. Patients in stage C can have either HFrEF or HFpEF. Most patients with heart failure are in stage C.

- *Stage D* includes patients with advanced structural heart disease, patients with marked symptoms of heart failure at rest despite maximal medical therapy, and patients who require specialized interventions. Patients in stage D include those who frequently are hospitalized for heart failure and cannot be discharged from the hospital safely, those who are in the hospital awaiting heart transplantation, and those who are supported with a mechanical circulatory assist device.

Acute Decompensated Heart Failure

Both the growing number of patients with heart failure and the progressive nature of the syndrome have led to substantial increases in hospitalizations for heart failure. *Acute decompensated heart failure* (ADHF) is defined as new or worsening signs or symptoms that are usually caused by (1) volume overload (pulmonary congestion, systemic congestion, or both); (2) hypoperfusion (hypotension, renal insufficiency, shock syndrome, or some combination); or (3) both volume overload and hypoperfusion. ADHF frequently requires hospitalization for acute treatment.

Causes of ADHF include medication and dietary noncompliance, atrial fibrillation or other arrhythmias, myocardial ischemia, uncontrolled high blood pressure, pulmonary embolus, concurrent illnesses (e.g., pneumonia), recent addition of negative inotropic drugs, nonsteroidal anti-inflammatory drugs (NSAIDs), excessive alcohol or illicit drug use, and progression of heart failure.

To determine the proper approach to therapy, patients are often assigned to one of four hemodynamic profiles:

- *Warm and dry:* Adequate perfusion (i.e., cardiac output) and no signs or symptoms of volume overload
- *Warm and wet:* Adequate perfusion but signs or symptoms of volume overload
- *Cold and dry:* Inadequate perfusion and no signs or symptoms of volume overload
- *Cold and wet:* Inadequate perfusion and signs or symptoms of volume overload

Most patients (about 70%) are assigned to the warm and wet classification.

Clinical Presentation

The primary manifestations of heart failure are (1) dyspnea and fatigue that may limit exercise tolerance and (2) fluid retention that may lead to pulmonary and peripheral edema. Both abnormalities can limit a patient's functional capacity and quality of life, but they do not necessarily occur at the same time. Some patients may have marked exercise intolerance but little evidence of fluid retention, whereas others may have prominent edema with few dyspnea or fatigue symptoms.

Other symptoms may include paroxysmal nocturnal dyspnea, orthopnea, tachypnea, cough, ascites, and nocturia. Other signs may include jugular venous distension, hepatojugular reflux, hepatomegaly, bibasilar rales, pleural effusion, tachycardia, pallor, and S_3 gallop. Patients with ADHF experience similar symptoms, but they may be more severe.

Pathophysiology

Heart failure can result from any disorder (see the next section on specific causes of heart failure) that impairs the heart's systolic function (i.e., pumping ability) or diastolic function (i.e., impaired cardiac relaxation). Many patients have manifestations of both abnormalities. In either case, the initiating event in heart failure is a decrease in cardiac output, which results in the activation of a number of compensatory mechanisms that attempt to maintain an adequate cardiac output.

The beneficial effects of angiotensin-converting enzyme inhibitors (ACEIs), β-blockers, and aldosterone antagonists on reducing mortality and slowing heart failure progression have resulted in the neurohormonal model of heart failure pathophysiology. The decrease in cardiac output leads to the activation of compensatory systems that release a number of neurohormones, including angiotensin II, norepinephrine, aldosterone, proinflammatory cytokines, and vasopressin. These neurohormones can increase renal sodium and water retention, vasoconstriction, and tachycardia and can stimulate ventricular hypertrophy and remodeling. Activation of the compensatory systems results in a systemic disorder that is not confined just to the heart and whose progression is largely mediated by these neurohormones.

Recent studies suggest that mutations in certain adrenergic receptors (β_1 and α_{2C}) and β-receptor signaling pathways may play an important role in the development of heart failure and the response to therapy.

Specific Causes of Heart Failure

Coronary artery disease is the cause of heart failure in about 65% of patients with HFrEF. Other causes include nonischemic cardiomyopathy (e.g., attributable to hypertension, thyroid disease, or valvular disease). Approximately 75% of patients with heart failure have antecedent hypertension.

Approximately 50% of patients have HFpEF, and their heart failure is secondary to impaired cardiac diastolic dysfunction. This type of heart failure is most often observed in elderly patients.

A number of drugs can precipitate or worsen heart failure:

- Drugs with negative inotropic effects include antiarrhythmics (disopyramide, flecainide, propafenone, and others); β-blockers; calcium channel blockers (verapamil and diltiazem); and oral antifungals (itraconazole and terbinafine).
- Cardiotoxic drugs include doxorubicin, daunorubicin, cyclophosphamide, ethanol, amphetamines (cocaine and methamphetamine), trastuzumab, bevacizumab, mitoxantrone, ifosfamide, lapatinib, sunitinib, and imatinib.
- Drugs that cause sodium and water retention can precipitate or worsen heart failure and include NSAIDs (which can also attenuate the efficacy, and increase the toxicity, of diuretics and ACEIs), glucocorticoids, rosiglitazone, and pioglitazone.
- Drugs with an uncertain mechanism for toxicity include infliximab, etanercept, and dronedarone.

Diagnostic Criteria

No single diagnostic test for heart failure exists; rather, the diagnosis is a clinical one based on history, signs and symptoms, and physical examination. A thorough history and physical examination are important for identifying cardiac and noncardiac disorders or behaviors (e.g., diet, adherence to medications) that may cause or hasten the progression of heart failure.

A rapid bedside assay for natriuretic peptides (B-type natriuretic peptide [BNP] or N-terminal proB-type natriuretic peptide [NT-proBNP]) is often used in acute care settings (e.g., emergency departments) as an aid in the diagnosis of suspected heart failure. These peptides are synthesized and released from the ventricles in response to pressure or volume overload and counteract increased sympathetic nervous system activity and renin–angiotensin–aldosterone system activity by increasing diuresis, renal sodium excretion, and vasodilation. The degree of elevation of natriuretic peptides correlates with prognosis. The assay is useful for differentiating between heart failure exacerbations and other causes of dyspnea, such as chronic obstructive pulmonary disease (COPD), asthma, or infection. Patients with dyspnea secondary

to heart failure will have elevated plasma natriuretic peptide concentrations.

The echocardiogram is one of the most useful diagnostic tests in patients with heart failure. It is useful for determining the LVEF as well as the presence of other structural or functional abnormalities that could be causing heart failure. Patients with an LVEF of < 40% generally are considered to have systolic dysfunction. LVEF can also be determined by nuclear imaging scans or during a cardiac catheterization. Note that, in general, there is a poor correlation between LVEF and symptoms.

Treatment Principles and Goals of Therapy

The goals of therapy include improving the patient's quality of life, minimizing symptoms, reducing hospitalizations for heart failure exacerbations, slowing progression of the disease, and improving survival.

The ACC–AHA guideline recommendations for treatment of stages A–D heart failure are available at http://circ.ahajournals.org/content/early/2013/06/03/CIR.0b013e31829e8776.citation. For stages A and B, therapy primarily is targeted toward prevention of heart failure development; in stages C and D, however, the focus is targeted toward treatment of patients with symptomatic heart failure.

An algorithm for treatment of patients with ADHF is shown in Figure 13-1.

13-4. Drug Therapy of Heart Failure

The following section on drug therapy focuses on the treatment of patients with stage C HFrEF (i.e., patients with known structural heart disease, current or prior heart failure signs and symptoms, and LVEF ≤ 40%). Patients with stage C HFrEF should be routinely managed with a diuretic (if needed to control volume retention), an ACEI or angiotensin II receptor blocker (ARB), a β-blocker, and an aldosterone antagonist. Drug therapies that can be considered in selected patients include digoxin, combination ACEI/ARB, and hydralazine-isosorbide dinitrate.

In contrast to patients with HFrEF, these same drug therapies have not been shown to improve important outcomes (e.g., mortality, hospitalizations, etc.) in patients with HFpEF. However, these same drugs are often used to treat HFpEF because these patients have many comorbidities (e.g., hypertension, diabetes, coronary artery disease) that require treatment with these drug classes.

Figure 13-1. Acute Decompensated Heart Failure

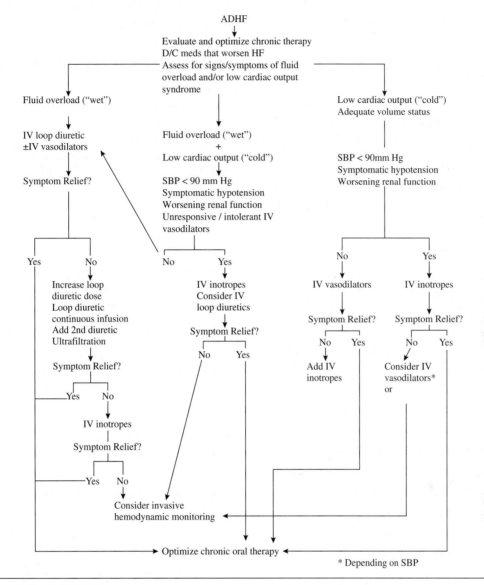

Parker RB, Rodgers JE, Cavallari LH, 2008.
SBP, systolic blood pressure; D/C, discontinue.

Loop Diuretics

Only patients with signs or symptoms of volume overload will need diuretic therapy. Most heart failure patients require use of the more potent loop diuretics instead of thiazide diuretics (Table 13-1).

Mechanism of action

Loop diuretics reduce the sodium and fluid retention associated with heart failure by inhibiting reabsorption of sodium and chloride in the loop of Henle.

Table 13-1. Loop Diuretics

Generic name	Trade name	Dosage form	Dosage range and frequency
Furosemide	Lasix	Oral tablet	20–160 mg qd bid
Bumetanide	Bumex	Oral tablet	0.5–5 mg qd bid
Torsemide	Demadex	Oral tablet	10–100 mg qd bid

Patient instructions and counseling

- Patients allergic to sulfa-containing medications also may be allergic to loop diuretics.
- Patients should take medication once a day in the morning or, if taking twice daily, in the morning and afternoon.
- Loop diuretics can cause frequent urination.
- Patients should weigh themselves daily (preferably in the morning, after urinating). Patients who gain more than 1 pound per day for several consecutive days or 3–5 pounds in a week should contact their health care provider.
- Patients should report muscle cramps, dizziness, excessive thirst, weakness, or confusion, as these may be signs of overdiuresis.
- Patients should avoid sun exposure or use sunscreen when taking loop diuretics.

Adverse drug events

- Electrolyte depletion: hypokalemia and hypomagnesemia
- Hypotension
- Renal insufficiency

Drug–drug and drug–disease interactions

- Food decreases the bioavailability of furosemide and bumetanide, so these agents should be taken on an empty stomach. Food does not affect torsemide absorption.
- The absorption of oral furosemide is slowed significantly in patients with ADHF, resulting in decreased diuretic response. Therefore, those individuals usually will require the use of intravenous (IV) furosemide.
- NSAIDs may diminish these agents' diuretic effects.
- Potassium supplementation may not be required in patients also receiving ACEIs, ARBs, or aldosterone antagonists.

Parameters to monitor

- Serum sodium, potassium, magnesium, creatinine, and blood urea nitrogen (BUN)
- Patient weight (a loss of 0.5–1 kg daily is desired until the patient achieves the desired dry weight)
- Urine output
- Blood pressure
- Jugular venous distension
- Improvement in heart failure symptoms (dyspnea and peripheral edema)

Kinetics

The bioavailability of torsemide is not affected by food and is less variable than that of furosemide.

Angiotensin-Converting Enzyme Inhibitors

ACEIs are recommended for all patients with HFrEF and current or prior symptoms of heart failure, unless contraindicated (Table 13-2). Clinical trials with more than 7,000 patients consistently demonstrate that ACEIs alleviate symptoms, improve clinical status and quality of life, and reduce mortality.

Mechanism of action

- ACEIs interfere with the renin–angiotensin system by inhibiting the angiotensin-converting enzyme, which is responsible for the conversion of angiotensin I to the potent vasoconstrictor angiotensin II. This inhibition results in a decrease in plasma angiotensin II and aldosterone concentrations, thus reducing the adverse effects of those neurohormones. Inhibition of the angiotensin-converting enzyme also prevents the breakdown of the endogenous vasodilator bradykinin.
- ACEIs reduce heart failure symptoms and decrease hospitalizations for heart failure.
- ACEIs reduce mortality by 20–30% and slow the progression of heart failure.

Patient instructions and counseling

- Patients who are pregnant or breast-feeding should not take ACEIs. If patients become pregnant while taking an ACEI, they should contact their physician immediately.

Table 13-2. Angiotensin-Converting Enzyme Inhibitors

Generic name	Trade name	Dosage form	Dosage range and frequency
Captopril	Capoten	Oral tablet	6.25–50 mg tid
Enalapril	Vasotec	Oral tablet	2.5–20 mg bid
Fosinopril	Monopril	Oral tablet	5–40 mg qd
Lisinopril	Zestril, Prinivil	Oral tablet	2.5–40 mg qd
Quinapril	Accupril	Oral tablet	5–40 mg bid
Ramipril	Altace	Oral capsule	1.25–5 mg bid
Perindopril	Aceon	Oral tablet	2–16 mg qd
Trandolapril	Mavik	Oral tablet	0.5–4 mg qd

- Captopril should be taken on an empty stomach, either 1 hour before or 2 hours after meals.
- Salt substitutes that contain potassium should be used cautiously.
- Patients should call their physician immediately if they experience swelling of the face, eyes, lips, tongue, arms, or legs or if they have difficulty breathing or swallowing.
- ACEIs may cause a cough.

Adverse drug events

- Hypotension
- Dizziness
- Renal insufficiency
- Cough
- Angioedema
- Hyperkalemia
- Rash
- Taste disturbances

Drug–drug and drug–disease interactions

- NSAIDs can increase the risk of renal insufficiency and attenuate the beneficial effects of ACEIs.
- Potassium supplements or potassium-sparing diuretics should be used with caution.
- Cyclosporine and tacrolimus may increase the risk of nephrotoxicity and hyperkalemia.
- Diuretics increase the risk of hypotension.

Parameters to monitor

- Blood pressure
- Renal function (i.e., serum BUN and creatinine)
- Serum potassium
- Heart failure symptoms
- Dose (initiate therapy at low doses; if lower doses are tolerated well, follow with gradual increases)

Other

ACEIs are pregnancy category C during the first trimester and pregnancy category D during the second and third trimesters. ACEIs can cause fetal and neonatal morbidity and death when administered to pregnant women.

Angiotensin II Receptor Blockers

ACEIs remain the drugs of choice for inhibiting the renin–angiotensin–aldosterone system in patients with HFrEF. Recent clinical trials confirm the efficacy and safety of candesartan and valsartan in this popu-

Table 13-3. Angiotensin II Receptor Blockers

Generic name	Trade name	Dosage form	Dosage range and frequency
Candesartan	Atacand	Oral tablet	4–32 mg qd
Losartan	Cozaar	Oral tablet	25–150 mg qd
Valsartan	**Diovan**	Oral tablet	20–160 mg bid

Boldface indicates one of top 100 drugs for 2012 by units sold at retail outlets, www.drugs.com/stats/top100/2012/units.

lation. Current guidelines recommend candesartan or valsartan for patients who are intolerant to ACEIs—both agents are approved for use in patients with heart failure. Intolerance to ACEIs is most often due to cough or angioedema, although caution is advised when using ARBs in patients who have angioedema secondary to an ACEI. Note that ARBs are just as likely as ACEIs to cause impaired renal function, hyperkalemia, or hypotension (Table 13-3).

Mechanism of action

- ARBs interfere with the renin–angiotensin system by blocking the angiotensin-1 receptor, thereby attenuating the detrimental effects of this hormone.
- Unlike ACEIs, ARBs do not affect the kinin system and thus are not associated with cough.
- ARBs reduce hospitalizations and improve survival.

Patient instructions and counseling

- Patients who are pregnant or breast-feeding should not take ARBs. If a patient becomes pregnant while taking an ARB, she should contact her physician immediately.
- Use salt substitutes that contain potassium cautiously.
- Dizziness or light-headedness may occur, especially in patients taking diuretics.

Adverse drug events

- Hypotension
- Dizziness
- Renal insufficiency
- Hyperkalemia

Drug–drug and drug–disease interactions

- Potassium supplements or potassium-sparing diuretics should be used with caution.
- Diuretics increase the risk of hypotension.

Parameters to monitor

- Blood pressure
- Renal function (i.e., serum BUN and creatinine)
- Serum potassium
- Heart failure symptoms
- Dose (initiate therapy at low doses; if lower doses are tolerated well, follow with gradual increases)

Other

- ARBs are pregnancy category C during the first trimester and pregnancy category D during the second and third trimesters. ARBs can cause fetal and neonatal morbidity and death when administered to pregnant women.

β-Blockers

Because of their negative inotropic effects, β-blockers were once considered to be contraindicated in patients with HFrEF. However, by inhibiting the deleterious effects of long-term activation of the sympathetic nervous system in heart failure, β-blockers repeatedly have been shown to provide hemodynamic, symptomatic, and survival benefits. Metoprolol succinate (extended-release metoprolol), bisoprolol, and carvedilol all have been shown to be effective, and one of these three agents should be used for the treatment of HFrEF (Table 13-4).

Mechanism of action

- Blockade of β-receptors antagonizes the increase in sympathetic nervous system activity, which is one of the significant mechanisms responsible for the progression of heart failure. Bisoprolol and metoprolol succinate are β_1-selective

Table 13-4. β-Blockers

Generic name	Trade name	Dosage form	Dosage range and frequency
Bisoprolol	Zebeta	Oral tablet	1.25–10 mg qd
Carvedilol	Coreg	Oral tablet	3.125–50 mg bid
Carvedilol	Coreg CR	Oral capsule	10–80 mg qd
Metoprolol succinate extended-release	Toprol-XL	Oral tablet	12.5–200 mg qd

Boldface indicates one of top 100 drugs for 2012 by units sold at retail outlets, www.drugs.com/stats/top100/2012/units.

agents, whereas carvedilol blocks β_1-, β_2-, and α_1-receptors. Whether these differences in pharmacologic actions have any important effects on outcomes remains uncertain.

- Treatment with β-blockers reduces symptoms, improves clinical status, and decreases the risk of death and hospitalization.
- One of the three β-blockers that have been shown to reduce mortality (bisoprolol, carvedilol, and extended-release metoprolol succinate) should be used in all stable patients with HFrEF and current or prior heart failure symptoms, unless contraindicated.
- In general, β-blockers should be used in combination with ACEIs or ARBs and diuretics.

Patient instructions and counseling

- β-blockers may cause fluid retention or worsening of heart failure upon initiation of therapy or after an increase in dose. Patients should report any cases of body or leg swelling or increased shortness of breath. Patients should weigh themselves daily; if they gain more than 1 pound per day for several consecutive days or 3–5 pounds in a week, they should contact their health care provider.
- Fatigue or weakness may occur in the first few weeks of treatment but usually will resolve spontaneously.
- Patients should report any cases of dizziness, lightheadedness, or blurred vision, which may be caused by the patient's blood pressure being too low or from bradycardia or heart block.
- Patients should take carvedilol with food.
- It is important not to miss doses or stop taking these medications abruptly.
- In patients with diabetes, β-blockers can increase blood sugar and may also mask the signs of hypoglycemia (except for sweating).

Adverse drug events

A list of adverse events most commonly observed in heart failure patients receiving β-blockers follows. For other adverse effects of β-blockers, see Chapter 12 on hypertension and Chapter 15 on ischemic heart disease.

- Fluid retention and worsening heart failure
- Fatigue
- Bradycardia and heart block
- Hypotension
- Abrupt withdrawal can lead to hypertension, tachycardia, or myocardial ischemia

Drug–drug and drug–disease interactions

- Amiodarone and calcium channel blockers (verapamil and diltiazem) can increase the risk of bradycardia, heart block, and hypotension.
- Quinidine, fluoxetine, paroxetine, and other inhibitors of cytochrome P4502D6 inhibit hepatic metabolism of metoprolol and carvedilol and may result in increased plasma concentrations and enhanced effects.
- Concomitant use of ophthalmic β-blockers may increase the risk of bradycardia, heart block, and hypotension.
- β-blockers may cause bronchoconstriction in patients with asthma or COPD.
- Do not use β-blockers in patients with symptomatic bradycardia or heart block unless a pacemaker is present.
- β-blockers may worsen blood glucose control in diabetics and mask the signs of hypoglycemia.

Parameters to monitor

- Blood pressure and heart rate
- Heart failure symptoms
- Weight (daily)

Kinetics

- Bisoprolol is eliminated about 50% by the kidneys, so dosage adjustment may be required in patients with renal insufficiency.
- Both metoprolol and carvedilol are metabolized by the liver.

Other

- Patients should be stable (i.e., minimal evidence of fluid overload or volume retention) before β-blocker treatment is initiated.
- Treatment should be initiated with low doses and titrated slowly upward until the target dose is reached. Doses usually are increased no more frequently than every 2 weeks, with close monitoring of symptoms required during the titration period.
- Fluid accumulation during dose titration usually can be managed by adjusting diuretic doses.
- Staggering the schedule of other heart failure medications that lower blood pressure (e.g., ACEIs and diuretics) may help reduce the risk of hypotension.
- A recent study comparing the effects of carvedilol with immediate-release metoprolol (metoprolol tartrate) in patients with heart failure found

that survival is improved in patients receiving carvedilol. Whether carvedilol is superior to extended-release metoprolol (metoprolol succinate) is unknown. However, these results strongly suggest that only β-blockers proven to improve survival (carvedilol, metoprolol succinate, and bisoprolol) should be used in patients with HFrEF as recommended by current guidelines.

Aldosterone Receptor Antagonists

Elevated plasma aldosterone plays an important detrimental role in the pathophysiology and progression of heart failure. Although short-term treatment with ACEIs or ARBs lowers circulating aldosterone concentrations, this suppression is not sustained with long-term therapy. In low doses, the aldosterone antagonists—spironolactone and eplerenone—reduce the risk of death and hospitalization in patients with moderate to severe heart failure. Current guidelines recommend the addition of aldosterone antagonists in patients with NYHA class II–IV HFrEF who can be monitored closely for renal function and serum potassium (Table 13-5). Aldosterone antagonists are also recommended for patients with acute myocardial infarction and an LVEF ≤ 40%, as well as heart failure symptoms or a history of diabetes.

Mechanism of action

Aldosterone plays an important role in heart failure pathophysiology. In addition to increasing renal sodium retention and potassium loss, aldosterone is also a key mediator of ventricular hypertrophy and remodeling, which drives the initiation and progression of heart failure. Antagonism of aldosterone receptors by spironolactone and eplerenone attenuates these detrimental effects.

Patient instructions and counseling

- Potassium-containing salt substitutes should be avoided.

Table 13-5. Aldosterone Antagonists

Generic name	Trade name	Dosage form	Dosage range and frequency
Spironolactone	Aldactone	Oral tablet	12.5–50 mg qd
Eplerenone	Inspra	Oral tablet	25–50 mg qd

- Patients should call their physician immediately if they experience muscle weakness or cramps; numbness or tingling in hands, feet, or lips; or slow or irregular heartbeat.
- Spironolactone may cause swollen or painful breasts in men.

Adverse drug events

- Hyperkalemia
- Gynecomastia (only with spironolactone)
- Irregular menses

Drug–drug and drug–disease interactions

- ACEIs, ARBs, and NSAIDs increase the risk of hyperkalemia.
- Spironolactone can increase digoxin plasma concentrations.
- Potassium supplements increase the risk of hyperkalemia. Supplements should not be used if serum potassium > 3.5 mEq/L.
- Elderly patients and patients with diabetes are at an increased risk of hyperkalemia.
- Erythromycin, clarithromycin, verapamil, keto-conazole, fluconazole, itraconazole, and other inhibitors of cytochrome P4503A4 inhibit hepatic metabolism of eplerenone and may result in increased plasma concentrations and enhanced effects.

Parameters to monitor

- Serum creatinine should be < 2.5 mg/dL in men or < 2 mg/dL in women (or estimated glomerular filtration rate > 30 ml/min for men and women) before therapy is initiated.
- Serum potassium should be < 5 mEq/L before therapy is initiated. Potassium should be evaluated 2–3 days after therapy is started, again 1 week after therapy is started, and then at least monthly for the first 3 months of therapy.

Digoxin

Unlike ACEIs or β-blockers, digoxin does not reduce mortality in patients with HFrEF but does appear to decrease hospitalizations for heart failure (Table 13-6).

Mechanism of action

- Digoxin inhibits the Na$^+$-K$^+$-ATPase pump, which results in an increase in intracellular calcium that, in turn, causes a positive inotropic effect.

Table 13-6. Digoxin

Generic name	Trade name	Dosage form	Dosage range and frequency
Digoxin	Lanoxin	Oral tablet, IV, elixir	0.125–0.25 mg qd
Digoxin	Lanoxicaps	Oral capsule	0.1–0.2 mg qd

- Recent evidence indicates that digoxin reduces sympathetic outflow from the central nervous system, thus blunting some of the excessive sympathetic activation that occurs in heart failure. These effects occur at low plasma concentrations, where little positive inotropic effect is seen.

Patient instructions and counseling

Patients should report any of the following to their health care provider:

- Dizziness, lightheadedness, or fatigue
- Changes in vision (blurred or yellow vision)
- Irregular heartbeat
- Loss of appetite
- Nausea, vomiting, or diarrhea

Adverse drug events

Major adverse effects involve three systems:

- Cardiovascular (cardiac arrhythmias, brady-cardia, and heart block)
- Gastrointestinal (anorexia, abdominal pain, nausea, and vomiting)
- Neurological (visual disturbances, disorientation, confusion, and fatigue)

Toxicity typically is associated with serum digoxin concentrations > 2 ng/mL but may occur at lower levels in elderly patients and in patients with hypokalemia or hypomagnesemia.

Drug–drug and drug–disease interactions

The following drugs increase serum digoxin concentrations:

- Quinidine, verapamil, dronedarone, and amiodarone (the dose of digoxin should be decreased by 50% if these medications are added)
- Propafenone
- Flecainide
- Macrolide antibiotics (erythromycin and clarithromycin)

- Itraconazole and ketoconazole
- Spironolactone
- Cyclosporine

Drugs that decrease serum digoxin concentrations include the following:

- Antacids
- Cholestyramine and colestipol
- Kaolin-pectin
- Metoclopramide

Diuretics increase the risk of digoxin toxicity in the presence of hypokalemia or hypomagnesemia.

Digoxin clearance is reduced in patients with renal insufficiency (see section on kinetics).

Parameters to monitor

- Digoxin serum concentration
  - There is little relationship between serum digoxin concentration and therapeutic effects in heart failure.
  - Current guidelines suggest a target digoxin serum concentration range of 0.5–1 ng/mL.
- Heart rate
- Serum potassium and magnesium
- Renal function (serum BUN and creatinine)
- Heart failure symptoms

Kinetics

See Table 13-7 for information about the pharmacokinetics of digoxin. Note the following:

- Approximately 60–80% of the dose is eliminated unchanged by the kidneys; therefore, dosage adjustment is required in patients with renal insufficiency.

Table 13-7. Digoxin Pharmacokinetics

Oral bioavailability

Tablets	0.5–0.9 (average 0.65)
Elixir	0.75–0.85 (average 0.8)
Capsules	0.9–1 (average 0.95)

Elimination half-life

Normal renal function	36 hours
Anuric patients	5 days
Volume of distribution	7 L/kg
Fraction excreted unchanged in urine	0.65–0.7

- Lower doses (0.125 mg daily or every other day) should be used in the elderly or in patients with a low lean body mass.
- No loading dose is needed in the treatment of heart failure.
- Because of the long distribution phase after either oral or intravenous digoxin administration, blood samples for determination of serum digoxin concentrations should be collected at least 6 hours, and preferably 12 hours or more, after the last dose.

Hydralazine–Isosorbide Dinitrate

Hydralazine and isosorbide dinitrate initially were combined because of complementary hemodynamic actions. An early clinical trial reported reduced mortality with this combination when compared with placebo. A comparison with an ACEI, however, showed that the ACEI was superior to hydralazine–isosorbide dinitrate. Adverse effects with the combination are common (primarily headache, dizziness, and gastrointestinal complaints), and these effects lead many patients to discontinue therapy. Current guidelines recommend the use of hydralazine–isosorbide dinitrate to reduce morbidity and mortality in self-described African-Americans with HFrEF and NYHA class III–IV symptoms, in addition to standard therapy with ACEI and β-blockers. Hydralazine-isosorbide dinitrate is also an option in patients with HFrEF who experience drug intolerance, hypotension, or renal insufficiency with ACEI or ARB treatment. A fixed-dose combination product is available (BiDil).

13-5. Drug Therapy for Acute Decompensated Heart Failure

Patients with ADHF usually are admitted to the hospital for aggressive treatment with IV diuretics, vasodilators (see Table 13-8), or positive inotropic drugs (see Table 13-9). When such patients have hypotension in addition to low cardiac output, they are said to be in cardiogenic shock. In these severe cases, therapy may be guided by invasive hemodynamic monitoring. Treatment goals include improving symptoms, reducing volume overload, improving cardiac output, identifying and addressing precipitating factors, and optimizing chronic therapy before hospital discharge. The approach to treatment is dictated by the patient's hemodynamic profile.

Table 13-8. Vasodilators

Generic name	Trade name	Mechanism of action	Dose[a]	Adverse effects and comments
Nitroprusside	Nipride	Arterial and venous dilator	Initial dose 0.1–0.25 mcg/kg/min and titrate to response	Hypotension, headache, tachycardia, cyanide and thiocyanate toxicity, myocardial ischemia
Nitroglycerin	Nitro-Bid, Nitrostat	Venous dilator but also an arterial dilator at higher doses	Initial dose 5–10 mcg/min and titrate to response	Hypotension, headache, tachycardia, tolerance to hemodynamic effects
Nesiritide	Natrecor	B-type natriuretic peptide that increases diuresis and is an arterial and venous dilator	Initially 2 mcg/kg bolus followed by 0.01 mcg/kg/min infusion; can increase to 0.03 mcg/kg/min	Hypotension, headache when used in combination with diuretics

a. All are given by continuous IV infusion.

Warm and Dry

- No specific therapy is needed.

Warm and Wet

- The goal is to reduce volume overload and minimize congestive symptoms.
- IV loop diuretics are often used. For patients who are unresponsive to loop diuretics, the addition of supplemental thiazide diuretics (e.g., metolazone) may be helpful.

- The addition of IV vasodilators (nitroglycerin, nitroprusside, and nesiritide) can also reduce symptoms.
- Inotropic therapy usually is not necessary, although it can be considered in patients not responding to IV loop diuretics or vasodilators.

Cold and Dry

- Patients may be clinically stable and often do not present with acute symptoms.

Table 13-9. Inotropes

Generic name	Trade name	Mechanism of action	Dose[a]	Adverse effects and comments
Dopamine	Intropin	Dose-dependent agonist of dopamine, β-, and α_1-receptors	0–3 mcg/kg/min: stimulates dopamine receptors; may improve urine output 3–10 mcg/kg/min: stimulates β_1- and β_2-receptors to increase cardiac output > 10 mcg/kg/min: stimulates α_1-receptors to increase blood pressure	Increases heart rate, contractility, myocardial oxygen demand, myocardial ischemia, arrhythmias, and systemic vascular resistance; should be used only in patients with marked systemic hypotension or cardiogenic shock
Dobutamine	Dobutrex	β_1- and β_2-receptor agonist and weak α_1 agonist; increases cardiac output and vasodilates	2.5–20 mcg/kg/min	Increases heart rate, contractility, myocardial oxygen demand, myocardial ischemia, arrhythmias; not useful to increase blood pressure in hypotensive patients
Milrinone	Primacor	Inhibits phosphodiesterase III, resulting in positive inotropic and vasodilating effects	0.125–0.75 mcg/kg/min	Arrhythmias, hypotension, and headache; alternative to patients not responding to dobutamine or dopamine; may be useful for patients receiving β-blockers because its positive inotropic effects are not mediated by β-receptors; adjust dose in patients with renal insufficiency

a. All are given by continuous IV infusion.

■ Rule out volume depletion from overdiuresis as the cause of decreased cardiac output.

■ Gradual introduction of β-blockers may be helpful.

Cold and Wet

■ Improve cardiac output first (i.e., before removing excess volume).

■ Cardiac output can be increased by IV vasodilators or inotropes, or both.

■ The relative roles of vasodilators and inotropes in this patient population are controversial.

Monitoring Parameters

■ Daily weight

■ Daily fluid intake and output

■ Vital signs, at least daily

■ Signs of heart failure, at least daily: edema, ascites, pulmonary rales, jugular venous pressure, hepatomegaly, and hepatojugular reflux

■ Symptoms of heart failure, at least daily: orthopnea, paroxysmal nocturnal dyspnea, cough, dyspnea, fatigue, and lightheadedness

■ Electrolytes, at least daily: sodium, potassium, and magnesium

■ Renal function, at least daily: BUN and serum creatinine

13-6. Nondrug Therapy

Nondrug therapies include the following:

■ Ultrafiltration

■ Intra-aortic balloon pump

■ Left ventricular assist devices

■ Cardiac resynchronization therapy

■ Biventricular pacing

■ Implantable cardioverter-defibrillator

■ Cardiac transplantation

13-7. Questions

1. Which of the following combinations represents optimal pharmacotherapy of patients with stage C HFrEF?

    A. Furosemide, clonidine, hydrochlorothiazide, and propranolol
    B. Furosemide, lisinopril, and carvedilol
    C. Carvedilol, verapamil, amlodipine, and nesiritide

D. Cardizem, hydrochlorothiazide, digoxin, and sotalol
E. Dobutamine, amiodarone, furosemide, and nitroglycerin

2. Which of the following mechanisms most likely contributes to the benefits of β-blockers in the treatment of heart failure?

    A. Stimulation of β_2-receptors
    B. Increased heart rate and decreased blood pressure
    C. Stimulation of β_1-receptors
    D. Blockade of increased sympathetic nervous system activity
    E. Blockade of angiotensin II receptors

3. Appropriate monitoring parameters for enalapril therapy in the treatment of heart failure include

    A. serum calcium.
    B. serum albumin.
    C. thyroid stimulating hormone.
    D. serum potassium.
    E. hemoglobin A1c.

4. Patients taking eplerenone for heart failure should avoid taking

    A. NSAIDs.
    B. ACEIs.
    C. β-blockers.
    D. Demadex.
    E. calcium supplements.

5. Which of the following is an adverse effect of digoxin?

    A. Hepatotoxicity
    B. Anorexia
    C. Stroke
    D. Pulmonary embolism
    E. Acute renal failure

6. Heart failure may be exacerbated by which of the following medications?

    A. Naproxen
    B. Glipizide
    C. Metformin
    D. Crestor (rosuvastatin)
    E. Fenofibrate

7. Cough is an adverse effect associated with which of the following medications?

    A. Ramipril
    B. Valsartan

C. Carvedilol
D. Torsemide
E. Eplerenone

8. Which of the following ACEIs has the shortest duration of action?

A. Ramipril
B. Captopril
C. Lisinopril
D. Monopril
E. Fosinopril

9. Which of the following adverse effects of lisinopril can be avoided by switching to candesartan?

A. Cough
B. Renal insufficiency
C. Hyperkalemia
D. Hypotension
E. Injury or death to developing fetus

10. Which of the following medications increases digoxin serum concentrations?

A. Biaxin (clarithromycin)
B. Hydralazine
C. Glyburide
D. Lipitor (atorvastatin)
E. Warfarin

11. Which of the following medications can cause bradycardia?

A. Carvedilol
B. Furosemide
C. Ramipril
D. Milrinone
E. Dobutamine

12. Which of the following is contraindicated in patients with a history of lisinopril-induced angioedema?

A. Captopril
B. Torsemide
C. Spironolactone
D. Milrinone
E. Carvedilol

13. Nesiritide would be indicated in

A. patients with asymptomatic left ventricular dysfunction.
B. patients with acute decompensated heart failure not responsive to IV diuretics.
C. patients with stage B heart failure.

D. patients with type 2 diabetes.
E. patients intolerant to digoxin.

14. Which of the following best describes the use of furosemide in heart failure?

A. Furosemide reduces mortality and slows heart failure progression.
B. Hypokalemia is a common adverse effect.
C. Response can be evaluated by monitoring hemoglobin A1c.
D. Oral absorption is increased in patients with acute decompensated heart failure.
E. Furosemide's bioavailability is not affected by food.

15. Which of the following is an important consideration when using β-blockers for treating HFrEF?

A. They are effective only in postmyocardial infarction patients.
B. All β-blockers are equally effective for the treatment of HFrEF.
C. Therapy should be initiated at the target dose.
D. Patients with fluid overload are the optimal candidates for initiating therapy.
E. Therapy should be initiated at low doses and titrated upward slowly.

16. The dose of which of the following medications should be reduced in patients with renal insufficiency?

A. Metoprolol
B. Carvedilol
C. Digoxin
D. Nitroglycerin
E. Dobutamine

17. Which of the following is true regarding digoxin therapy in patients with HFrEF?

A. Digoxin reduces mortality.
B. Concomitant amiodarone therapy decreases digoxin plasma concentrations.
C. Digoxin is contraindicated in patients with HFrEF and atrial fibrillation.
D. The target digoxin plasma concentration is 0.5–1 ng/mL.
E. Concomitant glyburide therapy increases digoxin plasma concentrations.

18. Which of the following β-blockers also blocks α_1-receptors and is effective for treating HFrEF?

A. Metoprolol
B. Carvedilol

C. Bisoprolol
D. Propranolol
E. Atenolol

19. Patients with HFrEF who experience fluid retention after β-blocker initiation should have

   A. the β-blocker dose increased.
   B. the digoxin dose increased.
   C. the β-blocker discontinued.
   D. the ACEI discontinued.
   E. the diuretic dose adjusted.

20. Which of the following is correct regarding the treatment of ADHF?

A. Nesiritide is the agent of choice in patients with ADHF and hypotension.
B. Milrinone is preferred over dobutamine in patients receiving concomitant β-blocker therapy.
C. Absorption of oral loop diuretics is increased.
D. Dobutamine and milrinone improve survival.
E. Verapamil reduces volume overload and improves cardiac output.

Use Patient Profile 13-1 to answer Questions 21 and 22.

Patient Profile 13-1

Patient Name:	William Johnson	**Height:**	5'11"	
Age:	64	**Weight:**	185 lb	
Sex:	Male			
Allergies:	NKA			

DIAGNOSIS Myocardial infarction 2008
Hypertension
Heart failure
Hyperlipidemia

LABORATORY AND DIAGNOSTIC TESTS

Echocardiogram in 12/08 showed LVEF 30%
Blood pressure on 4/1/09: 145/90 mm Hg
Heart rate on 4/1/09: 88 bpm
Lipid profile on 4/1/09:
   Total cholesterol, 160 mg/dL
   LDL cholesterol, 95 mg/dL
   HDL cholesterol, 50 mg/dL
   Triglycerides, 100 mg/dL
   Serum potassium, 2 mEq/L

MEDICATION RECORD

Date	Rx#	Physician	Drug and strength	Quantity	Sig	Refills
4/1	1000	Smith	Lanoxin 0.125 mg	90	1 tab qd	2
4/1	1001	Smith	Lasix 40 mg	60	1 tab q am	3
4/1	1002	Smith	KCl 20 mEq	90	1 tab q am	1
4/1	1003	Smith	Zocor 40 mg	90	1 tab qhs	3
4/1	1004	Smith	EC aspirin 325 mg	90	1 tab q am	2
4/1	1005	Smith	Plavix 75 mg	90	1 tab q am	3

21. Which of the following medications should be added to Mr. Johnson's regimen?

    A. Lisinopril and carvedilol
    B. Valsartan and prazosin
    C. Torsemide and amlodipine
    D. Verapamil and amiodarone
    E. Clonidine and hydrochlorothiazide

22. Mr. Johnson's serum potassium level of 2 mEq/L (normal 4–5 mEq/L) could

    A. increase the risk of Lanoxin (digoxin) toxicity.
    B. be treated by increasing the dose of Lasix (furosemide).
    C. be considered a side effect of therapy with EC aspirin.
    D. be caused by an interaction between Zocor (simvastatin) and Lanoxin.
    E. increase the risk of bleeding from Plavix.

Use Hospital Inpatient Profile 13-2 to answer Questions 23–25.

23. According to her profile, the recent worsening of Mrs. Smith's heart failure most likely is related to

    A. Zestril (lisinopril).
    B. naproxen.
    C. subtherapeutic serum digoxin concentration.
    D. furosemide.
    E. drug interaction between Zestril and furosemide.

24. Toprol-XL is an agent that

    A. is contraindicated in heart failure.
    B. blocks β_1-, β_2-, and α_1-receptors.
    C. blocks only β_1-receptors.
    D. should not be used in combination with Zestril.
    E. increases the serum digoxin concentration.

Hospital Inpatient Profile 13-2

Patient Name:	Ellen Smith	**Height:**	5′4″
Age:	71	**Weight:**	150 lb
Sex:	Female		
Allergies:	NKA		

DIAGNOSIS   Heart failure exacerbation with 20-lb weight gain over past 3–4 weeks

Hypertension

Osteoarthritis

LABORATORY AND DIAGNOSTIC TESTS

Echocardiogram in 2/09 showed LVEF 25%

Blood pressure on 4/1/09: 130/85 mm Hg

Heart rate on 4/1/09: 80 bpm

Serum digoxin concentration on 4/1/09: 0.8 ng/mL

MEDICATION RECORD

Date	Rx #	Physician	Drug and strength	Quantity	Sig	Refills
2/1	100	Jones	Lanoxin 0.125 mg	90	1 tab qd	2
3/1	101	Jones	Furosemide 80 mg	60	1 tab q am	3
1/4	102	Jones	Zestril 20 mg	90	1 tab q am	1
1/4	103	Jones	Toprol-XL 50 mg	90	1 tab qd	3
3/1	104	Nelson	Naproxen 500 mg	90	1 tab bid with food	3

25. Which of the following medications could improve this patient's symptoms and survival?

    A. Spironolactone
    B. Amlodipine
    C. Verapamil
    D. Dobutamine weekly infusion
    E. Warfarin

13-8. Answers

1. **B.** Furosemide, lisinopril (an ACEI), and carvedilol (a β-blocker) in combination should be used routinely in patients with heart failure.

2. **D.** Activation of the sympathetic nervous system plays an important role in the initiation and progression of heart failure. The benefits of β-blockers are thought to be due to the blockade of the sympathetic nervous system's increased activity.

3. **D.** Enalapril, as well as other ACEIs, can increase serum potassium. Thus, serum potassium, as well as serum creatinine, should be monitored.

4. **A.** Use of eplerenone is associated with renal potassium retention. Concomitant use of NSAIDs significantly increases the risk of hyperkalemia.

5. **B.** Anorexia is a common symptom of digoxin toxicity. Digoxin is not associated with hepatotoxicity, stroke, and pulmonary embolism, and it does not affect renal function.

6. **A.** Naproxen, an NSAID, can worsen heart failure (1) by increasing renal sodium and water retention and (2) by attenuating the efficacy and enhancing the toxicity of ACEIs and diuretics. Glipizide, metformin, fenofibrate, and Crestor do not affect heart failure.

7. **A.** Cough is frequently encountered as an adverse effect of ACEIs and is believed to be due to bradykinin accumulation.

8. **B.** Captopril must be given three times daily in patients with heart failure. The other agents can be given once daily.

9. **A.** The angiotensin receptor blocker candesartan is just as likely to cause hypotension, hyperkalemia, renal insufficiency, and fetal injury as is lisinopril (or any other ACEI). Candesartan is an alternative agent for patients intolerant to ACEIs because of cough.

10. **A.** The macrolide antibiotic Biaxin (clarithromycin) is associated with a 50–100% increase in serum digoxin concentrations.

11. **A.** Carvedilol is a β-blocker and is associated with a decreased heart rate (bradycardia). The other choices all increase (milrinone and dobutamine) or do not affect heart rate (furosemide and ramipril).

12. **A.** Lisinopril is an ACEI, and angioedema is a known adverse effect of all agents in that class. Thus, captopril, which also is an ACEI, should not be used in this situation.

13. **B.** Nesiritide is indicated for use only in patients with severe or decompensated heart failure. It must be given intravenously.

14. **B.** Furosemide causes renal potassium loss and thus is associated with hypokalemia. It does not improve mortality or affect heart failure progression. Its oral absorption is slowed in patients with ADHF, and its bioavailability is reduced by food. Hemoglobin A1c is not useful for monitoring furosemide therapy.

15. **E.** When used to treat heart failure, β-blocker therapy should be started at low doses and gradually titrated upward to the target dose that was shown in clinical trials to improve survival. Starting at the target dose or initiating treatment in patients with fluid overload increases the risk of worsening heart failure. Only carvedilol, bisoprolol, and metoprolol succinate extended-release are proven to be effective in heart failure.

16. **C.** Only digoxin is eliminated by the kidneys.

17. **D.** Current guidelines suggest a target digoxin plasma concentration of 0.5–1 ng/mL. Digoxin does not improve survival in patients with heart failure—it only improves symptoms. Amiodarone increases digoxin plasma concentrations, and glyburide does not affect digoxin concentrations. Digoxin is useful in the management of patients with heart failure who also have atrial fibrillation.

18. **B.** Only carvedilol blocks α_1-receptors and has been shown to be effective in patients with heart failure.

19. **E.** Some patients with heart failure may experience increases in fluid retention after initiation of β-blocker therapy. Fluid retention typically is managed best by adjusting the diuretic dose and closely monitoring the patient's weight.

20. **B.** The positive inotropic effects of milrinone are not mediated through the β-receptor; therefore, its effects are not diminished by concomitant β-blocker therapy. Nesiritide is associated with an increased risk of hypotension. No inotropic agents are shown to improve survival. Absorption of oral loop diuretics is decreased in ADHF. Verapamil has negative inotropic effects and would worsen volume overload.

21. **A.** An ACEI and β-blocker are indicated in this patient with heart failure to improve survival and slow disease progression.

22. **A.** Hypokalemia increases the risk of digoxin toxicity.

23. **B.** The addition of the NSAID naproxen approximately 3–4 weeks before admission likely is the cause of this episode of ADHF. NSAIDs can increase sodium and water retention and negate the effects of diuretics and ACEIs.

24. **C.** Toprol-XL (metoprolol succinate extended-release) is a cardioselective β-blocker. It blocks only the β_1-receptor at usual therapeutic doses.

25. **A.** The addition of an aldosterone antagonist, either spironolactone or eplerenone, has now been shown to improve survival and decrease symptoms in patients with HFrEF. Amlodipine would have no effect, and verapamil would likely worsen heart failure because of its negative inotropic effects. Weekly dobutamine infusions do not improve survival.

13-9. References

Butler J, Ezekowitz JA, Collins SP, et al. Update on aldosterone antagonists use in heart failure with reduced left ventricular ejection fraction. Heart Failure Society of America Guidelines Committee. *J Cardiac Fail*. 2012;18:265–81.

Carlson MD, Eckman PM. Review of vasodilators in acute decompensated heart failure: The old and the new. *J Cardiac Fail* 2013;19(7):478–93.

Gislason GH, Rasmussen JN, Abildstrom SZ, et al. Increased mortality and cardiovascular morbidity associated with use of nonsteroidal anti-inflammatory drugs in chronic heart failure. *Arch Int Med*. 2009;169:141–9.

Lindenfeld J, Albert NM, Boehmer JP, et al. Executive summary: HFSA 2010 Comprehensive Heart Failure Practice Guideline. *J Card Fail*. 2010; 16:475–539.

McMurray JJV. Systolic heart failure. *N Engl J Med*. 2010;362:228–38.

Parker RB, Nappi JM, Cavallari LH. Chronic heart failure. In: DiPiro JT, Talbert RL, Yee GC, et al., eds. *Pharmacotherapy: A Pathophysiologic Approach*. 9th ed. New York, NY: McGraw-Hill; 2014:85–122.

Parker RB, Rodgers JE, Cavallari LH. Heart failure. In: DiPiro JT, Talbert RL, Yee GC, et al., eds. *Pharmacotherapy: A Pathophysiologic Approach*. 7th ed. New York, NY: McGraw-Hill; 2008: 173–216.

Petersen JW, Felker GM. Inotropes in the management of acute heart failure. *Crit Care Med*. 2008;36:S106–11.

Rodgers JE, Reed BN. Acute Decompensated Heart Failure. In: DiPiro JT, Talbert RL, Yee GC, et al., eds. *Pharmacotherapy: A Pathophysiologic Approach*. 9th ed. New York, NY: McGraw-Hill; 2014:123–40.

Schentag J, Bang A, Kozinski-Tober J. Digoxin. In: Burton M, Shaw L, Schentag J, Evans W, eds. *Applied Pharmacokinetics and Pharmacodynamics*. 4th ed. Baltimore, MD: Lippincott Williams and Wilkins; 2006:411–39.

Taylor AL, Ziesche S, Yancy C, et al. Combination of isosorbide dinitrate and hydralazine in blacks with heart failure. *N Engl J Med*. 2004;351:2049–57.

von Leuder TG, Atar D, Krum H. Diuretic use in heart failure and outcomes. *Clin Pharmacol Ther* 2013;94(4):490–8.

Wong J, Patel RA, Kowey PR. The clinical use of angiotensin-converting enzyme inhibitors. *Prog Cardiovasc Dis*. 2004;47:116–30.

Yancy CW, Jessup M, Bozkurt B, et al. 2013 ACCF/AHA guideline for the management of heart failure: A report of the American College of Cardiology Foundation/American Heart Association Task Force on Practice Guidelines. *Circulation*. 2013;128:e240–e327.

Zannad F, McMurray JJV, Krum H, et al. Eplerenone in patients with systolic heart failure and mild symptoms. *N Engl J Med*. 2011;364:11–21.

Cardiac Arrhythmias

Robert B. Parker

Cardiac arrhythmias are abnormal heart rhythms resulting from alterations in impulse formation or conduction.

14-1. Key Points

- All antiarrhythmic drugs (AADs) are proarrhythmic.
- Cardiac arrhythmias range from benign to lethal.
- Antiarrhythmic drug therapy should be individualized to patient response while minimizing adverse effects.
- Most AADs are hepatically eliminated and are associated with significant drug interactions.
- Nonpharmacologic therapy is an important treatment modality, particularly for life-threatening ventricular tachycardia and ventricular fibrillation.
- Treatment of atrial fibrillation should always include an assessment of antithrombotic therapy.
- Direct-current cardioversion is typically the treatment of choice for severely symptomatic arrhythmias.
- Anticoagulant response to warfarin therapy is influenced by numerous factors, including diet, drug interactions, genetics, and concomitant diseases.
- The treatment of excessive anticoagulation secondary to warfarin should be based on the international normalized ratio (INR), the presence of active bleeding, and the risk of recurrent thromboembolism.
- Dabigatran, rivaroxaban, and apixaban are alternative anticoagulants to warfarin in patients with nonvalvular atrial fibrillation.
- Patient education and appropriate monitoring are important aspects of successful therapy that can minimize adverse effects.

14-2. Study Guide Checklist

The following topics may guide your study of this subject area:

- Risk factors for developing arrhythmias, especially atrial fibrillation
- AADs not proven to improve survival
- Selection of appropriate pharmacotherapy for atrial fibrillation including medications used for rate control, prevention of thromboembolism, and conversion to and maintenance of sinus rhythm, based on treatment guidelines and patient characteristics
- Mechanisms of action of classes of drugs used to treat arrhythmias
- Major adverse drug reactions of drugs used to treat arrhythmias
- Significant drug interactions involving medications used to treat arrhythmias
- Trade names and generic names of medications used to treat arrhythmias
- Patient-counseling points for drugs used to treat arrhythmias

14-3. Electrophysiology

Impulse Generation (Automaticity) and Conduction

- Initiation and propagation of the electrical impulse in cardiac cells are dependent on regulation of the action potential.
- Conduction velocity is determined by regulation of action potential, specifically the slope

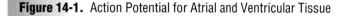
Figure 14-1. Action Potential for Atrial and Ventricular Tissue

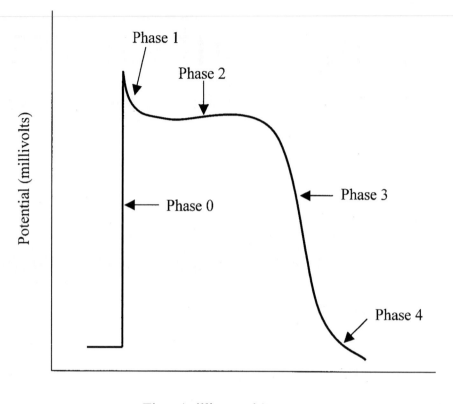

of phase 0 depolarization (Figure 14-1 and Table 14-1).

- The *absolute refractory period* is the time during which cardiac cells cannot conduct or propagate an action potential (Figure 14-1 and Table 14-1).
- The *relative refractory period* is the time during which cardiac cells may conduct and propagate action potentials secondary to strong electrical stimuli.

Normal Conduction System

The sinoatrial (SA) node, located in the right atrium, initiates an impulse that

- Stimulates the left atrium and atrioventricular (AV) node, which
- Stimulates the left and right bundle branches via the bundle of His, which then
- Stimulates Purkinje fibers and causes ventricular contraction.

Table 14-1. Phases of Atrial and Ventricular Tissue Action Potential

Phase	Process	Ion flow	Corresponding electrocardiogram
0	Depolarization	Na⁺ fast channel opens; Na⁺ enters cell.	Atrial: P wave; ventricular: QRS
1	Initial repolarization	Na⁺ channel closes; passive Cl⁻ influx.	
2	Prolongs depolarized state	Predominantly Ca²⁺ enters cell.	ST segment
3	Repolarization	Rapid efflux of K⁺ out of cell.	T wave, QT interval
4	Repolarization	Na⁺ leaks into cell; K⁺ pumped out of cell.	

14-4. Mechanisms of Arrhythmia

Cardiac arrhythmias arise secondary to the following disorders:

- Automaticity (impulse generation)
- Latent pacemaker (non-SA node pacemaker)
- Triggered automaticity (early or late after-depolarizations)
- Reentry
- Impulse conduction
- Automaticity and impulse conduction

14-5. Clinical Manifestations

Symptoms

Symptoms associated with ventricular arrhythmias range from asymptomatic to loss of consciousness and death. Patients with ventricular tachycardia (VT) may be asymptomatic, but VT can result in hypotension, syncope, or death. Ventricular fibrillation produces no cardiac output and causes most cases of sudden cardiac death.

Both bradyarrhythmias and tachyarrhythmias can be associated with reduced cardiac output, producing symptoms that include dizziness, syncope, chest pain, fatigue, confusion, and exacerbation of heart failure. Patients with tachyarrhythmias may report palpitations. With atrial fibrillation or flutter, patients may also experience dizziness, palpitations, light-headedness, dyspnea, and worsening heart failure, as well as symptoms of transient ischemic attack (TIA) or stroke.

Signs

- Electrocardiogram (ECG) abnormalities may be present.
- Ventricular rate can be assessed by documenting the heart rate from the radial artery or by carotid palpation.

14-6. Diagnostic Criteria and Therapy According to Arrhythmia Classification

Arrhythmias are defined by the following:

- Anatomic location
  - Supraventricular arrhythmias arise from abnormalities in the SA node, the atrial tissue, the AV node, or the bundle of His.

- Ventricular arrhythmias originate from below the bundle of His.
- Ventricular rate
  - *Bradyarrhythmias:* Heart rate < 60 beats per minute (bpm).
  - *Tachyarrhythmias:* Heart rate > 100 bpm.

Bradyarrhythmias

Sinus bradycardia

Diagnostic criteria and characteristics
Heart rate is less than 60 bpm; otherwise, the ECG is normal.

Mechanism of arrhythmia
The mechanism of arrhythmia is decreased SA node automaticity.

Clinical etiology
Causes include acute myocardial infarction (MI); hypothyroidism; drug-induced causes (β-blockers including ophthalmic agents, digoxin, calcium channel blockers [diltiazem, verapamil], clonidine, amiodarone, and cholinergic agents); and hyperkalemia.

Treatment goals
Restore normal sinus rhythm if the patient is clinically symptomatic.

Drug and nondrug therapy
For intermittent symptomatic episodes: administer atropine 0.5–1 mg intravenously, repeated up to maximum dose of 3 mg.

For persistent episodes or if there is no response to atropine, place transvenous or transcutaneous pacemaker.

Atrioventricular block

Diagnostic criteria and characteristics
Criteria are as follows:

- *First-degree:* Prolonged PR interval > 0.20 seconds, 1:1 atrioventricular conduction
- *Second-degree Mobitz type I:* Gradual prolongation of PR interval followed by P wave without ventricular conduction
- *Second-degree Mobitz type II:* Constant PR interval with intermittent P wave without ventricular conduction; may have widened QRS complex
- *Third-degree:* Heart rate 30–60 bpm; no temporal relation between atrial and ventricular contraction; ventricular contraction initiated by AV junction or ventricular tissue

Mechanism of arrhythmia

The mechanism of arrhythmia is prolonged conduction.

Clinical etiology

Causes include AV nodal disease; acute MI; myocarditis; increased vagal tone; drug-induced causes (β-blockers, digoxin, calcium channel blockers [diltiazem, verapamil]; clonidine, amiodarone, cholinergic agents); and hyperkalemia.

Treatment goals

Restore sinus rhythm if the patient is symptomatic.

Drug and nondrug therapy

If the cause is reversible, treat with a temporary pacemaker or intermittent atropine.

If the condition is chronic, implant a permanent pacemaker.

Supraventricular Arrhythmias

Atrial fibrillation and atrial flutter

Diagnostic criteria and characteristics

Criteria are as follows:

- *Atrial fibrillation:* No P waves; irregularly irregular QRS pattern
- *Atrial flutter:* Sawtooth P wave pattern; regular QRS pattern
- *Ventricular response:* Usually fast but can also be slow or normal

Mechanism of arrhythmia

The mechanism of arrhythmia is enhanced automaticity and reentry.

Clinical etiology

Causes include rheumatic heart disease, heart failure, hypertension, ischemic heart disease, diabetes, obesity, obstructive sleep apnea, pericarditis, cardiomyopathy, mitral valve prolapse, cardiac surgery, infection, alcohol abuse, hyperthyroidism, chronic obstructive pulmonary disease, pulmonary embolism, and idiopathic causes (lone atrial fibrillation).

Atrial fibrillation and flutter are the most commonly occurring arrhythmias, and risk increases with age.

Complications include stroke and heart failure exacerbation.

Specific treatment goals for atrial fibrillation

Figure 14-2 illustrates a treatment algorithm for atrial fibrillation.

Control the ventricular rate

Digoxin can be useful in patients with left ventricular systolic dysfunction (e.g., left ventricular ejection fraction < 40%), especially when combined with a β-blocker; digoxin slows the ventricular rate but has poor control in hyperadrenergic-induced atrial fibrillation.

The most effective agents are β-blockers (esmolol, metoprolol, propranolol, others) and calcium channel blockers (diltiazem, verapamil). Calcium channel blockers should not be used in patients with left ventricular systolic dysfunction.

For rapid control of ventricular rate, the intravenous (IV) route of administration should be used.

Digoxin, calcium channel blockers, and β-blockers do not restore sinus rhythm.

The target resting heart rate remains controversial, but current guidelines recommend a resting rate of < 80–110 bpm.

Restore and maintain sinus rhythm

Acute conversion to sinus rhythm may be required in patients with atrial fibrillation who are hemodynamically unstable (e.g., hypotensive).

Restoration of sinus rhythm is usually accomplished by electrical cardioversion or administration of antiarrhythmic drugs (AADs).

An important area of controversy centers on whether chronic AAD therapy should be administered to maintain sinus rhythm after cardioversion (*rhythm control approach*) or whether patients should simply be treated with agents to control ventricular response and anticoagulants to prevent thromboembolic stroke (*rate control approach*).

Historically, AADs were frequently used to restore and maintain sinus rhythm in patients with atrial fibrillation (rhythm control approach). With chronic therapy, AADs approximately double the chances of a patient remaining in sinus rhythm. However, this approach exposes patients to the large number of adverse effects associated with AADs. The rationale for this approach includes the possibility of fewer symptoms, lower risk of stroke, improved quality of life, and reduced mortality. Nevertheless, these benefits have never been proven in large clinical trials.

The alternative approach, so-called rate control, involves using drugs to control the ventricular response and chronic anticoagulation for stroke prevention.

The rate control and rhythm control approaches have recently been compared in a number of large clinical trials, and the studies demonstrate no advantage for rhythm control over rate control for improving cardio-

Figure 14-2. Treatment Algorithm for Atrial Fibrillation[a]

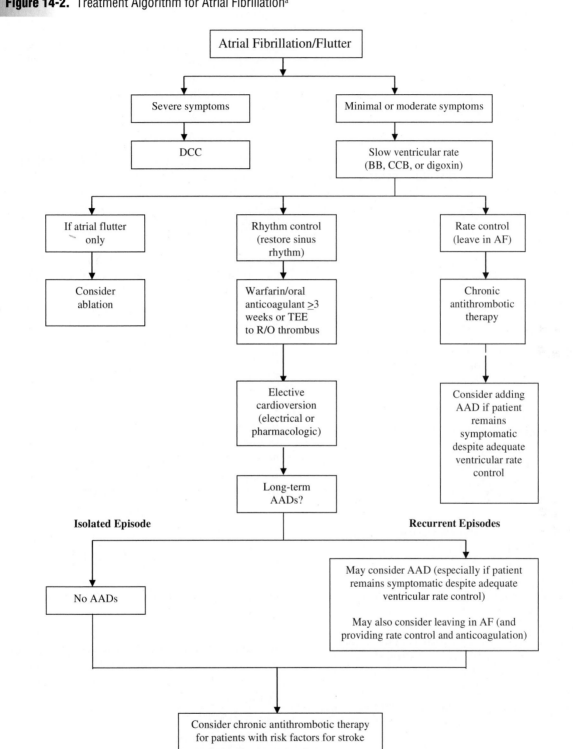

Reproduced with permission from Sanoski, Bauman, 2011.

AADs, antiarrhythmic drugs; AF, atrial fibrillation; BB, β-blocker; CCB, nondihydropyridine calcium channel blocker; DCC, direct-current cardioversion; R/O, rule out; TEE, transesophageal echocardiography.

a. Selection of the most appropriate antithrombotic therapy is based on the presence of risk factors for stroke, regardless of whether the rhythm or rate control approach is selected.

vascular outcomes. Rhythm control is reasonable to consider with patients in whom the ventricular rate cannot be controlled or with those who continue to have symptoms despite adequate control of ventricular response. The current American Heart Association–American College of Cardiology guideline recommendations for the use of AADs to maintain sinus rhythm can be found at http://circ.ahajournals.org/content/early/2014/04/10/CIR.000000000000041.citation. Regardless of the approach, appropriate anticoagulation based on the presence of stroke risk factors is needed.

Even when chronic antiarrhythmic therapy is used to maintain sinus rhythm, it is not 100% effective. Therefore, this approach is usually reserved for patients with recurrent, symptomatic episodes.

Nonpharmacologic therapy, particularly catheter ablation to abolish the reentrant focus causing atrial fibrillation, is now being used frequently.

Prevent thromboembolism

Prior to use of pharmacologic or direct-current cardioversion: If atrial fibrillation is present for ≥ 48 hours or of an unknown duration, anticoagulate with warfarin (INR [international normalized ratio] 2–3), dabigatran, rivaroxaban, or apixaban for at least 3 weeks prior to cardioversion, and continue for at least 4 weeks after sinus rhythm has been restored.

If atrial fibrillation is present for ≥ 48 hours or of an unknown duration and there is no anticoagulation in the preceding 3 weeks, transesophageal echocardiography (TEE) is often used to determine the presence of atrial thrombus. If no thrombus is seen, cardioversion can be attempted provided anticoagulation is achieved before TEE and continued for at least 4 weeks afterward. If atrial thrombus is seen on TEE, anticoagulation should be initiated and a repeat TEE performed before attempting later cardioversion.

Recommended chronic antithrombotic therapy

The choice of the optimal antithrombotic agent is based on the patient-specific risks of stroke and bleeding and should also involve shared decision making with patients based on their values and preferences. Current guidelines now recommend the use of the CHA_2DS_2-VASc score to calculate stroke risk in patients with nonvalvular atrial fibrillation instead of the $CHADS_2$ score, although some clinicians continue to use the $CHADS_2$. Each stroke risk factor is assigned a point value, and the total number of points is associated with an annual risk of stroke. The CHA_2DS_2-VASc risk factors for stroke are as follows:

- **C**ongestive heart failure or impaired left ventricular systolic function = 1 point
- **H**ypertension = 1 point
- **A**ge ≥ 75 years = 2 points
- **D**iabetes = 1 point
- **S**troke/TIA/thromboembolism = 2 points
- **V**ascular disease (MI, peripheral artery disease, or aortic plaque) = 1 point
- **A**ge 65–74 years = 1 point
- **S**ex category (female) = 1 point

The treatments below are recommended according to a CHA_2DS_2-VASc score:

- CHA_2DS_2-VASc score = 0: omitting antithrombotic therapy is reasonable.
- CHA_2DS_2-VASc score = 1: no antithrombotic therapy or treatment with oral anticoagulation (warfarin INR 2–3, dabigatran, rivaroxaban, or apixaban) or aspirin can be considered.
- CHA_2DS_2-VASc score ≥ 2: oral anticoagulation (warfarin INR 2–3, dabigatran, rivaroxaban, or apixaban) is recommended.
- For patients undergoing coronary revascularization (e.g., drug-eluting stent) with atrial fibrillation and a CHA_2DS_2-VASc score ≥ 2, the use of clopidogrel 75 mg daily together with oral anticoagulants but without aspirin may be reasonable.
- For patients with atrial fibrillation that have mechanical heart valves, warfarin therapy is recommended with an INR target based on the type and location of the prosthetic valve.
- Dabigatran and rivaroxaban are not recommended for patients who have atrial fibrillation and end-stage chronic kidney disease or who are on hemodialysis.
- Dabigatran, rivaroxaban, or apixaban should not be used in patients with atrial fibrillation and a prosthetic heart valve.

Warfarin (Coumadin)
Dosage forms
- Tablets: 1 mg (pink), 2 mg (lavender), 2.5 mg (green), 3 mg (tan), 4 mg (blue), 5 mg (peach), 6 mg (teal), 7.5 mg (yellow), 10 mg (white)
- Injections (IV): 5 mg powder for reconstitution (2 mg/mL)

Mechanism of action
Warfarin inhibits vitamin K epoxide-reductase and vitamin K reductase, preventing the conversion of vitamin K epoxide to vitamin K. It ultimately inhibits formation of vitamin K–dependent coagulation factors II, VII, IX, and X, as well as proteins C and S.

Absorption
Bioavailability of warfarin is 80–100% following oral administration. It is absorbed in the upper gastro-

intestinal tract. Food or enteral feedings may decrease the rate and extent of absorption.

Distribution
Warfarin is 99–99.5% protein bound, primarily to albumin.

Metabolism and elimination
Warfarin is administered as a racemic mixture of S- and R-warfarin; the S-isomer is five times more potent than the R-isomer. The S-isomer is primarily metabolized in the liver via cytochrome P450 2C9 (CYP2C9). The R-isomer is metabolized by several other enzymes of the cytochrome P450 system.

Warfarin has low-extraction pharmacokinetic characteristics.

Clearance decreases with increasing age.

The half-life of the R-isomer is 45 hours; for the S-isomer, it is 33 hours.

Pharmacogenomics
Recent studies show that genetic polymorphisms can markedly influence the metabolism and response to warfarin. Mutations in two genes—CYP2C9, which codes for the hepatic enzyme that metabolizes S-warfarin, and VKORC1, which regulates the vitamin K epoxide-reductase enzyme—can account for up to 50% of the variability in the dose of warfarin. The current package insert contains information regarding altered responses caused by polymorphisms in the CYP2C9 and VKORC1 genes. However, the use of genetic testing to prospectively determine the dose of warfarin remains controversial.

Pharmacodynamics
The S-isomer is approximately five times more potent than the R-isomer in inhibiting vitamin K reductase. Its pharmacodynamic effect (change in INR) is an indirect effect of the decreased formation of the vitamin K–dependent coagulation factors II, VII, IX, and X. The long half-lives of these factors result in delayed onset of action and delayed response to dosage changes.

Adverse effects
Several adverse effects are possible:

- Bleeding can occur, roughly proportional to the degree of anticoagulation.
- Skin necrosis, related to depletion or deficiency of protein C, is possible. This effect usually occurs within 10 days of warfarin initiation. Incidence is low.
- Purple-toe syndrome may occur. This syndrome usually occurs 3–8 weeks after warfarin initiation. Incidence is low.
- Birth defects and fetal hemorrhage are possible. Therefore, warfarin is pregnancy category X.

Some common drug–drug interactions
Medications decreasing warfarin anticoagulant response are as follows:

- Barbiturates
- Carbamazepine
- Cholestyramine
- Griseofulvin
- Nafcillin
- Phenytoin (chronic therapy)
- Rifampin

Medications that can increase warfarin anticoagulant response include the following (not a complete list):

- Acetaminophen
- Allopurinol
- Amiodarone
- Azole antifungal agents
- Cimetidine
- Ciprofloxacin, levofloxacin
- Diltiazem
- Erythromycin, clarithromycin
- Fenofibrate
- Fish oil
- Metronidazole
- Omeprazole (R-enantiomer)
- Phenytoin (acute therapy)
- Propafenone
- Simvastatin, fluvastatin
- Sulfinpyrazone
- Trimethoprim-sulfamethoxazole

Dosing management
Patients should take a once-daily dose of 1–10 mg orally. Patient response is highly variable. Management of elevated INR is described in Table 14-2.

Monitoring
The standard for assessing the degree of anticoagulation is the INR = (observed prothrombin ratio)^{ISI}, where ISI is the International Sensitivity Index, which corrects for variability in thromboplastin sensitivity.

Initially, the INR is monitored every 1–2 days until the desired INR is achieved and has stabilized at a given dose. Periodic INR monitoring (i.e., monthly) is recommended thereafter unless dosage changes are made.

Dabigatran (Pradaxa)
Dabigatran etexilate is a pro-drug (inactive) that after oral administration is converted to the active form dabigatran, which exerts its anticoagulant effect by direct inhibition of thrombin. It was recently approved by the U.S. Food and Drug Administration (FDA)

Table 14-2. Management of Elevated International Normalized Ratio

INR	Significant bleeding	Recommendations
< 4.5 but above therapeutic range	No	Lower dose or omit single dose and restart at lower dose when INR is therapeutic.
≥ 4.5 and ≤ 10	No	Omit several doses and resume at lower dose when INR is therapeutic; the routine use of vitamin K is not recommended.
> 10	No	Hold warfarin and administer vitamin K 2.5–5 mg orally; use additional vitamin K if necessary; resume warfarin at lower dose when INR is therapeutic.
Major bleeding at any elevation of INR	Yes	Hold warfarin; administer four-factor prothrombin complex concentrate (PCC) and give 5–10 mg vitamin K IV via slow infusion (over at least 10 minutes); can repeat vitamin K 10 mg IV q12h if necessary.

to reduce the risk of stroke and systemic embolism in patients with nonvalvular atrial fibrillation. The medication guide enclosed in the packaging should always be given to the patient each time dabigatran is dispensed.

Dosage forms
Capsules: 75, 150 mg

Mechanism of action
Dabigatran is a competitive reversible direct inhibitor of thrombin (factor IIa). By inhibiting thrombin, dabigatran blocks the conversion of fibrinogen to fibrin, thus preventing thrombus development.

Absorption
Bioavailability of dabigatran following oral administration of dabigatran etexilate is 3–7%. It may be administered with or without food. The capsules should not be broken, chewed, or opened before administration because this may result in a significant increase in bioavailability. Dabigatran is a substrate of the drug efflux transporter P-glycoprotein (P-gp).

Distribution
Dabigatran is approximately 35% protein bound.

Metabolism and elimination
The inactive dabigatran etexilate ester is hydrolyzed by esterases in the gut and liver to the active dabigatran moiety. Dabigatran then undergoes glucuronidation to several metabolites that are active. Dabigatran is primarily (80%) eliminated in the urine. The dose of dabigatran for patients with a creatinine clearance of > 30 mL/min is 150 mg orally twice daily. The dose should be reduced to 75 mg twice daily in

patients with a creatinine clearance of 15–30 mL/min. Dabigatran is not a substrate, inhibitor, or inducer of cytochrome P450 enzymes. The half-life ranges from 12 to 17 hours.

Pharmacodynamics
Dabigatran prolongs the activated partial thromboplastin time (aPTT), the thrombin clotting time (TT), and the ecarin clotting time. At clinically used doses, dabigatran has little effect on the INR. However, no clinical tests are used to monitor the intensity of anticoagulation with dabigatran.

Adverse effects
■ The risk of bleeding is increased in patients receiving dabigatran. Unlike warfarin, no specific agent is available to reverse dabigatran's anticoagulant effect.
■ Gastrointestinal adverse reactions including dyspepsia, nausea, abdominal pain or discomfort, or gastroesophageal reflux disease (GERD) can occur in up to 35% of patients.

Drug–drug interactions
The exposure to dabigatran is significantly reduced when administered with rifampin, a potent P-gp inducer. Therefore, the concomitant use of dabigatran with rifampin or other P-gp inducers should be avoided.

Dabigatran does not require dosage adjustment when administered with P-gp inhibitors such as ketoconazole, verapamil, amiodarone, quinidine, and clarithromycin. However, in patients with creatinine clearance of 15–30 mL/min, dabigatran should not be used in combination with P-gp inhibitors.

Monitoring

Unlike warfarin, in which close monitoring of the INR is required, with dabigatran no laboratory monitoring of the intensity of anticoagulation is required.

Rivaroxaban (Xarelto)

Rivaroxaban (Xarelto) is a factor Xa inhibitor recently approved by the FDA to reduce the risk of stroke and systemic embolism in patients with nonvalvular atrial fibrillation. Although approved for this indication, its use is not included in current guidelines for antithrombotic therapy of atrial fibrillation. The medication guide enclosed in the packaging should always be given to the patient each time rivaroxaban is dispensed.

Dosage forms

Tablets: 10, 15, 20 mg

Mechanism of action

Rivaroxaban is a factor Xa inhibitor that selectively blocks the factor Xa active site and does not require a cofactor (e.g., antithrombin III) for activity. Activation of factor X to factor Xa plays an important role in the clotting cascade.

Absorption

Bioavailability of the rivaroxaban 20 mg dose is 66% in the fasting state. Co-administration with food increases bioavailability by approximately 40–75%. Rivaroxaban should be administered with food at the evening meal.

Distribution

Rivaroxaban is approximately 92–95% protein bound.

Metabolism and elimination

Approximately 40–45% of rivaroxaban is eliminated unchanged by the kidneys. It also undergoes oxidative metabolism by CYP3A4 and possibly other cytochrome P450 enzymes. The dose of rivaroxaban for patients with a creatinine clearance of > 50 mL/min is 20 mg orally once daily with the evening meal. The dose should be reduced to 15 mg once daily in patients with a creatinine clearance of 15–50 mL/min. Rivaroxaban should not be used in patients with a creatinine clearance of < 15 mL/min. The drug does not inhibit or induce cytochrome P450 enzymes or drug transporters. Rivaroxaban is transported by P-gp. The half-life ranges from 5 to 9 hours.

Pharmacodynamics

Rivaroxaban produces dose-dependent inhibition of factor Xa activity. It also prolongs the aPTT and the prothrombin time (PT). However, no clinical tests are used to monitor the intensity of anticoagulation with rivaroxaban.

Adverse effects

- The risk of bleeding is increased in patients receiving rivaroxaban.
- Discontinuing rivaroxaban places patients at increased risk of thromboembolic events. If rivaroxaban is discontinued for reasons other than bleeding, administration of another anticoagulant should be considered.
- Epidural and spinal hematomas can occur in patients receiving rivaroxaban who undergo neuraxial anesthesia or spinal puncture. These hematomas can result in long-term or permanent paralysis.
- Other adverse reactions include extremity pain, muscle spasm, syncope, and pruritus.

Drug–drug interactions

Rivaroxaban should not be administered with agents that are combined P-gp and strong CYP3A4 inhibitors (e.g., ketoconazole, fluconazole, itraconazole, ritonavir, clarithromycin, erythromycin).

Rivaroxaban should not be administered with agents that are combined P-gp and strong CYP3A4 inducers (carbamazepine, phenytoin, rifampin, St. John's wort).

Monitoring

Unlike warfarin, in which close monitoring of the INR is required, no laboratory monitoring of the intensity of anticoagulation with rivaroxaban is required.

Apixaban (Eliquis)

Apixaban (Eliquis) is a factor Xa inhibitor indicated to reduce the risk of stroke and systemic embolism in patients with nonvalvular atrial fibrillation and for the prophylaxis of deep vein thrombosis in patients who have undergone hip or knee replacement surgery. The medication guide enclosed in the packaging should always be given to the patient each time apixaban is dispensed.

Dosage forms

Tablets: 2.5, 5 mg

Mechanism of action

Apixaban is a factor Xa inhibitor that selectively blocks the factor Xa active site and does not require a cofactor (e.g., antithrombin III) for activity. Activation of factor X to factor Xa plays an important role in the clotting cascade.

Absorption
Bioavailability of apixaban is approximately 50% and is not affected by food.

Distribution
Apixaban is approximately 87% protein bound.

Metabolism and elimination
Approximately 25% of apixaban is eliminated unchanged by the kidneys. It is primarily metabolized by CYP3A4 and possibly other cytochrome P450 enzymes. The recommended dose is 5 mg twice daily. The recommended dose is 2.5 mg twice daily in patients with any two of the following characteristics: age ≥ 80 years, weight ≤ 60 kg, or serum creatinine ≥ 1.5 mg/dL. The drug does not inhibit or induce cytochrome P450 enzymes or drug transporters. Apixaban is transported by P-gp. The half-life is approximately 12 hours.

Pharmacodynamics
Apixaban inhibits factor Xa, resulting in prolongation of the aPTT, PT, and INR. However, no clinical tests are used to monitor the intensity of anticoagulation with apixaban.

Adverse effects
- The risk of bleeding is increased in patients receiving apixaban. A specific antidote to reverse the drug's anticoagulant effect is not available.
- Discontinuing apixaban places patients at increased risk of thromboembolic events, including stroke. If apixaban is discontinued for reasons other than bleeding, administration of another anticoagulant should be strongly considered.
- Epidural and spinal hematomas can occur in patients receiving apixaban who undergo neuraxial anesthesia or spinal puncture. These hematomas can result in long-term or permanent paralysis.
- The use of apixaban in patients with mechanical heart valves is not recommended.

Drug–drug interactions
Apixaban is a substrate of both CYP3A4 and P-gp. In patients taking apixaban 5 mg twice daily, the dose should be decreased to 2.5 mg twice daily when administered with drugs that are strong combined P-gp and CYP3A4 inhibitors (e.g., ketoconazole, itraconazole, ritonavir, clarithromycin). In patients already taking apixaban 2.5 mg twice daily, co-administration of strong inhibitors of both CYP3A4 and P-gp (e.g., ketoconazole, itraconazole, ritonavir, clarithromycin) should be avoided.

Apixaban should not be administered with agents that are combined strong P-gp and CYP3A4 inducers (carbamazepine, phenytoin, rifampin, St. John's wort).

Co-administration of antiplatelet agents (e.g., aspirin, nonsteroidal anti-inflammatory drugs), fibrinolytics, and heparin increases bleeding risk.

Monitoring
Unlike warfarin, in which close monitoring of the INR is necessary, no laboratory monitoring of the intensity of anticoagulation with apixaban is required.

Paroxysmal supraventricular tachycardia

Diagnostic criteria and characteristics
Criteria for paroxysmal supraventricular tachycardia (PSVT) are as follows:

- Heart rate of 160–240 bpm that is abrupt in onset and termination with a normal QRS interval
- 1:1 AV conduction

Mechanism of arrhythmia
The mechanism of arrhythmia is reentry.

Clinical etiology
Causes include idiopathic causes, fever, and drug-induced causes (sympathomimetics, anticholinergics, β-agonists).

Treatment goals
See Figure 14-3 for the treatment algorithm for PSVT. Treatment goals are as follows:

- *Acute:* Terminate reentry circuit by prolonging refractoriness and slowing conduction.
- *Chronic:* Prevent or minimize the number and severity of episodes. AADs are no longer the treatment of choice to prevent recurrences. Most patients undergo radiofrequency catheter ablation of the reentrant substrate, which is curative and is associated with a low complication rate.

Acute nonpharmacologic therapy
Vagal maneuvers may terminate PSVT: carotid massage and Valsalva maneuver (most common), squatting, deep breathing, coughing, inducing eyeball pressure, and diving reflex (less common).

Ventricular Arrhythmias

Major classifications and diagnostic criteria

- Premature ventricular contractions (PVCs)
  - PVCs are extra abnormal heartbeats that originate in the ventricles. They are termed *premature* because they occur before the normal heartbeat.

Figure 14-3. Treatment Algorithm for Paroxysmal Supraventricular Tachycardia

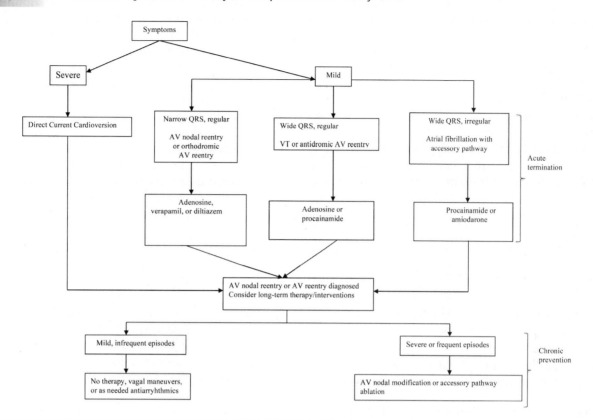

- PVCs often are asymptomatic or cause only mild palpitations.
- Ventricular tachycardia (VT)
  - VT is defined as three or more consecutive PVCs at a rate exceeding 100 bpm and a wide QRS interval (> 0.12 seconds), usually with a regular pattern.
  - Nonsustained VT (NSVT) is defined as an episode that lasts less than 30 seconds.
  - Sustained VT is defined as an episode that lasts more than 30 seconds.
- Ventricular fibrillation
  - Ventricular fibrillation is defined as an absence of organized cardiac electrical or mechanical activity and no recognizable P waves, QRS complexes, or T waves on the ECG.
  - Ventricular fibrillation rapidly results in no effective cardiac output, blood pressure, or pulse.

Clinical etiology

Causes include acute MI, electrolyte disturbances, catecholamines, and drug-induced causes.

Treatment goals

- Treat acute symptoms and precipitating causes.
- Restore sinus rhythm.
- Prevent or minimize recurrences.

14-7. Drug and Nondrug Therapy

Premature Ventricular Contractions

Apparently healthy patients without underlying structural heart disease are not at increased risk for VT or sudden cardiac death; therefore, no drug therapy is necessary.

Patients with PVCs and underlying heart disease (e.g., previous MI) are at increased risk for more serious arrhythmias. However, AADs do not reduce this risk, and in fact, their use is associated with increased risk of lethal arrhythmias. All such patients should receive medications proven to improve survival, including β-blockers, antiplatelet agents, statins, angiotensin-converting enzyme (ACE) inhibitors or angiotensin receptor blockers (ARBs), and aldosterone antagonists if appropriate. An implantable cardioverter defibrillator (ICD) is indicated in such patients with a left ventricular ejection fraction (LVEF) ≤ 30–40% to reduce mortality.

Nonsustained Ventricular Tachycardia

For patients with heart disease and LVEF > 40%, maximize other cardiovascular medications with proven effects on survival (see previous paragraph).

For patients with heart disease and LVEF ≤ 30–40%, recent studies indicate that they are at increased risk for sudden cardiac death (usually from ventricular fibrillation). Use of an ICD improves survival in this group, whereas amiodarone does not affect survival. Even in the absence of PVCs or NSVT in this patient group, these patients are at increased risk for sudden cardiac death, and an ICD is indicated to improve survival.

Unless contraindicated, these patients should also receive standard background therapy, which includes aspirin, ACE inhibitors or ARBs, β-blockers, statins, and aldosterone antagonists.

Sustained Ventricular Tachycardia or Ventricular Fibrillation (Postresuscitation)

If the event occurs within 24–48 hours of MI or because of other reversible causes, no antiarrhythmic drug therapy is needed except β-blockers.

If the event is not secondary to MI or another reversible cause, ICD placement is recommended.

AADs (i.e., amiodarone) may still be required to decrease the number of defibrillator discharges, increase patient comfort, and prolong ICD battery life.

Amiodarone can be considered if the patient refuses ICD placement.

Torsades de Pointes

This is a specific type of ventricular tachycardia with QRS complexes that appear to twist around the ECG baseline. It is associated with a prolonged QT interval.

Clinical etiology

Causes are as follows:

■ Genetic abnormalities in cardiac potassium channels
■ Acquired
  • Hypokalemia or hypomagnesemia
  • Myocardial ischemia or infarction
  • Subarachnoid hemorrhage
  • Hypothyroidism
  • Myocarditis or cardiomyopathy

• Arsenic poisoning
• Drug-induced causes (known association with torsades de pointes)
  ▪ *Antiarrhythmics:* quinidine, procainamide, disopyramide, sotalol, ibutilide, dofetilide, amiodarone
  ▪ *Antipsychotics:* chlorpromazine, haloperidol, mesoridazine, thioridazine, pimozide, atypical antipsychotics (e.g., quetiapine, ziprasidone)
  ▪ *Antidepressants:* amitriptyline, desipramine, doxepin, imipramine, nortriptyline
  ▪ *Antibiotics:* erythromycin, clarithromycin, azithromycin, gatifloxacin, moxifloxacin, sparfloxacin, pentamidine, trimethoprim-sulfamethoxazole
  ▪ *Others:* methadone, droperidol

Treatment

▦ Stop the offending drug if possible.
▦ Administer direct-current cardioversion for hemodynamically unstable patients.
▦ Administer magnesium sulfate 2 g over 1 minute IV.
▦ Use a pacemaker or isoproterenol infusion to increase heart rate.
▦ Correct hypokalemia or hypomagnesemia.

Drug therapy

See Tables 14-3, 14-4, and 14-5 for information about antiarrhythmic drugs. AADs terminate or minimize

Table 14-3. Effects of Antiarrhythmic Drugs on Cardiac Electrophysiology

Drug class	Ion block	Conduction	Refractory period	Automaticity
Ia	Sodium	↓	↑	↓
Ib	Sodium	0/↓	↓	↓
Ic	Sodium	↓↓	↑	↓
II	Calcium (indirect effect)	↓	↑	↓
III[a]	Potassium	0	↑↑	0
IV	Calcium	↓	↑	↓

↓, decreases; ↑, increases.
a. Sotalol also possesses β-blocking activity. Amiodarone also possesses sodium and calcium channel blockade.

Table 14-4. Antiarrhythmic Drug Availability and Standard Dosing Regimens

Generic name	Trade name	Dosage forms	Loading dose	Maintenance dose
Class Ia				
Quinidine gluconate	Quinaglute Dura-Tabs, Duraquin, Quinalan, Quinatime	324, 330 mg tablets 80 mg/mL injection	IV: not recommended	po: 328–648 mg tid
Quinidine sulfate	Quinidex Extentabs, Cin-Quin, Quinora	100, 200, 300 mg tablets	200 mg q 2–3 h for 5–8 doses (sulfate salt only)	200–400 mg qid
Procainamide	Pronestyl	100, 500 mg/mL injection Oral procainamide no longer available	IV: 15–18 mg/kg at 20–50 mg/min	IV: 1–6 mg/min
Disopyramide	Norpace, Norpace CR	100, 150 mg capsules 100, 150 mg capsules		150–300 mg q6h 300–600 mg q12h
Class Ib				
Lidocaine		10 mg/mL (5 mL and 10 mL) 20 mg/mL (5 mL) IV infusion: 2 (500 mL), 4 (250, 500, 1,000 mL), 8 (250, 500 mL) mg/mL in D₅W	IV: 100 mg repeat up to 2 times	IV: 1–4 mg/min
Mexiletine	Mexitil	150, 200, 250 mg capsules		100–300 mg q8h
Class Ic				
Flecainide	Tambocor	50, 100, 150 mg tablets	600 mg for conversion of atrial fibrillation to sinus rhythm	50–200 mg q12h
Propafenone	Rythmol, Rythmol-SR	150, 225, 300 mg tablets 225, 325, 425 mg capsules		150–300 mg q8h 225–425 mg q12h
Class II: β-blockers				
Metoprolol	Lopressor, Toprol XL	25, 50, 100 mg tablets 25, 50, 100, 200 mg tablets; 1 mg/mL injection	IV: 2.5–5 mg up to 3 doses	po: 25–450 mg daily
Propranolol	Inderal, Inderal LA	10, 20, 40, 60, 80 mg tablets 60, 80, 120, 160 mg capsules 20, 40 mg/mL oral solution 1 mg/mL (5 mL) injection	IV: 0.15 mg/kg IV: 0.5 mg/kg	po: 80–240 mg daily
Esmolol	Brevibloc	10 and 250 mg/mL injection	0.5 mg/kg/min × 1 min	IV: 0.05–0.2 mg/kg/min

(continued)

Table 14-4. Antiarrhythmic Drug Availability and Standard Dosing Regimens *(Continued)*

Generic name	Trade name	Dosage forms	Loading dose	Maintenance dose
Class III				
Amiodarone	Cordarone, Pacerone, Nexterone (premixed IV injection)	100, 200, 400 mg tablets	800–1,600 mg/day in divided doses × 2–4 weeks	po: 100–400 mg qd
		50 mg/mL IV solution, premix: 150 mg/100 mL and 360 mg/200 mL	IV (VT/VF): 150 mg/ 10 min or 900 mg in 500 mL D$_5$W at 1 mg/min × 6 h	IV: 0.5 mg/min
			IV (cardiac arrest): 300 mg	
Sotalol	Betapace, Betapace AF	80, 120, 160, 240 mg tablets		80–160 mg q12h
Ibutilide	Corvert	0.1 mg/mL (10 mL) injection	IV: 1 mg over 10 min; repeat × 1 if needed	Not applicable
Dofetilide	Tikosyn	125, 250, 500 mcg capsules		CrCl > 60 mL/min = 500 mcg bid; 40–60 mL/min = 250 mcg bid; 20–39 mL/ min = 125 mcg bid; < 20 mL/min = not recommended
Class IV: calcium channel blockers				
Verapamil	Calan, Calan SR, Isoptin SR, Covera-HS, Verelan, Verelan-PM	40, 80, 120 mg tablets	IV: 2.5–10 mg over 2 min	po: 120–360 mg/day
		120, 180, 240 mg tablets		IV: 5–15 mg/h
		180, 240 mg tablets		Calan, Isoptin: tid-qid
		120, 180, 240, 360 mg capsules		Calan SR, Isoptin SR, Covera-HS, Verelan: qd
		100, 200, 300 mg capsules		
		2.5 mg/mL injection		
Diltiazem	Cardizem, Cardizem CD, Cardizem Monovial, Cardizem Lyo-Ject, Cardizem SR, Cartia XT, Dilacor XR, Diltia XT, Tiazac, Cardizem LA	30, 60, 90, 120 mg tablets	IV: 20 mg over 2 min	IV: 5–15 mg/h
		5 mg/mL injection		po: 120–360 mg/day
		120, 180, 240, 300, 360 mg capsules		Cardizem: qid
		100 mg/mL injection		Cardizem SR: bid
		25 mg injection		Cardizem CD, Cardizem LA, Dilacor XR, Tiazac: qd
		60, 90, 120 mg capsules		
		120, 180, 240, 300 mg capsules		
		120, 180, 240 mg capsules		
		120, 180, 240, 300 mg capsules		
		120, 180, 240, 300, 360, 420 mg tablets		
Miscellaneous				
Atropine		0.1, 0.3, 0.4, 0.5, 0.6, 0.8, 1 mg/mL injection	0.5–1 mg q 5 min up to 3 mg total	
Adenosine	Adenocard	3 mg/mL injection		Initial dose: 6 mg IV bolus; if necessary, can be followed by 12 mg q 2 min as IV bolus; flush IV line after each administration

Table 14-4. Antiarrhythmic Drug Availability and Standard Dosing Regimens *(Continued)*

Generic name	Trade name	Dosage forms	Loading dose	Maintenance dose
Digoxin	Lanoxin, Lanoxicaps	125, 250, 500 mcg tablets 50 mcg/mL elixir 100, 250 mcg/mL injection 50, 100, 200 mcg capsules	IV and po: 0.25 mg q2h up to 1.5 mg	IV and po: 0.125–0.375 mg qd
Dronedarone	Multaq	400 mg tablets		400 mg bid

Table 14-5. Pharmacokinetics of Antiarrhythmic Drugs

Drug	Bioavailability (%)	Protein binding (%)	Primary route of elimination	Substrate for	Inhibitor of	Half-life	Therapeutic range (mg/L)
Quinidine	70–80	80–90	Hepatic	CYP3A4	CYP2D6, CYP3A4, P-gp	5–9 h	2–6
Procainamide	75–95	10–20	Hepatic and renal	NAT		2.5–5 h	4–15
Disopyramide	70–95	50–80	Hepatic and renal	CYP3A4		4–8 h	2–6
Lidocaine	20–40	65–75	Hepatic	CYP3A4, CYP2D6, CYP1A2	CYP1A2	60–180 min	1.5–5
Mexiletine	80–95	60–75	Hepatic	CYP2D6, CYP1A2	CYP1A2	6–12 h	0.8–2
Flecainide	90–95	35–45	Hepatic and renal	CYP2D6	CYP2D6	13–20 h	0.2–1
Propafenone	11–39	85–95	Hepatic	CYP2D6, CYP1A2, CYP3A4	CYP2D6	3–25 h	
Amiodarone	22–88	95–99	Hepatic	CYP3A4, CYP1A2, CYP2C19, CYP2D6	CYP1A2, CYP2C9, CYP2D6, CYP3A4, CYP2C19, P-gp	15–100 days	1–2.5
Sotalol	90–95	30–40	Renal			12–20 h	
Ibutilide		40	Hepatic			3–6 h	
Dofetilide	> 90	60–70	Renal	CYP3A4		6–10 h	
Digoxin	60–85 (90–100) for Lanoxicaps	20–30	Renal	P-gp		34–44 h	0.5–1 ng/mL
Diltiazem	35–50	70–85	Hepatic	CYP3A4, CYP2C9, CYP2D6	CYP3A4, CYP2C9, CYP2D6, P-gp	4–10 h	
Verapamil	20–40	95–99	Hepatic	CYP3A4, CYP1A2, CYP2C9	CYP3A4, CYP1A2, CYP2C9, CYP2D6, P-gp	4–12 h	
Dronedarone	4–15	> 98	Hepatic	CYP3A4	CYP3A4, CYP2D6, P-gp	13–19 h	

CYP, cytochrome P450 isoenzyme; NAT, N-acetyltransferase; P-gp, P-glycoprotein.

arrhythmias by

- Decreasing automaticity of abnormal pacemaker tissues
- Altering conduction characteristics of reentry
- Increasing refractory period
- Eliminating premature impulses that trigger reentry

Patient counseling

Patients should be counseled to take medication as prescribed. If a dose is missed, have the patient take the dose as soon as it is remembered, unless close to the next scheduled dose. In this case, the patient should skip the missed dose and continue the regular regimen; doses should not be doubled.

Many drug interactions are possible. Patients should inform health care providers of medications prescribed prior to starting new medications, including over-the-counter medications (Table 14-6).

Periodic ECG and laboratory assessments may be required to minimize or prevent adverse effects.

Patients should be educated that complete remission of their arrhythmia is unlikely. However, symptomatic arrhythmias that have increased in frequency or severity should be reported to the physician immediately.

Patients with atrial fibrillation or flutter should be educated about the importance of antithrombotic therapy as well as the signs and symptoms of stroke. Patients with symptoms including sudden onset of slurred speech, facial drooping, or muscle weakness should seek emergency care.

AADs that are administered as extended-release formulations should not be crushed, opened, or chewed. Advise patients to swallow the dose whole.

Drug-specific information

Amiodarone

The FDA now requires that a medication guide be distributed directly to each patient to whom amiodarone is dispensed.

Visual disturbances are rare but should be reported immediately to the physician.

Difficulty breathing, shortness of breath, wheezing, or persistent cough should be reported immediately to the physician.

If the patient experiences nausea or vomiting, passes brown or dark-colored urine, feels more tired than usual, or experiences stomach pain or if the patient's skin or whites of the eyes turn yellow, the symptoms should be reported immediately to the physician.

Cardiac symptoms such as pounding heart, skipping a beat, or very rapid or slow heartbeats, as well as lightheadedness or feeling faint, should be reported immediately to the physician.

Periodic laboratory tests to evaluate thyroid function, liver function, and pulmonary function, as well as diagnostic tests such as chest x-ray, ECG, and eye exams, may be necessary to assess and prevent adverse events (Table 14-7).

Amiodarone may cause skin photosensitivity. Patients should be advised to wear protective clothing and sunscreen when exposed to sunlight or ultraviolet light.

Prolonged use may cause blue-gray skin discoloration.

Patients should tell their doctor and pharmacist about all other medications they take, including prescription and nonprescription medications, vitamins, and herbal supplements.

Frequent administration with grapefruit juice may increase oral absorption. Encourage patients to drink water with amiodarone or to separate grapefruit juice consumption by at least 2 hours.

β-blockers (including sotalol)

Patients with asthma and chronic obstructive pulmonary disease should be advised that β-blockers may worsen their symptoms of airway disease. Advise patients to notify a physician immediately if this occurs.

Patients with diabetes should be advised that β-blockers may mask symptoms of hypoglycemia.

Patients should avoid abrupt withdrawal of β-blocker therapy. If withdrawal of β-blocker therapy is desired, the patient should contact the physician for the dosage-tapering regimen, if necessary.

Digoxin

Refer to chapter 13.

Warfarin

Warfarin should be avoided at any time during pregnancy.

To determine the correct dosage, the clinician will check the patient's INR regularly.

Encourage patients to maintain consistency in their diet. Abrupt changes, particularly in the intake of green leafy vegetables, may alter the effectiveness of warfarin.

Minor cuts may take longer to stop bleeding. If a cut or injury fails to stop bleeding, patients should be advised to contact their health care provider.

Excessive alcohol intake may alter the effectiveness of this medication.

Patients should tell their doctor and pharmacist about all other medications they take, including

Table 14-6. Antiarrhythmic Drug Interactions and Significant Adverse Effects

Drug	Effect of disease/drugs on antiarrhythmic drug concentrations	Effect of antiarrhythmic drug on other drug concentrations	Common or severe adverse effects
Quinidine	*Elevated:* cimetidine, amiodarone, verapamil, diltiazem, ketoconazole, urine alkalinization *Reduced:* enzyme inducers	*Elevated:* warfarin, digoxin, β-blockers, disopyramide, procainamide, propafenone, mexiletine, flecainide	QTc prolongation, torsades de pointes, diarrhea, fever, hepatitis, thrombocytopenia
Procainamide	*Elevated:* cimetidine, trimethoprim, amiodarone		Lupus-like syndrome, QTc prolongation, torsades de pointes, hypotension, gastrointestinal (GI) distress, agranulocytosis
Disopyramide	*Reduced:* enzyme inducers *Elevated:* erythromycin, protease inhibitors, cimetidine		Anticholinergic side effects, decreased cardiac contractility, heart failure, QTc prolongation, torsades de pointes, hypoglycemia
Lidocaine	*Increased:* with decreased cardiac output		Central nervous system (CNS) toxicity: paresthesias, dizziness, muscle twitching, confusion, nausea and vomiting, slurred speech, seizures, sinus arrest
Mexiletine	*Reduced:* enzyme inducers *Elevated:* quinidine, amiodarone, ritonavir	*Elevated:* theophylline	GI distress; CNS: tremor, dizziness, confusion, vertigo, nystagmus, diplopia, tremor, ataxia; hypotension; sinus bradycardia; AV block
Flecainide	*Elevated:* cimetidine, amiodarone	*Elevated:* digoxin	Proarrhythmia, prolonged PR interval and QRS complex, dizziness, blurred vision, headache, tremor, heart failure
Propafenone	*Reduced:* enzyme inducers *Elevated:* cimetidine, quinidine	*Elevated:* warfarin, digoxin, cyclosporine, theophylline	Metallic/bitter taste; CNS: dizziness, paresthesias, fatigue; GI distress; heart failure; liver injury; bradycardia; AV block; proarrhythmia
Amiodarone[a]		*Elevated:* quinidine, procainamide, warfarin, digoxin, phenytoin, cyclosporine, lovastatin, simvastatin, atorvastati	IV: phlebitis; general: corneal microdeposits, photophobia, increased liver enzymes, photosensitivity, bluegray skin discoloration, pulmonary fibrosis, hyper- and hypothyroidism, polyneuropathy
Sotalol			β-blocking effects: bradycardia, fatigue, dyspnea, bronchospasm, heart failure; QTc prolongation; torsades de pointes
Ibutilide			QTc prolongation, torsades de pointes
Dofetilide	*Elevated:* verapamil, cimetidine, ketoconazole, trimethoprim, megestrol, prochlorperazine		QTc prolongation, torsades de pointes
Digoxin	*Elevated:* quinidine, amiodarone, verapamil, diltiazem		

(continued)

Table 14-6. Antiarrhythmic Drug Interactions and Significant Adverse Effects *(Continued)*

Drug	Effect of disease/drugs on antiarrhythmic drug concentrations	Effect of antiarrhythmic drug on other drug concentrations	Common or severe adverse effects
Diltiazem	***Elevated:*** cimetidine	***Elevated:*** cyclosporine, carbamazepine, digoxin	Hypotension, bradycardia, heart failure
Verapamil	***Reduced:*** rifampin, phenobarbital	***Elevated:*** theophylline, digoxin, carbamazepine, cyclosporine, simvastatin, lovastatin	Hypotension, bradycardia, heart failure, constipation
Dronedarone	***Elevated:*** nefazodone, ritonavir, ketoconazole, itraconazole, voriconazole, telithromycin, clarithromycin, cyclosporine, grapefruit juice, verapamil, diltiazem ***Reduced:*** rifampin, phenobarbital, carbamazepine, phenytoin, St. John's wort	***Elevated:*** simvastatin, verapamil, diltiazem, nifedipine, sirolimus, tacrolimus, β-blockers, tricyclic antidepressants, selective serotonin reuptake inhibitors that are CYP2D6 substrates, digoxin, dabigatran	Contraindicated in patients with NYHA (New York Heart Association) class IV heart failure or NYHA class II–III heart failure with a recent decompensation requiring hospitalization or in patients with permanent atrial fibrillation, new or worsening heart failure, hepatocellular liver injury and acute liver failure, QTc prolongation, bradycardia, hypokalemia and hypomagnesemia when used with potassium-depleting diuretics; diarrhea, nausea, vomiting, abdominal pain, indigestion, weakness, fatigue, rash, itching

a. See Table 14-7.

prescription and nonprescription medications, vitamins, and herbal supplements.

Dabigatran

The FDA requires that the medication guide be distributed to patients when they start dabigatran and with each refill.

Dabigatran should be kept in the original bottle for protection from moisture. Once the bottle is opened, the medication should be used within 30 days. Only one capsule should be removed from the bottle at a time. Keep the bottle tightly closed when not in use.

Swallow the capsules whole. Do not break, chew, or empty the pellets from the capsule.

If a dose is missed, take it as soon as remembered. If the next dose is less than 6 hours away, skip the missed dose. Do not take two doses at the same time.

Dabigatran can be taken with or without food.

Bleeding is the most important adverse effect of dabigatran. Patients may bruise more easily and take longer for bleeding to stop. Patients should call their health care provider if any of the following occur:

- Bleeding is severe or cannot be controlled.
- Urine is pink or brown.

Table 14-7. Suggested Monitoring Guidelines for Amiodarone

Test	Baseline		6 months	12 months
Electrocardiogram	•		•	•
Pulmonary function tests	•	Routine monitoring is controversial; may repeat tests if patient becomes symptomatic.		
Ophthalmologic examination	•	Periodic exam is recommended.	•	•
Chest x-ray	•	Repeat earlier if patient becomes symptomatic.	•	•
Thyroid function tests	•		•	•
Liver enzymes	•		•	•

- Stools are red or black and tarry.
- Bruises that appear without a known cause get larger.
- Patient coughs up blood or blood clots.
- Patient vomits blood, or vomit looks like coffee grounds.
- Unexpected pain, swelling, or joint pain occurs.
- Patient has headaches, dizziness, or weakness.

Indigestion, upset stomach, or stomach pain may occur.

Patients should tell all of their health care providers, including dentists, that they are taking dabigatran. This is especially important if surgery or a medical or dental procedure is planned. Also, patients should tell their health care providers about other medications they are taking, including prescription and nonprescription medications, vitamins, and herbal supplements.

Do not run out of dabigatran. Refill the prescription before it runs out.

Rivaroxaban

The FDA requires that the medication guide be distributed to patients when they start rivaroxaban and with each refill.

Rivaroxaban is indicated to reduce the risk of stroke in patients with atrial fibrillation. Patients should not stop taking rivaroxaban without talking to their health care provider because stopping the medication can increase the risk of stroke.

Rivaroxaban should be taken once daily with the evening meal. If a dose is missed, take it as soon as remembered on the same day.

Bleeding is the most important adverse effect of rivaroxaban. Patients may bruise more easily and take longer for bleeding to stop. Patients should call their health care provider if any of the following occur:

- Bleeding is severe or cannot be controlled, such as nose bleeds that happen often, unusual gum bleeding, or menstrual bleeding that is heavier than normal.
- Urine is red, pink, or brown.
- Stools are red or black and tarry.
- Bruises that appear without a known cause get larger.
- Patient coughs up blood or blood clots.
- Patient vomits blood, or vomit looks like coffee grounds.
- Unexpected pain, swelling, or joint pain occurs.
- Patient has headaches, dizziness, or weakness.

Patients should tell all of their health care providers, including dentists, that they are taking rivaroxaban.

This is especially important if surgery or a medical or dental procedure is planned. Also, patients should tell their health care providers about other medications they are taking, including prescription and nonprescription medications, vitamins, and herbal supplements.

Do not run out of rivaroxaban. Refill the prescription before it runs out.

Apixaban

The FDA requires that the medication guide be distributed to patients when they start apixaban and with each refill.

Apixaban is indicated to reduce the risk of stroke in patients with atrial fibrillation and for prophylaxis of deep vein thrombosis after hip or knee replacement surgery. Patients should not stop taking apixaban without talking to their health care provider because stopping the medication can increase the risk of stroke.

Apixaban should be taken twice daily with or without food. If a dose is missed, take it as soon as remembered on the same day. Do not take more than one dose at the same time to make up for a missed dose.

Bleeding is the most important adverse effect of apixaban. Patients may bruise more easily and take longer for bleeding to stop. Patients should call their health care provider if any of the following occur:

- Bleeding is severe or cannot be controlled, such as nose bleeds that happen often, unusual gum bleeding, or menstrual bleeding that is heavier than normal.
- Urine is red, pink, or brown.
- Stools are red or black and tarry.
- Bruises that appear without a known cause get larger.
- Patient coughs up blood or blood clots.
- Patient vomits blood, or vomit looks like coffee grounds.
- Unexpected pain, swelling, or joint pain occurs.
- Patient has headaches, dizziness, or weakness.

Patients should tell all of their health care providers, including dentists, that they are taking apixaban. This is especially important if surgery or a medical or dental procedure is planned. Also, patients should tell their health care providers about other medications they are taking, including prescription and nonprescription medications, vitamins, and herbal supplements.

Do not run out of apixaban. Refill the prescription before it runs out.

Dronedarone

Dronedarone is indicated to reduce the risk of cardiovascular hospitalization in patients with paroxysmal or persistent atrial fibrillation or atrial flutter who are in sinus rhythm or who will be cardioverted.

Dronedarone should not be used in patients with permanent atrial fibrillation (i.e., heart rhythm remains in atrial fibrillation and cannot be changed back to normal rhythm).

Dronedarone should not be used in patients with severe heart failure because it may increase the risk of death. If patients were hospitalized for heart failure within the past month, they should not take dronedarone even if they feel better now.

Patients should be counseled to call their health care provider immediately if they experience signs and symptoms of worsening heart failure:

- Shortness of breath or wheezing at rest
- Wheezing, chest tightness, or coughing up of frothy sputum at rest, nighttime, or after minor exercise
- Trouble sleeping at night or waking up at night with problems breathing
- Use of more pillows to prop themselves up at night to breathe easier
- Rapid weight gain of more than 5 pounds
- Increased swelling in feet or legs

Dronedarone can be hepatotoxic including causing liver failure. Advise patients to report any symptoms of potential liver injury:

- Anorexia, nausea, or vomiting
- Fever or malaise
- Right upper quadrant abdominal pain or discomfort
- Jaundice, dark urine, or itching

Dronedarone can interact with many other medications. Patients should report to their health care provider and pharmacist all prescription and non-prescription medications, vitamins, or herbal supplements they are taking.

Dronedarone should be taken twice daily with food, once with the morning meal and once with the evening meal. If a dose is missed, wait and take the next dose at the regular time. Do not take two doses at the same time.

Do not drink grapefruit juice while taking dronedarone. Grapefruit juice can increase dronedarone plasma concentrations.

The most common adverse effects are diarrhea, nausea, vomiting, abdominal pain and indigestion, weakness, fatigue, rash, and itching.

A medication guide should be dispensed with dronedarone.

14-8. Questions

1. Which of the following is an adverse effect of oral amiodarone?

   A. Photosensitivity
   B. Pulmonary embolus
   C. Phlebitis
   D. Hyperkalemia
   E. Acute renal failure

2. Which of the following antiarrhythmic agents' mechanism of action is primarily the result of sodium ion transport blockade?

   A. Propafenone
   B. Ibutilide
   C. Sotalol
   D. Verapamil
   E. Diltiazem

3. First-degree atrioventricular heart block can be categorized as a disorder of

   A. automaticity.
   B. reentry.
   C. conduction.
   D. increased ventricular excitation.
   E. slowed sinus node firing.

4. Each of the following can be symptoms of atrial fibrillation *except*

   A. dizziness.
   B. palpitations.
   C. angina.
   D. hypertension.
   E. sudden-onset slurred speech.

5. Each of the following is recommended for monitoring patients requiring chronic amiodarone therapy *except*

   A. electrocardiogram.
   B. coagulation tests.
   C. thyroid function tests.
   D. liver function tests.
   E. chest x-ray.

6. For the treatment of chronic atrial fibrillation, warfarin therapy with a target INR of 2–3

would be appropriate for each of the following patients *except*

A. patients with heart failure and diabetes.
B. patients over 75 years old with hypertension.
C. a 50-year-old male with no risk factors for thromboembolism.
D. a 77-year-old female with diabetes and hypertension.
E. a 63-year-old male who has had a previous stroke.

7. The anticoagulant effect of dabigatran is mediated by

A. inhibiting synthesis of vitamin K–dependent clotting factors.
B. blocking the platelet P2Y12 receptor.
C. inhibiting clotting factor Xa.
D. direct thrombin inhibition.
E. inhibiting the VKORC1 enzyme.

8. Which of the following medications would be preferred for control of ventricular response in patients with atrial fibrillation and heart failure?

A. Digoxin
B. Verapamil
C. Diltiazem
D. Amlodipine
E. Dofetilide

9. Which of the following medications is associated with torsades de pointes?

A. Erythromycin
B. Ampicillin
C. Atenolol
D. Verapamil
E. Propafenone

10. Which of the following is an important determinant of the anticoagulant response to warfarin?

A. CYP2C19 genotype
B. CYP2D6 genotype
C. VKORC1 genotype
D. P-glycoprotein
E. Creatinine clearance

11. What is the recommended dosage regimen for dofetilide in a patient with a calculated creatinine clearance of 30 mL per minute?

A. Dofetilide therapy is not recommended.
B. 125 mcg po bid

C. 125 mg po bid
D. 500 mcg po bid
E. 500 mg po bid

12. A patient with atrial fibrillation receiving rivaroxaban should avoid which of the following?

A. Calcium supplements
B. Orange juice
C. Digoxin
D. Clarithromycin
E. Pravastatin

13. Which of the following will increase dronedarone plasma concentrations and should be avoided in patients taking this medication?

A. Grapefruit juice
B. Ranitidine
C. Atenolol
D. Nitroglycerin
E. Warfarin

14. A 66-year-old male with a past medical history of congestive heart failure and hypertension is receiving lisinopril 10 mg po qd, digoxin 0.25 mg po qd, carvedilol 25 mg bid, and spironolactone 25 mg po qd at home. He now presents to the emergency room with a 1-week history of intermittent palpitations and dizziness. The ECG reveals atrial fibrillation with a ventricular rate of 130 bpm. The decision is made to attempt to restore normal sinus rhythm. Which of the following represents the best therapeutic approach to cardioverting the patient?

A. Perform TEE; if no thrombus is present, cardiovert; there is no need for anticoagulation.
B. Perform TEE; if no thrombus is present, cardiovert; anticoagulate for at least 4 weeks postcardioversion.
C. Anticoagulate for 4 weeks prior to cardioversion; discontinue anticoagulation postcardioversion.
D. Anticoagulate for 2 weeks prior to cardioversion; continue anticoagulation for at least 4 weeks postcardioversion.
E. Direct-current cardiovert immediately.

15. After the initial successful cardioversion, the patient in the previous question continues to have recurrent symptomatic atrial fibrillation episodes. Chronic therapy to maintain sinus rhythm is to be initiated. Which of the

following antiarrhythmic drugs would be the best choice to maintain sinus rhythm?

A. Flecainide
B. Amiodarone
C. Sotalol
D. Ibutilide
E. Dronedarone

16. In a patient with mildly symptomatic PSVT, verapamil should be used for which of the following rhythms?

A. Narrow QRS complex, regular interval
B. Wide QRS complex, regular interval
C. Wide QRS complex, irregular interval
D. All wide QRS complex rhythms
E. Narrow QRS complex and hypotension

17. A 53-year-old male has a past medical history of MI and hypertension. He presents to his physician complaining of short (about 10 seconds in duration), intermittent palpitations during the past 2 days. Tests rule out an acute MI, and an echocardiogram shows a left ventricular ejection fraction of 25%. The patient is sent home with a Holter monitor to identify any arrhythmias. The Holter monitor reveals episodes of PVCs and nonsustained ventricular tachycardia. What is the most appropriate intervention for this patient?

A. No therapy is indicated.
B. Place an implantable cardioverter defibrillator.
C. Start propafenone.
D. Start verapamil.
E. Use direct-current cardioversion.

18. Treatment of torsades de pointes may include all of the following *except*

A. discontinuation of any drugs associated with prolonged QT interval.
B. isoproterenol infusion.
C. adenosine.
D. magnesium sulfate.
E. atrial–ventricular pacing.

19. Which of the following antiarrhythmic agents requires dosage adjustment in patients with impaired renal function?

A. Digoxin
B. Amiodarone

C. Lidocaine
D. Verapamil
E. Propafenone

20. Which of the following is *not* a characteristic of atrial fibrillation?

A. No discernable P waves
B. Ventricular rate of 100–130 bpm
C. Regular QRS pattern
D. Narrow QRS complex
E. Chaotic atrial contractions

21. Which of the following would be the best choice for ventricular rate control in atrial fibrillation secondary to hyperthyroidism?

A. Adenosine
B. Digoxin
C. Apixaban
D. Propranolol
E. Atropine

22. A dose-limiting adverse effect of sotalol is

A. bradycardia.
B. polyneuropathy.
C. metallic taste.
D. agranulocytosis.
E. lupus-like syndrome.

23. Which of the following is *not* available in both intravenous and oral dosage forms?

A. Metoprolol
B. Amiodarone
C. Verapamil
D. Digoxin
E. Ibutilide

24. Dosage adjustment should be considered when warfarin is administered with the following drugs *except*

A. amiodarone.
B. sotalol.
C. quinidine.
D. propafenone.
E. diltiazem.

25. The anticoagulant effect of apixaban is mediated by

A. inhibiting synthesis of vitamin K–dependent clotting factors.
B. blocking the platelet P2Y12 receptor.

C. inhibiting clotting factor Xa.

D. direct thrombin inhibition.

E. inhibiting the VKORC1 enzyme.

14-9. Answers

1. **A.** Photosensitivity is a common adverse effect of oral amiodarone. Patients should be counseled to limit sun exposure and use sunscreen. Phlebitis would be expected to occur only during intravenous amiodarone infusion, particularly through a peripheral intravenous line.

2. **A.** Propafenone blocks sodium entry into the cardiac cell, slowing depolarization. Ibutilide and sotalol act primarily by blocking potassium transport, whereas verapamil and diltiazem inhibit the calcium channel.

3. **C.** Atrioventricular heart block is caused by slowed conduction through the atrioventricular node.

4. **D.** Because of loss of functional atrial contraction and rapid ventricular rate (producing palpitations), cardiac output may decrease, resulting in decreased perfusion of major organs, particularly the brain (dizziness, confusion, etc.) and heart (angina and heart failure exacerbation). Depending on the vascular tone, blood pressure may remain stable or fall as a direct result of decreased cardiac output; however, hypertension would not be expected. Patients with atrial fibrillation are at increased risk of thrombosis, particularly stroke, secondary to pooling of blood in the left atrium and subsequent thrombus formation.

5. **B.** See Table 14-7 for recommended monitoring parameters and schedule. Coagulation tests are not routinely recommended for patients receiving amiodarone therapy. Coagulation tests may be required if a patient develops severe hepatotoxicity secondary to amiodarone or simply requires concomitant warfarin therapy for atrial fibrillation.

6. **C.** Patients under age 75 with no thromboembolic risk factors are at low risk of stroke, and no antithrombotic therapy is recommended by current guidelines.

7. **D.** Dabigatran is a direct thrombin inhibitor. It does not affect synthesis of the vitamin K–dependent clotting factors or affect platelet activity.

8. **A.** Digoxin would be the drug of first choice because it will help slow the ventricular rate and it does not have negative inotropic effects. Both verapamil and diltiazem are negative inotropes and should not be used in patients with heart failure and low LVEF. Although it is a calcium channel blocker, amlodipine does not affect AV nodal conduction. Dofetilide is used for conversion to and maintenance of sinus rhythm, not rate control.

9. **A.** Erythromycin can prolong the QTc interval and increase the risk of torsades de pointes.

10. **C.** The VKORC1 gene determines the activity of the vitamin K epoxide-reductase enzyme, which is the target for warfarin. Warfarin is not affected by mutations in the CYP2D6 or CYP2C19 genes. Warfarin is not a substrate for P-glycoprotein, and its elimination is not affected by renal function.

11. **B.** Dofetilide is renally eliminated and therefore must be adjusted according to creatinine clearance to decrease the significant risk of torsades de pointes. See Table 14-4.

12. **D.** Patients receiving rivaroxaban should avoid clarithromycin because it is a combined P-gp inhibitor and strong CYP3A4 inhibitor. Concomitant administration increases rivaroxaban plasma concentrations and increases bleeding risk.

13. **A.** Dronedarone is metabolized by CYP3A4, and grapefruit juice is a potent CYP3A4 inhibitor. Grapefruit juice should not be used by patients taking dronedarone. This combination results in significant increases in dronedarone plasma concentrations and the risk of adverse effects.

14. **B.** Because the patient appears to have been in atrial fibrillation for 1 week by history, there is a significant risk of thromboembolism during conversion to sinus rhythm. Proper treatment would require at least 3–4 weeks of anticoagulation (warfarin INR 2–3) prior to cardioversion, followed by at least 4 weeks of anticoagulation postcardioversion. Alternatively, a TEE can be used to rule out an atrial thrombus, allowing immediate cardioversion. Because the atria will require time to recover normal contractile activity, anticoagulation will be required for at least 4 weeks postconversion.

15. **B.** Because the patient has heart failure, the results of the Cardiac Arrhythmia Suppression Trial (CAST) indicate that class Ic agents should be avoided because of increased risk of death. Sotalol may worsen heart failure. Ibutilide is indicated for conversion only, not for maintenance of sinus rhythm. Dronedarone is contraindicated in patients with heart failure because of an increased risk of mortality.

16. **A.** A wide QRS complex signifies conduction via an accessory pathway other than the AV node. Because calcium channel blockers prolong conduction in the AV node and not in the accessory pathways, administration of these agents will block the AV node and force impulses to be conducted via the accessory pathways, which have shorter refractory periods. Consequently, the ventricular response will significantly increase. In the presence of hypotension, direct-current cardioversion should be used; verapamil will worsen hypotension.

17. **B.** Patients with LVEF ≤ 30–40% and previous MI are at increased risk of sudden cardiac death, usually from ventricular fibrillation. Implantation of an ICD in these patients reduces the risk of mortality. Propafenone has negative inotropic effects and may worsen heart failure. The risk of ventricular proarrhythmia is significantly increased if propafenone is used in this patient. Verapamil also would worsen heart failure and not reduce the risk of mortality. Direct-current cardioversion is not indicated because the patient is stable. All standard heart failure medications should be optimized.

18. **C.** Adenosine is typically used only to terminate PSVT. Discontinuation of drugs that prolong the QT interval is essential to terminate torsades de pointes and prevent recurrences. Treatment should consist of intravenous magnesium sulfate and electrical pacing. An isoproterenol infusion can be used while waiting for electrical pacing.

19. **A.** Digoxin requires dosage adjustment in patients with impaired renal function.

20. **C.** Atrial fibrillation represents chaotic atrial activity resulting in no identifiable P wave. Because atrial fibrillation originates above the AV node, the QRS complex is narrow and the ventricular rate is typically greater than 100 bpm.

21. **D.** β-blockers are the preferred rate-controlling agent for hyperthyroidism because they inhibit the adrenergic response and decrease thyroid hormone conversion (especially propranolol). Digoxin is not as effective in controlling the ventricular rate related to a hyperadrenergic state (hyperthyroidism).

22. **A.** Sotalol possesses significant β-blocking activity, and therefore the patient may experience adverse effects similar to traditional β-blockers.

23. **E.** All of these medications except ibutilide are available in both intravenous and oral dosage forms.

24. **B.** Warfarin is metabolized by multiple cytochrome P450 isoenzymes, including CYP2C9, CYP1A2, and CYP3A4. Amiodarone inhibits by CYP2C9, CYP1A2, and CYP3A4; quinidine by unknown mechanisms; propafenone by CYP1A2 and CYP3A4; and diltiazem by CYP3A4. Sotalol is primarily renally eliminated and does not result in cytochrome P450–mediated drug interactions.

25. **C.** Apixaban inhibits factor Xa. It does not affect synthesis of the vitamin K–dependent clotting factors or platelet activity.

14-10. References

Ageno W, Gallus AS, Wittkowsky A, et al. Oral anticoagulant therapy. *Chest*. 2012;141:e44S–88S.

Atrial Fibrillation Follow-up Investigation of Rhythm Management (AFFIRM) Investigators. A comparison of rate control and rhythm control in patients with atrial fibrillation. *N Engl J Med*. 2002;347: 1825–33.

Blomstrom-Lundqvist C, Scheinman MM, Aliot EM, et al. ACC/AHA/ESC guidelines for the management of patients with supraventricular arrhythmias: Executive summary. *J Am Coll Cardiol*. 2003;42:1493–531.

Cheng JWM, Dopp AL, Kalus JS, et al. Key articles and guidelines in the management of arrhythmias. *Pharmacotherapy*. 2011;31:1e–32e.

Connolly SJ, Ezekowitz MD, Yusuf S, et al., and the RE-LY Steering Committee and Investigators. Dabigatran versus warfarin in patients with atrial fibrillation. *N Engl J Med*. 2009;361:1139–51.

Echt DS, Liebson PR, Mitchell LB, et al. Mortality and morbidity in patients receiving encainide, flecainide, or placebo. *N Engl J Med*. 1991;324:781–88.

Gonsalves WI, Pruthi RK, Patnaik MM. The new oral anticoagulants in clinical practice. *Mayo Clin Proc.* 2013;88:495–511.

Granger CB, Alexander JH, McMurray JJ, et al. Apixaban versus warfarin in patients with atrial fibrillation. *N Engl J Med.* 2011;365:981–992.

Holbrook A, Schulman S, Witt DM, et al. Evidence-based management of anticoagulant therapy. *Chest.* 2012;141:e152S–184S.

January CT, Wann LS, Alpert JS, et al. 2014 AHA/ACC/HRS guideline for the management of patients with atrial fibrillation: A report of the American College of Cardiology/American Heart Association Task Force on Practice Guidelines and the Heart Rhythm Society. *Circulation.* 2014;129:1–123.

Katsnelson M, Sacco RL, Moscussi M. Progress for stroke prevention with atrial fibrillation: Emergence of alternative oral anticoagulants. *Circulation.* 2012;125:1577–83.

Limdi NA, Veenstra DL. Warfarin pharmacogenetics. *Pharmacotherapy.* 2008;28:1084–97.

Sanoski CA, Bauman JL. The Arrhythmias. In: Dipiro JT, Talbert RL, Yee GC, et al., eds. *Pharmacotherapy: A Pathophysiologic Approach.* 8th ed. New York, NY: McGraw-Hill; 2011:273–309.

Sanoski CA, Bauman JL. The Arrhythmias. In: Dipiro JT, Talbert RL, Yee GC, et al., eds. *Pharmacotherapy: A Pathophysiologic Approach.* 9th ed. New York, NY: McGraw-Hill; 2014:207–44.

Trujillo TC, Nolan PE. Antiarrhythmic agents: Drug interactions of clinical significance. *Drug Safety.* 2000;23:509–12.

You JJ, Singer DE, Howard PA, et al. Antithrombotic therapy for atrial fibrillation. *Chest.* 2012;141:e531S–75S.

Zipes DP, Camm AJ, Borggrefe M, et al. ACC/AHA/ESC 2006 guidelines for management of patients with ventricular arrhythmias and the prevention of sudden cardiac death: A report of the American College of Cardiology/American Heart Association Task Force and the European Society of Cardiology Committee for Practice Guidelines (Writing Committee to Develop Guidelines for Management of Patients with Ventricular Arrhythmias and the Prevention of Sudden Cardiac Death). *Circulation.* 2006;114:e385–484.

Ischemic Heart Disease and Acute Coronary Syndrome

15

Kelly C. Rogers
Carrie S. Oliphant
Shannon W. Finks

15-1. Key Points

- Angina is a syndrome described as discomfort or pain in the chest, arm, shoulder, back, or jaw. Angina is frequently worsened by physical exertion or emotional stress and is usually relieved by sublingual (SL) nitroglycerin (NTG). Patients with angina usually have coronary artery disease (CAD).
- Anginal symptoms are caused by a decrease in oxygen supply because of reduced blood flow.
- The goals for treating stable ischemic heart disease (SIHD) are to prevent death, reduce symptoms, and improve quality of life.
- Patients with SIHD should receive aspirin, β-blockers, and statin therapy. Additional anginal control can be obtained by adding on a nitrate, calcium channel blockers (CCBs), or ranolazine (Ranexa). CCBs can be combined with β-blockers (with caution) or used as a substitute because of intolerance.
- Angiotensin-converting enzyme inhibitors (ACEIs) should be prescribed to SIHD patients with reduced left ventricular ejection fraction (LVEF) ≤ 40%, hypertension (HTN), diabetes mellitus (DM), or chronic kidney disease (CKD). Angiotensin II receptor blockers (ARBs) can be used as an alternative for ACEI intolerance.
- Aspirin has been shown to decrease the incidence of myocardial infarction (MI), adverse cardiovascular events, and sudden death in patients with CAD.
- β-blockers are first-line therapy for treatment of angina in patients with or without a history of MI.
- Patients prescribed nitrates for treatment of angina need to be counseled on their appropriate use.

- Ranolazine is a novel antianginal medication that minimally affects blood pressure (BP) or heart rate (HR). It can be used as initial therapy or in combination with other antianginal medications.
- Upon hospital presentation with unstable angina (UA), non-ST-segment elevation myocardial infarction (NSTEMI), or ST-segment elevation myocardial infarction (STEMI), initial therapy includes morphine, oxygen, nitroglycerin, and aspirin. If there are no contraindications, patients should be given aspirin therapy for life.
- The first-line anti-ischemic therapy for the treatment of acute coronary syndrome (ACS) is a β-blocker and should be given orally within the first 24 hours. If chest pain continues, intravenous NTG can be considered.
- Patients who receive a stent will need dual antiplatelet therapy (DAPT). For a non-ACS indication with bare metal stent (BMS), at least 1 month of DAPT is required. For ACS indications or for drug-eluting stent (DES) placement, 12 months of DAPT is recommended. Patients treated medically following an ACS event will need aspirin indefinitely and DAPT with clopidogrel or ticagrelor for a minimum of 12 months. Prasugrel (Effient) is not recommended in patients not receiving a stent. DAPT may be considered beyond 15 months following DES in some patients.
- To reduce the risk of major bleeding, clopidogrel (Plavix) and ticagrelor (Brilinta) should be held for 5 days and prasugrel for 7 days prior to major surgery (e.g., coronary artery bypass graft [CABG]).

- All medically managed patients presenting with UA or NSTEMI should receive anticoagulation with unfractionated heparin (UFH), enoxaparin (Lovenox), or fondaparinux (Arixtra). If a percutaneous coronary intervention (PCI) is planned, acceptable options include UFH, enoxaparin, or bivalirudin (Angiomax).
- All patients presenting with STEMI who are undergoing primary PCI should receive anticoagulation with UFH or bivalirudin. If thrombolytic therapy is the chosen reperfusion strategy, anticoagulant options include UFH, enoxaparin, or fondaparinux.
- Following presentation for ACS, all patients with pulmonary congestion or an LVEF ≤ 40% should receive an ACEI within 24 hours unless contraindicated. Therapy should be continued indefinitely for patients with heart failure, LVEF ≤ 40%, HTN, or DM. An ARB can be used if the patient is ACE intolerant. Aldosterone blockade should be considered post-MI in patients with an LVEF ≤ 40% and either symptomatic HF or DM.
- Secondary prevention of MI should include DAPT, β-blockers, ACEIs, and statin therapy in all patients who have no contraindications.

15-2. Study Guide Checklist

The following topics may guide your study of this subject area:

- Risk factors for ischemic heart disease (IHD)
- Optimal acute and chronic medical treatment for SIHD and ACS
- Actions of medications used to treat patients with SIHD, ACS, and PCI
- Indications for medications used to treat SIHD, UA, NSTEMI, and STEMI
- Trade names, available dosage forms, and dosing frequency, particularly the "Top 100 Drugs" for 2012
- Major adverse drug reactions of medications used to treat SIHD and ACS
- Significant drug interactions of medications used to treat SIHD and ACS
- Differences in therapy between UA, NSTEMI, and STEMI
- Secondary prevention strategies and post-ACS discharge medications
- Any unique counseling points for patients discharged with SIHD, ACS, or post-PCI

15-3. Introduction

Definitions

- *Ischemia:* Lack of oxygen from inadequate perfusion caused by an imbalance between oxygen supply and demand.
- *Ischemic heart disease (IHD):* Disease caused most frequently by atherosclerosis. IHD may present as silent ischemia, chest pain (at rest or on exertion), or myocardial infarction (MI).
- *Angina:* Syndrome classically described as discomfort or pain in the chest, arm, shoulder, back, or jaw. Angina is frequently worsened by physical exertion or emotional stress and usually relieved by sublingual (SL) nitroglycerin (NTG). Patients with angina usually have coronary artery disease (CAD).
- *Atypical angina:* Transient pain or discomfort lacking one or more of the criteria of classic angina. Atypical angina is more common in women, elderly patients, and diabetics.
- *Acute coronary syndrome (ACS):* Syndrome encompassing the following:
  - Unstable angina (UA)
  - Non-ST-segment elevation myocardial infarction (NSTEMI)
  - ST-segment elevation myocardial infarction (STEMI)
- *Coronary artery disease:* An atherosclerotic disease of the coronary arteries that typically cycles in and out of the clinically defined phases of ACS and asymptomatic, stable, or progressive angina.
- *Percutaneous coronary intervention (PCI):* Procedure to reopen a partially or completely occluded coronary vessel to restore blood flow.
- *Coronary artery bypass graft (CABG):* Surgical procedure in which an artery such as the left internal mammary or a vein from the leg is attached to the heart as a new coronary vessel in order to bypass a diseased vessel.

Epidemiology of IHD

Cardiovascular disease (CVD) is the major cause of death in the United States. Approximately 82.6 million adult Americans have some type of CVD, which includes IHD, high blood pressure (BP), heart failure (HF), stroke, and congenital defects.

According to the American Heart Association (AHA) Heart Disease and Stroke 2014 Statistical Update, coronary heart disease is a cause of one in every six deaths in the United States. Evidence suggests that 47% of the decrease in CAD deaths over the past four to five decades is due to increased use of evidence-based medical therapy and improvements in lifestyle modification strategies.

15-4. Normal Physiology and Pathophysiology

Coronary arterioles change their resistance and dilate as needed to enable the heart to receive a fixed amount of oxygen (O_2). Increases in myocardial O_2 demand (MVO_2) such as physical exertion or an increase in BP causes the arterioles to dilate to maintain O_2 supply to the heart. In atherosclerosis, plaque narrows the larger conductance vessels, causing the arterioles to dilate under normal or resting conditions to prevent ischemia. Stress, exercise, or any increase in MVO_2 in the setting of limited O_2 supply results in ischemia and angina. Pharmacotherapy for IHD may target determinants of MVO_2 (heart rate [HR], myocardial wall tension, contractility) or myocardial O_2 supply (coronary flow, vasospasm, diastole).

15-5. Stable Ischemic Heart Disease (SIHD) and Prinzmetal's or Variant Angina

Clinical Presentation

SIHD

Symptoms are caused by decreased O_2 supply secondary to reduced flow. Angina is considered stable if symptoms have been occurring for several weeks without worsening. Characteristics of stable angina are as follows:

- Pain located over sternum that may radiate to left shoulder or arm, jaw, back, right arm, or neck
- Pressure or heavy weight on chest, burning, tightness, deep, squeezing, aching, viselike, suffocating, crushing
- Duration of 0.5–30 minutes
- Symptoms often precipitated by exercise, cold weather, eating, emotional stress, or sexual activity
- Pain relieved by SL NTG or rest

Prinzmetal's or variant angina

- This uncommon form of angina is usually caused by spasm without increased MVO_2.
- Most patients have atherosclerosis.
- Recurrent, prolonged attacks of severe ischemia are characteristic.
- Patients are often between 30 and 40 years old.
- Pain usually occurs at rest or awakens the patient from sleep.
- Electrocardiogram (ECG) shows ST-segment elevation, which returns to baseline when the patient is given NTG.

Pharmacologic Management

SIHD

Goals of therapy are as follows:

- To prevent MI and death
- To reduce symptoms of angina and occurrence of ischemia to improve quality of life

Antiplatelets

- Aspirin (acetylsalicylic acid) decreases the incidence of MI, adverse cardiovascular events, and sudden death.
- Clopidogrel has been used as an alternative when aspirin is contraindicated or in combination with aspirin in certain high-risk individuals. Ticlopidine is not recommended because of its poor side effect profile.
- Newer antiplatelet agents such as prasugrel and ticagrelor have not been studied in the setting of chronic stable angina at this time and are therefore not indicated.
- Indications for therapy are as follows:
  - Aspirin (75–162 mg daily) is recommended in all patients with SIHD (with or without symptoms) in the absence of contraindications.
  - Clopidogrel (75 mg daily) is chosen when aspirin is absolutely contraindicated.
  - The combination of clopidogrel plus aspirin is reasonable in certain high-risk patients.

Anti-ischemic therapy
β-blockers

- Effects on MVO_2 are as follows:
  - Inhibit catecholamine effects, thereby decreasing MVO_2
  - Decrease HR (negative chronotrope effects cause a decrease in conduction through the atrioventricular [AV] node)

- Decrease contractility (negative inotrope effects cause a decrease in force of contraction)
- Reduce BP
- Effects on oxygen supply are as follows:
  - β-blockers cause no direct improvement of oxygen supply.
  - They increase diastolic perfusion time (coronary arteries fill during diastole) secondary to decreased HR, which may enhance left ventricle (LV) perfusion.
  - Ventricular relaxation causes increased subendocardial blood flow.
  - Unopposed alpha stimulation may lead to coronary vasoconstriction.
- Dosing recommendations:
  - Start low, go slow.
  - Titrate to resting HR of 55–60 bpm, maximal exercise HR ≤ 100 bpm.
  - Avoid abrupt withdrawal, which can precipitate more severe ischemic episodes and MI; taper over 2 days.
- Selection of β-blockers is based on the following factors:
  - β-blockers with cardioselectivity have fewer adverse effects; they lose cardioselectivity at higher doses.
  - The intrinsic sympathomimetic activity (ISA) with acebutolol and pindolol may not be as effective because the reduction in HR would be minimal; therefore, the reduction in MVO_2 is small. β-blockers with ISA are generally reserved for patients with low resting HR who experience angina with exercise.
  - Lipophilicity is associated with more central nervous system (CNS) side effects.
  - β-blockers are preferred in patients with a history of MI, chronic heart failure, high resting HR, and fixed angina threshold.
- Indications for therapy are as follows:
  - β-blockers are used as first-line therapy if not contraindicated in patients with prior MI, ACS, or history of heart failure.
  - They are often used as initial therapy in SIHD patients without prior MI.
  - They are more effective than nitrates and calcium channel blockers (CCBs) in silent ischemia.
  - They are effective as monotherapy or with nitrates, CCBs, ranolazine, or a combination thereof.
  - β-blockers should be avoided in patients with primary vasospastic or Prinzmetal's angina.
  - They improve symptoms 80% of the time.

Nitrates
- Effects on MVO_2 are as follows:
  - Peripheral vasodilation leads to decreased blood return to the heart (preload), which leads to decreased LV volume, decreased wall stress, and decreased O_2 demand.
  - Arterial vasodilation (occurring after high doses) leads to decreased peripheral resistance (afterload), decreased systolic BP, and decreased O_2 demand.
  - Nitrates can cause a reflex increase in sympathetic activity, which may increase HR or contractility and lead to an increase in O_2 demand in some patients. This problem can be overcome with the use of a β-blocker.
- Effects on O_2 supply: Dilation of large epicardial coronary arteries and collateral vessels in areas with or without stenosis leads to increased O_2 supply.
- Indications for therapy are as follows:
  - SL NTG or NTG spray can be used for the immediate relief of angina.
  - Long-acting nitrates should be used as initial therapy to reduce symptoms only if β-blockers or CCBs are contraindicated.
  - Long-acting nitrates in combination with β-blockers can be used when initial treatment with β-blockers is ineffective.
  - Long-acting nitrates can be used as a substitute for β-blockers if β-blockers cause unacceptable side effects.
  - Nitrates are used in patients with CAD or other vascular disease.
  - Nitrates are preferred agents in the treatment of Prinzmetal's or vasospastic angina.
  - Nitrates improve exercise tolerance.
  - They produce greater effects in combination with β-blockers or CCBs.

Calcium channel blockers
- Effects on MVO_2 are as follows:
  - CCBs act primarily by decreasing systemic vascular resistance and arterial BP by vasodilation of systemic arteries.
  - They cause decreased contractility and O_2 requirement (all CCBs exert varying degrees of negative inotropic effects): verapamil (Calan, Isoptin SR, Verelan) > diltiazem (Cardizem, Cartia, Dilacor XR, Dilt-XR, Tiazac) > nifedipine (Adalat, Procardia)
  - Verapamil and diltiazem promote additional decreases in MVO_2 by decreasing conduction through the AV node, thereby decreasing HR.

- Effects on O_2 supply are as follows:
  - Increased diastolic perfusion time secondary to decreased HR, which may enhance LV perfusion
  - Decreased coronary vascular resistance and increased coronary blood flow by vasodilation of coronary arteries
  - Coronary vasodilation at sites of stenosis
  - Prevention or relief of vasospastic angina by dilation of the epicardial coronary arteries
- Indications for therapy are as follows:
  - CCBs can be used as initial therapy for reduction of symptoms. They are usually second line when β-blockers are contraindicated.
  - They are used in combination with β-blockers when initial treatment with β-blockers is not successful.
  - They are used as a substitute for β-blockers if initial treatment with β-blockers causes unacceptable side effects.
  - Slow-release, long-acting dihydropyridines and nondihydropyridines are effective in stable angina.
  - Avoid using short-acting dihydropyridines.
  - Newer-generation dihydropyridines, such as amlodipine or felodipine, can be used safely in patients with depressed LV systolic function and can be used in combination with β-blockers.

Combination therapy: β-blockers and nitrates

- β-blockers can potentially increase LV volume and LV end-diastolic pressure. Nitrates attenuate this effect.
- Nitrates increase sympathetic tone and may cause a reflex tachycardia. β-blockers attenuate this response.

Combination therapy: β-blockers and CCBs

- β-blockers and long-acting dihydropyridine CCBs are usually efficacious and well tolerated.
- CCBs, especially the dihydropyridines, increase sympathetic tone and may cause reflex tachycardia. β-blockers attenuate this effect.
- β-blockers and nondihydropyridine CCBs should be used together cautiously because the combination can lead to excessive bradycardia or AV block. The combination can also precipitate symptoms of heart failure in susceptible patients.

Ranolazine

- Unlike β-blockers and CCBs, ranolazine's anti-anginal and anti-ischemic effects occur without causing any significant hemodynamic changes in BP or HR.
- The mechanism of action is not clearly understood, but it appears to inhibit the late Na current (I_{Na}) during ischemic conditions, preventing Ca overload and ultimately blunting the effects of ischemia by improving myocardial function and perfusion.
- Ranolazine is indicated for the treatment of chronic angina and can be used in combination with β-blockers, CCBs, or nitrates.

Angiotensin-converting enzyme inhibitors

- Angiotensin-converting enzyme inhibitors (ACEIs) reduce the incidence of MI, cardiovascular death, and stroke in patients at high risk for vascular disease.
- Low-risk patients with SIHD and normal or slightly reduced LV function may not benefit from ACEI therapy as greatly as high-risk patients.
- Indications for therapy are as follows:
  - ACEIs should be used in patients with SIHD who also have left ventricular ejection fraction (LVEF) ≤ 40%, hypertension, diabetes, or chronic kidney disease (CKD) unless contraindicated.
  - They are used in high-risk patients with CAD (by angiography or previous MI) or other vascular disease.
  - It is reasonable to consider angiotensin receptor blockers (ARBs) for patients who have LVEF ≤ 40%, hypertension, diabetes, or CKD but are intolerant of ACEIs.

Lipid-lowering therapy

- Lipid-lowering therapy is recommended in patients with established CAD, including SIHD, even if only mild or moderate elevations of low-density lipoprotein (LDL) cholesterol are present.
- Omega-3 fatty acids can be encouraged in either dietary consumption or capsule form (1 g daily) for risk reduction; higher doses are recommended for treatment of elevated triglycerides.
- Therapeutic options to treat triglycerides or non-high-density lipoprotein (non-HDL) cholesterol include niacin and fibrates (after appropriate LDL-lowering therapy with statins).
- Indications for therapy are as follows:
  - Moderate- to high-intensity statins are indicated in patients with documented or suspected CAD.

- A combination of statins with other lipid-lowering therapy requires careful monitoring for the development of myopathy and rhabdomyolysis.

Prinzmetal's or variant angina

- β-blockers have no role in management and may increase painful episodes.
- β-blockers may induce coronary vasoconstriction and prolong ischemia.
- Nitrates are often used for acute attacks.
- CCBs, such as nifedipine, amlodipine (Norvasc), diltiazem, or verapamil, may be more effective, may be dosed less frequently, and have fewer side effects than nitrates.
- Nitrates can be added if there is no response to CCBs.
- Combination therapy with nifedipine + diltiazem or nifedipine + verapamil has been reported to be useful.
- Dose titration is recommended to obtain efficacy without unacceptable side effects.
- Treat acute attacks, and provide prophylactic treatment for 6–12 months.

15-6. Acute Coronary Syndrome

ACS is composed of UA, NSTEMI, and STEMI.

Pathophysiology

Tissue ischemia is a result of a mismatch between O_2 supply and demand. Most commonly, the process of ischemic syndromes involves two essential events:

- Disruption of an atherosclerotic plaque resulting in platelet aggregation
- Formation of a platelet-rich thrombus

The clinical manifestation depends on the extent and duration of the thrombotic occlusion. In UA or NSTEMI, the thrombus does not completely occlude the vessel. UA and NSTEMI are often indistinguishable by symptoms or ECG changes alone but can be differentiated by the presence or absence of positive biomarkers (Table 15-1).

UA and NSTEMI may evolve into STEMI without treatment. In STEMI, the thrombus completely occludes the coronary artery. If left untreated, this occlusion can result in sudden cardiac death.

Table 15-1. Cardiac Enzymes and ECG Changes: UA versus NSTEMI/STEMI

Biomarkers	UA	NSTEMI/STEMI
Troponin I or T	Negative	Positive
ECG changes: ST-segment, T-wave changes	ST depression or T-wave inversion; if present, may be transient or nonspecific	Abnormal changes/ST elevation

Presentation

- Central or substernal or crushing chest pain can radiate to the neck, jaws, back, shoulders, and arms.
- Patients may present with diaphoresis, nausea, vomiting, arm tingling, weakness, shortness of breath, or syncope.
- Pain may be similar to typical angina except that the occurrences are more severe, may occur at rest, and may be caused by less exertion than typical angina.
- ACS symptoms may be incorrectly interpreted as dyspepsia or indigestion.
- Pain is not usually relieved by SL NTG or rest.

Diagnosis

UA and NSTEMI

- Angina occurring at rest and persisting longer than 20 minutes; new onset angina resulting in marked limitations of normal activity; or angina that occurs more frequently, lasts longer, or occurs at a lower threshold of activity
- Cardiac enzymes (positive in NSTEMI) and ECG changes (ST depression, T-wave inversions, or transient ST elevation)

STEMI

- Similar clinical presentation as UA, NSTEMI, or both; ST-segment elevation on the ECG and elevations of cardiac enzymes
- New left bundle branch block is considered a STEMI equivalent.

See Table 15-1 for a comparison of ECG changes and cardiac enzymes in ACS.

Goals of Therapy

- Limit size of infarction or prevent progression to infarction in UA.
- Completely restore blood flow to the myocardium, resulting in tissue salvage.
- Prevent MI, arrhythmias, and ischemia.
- Reduce mortality.

See Table 15-2 for a comparison of UA/NSTEMI and STEMI.

Reperfusion therapy (STEMI)

- The goal is to open the occluded coronary artery to reestablish blood flow through the use of primary PCI (percutaneous transluminal coronary angioplasty [PTCA] with coronary stenting) or with fibrinolytic therapy.
- Mechanical reperfusion with PCI has been shown to be more successful and is preferred over fibrinolysis when the patient can be transported to a center with expert capability within 120 minutes of presentation. Primary PCI is discussed in section 15-7.

Fibrinolytic therapy (also known as thrombolytic therapy)
- Agents (see Table 15-16)
  - Reteplase (rPA; Retavase)
  - Streptokinase (Streptase)
  - Tenecteplase (TNKase)
  - Tissue plasminogen activator (tPA; Alteplase)
- Fibrinolytic therapy improves myocardial O_2 supply, limits infarct size, and decreases mortality.
- Fibrinolytic therapy achieves patency of infarcted artery in less than 60% of cases as compared to 90–100% with primary PCI and thus is not preferred when PCI is available.
- Fibrin-specific agents (alteplase, reteplase, tenecteplase) are preferred over the non-fibrin-specific agent, streptokinase.
- Fibrin-specific agents require concomitant anti-coagulation for at least 48 hours after and up to 8 days after fibrinolytic therapy or until revascularization is performed.
- Door-to-needle time of < 30 minutes is an important goal.
- Signs of successful reperfusion include relief of chest pain, resolution of ST-segment changes, and reperfusion arrhythmias, usually ventricular in nature.
- Indications for fibrinolytic therapy are as follows:
  - ST-segment elevation is > 1 mm in two or more contiguous leads or left bundle branch block is present (obscuring ST observational changes).
  - Presentation is within 12 hours of symptom onset and primary PCI is unlikely to be performed within 120 minutes of first medical contact.
  - Fibrinolytic therapy can be administered to patients with ongoing ischemia within 12–24 hours of symptom onset.
  - It should not be used in UA or NSTEMI patients.

Table 15-2. Pathophysiology: STEMI versus UA/NSTEMI

STEMI	UA/NSTEMI
Totally occlusive thrombus is present.	Platelet-rich thrombi, which do not completely block coronary blood flow, are present.
More extensive myocardial damage occurs.	Smaller, less extensive myocardial damage occurs.
STEMI results in an injury that affects the entire thickness of the myocardial wall.	NSTEMI involves only the subendocardial myocardium.
Occlusion persists long enough to compromise myocardial function and leads to myocardial necrosis.	UA is ischemia; NSTEMI may still result in necrosis, but not to the extent of STEMI.
ST-segment elevation is present on ECG.	ST depression or no ST elevation on ECG is present.
Reperfusion therapy with primary PCI or lytic therapy is a main treatment strategy.	An early invasive strategy (PCI) may be chosen for those at highest risk.

Early Hospital Management of ACS

Morphine, oxygen, nitrates, and aspirin (MONA)

Indications for therapy are shown in Table 15-3.

Anti-ischemic therapy

β-adrenergic blockade
- In STEMI patients, β-blockers have been shown to reduce the incidence of reinfarction and ventricular arrhythmias.
- Preference is for an agent without ISA.
- Agents with $β_1$ selectivity are preferred in patients with bronchoconstrictive disease.
- No evidence indicates that one agent is superior to another.

Table 15-3. Morphine, Oxygen, Nitrates, and Aspirin Therapy

Medication	Details
Morphine	Vasodilatory properties on both arterial and venous sides decrease both preload and afterload. Pain relief decreases tachycardia, along with decrease in preload and afterload; all work to decrease MVO_2.
	Increments of 2–4 mg IV are given every 5–15 minutes until pain is relieved.
	Nausea, vomiting, hypotension, sedation, and respiratory depression may occur.
	Morphine produces a vagotonic effect that may be contraindicated in patients with bradycardia. Monitor for hypotension, respiratory depression, and allergic reactions.
Oxygen	Supplemental O_2 2–4 L/min by nasal cannula is recommended to correct and avoid hypoxia, particularly within the first 2–3 hours. More aggressive ventilatory support should be considered and given as needed.
Nitrates	All patients should receive NTG as a sublingual tablet or spray 0.4 mg, if not contraindicated. If pain is unrelieved after one dose, call 911.
	IV NTG may be used in the first 48 hours in the setting of ongoing chest pain, pulmonary congestion, or hypertension.
	NTG should not be administered to patients with hypotension (SBP < 90 mm Hg), severe bradycardia, or suspected right ventricular infarction. Patients with right ventricular infarction are dependent on preload to maintain cardiac output, and the use of NTG could cause profound hypotension.
	Long-acting nitrates should be used as secondary prevention in patients who do not tolerate β-blockers and CCBs. These nitrates can be used in patients who have continual chest pain despite the use of β-blockers and CCBs. Nitrates are contraindicated if sildenafil or vardenafil has been used within 24 hours or within 48 hours of tadalafil administration.
Aspirin	Nonenteric-coated aspirin 162–325 mg should be given at the onset of chest pain unless contraindicated. Chew and swallow the first dose.
	A dose of 81–162 mg should be taken daily for life thereafter.
	Aspirin 81 mg daily after PCI is preferred over higher maintenance doses.
	Clopidogrel may be substituted if a true aspirin allergy is present or if the patient is considered unresponsive to aspirin.

- Initial choices include metoprolol and atenolol.
- Indications for therapy are as follows:
  - β-blockers should be used in all patients without contraindications.
  - The first dose should be given orally within the first 24 hours unless contraindications exist, including signs of heart failure, symptoms of low output state, increased risk of cardiogenic shock, or other relative contraindications (e.g., bradycardia, hypotension, heart block, active asthma, reactive airway disease). In patients who are hypertensive at the time of presentation, the intravenous (IV) route can be used.

Nitrates
Nitrates are discussed in Table 15-3.

Calcium channel blockers
- There is no mortality benefit from the use of CCBs; therefore, they are not recommended as first-line therapy.

- Indications for therapy are as follows:
  - In patients with contraindications to β-blockers or with recurrent ischemia receiving β-blockers and nitrates, a nondihydropyridine CCB (verapamil, diltiazem) can be used in the absence of significant LV dysfunction or other contraindications.
  - Oral long-acting dihydropyridine CCBs can provide additional control of hypertension or anginal symptoms in patients who are already receiving β-blockers and nitrates.
  - In general, short-acting dihydropyridines should be avoided. If used, combine with a β-blocker.

Antiplatelet therapy or dual antiplatelet therapy

Antiplatelet and anticoagulant strategies for ACS and PCI are outlined in Table 15-4.

Oral antiplatelet therapy
- Aspirin plus a $P2Y_{12}$ receptor antagonist (thienopyridines or ticagrelor, a cyclopentyltriazolopy-

Table 15-4. Recommendations for Evidenced-Based Antiplatelet and Anticoagulant Therapies for the Management of ACS

Recommended therapy	UA/NSTEMI	STEMI	PCI
Antiplatelet therapy			
Aspirin	Chew and swallow nonenteric-coated aspirin 162–325 mg at the onset of chest pain unless contraindicated.		Pre-PCI, if patient is already on aspirin therapy, give additional 81–325 mg. If not, give 325 mg before procedure.
	Aspirin should be continued indefinitely after ACS (with or without stenting).		Aspirin should be 81 mg daily after PCI.
P2Y$_{12}$ receptor antagonists			
	DAPT with aspirin and a P2Y$_{12}$ receptor antagonist is recommended after ACS (with or without PCI) and after PCI (with or without ACS indication).		
	If risk of morbidity from bleeding outweighs anticipated benefit, early discontinuation (< 12 months) of P2Y$_{12}$ inhibitor therapy can be considered.		
	Hold clopidogrel and ticagrelor for 5 days and prasugrel for 7 days prior to CABG surgery.		
Clopidogrel	Loading dose is 600 mg followed by 75 mg daily with aspirin for 12 months. Clopidogrel 600 mg, then 150 mg daily for 6 days, then 75 mg daily (if not at high risk of bleeding) is an alternative strategy.	Loading dose is 600 mg. For patients undergoing PCI after fibrinolytic therapy, dose is 300 mg within 24 hours and 600 mg if > 24 hours followed by 75 mg daily.	Loading dose is 600 mg (ACS and non-ACS patients) followed by 75 mg daily.
	Maintenance dose is 75 mg daily with aspirin for the following indications: • Medical management of ACS: for up to 1 year • BMS or DES for ACS: at least 12 months • DES for a non-ACS indication: at least 12 months • BMS for a non-ACS indication: minimum of 1 month and ideally up to 12 months (unless patient is at increased risk of bleeding; then minimum of 2 weeks)		
Prasugrel	Prasugrel is not recommended in ACS patients who do not undergo PCI.		Loading dose is 60 mg; continue 10 mg daily for at least 12 months. Use 5 mg daily dose for patients weighing < 60 kg.
Ticagrelor	Loading dose is 180 mg (ACS patients with or without PCI). Continue 90 mg twice daily for at least 12 months. Do not exceed 100 mg aspirin daily.		
Glycoprotein IIb/IIIa inhibitors (GPIs)			
	See Tables 15-13 and 15-14.		
Anticoagulant therapy			
Unfractionated heparin	Give 60 unit/kg bolus (maximum 4,000 units), 12 units/kg/h (maximum 1,000 units/h) for 48 hours or end of PCI with a goal aPTT of 50–70 seconds.	STEMI with fibrinolysis: Give 60 units/kg bolus (maximum 4,000 units), 12 units/kg/h (maximum 1,000 units/h) for 48 hours or end of PCI, with a goal aPTT of 50–70 seconds. STEMI with primary PCI: With GPI, give 50–70 units/kg bolus. If no GPI, give 70–100 units/kg IV. Give supplemental doses to target goal ACT.	Give supplemental doses to achieve target ACT.

(continued)

Table 15-4. Recommendations for Evidenced-Based Antiplatelet and Anticoagulant Therapies for the Management of ACS *(Continued)*

Recommended therapy	UA/NSTEMI	STEMI	PCI
Enoxaparin	Give 1 mg/kg q12h subcutaneously for duration of hospitalization (up to 8 days) or until end of PCI.	If patient < 75 years, give 30 mg IVP, followed immediately by 1 mg/kg q12h subcutaneously (first two doses maximum: 100 mg). If patient > 75 years, give no bolus, 0.75 mg/kg q12h subcutaneously (first two doses maximum: 75 mg).	If last dose < 8 hours, no additional dose is needed. If last dose 8–12 hours before PCI, or if fewer than two therapeutic doses received, give 0.3 mg/kg IVP.
	If CrCl < 30 mL/min, dose at 1 mg/kg subcutaneously daily.		
	Avoid if history of heparin-induced thrombocytopenia.		
Bivalirudin	Give 0.75 mg/kg IVP, then 1.75 mg/kg/h IV.	Give 0.75 mg/kg IVP, then 1.75 mg/kg/h IV.	Give 0.75 mg/kg IVP, then 1.75 mg/kg/h IV. Discontinue at end of PCI or continue for up to 4 hours.
	Adjust infusion in severe renal dysfunction. If CrCl < 30 mL/min, reduce infusion to 1 mg/kg/h. If patient is on hemodialysis, reduce infusion to 0.25 mg/kg/h.		
Fondaparinux	Give 2.5 mg subcutaneously daily.	Give 2.5 mg IV push, then 2.5 mg subcutaneously daily.	Fondaparinux should not be used as the sole anticoagulant for PCI. Add UFH or bivalirudin at time of PCI if fondaparinux was given before PCI.
	Therapy is continued for the duration of the hospitalization (up to 8 days).		
	Fondaparinux is contraindicated in patients with CrCl < 30 mL/min.		

ACT, activated clotting time; BMS, bare metal stents; CrCl, creatinine clearance; DES, drug-eluting stents; IVP, IV push.
Boldface indicates one of top 100 drugs for 2012 by units sold at retail outlets, www.drugs.com/stats/top100/2012/units.

rimidine) reduces rates of atherothrombotic events in patients with ACS and reduces risk of stent thrombosis after PCI.

■ The mechanism of platelet aggregation for the P2Y$_{12}$ receptor antagonists and aspirin differ; therefore, their effects are additive; bleeding risk is higher with dual antiplatelet therapy (DAPT) over aspirin alone.

P2Y$_{12}$ receptor antagonists
Thienopyridines
■ Clopidogrel and prasugrel are the members of this class.
■ Inhibition of platelet aggregation is irreversible.
■ Therapy is initiated with a loading dose for a more rapid effect.

Cyclopentyltriazolopyrimidine
■ Ticagrelor is the only medication in this class.
■ Inhibition of platelet aggregation is reversible, although it should still be held 5 days before major surgery to reduce the risk of bleeding.

■ The drug has a unique side effect profile compared to the other P2Y$_{12}$ receptor antagonists because of inhibition of adenosine reuptake.
■ A loading dose is given to initiate therapy for a more rapid effect.
■ Twice-daily dosing is different from other P2Y$_{12}$ receptor antagonists and is an important consideration for patient adherence.

Indications for antiplatelet therapy
Clopidogrel
■ Reduces rate of atherothrombotic events (MI, stroke, vascular deaths) in patients with recent MI or stroke or with established peripheral arterial disease
■ Reduces rate of atherothrombotic events in patients with UA or NSTEMI managed medically or with PCI (with or without stent)

■ Reduces rate of death and atherothrombotic events in patients with STEMI managed medically

Prasugrel

■ Prasugrel is used to reduce thrombotic cardiovascular events (including stent thrombosis) in patients with ACS who are to be managed with PCI.

■ Prasugrel is contraindicated in patients with previous stroke or TIA.

Ticagrelor

■ Ticagrelor is used in conjunction with aspirin (< 100 mg daily) to reduce the rate of death and atherothrombotic events in patients with ACS managed medically or with PCI.

Glycoprotein IIb/IIIa receptor inhibitors

Glycoprotein IIb/IIIa receptor inhibitors (GPIs) are discussed in section 15-7. Also refer to Tables 15-4, 15-13, and 15-14.

Agents

■ Abciximab (ReoPro)
■ Eptifibatide (Integrilin)
■ Tirofiban (Aggrastat)

Indications for therapy

All of these agents can be used as adjunctive therapy in patients undergoing PCI. Use of these agents in the setting of PCI is covered in Table 15-4.

Anticoagulant therapy

Anticoagulant therapy should be added to antiplatelet therapy as soon as possible following presentation of ACS. Acceptable options include unfractionated heparin (UFH), enoxaparin, bivalirudin, and fondaparinux (see Table 15-4).

Agent selection depends on type of ACS, management strategy (invasive versus conservative), and the need for a surgical procedure (CABG).

Indications for anticoagulant therapy are as follows:

■ UA and NSTEMI
  • In patients with a planned conservative strategy (i.e., medical management), enoxaparin, UFH, and fondaparinux are options.
  • Fondaparinux is preferred in patients who are considered a high bleeding risk.
  • For patients with a planned PCI procedure, the preferred agents include UFH, enoxaparin, and bivalirudin.

■ STEMI
  • For patients with a planned PCI procedure, the preferred agents include UFH, enoxaparin, and bivalirudin.
  • UFH, enoxaparin, or fondaparinux can be used in patients receiving fibrinolytic therapy.

Unfractionated heparin

■ UFH indirectly inhibits thrombin by accelerating the body's own natural antithrombin.

■ UFH is continued for 48 hours or until a PCI procedure is completed.

Enoxaparin

■ Enoxaparin is a low molecular weight heparin (LMWH).

■ LMWH differs from UFH in size and affinity for thrombin.

■ Advantages of LMWH over UFH include better bioavailability, more predictable response, ease of administration, fewer side effects, and no recommended routine monitoring.

■ Enoxaparin is continued for the duration of the hospitalization (up to 8 days) or until a PCI procedure is completed.

Bivalirudin

■ Bivalirudin is a direct thrombin inhibitor.

■ Bivalirudin differs from UFH in that it can inhibit both clot-bound and free thrombin.

■ Studies have shown that bivalirudin is noninferior to heparin plus GPI, but with less bleeding.

■ Bivalirudin is continued until the angiography or PCI procedure is completed.

Fondaparinux

■ Fondaparinux is an indirect factor Xa inhibitor.
■ Fondaparinux has no effect on thrombin.
■ Fondaparinux has been found to be noninferior to enoxaparin in reducing the risk of ischemic events and has a lower incidence of major bleeding events in NSTEMI patients.
■ Therapy is continued for the duration of the hospitalization (up to 8 days).
■ Fondaparinux is not indicated in patients who undergo PCI because of an increase in catheter-related thrombosis.

Statin therapy

■ HMG-CoA (3-hydroxy-3-methyl-glutaryl-coenzyme A) reductase inhibitors (statins) should be started in all ACS patients without contraindications.

- Among patients with ACS, high-intensity statin therapy reduces major adverse cardiovascular events compared with moderate-intensity statin therapy.
- Administration of a high-intensity statin is reasonable before PCI to reduce risk of peri-procedural MI in both statin-naïve patients and those already receiving statins.

Inhibition of the renin–angiotensin–aldosterone system

- ACEIs, ARBs, and aldosterone antagonists (spironolactone, eplerenone [Inspra]) are agents that inhibit the renin–angiotensin–aldosterone (RAA) system.
- Indications for therapy are as follows:
  - ACEIs should be started orally within the first 24 hours in all patients with STEMI in anterior location, HF, or LVEF ≤ 40% unless contraindicated.
  - ACEIs should be given to patients with UA/NSTEMI with HF, LV dysfunction, hypertension, or diabetes, unless contraindicated.
  - It is reasonable to use ACEIs orally within the first 24 hours in all patients with ACS unless contraindicated.
  - An intravenous ACEI should not be used within the first 24 hours because of hypotension risk.
  - ARBs should be given to those patients with ACS who have indications for but are intolerant of an ACEI.

Analgesia in Patients with ACS

- Discontinue nonsteroidal anti-inflammatory drugs (NSAIDs) except for aspirin at time of ACS presentation.
- NSAIDs should not be started during hospitalization for ACS.
- If pain management is required at discharge, a stepped-care approach should be taken, starting with acetaminophen or aspirin, small doses of narcotics, or nonacetylated salicylates and nonselective NSAIDs (e.g., naproxen).

Secondary Prevention of ACS

Dual antiplatelet therapy

DAPT is indicated post-ACS in all patients. (Refer to Table 15-4 for dosing strategies.)

β-blockers

β-blockers are indicated long term following ACS in patients with LVEF < 40% with heart failure, unless contraindicated.

β-blockers are recommended for 3 years post-MI in patients with normal LVEF. Evidence indicates treatment beyond 3 years may be reasonable in some patients.

Inhibition of the RAA system

- ACEIs are recommended long term for patients with LVEF < 40%, hypertension, CKD, or diabetes, unless contraindicated.
- It is also appropriate to administer an ACEI or ARB to patients without LV dysfunction, diabetes, or hypertension, unless contraindicated.
- Consider ACEI in all high-risk patients with CAD.
- ARBs are recommended in patients who are intolerant of ACEIs.
- Unless contraindicated, long-term aldosterone blockade should be prescribed for patients who are already receiving therapeutic doses of ACEIs and β-blockers and who have an LVEF ≤ 40% and either symptomatic heart failure or diabetes. Creatinine clearance (CrCl) should be > 30 mL/min, and potassium should be < 5 mEq/L.

Lipid-lowering therapy

Moderate- to high-intensity statin therapy is indicated for all patients post-ACS unless contraindicated.

Nitroglycerin

Upon discharge from the hospital for an ACS event, patients should receive a prescription for SL NTG and be instructed on its proper use.

15-7. Revascularization

Percutaneous Coronary Intervention

Procedure types include balloon angioplasty (PTCA), coronary stenting, and ablative technologies (laser, atherectomy).

Potential complications of invasive PCI include problems with the arterial access site, technical complications, acute vessel closure, restenosis, and acute renal failure secondary to nephrotoxic dye.

Indications are as follows:

- STEMI
  - Primary PCI is the preferred method over fibrinolytic therapy for reestablishing coronary perfusion.
  - Primary PCI should be performed as quickly as possible with the goal of first medical contact-to-device time of 90 minutes.
- UA and NSTEMI
  - If an invasive strategy is selected, the PCI procedure is typically done within the first 48 hours of hospital admission.

Bare Metal Stents and Drug-Eluting Stents

Restenosis is the loss of 50% or more of the diameter of the in-stent lumen at the site of an initially successful intervention; it usually occurs within the first 3–6 months after PCI.

Drug-eluting stents (DES) were introduced in 2003 and have the principal advantage of reducing restenosis to less than 5% over angioplasty alone and bare metal stents (BMS).

DES have pharmacologic agents, such as sirolimus, paclitaxel, zotarolimus, and everolimus, embedded in the stent and released over time.

Anticoagulation during PCI

Anticoagulation is mandatory because the vessel manipulation during PCI is inherently thrombogenic. See Table 15-4 for specific differences in antiplatelet and anticoagulant recommendations.

Antiplatelet therapy surrounding PCI

Dual antiplatelet therapy (aspirin plus a P2Y$_{12}$ receptor antagonist)
- Nonenteric aspirin 162–325 mg should be administered prior to PCI for patients already taking aspirin.
- A loading dose of clopidogrel 600 mg, prasugrel 60 mg, or ticagrelor 180 mg is recommended as early as possible or at the time of PCI.
- After PCI for ACS, clopidogrel, ticagrelor, or prasugrel, in combination with aspirin, is used to reduce in-stent thrombosis and for a minimum of 12 months regardless of type of stent received. Continuation of DAPT beyond 15 months may be considered in select patients who receive a DES.
- After PCI with a DES for a non-ACS indication, clopidogrel is the preferred agent and is recommended for at least 12 months.

- After PCI with a BMS for a non-ACS indication, clopidogrel is recommended for a minimum of 1 month and ideally up to 12 months, unless the patient has a high bleeding risk (can use for a minimum of 2 weeks).
- After PCI, aspirin 81 mg daily should be continued indefinitely.

Glycoprotein IIb/IIIa inhibitors
- GPIs are considered before or during PCI for UA and NSTEMI patients receiving UFH who have high-risk features such as elevated cardiac biomarkers.
- GPIs are of uncertain benefit in those adequately pretreated with a P2Y$_{12}$ inhibitor.
- Although not routine, it is reasonable to administer GPIs during primary PCI in select patients with STEMI, especially if they have a large anterior MI or a large thrombus burden.
- Special attention should be focused on proper dosage adjustments of renally cleared agents, especially in elderly patients, women, and those with renal insufficiency.
- Indications for therapy are as follows:
  - Routine use of upstream GPIs in patients with STEMI undergoing primary PCI is not recommended.
  - GPIs are reasonable in ACS patients undergoing PCI treated with UFH whether or not pretreatment with clopidogrel was given.
  - In patients undergoing elective PCI who are treated with UFH and not pretreated with clopidogrel, it is reasonable to administer GPIs.

Coronary Artery Bypass Graft Surgery

- CABG is indicated in patients with multivessel disease, severe left main coronary artery disease, or significant disease of a major coronary vessel that is not amenable to PCI.
- P2Y$_{12}$ receptor antagonists should be discontinued for a minimum of 5 days (clopidogrel and ticagrelor) and 7 days (prasugrel) before CABG to reduce the risk of bleeding.
- In an emergency CABG, clopidogrel and ticagrelor should be held for at least 24 hours to minimize risk of CABG-related bleeding.
- For UA and NSTEMI patients when CABG is selected as a postangiography management strategy, discontinue long-acting anticoagulant (enoxaparin 12–24 hours and fondaparinux 24 hours) and injectable antiplatelet agents

(eptifibatide or tirofiban 2–4 hours and abciximab 12 hours) prior to surgery. UFH can be used and continued up until time of surgery.

15-8. Primary Prevention: Risk Factor Modification

The majority of the causes of CVD are known and modifiable. Therefore, risk factor screening should begin at age 20 with the hope that all adults know the levels and significance of risk factors as routinely assessed by their primary care provider.

Nonmodifiable Risk Factors

Age

- Men > 45
- Women > 55 (or those who had an early hysterectomy regardless of age)

Race

Higher risk exists in African American males and females than in Caucasian males and females.

Family history

- Father or brother with a coronary event before age 55
- Mother or sister with a coronary event before age 65

Modifiable Risk Factors

- Smoking
- Hypertension
- Hyperlipidemia (low HDL-cholesterol; high LDL-cholesterol)
- Diabetes
- Metabolic syndrome
- Obesity or physical inactivity
- Alcohol consumption
- Other emerging inflammatory markers

Pharmacologic Therapy

Aspirin

The Ninth American College of Clinical Pharmacy Evidence-Based Clinical Practice Guidelines on Antithrombotic and Thrombolytic Therapy (Chest Guidelines) recommends that aspirin (75–100 mg/day) be considered for individuals who are without contraindications and 50 years of age or older (regardless of cardiac risk profile, gender, or other patient characteristics).

The recommendation for aspirin use for primary prevention is stronger in men than in women. The primary prevention guidelines in women recommend that aspirin be prescribed according to the risk profile (stroke or MI) and age:

- For women < 65 years of age who are at risk for ischemic stroke and have low bleeding risk, 75–100 mg/day is recommended to prevent stroke.
- For women > 65 years of age who are at risk for ischemic stroke or MI and have low bleeding risk, 75–100 mg/day is recommended to prevent stroke and MI.
- The routine use of aspirin in healthy women < 65 years is not recommended to prevent MI.

For the diabetic patient, the American Diabetes Association recommends considering aspirin therapy (75–162 mg/day) to prevent cardiovascular events in patients with diabetes who have a greater than 10% risk of a cardiac event over 10 years and who are without contraindications to aspirin. (Those adults with diabetes who fit this increased risk category include most men over age 50 and women over age 60 who have one or more of the additional following risk factors: smoking, hypertension, dyslipidemia, family history, CVD, and albuminuria.)

ACEIs and ARBs

- Based on clinical trials, the use of ACEIs in high-risk patients has been shown to reduce the risk of MI, stroke, and death from cardiovascular causes.
- Chronic ACEI therapy may be most beneficial in high-risk patients (uncontrolled hyperlipidemia, hypertension, smoking, proteinuria, vascular disease).

Lipid lowering

- Consider moderate- to high-intensity statins along with lifestyle therapy in all patients with a 10-year risk of arteriosclerotic cardiovascular disease ≥ 7.5%.

Nonpharmacologic Therapy for IHD

Smoking cessation

- Smoking cessation is one of the most important risk-modifying behaviors. Evidence suggests that the best adherence to a cessation program combines pharmacotherapy with behavioral modification.

- A wide range of smoking cessation aids (prescription and nonprescription) and products is available.
- Nicotine replacement alone is not an effective management strategy for smoking cessation. Behavioral modifications (i.e., counseling, smoking cessation programs) combined with pharmacotherapy have been the most successful.

Diet

- Diets low in saturated fat and high in fruits, vegetables, whole grains, and fiber should be considered heart healthy.
- For omega-3 fatty acids, the AHA Dietary Guidelines recommend inclusion of at least two servings of fish per week (particularly fatty fish).
- Evidence supports a strong link between an overall healthy dietary pattern, in particular the Mediterranean diet, and a reduction in CVD mortality.

Exercise

- Exercise plays a role in both primary and secondary prevention of CVD.
- Current guidelines from the U.S. Centers for Disease Control and Prevention and National Institutes of Health recommend that Americans should accumulate at least 30 minutes of moderate-intensity physical activity on most, preferably all, days of the week to prevent risk of chronic disease in the future.
- The Institute of Medicine recommends 60 minutes of physical activity per day.
- A combination of aerobic exercise with flexibility and weight training is recommended at least twice weekly to increase lean muscle tissue.

Weight loss

- Weight loss can reduce blood pressure, lower blood glucose levels, and improve blood lipid abnormalities. A goal of 5–10% of body weight loss is associated with decreased morbidity and mortality.
- Pharmacotherapy used for weight loss should be reserved for (1) those with a body mass index exceeding 30 and (2) those with a body mass index exceeding 27 plus other risk factors for comorbid diseases.

Alcohol consumption

- Lowest cardiovascular mortality occurs in those who consume one or two drinks per day. People with no alcohol consumption have higher total mortality than those drinking one or two drinks per day.
- In the absence of alcohol-related illnesses, one or two drinks per day in males and one alcoholic drink per day in females may be considered for high-risk patients.
- A drink equivalent amounts to a 12-ounce bottle of beer, a 5-ounce glass of wine, or a 1.5-ounce shot of 80 proof spirits.
- A general increase in alcohol consumption at the population level is not recommended.

15-9. Pharmacology

Anti-ischemic Drug Therapy

β-blockers

See Chapter 12 for specific pharmacology information about β-blockers.

Nitrates

Mechanism of action
- Organic nitrates are pro-drugs that must be transformed to exert pharmacological effect.
- Denitration of NTG leads to liberation of NO, which results in guanylate cyclase stimulation, leading to an increase in cyclic guanosine monophosphate, ultimately causing vasodilation.
- NO also reduces platelet adhesion and aggregation and affects endothelial function and vascular growth.

Properties
- ***Oral:*** Isosorbide dinitrate and NTG undergo extensive first-pass metabolism when given orally. Isosorbide mononitrate does not; it is completely bioavailable. Oral NTG requires a nitrate-free interval of 8–12 hours between doses to prevent tolerance.
- ***IV:*** IV use achieves the highest concentrations. Usually, IV is used for only 24–48 hours to avoid developing tolerance.
- ***SL tablet or spray for immediate release:*** Unlike tablets, spray does not degrade when exposed to air. The half-life is 1–5 minutes regardless of route.

Table 15-5. Pharmacologic Properties and Doses of Nitrates

Drug	Route	Onset	Duration of action	Dose
Nitroglycerin sublingual tablet (Nitrostat, Nitroquick)	Sublingual	1–3 min	30–60 min	0.2–0.6 mg every 5 min. Seek emergency treatment if chest pain is unrelieved after one dose.
Nitroglycerin spray (Nitrolingual, Nitromist)	Translingual	2 min	30–60 min	0.4 mg every 5 min. Seek emergency treatment if chest pain is unrelieved after one spray.
Nitroglycerin ointment (Nitro-Bid, Nitrol)	Topical	30–60 min	2–12 hours	1–2 inches every 8 hours up to 4–5 inches every 4 hours. Allow a 10–12 hour nitrate-free interval.
Nitroglycerin transdermal patches (Nitro-Dur, Minitran)	Topical	30–60 min	Up to 24 hours	Starting dose: 0.2–0.4 mg/h. Apply, and allow patch to stay in place for 12 hours. Remove the patch after 12 hours to allow a nitrate-free interval.
Nitroglycerin sustained-release tablets or capsules	Oral	20–45 min	3–8 hours	Starting dose: 2.5 mg tid–qid. Increase the dose by 2.5 mg two to four times daily to reach effective dose. Allow a 10–12 hour nitrate-free interval.
Nitroglycerin intravenous	IV	1–2 min	3–5 min	Starting dose: 5 mcg/min. Titrate every 3–5 minutes to response. Tachyphylaxis will develop within 24 hours.
Isosorbide mononitrate (Ismo, Monoket)	Oral	30–60 min	No data	20 mg bid (given 7 hours apart). May need to start with 5 mg bid for low-weight patients.
Isosorbide mononitrate, extended-release (Imdur)	Oral	30–60 min	No data	Starting dose: 30–60 mg daily. Maximum dose: 240 mg daily.
Isosorbide dinitrate (Isordil Titradose)	Oral	20–40 min	4–6 hours	Starting dose: 5–20 mg q6h. Maintenance dose: 10–40 mg q6h. Allow a 10–12 hour nitrate-free interval.
Isosorbide dinitrate, sustained-release tablets or capsules (Dilatrate-SR)	Oral	Up to 4 hours	6–8 hours	Initial dose: 40 mg q8h. Maintenance dose: 40–80 mg q8–12h. Allow a 10–12 hour nitrate-free interval.

Doses
See Table 15-5 for dosing information.

Monitoring parameters
Blood pressure and heart rate should be monitored.

Adverse drug reactions
Adverse drug reactions to nitrate are described in Table 15-6.

Drug–drug interactions
Nitrate drug–drug interactions are described in Table 15-7.

Drug–disease interactions
- Glaucoma
  - Intraocular pressure may increase.
  - Use with caution in patients with glaucoma.
- Hypertrophic obstructive cardiomyopathy

Table 15-6. Nitrate Adverse Reactions

Type	Reaction
Tolerance	Can develop if dosing does not allow for a nitrate-free interval (10–12 hours)
CNS	Headache (up to 50%), dizziness, anxiety, nervousness
Cardiovascular	Hypotension, tachycardia, palpitations, syncope
Gastrointestinal	Nausea, vomiting, dyspepsia
Dermatologic	Rash or dermatitis
Other	Blurred vision, muscle twitching, perspiration, edema, arthralgia

Table 15-7. Nitrate Drug–Drug Interactions

Interacting medication	Effect
Sildenafil, vardenafil, tadalafil	Significant reduction of blood pressure may occur.
	Do not give sildenafil or vardenafil within 24 hours and tadalafil within 48 hours of nitrate use.
Calcium channel blockers	Symptomatic hypotension may occur.
Alcohol	Symptomatic hypotension may occur.

■ Severe aortic stenosis: Can cause hypotension and syncope

Contraindications
■ Sildenafil (Viagra) or vardenafil (Levitra) use within 24 hours
■ Tadalafil (Cialis) use within 48 hours
■ Hypersensitivity to nitrates

Patient instructions and counseling
■ General instructions:
  • Avoid alcohol consumption.
  • May cause dizziness; use caution when driving or engaging in hazardous activities until drug effect is known.
  • When standing from a sitting position, rise slowly to avoid an abrupt drop in blood pressure.
  • Notify physician of acute headache, dizziness, or blurred vision.
■ Instructions for SL tablets:
  • Keep tablets in their original container.
  • Dissolve tablet under the tongue. Lack of tingling does not indicate a lack of potency.
  • Take one tablet at the first sign of chest pain. If chest pain is unrelieved after one tablet, seek emergency medical attention.
■ Instructions for translingual spray:
  • Spray under tongue or onto tongue.
  • Hold spray nozzle as close to the mouth as possible, and spray medicine onto or under the tongue.
  • Do not inhale the spray, use near heat or open flame, or use while smoking.
  • Close mouth immediately after spraying.
  • Avoid eating, drinking, or smoking for 5–10 minutes.
  • If the pain does not go away after one spray, seek emergency medical attention.
■ Instructions for ointment:
  • Measure the correct amount using the papers provided with the product.
  • Use papers for the application, not fingers.
  • Apply to the chest or back.
  • Wipe off any residual ointment before applying another dose.
■ Instructions for transdermal patches:
  • Tear the wrapper open carefully. Never cut the wrapper or patch with scissors. Do not use any patch that has been cut by accident.
  • Apply to a hairless area, and rotate sites to avoid irritation.

  • Do not put the patch over burns, cuts, or irritated skin.
  • Remove the patch approximately 12–14 hours after placing it on every day. This prevents tolerance to the beneficial effects of NTG.
  • Used patches may still contain residual medication; use caution when disposing around children and pets.
  • Store the patches at room temperature in a closed container, away from heat, moisture, and direct light. Do not refrigerate.
■ Instructions for sustained-release tablets:
  • Take at the same time each day as directed.
  • Do not chew or crush tablets or capsules.

Calcium channel blockers

See Chapter 12 for specific pharmacology information about CCBs.

Ranolazine

Mechanism of action
The mechanism of action of ranolazine is not clearly understood but appears to inhibit the late Na current (I_{Na}), preventing Ca overload and ultimately blunting the effects of ischemia by improving myocardial function and perfusion.

Dose
■ Initiate at 500 mg po bid, and titrate to a maximum dose of 1 g po bid as tolerated.
■ Take without regard to meals. Do not crush, break, or chew tablet.

Monitoring parameters
■ Monitor anginal symptoms.
■ Perform baseline and follow-up ECGs to evaluate QT interval.
■ Monitor BP regularly in patients with severe renal insufficiency.

Adverse drug reactions
Adverse reactions to ranolazine are described in Table 15-8.

Drug–drug interactions
Drug–drug interactions are described in Table 15-9.

Contraindications
■ Use with strong CYP3A (cytochrome P450 3A) inhibitors or inducers.
■ Use in patients with clinically significant hepatic impairment.

Table 15-8. Ranolazine Adverse Drug Reactions

Type	Reaction
CNS	Dizziness, headache, asthenia
Cardiovascular	Bradycardia, palpitations, hypotension, orthostatic hypotension
Gastrointestinal	Nausea, abdominal pain, vomiting, dry mouth, constipation
Other	Tinnitus, vertigo, dyspnea, peripheral edema

Table 15-9. Ranolazine Drug–Drug Interactions

Interacting medication	Effect
Strong CYP3A inhibitors: Ketoconazole, itraconazole, clarithromycin, nefazodone, ritonavir, nelfinavir, indinavir, saquinavir	Medication increases average steady-state plasma concentration of ranolazine threefold, which can precipitate QTc prolongation. Concomitant use is contraindicated.
Moderated CYP3A inhibitors: Diltiazem, verapamil, erythromycin, fluconazole, grapefruit juice	Medication increases ranolazine steady-state plasma concentrations twofold, which can precipitate QTc prolongation. Limit the dose of ranolazine to 500 mg twice daily.
P-glycoprotein inhibitors: Cyclosporine	Increased ranolazine concentrations can occur; use lower doses of ranolazine.
CYP3A inducers: Rifampin, rifabutin, phenobarbital, phenytoin, carbamazepine, St. John's Wort	Medication decreases plasma concentrations of ranolazine by up to 95%. Concomitant use is contraindicated.
CYP3A substrates: Simvastatin, lovastatin, cyclosporine, tacrolimus, sirolimus	Ranolazine may increase plasma concentrations. Plasma levels of simvastatin are increased approximately twofold. Do not exceed 20 mg of simvastatin. Dose adjustment of other substrates may be necessary.
Drugs transported by P-glycoprotein: Digoxin	Concomitant use may result in increased digoxin concentrations.
CYP2D6 substrates: TCAs, antidepressants, antipsychotics	Concomitant use may result in increased concentration of these substrates, and lower doses may be required.
Drugs transported by OCT2: Metformin	Increased levels of metformin can occur. Do not exceed metformin 1,700 mg daily when ranolazine 1,000 mg twice daily is co-administered. Monitor blood glucose carefully.

CYP, cytochrome P450; OCT2, organic cation transporter 2; TCA, tricyclic antidepressant.

Patient instructions and counseling
- Ranolazine is not for use with acute anginal symptoms.
- Notify physician if you take any other medications, including over-the-counter medications.
- Notify physician if you have any history or family history of QTc prolongation or congenital long-QT syndrome or if you are receiving drugs that prolong the QTc interval, such as antiarrhythmic agents, erythromycin, and certain antipsychotics (thioridazine, ziprasidone).
- Notify physician if you start any new medications.
- Ranolazine can be taken with or without meals.
- Ranolazine should be swallowed whole; do not crush, break, or chew tablets.
- Ranolazine may cause dizziness or lightheadedness; therefore, notify physician if you experience fainting spells, and know how you react to this drug before operating heavy machinery.

Inhibition of the RAA system

See Chapter 12 for specific pharmacology information about ACEIs, ARBs, and aldosterone antagonists.

Antiplatelet Drug Therapy

Aspirin

Mechanism of action
Aspirin blocks prostaglandin synthesis, which prevents the formation of thromboxane A_2.

Dose
- At the onset of chest pain: 162–325 mg chewed and swallowed
- Maintenance dose:
  - Aspirin 325 mg given at least 2 hours and preferably 24 hours before PCI is recommended, after which aspirin 81 mg daily should be continued indefinitely.
  - The maximum dose of aspirin is 100 mg daily when used in combination with ticagrelor.
  - Following CABG surgery, aspirin should be started within 6 hours of surgery at a dose of 100–325 mg daily and administered indefinitely.
- Monitoring parameters: Signs of bleeding, gastrointestinal intolerance, renal function, and tinnitus

Table 15-10. Aspirin Adverse Reactions

Type	Reaction
Cardiovascular	Hypotension, edema, tachycardia
CNS	Fatigue, nervousness, dizziness
Dermatologic	Rash, urticaria, angioedema
Gastrointestinal	Nausea, vomiting, dyspepsia, gastrointestinal ulceration, gastric erosion, duodenal ulcers
Hematologic	Bleeding, anemia
Otic	Hearing loss, tinnitus
Renal	Renal impairment, increased serum creatinine, proteinuria
Respiratory	Asthma, bronchospasm, dyspnea, tachypnea, respiratory alkalosis

Adverse drug reactions

Adverse reactions to aspirin are described in Table 15-10.

Drug–drug interactions

Antiplatelet agents, anticoagulants, and NSAIDs may all increase the risk of bleeding if used in combination with aspirin.

Drug–disease interactions

- Peptic ulcer disease (PUD).
- Other active bleeding.
- Aspirin may cause gastric ulceration or gastritis.
- An enteric-coated tablet may reduce gastrointestinal intolerance.

Patient instructions and counseling

- Avoid additional over-the-counter products containing aspirin, NSAIDs, or salicylate ingredients without the direction of a physician.
- Patients who receive a stent for an ACS indication will need aspirin indefinitely and DAPT consisting of clopidogrel, prasugrel, or ticagrelor for a minimum of 1 year. Patients who received a stent for a non-ACS indication will need aspirin indefinitely and DAPT consisting of clopidogrel for a minimum of 1 month (BMS) and up to 1 year (DES). Patients treated medically following an ACS event will need aspirin indefinitely and DAPT with clopidogrel or ticagrelor therapy for 12 months.
- Notify physician of dark, tarry stools; persistent stomach pain; difficulty breathing; unusual bruising or bleeding; or skin rash.
- Do not crush an enteric-coated product.

P2Y$_{12}$ receptor antagonists

Mechanism of action

These drugs inhibit platelet activation and aggregation mediated by the P2Y$_{12}$ adenosine diphosphate receptor.

Dose

Clopidogrel

- Loading dose: 300–600 mg orally
- Maintenance dose:
  - 75 mg daily combined with aspirin for a minimum of 14 days (STEMI) and up to 12 months (UA/NSTEMI, STEMI) in patients who were treated medically and did not undergo PCI
  - 75 mg daily combined with aspirin for a minimum of 12 months post-PCI following an ACS event (regardless of stent type)
  - 75 mg daily combined with aspirin for a minimum of 1 month (BMS) and up to 12 months (DES) post-PCI for a non-ACS indication
  - 75 mg daily for life in patients who cannot tolerate aspirin, including patients with chronic stable angina (Prasugrel and ticagrelor are not recommended as alternatives to aspirin in this setting.)

Prasugrel

- Loading dose: 60 mg orally at time of PCI
- Maintenance dose: 10 mg daily combined with aspirin for a minimum of 12 months post-PCI (5 mg dose recommended for patients weighing < 60 kg)

Ticagrelor

- Loading dose: 180 mg orally
- Maintenance dose: 90 mg po bid daily combined with aspirin (maximum dose 100 mg) for a minimum of 12 months post-PCI; also indicated as DAPT for patients medically managed (no PCI) post-ACS

Monitoring parameters

Clopidogrel, prasugrel, and ticagrelor

Monitor for signs of bleeding.

Adverse drug reactions

Adverse reactions are described in Table 15-11.

Drug–drug interactions

Drug–drug interactions are described in Table 15-12.

Table 15-11. P2Y$_{12}$ Receptor Antagonist Adverse Reactions

Drug	Reaction
Clopidogrel	Bleeding, chest pain, headache, dizziness, abdominal pain, vomiting, diarrhea, arthralgia, back pain, upper respiratory infections, flu-like symptoms, blood dyscrasias, rash, thrombotic thrombocytopenic purpura
Prasugrel	Bleeding, chest pain, headache, dizziness, rash, dyspnea, nausea, hypertension, back pain, anemia, thrombocytopenia, leucopenia, thrombotic thrombocytopenic purpura
Ticagrelor	Bleeding, chest pain, back pain, headache, fatigue, syncope, ventricular pauses, dyspnea, cough, dizziness, nausea, diarrhea, hypertension, elevated serum creatinine, elevated uric acid levels, blood dyscrasias

Drug–disease interactions
PUD or other active bleeding

Contraindications
- Hypersensitivity to an individual product
- Active bleeding (e.g., gastrointestinal or intra-cranial hemorrhage)
- Severe liver disease
- Neutropenia, thrombocytopenia
- Prasugrel only: History of stroke or transient ischemic attack; use in patients ≥ 75 years is not generally recommended unless considered high risk (history of diabetes or prior MI).

Patient instructions and counseling
Following stent implantation, patients will receive DAPT with a P2Y$_{12}$ receptor antagonist and aspirin for a minimum of 1 month (non-ACS indication with BMS) to 12 months following PCI (DES).

Table 15-12. P2Y$_{12}$ Receptor Antagonist Drug–Drug Interactions

Interacting medication	Effect
Antiplatelet agents, anticoagulants, and NSAIDs	Combination may increase the risk of bleeding.
Clopidogrel	
CYP2C9 substrates (phenytoin, fluvastatin, NSAIDs, losartan, irbesartan, valsartan)	Clopidogrel may increase serum levels and cause toxicity.
CYP2C19 inhibitors such as proton pump inhibitors (omeprazole, esomeprazole)	Reduced plasma concentrations of the active metabolite of clopidogrel and a reduction in platelet inhibition may occur. It may be reasonable to avoid strong inhibitors of CYP2C19 (omeprazole, esomeprazole). No drug–drug interaction is apparent with prasugrel or ticagrelor.
Ticagrelor	
Strong CYP3A inhibitors (ketoconazole, itraconazole, voriconazole, clarithromycin, nefazodone, ritonavir, select protease inhibitors)	Increased serum concentrations of ticagrelor may occur, which may increase risk of adverse events.
Strong CYP3A inducers (rifampin, dexamethasone, phenytoin, carbamazepine, phenobarbital)	Decreased serum concentrations of ticagrelor may occur, which may result in a reduction in platelet inhibition.
Simvastatin, lovastatin	Increased concentration of simvastatin or lovastatin may occur, which may increase the risk of myopathy with statin therapy. Maximum dose of these statins is 40 mg.
Digoxin	Inhibition of the P-glycoprotein transporter may occur, which may result in increased digoxin serum concentration. Monitor digoxin levels closely during initiation or discontinuation of ticagrelor.
Aspirin	Doses of aspirin > 100 mg result in reduced effectiveness of ticagrelor. Maximum dose of aspirin is 100 mg.

Table 15-13. Pharmacologic Properties of GPIs

Drug	Chemical nature	Duration of effect (hours)	Renal elimination	Renal dosing adjustment
Abciximab	Antibody	>12[a]	No	No
Eptifibatide	Nonpeptide	4–8	Yes	Yes
Tirofiban	Peptide fragment	4	Yes	Yes

a. Action can be reversed by a platelet infusion.

Patients treated medically following an ACS event will need the combination of clopidogrel or ticagrelor and aspirin for up to 1 year.

The lowest dose of aspirin (i.e., 81 mg) should be administered.

Patients should be counseled as follows:

- Avoid additional aspirin, salicylates, and NSAID products unless under the direction of a physician.
- Notify physician for unusual bleeding or bruising; blood in the urine, stool, or emesis; skin rash; or yellowing of the skin or eyes.
- Patients taking ticagrelor should notify their physician if they experience new or unexpected shortness of breath.
- Do not stop taking these medications without discussing with physician.
- Discontinue clopidogrel and ticagrelor at least 5 days and prasugrel at least 7 days prior to major surgery.

Glycoprotein IIb/IIIa receptor inhibitors

Mechanism of action
Blockade of the glycoprotein IIb/IIIa receptor prevents fibrinogen binding, thus inhibiting platelet aggregation, the final common pathway for platelet aggregation.

Properties of individual agents
See Table 15-13 for properties of GPIs.

Indications and doses
Table 15-14 provides information about indications and doses.

Monitoring parameters
- Signs and symptoms of bleeding
- Laboratory monitoring: Hematocrit and hemoglobin, platelet count, activated clotting time (during PCI), serum creatinine

Adverse drug reactions
Adverse drug reactions include bleeding, thrombocytopenia, and allergic reaction from repeated exposure (abciximab).

Table 15-14. Indications and Doses of GPIs

Drug	Indication	Dose
Abciximab	Adjunct to PCI or when PCI is planned within 24 hours	0.25 mg/kg IV bolus, 0.125 mcg/kg/min infusion continued for 12 hours postprocedure; maximum length of infusion: 18–24 hours
Eptifibatide	Adjunct to PCI	180 mcg/kg IV bolus × 2, 10 min apart; 2 mcg/kg/min infusion (CrCl < 50 mL/min; 1 mcg/kg/min) started after the first bolus and continued for 18–24 hours postprocedure (minimum of 12 hours)
	ACS medical management	180 mcg/kg IV bolus, 2 mcg/kg/min infusion (CrCl < 50 mL/min; 1 mcg/kg/min) continued until discharge, up to 72 hours; or if post-PCI, for 18–24 hours
Tirofiban	Adjunct to PCI	25 mcg/kg IV bolus over 3 min, followed by 0.15 mcg/kg/min infusion for 12–24 hours (CrCl < 30 mL/min; bolus and infusion reduced by 50%)
	ACS medical management or if significant delay to PCI	0.4 mcg/kg/min IV bolus for 30 min, 0.1 mcg/kg/min infusion (CrCl < 30 mL/min; bolus and infusion reduced by 50%) for 12–24 hours postprocedure

Drug–drug interactions

Antiplatelet agents, anticoagulants, and NSAIDs may all increase the risk of bleeding if used in combination with GPIs.

Drug–disease interactions

PUD or other active bleeding

Contraindications

■ Active bleeding
■ Platelet count < 100,000
■ History of intracranial hemorrhage, neoplasms, AV malformations, or aneurysm
■ History of stroke within the past 30 days or any history of hemorrhage stroke
■ Severe hypertension (BP > 180/110 mm Hg)
■ Major surgery within past 6 weeks
■ Dialysis dependent (eptifibatide only)

Anticoagulants

Heparin

Mechanism of action

UFH enhances the action of antithrombin, thereby inactivating thrombin and preventing the conversion of fibrinogen to fibrin.

Dose

■ **UA and NSTEMI:** 60 units/kg (maximum 4,000 units) IV bolus, 12 units/kg/h (maximum 1,000 units/h) infusion titrated to an activated partial thromboplastin time (aPTT) range of 50–70 seconds for 48 hours or end of PCI
■ **STEMI (in combination with fibrinolytic):** 60 units/kg (maximum 4,000 units) IV bolus, 12 units/kg/h (maximum 1,000 units/h) infusion titrated to an aPTT range of 50–70 seconds for 48 hours
■ **PCI:** Supplemental doses to target activated clotting time (ACT)

Monitoring parameters

Monitor aPTT or heparin anti-Xa level, platelet count, hemoglobin and hematocrit, signs of bleeding, and ACT (during PCI).

Adverse drug reactions

Bleeding, thrombocytopenia, hemorrhage, epistaxis, allergic reactions, and osteoporosis may occur.

Protamine can be used to reverse the effects of heparin; 1 mg of protamine neutralizes 100 units of heparin.

Drug–drug interactions

Antiplatelet agents, anticoagulants, and NSAIDs may all increase the risk of bleeding if used in combination with UFH. Switching from heparin to LMWH without an appropriate washout period may increase the risk of bleeding.

Drug–disease interaction

PUD or other active bleeding

Contraindications

■ History of heparin-induced thrombocytopenia
■ Severe thrombocytopenia
■ Active bleeding
■ Suspected intracranial hemorrhage

LMWH (enoxaparin)

Mechanism of action

The mechanism of action is similar to that of heparin; however, molecules are smaller and have a stronger affinity for factor Xa than thrombin.

Properties

Properties are described in Table 15-15.

Dose

■ **UA and NSTEMI:** 1 mg/kg q12h subcutaneously (CrCl < 30 mL/min: 1 mg/kg q24h subcutaneously)
■ **STEMI:** 30 mg IV, then 1 mg/kg q12h subcutaneously (CrCl < 30 mL/min: 1 mg/kg q24h subcutaneously); for patients > 75 years of age, eliminate the IV bolus and give 0.75 mg/kg q12h subcutaneously

Monitoring parameters

Serum creatinine, platelet count, hemoglobin and hematocrit, anti-Xa levels (optional use of enoxaparin as calibrator), signs of bleeding, and neurologic functions should be monitored.

Table 15-15. Properties of Enoxaparin versus UFH

Drug	Half-life (hours)	Molecular weight (daltons)	Anti-Xa: anti-IIa	Renal elimination
Enoxaparin	4.5	4,500	2.7:1	Yes
UFH	1	15,000	1:1	No

Boldface indicates one of top 100 drugs for 2012 by units sold at retail outlets, www.drugs.com/stats/top100/2012/units.

Adverse drug reactions

Adverse reactions include bleeding, thrombocytopenia (decreased incidence compared to UFH), hemorrhage, and epistaxis.

Drug–drug interactions

Antiplatelet agents, anticoagulants, and NSAIDs may all increase the risk of bleeding if used in combination with LMWH.

Switching from LMWH to UFH without an appropriate washout period may increase the risk of bleeding.

Drug–disease interactions

PUD or any active bleeding

Warnings

Patients with recent or anticipated epidural or spinal anesthesia are at risk of hematoma and subsequent paralysis. Neurological impairment requires immediate treatment.

Contraindications

- Severe thrombocytopenia
- Active bleeding
- Suspected intracranial hemorrhage

Fondaparinux

Mechanism of action

Direct inhibition of factor Xa occurs, thereby inhibiting thrombin formation.

Properties

Half-life is 17–21 hours. The drug is excreted primarily unchanged in urine.

Dose

- **UA and NSTEMI (conservative strategy only):** 2.5 mg subcutaneously daily up to 8 days
- **STEMI (with or without fibrinolytics):** 2.5 mg IV, then subcutaneously daily up to 8 days; not recommended if patient is undergoing primary PCI

Monitoring parameters

Serum creatinine, platelet count, hemoglobin and hematocrit, anti-Xa levels (optional, use of fondaparinux as calibrator), and signs of bleeding should be monitored.

Adverse drug reactions

Adverse reactions include bleeding, thrombocytopenia (decreased incidence compared to UFH), hemorrhage, and epistaxis.

Drug–drug interactions

Antiplatelet agents, anticoagulants, and NSAIDs may all increase the risk of bleeding if used in combination with fondaparinux.

Drug–disease interactions

- PUD or any active bleeding
- Not preferred anticoagulant when PCI is planned

Warnings

Patients with recent or anticipated epidural or spinal anesthesia are at risk of hematoma and subsequent paralysis.

Contraindications

- Severe thrombocytopenia
- Active bleeding
- Suspected intracranial hemorrhage
- CrCl < 30 mL/min
- When PCI is planned, use alternative anticoagulant.

Bivalirudin

Mechanism of action

Bivalirudin is a direct thrombin inhibitor. The mechanism of direct thrombin inhibition differs from UFH in that bivalirudin is able to inhibit both bound and free thrombin.

Dose

- **ACS and PCI:** 0.75 mg/kg IV bolus then 1.75 mg/kg/h IV infusion for the duration of the PCI procedure. The infusion may be continued for up to 4 hours following completion of the procedure.
- In patients with CrCl < 30 mL/min, reduce infusion to 1 mg/kg/h; dose for hemodialysis is 0.25 mg/kg/h.

Monitoring parameters

ACT (during PCI), aPTT, and signs of bleeding should be monitored.

Adverse drug reactions

Adverse reactions include bleeding, back pain, hypotension, and nausea.

Drug–drug interactions

Antiplatelet agents, anticoagulants, and NSAIDs may all increase the risk of bleeding if used in combination with bivalirudin.

Drug–disease interactions
PUD or any active bleeding

Contraindications
Severe, active bleeding

Fibrinolytic Therapy

Mechanism of action

Fibrinolytic or thrombolytic therapy acts either directly or indirectly to activate or convert plasminogen to plasmin to lyse a formed clot. The conversion of plasminogen to plasmin activates the body's natural thrombolytic–fibrinolytic system, which lyses the clot and releases fibrin degradation products.

Dose

Fibrinolytic doses are given in Table 15-16.

Monitoring parameters

CBC (complete blood count), ECG, aPTT, signs of bleeding, BP, and signs of reperfusion should be monitored.

Adverse drug reactions

Adverse reactions include bleeding, intracranial hemorrhage (< 1%), stroke (< 2%), and epistaxis.

Drug–drug interactions

Antiplatelet agents, anticoagulants, and NSAIDs may all increase the risk of bleeding if used in combination with thrombolytics.

Table 15-16. Fibrinolytic Doses

Drug	Dose
Streptokinase	1.5 million units in 50 mL of normal saline or D5W given over 60 min
Tissue plasminogen activator	15 mg IV bolus, followed by 0.75 mg/kg IV infusion over 30 min (not to exceed 50 mg); then 0.5 mg/kg IV infusion over 1 h (not to exceed 35 mg)
Reteplase	10 units IV push over 2 min, followed in 30 min by a repeat 10 units IV bolus over 10 min
Tenecteplase	Patient weighs < 60 kg, give 30 mg IV bolus; 60–69.9 kg, give 35 mg IV bolus; 70–79.9 kg, give 40 mg IV bolus; 80–89.9 kg, give 45 mg IV bolus; > 90 kg, give 50 mg IV bolus; each bolus given over 5 seconds

Contraindications

Contraindications
- Any prior intracranial hemorrhage
- Known structural cerebrovascular lesion
- Ischemic stroke within 3 months, except acute ischemic stroke within 4.5 hours
- Known intracranial neoplasm (primary or metastatic)
- Active internal bleeding or bleeding diathesis (does not include menses)
- Suspected aortic dissection
- Significant closed head or facial trauma within 3 months
- Intracranial or intraspinal surgery within 2 months

Relative contraindications
- Severe uncontrolled hypertension (BP > 180/110 mm Hg) or chronic, poorly controlled hypertension
- History of prior ischemic stroke greater than 3 months, dementia, or known intracerebral pathology not covered in contraindications
- Current use of anticoagulants in therapeutic doses
- Traumatic or prolonged (> 10 min) cardiopulmonary resuscitation or major surgery (< 3 weeks)
- Noncompressible vascular punctures
- Recent (within 2–4 weeks) internal bleeding
- For streptokinase, prior exposure or prior allergic reaction
- Pregnancy
- Active peptic ulcer

15-10. Questions

Use the following case study to answer Questions 1–3:

Mr. Smith is a 66-year-old white male who presented to his local physician with complaints of chest pain. He described the pain as sharp, aching, and nonradiating. The pain, which he has had for the past few weeks, has occurred mainly during his daily walk and is usually relieved when he stops to rest.

Past medical history: Hypertension, PUD, asthma, CAD
Family history: Father died of a stroke at age 86; mother died at age 82 with diabetes mellitus and heart failure; sister died of MI at 52
Social history: Smokes 1 pack per day × 40 years; drinks alcohol socially 1–2 times a week

Medications:

- Proventil MDI 2 puffs prn
- Flovent 44 mcg 2 puffs bid
- Prilosec 20 mg daily
- Aspirin 81 mg daily
- HCTZ 25 mg daily

Vital signs: BP 148/92; HR 82; RR 18; height 72 inches; weight 200 lb

Labs: (fasting) total cholesterol 246 mg/dL; TG 110 mg/dL; HDL 38 mg/dL; LDL 196 mg/dL; Chem 12 within normal limits; troponin negative × 3

ECG: Normal (patient currently pain free)

Cath 2 years ago: Minimal two-vessel disease

1. Which treatment algorithm should be considered given Mr. Smith's current symptoms and presentation?

   A. Unstable angina
   B. Stable angina
   C. Variant angina
   D. Silent ischemia
   E. NSTEMI

2. Considering Mr. Smith's comorbidities, which of the following would be the most appropriate therapeutic intervention at this time?

   A. SL NTG prn
   B. Inderal
   C. Zestril and SL NTG prn
   D. Cardizem and SL NTG prn
   E. Coreg and SL NTG

3. What additional medication should be considered for Mr. Smith?

   A. Ticagrelor
   B. Atorvastatin
   C. Clopidogrel
   D. Prasugrel
   E. Reteplase

4. Which of the following effects on myocardial oxygen demand is *not* affected by β-blockers?

   A. Decreased HR
   B. Decreased BP
   C. Decreased contractility
   D. Peripheral vasodilation
   E. Decreased conduction through the AV node

5. Which of the following statements is most accurate regarding the use of calcium channel blockers in IHD?

   A. Amlodipine and felodipine reduce MVO_2 by decreasing conduction through the AV node.
   B. Calcium channel blockers should be used as first-line therapy in patients with stable angina.
   C. Newer-generation dihydropyridines like nifedipine immediate release are safe in the treatment of IHD.
   D. Calcium channel blockers can be used in combination with β-blockers to attenuate the effect of increased sympathetic tone that some dihydropyridines may cause.
   E. The combination of verapamil and metoprolol in a patient with reduced LV systolic function is safe and well tolerated by most patients.

6. Which of the following is *not* considered a potential cardiovascular benefit of ACEIs in IHD?

   A. ACEIs reduce the incidence of MI.
   B. ACEIs reduce the incidence of cardiovascular death and stroke in patients at high risk for vascular disease.
   C. ACEIs have been proven to be superior and provide more antianginal effects than do β-blockers.
   D. ACEIs should be used in all stable angina patients with known CAD who also have diabetes.
   E. ACEIs have shown greater benefit post-MI in higher-risk patients.

7. A 64-year-old male with stable ischemic heart disease complains of angina that occurs after walking 2–3 blocks. No lesions detected on his coronary angiogram (cardiac cath) are amenable to intervention (stent or CABG). His HR is 58–62 and BP is 130/68. Current medications include aspirin 81 mg daily, rosuvastatin 40 mg at bedtime, metoprolol 50 mg twice daily, ramipril 10 mg daily, and tadalafil as needed. Which of the following interventions will be of most benefit to treat this patient's angina?

   A. Add isosorbide mononitrate 60 mg daily.
   B. Add diltiazem 180 mg every morning.
   C. Increase metoprolol to 100 mg twice daily.
   D. Add amlodipine 5 mg daily.
   E. Add ranolazine 1,000 mg twice daily.

8. Ideal properties for a β-blocker in the treatment of ACS include which of the following?

    A. Available as an IV product, cardioselectivity
    B. Low lipophilicity, has ISA
    C. Has ISA, cardioselectivity
    D. Cardioselectivity, low lipophilicity, does not have ISA
    E. Noncardioselective, high lipophilicity

9. The possible benefits of LMWH over UFH include all of the following *except*

    A. predictable response.
    B. ease of administration.
    C. no recommended routine monitoring.
    D. lower incidence of heparin-induced thrombocytopenia.
    E. no renal adjustment necessary.

10. Which of the following β-blockers has ISA activity?

    A. Tenormin
    B. Sectral
    C. Inderal
    D. Lopressor
    E. Coreg

11. Which of the following medications is contraindicated within 24 hours of a nitrate?

    A. Metoprolol
    B. Quinapril
    C. Verapamil
    D. Sildenafil
    E. Felodipine

12. Which of the following is the preferred narcotic to relieve chest pain after the use of SL NTG?

    A. Meperidine
    B. Oxycodone
    C. Morphine
    D. Hydromorphone
    E. Fentanyl

Use the following case study to answer Questions 13 and 14:

A 54-year-old male presents to the hospital with crushing substernal chest pain and radiation to his left arm. Past medical history is significant for hypertension, COPD, and gout. The patient has a history of smoking × 30 years and occasionally consumes alcohol. Vital signs on admission include BP 170/85 mm Hg, pulse 72, RR 18, and temp 97°F. Before admission, the patient was taking enteric-coated aspirin 81 mg daily, Combivent inhaler 2 puffs qid, Tiazac 240 mg daily, and Zyloprim 300 mg daily.

Allergies: Sulfa

Lab/diagnostic tests:

- ECG: ST-segment depression, T-wave changes in leads II, III, and aVF
- Troponin: positive × 3
- Ejection fraction: < 35%
- LDL: 135 mg/dL

Diagnosis:

- NSTEMI
- Heart failure

13. What is the preferred β-blocker for this patient?

    A. Propranolol
    B. Carvedilol
    C. Labetalol
    D. Metoprolol
    E. Nadolol

14. Which of the following therapies should be avoided in this patient?

    A. Reteplase
    B. Clopidogrel
    C. Enalapril
    D. Atorvastatin
    E. Unfractionated heparin

Use the following case study to answer Questions 15 and 16:

A 56-year-old female presents to the local emergency room complaining of crushing, substernal chest pain × 3 hours, which has been unrelieved by SL NTG. Past medical history is significant for hypertension, type 2 diabetes mellitus, TIA × 2, hypercholesterolemia, and metabolic syndrome. Heart rate and rhythm are regular, and no S₃ or S₄ sounds are present. Vital signs include BP 184/119 mm Hg, HR 100, and RR 32/min. ECG shows ST-segment elevation > 1 mm in leads II, III, and aVF. She is immediately admitted to the chest pain center and started on oxygen. The cath lab personnel have been notified that she is being transported to the cath lab for primary PCI.

15. Which of the following regimens is appropriate for this patient at this time?

    A. Aspirin 81 mg, clopidogrel 600 mg, and enoxaparin 1 mg/kg subcutaneous twice daily
    B. Aspirin 81 mg, clopidogrel 600 mg, and heparin 60 unit/kg bolus followed by heparin 12 units/kg/h
    C. Ticagrelor 180 mg and eptifibatide 180 mg/kg/IV bolus followed by eptifibatide 2 mcg/kg/h infusion
    D. Aspirin 325 mg, prasugrel 60 mg, and bivalirudin 0.75 mg/kg IV bolus followed by bivalirudin 1.75 mg/kg/h
    E. Aspirin 325 mg, ticagrelor 180 mg, and bivalirudin 0.75 mg/kg IV bolus followed by bivalirudin 1.75 mg/kg/h

16. Which of the following agents would be beneficial to this patient?

    A. tPA 100 mg IV over 90 minutes
    B. IV magnesium
    C. Prophylactic lidocaine
    D. Metoprolol 12.5 mg po
    E. Diltiazem 240 mg po

17. Of the following, which medication regimen is the best choice as discharge therapy for a 65-year-old patient weighing 70 kg who is post-ACS with DES placement and preserved LVEF?

    A. Aspirin 325 mg daily, clopidogrel 75 mg daily, diltiazem 240 mg daily, and simvastatin 40 mg daily
    B. Aspirin 81 mg daily, atorvastatin 80 mg daily, ticagrelor 90 mg twice daily, and metoprolol tartrate 50 mg twice daily
    C. Prasugrel 5 mg daily, enalapril 10 mg twice daily, metoprolol succinate 100 mg daily, and simvastatin 40 mg daily
    D. Aspirin 81 mg daily, metoprolol tartrate 100 mg twice daily, prasugrel 10 mg daily, and SL NTG
    E. Aspirin 325 mg daily, morphine 2–4 mg IV as needed, oxygen, and SL NTG

18. The anticoagulant effect of unfractionated heparin requires the binding to which plasma cofactor?

    A. Thrombospondin
    B. Antithrombin

    C. Plasminogen
    D. Factor XIIa
    E. Factors II, VII, IX, and X

Use the following case study to answer Question 19:
A 45-year-old marathon runner presents to the emergency department with complaints of chest pain during his morning run. His father died of an MI at age 48. His past medical history is positive for angina, hyperlipidemia, and hypertension. His current medications include aspirin, rosuvastatin, nifedipine, and clonidine. His ECG is consistent with acute ischemia. His HR is 52 and BP is 170/100 mm Hg. CBC and Chem-7 are within normal limits.

19. Which of the following interventions is the *least* appropriate for this patient at this time?

    A. Enoxaparin 1 mg/kg bid subcutaneously
    B. Metoprolol 50 mg bid po
    C. Nitroglycerin SL prn and IV drip titrated to pain and blood pressure
    D. Continuation of aspirin
    E. Morphine if NTG does not control the pain

20. Which one of the following agents is *not* indicated in the setting of STEMI when pharmacologic reperfusion is the planned strategy?

    A. Eptifibatide
    B. LMWH
    C. Aspirin
    D. tPA
    E. Metoprolol

21. Which of the following agents would *not* be administered at the same time as heparin?

    A. tPA
    B. Reteplase
    C. Eptifibatide
    D. TNKase
    E. Streptokinase

22. Which of the following statements about the GPIs is *least* accurate?

    A. Abciximab, eptifibatide, and tirofiban are all administered as a bolus followed by a continuous infusion.
    B. It is possible to experience an allergic reaction after repeated exposure to abciximab.
    C. Eptifibatide, tirofiban, and abciximab can all be reversed by a platelet infusion.

D. Tirofiban and eptifibatide are renally eliminated; therefore, dosage adjustment is required for patients with renal dysfunction.

E. Abciximab, eptifibatide, and tirofiban are all indicated as adjuncts to PCI.

15-11. Answers

1. **B.** Angina is considered stable if symptoms have been occurring for several weeks without worsening, it lasts < 30 minutes, and it is relieved by rest or SL NTG. Mr. Smith's chest pain symptoms are not variant or silent; therefore, C and D are not correct. A and E are incorrect because the patient did not have positive cardiac enzymes and EKG changes significant for myocardial infarction.

2. **D.** All patients with chronic chest pain need SL NTG for acute use. However, SL NTG alone is not appropriate antianginal therapy; Answer A is incorrect. A calcium channel blocker regimen (Answer D) will help control his angina as well as lower his BP. Although β-blockers should be considered first-line therapy in patients with stable angina for anti-ischemic effects, calcium channel blockers can be additive or used in settings where a contraindication to a β-blocker exists. In this case, the calcium channel blocking regimen will avoid β2-blocking effects in this asthmatic patient. B and E are incorrect because Inderal (propranolol) and Coreg (carvedilol) are not β1-selective and could worsen his asthma. C is incorrect because this patient needs an agent to control angina symptoms and ACEIs are not effective as antianginal agents.

3. **B.** Mr. Smith has an elevated LDL with known heart disease, and he needs to be treated with a statin. A and D are incorrect because ticagrelor and prasugrel are not indicated in stable angina. C is incorrect because clopidogrel is not indicated for treating stable angina unless a patient cannot tolerate aspirin. E is incorrect because thrombolytics are not indicated in stable angina.

4. **D.** Unlike nitrates or calcium channel blockers, β-blockers do not cause peripheral vasodilation. However, they do decrease heart rate (Answer A), blood pressure (Answer B), contractility (Answer C), and conduction through the AV node (Answer E).

5. **D.** The increased sympathetic tone caused by some dihydropyridines can lead to a reflex tachycardia, which would be detrimental in an IHD patient. Therefore, using a β-blocker to block this effect is desirable. A is incorrect; unlike verapamil or diltiazem, the dihydropyridines do not decrease conduction through the AV node. B is incorrect; CCBs are not indicated as first-line therapy unless a patient has a contraindication to a β-blocker. C is incorrect because immediate-release nifedipine can lead to increased side effects if not combined with a β-blocker. E is incorrect because both verapamil and metoprolol can lead to worsening systolic function, and used in combination, they would be unsafe.

6. **C.** ACEIs are not antianginal agents and have not been shown to be superior to β-blockers for control of angina symptoms. ACEIs are protective and reduce the incidence of MI, cardiovascular death, and stroke in patients at high risk for vascular disease; Answers A and B are incorrect. Because of their protective effect in high-risk patients, they should be used in all stable angina patients with known CAD who also have diabetes if no contraindication exists; Answers D and E are incorrect.

7. **D.** Adding a calcium channel blocker will give additional antianginal effects. Using amlodipine (Answer D) rather than a stronger AV nodal blocker such as diltiazem is important given this patient's heart rate; Answer B is incorrect. Adding nitrates to this patient who occasionally takes tadalafil is an absolute contraindication because concomitant use can cause dangerously low blood pressure; Answer A is incorrect. β-blockers should be titrated for antianginal effects, but this patient's heart rate and blood pressure may not tolerate a doubling of dose; Answer C is incorrect. Finally, ranolazine is an option in patients with low heart rate and blood pressure who need additional antianginal effects, but the starting dose should be limited to 500 mg twice daily; Answer E is incorrect.

8. **D.** Ideally, a β-blocker used for the treatment of UA or NSTEMI would have β1-receptor selectivity and no ISA and low lipophilicity. Being available as an IV agent is not an advantage because oral initiation of β-blockers is preferred to avoid adverse effects; Answer A is incorrect. β1-receptor selectivity would reduce the chance for bronchospasm, and low lipophilicity would reduce the neurological side

effects; Answer E is incorrect. β-blockers with ISA reduce heart rate to a lesser degree than non-ISA β-blockers, thus producing a smaller decrease in oxygen demand; Answers B and C are incorrect.

9. **E.** Renal adjustment is necessary with LMWH in patients with a CrCl < 30 mL/min whereas UFH does not require dosage adjustment. LMWH has advantages over UFH in ease of administration (Answer B), reduced incidence of heparin-induced thrombocytopenia (Answer D), more predictable therapeutic response (Answer A), and lack of required monitoring (Answer C).

10. **B.** β-blockers with ISA activity include Sectral (acebutolol) (Answer B) and Visken (pindolol). Tenormin (atenolol) (Answer A), Inderal (propranolol) (Answer C), Lopressor (metoprolol) (Answer D), and Coreg (carvedilol) (Answer E) do not have ISA activity.

11. **D.** Sildenafil use is contraindicated within 24 hours of a nitrate. β-blockers (metoprolol) (Answer A), ACEIs (quinapril) (Answer B), and calcium channel blockers (verapamil and felodipine) (Answers C and E) can be safely combined with nitrates.

12. **C.** Morphine has vasodilator properties, thereby decreasing both preload and afterload, which decreases oxygen demand. In addition, morphine lowers heart rate by relieving pain and anxiety. If a true morphine allergy exists, meperidine may be used as an alternate agent, but it is not preferred over morphine; Answer A is incorrect. Oxycodone (Answer B), hydromorphone (Answer D), and fentanyl (Answer E) are not recommended for the treatment of anginal pain.

13. **D.** With the patient's history of COPD, a β-blocker with β_1-receptor selectivity is preferred. The only agent with β_1-selectivity in this list is metoprolol. All of the remaining agents are nonselective and are incorrect choices. In addition, metoprolol succinate would be an appropriate β-blocker to use in this patient with heart failure. It would be also important to discontinue Tiazac (or Cardizem) in this patient with an ejection fraction of < 40%.

14. **A.** Reteplase is a thrombolytic agent, which does not have a role in the treatment of NSTEMI. Thrombolytic therapy is indicated for the treatment of STEMI when PCI is not possible within 120 minutes. When PCI is not available, clopidogrel (or ticagrelor) should be considered in all patients with NSTEMI; Answer B is incorrect. High-intensity statin therapy (e.g., atorvastatin 40–80 mg or rosuvastatin 20–40 mg) should be initiated in this patient because patients with ACS are a group who have shown benefit from statin therapy (Answer D is incorrect). This patient has a clear indication for an ACEI (enalapril) because of his ejection fraction of < 40%; Answer C is incorrect. An anticoagulant should be started on presentation; options include UFH, enoxaparin, fondaparinux, or bivalirudin if PCI is planned; Answer E is incorrect.

15. **E.** Antiplatelet therapy during PCI includes aspirin, a $P2Y_{12}$ receptor antagonist, and an appropriate antithrombotic agent. Dosing of aspirin during an acute event should be at least 162 mg; Answers A and B are incorrect. Answer D is not correct because patients with history of TIA or stroke are not to receive prasugrel (absolute contraindication). Answer C is incorrect because aspirin is not used, and this option is missing an anticoagulant agent.

16. **D.** This patient is going immediately to the cath lab where primary PCI is preferred over lytic therapy for STEMI. In centers where PCI is not available within 120 minutes, lytics should be considered. However, one of the relative contraindications to fibrinolytic therapy is severe uncontrolled hypertension (BP > 180/110 mm Hg). Answer A is not appropriate in this patient for these reasons. Routine use of magnesium (Answer B) post-MI is not recommended and should be reserved only for patients with hypomagnesemia or torsades de pointes. No labs were given for this patient and no life-threatening arrhythmias were noted, so answer B is not appropriate at this time. Prophylactic lidocaine (Answer C) has been shown to increase all-cause mortality and is not recommended in the early management of STEMI for prevention of VF. β-blockers reduce the incidence of ventricular arrhythmias, recurrent ischemia, reinfarction, infarct size, and mortality in patients with STEMI. Because this patient does not have any contraindications to β-blockade, D is the correct choice. Calcium channel blockers do not have a role in STEMI when a β-blocker can be given; Answer E is incorrect.

17. **B.** β-blockers, dual antiplatelet therapy with aspirin and a P2Y$_{12}$ receptor antagonist, and statin therapy should be given to all patients without contraindications post-MI. Clopidogrel can be combined with aspirin and can be continued for at least 12 months regardless of whether the patient underwent PCI. Answer A is not correct because although calcium channel blockers can be given if a patient has contraindications to β-blockade, they are not recommended as first-line treatment. Further, the dosing of aspirin is too high and the dosing of statin not intense enough for chronic administration after ACS. Answer C is incorrect because aspirin is omitted and the dosing of prasugrel is incorrect given that the patient weighs > 60 kg. Answer D is incorrect because high-intensity statin therapy is not included. Answer E would be a correct choice for the immediate treatment of someone who presents with ACS, but not as discharge therapy.

18. **B.** Heparin's anticoagulant effect requires binding to antithrombin (previously antithrombin III), and that binding converts antithrombin from a slow, progressive thrombin inhibitor to a very rapid inhibitor of thrombin and factor Xa.

19. **B.** One of the contraindications to β-blockade is an HR < 55 bpm. Because the patient has an HR of 52 bpm, metoprolol should not be given at this time. Enoxaparin, NTG, aspirin, and morphine are all therapies that should be continued.

20. **A.** Glycoprotein IIb/IIIa inhibition can be given in the setting of STEMI, but it is not preferred when a fibrinolytic agent is administered. Trials to date in combination with full- and half-dose fibrinolytic agents have shown a more complete reperfusion at the price of higher bleeding rates.

21. **E.** A combination of UFH with streptokinase is not desirable because streptokinase is a nonspecific fibrinolytic, and UFH may increase the risk of bleeding because of streptokinase's long half-life. Therefore, answer E is the correct choice. Heparin should be administered for at least 48 hours with the other lytic choices (Answers A, B, and D) to reduce risk of re-occlusion. A GPI should be administered with heparin, and therefore C is not the correct answer.

22. **C.** The only GPI that is reversed by a platelet infusion is abciximab, making C the least accurate statement. All of the remaining selections are true statements. All of the available GPI agents are administered as a bolus and infusion (Answer A). Abciximab is a monoclonal antibody; therefore, it is possible to develop an allergic reaction upon rechallenge (Answer B). Only two GPIs are renally eliminated: eptifibatide and tirofiban (Answer D). All of the agents are indicated as adjuncts to PCI (Answer E).

15-12. References

Eckel RH, Jakicic JM, Ard JD, et al. 2013 AHA/ACC guideline on lifestyle management to reduce cardiovascular risk: A report of the American College of Cardiology/American Heart Association Task Force on Practice Guidelines. *Circulation.* 2013. doi:10.1161/01.cir.0000437740.48606.d1.

Fihn SD, Gardin JM, Abrams J, et al. 2012 ACCF/AHA/ACP/AATS/PCNA/SCAI/STS guideline for the diagnosis and management of patients with stable ischemic heart disease: A report of the American College of Cardiology Foundation/American Heart Association Task Force on Practice Guidelines, and the American College of Physicians, American Association for Thoracic Surgery, Preventive Cardiovascular Nurses Association, Society for Cardiovascular Angiography and Interventions, and Society of Thoracic Surgeons. *J Am Coll Cardiol.* 2012;60:e44–e164.

Go AS, Mozaffarian D, Roger VL, et al.; on behalf of the American Heart Association Statistics Committee and Stroke Statistics Subcommittee. Heart disease and stroke statistics—2014 update: A report from the American Heart Association. *Circulation.* 2014;129:e28–e292.

Hillis LD, Smith PK, Anderson JL, et al. 2011 ACCF/AHA guideline for coronary artery bypass graft surgery: A report of the American College of Cardiology Foundation/American Heart Association Task Force on Practice Guidelines. *Circulation.* 2011;124:e652–e735.

Jensen MD, Ryan DH, Apovian CM, et al. 2013 AHA/ACC/TOS guideline for the management of overweight and obesity in adults: A report of the American College of Cardiology/American Heart Association Task Force on Practice Guidelines and The Obesity Society. *Circulation.* 2013. doi:10.1161/01.cir.0000437739.71477.ee.

Jneid H, Anderson JL, Wright RS, et al. 2012 ACCF/AHA focused update of the guideline for the management of patients with unstable angina/non-ST-elevation myocardial infarction (updating the 2007 guideline and replacing the 2011 focused update): A report of the American College of Cardiology Foundation/American Heart Association Task Force on Practice Guidelines. doi:10.1161/CIR.0b013e318256f1e0. http://circ.ahajournals.org/content/126/7/875.

Levine GN, Bates ER, Blankenship JC, et al. 2011 ACCF/AHA/SCAI guideline for percutaneous coronary intervention: A report of the American College of Cardiology Foundation/American Heart Association Task Force on Practice Guidelines and the Society for Cardiovascular Angiography and Interventions. *J Am Coll Cardiol.* 2011;58:e44–e122.

Mosca L, Benjamin EJ, Berra K, et al. Effectiveness-based guidelines for the prevention of cardiovascular disease in women—2011 update: A guideline from the American Heart Association. *Circulation.* 2011;123:1243–62.

O'Gara PT, Kushner FG, Ascheim DD, et al. 2013 ACCF/AHA guideline for the management of ST-elevation myocardial infarction: A report of the American College of Cardiology Foundation/American Heart Association Task Force on Practice Guidelines. *J Am Coll Cardiol.* 2013;61:e78–e140.

Pignone M, Alberts MJ, Colwell JA, et al. Aspirin for primary prevention of cardiovascular events in people with diabetes: A position statement of the American Diabetes Association, a scientific statement of the American Heart Association, and an expert consensus document of the American College of Cardiology Foundation. *Circulation.* 2010;121:2694–701.

Smith SC Jr, Benjamin EJ, Bonow RO, et al. AHA/ACCF secondary prevention and risk reduction therapy for patients with coronary and other atherosclerotic vascular disease: 2011 update: A guideline from the American Heart Association and American College of Cardiology Foundation. *Circulation.* 2011;113:2458–73.

Stone NJ, Robinson J, Liechtenstein AH, et al. 2013 ACC/AHA Guideline on the treatment of blood cholesterol to reduce atherosclerotic cardiovascular risk in adults. A report of the American College of Cardiology/American Heart Association Task Force on Practice Guidelines. *Circulation.* 2013. doi:01.cir.0000437738.63853.7a. http://circ.ahajournals.org/content/early/2013/11/11/01.cir.0000437738.63853.7a.

Vandvik PO, Lincoff AM, Gore JM, et al. Primary and secondary prevention of cardiovascular disease: Antithrombotic Therapy and Prevention of Thrombosis, 9th ed.: American College of Chest Physicians Evidence-Based Clinical Practice Guidelines. *Chest.* 2012;141:e637S–e68S.

Dyslipidemia

Anita Airee

16-1. Key Points

- Dyslipidemia is a disorder of lipid metabolism manifested primarily by an elevation of total cholesterol, low-density lipoprotein (LDL) cholesterol, or triglycerides, or a decrease in high-density lipoprotein (HDL).
- Disorders of lipid metabolism can lead to atherosclerotic vascular disease (ASCVD).
- Dyslipidemia can be caused by genetic or environmental factors.
- Screening is recommended every 4–6 years in patients without ASCVD or diabetes and with LDL of 70–189 mg/dL.
- Lifestyle modifications are recommended for all patients with dyslipidemia.
- Though target LDL levels have historically been the mainstay of goal-directed therapy, the 2013 American College of Cardiology/American Heart Association (ACC/AHA) guidelines recommend fixed-dose statins for primary and secondary prevention of ASCVD.
- High-intensity statins are those that reduce LDL by ≥ 50%; moderate-intensity statins are those that lower LDL by 30–49%.
- The 2013 ACC/AHA guidelines suggest treatment with statins within four major groups for whom the benefit outweighs the risk (adverse effect risk, medication interactions) and when patient preference is considered.

- The Pooled Cohort Risk calculator is used to determine the 10-year ASCVD risk.
- High-intensity statins are recommended for all patients with existing ASCVD; moderate-intensity statins can be used if high intensity is not tolerated.
- High-intensity statins are recommended for all patients ≥ 21 years of age with an LDL > 190 mg/dL; moderate-intensity statins can be used if high intensity is not tolerated.
- Both moderate- and high-intensity statins are recommended for all diabetic patients age 40 to 75; consider a high-intensity statin when the ASCVD risk is > 7.5%.
- Use of statins in primary prevention of nondiabetic patients > 21 years depends on ASCVD risk score.
- Secondary causes of dyslipidemia can include medications (diuretics, cyclosporine, glucocorticoids, amiodarone), diseases (biliary obstruction, nephrotic syndrome, hypothyroidism), and altered metabolic states (obesity, pregnancy).
- Nonstatin medications should be used for patients unable to tolerate any statin or the recommended doses of statin or for high-risk patients who have less than the anticipated response to statins.
- Cholesterol screenings are recommended for children age 2–8 years if they have a family history of dyslipidemia or heart disease or if the child has other risk factors for heart disease such as obesity, hypertension, diabetes, or exposure to cigarette smoke. Universal screening is recommended for all children ages 9–11.

Editor's Note: This chapter is based on the 10th edition chapter written by Lawrence M. Brown.

16-2. Study Guide Checklist

The following topics may guide your study of this subject area:

- Pathophysiology of atherosclerosis and lipid metabolism
- Risk factors for atherosclerotic vascular disease
- Lifestyle modifications recommended for risk reduction (Dietary Approaches to Stop Hypertension diet, exercise).
- Mechanism of action and adverse effects of categories of drugs for dyslipidemia
- Doses of statins that are considered high intensity versus moderate intensity
- Trade names and dosage forms of medications, particularly those in the "Top 100 drugs" list
- Combinations of medications for dyslipidemia including benefit and risk
- Unique counseling points for medications used in dyslipidemia
- Purpose of the new ACC/AHA guidelines and their role in the management of dyslipidemia

16-3. Introduction

Lipoproteins are the means by which lipids are transported through the blood. They are composed of a central core of esterified cholesterol and triglycerides (TG), an outer layer of phospholipids, and an associated apolipoprotein. The three major forms of lipoproteins are low-density lipoprotein (LDL), high-density lipoprotein (HDL), and VLDL (very low-density lipoprotein). The VLDL component could also be equated with the TG content divided by 5. A simplified way to view total cholesterol (TC) is TC = LDL + HDL + VLDL (see Table 16-1). If VLDL can be estimated as TG/5, the Friedewald equation for calculating LDL is more easily understood:

$$LDL = TC - (HDL + TG/5)$$

This calculated formula is most accurate when TG < 200 mg/dL and should not be used when TG > 400 mg/dL. When TG > 200 mg/dL, a direct LDL or non-HDL measurement most accurately represents the LDL level.

Lipids enter the bloodstream though either the exogenous pathway or the endogenous pathway.

Table 16-1. Classification of Lipids

Type	Classification
LDL cholesterol	
< 100 mg/dL	Optimal
100–129 mg/dL	Near optimal or above optimal
130–159 mg/dL	Borderline high
160–189 mg/dL	High
≥ 190 mg/dL	Very high
Total cholesterol	
< 200 mg/dL	Desirable
200–239 mg/dL	Borderline high
≥ 240 mg/dL	High
HDL cholesterol	
< 40 mg/dL	Low
≥ 60 mg/dL	High
Triglycerides	
< 150 mg/dL	Normal
150–199 mg/dL	Borderline high
200–499 mg/dL	High
≥ 500 mg/dL	Very high

The exogenous pathway involves ingestion of dietary fat, emulsification by bile acids, and absorption via chylomicrons (TG and cholesterol esters). Triglycerides are hydrolyzed to free fatty acids to be used by muscle or stored in adipose tissue. The endogenous pathway is a complex method of cholesterol production via hepatic secretion of VLDL, which is then processed to LDL and HDL. LDL and its permeation into the endothelium and subsequent oxidation to foam cells is linked to atherosclerotic vascular disease (ASCVD). Endothelial inflammation also plays a role in plaque formation, and rupture may lead to coronary and cerebrovascular events. Reverse cholesterol transports cholesterol via HDL back to the liver. Several randomized controlled trials have independently associated low HDL, elevated LDL, and elevated TG with ASCVD.

Diagnostic Criteria

Screening of adults > 20 years of age is recommended every 4–6 years in patients without ASCVD or diabetes and with LDL of 70–189 mg/dL. Children ages 2–8 should be screened if they have a family history of dyslipidemia or heart disease, or if the child has other risk factors for heart disease such as obesity, hypertension, diabetes, or exposure to cigarette smoke. Universal screening is recommended for all children ages 9–11. LDL levels in excess of 160 mg/dL may indicate a familial dyslipidemia.

Secondary causes of dyslipidemia should be investigated. Common causes of elevated LDL are diet (excess saturated or trans fats, weight gain, anorexia), diseases (biliary obstruction, nephrotic syndrome), or disorders and altered metabolic states (hypothyroidism, obesity, pregnancy). Elevated TG may be caused by diet (weight gain, very low-fat diets, high intake of refined carbohydrates, excessive alcohol). See Table 16-2 for medication-related causes of dyslipidemia.

Familial hypercholesterolemia

Familial hypercholesterolemia (FH) is associated with a mutation in the LDL receptor gene, the apolipoprotein B (Apo B) gene, or the proprotein convertase subtilisin/kexin type 9 (PCSK9) gene. Patients who are homozygous for this mutation may have LDL cholesterol > 800 mg/dL in infancy, and those with heterozygous FH often have LDL cholesterol > 160 mg/dL. Cardiovascular mortality in patients age 20–39 is 100-fold that of the general population, if the condition is untreated. FH treatment in children should target LDL values < 130 mg/dL or a 50% LDL reduction with a high-intensity statin.

Table 16–2. Medications That Cause Dyslipidemia

Secondary Cause	Elevated LDL	Elevated Triglycerides
Medications	Diuretics	Thiazide diuretics
	Glucocorticoids	Glucocorticoids
	Amiodarone	Oral estrogens
	Cyclosporine	Bile acid sequestrants
		Protease inhibitors
		Retinoic acid
		Anabolic steroids
		Sirolimus
		Raloxifene
		Tamoxifen
		Beta blockers (except carvedilol)

Children and adolescents

Children age 8 and older with LDL levels > 190 mg/dL should be considered for medication therapy (> 160 mg/dL for children with family history of heart disease or more than two other risk factors and > 130 mg/dL for children with diabetes). First-line medication options include bile acid sequestrants, cholesterol absorption inhibitors, and statins. Niacin products are not recommended for children, and fibrates should be used with caution and under the supervision of a pediatric lipid specialist.

Children age 2 and older who are overweight or obese and who have a high TG level or low HDL level should receive a recommendation of weight management and increased physical activity as the primary treatment.

Clinical Presentation

Dyslipidemias are usually asymptomatic, except in some familial lipid disorders in which patients may develop cutaneous manifestations of lipid deposition (e.g., tendon xanthomas, planar xanthomas, xanthelasmas, and eye manifestations [corneal arcus]).

Treatment Principles

Prior to November 2013, the Adult Treatment Panel (ATP) III (published in 2001) and Update to ATP III (published in 2004) served as the standard of care for lipid management. Within these guidelines, assessment of risk factors and titration of medication therapy to target LDL levels were the mainstay of treatment. In 2013, the American College of Cardiology/American Heart Association (ACC/AHA) issued updated recommendations for the treatment of blood cholesterol that were markedly different from previous guidelines. Though ACC/AHA explicitly stated that these were not meant to be a comprehensive guide to lipid management, they are a recommendation for treatment of lipids using fixed-dose statins to prevent ASCVD.

ASCVD is defined as follows:

- Acute coronary syndromes
- Myocardial infarction
- Stable or unstable angina
- Coronary or other arterial revascularization
- Stroke or transient ischemic attack (TIA)
- Peripheral arterial disease

Consider potential ASCVD risk and benefit, taking into consideration adverse effects, drug–drug interactions, and patient preferences for statins.

Lifestyle modification

All patients with dyslipidemia should undertake lifestyle modifications. For the purposes of ASCVD prevention, the 2013 ACC/AHA guidelines recommended the Dietary Approaches to Stop Hypertension (DASH) diet because evidence shows that it can reduce the risk of ASCVD. The DASH diet consists of dietary intake patterns that emphasize vegetables, fruits, whole grains, low-fat dairy products, poultry, fish, legumes, nontropical vegetable oils, and nuts. Intake of sweets, sugar-sweetened beverages, and red meats should be limited. Daily intake from saturated fats should be 5–6% of total calories. Sodium in the diet should be limited to no more than 2,400 mg/day, with reduction to 1,500 mg sodium/day producing the maximum blood pressure reduction. Exercise should consist of moderate to vigorous aerobic activity 3–4 times per week, lasting an average of 40 minutes per session.

Other dietary interventions that can lower LDL cholesterol (but are not included in the new recommendations) include viscous fiber (10–25 g/day) and plant stanols or sterols (2 g/day). Plant sterols and stanols interfere with micellar absorption of cholesterol. Viscous fiber, found in oats, pectin, and psyllium, also interferes with cholesterol absorption. Soy protein (25–40 g/day), when replacing animal food products, can also lower cholesterol. Though there is less evidence to support such measures in ASCVD prevention in adults, these dietary interventions are still recommended for children and adolescents who do not achieve their LDL goals.

Risk evaluation

The Pooled Cohort Risk Score takes into account age, gender, race (non-Hispanic white or African American), total cholesterol, HDL cholesterol, systolic blood pressure, blood pressure medication use, diabetes, and smoking status to determine a percent risk for an atherosclerotic event at 10 years. The equation may be used for other ethnic groups; however, it may underestimate risk in subgroups such as Native Americans, South Asians, and Puerto Ricans and overestimate risk for East Asians and Mexican Americans. Cut-points of ≥ 7.5.% or < 7.5% have been established to guide therapy.

Treatment

Patients are stratified by presence or absence of existing ASCVD disease, baseline LDL level, presence of diabetes, and age. See Table 16-3 to delineate statin therapy for patients with associated risk. Four major benefit groups are outlined.

Though these statin benefit groups are identified, patients may not completely fit into one of the categories. The following risk factors should also be considered when evaluating individual patient risk:

- Primary LDL > 160 mg/dL or other evidence of genetic dyslipidemia
- Family history of premature ASCVD onset (< 55 years of age in a first-degree male relative, < 65 years of age in a first-degree female relative)
- High-sensitivity C-reactive protein
- Coronary artery calcium (CAC) score > 300 Agatston units or ≥ 75th percentile for age, gender, and ethnicity
- Ankle-brachial index < 0.9
- Elevated lifetime risk of ASCVD.

16-4. Drug Therapy

Prior to initiation of therapy, a baseline fasting lipid panel (FLP) should be obtained and then reevaluated at 4–12 weeks to assess adherence. Following this initial test, FLP should be assessed every 3–12 months to assess adherence and response to treatment. Other laboratory parameters specific to each medication will be included separately.

HMG-CoA Reductase Inhibitors (statins)

These agents competitively inhibit HMG-CoA (3-hydroxy-3-methyl-glutaryl-coenzyme A) reductase, which is the enzyme responsible for conversion of HMG-CoA to mevalonate.

Mevalonate is an early precursor to and a rate-limiting step in cholesterol synthesis. This reduction in liver cholesterol synthesis results in upregulation of liver LDL receptors and increased clearance of LDL and VLDL particles in the blood. These actions induce a decrease in total cholesterol and LDL cholesterol, promote a slight increase in HDL cholesterol, and effect a modest decrease in TG.

Monitoring

- Conduct baseline liver function tests (LFTs), A1c, thyroid function tests (thyroid-stimulating hormone [TSH] tests), serum creatinine (SCr), and creatine phosphokinase (CPK) in patients

Table 16-3. Reduction of ASCVD Risk with Statins: Daily Doses and Associated Risk Categories

Risk Category	High-intensity statin (Lowers LDL ~> 50)	Moderate-intensity statin (Lowers LDL ~30–49%)	Low-intensity statin (Lowers LDL < 30%)
	Atorvastatin 40–80 mg	**Atorvastatin** 10–20mg	Fluvastatin 20–40 mg
	Rosuvastatin 20–40 mg	Fluvastatin 40mg bid	Lovastatin 20 mg
		Fluvastatin XL 80 mg	Pitavastatin 1 mg
		Lovastatin 40 mg	Pravastatin 10–20 mg
		Pitavastatin 2–4 mg	Simvastatin 10 mg
		Pravastatin 40–80 mg	
		Simvastatin 20–40 mg	
		Rosuvastatin 5–10 mg	
1) Existing ASCVD			
Age ≤ 75	Preferred	Preferred if high-intensity statin is contraindicated	
		If characteristics predisposing to adverse effects are present	
Age > 75	Continue current statin therapy if tolerating; otherwise, evaluate patient preferences, drug–drug interactions, and risk of adverse effects before starting a moderate- or high-dose statin.		
No ASCVD			
2) Age ≥ 21 and LDL ≥ 190 mg/dL	Preferred	Preferred if unable to tolerate high-intensity statin	
	(Once 50% LDL reduction is achieved, it is reasonable to add nonstatin drug to further lower LDL. Evaluate patient preferences, drug–drug interactions, and risk of adverse effects.)		
3) Age 40–75 Diabetes mellitus LDL 70–189 mg/dL	Preferred if ASCVD risk is > 7.5%	Preferred	
4) Age 40–75 No diabetes mellitus LDL 70–189 mg/dL	Preferred if ASCVD risk is > 7.5%	Preferred if ASCVD risk is 5–7.5%	

Boldface indicates one of top 100 drugs for 2012 by units sold at retail outlets, www.drugs.com/stats/top100/2012/units.

with a personal or family history of muscle side effects from statins.
- LFTs should be repeated only when clinically indicated.
- CPK needs to be monitored only if the patient has suspected muscle damage.
- Patients with LDL cholesterol < 40 mg/dL on two separate readings should have their statin dose decreased.

Dosage and administration

See Tables 16-4 and 16-5 for detailed information regarding dosing.

Short-acting statins (pravastatin, simvastatin, fluvastatin) are administered at bedtime because most hepatic cholesterol production occurs overnight. Atorvastatin, rosuvastatin, and pitavastatin may be given any time of the day because of their longer half-life. Lovastatin conventional tablets should be given with the evening meal because absorption is better with food; however, the extended-release lovastatin products should be taken at bedtime. The lovastatin plus Niaspan combination product should be taken at bedtime with a low-fat snack. Administration of simvastatin 80 mg is limited to patients who have been taking this dose for ≥ 12 consecutive months without evidence of myopathy. Initiation of simvastatin 80 mg is no longer recommended because of risk of myopathy. All statins are approved for use in children ages 10–18. Only pravastatin is approved for children ≥ 8 years of age.

Table 16–4. Statin Dosing Considerations

Statin	Drug–drug Interactions	Dosing considerations
Atorvastatin	Amiodarone, boceprevir, clarithromycin	
Fluvastatin	Cyclosporine, danazol, delavirdine	Dose adjust if CrCl < 30 mL/min.
Lovastatin	Erythromycin, fluoxetine, fluvoxamine, verapamil	Maximum dose is 20 mg if danazol or diltiazem. Maximum dose is 40 mg if amiodarone.
Pitavastatin	Grapefruit juice, indinavir, itraconazole	
Simvastatin	Strong CYP3A4 inhibitors (ketoconazole, nefazodone, nelfinavir) contraindicated with simvastatin	Maximum dose is 20 mg if amiodarone, amlodipine, or ranolazine. Maximum dose is 10 mg if verapamil, diltiazem, or dronedarone. Dose adjust if CrCl < 30 mL/min.
Rosuvastatin	Nicardipine, pimozide, posaconazole, quinidine, ritonavir, saquinavir, sildenafil, tacrolimus, telaprevir, testosterone, verapamil, zafirlukast	Initiate at 5 mg daily in Asians. Dose adjust if CrCl < 30 mL/min.
Pravastatin	Metabolized by 2D6	

Boldface indicates one of top 100 drugs for 2012 by units sold at retail outlets, www.drugs.com/stats/top100/2012/units.

Table 16-5. Drug Products and Dosage

Generic name	Trade name	Dosage range and schedule	Dosage form and strength
Statins			
Atorvastatin	**Lipitor**	10–80 mg/day	10, 20, 40, 80 mg tablets
Fluvastatin	Lescol	20–80 mg nightly	20, 40 mg capsules; 80 mg XL tablet
Lovastatin	Mevacor	20–80 mg nightly	10, 20, 40 mg tablets
Lovastatin extended-release	Altoprev	10–60 mg nightly	10, 20, 40, 60 mg tablets
Pitavastatin	Livalo	1–4 mg/day	1, 2, 4 mg tablets
Pravastatin	Pravachol	20–80 mg nightly	10, 20, 40, 80 mg tablets
Simvastatin	Zocor	20–80 mg nightly	5, 10, 20, 40, 80 mg tablets
Rosuvastatin	**Crestor**	5–40 mg/day	5, 10, 20, 40 mg tablets
Bile acid sequestrants			
Cholestyramine	Questran	4–16 g/day divided	Powder
Colestipol	Colestid	5–20 g/day divided	Powder or tablet
Colesevelam	Welchol	2.6–3.8 g/day (daily or bid)	625 mg tablet
Nicotinic acid			
Immediate release	Niacor	1.5–3 g/day (divided tid)	500 mg tablet
Sustained release	Slo-Niacin	1–2 g nightly	250, 500, 750 mg tablets
Extended release	**Niaspan**	1–2 g nightly	500, 750, 1,000 mg tablets
Fibric acids			
Gemfibrozil	Lopid	600 mg before meals bid	600 mg tablet
Fenofibrate	**Tricor**	48–145 mg/day	48, 145 mg tablets
Fenofibric acid	Fibricor	35–105 mg/day	35, 105 mg tablets
	Trilipix	45–135 mg/day	45, 135 mg capsules

Table 16-5. Drug Products and Dosage *(Continued)*

Generic name	Trade name	Dosage range and schedule	Dosage form and strength
Cholesterol inhibitors			
Ezetimibe	**Zetia**	10 mg/day	10 mg tablet
Omega-3 fatty acids			
Omega-3 fatty acid	**Lovaza**	4 g qd or 2 g bid	1 g capsule
Combinations			
Aspirin + pravastatin[a]	Pravigard PAC	81/20–325/80 mg qhs	81/20, 81/40, 81/80 mg tablets; 325/20, 325/40, 325/80 mg tablets
Ezetimibe + simvastatin	**Vytorin**	10/10–10/80 mg qhs	10/10, 10/20, 10/40, 10/80 mg tablets
Ezetimibe + atorvastatin	Liptruzet	10/10–10/80 mg/day	10/10, 10/20, 10/40, 10/80
Lovastatin + **Niaspan**	Advicor	20/500–40/2,000 mg/day	20/500, 20/750, 20/1,000 mg tablets
Simvastatin + Niacin	Simcor	500/20–2,000/40 mg/day	500/20, 500/40, 750/20, 1,000/20, 1,000/40 mg tablets
Other			
Mipomersen	Kynamro	200 mg subcutaneously once weekly	200 mg/mL

Boldface indicates one of top 100 drugs for 2012 by units sold at retail outlets, www.drugs.com/stats/top100/2012/units.
a. Aspirin tablets and pravastatin tablets are separate tablets within the Pravigard PAC.

Doubling the dose of statin lowers LDL levels only by an additional 6%.

Adverse effects

- Myopathy (muscle damage) may occur.
- Myalgia (muscle pain, soreness, or tenderness) may occur.
- Myositis occurs in 0.2% of patients. Myositis is myalgia combined with CPK elevated 3–10 times the upper limit of normal (ULN).
- Rhabdomyolysis occurs rarely, but it can cause acute renal failure. The statin or other offending drug should be discontinued immediately. Rhabdomyolysis is the combination of severe muscle symptoms plus CPK elevated 10 times the ULN with increased serum creatinine and urine myoglobin.
- Elevated liver enzymes occur in 0.1–2.3% of patients.
- Cognitive impairment, such as memory loss, forgetfulness, and confusion, has been reported by some statin users.
- Statins may be associated with a slightly increased rate of incident type 2 diabetes.
- Flu-like symptoms and headache may occur.
- Patients may have mild gastrointestinal (GI) complaints.
- Active liver disease is a contraindication to statin therapy; caution should be used in patients with chronic liver disease or unexplained elevations in transaminases ($> 3 \times$ ULN). Statins may be beneficial in fatty liver disease.

Drug interactions

See Table 16-4 for dosing considerations with statins. Patients taking pitavastatin who are also taking erythromycin should not take more than 1 mg/day of pitavastatin. Patients taking pitavastatin who are also taking rifampin should not take more than 2 mg/day of pitavastatin. Dosing of simvastatin 80 mg should be avoided except in patients who have been stable on this dose for the past 12 months.

Bile Acid Sequestrants (Resins)

Nonabsorbable anion exchange resins exchange chloride ions for bile acids and other anions in the intestine. This action inhibits enterohepatic recycling, which results in bile excretion and a decrease in the cholesterol pool in the liver. LDL receptors are upregulated, increased LDL is cleared, and LDL is lowered.

Monitoring

- Evaluate baseline FLP for hypertriglyceridemia:
  - If TG > 200 mg/dL, use resins with caution.
  - If TG > 400 mg/dL, resins are contraindicated.

Dosing and administration

Cholestyramine and colestipol should be titrated slowly to avoid GI side effects. They may be started with one dose daily with the largest meal. They may be increased (after the patient adjusts to the resin) to two doses daily with the largest meals or divided between breakfast and dinner. Powdered doses can be mixed with food such as soup, oatmeal, nonfat yogurt, and applesauce. The mixture can also be chilled overnight to improve palatability. To prevent constipation, resins may be mixed with psyllium; however, this mixture should be ingested immediately after mixing to prevent a gel from forming. Counsel the patient to rinse the glass and drink the remains to ensure ingestion of all resin. Colesevelam is a tablet formulation, which may be easier for some patients to self-administer. However, the tablets are large, and some patients may not be able to swallow them. Separate other medications 1 hour before and 4 hours after administration to prevent binding of medications.

Adverse effects

- GI distress may occur.
- Patients may experience palatability problems with the resin slurry.
- Constipation may occur that increases with the dose and in the elderly.
- Decreased absorption of other drugs may occur. Dose other drugs 1 hour before or 4 hours after ingestion of resin.
- Contraindication is absolute in history of bowel obstruction, hypertriglyceridemia-induced pancreatitis, or TG > 500 mg/dL.

Drug interactions

Avoid concomitant administration with all other drugs, especially digoxin, levothyroxine, tetracycline, warfarin, fat-soluble vitamins, and minerals.

Niacin

Niacin reduces LDL cholesterol and TG and increases HDL cholesterol. It may decrease VLDL synthesis, thereby leading to decreased LDL cholesterol and TG. It may inhibit metabolism of apolipoprotein A-I, which increases HDL cholesterol.

Nicotinic acid

- Evaluate baseline fasting glucose, LFTs, and serum uric acid levels.
- For immediate-release niacin, repeat these tests 4–6 weeks after each dose titration.
- For sustained-release niacin, evaluate monthly LFTs while dosage is titrated; then every 12 weeks for the first year; and then periodically.
- Patients with diabetes require periodic fasting glucose tests, especially when higher doses of nicotinic acid are used.
- Following achievement of target dose, monitor serum uric acid in patients with a history of hyperuricemia or gout.

Patient counseling

Immediate-release niacin should be started at a low dose and slowly titrated upward:

- Start with 100 mg tid, and titrate upward the second week to 200 mg tid. The next week, increase to 350 mg tid; and the following week, increase to 500 mg tid. When 1,500 mg/day is reached and maintained for 4 weeks, assess efficacy before further increasing the dose.
- If further titration is needed, increase to 750 mg tid and assess effectiveness after 4 weeks before increasing titration.
- The usual dose is 1,000–2,000 mg tid. The dose should not exceed 6 g/day.

Extended-release niacin should be started with 500 mg at bedtime and titrated weekly to a maximum dose of 2,000 mg/day.
- Take with food to minimize GI upset.
- Avoid alcohol, hot drinks, or spicy foods at time of ingestion to minimize flushing and pruritus.

Adverse effects

- Flushing is common. Pretreat with aspirin (325 mg) or ibuprofen 200 mg 30 minutes before the first niacin dose of the day.
- Hyperglycemia is a risk. Use with caution in diabetics.

- Hyperuricemia (or gout) may occur:
- Upper GI distress
- Hepatotoxicity
- Absolute contraindication in chronic liver disease and severe gout
- Relative contraindication in diabetes, hyperuricemia, severe gout, or active peptic ulcer disease

Use caution in combination with resins. Combination therapy with statins and gemfibrozil may cause an increased risk of myopathy.

Fibric Acids (Fibrates)

Fibrates reduce TG by reduction of apolipoproteins B, C-III, and E. They increase HDL cholesterol by increasing apolipoproteins A-I and A-II.

Monitoring

Evaluate baseline renal function.

Patient counseling

Gemfibrozil should be taken twice daily 30 minutes before meals. Tricor and fenofibric acid can be taken with or without food once daily.

Reduce the dose in patients with renal insufficiency, and monitor for muscle toxicity, especially when used in combination with statins and niacin.

Adverse effects

- Dyspepsia may occur.
- Gallstones may occur.
- Risk for myopathy increases when combined with statins.
- Fibrates are contraindicated in severe renal or severe hepatic disease.

Drug interactions

- These agents are highly protein bound, and they are metabolized by the cytochrome P450 (CYP450) 3A4 enzyme system.
- The effect of warfarin may be increased.
- Cyclosporine may increase gemfibrozil concentrations.
- Fenofibrate may have less interaction potential with warfarin and cyclosporine.
- Bile acid sequestrants (resins) decrease fibrate absorption.
- Combinations with statins and niacin may increase the risk of myopathy.

Cholesterol Inhibitors (Ezetimibe)

Cholesterol inhibitors selectively inhibit intestinal absorption of dietary and biliary cholesterol at the brush border of the small intestine, which results in a decrease in the absorption of cholesterol and a decrease in cholesterol in the blood. When added to statin therapy, ezetimibe provides an additional 15% reduction in LDL levels.

Dosing and administration

Cholesterol inhibitors are dosed once daily without regard to food. They can be taken simultaneously in combination with statins.

Adverse effects

- GI distress (less than with resins) may occur.
- Use with caution in moderate to severe hepatic disease.

Drug interactions

Combination with a resin may decrease absorption. Combination with a fibric acid may predispose to gallbladder disease.

Cyclosporine may increase ezetimibe concentrations.

Omega-3 Fatty Acids

The mechanism of action for omega-3 fatty acids is not completely understood. Possible mechanisms of action include the following:

- Inhibition of acyl CoA: 1,2-diacylglycerol acyltransferase
- Increased mitochondrial and peroxisomal β-oxidation in the liver
- Decreased lipogenesis in the liver
- Increased lipoprotein lipase activity

Dosing and administration

The daily dose (4 g) can be taken in a single or divided dose (2 g bid). These agents should be taken with meal(s).

Monitoring

- Omega-3 fatty acids are not for use in patients with a history of allergy or sensitivity to fish.
- Assess effectiveness at 2 months. Discontinue use if the decrease in TG level is not adequate.

- Evaluate baseline FLP for TG ≥ 500 mg/dL.
- Periodic monitoring of alanine aminotransferase levels is recommended.
- Periodic monitoring is recommended for increase in LDL cholesterol levels.

Adverse effects

- Burping
- Indigestion
- Taste sense alteration
- Possible prolonged bleeding time when used with anticoagulants

Other Agent

Mipomersen

Mipomersen is an oligonucleotide inhibitor of apo B synthesis via binding to mRNA (messenger ribonucleic acid). Apo B is the principal lipoprotein associated with VLDL and LDL; therefore, inhibition of production results in lower LDL and VLDL levels.

Dosage and administration

For adults with homozygous familial hypercholesterolemia, mipomersen is to be used as an adjunct to lipid-lowering medications: 200 mg subcutaneously once weekly on the same day every week. Safety and efficacy in pediatric patients have not yet been established.

Monitoring

Mipomersen is contraindicated in moderate or severe hepatic impairment.

Monitor lipid levels every 3 months during the first year of therapy.

Monitor LDL cholesterol after 6 months to weigh benefit of LDL reduction versus risk of hepatotoxicity.

Monitor baseline alanine aminotransferase (ALT) and aspartate aminotransferase (AST), alkaline phosphatase, total bilirubin, then ALT and AST monthly during first year of therapy, then every 3 months or more often if clinically indicated.

Adverse effects

- Mipomersen may cause elevations of ALT and AST, abnormal liver function tests.
- Injection site reactions (pain, erythema, hematoma, edema, pruritus) are common.

Table 16-6. Efficacy of Drugs Used to Treat Dyslipidemia

Drug class	Lipid and lipoprotein effect
Statins	LDL ↓18–55%
	HDL ↑5–15%
	TG ↓7–30%
Resins	LDL ↓15–30%
	HDL ↑3–5%
	TG (no change)
Nicotinic acid	LDL ↓5–25%
	HDL ↑15–35%
	TG ↓20–50%
Fibric acids	LDL ↓5–20%
	HDL ↑10–20%
	TG ↓20–50%
Cholesterol inhibitors	LDL ↓17%
	HDL ↓1.3%
	TG ↓6%
Omega-3 fatty acid (**Lovaza**)	LDL ↑25–31%
	HDL ↑4–13%
	TG ↓45%

Boldface indicates one of top 100 drugs for 2012 by units sold at retail outlets, http://www.drugs.com/stats/top100/2012/units.

- It may cause fatigue, flu-like illness, shivering, or fever.
- Antibodies may develop to injection.

See Tables 16-6 and 16-7 for summaries of use and for a summary of lipid-lowering agents and their effect on lipid parameters.

Table 16-7. Pharmacotherapeutic Options for Treatment of Dyslipidemia

Lipid target	Pharmacotherapy
LDL	Statin most potent and effective for large LDL reductions
	Niacin and resins effective for moderate LDL reductions
	Combination of statin + ezetimibe
	Combination of statin + resin
LDL + TG	Combination of statin + fibric acid
TG	Fibric acid or niacin

16-5. Questions

Use the following case study to answer Questions 1–5.

A 50-year-old man comes to your pharmacy for cholesterol and medication monitoring. His medical history is notable for hypertension, recent-onset type 2 diabetes, and hypercholesterolemia. Family history is noncontributory. Social history indicates that he neither smokes nor uses alcohol. He has no known allergies. His medication history reveals that he occasionally takes acetaminophen for headaches and no other OTC medications or herbal products. Current medications include hydrochlorothiazide 25 mg/day (for 4 years) and a new prescription today for atorvastatin 10 mg/day. Your physical assessment reveals the following: BP 144/90 mm Hg; pulse, 70 and regular; weight, 185 lb; height, 5'9''. Other pertinent labs include an A1c of 7.3%. A FLP today reveals the following: total cholesterol = 250 mg/dL, HDL = 40 mg/dL, and TG = 145 mg/dL.

1. What is the patient's LDL cholesterol?

   A. 130 mg/dL
   B. 153 mg/dL
   C. 162 mg/dL
   D. 178 mg/dL
   E. 181 mg/dL

2. What medication changes, if any, are recommended for this patient?

   A. No changes should be made.
   B. Change atorvastatin to 40 mg daily.
   C. Add niacin to atorvastatin 10 daily.
   D. Discontinue hydrochlorothiazide.
   E. Add Welchol to the treatment regimen.

3. At what time point should you assess the effectiveness of therapy?

   A. 3 weeks
   B. 4 weeks
   C. 6 months
   D. Only if adverse events are noted
   E. Annually

4. Which of the following baseline labs would be optimal to assess prior to initiation of this patient's medication for dyslipidemia?

   A. CBC, SCr, LFTs
   B. SCr, LFTs
   C. SCr, LFTs, CPK, TSH

   D. CBC, LFTs
   E. SCr, LFTs, CPK

5. The patient returns for reassessment at the appropriate time. His FLP shows that his LDL cholesterol is now 115 mg/dL. What is your assessment?

   A. Stop the statin because the patient has achieved optimal LDL levels.
   B. The optimal dose reduction for this patient has been achieved.
   C. The optimal dose reduction for this patient has not been achieved.
   D. Fenofibrate needs to be added to the regimen.
   E. Add cholestyramine.

6. Which of the following statins must be dosed with the evening meal?

   A. Atorvastatin
   B. Simvastatin
   C. Pitavastatin
   D. Lovastatin
   E. Rosuvastatin

7. Which of the following is *not* a secondary cause of dyslipidemia?

   A. High LDL cholesterol
   B. Hypothyroidism
   C. Diabetes
   D. Renal disease
   E. β-blockers

8. Cholesterol biosynthesis can be decreased by which of the following?

   A. Statins
   B. Oat bran
   C. Bile acid sequestrants (resins)
   D. Zetia
   E. Aspirin

9. Which of the following medications has the greatest efficacy in raising HDL levels?

   A. Lovastatin
   B. Pravastatin
   C. Gemfibrozil
   D. Nicotinic acid
   E. Colesevelam

10. Which of the following has the most potent LDL-lowering effect?

   A. Nicotinic acid
   B. Fibric acids
   C. Omega-3 fatty acids
   D. Cholesterol inhibitors
   E. HMG-CoA reductase inhibitors

11. Which of the following could be an adjunct medication to statins and diet in a child with homozygous familial hypercholesterolemia?

   A. Niacin
   B. Fibrate
   C. Ezetimibe
   D. Mipomersen
   E. No adjunct is available.

12. Which of the following most accurately describes a medication and its corresponding effect?

   A. Diabetes is an absolute contraindication to the use of nicotinic acid.
   B. Aspirin is dosed three times per day to prevent flushing from niacin.
   C. Gemfibrozil may reduce triglycerides by as much as 50%.
   D. Colesevelam has similar patient tolerability problems as cholestyramine.
   E. Ezetimibe frequently causes muscle toxicity.

13. A 45-year-old patient has a past medical history of diabetes, hypertension, depression, and tobacco abuse. He had a history of TIA 3 years ago, and his LDL cholesterol is 140 mg/dL. The decision is made to initiate statin therapy. Which of the following doses of statin would be most appropriate?

   A. Lipitor 10 mg
   B. Lipitor 40 mg
   C. Zocor 40 mg
   D. Pravachol 80 mg
   E. Lescol XL 80 mg

14. Which of the following agents would be most likely to produce myalgias when combined with a statin?

   A. Fibrate
   B. Aspirin

   C. ACE inhibitor
   D. Levothyroxine
   E. Colesevelam

15. Which of the following patient conditions would affect the decision to initiate therapy with nicotinic acid?

   A. Concomitant therapy with a diuretic
   B. Concomitant therapy with renally toxic medications
   C. Active liver disease
   D. Baseline elevation of serum creatinine
   E. Uncontrolled hypertension

16. Identify a baseline laboratory test that is required before initiating a statin.

   A. Serum potassium
   B. Complete blood cell count
   C. Liver function tests
   D. hs-CRP
   E. Platelet function tests

17. The major troublesome side effect in nicotinic acid therapy is

   A. diarrhea.
   B. vomiting.
   C. hair growth.
   D. flushing.
   E. dizziness.

18. Which of the following medications has this warning: "For patients switching from immediate-release niacin, therapy with this drug should be initiated with a low dose and then titrated to the desired therapeutic response"?

   A. Pravigard
   B. Vytorin
   C. Advicor
   D. Atorvastatin
   E. Ezetimibe

19. Identify the drug interaction that involves the CYP450 system.

   A. Ezetimibe + niacin
   B. Colestipol + simvastatin
   C. Gemfibrozil + cholestyramine
   D. Fenofibrate + ezetimibe
   E. Lovastatin + itraconazole

20. Which of the following agents produces an additional 15% LDL reduction when combined with a statin?

    A. Colesevelam
    B. Nicotinic acid
    C. 15 grams of soluble fiber
    D. Fenofibrate
    E. Ezetimibe

16-6. Answers

1. **E.** Use the Friedewald equation to calculate LDL:

$$LDL = total\ cholesterol - (HDL + TG/5)$$

$$LDL = 250 - (40 + 145/5) = 181$$

2. **A.** The new guidelines recommend a moderate-dose statin in a diabetic patient between the ages of 40 and 75 with no other contraindications unless the ASCVD risk is greater than 7.5%. Because the ASCVD risk is not known, a moderate-dose statin is acceptable.

3. **B.** A repeat FLP should be drawn after 4–12 weeks to assess adherence to therapy. Atorvastatin 40 mg would be expected to produce ~50% decrease in LDL cholesterol.

4. **C.** In addition to baseline SCr (for renally adjusted statins), CPK, and LFTs, measuring TSH is optimal because hypothyroidism is a factor in statin-induced myalgias.

5. **B.** The dose of statin has achieved a 36% reduction in LDL cholesterol. The expected reduction for atorvastatin 10 mg daily would approximate 30–49%. Had that dose reduction not been achieved, a recommendation would have been to investigate possible nonadherence to therapy with the patient.

6. **D.** Lovastatin is the only statin that must be dosed with the evening meal to increase its absorption.

7. **A.** Causes of dyslipidemia must be ruled out. The common secondary causes are renal failure; hypothyroidism; obstructive liver disease; diabetes; and drugs such as β-blockers, thiazide diuretics, oral contraceptives, oral estrogens, glucocorticoids, and cyclosporine.

8. **A.** Statins competitively inhibit HMG-CoA reductase, which is the enzyme responsible for converting HMG-CoA to mevalonate. Inhibition of mevalonate reduces cholesterol synthesis.

9. **D.** Nicotinic acid (Niaspan) has the most efficacy in raising HDL cholesterol compared with other therapies. HDL cholesterol may be raised 15–35%.

10. **E.** Statins (HMG-CoA reductase inhibitors) have the most efficacy in lowering LDL cholesterol. LDL cholesterol may be lowered 18–55%.

11. **C.** Ezetimibe could be added to statins and diet in a pediatric patient. Niacin and fibrates are not recommended. Safety and efficacy of mipomersen in pediatric patients has not been established.

12. **C.** Gemfibrozil can reduce TG by 20–50%. Diabetes is a relative contraindication to the use of nicotinic acid. Aspirin is dosed once daily, before the first nicotinic acid dose of the day. Colesevelam is a tablet and avoids most of the palatability problems of other resins. Ezetimibe does not cause muscle toxicity.

13. **B.** The patient has a history of TIA; therefore, he has existing ASCVD. He is less than 75 years of age, so a high-intensity statin is preferred.

14. **A.** Use of fibrates in combination with statins increases the risk for myalgias. Though hypothyroidism can also contribute to myalgias, treatment with levothyroxine would not have any effect.

15. **C.** Active liver disease would be a contraindication to initiating therapy with nicotinic acid. Because nicotinic acid is hepatically metabolized, baseline elevations of creatinine and other renally toxic medications would not affect a decision to initiate therapy. Because of niacin's effect on blood glucose, uncontrolled diabetes may warrant consideration of use of another medication.

16. **C.** Baseline tests before statin use include LFTs and CPK.

17. **D.** The most common side effect is flushing, which may occur in many patients. To decrease flushing intensity, a patient should take aspirin 325 mg 30 minutes prior to the first dose of nicotinic acid. Itching may also occur with flushing.

18. **C.** Advicor (Niaspan + lovastatin) contains Niaspan, which is not dose equivalent to immediate-release or modified-release (sustained-release or time-release) niacin preparations.

19. **E.** Lovastatin is metabolized by CYP450 3A4 enzymes, and itraconazole will inhibit this enzyme system. Inhibition causes lovastatin blood and tissue concentrations to rise, thus predisposing the patient to muscle or liver toxicity.

20. **E.** Ezetimibe, when used in combination with a statin, produces an additional 15% reduction in LDL cholesterol.

16-7. References

Daniels SR, Greer FR, Committee on Nutrition. Lipid screening and cardiovascular health in childhood. *Pediatrics.* 2008;122:198–208.

Expert Panel on Detection, Evaluation, and Treatment of High Blood Cholesterol in Adults. Executive summary of the Third Report of the National Cholesterol Education Program (NCEP) Expert Panel on Detection, Evaluation, and Treatment of High Blood Cholesterol in Adults (Adult Treatment Panel III). *JAMA.* 2001;285:2486–97.

Expert Panel on Integrated Guidelines for Cardiovascular Health and Risk Reduction in Children and Adolescents summary report. *Pediatrics.* 2011; 128:S213–56.

Long-Term Intervention with Pravastatin in Ischaemic Disease (LIPID) Study Group. Prevention of cardiovascular events and death with pravastatin in patients with coronary heart disease and a broad range of initial cholesterol levels. *N Engl J Med.* 1998;339:1349–57.

Myśliwiec M, Walczak M, Małecka-Tendera E, et al. Management of familial hypercholesterolemia in children and adolescents. Position paper of the Polish Lipid Expert Forum. *J Clin Lipidology.* 2014; 8:173–80.

Pasternak RC, Smith SC Jr, Bairey-Merz CN, et al. ACC/AHA/NHLBI clinical advisory on the use and safety of statins. *J Am Coll Cardiol.* 2002;40: 568–73.

Stone NJ, Robinson J, Lichtenstein AH, et al. 2013 ACC/AHA guideline on treatment of blood cholesterol to reduce atherosclerotic cardiovascular risk in adults: A report of the American College of Cardiology/American Heart Association Task Force on Practice Guidelines. *Circulation.* 2013: doi:10.1161/01.cir.0000437738.63853.7a. http://circ.ahajournals.org/content/early/2013/11/11/01.cir.0000437738.63853.7a.citation. Accessed April 29, 2014.

Talbert RL. Hyperlipidemia. In: DiPiro JT, Talbert RL, Yee GC, et al., eds. *Pharmacotherapy: A Pathophysiologic Approach.* 8th ed. New York, NY: McGraw-Hill; 2008:365–88.

Diabetes Mellitus

17

Michelle Z. Farland

17-1. Key Points

- Diabetes mellitus (DM) is a group of chronic metabolic diseases exhibiting hyperglycemia resulting from defects in insulin secretion, insulin action, or both.
- Type 1 diabetes results from immune-mediated β-cell destruction, which leads to absolute insulin deficiency.
- Type 2 diabetes is characterized by relative insulin deficiency, insulin resistance, or both.
- The principal treatment goals include maintaining blood glucose levels in the normal or near-normal range and preventing acute and chronic complications.
- Goals of diabetes therapy include achieving and maintaining glycemic control and reaching recommended blood pressure and lipid goals.
- Complications of diabetes include cardiovascular disease, nephropathy, neuropathy, and retinopathy.
- Pharmacotherapy should be individualized to each patient, considering factors such as glucose goals; length of time with DM; concomitant diseases; and psychosocial issues, including available support for the patient, cost for medications and supplies, and the level of risk for acute and chronic complications.
- Multiple studies have shown improved glycemic control delays the onset, slows the progression, and lowers the risk of long-term microvascular complications.

- Metformin should be the backbone of pharmacotherapy for patients with type 2 DM unless contraindicated (severe or unstable renal dysfunction, uncontrolled heart failure) or not tolerated.
- Combination therapy of two or more oral medications, oral medications *plus* insulin, or oral medications *plus* glucagon-like peptide-1(GLP-1) analogs will be required in most patients to maintain continued type 2 DM control.
- Patients with type 1 DM require basal/bolus insulin for glycemic management.
- Metformin
  - Is considered first-line therapy in newly diagnosed type 2 DM
  - Is contraindicated in renal dysfunction patients
  - Has low or minimal risk of hypoglycemia with monotherapy
  - Has gastrointestinal (GI) side effects (flatulence, GI upset, abdominal pain, diarrhea, bloating), which are dose-limiting problems
  - Causes no weight gain
- Secretagogues
  - Are helpful in combination with other oral agents and injectable products
  - Increase risk of hypoglycemia (sulfonylureas > meglitinides)
  - Increase weight (sulfonylureas > meglitinides)
  - Have high rate of failure over time
  - Must be used with caution in renally impaired and elderly patients
- Thiazolidinediones
  - Help improve peripheral insulin resistance
  - Increase weight and edema
  - Have low or minimal risk of hypoglycemia with monotherapy

---

Editor's Note: This chapter is based on the 10th edition chapter with the same title, written by Joni Foard and Benjamin N. Gross.

- Are contraindicated in patients with congestive heart failure
- Have delayed time to see full effects on DM control
- May decrease the progression to DM in high-risk patients
- Alpha-glucosidase inhibitors
  - Block absorption of carbohydrates in the small intestine
  - Have low or minimal risk of hypoglycemia with monotherapy
  - Have GI side effects (flatulence, GI upset, abdominal pain, diarrhea, bloating), which are dose-limiting problems
  - Are more effective for postprandial hyperglycemia
  - Have minimal effect on weight
- GLP-1 agonists and amylin-based medications
  - Increase insulin production in a glucose-dependent fashion
  - Decrease production of glucagon
  - Improve β-cell functioning
  - Slow gastric emptying
  - Increase satiety and possible weight loss
  - Have a dose-limiting side effect of nausea
  - Are injectable products
  - Are for use in type 2 DM
  - Are high cost
- Dipeptidyl peptidase–4 (DPP-4) inhibitors
  - Increase insulin production in a glucose-dependent fashion
  - Decrease production of glucagon
  - Improve β-cell functioning
  - Have no effect on weight
  - Are well tolerated with few side effects
  - Are for use in type 2 DM
  - Are high cost
- Amylin mimetic (Symlin)
  - Decreases production of glucagons
  - Slows gastric emptying
  - Increases satiety and possible weight loss
  - Has significant risk of hypoglycemia in combination with insulin in type 1 DM
  - Has the dose-limiting side effect of nausea
  - Is for use in type 1 and type 2 DM
  - Is high cost
- Insulin
  - Is essential for type 1 DM
  - Is often used in type 2 DM in combination with other therapies
  - Should be considered initial agent for type 2 DM if glucose is > 250 mg/dL or A_{1C} > 10%
  - Is often started as basal therapy (0.1–0.2 units/kg/day) added to an existing oral regimen

- Should be individualized to the patient's goals and motivation: intensive insulin therapy (> 3 doses/day or use of continuous subcutaneous insulin infusion) is replacing conventional insulin therapy (split-mix dosing: two-thirds of total daily dose)
- Varies principally by source; appearance; time-activity profiles (onset, peak, and duration); dosing; and route of administration
- May have these adverse events: hypoglycemia, weight gain, and lipodystrophies
- Patient education is essential for the management of DM because it provides a means for persons with this chronic disease to become empowered, cope effectively, and engage in appropriate self-care.
- Recommended lifestyle modifications include weight management, increased physical activity, and smoking cessation.

17-2. Study Guide Checklist

The following topics may guide your study of this subject area:

- Summarize diagnostic criteria for patients at risk for diabetes (prediabetes) and diabetes.
- Differentiate mechanism of action, adverse events, efficacy, and contraindications for non-insulin antihyperglycemic agents for type 2 diabetes.
- Differentiate the pharmacokinetics of available insulin products.
- Design an initial insulin regimen for patients with type 1 and type 2 diabetes.
- Identify key patient-counseling points for specific antihyperglycemic agents.
- Identify components of diabetes self-management education to assist patients with lifestyle modifications to improve glycemic control.

17-3. Overview

Diabetes mellitus (DM) is a group of chronic metabolic diseases caused by defects in insulin secretion, insulin action, or both that result in hyperglycemia. DM is associated with long-term macrovascular and microvascular complications. It affects 25.8 million people in the United States, or approximately 8.3% of the population: 18.8 million diagnosed and 7 million undiagnosed. DM is the seventh leading cause of death. Risk of death is two times that of people without DM of similar age.

Classification (Table 17-1)

Type 1 diabetes

Type 1 DM comprises 5–10% of all diagnosed cases and requires exogenous insulin for survival.

Type 2 diabetes

Type 2 DM comprises 90–95% of all diagnosed cases.

Gestational diabetes mellitus

Gestational diabetes mellitus (GDM) involves glucose intolerance with onset of pregnancy or first recognition during pregnancy (second and third trimesters). Approximately 7% of pregnant women develop GDM, which is more than 200,000 annually. Women with GDM have a 40–60% chance of developing type 2 DM later.

Other types of diabetes

Secondary types of DM may be attributed to genetic defects of β-cell function (e.g., maturity-onset diabetes of the young); genetic defects in insulin action; diseases of the exocrine pancreas (e.g., pancreatitis, trauma, pancreatic cancer); endocrinopathies (e.g., acromegaly, Cushing's syndrome); drug-induced DM (e.g., glucocorticoids); infections; and other genetic syndromes. Secondary types of DM constitute 1–5% of all diagnosed cases.

Categories of increased risk for diabetes

Also referred to as having prediabetes, this group of individuals has plasma glucose levels that are higher than normal but lower than those diagnostic for DM. Prediabetes has also been characterized as *impaired fasting glucose* (IFG) and *impaired glucose tolerance* (IGT). It is a risk factor for future DM and cardiovascular disease (CVD).

Categories of increased risk for DM include a fasting plasma glucose (FPG) of 100 mg/dL to 125 mg/dL, a 75 g oral glucose tolerance test 2-hour glucose of 140 mg/dL to 199 mg/dL, or an A_{1C} of 5.7–6.4%. Once a patient is identified as having increased risk for DM, screening for DM using one of the above tests should be completed at least annually.

Table 17-1. Comparison of Type 1 and Type 2 Diabetes Mellitus

	Type 1	Type 2
Previous names	Insulin-dependent diabetes mellitus; juvenile-onset diabetes	Non-insulin-dependent diabetes mellitus; adult-onset diabetes
Percentage of DM cases	5–10	90–95
Age of occurrence	< 30 years (usually childhood or adolescence); at any age following autoimmune stimulus (e.g., virus)	> 30 years; increasing in childhood and adolescence in association with obesity and inactivity
Onset	Rapid	Gradual
Primary etiology	Autoimmune-mediated mechanism with genetic predisposition	Genetic and environmental (e.g., family history, ethnicity, obesity, inactivity)
Pathogenesis	Destruction of β-cells resulting in absolute insulin deficiency and abnormal glucose control	Increasing resistance of tissue (liver and skeletal muscle) to insulin; impaired insulin secretion resulting in relative deficiency of insulin; increased hepatic glucose production
Signs and symptoms	Polyuria, polydipsia, polyphagia, unexplained weight loss, fatigue, blurred vision, possibly ketoacidosis	Polyuria, polydipsia, polyphagia, obesity, fatigue, blurred vision, possibly asymptomatic
Ketoacidosis	Ketosis prone (DKA)	Not ketosis prone because of residual insulin (hyperglycemic hyperosmolar nonketotic syndrome)
Treatment:		
Nondrug therapy	Medical nutrition therapy and physical activity approved by physician	Essential adjunct to oral antidiabetic therapy; may be sufficient as monotherapy to control blood glucose
Drug therapy	Insulin monotherapy *or,* rarely, oral antidiabetic drugs as adjunct to insulin therapy (if accompanied by insulin resistance)	MNT monotherapy *or* oral antidiabetic drugs *or* oral antidiabetic drugs in combination therapy *or* insulin monotherapy *or* insulin and oral antidiabetic drugs in combination therapy

Clinical Presentation

Classic signs and symptoms include polydipsia, polyuria, and polyphagia. Other common findings include fatigue, blurred vision, and frequent infections.

Type 1 diabetes

Onset is rapid. In addition to the signs above, it may also include unexplained weight loss. Patients may be ketonuric or experience ketoacidosis. They may experience a "honeymoon" period, a phase of erratic insulin secretion lasting months to a year during destruction of β-cells.

Type 2 diabetes

Onset is gradual and progressive. Patients may be asymptomatic or experience classic signs and symptoms. Most are obese or have a history of obesity. Patients may present with existing microvascular or macrovascular chronic complications, or both.

Pathophysiology and Etiology

Type 1 diabetes

- β-cell destruction leads to absolute insulin deficiency.
- Patients are prone to ketoacidosis.
- Peak onset occurs at the time of puberty but may occur at any age.

Type 2 diabetes

- Insulin resistance and progressive β-cell dysfunction occur.
- It often involves a strong genetic predisposition.
- It is associated with environmental factors such as excessive caloric intake, decreased activity, weight gain, and obesity.
- Insulin resistance may be present years before the onset of DM.
- Initially normal glucose levels are maintained by increased insulin secretion by β-cells.
- Increasing insulin resistance or a failure of β-cells to maintain insulin secretion eventually leads to the development of DM.
- Insulin resistance is influenced by age, ethnicity, physical activity, medications, and weight.
- It is usually diagnosed in adulthood but can occur at any age with recent increases in diagnosis in children and adolescents.

- Incidence is higher among certain ethnic populations (American Indians/Alaska Natives, non-Hispanic blacks, Hispanic/Latinos, and non-Hispanic whites).

Diagnostic Criteria

Box 17-1 shows the criteria for the diagnosis of DM.

Type 1 and type 2 DM

Diagnosis can be made on the basis of an A_{1C}, an FPG test, a random plasma glucose test, or an oral glucose tolerance test (OGTT). The A_{1C} may be more convenient because fasting is not required, and daily changes are possible during stress or illness in an FPG. These advantages may be balanced by greater cost and limited availability of A_{1C} testing in certain regions of the world. The A_{1C} may not be as accurate with certain forms of anemia (e.g., iron deficiency, hemolysis) and hemoglobinopathies (e.g., sickle cell trait).

Gestational diabetes mellitus

There are two methods to test for gestational diabetes. Women not known to have DM prior to pregnancy should undergo testing between 24 and 28 weeks of gestation.

Box 17-1. Criteria for the Diagnosis of Diabetes Mellitus

Hemoglobin $A_{1C} \geq 6.5\%$[a]

OR

Fasting plasma glucose (FPG) ≥ 126 mg/dL (7.0 mmol/L). Fasting is defined as no caloric intake for at least 8 hours.[a]

OR

Two-hour plasma glucose ≥ 200 mg/dL (11.1 mmol/L) during an oral glucose tolerance test (OGTT) using a glucose load containing the equivalent of 75 g anhydrous glucose dissolved in water.[a]

OR

In a patient with classic symptoms of hyperglycemia or hyperglycemic crisis, a random plasma glucose ≥ 200 mg/dL (11.1 mmol/L).

American Diabetes Association. Diagnosis and classification of diabetes mellitus. *Diabetes Care.* 2014;37(suppl 1):S81–S90.

a. In the absence of unequivocal hyperglycemia, the first three criteria should be confirmed by repeat testing of the same test.

The one-step approach includes administration of a 75 g OGTT with glucose measurements fasting (overnight fast at least 8 hours), 1 hour and 2 hours post-glucose load.

The diagnosis of GDM is made when any of the following glucose values is exceeded:

- Fasting: ≥ 92 mg/dL (5.1 mmol/L)
- 1 hour: ≥ 180 mg/dL (10 mmol/L)
- 2 hours: ≥ 153 mg/dL (8.5 mmol/L)

The two-step approach includes administration of a nonfasting 50 g glucose challenge test with glucose assessment 1 hour after glucose administration. If the plasma glucose value at 1 hour is ≥ 140 mg/dL, then the patient proceeds to a 3-hour 100g OGTT. The diagnosis of GDM is made when the plasma glucose is ≥ 140 mg/dL 3 hours after the glucose load.

Treatment Principles and Goals

- To achieve and maintain glycemic control. Treatment goals should be individualized on the basis of patient characteristic such as duration of DM, age, life expectancy, comorbid conditions, known CVD, presence of microvascular complications, hypoglycemic unawareness, and other individual patient considerations. In general, the glycemic goals include $A_{1C} < 7\%$, preprandial capillary plasma glucose 70–130 mg/dL, and 1–2 hour postprandial capillary plasma glucose < 180 mg/dL. Individual patient goals may be more or less stringent than these parameters.
- To attain recommended blood pressure and lipid goals (see chapters 12 and 16 for disease goals and management)
- To modify lifestyle to promote general health and achieve weight management goals
- To prevent or slow progression of chronic complications
- To prevent or resolve acute complications
- To achieve an acceptable quality of life and satisfaction with care

Prevention of complications

The following activities can prevent complications from arising:

- Cessation of tobacco use
- Aspirin or anti platelet therapy
  - Consider aspirin (75–162 mg/day), or clopidogrel if patient is allergic to aspirin, as secondary prevention for diabetics with a history of CVD.

- Use as primary prevention with 10-year cardiovascular risk > 10%. It should not be recommended for primary prevention for diabetics with low CVD risk (10-year risk < 5%) because of potential adverse effects. If 10-year risk is between 5% and 10%, clinical judgment should be used regarding antiplatelet therapy.
- Immunization
  - Annual influenza vaccine if patient is 6 months of age or older and no contraindications
  - At least one lifetime pneumococcal polysaccharide vaccine for patients ≥ 2 years of age with no contraindications
  - One-time pneumococcal polysaccharide revaccination if the patient is > 65 years of age and was previously immunized > 5 years ago
  - Hepatitis B vaccination for previously unvaccinated adults 19–59 years of age
- Foot care: self-inspection daily, visual inspection at each office visit, and an annual comprehensive exam (i.e., foot pulses, testing for loss of protective sensation) by a medical provider
- Skin care: self-inspection and care daily
- Dental care: annual examination
- Eye care: annual dilated eye examination starting at the time of diagnosis of type 2 DM or 5 years after the diagnosis of type 1 DM
- Nephropathy screening: annual serum creatinine for estimated glomerular filtration rate (eGFR); annual evaluation of urine albumin excretion starting at the time of diagnosis of type 2 DM or 5 years after the diagnosis of type 1 DM

Complications of diabetes

Macrovascular disease
- **Coronary atherosclerosis:** Rate is two to four times higher in adults with DM.
- **Cerebrovascular atherosclerosis:** Stroke risk is two to four times higher among people with DM.
- **Peripheral vascular disease:** Insufficient circulation impairs healing and increases risk of amputation.

Microvascular disease
- Retinopathy
  - DM is the leading cause of new cases of blindness in adults 20–74 years of age.
  - Retinopathy may develop without symptoms; annual dilated eye examination is recommended for detection.
  - Treatment includes glycemic control, blood pressure control, and laser photocoagulation.

■ Nephropathy
  • It occurs in 20–40% of diabetics and is the leading cause of end-stage renal disease.
  • Treatment includes glycemic and blood pressure control; angiotensin-converting enzyme (ACE) inhibitors or angiotensin II receptor blockers should be used except during pregnancy.
■ Distal symmetric polyneuropathy
  • Sensorimotor nervous system dysfunction occurs.
  • Pain and diminished sensation occur, with potential for poor detection of trauma; polyneuropathy increases risk for ulceration and infection.
  • See chapter 27 (Pain Management and Migraines) for information about treatment of distal symmetric polyneuropathy.
■ Autonomic neuropathy
  • Gastrointestinal (GI) effects include gastroparesis, constipation, and diarrhea.
  • Genitourinary effects include neurogenic bladder and sexual dysfunction in men.
  • Cardiovascular effects include orthostatic hypotension and resting tachycardia.
■ Diabetic foot problems
  • DM accounts for > 60% of nontraumatic amputations in the United States.
  • Prevention, early detection with regular foot exams, and prompt treatment of lesions are essential to avoid complications.

Acute complications
■ Hypoglycemia
  • Definition is plasma glucose < 70 mg/dL.
  • Glucose (15–20 g) is the preferred treatment.
  • Other sources to provide 15–20 g of carbohydrates can be used (e.g., 4 oz fruit juice, 4 oz regular soda).
  • Treatment effects should be seen in approximately 15 minutes.
  • Symptoms can range from mild (tremor, palpitations, sweating) to severe (unresponsiveness, unconsciousness, or convulsions).
  • Severe hypoglycemia may require assistance from another individual for treatment with subcutaneous glucagon injection or intravenous glucose.
■ Diabetic ketoacidosis (DKA)
  • In type 1 DM, DKA is a medical emergency caused by absolute or relative insulin deficiency.
  • Omission of insulin, major stress, infection, or trauma may precipitate DKA.
  • DKA is characterized by glucose > 250 mg/dL, elevated ketones, arterial pH < 7.2, and plasma bicarbonate < 15 mEq/L.
  • Ketone bodies are formed in excess because of fatty acid metabolism in the liver, leading to ketonuria and ketonemia and ultimately diabetic ketoacidosis.
  • Kussmaul respirations (deep and rapid) are characteristic in an attempt to compensate for metabolic acidosis.
  • DKA requires prompt intervention with insulin, fluids, and electrolytes to prevent coma and death.
■ Hyperglycemic hyperosmolar state
  • A complication of type 2 DM, this is also known as *hyperglycemic hyperosmolar nonketotic coma*.
  • It is characterized by elevated plasma glucose (typically > 500 mg/dL), dehydration, and hyperosmolarity in the absence of significant ketoacidosis.
  • It may be triggered by infection or other stressors such as stroke or myocardial infarction.
  • Treatment includes fluid and electrolyte replacement as well as insulin.

17-4. Drug Therapy

Oral Medications for DM Treatment

Biguanides (Table 17-2)

Mechanism of action
The primary mechanism is seen through decreased hepatic gluconeogenesis as well as improved glucose utilization and uptake in peripheral tissues and decreased intestinal absorption of glucose.

Clinical considerations
■ Biguanides are considered the first choice when beginning drug treatment in newly diagnosed type 2 DM unless they are contraindicated or the patient is not able to tolerate them.
■ They pose minimal risk of hypoglycemia unless combined with secretagogues or insulin.
■ They may decrease weight up to 5 kg.
■ They decrease triglycerides, decrease low-density lipoprotein (LDL), and increase high-density lipoprotein (HDL).
■ GI symptoms (nausea, vomiting, bloating, flatulence, anorexia, and diarrhea) are the most common adverse effects.
  • Take doses with or after meals to reduce GI symptoms.
  • GI symptoms are transient and improve in most patients over time.

Table 17-2. Biguanides

Drug	Trade name	Strength	Daily dose	Duration of action	Comments
Metformin	Glucophage	500, 850, 1,000 mg; solution 500 mg/5mL	1,000–2,550 mg (adult); up to 2,000 mg (10 years of age and older)	≥ 24 hours	
Metformin extended release	Glucophage XR Glumetza Fortamet	500, 750 mg 500, 1,000 mg 500, 1,000 mg	2,000 mg qpm; may take 1 g bid if daily dosing causes GI symptoms		*Do not* cut, crush, or chew

- Titrate the dose up slowly to minimize GI symptoms: 500 mg daily with the largest meal × 1 week; then increase to 500 mg twice daily with the two largest meals × 1 week; then increase to 1 g (two 500 mg tablets) with the largest meal and 500 mg with the second-largest meal × 1 week; and then increase to 1 g twice daily with the two largest meals of the day.
- Biguanides interfere with vitamin B_{12} absorption. B_{12} deficiency may cause symptoms of peripheral neuropathy that are similar to symptoms of diabetes-related peripheral neuropathy. B_{12} deficiency may also cause macrocytic anemia. Monitor vitamin B_{12} concentrations annually.
- They may require as much as 8 weeks of therapy before effectiveness can be assessed.
- Biguanides can be used in patients with type 2 diabetes who are pregnant, but they do not have an indication for use approved by the U.S. Food and Drug Administration (FDA). They are considered safe to use during breast-feeding.
- They are indicated for the treatment of type 2 DM in children 10 years of age and older.
- They may decrease the progression to DM from IGT and IFG (prediabetes).
- They have positive cardiovascular benefits when used in obese patients with DM.

A_{1C} reduction
A reduction of 1–2% is expected.

Cautions and contraindications
Most cautions and contraindications are related to the ability of biguanides to increase the risk of lactic acidosis with metformin (less than one case per 100,000 treated patients).

Contraindications
- Renal insufficiency (serum creatinine [SCr], or SCr ≥ 1.4 females and SCr ≥ 1.5 males) is a contraindication; recent studies have suggested that metformin is safe unless the eGFR falls to < 30 mL/min.
- Hepatic dysfunction is a contraindication.
- Excessive alcohol use (binge or chronic use of more than two drinks per day or at one sitting) is a contraindication.
- Medication should be avoided in patients with unstable symptomatic congestive heart failure (New York Heart Association classifications III and IV).

Cautions
- Medication should be discontinued in situations of increased risk for lactic acidosis, including acute myocardial infarction, congestive heart failure exacerbation, severe respiratory disease, shock, and septicemia.
- Medication should be discontinued before procedures that require iodinated contrast media and major surgeries. It can be resumed 2–3 days after renal function has returned to baseline and remains stable.

Secretagogues (Table 17-3)

Mechanism of action
The primary mechanism of secretagogues is to cause a reduction in blood glucose by stimulating the release of insulin from the pancreas. This mechanism may in turn cause a decrease in hepatic gluconeogenesis and a slight decrease in insulin resistance at the muscle level. Effectiveness depends on pancreatic β-cell function.

Clinical and counseling considerations
- Medication should be taken before meals: sulfonylureas, once or twice daily; meglitinides, before each meal.
- Medication causes a 1–2 kg weight gain.
- A positive risk of hypoglycemia exists, which is greater with sulfonylureas than with meglitinides, because of differences in duration of action.

Table 17-3. Secretagogues

Drug	Trade name	Strength	Daily dose	Duration of action	Comments
First generation sulfonylureas					
Acetohexamide	Dymelor	250, 500 mg	250–1,500 mg	Up to 16 hours	Active metabolite excreted by kidney
Chlorpropamide	Diabinese	100, 250 mg	100–500 mg	Up to 72 hours	Contraindicated in renal insufficiency
Tolazamide	Tolinase	100, 250, 500 mg	100–1,000 mg	Up to 10 hours	
Tolbutamide	Orinase	250, 500 mg	500–3,000 mg daily–bid	Up to 10 hours	
Second generation sulfonylureas					
Glipizide	Glucotrol, Glucotrol XL	5, 10 mg	5–40 mg daily–bid 5–20 mg daily (XL)	Up to 20 hours	Given with or without meal; do not cut XL tab
Glyburide	DiaBeta, Micronase	1.25, 2.5, 5 mg	1.25–20 mg daily–bid	Up to 24 hours	3 mg Glynase = 5 mg glyburide
Glyburide micronized	Glynase	1.5, 3, 4.5, 6 mg	1.5–12 mg daily	Up to 24 hours	
Glimepiride	Amaryl	1, 2, 4 mg	1–8 mg daily	24 hours	Begin with 1 mg in renal insufficiency
Meglitinides and phenylalanines					
Repaglinide	Prandin	0.5, 1, 2 mg	0.5–4 mg before each meal; maximum dose = 16 mg/day	Peak effect: ~1 hour; duration: ~2–3 hours	Skip dose if meal skipped; do not give in combination with sulfonylureas
Nateglinide	Starlix	60, 120 mg	60–120 mg before each meal	Peak effect: ~1 hour; duration: ~4 hours	Efficacy: Prandin > Starlix

- Secretagogues are typically not indicated during pregnancy, when breast-feeding, or in children. However, glyburide can be used during pregnancy and breast-feeding.
- A fast-acting oral carbohydrate should be carried for emergency use.

A_{1C} reduction
- 1–2% (sulfonylureas)
- 0.5–2% (meglitinides)

Cautions and contraindications
- Use with caution in elderly patients; do *not* use chlorpropamide.
- Use with caution in cases of renal and hepatic insufficiency; glipizide and glimepiride are safer.
- Avoid in patients with significant alcohol use.
- Drug interactions (worse with first-generation sulfonylureas) may cause increased risk of hypoglycemia: anticoagulants, fluconazole, salicylates, gemfibrozil, sulfonamides, tricyclic antidepressants, digoxin.
- Use is contraindicated in patients with DKA, severe infection, surgery, or trauma.
- Patients should wear medical identification.
- Store drug in a cool, dry place (not the bathroom or kitchen).
- Syndrome of inappropriate antidiuretic hormone secretion, disulfiram-like reaction with alcohol, and sun-sensitivity reactions are more common in first-generation sulfonylureas than in second-generation sulfonylureas.

Thiazolidinediones (Table 17-4)

Mechanism of action
Thiazolidinediones (also called *glitazones* or *TZDs*) are agonists of the PPARγ (peroxisome proliferators-activated receptor-γ) receptor, which, when stimulated, improves peripheral muscle and adipose tissue

Table 17-4. Thiazolidinediones

Drug	Trade name	Strength	Daily dose	Duration of action	Comments
Rosiglitazone	Avandia	2, 4, 8 mg	4–8 mg daily or 2–4 mg bid	24 hours	May be more effective when given bid
Pioglitazone	**Actos**	15, 30, 45 mg	30–45 mg daily	24 hours	

Boldface indicates one of top 100 drugs for 2012 by units sold at retail outlets, www.drugs.com/stats/top100/2012/units.

insulin sensitivity as well as suppresses hepatic glucose output.

Clinical considerations
- Minimal risk of hypoglycemia exists unless combined with secretagogues or insulin.
- TZDs may cause a 5 kg weight gain—more if combined with secretagogues or insulin.
- They decrease triglycerides (pioglitazone > rosiglitazone), increase HDL (pioglitazone = rosiglitazone), and increase LDL (rosiglitazone).
- They are dosed daily, though rosiglitazone may be slightly more effective when dosed twice daily.
- As much as 16 weeks of therapy may be required before assessing effectiveness.
- Generally, they are not indicated during breast-feeding or pregnancy.
- They may decrease the progression to DM from IGT and IFG.
- Edema may best be treated by aldosterone antagonists.
- They are not indicated by the FDA for treatment of type 2 DM in children, though they have been used.
- They may be helpful in nonalcoholic fatty liver disease.
- Conflicting data exist regarding risk of ischemic cardiovascular events caused by rosiglitazone.

A_{1c} reduction
A reduction of 1–2% is expected.

Cautions and contraindications
- Edema—with oral therapies (approximately 5%) and with insulin (approximately 15%)—may occur in patients with *no* history of heart problems. (The condition may be dose related.) Recommendation: Discontinue therapy if the problem is significant, decrease the dose if the problem is minor, and consider further cardiac workup.
- They are contraindicated in patients with congestive heart failure.

- Hepatotoxicity incidence is approximately 0.2% of alanine aminotransferase (ALT) > three times upper limit of normal (ULN) for both agents. Recommendation: Liver function tests (LFTs) every other month for first 12 months and periodically thereafter. If ALT > 2.5 ULN, do not start; if ALT = 1–2.5 ULN, monitor closely; if ALT = 3 × ULN, discontinue medication.
- Pioglitazone has been linked to increased incidence of bladder cancer.
- Medication may cause resumption of ovulation in anovulatory women.
- Medication decreases oral contraceptive effectiveness.
- The FDA proposed changes to rosiglitazone in the Risk Evaluation and Mitigation Strategy (REMS) in November 2013:
  - Distribution is no longer restricted.
  - Patients, pharmacies, and health care providers no longer need to complete the REMS program to use the medications.
  - Manufacturers of rosiglitazone-containing medications will provide training to health care professionals who are likely to prescribe the medications and send a Dear Health Care Provider letter to educate prescribers about the updated information.
  - It must be dispensed with a medication guide. Medication guides are available through the FDA for rosiglitazone-containing products.

Alpha-glucosidase inhibitors (Table 17-5)
Mechanism of action
Alpha-glucosidase inhibitors delay the digestion of carbohydrates into simple sugars and their subsequent absorption in the small intestine.

Clinical considerations
- Minimal risk of hypoglycemia exists unless the drug is combined with secretagogues or insulin.

Table 17-5. Alpha-Glucosidase Inhibitors

Drug	Trade name	Strength	Daily dose	Duration of action	Comments
Acarbose	Precose	50, 100 mg	25–100 mg tid	1–3 hours	Maximum dose: < 60 kg = 50 mg tid; > 60 kg = 100 mg tid
Miglitol	Glyset	25, 50, 100 mg	25–100 mg tid	1–3 hours	

- Alpha-glucosidase inhibitors have minimal effect on weight but can cause possible decrease in weight secondary to side effects.
- Main target of therapy is postprandial hyperglycemia.
- GI symptoms (flatulence, GI upset, abdominal pain, diarrhea, bloating) are the most common side effects. These side effects tend to dissipate over time with continued treatment. Dosing for both agents in the class must be individualized and slowly titrated up as tolerated: 25 mg daily × 1 week; then 25 mg twice daily × 1 week; then 25 mg three times daily × 1 week; and then continued increased dose as tolerated up to 50 mg three times daily.
- Patient should be counseled to increase complex carbohydrate intake and decrease intake of simple sugars.
- Treatment of hypoglycemia:
  - Patient should use glucose (tablets, gel, liquid), but milk (lactose) or fruit juice (fructose) can also be used if glucose is not available. Do *not* use sucrose.
  - Any carbohydrate can be used if > 2–3 hours since last dose of alpha-glucosidase inhibitor agent.
- Alpha-glucosidase inhibitors are generally not indicated during pregnancy, while breast-feeding, or in children.
- Alpha-glucosidase inhibitors decrease the bioavailability of digoxin, propranolol, and ranitidine.

A$_{1C}$ reduction
A reduction of 0.5–1% is expected.

Cautions and contraindications
- Avoid use in patients with GI disorders such as ulcerative colitis, Crohn's disease, possible bowel obstruction, and short bowel syndrome.
- Avoid use in patients with SCr > 2 mg/dL or creatinine clearance (CrCl) of ≤ 25mL/min.
- Increased LFTs may be seen with acarbose, depending on the dose (> 300 mg/day) and the weight of the patient. Avoid use in patients with cirrhosis.

Dipeptidyl peptidase–4 inhibitors (Table 17-6)

Mechanism of action
Dipeptidyl peptidase–4 (DPP-4) inhibitors inhibit the degradation of endogenous glucagon-like peptide-1 (GLP-1) and glucose-dependent insulinotropic polypeptide, which in turn causes increased insulin production in a glucose-dependent fashion, and decreased production of glucagon.

Table 17-6. Dipeptidyl Peptidase–4 Inhibitors

Drug	Trade name	Strength	Daily dose	Duration of action	Comments
Saxagliptin	Onglyza	2.5, 5 mg	5 mg daily	24 hours	CrCl ≤ 50 mL/min; 2.5 mg daily
Linagliptin	Tradjenta	5 mg	5 mg daily	24 hours	
Sitagliptin	**Januvia**	25, 50, 100 mg	100 mg daily	24 hours	CrCl 30–50: 50 mg daily; CrCl < 30: 25 mg daily
Alogliptin	Nesina	6.25, 12.5, 25 mg	25 mg daily	24 hours	CrCl 30–<60 mL/min: 12.5 mg daily; CrCl 15–< 30 mL/min: 6.25 mg daily; CrCl < 15 or requiring hemodialysis: 6.25 mg daily without regard to timing of hemodialysis

Boldface indicates one of top 100 drugs for 2012 by units sold at retail outlets, www.drugs.com/stats/top100/2012/units.

Clinical considerations

- Minimal risk of hypoglycemia exists unless drug is combined with secretagogues or insulin.
- These drugs have minimal or no effect on weight.
- They can be used either as monotherapy or in combination with metformin, thiazolidinediones, or insulin.
- This is the only drug class affecting the GLP-1 system administered orally.
- Generally, DPP-4 inhibitors are very well tolerated. The most common side effects include nasopharyngitis and upper respiratory tract infections, headache, and urinary tract infections (saxagliptin).
- There have been reports of acute pancreatitis in patients who have taken these medications.
- Secondary to newness of the drugs, no significant long-term outcome data are available.

A_{1C} reduction

A reduction of 0.6–0.9% is expected.

Cautions and contraindications

- The dose should be adjusted for renal insufficiency except for linagliptin (Tradjenta).
- The drugs may cause adverse immunologic reactions through T-cell inhibition.
- The drugs should not be used in patients with DKA or type 1 DM.
- Co-administration with strong cytochrome P450 (CYP) 3A4/5 inhibitors (ketoconazole, atazanavir, clarithromycin, indinavir, itraconazole, nefazodone, nelfinavir, ritonavir, saquinavir, and telithromycin) significantly increases saxagliptin concentrations. Limit dose to 2.5 mg once daily.

Sodium-glucose co-transporter 2 inhibitors (Table 17-7)

Mechanism of action

These medications inhibit the sodium-glucose co-transporter 2 (SGLT-2) in the proximal renal tubule, which reduces reabsorption of glucose filtered in the tubular lumen and lowers the renal threshold for glucose. This results in increased urinary glucose excretion and decreased plasma glucose.

Clinical considerations

- Minimal risk of hypoglycemia unless used in combination with other agents that increase risk of hypoglycemia (e.g., secretagogues, insulin)
- These agents can cause weight loss.
- These agents may lower blood pressure and can increase risk of hypotension.
- These agents increase risk for genital fungal infections and urinary tract infections.

A_{1C} reduction

A reduction of 0.7–1% is expected.

Cautions and contraindications

- Avoid use of these medications in renal insufficiency: canagliflozin (eGFR < 45 mL/min/1.73 m²) and dapagliflozin (eGFR < 60 mL/min/1.73m²).
- Canagliflozin may be associated with increased risk of stroke.
- Dapagliflozin may be associated with increased risk of bladder cancer. Do not use in patients with active bladder cancer. Use caution in patients with history of bladder cancer.

Table 17-7. Sodium-Glucose Co-transporter 2 (SGLT-2) Inhibitors

Drug	Trade name	Strength	Daily dose	Duration of action	Comments
Canagliflozin	Invokana	100, 300 mg	100–300 mg daily	24 hours	Take prior to first meal of the day; eGFR 45–< 60 mL/min/1.73m²: 100 mg daily; eGFR 30–45: use not recommended; eGFR < 30 and ESRD on hemodialysis: contraindicated
Dapagliflozin	Farxiga	5, 10 mg	5–10 mg daily	24 hours	eGFR < 60: use not recommended; eGFR < 30, ESRD, or hemodialysis: contraindicated
Empagliflozin	Jardiance	10, 25 mg	10–25 mg daily	24 hours	Take in the morning with or without food; eGFR <30, ESRD, or dialysis: contraindicated

ESRD, end-stage renal disease.

Miscellaneous

Colesevelam (Welchol)
Mechanism of action
Colesevelam is a bile acid sequestrant. The exact mechanism of effect on plasma glucose levels is unknown but may be caused by decreased hepatic glucose production and increased incretin levels.

Clinical considerations
- The medication has no effect on weight.
- It may reduce LDL cholesterol by 12–16% in type 2 DM and can increase triglycerides.
- Absorption-related drug–drug interactions occur. Take interacting medications 4 hours prior to administering the colesevelam.
  - Medications with known interaction include levothyroxine, glyburide, and oral contraceptives with ethinyl estradiol and norethindrone.
  - They also may include phenytoin, warfarin, digoxin, and fat-soluble vitamins (A, D, E, K).
- Most common side effects include constipation and dyspepsia; take with a large amount of water.
- Hypoglycemia is rare, but use caution with insulin and sulfonylureas.

A_{1C} reduction
A reduction of 0.3–0.5% is expected.

Cautions and contraindications
- The medication is contraindicated in patients with history of bowel obstruction or evidence of gastroparesis.
- It is contraindicated in hypertriglyceridemia-induced pancreatitis.
- It is contraindicated in patients with serum triglyceride levels > 500 mg/dL. Use caution in patients with serum triglyceride levels > 300 mg/dL.

Dosing
Colesevelam is dosed in three 625 mg tablets twice daily or 1.875 g single-dose packet twice daily with meals.

Dopamine agonists
Mechanism of action
Bromocriptine (Cycloset) is a dopamine agonist, and the exact mechanism of glycemic improvement is unknown but may increase insulin sensitivity when administered in the morning.

Clinical considerations
- In clinical trials, adverse reactions leading to discontinuation occurred more in patients receiving bromocriptine compared to those receiving a placebo.
  - Nausea (25–35%), vomiting, headache, and dizziness were the most common adverse events.
  - Orthostatic hypotension or syncope is rare but can be seen with use and is more common during dose titration.
- The drug is extensively metabolized by CYP3A4; levels may be changed by strong inhibitors and inducers.
- It has decreased effectiveness in combination with atypical antipsychotics.
- Increased migraine and ergot-related nausea and vomiting may occur with ergot-based therapies.

A_{1C} reduction
A reduction of 0.1–0.4% is expected.

Cautions and contraindications
- Medication may inhibit lactation in breast-feeding women.
- It is contraindicated in patients with syncope migraine because of increased risk of hypotensive episode.

Dosing
- Starting dose is 0.8 mg daily within 2 hours of awakening; titrate weekly by 0.8 mg up to a maximum of 4.8 mg daily.
- Minimal effective dose is 1.6 mg daily.

Combination oral agents for DM

Figure 17-1 shows the combination oral agents for DM. See individual agents for details.

Injectable Medications for DM Treatment
Insulin products (Table 17-8)

Mechanism of action
At low levels, insulin causes suppression of endogenous hepatic glucose production. At higher levels, insulin promotes glucose uptake by muscle tissue.

Clinical considerations
- Insulin carries a risk of hypoglycemia.
- It causes an increase in weight.
- Insulin should be considered as initial agent if glucose is > 250 mg/dL or A_{1C} is > 10%.
- There is no dosage limit.

Figure 17-1. Combination Oral Agents

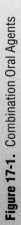

Product			
Kazano	Metformin 500 mg → Alogliptin 12.5 mg	Metformin 1,000 mg → Alogliptin 12.5 mg	
Glipizide/ metformin	Metformin 250 mg → Glipizide 2.5 mg	Metformin 500 mg → Glipizide 2.5 mg	Metformin 500 mg → Glipizide 5 mg
Glucovance	Metformin 250 mg → Glyburide 1.25 mg	Metformin 500 mg → Glyburide 2.5 mg	Metformin 500 mg → Glyburide 5 mg
Jentadueto	Metformin 500 mg → Linagliptin 2.5 mg	Metformin 850 mg → Linagliptin 2.5 mg	Metformin 1,000 mg → Linagliptin 2.5 mg
Actoplus Met	Metformin 500 mg → Pioglitazone 15 mg	Metformin 850 mg → Pioglitazone 15 mg	
Actoplus Met XR	Metformin 1,000 mg → Pioglitazone 15 mg	Metformin 1,000 mg → Pioglitazone 30 mg	
PrandiMet	Metformin 500 mg → Repaglinide 1 mg	Metformin 500 mg → Repaglinide 2 mg	
Avandamet	Metformin 500 mg → Rosiglitazone 2 mg	Metformin 500 mg → Rosiglitazone 4 mg	Metformin 1,000 mg → Rosiglitazone 2 mg; Metformin 1,000 mg → Rosiglitazone 4 mg
Kombiglyze XR	Metformin 1,000 mg → Saxagliptin 2.5 mg	Metformin 500 mg → Saxagliptin 5 mg	Metformin 1,000 mg → Saxagliptin 5 mg
Janumet	Metformin 500 mg → Sitagliptin 50 mg	Metformin 1,000 mg → Sitagliptin 50 mg	
Janumet XR	Metformin 500 mg → Sitagliptin 50 mg	Metformin 1,000 mg → Sitagliptin 50 mg	Metformin 1,000 mg → Sitagliptin 100 mg
Duetact	Glimepiride 2 mg → Pioglitazone 30 mg	Glimepiride 4 mg → Pioglitazone 30 mg	
Avandaryl	Glimepiride 1 mg → Rosiglitazone 4 mg; Glimepiride 2 mg → Rosiglitazone 4 mg	Glimepiride 4 mg → Rosiglitazone 4 mg; Glimepiride 2 mg → Rosiglitazone 8 mg	Glimepiride 4 mg → Rosiglitazone 8 mg
Oseni	Alogliptin 12.5 mg → Pioglitazone 15 mg; Alogliptin 12.5 mg → Pioglitazone 30 mg; Alogliptin 12.5 mg → Pioglitazone 45 mg	Alogliptin 25 mg → Pioglitazone 15 mg; Alogliptin 25 mg → Pioglitazone 30 mg; Alogliptin 25 mg → Pioglitazone 45 mg	
Juvisync	Sitagliptin 50 mg → Simvastatin 10 mg; Sitagliptin 50 mg → Simvastatin 20 mg; Sitagliptin 50 mg → Simvastatin 40 mg	Sitagliptin 100 mg → Simvastatin 10 mg; Sitagliptin 100 mg → Simvastatin 20 mg; Sitagliptin 100 mg → Simvastatin 40 mg	

Table 17-8. Insulin Products

Insulin type	Trade name	Device availability	Onset of action	Time of peak	Duration of action
Rapid acting					
Glulisine	Apidra	OptiClik pen, **SoloSTAR**	15–30 min	30–90 min	1–3 hours
Aspart	**NovoLog**	NovoPen	10–15 min	30–90 min	3–5 hours
Lispro	**Humalog**	Lilly pen, HumaPen Memoir, HumaPen Luxura HD	10–15 min	30–90 min	3–4 hours
Short acting					
Regular	Novolin R		0.5–1 hour	2–3 hours	4–6 hours
	Humulin R				
Intermediate acting					
Human NPH	Novolin N	NovoPen, InnoLet	1–3 hours	4–12 hours	10–18 hours
	Humulin N	Lilly pen	1–3 hours	4–12 hours	10–18 hours
Long acting					
Glargine	**Lantus**	**SoloSTAR**	1–2 hours	No peak	24 hours
Detemir	**Levemir**	FlexPen	1–2 hours	6–8 hours	18–24 hours
Premixed[a]					
NPH + regular	Novolin 70/30	FlexPen			
	Humulin 70/30	Lilly pen			
	Humulin 50/50	Lilly pen			
Insulin protamine + analogs	NovoLog Mix 70/30	FlexPen			
	Humalog Mix 75/25	KwikPen			
	Humalog Mix 50/50	KwikPen			

Boldface indicates one of top 100 drugs for 2012 by units sold at retail outlets, www.drugs.com/stats/top100/2012/units.

Most common available concentration = 100 units per mL. Concentration used in severe insulin resistance = 500 units per mL (Humulin R U–500, available in 20 mL vial).

a. The onset of action, time to peak, and duration of action for mixed insulin is a combination of the two agents included in the mixture. Refer to information on individual agents to assess approximate onset of action, time to peak, and duration of action.

- Educate patients to rotate injection sites for insulin to avoid lipohypertrophy.
- Dosing for type 2 DM is often started with a basal insulin (0.1–0.2 units/kg/day) and added to an existing oral regimen of two or more agents.
- Dosing for type 1 DM is often started with 0.4–0.5 units/kg/day divided as 50% basal insulin and 50% bolus insulin (divided between meals).
- Insulin pharmacokinetics can be altered by site of administration, total dose administered, concentration of insulin, and increased blood flow to site of injection (e.g., rubbing, exercising, heat application).

- Insulin regimen should be individualized to the patient accounting for
  - Glucose readings
  - Renal function
  - Patient schedule and preferences
  - Patient education and health literacy and numeracy level
  - Intensity of glucose control desired
  - Cost to patient
- Consider patient with type 2 DM for prandial insulin coverage when
  - Patient has fasting blood glucose target (70–130 mg/dL), but A_{1C} is above treatment goal.

- A_{1C} is above treatment goal with evidence of frequent 2-hour postprandial glucose values > 160 mg/dL.
- Nighttime or daytime hypoglycemia occurs with skipped or delayed meals.
- The basal insulin dose has been titrated to 0.4–0.6 units/kg, and A_{1C} is above treatment goal.

A_{1C} reduction
A reduction of 2.5% is expected.

Cautions and contraindications
- Dose cautiously in patients with renal and hepatic insufficiency.
- Dose cautiously in elderly patients.
- When insulins in different vials are mixed into the same syringe for administration, the clear insulin should be drawn up first, then add the cloudy neutral protamine Hagedorn (NPH) insulin. Lantus, Levemir, and insulins contained in a cartridge or pen device should not be mixed with other insulin products for administration.
- Counsel patients on signs and symptoms of hypoglycemia and how to appropriately treat.
- Most insulin products are stable at room temperature for 28–30 days, other than premixed insulin pen products (10–14 days) and Levemir (42 days).
- Pregnancy Risk Factor for insulin is category B, except for Lantus and glulisine (category C) and NPH (not categorized).

Incretin mimetics (Table 17-9)

Mechanism of action
Incretin mimetics are receptor agonists of endogenous GLP-1 that cause (1) increased insulin production in a glucose-dependent fashion, (2) decreased postprandial release of glucagon, (3) slowing of gastric emptying, and (4) early satiety and weight loss.

Clinical considerations
- Minimal risk of hypoglycemia exists unless the drug is combined with secretagogues (consider initial reduction in secretagogue). There is a minor increase in hypoglycemia risk if the drug is combined with TZDs.
- Moderate weight loss of about 10 pounds is seen after sustained use.
- A dose-limiting side effect is nausea. Approximately 30–50% of patients report some degree of nausea but stop the drug secondary to the problem. Nausea is worse with initiation and dose titration, but seems to lessen with time. Incidence of nausea can be decreased by educating patients to eat more slowly.
- Patients should decrease meal size and carbohydrate content of meals prior to use of exenatide to lessen problem of nausea.
- Exenatide (Byetta) dose should be given 10–15 minutes prior to the two largest meals of the day, which should be spaced at least 6 hours apart.
- Liraglutide (Victoza) can be given once daily regardless of meals.
- Exenatide extended release (Bydureon) can be given once weekly regardless of meals.
- Exenatide and liraglutide can be stored at room temperature for 30 days after first dose is given.
- Bydureon must be administered immediately after reconstitution; 2 mg injected every 7 days.
- Drugs can be combined with sulfonylurea, metformin, sulfonylurea + metformin, TZDs, or metformin + TZD. Exenatide and liraglutide currently have FDA indication in combination with basal insulin.
- For exenatide, begin with 5 mcg injected bid for 1 month; then increase to 10 mcg bid as tolerated.
- For liraglutide, begin with 0.6 mg injected once daily for 1 week; then increase to 1.2 mg daily for one week; then increase to 1.8 mg daily as tolerated. Minimum effective dose is 1.2 mg daily.

Table 17-9. Incretin Mimetics

Drug	Trade name	Strength	Daily dose	Duration of action
Albiglutide	Tanzeum	30, 50 mg	30–50 mg weekly	5 days, steady state 4–5 weeks
Liraglutide	**Victoza**	0.6, 1.2, 1.8 mg	0.6–1.8 mg daily	~24 hours
Exenatide	Byetta	5, 10 mcg	5–10 mcg bid	~8–10 hours
Exenatide extended release	Bydureon	2 mg	2 mg once weekly	~2 weeks initial peak, steady state 6–7 weeks

Boldface indicates one of top 100 drugs for 2012 by units sold at retail outlets, www.drugs.com/stats/top100/2012/units.

- Exenatide is supplied as a pen device that contains 60 doses (1-month supply).
- Liraglutide is supplied as a 3 mL pen (6 mg/mL) device that contains 0.6 mcg, 1.2 mcg, and 1.8 mcg doses in the same pen. At 0.6 mcg dose, one pen lasts 30 days; at 1.2 mg dose, one pen lasts 15 days; at 1.8 mg dose, one pen lasts 10 days.
- Incretin mimetics are most effective in lowering postprandial glucose elevations.
- Initial peak with Bydureon is 2 weeks, with steady-state reached in 6 to 7 weeks. Dose titration is not needed.
- Pancreatitis has been associated with use of GLP agonists; however, whether the relationship is causal or coincidental is not yet clear. Avoid use in patients with history of pancreatitis.

A_{1C} reduction
A reduction of 0.5–1.5% is expected.

Cautions and contraindications
- Exenatide should *not* be given to patients with CrCl ≤ 30 mL/min.
- The drug class should *not* be given to patients with severe GI disease, including gastroparesis.
- The drug class should not be used in patients with DKA or type 1 DM.
- Liraglutide, Bydureon, and Albiglutide should not be used in, patients with a personal or family history of medullary thyroid carcinoma or in patients with multiple endocrine neoplasia syndrome type 2.

Amylin mimetics (Table 17-10)

Mechanism of action
The medication is an analog of endogenous amylin that when dosed at therapeutic levels causes (1) decreased production of glucagon, (2) slowing of gastric emptying, and (3) early satiety and weight loss.

Clinical considerations
- Drug can be used in combination with insulin therapy in both type 1 and type 2 DM patients who have failed to achieve desired glucose control.

- Because of significant risk of severe hypoglycemia, prandial insulin dose should be decreased by 50% when starting pramlintide.
- A dose-limiting side effect is nausea, which seems to lessen over time.
- For type 2 DM, start with 60 mcg before meals; increase to 120 mcg before meals when no significant nausea has occurred for 3–7 days.
- For type 1 DM, start with 15 mcg before meals; titrate in 15 mcg increments every 3 days if no significant nausea has occurred to a target dose of 30–60 mcg before meals.
- Pens may be stored at room temperature for 28 days after first use.
- Do not mix with insulin. Administer in the abdomen or thigh in a location different from insulin injection (e.g., insulin administered on right side of abdomen and incretin mimetic administered on left side of abdomen).

A_{1C} reduction
A reduction of 0.5–1% is expected.

Cautions and contraindications
The medication should *not* be used in patients with

- Severe GI disease, including gastroparesis
- Poor adherence with current insulin regimen or self-monitoring of blood glucose
- Recurrent severe hypoglycemia requiring assistance in the past 6 months
- $A_{1C} \geq 9\%$
- Hypoglycemia unawareness

17-5. Nondrug Therapy

Lifestyle changes through diet and exercise should be emphasized. Weight loss is recommended for all patients with DM who are overweight or obese. Modest weight loss (5%) has been shown to improve insulin resistance in type 2 DM.

Patient education is an essential component of successful DM management.

Table 17-10. Amylin Mimetics

Drug	Trade name	Strength	Daily dose	Duration of action	Comments
Pramlintide	SymlinPen 60, SymlinPen 120	0.6 mg/mL–5 mL vial	Type 1 DM: 15–60 mcg tid with meals; type 2 DM: 60–120 mcg tid with meals	4–6 hours	Do NOT mix with insulin. Reduce prandial insulin dose by 50% when initiating to avoid hypoglycemia.

Medical Nutrition Therapy

Medical nutrition therapy (MNT) should be individualized to achieve treatment goals with consideration of usual dietary habits, metabolic profile, and lifestyle.

Carbohydrate intake should be monitored by exchanges, carbohydrate counting, or experience-based estimation. The mix of carbohydrates, protein, and fat should be adjusted to meet the weight and metabolic goals of the patient.

Protein intake may need to be modified if renal function is reduced. Saturated fat should be < 7% of total daily calories. Fiber intake should be encouraged, but there is no reason to recommend a greater amount than that recommended for persons without DM (14 g fiber/1,000 kcal). Alcohol intake should be limited (adult females: one drink or fewer per day; adult males: two drinks or fewer per day).

Physical Activity and Exercise

Regular exercise improves blood glucose control, reduces cardiovascular risk factors, and contributes to weight loss. An exercise regimen should be individualized. The patient's history and a detailed medical examination are essential.

For most patients, a program of 150 min/week of moderate-intensity aerobic exercise is recommended. The program should be adjusted in the presence of macro- and microvascular complications that may be worsened:

- *Retinopathy:* Vigorous exercise may be contraindicated because of the risk of triggering vitreous hemorrhage or retinal detachment.
- *Peripheral neuropathy:* Non-weight-bearing activities may be best because decreased pain sensation in the extremities increases the risk of skin breakdown and infection.

- *Autonomic neuropathy:* Patients should undergo cardiac evaluation before increasing physical activity, which may lead to decreased cardiac responsiveness to exercise or postural hypotension.

Blood glucose monitoring may be necessary before, during, and after exercise. Fast-acting oral carbohydrates (e.g., glucose tablets, gel, solution) should be available during and after exercise.

Diabetes Self-Management Education

Diabetes self-management education (DSME) provides a means for those with DM to become empowered with the knowledge of self-care. Education content includes the DM disease process; acute and long-term complications; drug and nondrug treatments; monitoring; preventive measures; decision-making skills; goal setting; psychosocial adjustment; and specific self-care measures relative to foot, skin, dental, and eye care.

DSME should be offered in a variety of settings, typically by a multidisciplinary team.

17-6. Questions

Use Patient Profile 17-1 to answer Question 1.

1. What is one of the most common adverse drug events caused by Ms. Even's oral antidiabetic agent?

   A. Flatulence
   B. Hypoglycemia
   C. Renal failure
   D. Hyperglycemia
   E. Weight gain

Patient Profile 17-1. Institution or Nursing Home Care

Patient Name:	Barbara Even	Lab/Diagnostic Tests:		
Address:	413 Summit Street		Date	Test
Age:	68	1)	2/1	LFTs
Height:	5' 5"	2)	2/1	Serum K
Weight:	190 lb	3)	5/1	LFTs
Sex:	Female	4)	5/1	Serum K
Race:	African American	5)	6/1	A$_{1c}$
Allergies:	Penicillin, sulfa drugs	6)	6/1	Serum creatinine
		7)	6/1	BUN
		8)	6/1	Serum K

(continued)

Patient Profile 17-1. Institution or Nursing Home Care *(Continued)*

Diagnosis:

Primary   1) Type 2 DM

Secondary   1) Hypertension

            2) Asthma

Additional Orders:

1) Referral to dietitian for weight reduction diet

2) Low-impact exercise 30 minutes 3 days per week

Dietary Considerations:

1) Dietary changes per dietitian consult

2) Enteral and parenteral

Pharmacist Notes and Other Patient Information:

	Date	Comment
1)	2/1	Advised patient to continue SMBG and to report any hypoglycemic episodes. Instructed patient to treat hypoglycemia with glucose or lactose products. Instructed patient to take acarbose with first bite of meal. Foot exam negative. Patient reports having 1–2 drinks of bourbon per day.
2)		Informed patient to report any changes in blood glucose.

Medication Orders:

Date	Rx #	Physician	Drug and strength	Quantity	Sig	Refills
2/1	834924	Jones	Propranolol 20 mg	30	1 po bid	3
2/1	834925	Jones	Albuterol inhaler	1	1–2 inhalations q4–6h	3
2/1	834926	Jones	Acarbose 25 mg	90	1 tab po w/meals	2
5/1	834927	Jones	Acarbose 50 mg	90	1 tab po w/meals	2
6/1	834928	Jones	Prednisone 10 mg	30	1 tab po daily	0
6/1	834929	Jones	Propranolol 20 mg	30	1 tab po bid	3
6/1	834930	Jones	Albuterol inhaler	1	1–2 inhalations q4–6h	3
6/1	834931	Jones	ASA 81 mg	30	1 tab po daily	3

Use Patient Profile 17-2 to answer Questions 2 and 3.

2. What is the highest priority drug-related problem in Mr. Right's medication record?

   A. Insulin therapy not indicated for persons with type 2 DM
   B. Therapeutic duplication of sulfonylurea therapy
   C. Potential decrease of blood glucose because of drug–drug interaction between phenytoin and tolazamide
   D. Potential increase of blood glucose because of drug–drug interaction between glimepiride and itraconazole
   E. Use of an ACE inhibitor for hypertension in type 2 DM

3. Which of the following laboratory tests is needed to monitor Mr. Right's drug therapy regimen?

   A. Hemoglobin A_{1C}
   B. Glimepiride serum concentration
   C. Insulin receptor substrate-1
   D. Insulin concentration
   E. Serum C-peptide concentration level

4. Which of the following is *not* an appropriate treatment for a hypoglycemic episode with a blood glucose reading of 64 mg/dL?

   A. 1/2 cup of diet soda
   B. 6–7 hard candies containing sugar
   C. 3 glucose tablets
   D. 4 oz of regular soda
   E. 4 oz of orange juice

Patient Profile 17-2. Community

Patient Name:	Tom Right	**Diagnosis:**	
Address:	20 Blue Ridge Drive	Primary	1) Type 2 DM
Age:	48		2) Epilepsy
Height:	5' 6"	Secondary	1) Hypertension
Weight:	135 lb		2) Fungal infection under toenails
Sex:	Male		
Race:	Caucasian	**Pharmacist Notes and Other Patient Information:**	
Allergies:	NKDA		

Pharmacist Notes and Other Patient Information:

	Date	Comment
1)	4/8	Patient should be monitored closely for hypoglycemia. Teach patient signs and symptoms of hypoglycemia and treatment measures.

Medication Orders:

Date	Rx #	Physician	Drug and strength	Qty	Sig	Refills
1/6	765321	Smith	Tolazamide 250 mg	90	1 tab po daily	0
4/8	765323	Smith	Glimepiride 2 mg	90	1 tab po daily	0
8/6	765324	Smith	Lisinopril 5 mg	90	1 tab po daily	0
8/6	765325	Thomas	Phenytoin extended	60	300 mg po daily	0
8/6	765366	Smith	Itraconazole	14	50 mg po daily	0
8/6	765367	Smith	Regular insulin	Trial	5 units SC before meals	0

5. Persons on insulin therapy should be advised to rotate their injection sites for which of the following reasons?

    A. It reduces the risk of infection.
    B. It reduces the risk of lipoatrophy.
    C. It reduces the risk of lipohypertrophy.
    D. It reduces the risk of generalized myalgia.
    E. This advice is outdated because of the use of human insulin.

6. Which of the following is the most appropriate treatment for a severe hypoglycemic episode when a patient is unconscious?

    A. 1/2 cup of diet soda
    B. 3 hard candies containing sugar
    C. 1 glucose tablet
    D. Glucagon injection
    E. 2–3 small sugar cubes

7. Insulin therapy is indicated in all of the following *except*

    A. newly diagnosed type 1 DM, A_{1C} 7.5%.
    B. GDM not controlled by diet.

    C. hyperglycemic hyperosmolar nonketotic syndrome.
    D. newly diagnosed type 2 DM, A_{1C} 7.9%.
    E. DKA.

8. Which of the following oral antidiabetic agents is a micronized formulation?

    A. Micronase
    B. Glynase
    C. Glucotrol XL
    D. Amaryl
    E. Orinase

9. Which of the following scenarios can alter the pharmacokinetics of insulin products?

    A. Rotating of injection site around the abdomen
    B. Rubbing of the injection site
    C. Needle size and length
    D. Administration time of day
    E. Administration just prior to a meal

10. When mixing rapid- or short-acting insulin with intermediate- or long-acting insulin,

which of the following insulins should be drawn up first?

A. Regular
B. NPH
C. Detemir
D. Degludec
E. Glargine

11. DM is the leading cause of which of the following microvascular complications?

A. Pancreatitis
B. Fatty liver
C. Blindness
D. Stroke
E. Deafness

12. Which of the following is an indication that a patient is developing a long-term complication from DM?

A. Tremor
B. Glucosuria
C. Leukocytosis
D. Proteinuria
E. Tinnitus

13. Which sulfonylurea has been associated with the greatest incidence of prolonged hypoglycemia in the elderly?

A. Tolazamide
B. Tolbutamide
C. Chlorpropamide
D. Glimepiride
E. Glipizide

14. Which of the following drugs taken with alcohol is most likely to cause a disulfiram-like reaction?

A. Chlorpropamide
B. Acarbose
C. NPH insulin
D. Glucagon
E. Pioglitazone

15. Metformin should be withheld for 48 hours prior to any procedure requiring the use of parenteral iodinated contrast medium because of the potential for which of the following adverse drug events?

A. Optic neuritis
B. Metabolic alkalosis

C. Lactic acidosis
D. Purple-toe syndrome
E. Tinnitus

16. All of the following are true of acarbose therapy *except*

A. it is contraindicated in inflammatory bowel disease.
B. it should be taken with the first bite of each meal.
C. it does not cause hypoglycemia or weight gain.
D. hypoglycemia attributable to combination therapy should be treated with sucrose.
E. LFTs are given every 3 months during the first year and periodically thereafter (if the dose is > 50 mg tid).

17. Which of the following is a common adverse effect of Tradjenta when used as monotherapy?

A. Upper respiratory infection
B. Weight gain
C. Hypoglycemia
D. Angioedema
E. Myopathy

18. Which one of the following antidiabetic agents does *not* require LFTs for monitoring?

A. Glargine
B. Miglitol
C. Rosiglitazone
D. Acarbose
E. Metformin

19. Which of the following is an adverse drug event reported for pioglitazone?

A. Heart failure
B. Myocardial infarction
C. Angioedema
D. Hypoglycemic unawareness
E. Atrial fibrillation

20. Pramlintide (Symlin)

A. is a basal insulin.
B. is an insulin analog.
C. is an oral insulin.
D. is an inhaled insulin.
E. is an amylin analog.

17-7. Answers

1. **A.** The most common adverse drug events for acarbose are flatulence, abdominal pain, and diarrhea. These adverse events may be decreased by titrating the dose gradually and taking the drug with the first bite of each meal.

2. **B.** Although tolazamide and glimepiride are first- and second-generation sulfonylureas, duplication of drug class is inappropriate. These agents are both intermediate acting and therefore might potentiate the adverse drug event of hypoglycemia. Insulin may be indicated in a person with type 2 DM as the disease progresses. The potential drug–drug interaction between phenytoin and tolazamide could result in an increased blood glucose level, and the potential drug–drug interaction between glimepiride and itraconazole could result in a decreased blood glucose level. An ACE inhibitor for hypertension in type 2 DM is appropriate because this drug is renal protective.

3. **A.** The A_{1C} is essential for monitoring the success of glucose control therapy. It gives an average reading over the previous 2–3 months (or 120 days, the lifespan of a red blood cell). Glimepiride serum concentrations do not need to be monitored. Insulin receptor substrate-1 and insulin concentrations are not routinely required to monitor drug therapy. A serum C-peptide might be diagnostic for the determination of functioning β-cells; however, it is not used to assess safety or efficacy of the medication regimen.

4. **A.** One-half cup of diet soda would not be appropriate because a hypoglycemic episode requires a fast-acting oral carbohydrate for resolution and diet soda has none. The other options would all be appropriate for resolution of the event.

5. **C.** Lipohypertrophy (a bulging of the injection site) is caused by nonrotation of injection sites. The risk of infection may be reduced by using aseptic injecting technique. Lipoatrophy (a pitting of the injection site) may be caused by an antigenic response to insulin. The advice regarding rotation of injection site has not changed with different types of insulin now available.

6. **D.** Glucagon, a pancreatic hormone that is given parenterally, is the most appropriate treatment for a severe hypoglycemic episode because the patient may be unconscious and not able to take a fast-acting carbohydrate by mouth. The other items represent inappropriate treatment for mild to moderate hypoglycemia (the amounts of items B, C, and E are inadequate, and the soda in item A should be regular soda).

7. **D.** Newly diagnosed type 2 DM with A_{1C} < 10% should first have a trial with MNT and exercise, and if this nondrug therapy fails, oral antidiabetic monotherapy should be added. Combination oral therapy would be indicated next with failure of monotherapy. Then, following the failure of oral therapy, insulin monotherapy or insulin therapy in combination with oral agents is indicated. Insulin is indicated in all the other situations.

8. **B.** Glynase is a micronized formulation of glyburide that is significantly absorbed (e.g., a 3 mg tablet provides blood levels similar to a 5 mg conventional tablet). Micronase is a trade name for nonmicronized glyburide. Glucotrol XL is the name of an extended formulation of glipizide. Orinase is the trade name for tolbutamide (the only first-generation sulfonylurea listed here), and Amaryl is the trade name for glimepiride.

9. **B.** Insulin pharmacokinetics can be altered by temperature of the site of administration, so activities such as rubbing the area will alter the temperature and therefore the pharmacokinetics. Rotating the administration site between the abdomen, arm, and leg can alter the pharmacokinetics, but rotation in the same general area does not significantly change the onset, peak, and duration. The needle size and length and the timing of administration do not alter the pharmacokinetics of insulin.

10. **A.** Regular or clear insulin is always drawn up first to ensure that all persons mixing insulins will use the same procedure and that no intermediate- or long-acting insulin will be placed in the regular insulin vial, potentially causing contamination and dose variance. Glargine and detemir are also clear insulins; however, they are never to be mixed with other insulins.

11. **C.** Diabetes is the leading cause of new cases of blindness among adults 20–74 years of age in the United States. There is also an increased incidence of stroke, but diabetes is not the leading cause of this problem. The other items are incorrect.

12. **D.** Proteinuria is an indication that a patient is developing the long-term complication of nephropathy. Items A, B, and C could be related to acute complications such as DKA (glucosuria and leukocytosis) and hypoglycemia tremor. Item E is incorrect.

13. **C.** Chlorpropamide has a half-life of 35 hours and a duration of action of 60 hours; therefore, it has been associated with prolonged hypoglycemia in the elderly. The other sulfonylureas have had fewer reports of hypoglycemia.

14. **A.** Chlorpropamide has had the greatest reporting of this drug interaction relative to the first-generation sulfonylureas. The remaining drugs listed have not had reports of this adverse drug event.

15. **C.** Lactic acidosis can result if metformin is given in this situation, and it can be potentially fatal. Renal function must be evaluated following such a procedure, and it must be stabilized before metformin may be resumed. The other items are incorrect.

16. **D.** Oral glucose instead of carbohydrate sources with sucrose (cane sugar) or fructose is used because absorption of these is inhibited. The remaining items are true of acarbose therapy.

17. **A.** Tradjenta is a dipeptidyl peptidase IV inhibitor. This class of medications can increase a patient's risk for upper respiratory tract infections. When used as monotherapy agents in this class, they do not cause hypoglycemia, weight gain, or myopathy. Angioedema can occur but is very rare.

18. **A.** The alpha-glucosidase inhibitors (e.g., acarbose), biguanides (e.g., metformin), and thiazolidinediones (e.g., rosiglitazone) all require LFTs for monitoring. Glargine, a long-acting insulin, does not require LFTs for monitoring; rather, it requires blood glucose monitoring.

19. **A.** Pioglitazone is a thiazolidinedione and has been associated with exacerbation of heart failure, which led to a black box warning against use in patients with this condition. Pioglitazone has not been linked to myocardial infarction, angioedema, hypoglycemic unawareness, or atrial fibrillation.

20. **E.** Pramlintide (Symlin) was approved in March 2005 as the first new type 1 diabetes treatment in more than 80 years. It is an injectable synthetic version of the human hormone amylin.

17-8. References

American Diabetes Association. Diagnosis and classification of diabetes mellitus. *Diabetes Care.* 2014; 37(suppl 1):S81–S90.

American Diabetes Association. Standards of medical care in diabetes—2014. *Diabetes Care.* 2014;37 (suppl 1):S14–S80.

Diabetes Control and Complications Trial Research Group. The effect of intensive treatment on the development and the progress of long-term complications in insulin-dependent diabetes mellitus. *N Engl J Med.* 1993;329:977–86. Available at: http://www.nejm.org/doi/full/10.1056/NEJM199309303291401.

Evert AB, Boucher JL, Cypress M, et al. Nutrition therapy recommendations for the management of adults with diabetes. *Diabetes Care.* 2014; 37(suppl 1):S120–S143.

Haas L, Maryniuk M, Beck J, et al. National Standards for Diabetes Self-Management Education and Support. *Diabetes Care.* 2014; 37(suppl 1):S144–S153.

Inzucchi SE, Bergenstal RM, Buse JB, et al. Management of hyperglycemia in type 2 diabetes: A patient-centered approach. Position statement of the American Diabetes Association (ADA) and the European Association for the Study of Diabetes (EASD). *Diabetes Care.* 2012;35:1364–79.

Skyler JS, Bergenstal R, Bonow RO, et al.; American Diabetes Association; American College of Cardiology Foundation; American Heart Association. Intensive glycemic control and the prevention of cardiovascular events: Implications of the ACCORD, ADVANCE, and VA diabetes trials; A position statement of the American Diabetes Association and a scientific statement of the American College of Cardiology Foundation and the American Heart Association. *Diabetes Care.* 2009;32:187–92.

Triplett CL, Repas T, Alvarez CA. Diabetes mellitus. In: Dipiro JT, Talbert RL, Yee GC, et al., eds. *Pharmacotherapy: A Pathophysiologic Approach.* 9th ed. New York: McGraw-Hill Education; 2014.

UK Prospective Diabetes Study (UKPDS) Group. Effect of intensive blood-glucose control with metformin on complications in overweight patients with type 2 diabetes (UKPDS 34). *Lancet.* 1998;352:854–65.

UK Prospective Diabetes Study (UKPDS) Group. Intensive blood-glucose control with sulphonylureas or insulin compared with conventional treatment and risks of complications in patients with type 2 diabetes (UKPDS 33). *Lancet.* 1998;352: 837–53.

Thyroid, Adrenal, and Miscellaneous Endocrine Drugs

Joyce E. Broyles

18

18-1. Key Points

- Levothyroxine is the drug of choice for hypothyroidism.
- Lower doses of levothyroxine are used in elderly and cardiac patients.
- Overtreatment with thyroid hormones causes osteoporosis and atrial fibrillation.
- Antacids, bile acid sequestrants, sucralfate, calcium, and iron supplements decrease absorption of levothyroxine and must be separated by at least 4 hours.
- Propylthiouracil and methimazole are thioamide derivatives used to treat hyperthyroidism.
- Thioamides may cause life-threatening agranulocytosis or hepatitis, so patients must report to their physician if they experience fever, sore throat, abdominal pain, or jaundice.
- Drugs used to treat Cushing's disease inhibit synthesis of cortisol.
- Corticosteroids should be used at the lowest dose for the shortest time to reduce the risk of hypothalamic-pituitary-adrenocortical (HPA) axis suppression and adrenal insufficiency.
- Patients with adrenal insufficiency must receive supplemental corticosteroids in times of physiologic stress.
- Vasopressin and desmopressin are antidiuretic hormones.
- Androgens and anabolic steroids are abused by some athletes seeking to enhance performance.

Editor's Note: This chapter is based on the 10th edition chapter written by Jeff Lewis.

18-2. Study Guide Checklist

The following topics may guide your study of this subject area:

- Regulation of endocrine system
- Signs and symptoms of thyroid disease
- Monitoring parameters for thyroid replacement
- Etiology of Cushing's disease
- Symptoms of Addison's disease
- Treatment strategies for Addison's disease, including those for Addisonian crisis

18-3. Thyroid

Hypothyroidism

Disease overview

Definition and epidemiology
- Hypothyroidism is a syndrome of deficient thyroid hormone production that results in a slowing down of all bodily functions.
- Retardation of growth occurs in infants and children.
- Prevalence of hypothyroidism is greater in women and increases with age; it affects 1.5% to 2% of women and 0.2% of men.

Types
- Most cases are caused by thyroid gland failure (primary hypothyroidism).
- Hashimoto's disease (autoimmune thyroiditis) is the cause of 90% of primary hypothyroidism.
- Pituitary failure from any cause will result in secondary hypothyroidism.

- Hypothalamic failure from any cause will result in tertiary hypothyroidism.
- Iatrogenic hypothyroidism follows exposure to radiation with radioiodine or external radiation.
- Other causes of hypothyroidism include thyroidectomy, iodine deficiency, enzymatic defects, iodine, lithium, and interferon-alfa.

Clinical presentation

- Symptoms include cold intolerance, fatigue, somnolence, constipation, menorrhagia, myalgia, and hoarseness.
- Signs include thyroid gland enlargement or atrophy, bradycardia, edema, dry skin, and weight gain.
- Myxedema coma is an end stage of hypothyroidism characterized by weakness, confusion, hypothermia, hypoventilation, hypoglycemia, hyponatremia, coma, and shock.

Pathophysiology

- Thyroxine (T_4) is the major hormone secreted by the thyroid; T_4 is converted to the more potent triiodothyronine (T_3) in tissues.
- Thyroxine secretion is stimulated by thyroid-stimulating hormone (TSH).
- TSH secretion is inhibited by T_4, forming a negative feedback loop.
- Hashimoto's disease is an autoimmune-mediated disease resulting from cell- and antibody-mediated thyroid injury.
- Antimicrosomal antibodies are directed against thyroid peroxidase.

Diagnosis

- Plasma TSH assay is the initial test of choice if hypothyroidism is suspected clinically.
- TSH levels are elevated in primary hypothyroidism.
- Low plasma-free T_4 (or T_4 index) confirms the diagnosis of hypothyroidism.

Treatment principles

- Synthetic thyroxine (levothyroxine) is the drug of choice for hypothyroidism because it is chemically stable, inexpensive, and free of antigenicity and because it has uniform potency.
- The typical maintenance dose is 125 mcg po once daily.
  - The starting dose in the elderly and in patients with coronary artery disease is reduced to 25 mcg to decrease the risk of precipitating angina.
  - Replacement dose should be based on ideal body weight rather than actual body weight.
  - Most adult patients will reach a levothyroxine dose of 1.7 mcg/kg/day at steady state.
- The goal of therapy is to maintain plasma TSH in the normal range.
- Dose changes are made at 6- to 8-week intervals until the TSH is normal.
- Overtreatment is detected by subnormal TSH and is associated with osteoporosis and atrial fibrillation.
- Failure to respond to appropriate doses is most often due to poor compliance.
- Patient compliance may be assessed by monitoring T_4 levels.
- Do not use thyroid hormones to facilitate weight loss in euthyroid patients.
- Thyroid hormones have a narrow therapeutic index; careful monitoring of clinical condition and thyroid function is required.

Drug therapy for hypothyroidism

Thyroid preparations for the treatment of hypothyroidism are described in Table 18-1.

Mechanism of action

Thyroid hormones enhance oxygen consumption by most tissues and increase basal metabolic rate and metabolism of carbohydrates, lipids, and proteins.

Patient counseling

- Take once daily, 30 minutes before breakfast, because food may decrease absorption.
- Replacement therapy is usually for life; do not discontinue without advice of the prescriber.
- Notify the prescriber if you experience rapid or irregular heartbeat, chest pain, shortness of breath, nervousness, irritability, tremors, heat intolerance, or weight loss.
- Antacids, calcium, bile acid sequestrants, sucralfate, and iron supplements decrease absorption of levothyroxine. Do not take these medications within 4 hours of levothyroxine.

Adverse effects

- ***Cardiovascular:*** Tachycardia, arrhythmia, angina, myocardial infarction
- ***Central nervous system (CNS):*** Tremor, headache, nervousness, insomnia, irritability, hyperactivity
- ***Gastrointestinal (GI):*** Diarrhea, vomiting, cramps
- ***Miscellaneous:*** Weight loss, fatigue, menstrual irregularities, excessive sweating, heat intolerance,

Table 18-1. Thyroid Preparations for the Treatment of Hypothyroidism

Trade name	Generic name	Dosage forms	Usual dosage range
Synthroid, Levothroid, Levoxyl, Unithroid, Thyro-Tabs	Levothyroxine sodium (T₄)	Tablet: 0.025, 0.05, 0.075, 0.088, 0.1, 0.112, 0.125, 0.137, 0.15, 0.175, 0.2, 0.3 mg	0.1–0.15 mg po daily for hypothyroidism (dosage is individualized); higher doses used in treating thyroid cancer
		Injection: 200, 500 mcg	
Armour Thyroid, Nature-Throid, Westhroid	Desiccated thyroid USP	Tablet: 15, 30, 32.4, 60, 64.8, 65, 90, 120, 129.6, 130, 180, 194.4, 195, 240, 300 mg	60–120 mg po daily for hypothyroidism (dosage is individualized); higher doses used in treating thyroid cancer
Cytomel, Triostat	Liothyronine (T₃)	Tablet: 5, 25, 50 mcg	25 mcg po daily for hypothyroidism
		Injection: 10 mcg	
Thyrolar	Liotrix (T₄ and T₃ in a 4:1 ratio)	Tablet: 3.1/12.5 mcg, 6.25/25 mcg, 12.5/50 mcg, 25/100 mcg, 37.5/150 mcg	60–120 mg po daily for hypothyroidism

Boldface indicates one of top 100 drugs for 2012 by units sold at retail outlets, www.drugs.com/stats/top100/2012/units.

fever, muscle weakness, hair loss, decreased bone mineral density, hypersensitivity

Drug interactions

- Amiodarone may cause hypothyroidism or hyperthyroidism.
- Antacids decrease absorption of levothyroxine. Separate administration by at least 4 hours.
- Antidiabetic agents may be less effective with levothyroxine. An increase in the insulin or oral hypoglycemic dose may be needed.
- Bile acid sequestrants reduce absorption of levothyroxine. Separate administration by at least 4 hours.
- Enzyme-inducing antiepileptic agents increase hepatic degradation of levothyroxine. The thyroxine dosage may need to be increased.
- Estrogens may decrease response to levothyroxine. The levothyroxine dosage may need to be increased.
- Lithium commonly causes hypothyroidism.
- Levothyroxine may enhance warfarin's effect. The warfarin dosage may need to be decreased.
- Levothyroxine supplementation may reduce digoxin levels.
- Sucralfate may decrease levothyroxine absorption. Separate administration by at least 4 hours.
- Soybean formula decreases levothyroxine absorption.
- Sympathomimetic drugs may potentiate the effects of levothyroxine.
- Levothyroxine may enhance theophylline clearance.

Monitoring parameters

- Plasma TSH should be done every 6–8 weeks until normalization.
- Signs and symptoms of hypothyroidism should improve within a few weeks.
- Once the optimum replacement dose is attained, a physical examination should be made and TSH level should be monitored every 6–12 months.
- Patients at risk for coronary artery disease should be monitored for angina.

Pharmacokinetics

- The U.S. Food and Drug Administration states that all levothyroxine products should be considered therapeutically inequivalent unless equivalence (AB rating) has been established and noted in the *Orange Book: Approved Drug Products with Therapeutic Equivalence Evaluations.*
- Levoxyl, Levothroid, Synthroid, Unithroid, and some generics are bioequivalent.
- Because of the narrow therapeutic index of levothyroxine, many experts recommend rechecking TSH concentrations 6–8 weeks after any change in formulation, even when bioequivalent.
- Oral absorption is improved by fasting but decreased by dietary fiber, drugs, and foods.
- A half-life of 7 days allows once-daily dosing.
- Average bioavailability of levothyroxine products ranges from 40% to 80%. When a switch is made from oral to intravenous levothyroxine, the dosage should be reduced by 25% to 50%.

Other

- Use of natural thyroid hormones such as desiccated thyroid USP is discouraged because their potency and stability are less predictable than synthetic levothyroxine.
- Synthetic T$_3$ (liothyronine) has a shorter half-life than levothyroxine, has a higher incidence of cardiac side effects, and is more difficult to monitor.

Hyperthyroidism

Disease overview

Definition and epidemiology

- Hyperthyroidism (thyrotoxicosis) is the clinical syndrome that results when tissues are exposed to high levels of thyroid hormone.
- Thyrotoxicosis is more common in women than men, occurring in 3 per 1,000 women.

Types

- Graves' disease is the most common cause of hyperthyroidism.
- Toxic multinodular goiter (MNG), toxic adenoma, and exogenous thyroid hormone ingestion may also cause hyperthyroidism.
- Thyroid storm is a life-threatening, sudden exacerbation of all the symptoms of thyrotoxicosis, characterized by fever, tachycardia, delirium, and coma.
- Hyperthyroidism may be caused by drugs such as amiodarone and iodine.

Clinical presentation

- Symptoms include heat intolerance, weight loss, weakness, palpitations, and anxiety.
- Signs include tremor; tachycardia; weakness and eyelid lag; and warm, moist skin.

- Other manifestations include atrial fibrillation and congestive heart failure in patients with documented cardiac history.

Pathophysiology

- Graves' disease is an autoimmune disease in which thyroid-stimulating antibodies are produced. These antibodies mimic the action of TSH on thyroid tissue.
- Toxic adenomas and MNGs are masses of thyroid tissue that secrete thyroid hormones independent of pituitary control.

Diagnosis

Elevated T$_4$ or T$_3$ in the presence of a decreased TSH confirms the diagnosis of hyperthyroidism.

Treatment principles

- The three primary methods for controlling hyperthyroidism are surgery, radioactive iodine (RAI), and antithyroid (thioamide) drugs.
- The goal is to minimize symptoms and eliminate excess thyroid hormone.
- RAI is often considered the treatment of choice in Graves' disease, toxic adenomas, and MNGs.
- Propylthiouracil is no longer preferred in pregnancy because of the increased risk of hepatoxicity; RAI is contraindicated.
- Thioamide drugs (propylthiouracil and methimazole) have no permanent effect on thyroid function.
- Adjunctive treatments for hyperthyroidism include β-adrenergic receptor blockers or nondihydropyridine calcium channel blockers to control tachycardia associated with hyperthyroidism.

Drug therapy of hyperthyroidism

Antithyroid medications are summarized in Table 18-2.

Table 18-2. Antithyroid Medications

Drug name	Drug contains	Dosage forms	Usual dosage range
PTU	Propylthiouracil	Tablet: 50 mg	150–300 mg po daily at 8-hour intervals
Tapazole	Methimazole	Tablet: 5, 10 mg	5–40 mg po in single daily dose or divided
Lugol's solution	Strong iodine solution	Solution: 5% iodine and 10% potassium iodide; delivers 6.3 mg iodine per drop	0.1–0.3 mL (3–5 drops) po tid
SSKI	Saturated solution of potassium iodide	Solution: 1 g/mL; delivers 38 mg iodine per drop of saturated solution	1–5 drops po tid in water or juice

Thioamides
Mechanism of action
- Propylthiouracil and methimazole inhibit the synthesis of thyroid hormones by preventing the incorporation of iodine into iodotyrosines and by inhibiting the coupling of monoiodotyrosine and diiodotyrosine to form T_4 and T_3.
- Propylthiouracil inhibits the peripheral conversion of T_4 to T_3.

Patient counseling
- This medication prevents excessive thyroid hormone production.
- It must be taken regularly to be effective.
- Do not discontinue use without first consulting your physician.
- Notify your physician if fever, sore throat, unusual bleeding, rash, abdominal pain, or yellowing of the skin occurs.

Adverse effects
- *CNS*: Fever, headache, paresthesias
- *General*: Rash, arthralgia, urticaria
- *GI*: Jaundice, hepatitis
- *Hematologic*: Agranulocytosis, leukopenia, bleeding
- *Black box warning*: Propylthiouracil should be used only in patients where other treatments are not tolerated because of potentially fatal cases of severe liver injury and acute liver failure.

Drug interactions
Potentiation of warfarin's effect may occur.

Monitoring parameters
- Monitor for improvement in signs and symptoms of hyperthyroidism.
- Perform thyroid function tests with periodic blood counts; watch for signs and symptoms of agranulocytosis (fever, malaise, sore throat).

Pharmacokinetics
Propylthiouracil and methimazole are typically dosed three to four times daily, but evidence exists that both drugs can be given once daily.

Iodides
Mechanism of action
- Medication blocks hormone release and inhibits thyroid hormone synthesis.
- Medication may be used to rapidly reduce thyroid hormone secretion when desired, such as in thyroid storm, or to decrease glandular vascularity prior to thyroidectomy.
- Because of its harsh taste, iodine is not used for long-term thyroid suppression.

Patient instructions
- Dilute with water or fruit juice to improve taste.
- Notify physician if fever, skin rash, metallic taste, swelling of the throat, or burning of the mouth occurs.

Adverse effects
Adverse effects include rash, swelling of salivary glands, metallic taste, burning of the mouth, GI distress, hypersensitivity, and goiter.

Drug interactions
Lithium potentiates the antithyroid effect of iodides.

Monitoring parameters
Monitor for improvement in signs and symptoms of hyperthyroidism and for adverse effects.

18-4. Adrenals

Cushing's Syndrome

Disease overview

Definition and epidemiology
- Cushing's syndrome results from chronic glucocorticoid excess.
- The incidence rate is 2–4 persons per million population each year.

Types
- Cushing's syndrome is usually iatrogenic, caused by therapy with glucocorticoid drugs.
- Endogenous Cushing's syndrome is usually caused by overproduction of adrenocorticotropic hormone (ACTH) by pituitary gland adenomas (Cushing's disease).

Clinical presentation
Patients may present with obesity involving the face, neck, trunk, and abdomen; hypertension; hirsutism; acne; amenorrhea; depression; thin skin; easy bruising; diabetes; and osteopenia.

Pathophysiology
The hypothalamus produces a corticotropin-releasing hormone, which stimulates the anterior pituitary gland

to release ACTH (corticotropin). Circulating ACTH stimulates the adrenal cortex to produce cortisol.

Diagnosis

- Diagnosis is usually based on signs and symptoms of hypercortisolism.
- Dexamethasone suppression test or 24-hour urine cortisol measurement may be used.

Treatment principles

- If the syndrome is iatrogenic, minimization of corticosteroid exposure is essential.
- Pharmacotherapy of Cushing's syndrome is aimed at reducing cortisol production or activity with drugs, radiation, or surgery.

Drug therapy of Cushing's syndrome

Drugs for Cushing's syndrome are described in Table 18-3.

Mechanism of action

- Drugs used to treat Cushing's disease suppress synthesis of cortisol.
- Ketoconazole inhibits cytochrome P450 (CYP450)–dependent enzymes and cortisol synthesis.
- Aminoglutethimide inhibits conversion of cholesterol to pregnenolone.
- Mitotane is a cytotoxic drug that suppresses ACTH secretion and reduces synthesis of cortisol.
- Metyrapone decreases cortisol synthesis by inhibition of 11-hydroxylase activity.

Patient counseling

Ketoconazole should be taken with food. Separate from antacids by at least 2 hours. Notify the physician if abdominal pain, yellow skin, or pale stool occurs.

Adverse effects

- Ketoconazole causes nausea, vomiting, headache, impotence, and hepatotoxicity.
- Aminoglutethimide causes drowsiness, rash, weakness, hypotension, nausea, loss of appetite, hypothyroidism, and blood dyscrasias.
- Metyrapone causes nausea, vomiting, dizziness, and sedation.
- Mitotane may cause nausea, vomiting, diarrhea, and tiredness.

Drug interactions

- Ketoconazole is a CYP450 3A4 enzyme inhibitor and may increase serum concentrations of cyclosporine, warfarin, cisapride, and triazolam. Drugs that lower gastric acidity will decrease ketoconazole absorption. Rifampin decreases ketoconazole levels.
- Aminoglutethimide may induce metabolism of warfarin.

Monitoring parameters

Cortisol monitoring is required with mitotane.

Adrenal Insufficiency

Disease overview

Definition and epidemiology

- Primary adrenocortical deficiency (Addison's disease) is caused by autoimmune-mediated destruction of the adrenal cortex and results in glucocorticoid and mineralocorticoid deficiency.
- Addison's disease occurs in 5–6 persons per million population per year.

Types

- Primary adrenal insufficiency (Addison's disease) involves autoimmune destruction of the adrenal cortex.

Table 18-3. Drugs for Cushing's Syndrome

Trade name	Generic name	Dosage forms	Usual dosage range
Nizoral	Ketoconazole	Tablet: 250 mg	800–1,200 mg po daily
Cytadren	Aminoglutethimide	Tablet: 250 mg	250 mg po q6h
Lysodren	Mitotane	Tablet: 500 mg	9–10 g/day po in divided doses
Metopirone	Metyrapone	Capsule: 250 mg	1–6 g/day po in 4–6 divided doses

- Secondary adrenal insufficiency occurs after cessation of chronic exogenous corticosteroid use.
- Acute adrenal insufficiency, or Addisonian crisis, is an endocrine emergency precipitated by severe stress.

Clinical presentation

- Glucocorticoid deficiency (weight loss, malaise, abdominal pain, depression)
- Mineralocorticoid deficiency (dehydration, hypotension, hyperkalemia, salt craving)

Pathophysiology

- Cortisol is synthesized in the adrenal cortex when cholesterol is converted to pregnenolone by ACTH.
- The adrenal cortex secretes aldosterone, cortisol, and androgenic hormones.
- Mineralocorticoids (e.g., aldosterone) enhance reabsorption of sodium and water from the distal tubule of the kidney and increase urinary potassium excretion.
- Glucocorticoids affect glucose, carbohydrate, and fat metabolism; produce anti-inflammatory and immunosuppressive effects; and affect other physiologic processes.
- Chronic administration of corticosteroids produces inhibition of pituitary ACTH secretion and reduced cortisol production (hypothalamic-pituitary-adrenocortical [HPA] axis suppression).

- Abrupt cessation of steroids may precipitate adrenal insufficiency.

Diagnosis

A cosyntropin (ACTH) stimulation test may be used to assess hypocortisolism.

Treatment principles

- Addison's disease requires lifelong glucocorticoid and mineralocorticoid replacement.
- Hydrocortisone 100 mg intravenous (IV) q8h is the drug of choice for acute adrenal crisis.
- "Stress doses" of corticosteroids are given for minor illness, injury, or surgery. If stress is severe, hydrocortisone 100 mg IV q8h is used.
- Gradual tapering of corticosteroids reduces the risk of adrenal insufficiency in patients with HPA axis suppression.
- Nonadrenal uses for corticosteroids are numerous, including allergic reactions; inflammatory conditions; hematologic disorders; rheumatic disorders; neurologic diseases; cancer; immunosuppression; pulmonary, renal, skin, and thyroid diseases; and hypercalcemia.
- Fludrocortisone has minimal anti-inflammatory activity and is used only when mineralocorticoid activity is needed, such as when increased blood pressure is desired.

Drug therapy of adrenal insufficiency

Information about corticosteroids is provided in Table 18-4.

Table 18-4. Corticosteroids and Dose Equivalents

Trade name	Generic name	Anti-inflammatory potency	Sodium-retaining potency	Equivalent dose (mg)	Half-life
Cortone	Cortisone	0.8	2	25	Short
Cortef, Hydrocortone, Solu-Cortef	Hydrocortisone	1	2	20	Short
Deltasone, Liquid Pred	Prednisone	4	1	5	Medium
Prelone, Pediapred, Delta-Cortef	Prednisolone	4	1	5	Medium
Medrol, Solu-Medrol, Depo-Medrol, A-Methapred	Methylprednisolone	5	0	4	Medium
Aristocort, Kenacort, Kenalog	Triamcinolone	5	0	4	Medium
Decadron, Dexameth, Dexone, Hexadrol	Dexamethasone	30	0	0.75	Long
Celestone	Betamethasone	25	0	0.75	Long
Florinef	Fludrocortisone	15	150	2	Medium

Mechanism of action

- Glucocorticoids increase blood glucose by stimulating gluconeogenesis and glycogenolysis; fat deposition is increased.
- Catabolic effects occur in lymphoid, connective tissue, bone, muscle, fat, and skin.
- Inhibition of inflammation and immuno-suppression, vasoconstriction, reduction in prostaglandin and leukotriene synthesis, decreased neutrophils at sites of inflammation, and inhibition of macrophage function result.

Patient counseling

- Steroids may cause stomach upset, so take them with food.
- It is preferable to take the dose before 9:00 am.
- Wear or carry identification if on chronic steroid therapy.
- Therapy may mask signs of infection.
- Drugs may increase insulin or oral hypoglycemic requirements if patient is diabetic.
- Notify the physician if weight gain, muscle weakness, sore throat, or infection occurs.
- Report tiredness, stomach pain, weakness, and high or low blood sugar to the physician.
- Do not discontinue abruptly if taking long term.

Adverse effects

- *Cardiac*: Hypertension, sodium and fluid retention, atherosclerosis
- *CNS*: Insomnia, anxiety, depression, psychosis
- *Metabolic*: Obesity, hyperglycemia, hypokalemia, amenorrhea, impotence
- *Ophthalmic*: Cataracts, glaucoma
- *Immune*: Infections, impaired wound healing, leukocytosis
- *Musculoskeletal*: Myopathy, osteoporosis

Drug interactions

- Rifampin and other enzyme-inducing drugs increase metabolism of corticosteroids and decrease their effectiveness.

- Concomitant use of nonsteroidal anti-inflammatory drugs (NSAIDs) and corticosteroids increases risk of peptic ulcer disease.
- Corticosteroids may impair immunologic response to vaccines in some patient populations.
- Estrogens may increase corticosteroid clearance.
- Ketoconazole, macrolides, and other CYP450 3A4 enzyme-inhibiting drugs may decrease clearance of corticosteroids.
- Corticosteroids increase insulin and oral hypoglycemic drug requirements.

Monitoring parameters

Patients should be monitored for weight gain, edema, increased blood pressure, electrolytes, blood glucose, and infection.

Pharmacokinetics

Many dosage forms, doses, and schedules are used, including tablets, topicals, enemas, oral liquids, injections, and depot injection forms for intra-articular or intramuscular use.

18-5. Miscellaneous Endocrine Drugs

ACTH and Cosyntropin

Table 18-5 provides information about ACTH and cosyntropin.

Therapeutic uses

ACTH and cosyntropin are used for diagnosis of adrenal insufficiency. ACTH is rarely used as an alternative to corticosteroids.

Mechanism of action

- ACTH stimulates the adrenal cortex to secrete adrenal hormones.

Table 18-5. ACTH and Cosyntropin

Trade name	Generic name	Dosage forms	Usual dosage range
Cortrosyn	Cosyntropin	Injection: 0.25 mg	0.25–0.75 mg for testing
Acthar (ACTH)	Corticotropin	Injection: 25, 40 units	10–25 units for testing
H.P. Acthar Gel		Repository injection: 40, 80 units/mL	40–80 units of repository injection every 1–3 days

- If ACTH fails to elicit an appropriate cortisol response, adrenal insufficiency is present.
- Cosyntropin is a synthetic peptide that is similar to human ACTH, but less allergenic.

Patient counseling and adverse effects

Patients should receive the same counseling as for corticosteroids. Adverse effects are the same.

Drug interactions

Enzyme-inducing drugs will decrease effects.

Monitoring parameters

Monitoring parameters are the same as for corticosteroids.

Vasopressin and Desmopressin

Table 18-6 describes the dosages for vasopressin and desmopressin.

Therapeutic uses

- *Vasopressin*: Diabetes insipidus, variceal hemorrhage, shock, ventricular fibrillation
- *Desmopressin*: Nocturnal enuresis, diabetes insipidus, hemophilia A, von Willebrand's disease

Mechanism of action

- Vasopressin is also known as antidiuretic hormone (ADH); it increases water resorption.
- Vasopressin causes vasoconstriction in portal and splanchnic vessels (GI tract).
- Desmopressin is a synthetic derivative of vasopressin with ADH activity and only minimal

vasoconstrictive properties; it increases clotting factor VIII levels.

Patient counseling

For intranasal desmopressin, the patient should be instructed on proper intranasal use. The following instructions should also be given:

- Discard the bottle after 25 or 50 doses.
- Do not transfer the solution to another bottle.
- The drug may cause nasal irritation.
- Notify the physician if bleeding is not controlled or if headache, shortness of breath, or severe abdominal cramps occur.

Adverse effects

- *Vasopressin*: Angina, myocardial infarction, vasoconstriction, hyponatremia, gangrene, abdominal cramps, tissue necrosis if extravasation occurs, hypersensitivity
- *Desmopressin*: Abdominal pain, headache, flushing, nausea, nasal irritation, vulvar pain, nosebleed, rhinitis, hypersensitivity

Drug interactions

- Drugs may enhance effects of other pressors.
- Carbamazepine and chlorpropamide potentiate the effect of desmopressin on ADH.

Monitoring parameters

- With diabetes insipidus, monitor urine volume and plasma osmolality.
- With von Willebrand's disease, monitor factor VIII levels and bleeding time.
- When IV vasopressin is used, monitor blood pressure and pulses.

Table 18-6. Vasopressin and Desmopressin

Trade name	Generic name	Dosage forms	Usual dosage range
Pitressin	Vasopressin	Injection: 20 units/mL	10–20 units intramuscular, subcutaneous, or IV daily at 3- to 4-hour intervals or as a continuous infusion
Stimate (DDAVP)	Desmopressin	Tablet: 0.1, 0.2 mg	Nocturnal enuresis: 0.2–0.6 mg po nightly
		Nasal solution: 0.1, 1.5 mg/mL	Diabetes insipidus: 0.1–0.2 mg po bid, 0.1–0.4 mL intranasally in single or divided doses
		Injection: 4 mcg/mL	

Androgens and Anabolic Steroids

Table 18-7 provides information about androgens and anabolic steroids.

Therapeutic uses

- Androgens and anabolic steroids are used to treat hypogonadism, delayed puberty, metastatic breast cancer, anemia, acquired immune deficiency syndrome (AIDS) wasting in human immunodeficiency virus (HIV)–infected men, corticosteroid-induced hypogonadism and osteoporosis, and moderate to severe vasomotor symptoms associated with menopause (when combined with estrogen).
- They are schedule C-III controlled substances because they are intentionally misused by those seeking performance-enhancing effects and enhanced muscular development and endurance.

Mechanism of action

- Androgens promote growth and development of male sex organs and maintenance of secondary sex characteristics.
- Androgens also cause retention of nitrogen, sodium, potassium, and phosphorus; increase protein anabolism; and decrease protein catabolism.
- Androgens are responsible for the growth spurt of adolescence and termination of linear growth by fusion of epiphyseal growth centers.
- Exogenous androgens stimulate production of red blood cells, suppress endogenous testosterone release through feedback inhibition of luteinizing hormone, and suppress spermatogenesis through feedback inhibition of follicle-stimulating hormone.

Patient counseling

- Medication may cause stomach upset.
- Notify a physician if swelling of the ankles or persistent erections occur.
- This product is a controlled substance; do not misuse or abuse it.
- For females, notify physician if deepening of the voice, increased facial hair, or menstrual irregularities occur.

Table 18-7. Androgens and Anabolic Steroids

Trade name	Generic name	Dosage forms	Usual dosage range
AndroGel 1.62%	Testosterone	Gel: 1.62%	40.5 mg once daily
Axiron	Testosterone	Solution: 30 mg/1.5 ml	30 mg once daily
Fortesta	Testosterone	Gel: 10 mg/0.5 g	40 mg once daily
Testoderm	Testosterone transdermal system	Patch: 2.5, 4, 5, 6 mg	Patch: 2.5–6 mg for 24 hours
Androderm	Testosterone transdermal system	Patch: 2, 2.5, 4, 5 mg	Patch: 2–7.5 mg for 24 hours
AndroGel 1%, Testim	Testosterone	Gel: 1%	5 g once daily
Depo-Testosterone	Testosterone cypionate (in oil)	Injection in oil: 100, 200 mg/mL	50–400 mg every 2–4 weeks
Delatestryl	Testosterone enanthate (in oil)	Injection in oil: 100, 200 mg/mL	50–400 mg every 2–4 weeks
Testopel	Testosterone	Pellet for subcutaneous implantation: 75 mg	150–450 mg every 3–6 months
Striant	Testosterone	Buccal tablet: 30 mg	30 mg every 12 hours
Methitest	Methyltestosterone	Tablet: 10, 25 mg	10–50 mg once daily
Testred, Android	Methyltestosterone	Capsule: 10 mg	10–50 mg once daily
Halotestin, Androxy	Fluoxymesterone	Tablet: 2, 5, 10 mg	5–10 mg once daily
Anadrol-50	Oxymetholone	Tablet: 50 mg	50–100 mg once daily
Winstrol	Stanozolol	Tablet: 2 mg	2 mg daily tid
Oxandrin	Oxandrolone	Tablet: 2.5, 10 mg	2.5–10 mg daily
Deca-Durabolin	Nandrolone decanoate	Injection: 100, 200 mg/mL (in oil)	100–200 mg once weekly

Boldface indicates one of top 100 drugs for 2012 by units sold at retail outlets, www.drugs.com/stats/top100/2012/units.

■ Patients receiving transdermal testosterone should be provided with the manufacturer's patient instructions and carefully counseled on use and disposal of the system.

Adverse effects

■ *General:* Jaundice, hepatitis, edema, high abuse potential in an effort to enhance athletic performance, hypercholesterolemia and atherosclerosis, increased aggression and libido
■ *Women:* Hirsutism, voice deepening, acne, decreased menses, clitoral enlargement
■ *Men:* Acne, sleep apnea, gynecomastia, azoospermia, prostate enlargement, decreased testicular size

18-6. Questions

Use Patient Profile 18-1 to answer Questions 1 and 2.

1. The Synthroid prescription dispensed to the patient on 3/21 requires advising her to

   A. take 4 hours before or 4 hours after Questran.

   B. take with food.
   C. watch for signs of infection.
   D. take as needed to keep her desired level of energy.
   E. discontinue if she experiences nausea.

2. Which of the following of the patient's conditions could the Synthroid exacerbate?

   A. Hypercholesterolemia
   B. Anemia
   C. Coronary artery disease
   D. Hypertension
   E. Constipation

3. Excessive doses of levothyroxine may cause

   A. weight gain.
   B. osteoporosis.
   C. cold intolerance.
   D. bradycardia.
   E. sedation.

4. Which of the following drugs may produce hypothyroidism?

   A. Amitriptyline
   B. Sertraline

Patient Profile 18-1. Corn State Community Pharmacy

Patient: 78-year-old female
Race: Hispanic

Height: 48″
Weight: 103 lb
Allergies: Cats
Pharmacist notes

Diagnosis:

		Date	Comment
Primary	1. Hypercholesterolemia	2/23	Patient reminded to continue taking aspirin 325 mg for CAD
	2. Anemia	2/23	Patient to take OTC ferrous sulfate 325 mg daily for 3 months for anemia
	3. Coronary artery disease		Advised patient to begin docusate 100 mg daily if constipation occurs
Secondary	1. Hypertension		

Medication orders

Date	Rx #	Physician	Drug and strength	Quantity	Sig	Refills
2/23	88768	Hooper	Zocor 40 mg	30	1 po nightly	5
2/23	88769	Hooper	Questran 4 g	60	1 packet bid, mix with juice	5
2/23	88770	Hooper	Tenormin 50 mg	30	1 po daily	5
2/23	88771	Hooper	Enalapril 5 mg	60	1 po bid	5
3/21	89995	Stubie	Synthroid 0.025 mg	30	1 po daily	0

C. Cholestyramine and ACTH
D. Lithium and amiodarone
E. Levothyroxine

5. All of the following may decrease the effect of thyroid hormone supplementation *except*

A. antacids.
B. bile acid sequestrants.
C. estrogens.
D. sucralfate.
E. theophylline.

6. A patient who is suffering from heat intolerance, weight loss, tachycardia, tremor, and anxiety may be treated with

A. acetaminophen.
B. mitotane.
C. cyproheptadine.
D. propylthiouracil.
E. diazepam.

7. A patient with atrial fibrillation may require a decreased warfarin dosage when which of the following drugs is initiated?

A. Liothyronine
B. Propylthiouracil
C. Methimazole
D. ACTH
E. Diphenhydramine

8. Which of the following drugs is used to treat Cushing's disease?

A. Clotrimazole
B. Propylthiouracil
C. Mitotane
D. Vasopressin
E. Prednisone

9. Which of the following drugs works by decreasing cortisol synthesis?

A. Cortrosyn
B. ACTH
C. Oxandrolone
D. Prednisone
E. Metyrapone

10. Decreased ketoconazole absorption may occur if it is administered concomitantly with which of the following?

A. Antacids
B. Food

C. Warfarin
D. Cyclosporine
E. CYP450 3A4 inhibitors

11. Close monitoring of adrenal hormone secretion may be required when administering which of the following?

A. Methyltestosterone
B. Mitotane
C. Desmopressin
D. Iodides
E. Propylthiouracil

12. Which of the following is used to treat adrenal crisis?

A. Cosyntropin
B. Aminoglutethimide
C. Fluoxymesterone
D. Vasopressin
E. Hydrocortisone

13. Which of the following is *not* an effect of glucocorticoids?

A. Immunosuppression
B. Decreased prostaglandin synthesis
C. Inhibition of glycogenolysis
D. Decreased neutrophils at sites of infection
E. Inhibition of macrophages

Use Patient Profile 18-2 to answer Questions 14 and 15.

14. Which of the following is *least* likely to contribute to the increased blood glucose seen in this patient?

A. Dextrose 5%/NaCl 0.9% solution
B. Captopril
C. Epinephrine
D. Methylprednisolone
E. Anaphylaxis

15. The patient is discharged on a new prescription for Deltasone 40 mg daily for 7 days. He should be instructed to

A. check feet closely for wounds.
B. take ibuprofen for musculoskeletal pain.
C. take on an empty stomach.
D. take at bedtime.
E. wear identification for steroid therapy.

Patient Profile 18-2. Big Sky Hospital

Patient: 28-year-old male

Race: White

Date of admission: 4/21 at 15:26

Height: 5'8"

Weight: 178 lb

Allergies: Aspirin

Diagnosis:

Admit diagnosis   1. Anaphylactic reaction to aspirin

Secondary   1. Type 2 diabetes mellitus

          2. Hypertension

Laboratory

Date	Time	Lab	Result	(Normal range)
4/21	15:29	Glucose	144	(60–110 mg/dL)
4/21	19:20	Glucose	181	(60–110 mg/dL)
4/22	06:00	Glucose	240	(60–110 mg/dL)
4/22	12:21	Glucose	289	(60–110 mg/dL)
4/22	19:15	Glucose	352	(60–110 mg/dL)
4/23	06:20	Glucose	391	(60–110 mg/dL)
4/23	12:32	Glucose	443	(60–110 mg/dL)

Active medication orders

Date	Time	Drug and strength	Route	Frequency or schedule
4/21	15:30	Solu-Medrol 125 mg	IV	q6h
4/21	15:30	Dextrose 5%/NaCl 0.9%	IV	200 mL/h
4/21	15:30	Diphenhydramine 50 mg	IV	q6h
4/21	17:03	Glipizide 5 mg	Po	bid
4/21	17:03	Glucophage 850 mg	Po	bid
4/21	17:03	Captopril 50 mg	Po	tid

Discontinued medication orders

Date	Time	Drug and strength	Route	Frequency or schedule
4/21	15:30	Epinephrine 0.1 mg	Subcutaneous	Stat
4/21	15:30	Diphenhydramine 50 mg	IV	Stat

Dietary

Date	
4/21	1,800 kcal American Diabetes Association diet

16. Chronic administration of glucocorticoids predisposes patients to which of the following?

    A. Arthritis
    B. Obesity
    C. Alzheimer's disease
    D. Osteoporosis
    E. Hepatitis

17. A patient is taking prednisone 40 mg daily for 6 months. On abrupt cessation, which of the following may occur?

    A. Myopathy
    B. Diabetes
    C. Infection
    D. Adrenal crisis
    E. Psychosis

18. An increased risk of peptic ulcer disease occurs when NSAIDs are combined with which of the following?

    A. Ranitidine
    B. Ferrous sulfate
    C. Dexamethasone
    D. Carbamazepine
    E. Acetaminophen

19. Which of the following drugs may be used to diagnose adrenal insufficiency?

    A. Desmopressin
    B. Clemastine
    C. Captopril
    D. Cosyntropin
    E. Aminoglutethimide

20. Decreased urine production is an effect of

    A. carmustine.
    B. propylthiouracil.
    C. ACTH.
    D. desmopressin.
    E. SSKI.

21. Which of the following hormones is secreted by the pituitary gland?

    A. Adrenocorticotropic hormone
    B. Testosterone
    C. Cortisol
    D. Thyroxine
    E. Corticotropin-releasing hormone

22. Chronic administration of Winstrol may produce all of the following complications *except*

    A. prostate enlargement.
    B. increased testicular size.
    C. gynecomastia in men.
    D. accelerated atherosclerosis.
    E. decreased menses in women.

23. Androderm is administered

    A. once daily.
    B. three times per week.
    C. once weekly.
    D. every 2 weeks.
    E. monthly.

24. Which of the following is *not* an acceptable indication for testosterone?

    A. Anemia
    B. Hypogonadism
    C. Delayed puberty
    D. Body building
    E. Metastatic breast cancer

18-7. Answers

1. A. Bile acid sequestrants reduce levothyroxine absorption and must be separated from levothyroxine administration by at least 4 hours. Levothyroxine should be administered before a meal on an empty stomach to maximize absorption.

2. C. Thyroid hormones enhance oxygen consumption and increase the oxygen demand. The patient has a past medical history of coronary artery disease and is elderly. Thyroid supplementation would actually lower her cholesterol in the long run but may precipitate angina acutely.

3. B. Levothyroxine decreases bone mineral density and when given in supratherapeutic doses may cause osteoporosis. For this reason, the lowest possible replacement dose should be administered.

4. D. Lithium and amiodarone have both been associated with hypothyroidism. Amiodarone contains iodine and may cause hypo- or hyperthyroidism.

5. **E.** Numerous drugs are known to decrease thyroid hormone absorption, including antacids that contain divalent and trivalent cations, calcium salts, magnesium, sucralfate, and bile acid sequestrants. Estrogens and enzyme-inducing drugs may decrease circulating thyroid hormone levels and necessitate a dose increase of thyroxine.

6. **D.** Heat intolerance, weight loss, tachycardia, tremor, and anxiety are cardinal features of hyperthyroidism. Propylthiouracil is effective at reducing the excessive thyroxine level.

7. **A.** Liothyronine (Cytomel) is T_3, a potent thyroid hormone. In states of hypothyroidism, metabolism is decreased. However, if thyroid hormone is supplemented, blood clotting factors will be metabolized more quickly, leading to decreased warfarin requirements.

8. **C.** Mitotane is used to treat Cushing's disease. Propylthiouracil is used to treat hyperthyroidism. Clotrimazole is a topical antifungal, and vasopressin is used to treat diabetes insipidus.

9. **E.** Metyrapone (Metopirone) inhibits 11 hydroxylase activity and thus decreases cortisol synthesis.

10. **A.** Ketoconazole requires the presence of stomach acid to be absorbed. Any drug that decreases gastric acidity will decrease the extent of ketoconazole absorption. Food increases ketoconazole absorption because food stimulates release of gastric acid.

11. **B.** Mitotane is cytotoxic to adrenal cells and thus reduces cortisol synthesis and release. ACTH increases cortisol release. Close monitoring of cortisol levels is important when mitotane is used.

12. **E.** Hydrocortisone is the drug of choice for adrenal crisis because it possesses both mineralocorticoid and glucocorticoid properties. Although cosyntropin increases cortisol release, patients with adrenal crisis may not have enough adrenal reserve to meet their increased demand.

13. **C.** Glucocorticoids have potent effects on glucose and carbohydrate metabolism. They promote glycogen breakdown, rather than inhibit it.

14. **B.** Captopril increases insulin sensitivity and would not be expected to contribute to increased blood glucose. This patient's blood glucose began rising shortly after admission. His IV fluids contain glucose; epinephrine increases blood glucose by increasing glycogen breakdown, methylprednisolone (Solu-Medrol) promotes glycogenolysis, and anaphylaxis would be expected to increase stress response, thereby leading to increased epinephrine release and increased blood glucose.

15. **A.** The patient has a history of diabetes and will be given prednisone (Deltasone), which would be expected to increase blood glucose. When diabetes is poorly controlled, infections are more likely to occur. For this reason, he should monitor more closely for wounds that may become infected. He will not be taking prednisone long enough to develop adrenal insufficiency, so there is no need for him to wear identification for steroid therapy.

16. **D.** Glucocorticoids have catabolic effects on a number of tissues, including muscle, fat, skin, and bone. Chronic administration leads to osteopenia and osteoporosis.

17. **D.** Chronic administration of glucocorticoids such as prednisone will lead to feedback inhibition of pituitary ACTH release and atrophy of the adrenal cortex. When prednisone is abruptly stopped, the adrenals will not be able to meet the body's demand for cortisol during severe stress, and adrenal crisis may occur.

18. **C.** Corticosteroids such as dexamethasone (Decadron) are known to increase the risk of peptic ulcers when used in combination with NSAIDs.

19. **D.** Cosyntropin (Cortrosyn) is a synthetic analogue of ACTH that is used to diagnose adrenal insufficiency. It works by stimulating the adrenal cortex to secrete cortisol. If cosyntropin administration does not result in an appropriate increase in cortisol release, adrenal insufficiency is present.

20. **D.** Desmopressin (DDAVP) is a synthetic analogue of vasopressin, or antidiuretic hormone. Thus, it decreases urine production by increasing water resorption.

21. **A.** Adrenocorticotropic hormone, or ACTH, is released by the pituitary and acts on the adrenal glands to increase cortisol release. Corticotropin-releasing hormone is released by the hypothalamus and acts on the pituitary to stimulate ACTH release.

22. **B.** Stanozolol (Winstrol) is an androgen that would be expected to promote growth and development of male sex organs. However, chronic administration leads to feedback inhibition of testosterone secretion, which leads to testicular atrophy.

23. **A.** Testosterone transdermal systems (Androderm, Testoderm) are applied once daily for 24 hours. Longer-acting androgens are available, such as nandrolone decanoate (Deca-Durabolin), for once-weekly administration.

24. **D.** Anabolic steroids may be abused by those who are seeking enhanced muscular development and endurance, such as athletes. For this reason, all of these agents are subject to the Controlled Substances Act.

18-8. References

Baskin HJ, Cobin RH, Duick DS. American Association of Clinical Endocrinologists Medical Guidelines for Clinical Practice for the evaluation and treatment of hyperthyroidism and hypothyroidism (AACE Thyroid Task Force). *Endocr Pract.* 2002; 8:457–69.

Chrousos GP. Adrenocorticosteroids and adrenocortical antagonists. In: Katzung BG, Masters S, Trevor T, eds. *Basic and Clinical Pharmacology.* 12th ed. New York, NY: McGraw-Hill; 2012: 697–714.

Chrousos GP. The gonadal hormones and inhibitors. In: Katzung BG, Masters S, Trevor T, eds. *Basic and Clinical Pharmacology.* 12th ed. New York, NY: McGraw-Hill; 2012:715–52.

Dayan CM, Daniels GH. Chronic autoimmune thyroiditis. *N Engl J Med.* 1996;335:99–106.

Dietrich E, Smith SM, Gums JG. Adrenal gland disorders. In: DiPiro J, Talbert R, Yee G, et al., eds. *Pharmacotherapy: A Pathophysiologic Approach.* 9th ed. New York, NY: McGraw-Hill; 2014: 1217–36.

Dong BJ, Greenspan FS. Thyroid and antithyroid drugs. In: Katzung BG, Masters S, Trevor T, eds. *Basic and Clinical Pharmacology.* 12th ed. New York, NY: McGraw-Hill; 2012:681–96.

Dong BJ, Hauck WW, Gambertoglio JG, et al. Bioequivalence of generic and brand name levothyroxine products in the treatment of hypothyroidism. *JAMA.* 1997;277:1205–13.

Garber JR, Cobin RH, Gharib H, et al. Clinical practice guidelines for hypothyroidism in adults: Cosponsored by the American Association of Clinical Endocrinologists and the American Thyroid Association. *Endocr Pract.* 2012;18:e2.

Jonklaas J, Talbert R. Thyroid disorders. In: DiPiro J, Talbert R, Yee G, et al., eds. *Pharmacotherapy: A Pathophysiologic Approach.* 9th ed. New York, NY: McGraw-Hill; 2014:1191–84.

Master SB, Rosenthal SM. Hypothalamic and pituitary hormones. In: Katzung BG, Masters S, Trevor T, eds. *Basic and Clinical Pharmacology.* 12th ed. New York, NY: McGraw-Hill; 2012: 659–80.

McEvoy GK, ed. *AHFS Drug Information 2009.* Bethesda, MD: American Society of Health-System Pharmacists; 2009.

Smith S, Gums J. Adrenal gland disorders. In: DiPiro J, Talbert R, Yee G, et al., eds. *Pharmacotherapy: A Pathophysiologic Approach.* 8th ed. New York, NY: McGraw-Hill; 2011:1327–44.

U.S. Food and Drug Administration. *Orange Book: Approved Drug Products with Therapeutic Equivalence Evaluations.* 32nd ed. Silver Spring, MD: U.S. Food and Drug Administration; 2012. http://www.accessdata.fda.gov/scripts/cder/ob/default.cfm.

Women's Health

19

Andrea S. Franks

19-1. Key Points

Postmenopausal Hormone Therapy

- Postmenopausal hormone therapy (HT) must be selected on an individual basis taking into account risks and benefits, concomitant diseases, and medications. Important patient factors to consider include menopause symptoms; coronary artery disease risk; osteoporosis risk; breast cancer risk; and thromboembolism risk or history, or both.
- The primary indication for initiating HT is to relieve vasomotor and other menopausal symptoms to improve quality of life.
- HT should be used at the lowest effective dose and for the shortest duration possible.
- Estrogen plus progestin therapy is indicated in patients with a uterus. Estrogen alone is indicated in women who no longer have a uterus.

Contraceptives

- Oral contraceptives are highly effective and safe when used properly according to the manufacturer's recommended dose and administration. Selection of prescription contraceptives requires careful consideration of patient medical history, lifestyle, adherence, and preference.
- In addition to the contraceptive benefit of these products, other menstrual-related health problems may be resolved or lessened (e.g., menstrual pain, irregular menses).
- Changes in dose or product are often necessary to achieve an appropriate balance of estrogen and progestin that minimizes undesirable adverse effects.

- Patients must be educated to immediately seek medical care if they experience severe abdominal pain, severe chest pain, shortness of breath, severe headache, visual disturbances, or severe pain and swelling in the leg or calf.

Osteoporosis

- Women should be counseled about the preventive measures to increase bone mineral density, including adequate calcium intake (1,000–1,200 mg/day for adults), adequate vitamin D intake (600–1,000 IU daily for adults), moderation in alcohol use, and smoking cessation. Regular weight-bearing and strengthening exercises that help reduce falls and prevent fractures should be encouraged.
- Bone mineral density testing should be recommended to all postmenopausal women 65 years of age or older and for postmenopausal women younger than 65 years who have one or more risk factors for osteoporosis.
- Osteoporosis therapy must be selected on an individual basis considering risks and benefits, concomitant diseases, and medications.
- Bisphosphonates are first-line pharmacologic options for osteoporosis prevention and treatment. Most oral formulations must be taken with a full glass of water 30–60 minutes prior to the first meal of the day or any other medications. The patient must remain upright for at least 30 minutes after taking an oral dose. Bisphosphonates are contraindicated in patients with significant kidney disease.

19-2. Study Guide Checklist

The following topics may guide your study of this subject area:

- Indications for HT
- Contraindications to HT
- Commonly prescribed dosage forms and regimens of HT
- Common adverse effects with oral contraceptives, and the way to manage them
- Medical conditions that determine which type of contraceptive, if any, is appropriate
- Commonly prescribed dosage forms and regimens for contraceptive agents
- Recommended intake of calcium for older adults
- Recommended intake of vitamin D for older adults
- Contraindications and potential adverse effects of osteoporosis agents, including bisphosphonates, calcitonin, raloxifene, and teriparatide

19-3. Hormone Therapy

Menopause, defined as 12 consecutive months of amenorrhea, is the permanent cessation of menses. The median age of onset in the United States is 51 years of age (range 40–55 years). Perimenopausal symptoms and changes may begin up to 8 years prior to the cessation of menses.

Perimenopause is the time before menopause and the first year following menopause. Ovarian function and production of estrogen decline during this time, menstrual cycles may be irregular, and women may experience vasomotor symptoms. It is important to consider contraception during the perimenopausal period.

Clinical Presentation

- Cessation of menses for at least 12 consecutive months
- Symptoms of perimenopause related to declining estrogen:
  - Anovulation
  - Irregular menstrual cycles
- Symptoms of menopause directly related to lack of estrogen:
  - Vaginal dryness and vulvar or vaginal atrophy
  - Vasomotor symptoms (night sweats, hot flashes)

- Symptoms associated with menopause, but without a proven link to estrogen deficiency:
  - Arthralgia
  - Depression
  - Insomnia
  - Migraines
  - Mood swings
  - Myalgia
  - Urinary frequency
  - Cognitive changes (memory, concentration)

Pathophysiology

- Loss of ovarian follicular activity results in endocrine, biologic, and clinical changes.
- Ovarian production of estradiol and progesterone diminishes.
- Follicle-stimulating hormone and luteinizing hormone concentrations increase.
- Primary estrogen available is now estrone (which is converted peripherally from androstenedione and is less potent), not estradiol.

Treatment Principles

- Women with an intact uterus must be treated with estrogen plus progestin to reduce the risk of endometrial hyperplasia and endometrial cancer.
- Women who have had a hysterectomy may safely take unopposed estrogen.
- Hormone therapy (HT) should be initiated on an individual basis with careful consideration of the individual's risks and benefits.
- Contraindications to estrogen therapy (ET) are
  - Abnormal, undiagnosed genital bleeding
  - Known, suspected, or history of breast cancer
  - History of deep-vein thrombosis or pulmonary embolism
  - Estrogen-dependent neoplasia
  - Pregnancy
  - Stroke or myocardial infarction in the past year
  - Liver dysfunction or disease

Drug Therapy

Table 19-1 provides an overview of selected HT products.

Estrogen and progestin

Mechanism of action
ET is used alone (if no uterus) or in combination with progestin to replace diminished levels of endogenous hormones.

Table 19-1. Selected Hormone Therapy Products

Medication	Available strengths and dosing
Oral estrogen products	
Conjugated equine estrogens (CEE) (Premarin)	0.3, 0.45, 0.625, 0.9, 1.25 mg daily
Synthetic conjugated estrogens (Cenestin, Enjuvia)	0.3, 0.45, 0.625, 0.9, 1.25 mg daily
Estradiol (Estrace, Gynodiol)	0.5, 1, 1.5, 2 mg daily
Estradiol acetate (Femtrace)	0.45. 0.9, 1.8 mg daily
Estropipate (Ortho-Est, Ogen)	0.625, 1.25, 2.5, 5 mg estrone sulfate daily
Esterified estrogens (Menest)	0.3, 0.625, 1.25, 2.5 mg daily
Transdermal products	
Estradiol transdermal patch (Estraderm, Alora, Vivelle-Dot, Minivelle)	Apply twice weekly
Estradiol transdermal patch (Climara, Menostar)	Apply once weekly
Estradiol and levonorgestrel (Climara Pro)	Apply once weekly
Estradiol and norethindrone (CombiPatch)	Apply twice weekly
Estradiol topical emulsion (Estrasorb)	Apply daily
Estradiol micronized gel (Estrogel, Divigel, Elestrin)	Apply daily
17-β-estradiol transdermal spray (Evamist)	Apply one spray daily
Vaginal estrogen products	
Estrace vaginal cream (local effects)	0.1 mg estradiol/g; dose: 2–4 g daily for 1–2 weeks; maintenance dose: 1 g 1–3 times/week
Premarin vaginal cream (local effects)	0.625 mg conjugated estrogen/g; dose: 0.5–2 g daily for 3 weeks, then 1 week off
Estring vaginal ring, 17-β-estradiol (local effects)	2 mg estradiol ring releases 7.5 mcg/24 h; ring remains in vagina for 3 months
Vagifem vaginal tablet (local effects)	10 mcg estradiol/tablet; dose: 1 tablet once daily for 2 weeks; maintenance dose: 1 tablet twice/week
Femring vaginal ring (systemic absorption)	0.05 mg daily, 0.1 mg daily estradiol acetate; ring remains in vagina for 3 months
Oral combination estrogen–progestin products	
Activella	Estradiol/norethindrone 1 mg/0.5 mg, 0.5 mg/0.1 mg
Angeliq	Estradiol/drospirenone 0.5 mg/0.25 mg, 1 mg/0.5 mg, 1 mg/1 mg
Femhrt	Norethindrone acetate/ethinyl estradiol 0.5 mg/2.5 mcg
Prempro	Conjugated estrogen/medroxyprogesterone 0.3 mg/1.5 mg, 0.45/1.5 mg, 0.625 mg/2.5 mg, 0.625 mg/5 mg
Premphase	0.625 mg conjugated estrogen, 5 mg medroxyprogesterone (2 weeks of estrogen alone, 2 weeks of combination)
Combination estrogen–androgen products	
Estratest HS, Covaryx HS	0.625 mg esterified estrogens/methyltestosterone 0.625 mg/1.25 mg
Estratest, EEMT, Covaryx	1.25 mg esterified estrogens/methyltestosterone 1.25 mg/2.5 mg

Adapted from Kalantaridou et al., 2014; Hester, 2014.

Combined estrogen–progestin therapy (EPT) includes progestin to prevent endometrial hyperplasia and cancer.

Patient instructions and counseling

- Side effects of estrogen may be diminished by starting with a low dose and may be alleviated by changing products. Most side effects improve with time.
- Side effects of progestin may be alleviated or diminished by changing products or changing from a continuous to a cyclic regimen.
- Patients should be instructed to immediately report any unusual vaginal bleeding.
- Patients should be instructed to contact their physician promptly if any of the following events occur:
  - Abdominal tenderness, pain, or swelling
  - Disturbances of vision or speech
  - Dizziness or fainting
  - Lumps in the breast
  - Numbness or weakness in an arm or leg
  - Severe vomiting or headache
  - Sharp chest pain or shortness of breath
  - Sharp pain or swelling in the calves

Adverse drug events

Increased risks for venous thromboembolism, stroke, coronary heart disease, and breast cancer were identified in the Women's Health Initiative (WHI) trial with postmenopausal women receiving HT. The beneficial effects may include reductions in fractures and colorectal cancer. Both ET and EPT should be used at the lowest doses and for the shortest possible time period for women who are experiencing moderate to severe vasomotor symptoms or vulvovaginal atrophy. Consider topical estrogen, particularly if the primary complaint is vulvovaginal atrophy.

The following adverse effects are most common with estrogen:

- Breast tenderness
- Heavy or irregular bleeding
- Headache
- Nausea

The following adverse effects are most common with progestin:

- Depression
- Headache
- Irritability

Drug–drug and drug–disease interactions

Estrogen may exacerbate illness in the following disease states:

- Depression
- Hypertriglyceridemia (avoid by using transdermal product)
- Thyroid disorder (patients may require an increased dose of thyroid supplement)
- Impaired hepatic function (poor metabolism of estrogens)
- Cardiovascular disorders (coronary heart disease and venous thromboembolism risk may be increased with estrogens)
- Cholelithiasis
- Gastroesophageal reflux disease

Interaction may result in decreased pharmacologic effect of estrogens:

- Cytochrome P450 (CYP450) 3A4 inducers:
  - Barbiturates
  - Carbamazepine
  - Rifampin
  - St. John's wort
  - Phenytoin

Interaction may result in increased pharmacologic effect of estrogens:

- CYP450 3A4 inhibitors:
  - Azole antifungals
  - Macrolide antibiotics
  - Ritonavir

Parameters to monitor

Laboratory monitoring is not recommended. Patients should be monitored for symptom improvement, adverse effects, and appropriate health maintenance (e.g., annual mammograms).

Androgens (testosterone)

Mechanism of action

Androgens are the precursor hormones to estrogen production by the ovaries and peripheral sites. Ovarian testosterone production declines with menopause.

Androgens act at androgen receptor sites or exhibit action following conversion to estrogen. Androgen replacement improves deficiency-related symptoms (i.e., decreased sexual desire, decreased energy, diminished well-being).

Patient instructions and counseling

- Testosterone therapy should be administered only to postmenopausal women who are receiving concurrent estrogen therapy.
- The following are relative contraindications to testosterone therapy:
  - Androgenic alopecia
  - Hirsutism
  - Moderate to severe acne

Adverse drug events

- Fluid retention
- Decreased high-density lipoprotein and triglycerides
- Hepatic dysfunction
- Hepatocellular carcinoma (prolonged use of high doses)

Parameters to monitor

Laboratory monitoring is not recommended.

Nondrug Therapy

Phytoestrogens

- Phytoestrogens are plant compounds (isoflavones, lignans, coumestans).
- Food sources of phytoestrogens include soy (milk, edamame, tofu); flaxseed; and alfalfa sprouts.
- Phytoestrogens may improve vaginal symptoms, lipids, weight, and blood pressure and may slow loss of bone mineral density.
- No evidence supports improvement in other symptoms of menopause (i.e., hot flashes, depression, anxiety, headache, myalgia).

19-4. Contraception

Contraception is the prevention of pregnancy by one of two methods:

- Preventing implantation of the fertilized ovum in the endometrium
- Inhibiting contact of sperm with mature ovum

Prescription Contraceptive Options

Combined hormonal contraception (CHC)

- Combined oral contraceptive (COC)
  - COC contains estrogen plus progestin.
  - It may be monophasic, biphasic, triphasic, or four-phasic.
    - Monophasic may be used in extended regimens.
- Transdermal contraceptive patch
  - Apply to skin once weekly.
  - Patch may be used for extended regimens.
- Contraceptive vaginal ring
  - Insert once monthly, leave in for 3 weeks, and then remove for 1 week.
  - Ring may be used for extended regimens.

Progestin-only hormonal contraception

- Progestin-only oral contraceptive (minipill)
  - Appropriate for breast-feeding women
  - Less efficacious than combined oral contraceptives
  - Free of cardiovascular risks associated with estrogen-containing products, but may cause weight gain
- Injectable depot medroxyprogesterone acetate (DMPA)
  - Intramuscular or subcutaneous
  - Injection every 3 months
  - Weight gain, menstrual irregularity, and osteoporosis
- Intrauterine device (IUD)
  - May contain copper (Paragard) or levonorgestrel (Mirena, Skyla)
  - Contraindicated in women who have pelvic inflammatory disease, are immuno-compromised, or have a history of ectopic pregnancy
- Subdermal progestin-releasing implant
  - Etonogestrel (Nexplanon)
  - Effective up to 3 years
  - Possible decrease in efficacy in women over 130% of ideal body weight
  - May cause menstrual irregularity

Estrogens and Progestins Used in Prescription Contraceptives (Table 19-2)

- Estrogens:
  - Ethinyl estradiol, estradiol valerate
  - Mestranol
- Progestins:
  - Desogestrel
  - Norgestrel, levonorgestrel
  - Ethynodiol diacetate
  - Norethindrone, norethindrone acetate, norethynodrel
  - Dienogest

Table 19-2. Prescription Contraceptive Products

Product	Estrogen	Progestin
Progestin-only oral contraceptives		
Micronor, Errin, Nor-QD, Nora-BE, Camila	n.a.	Norethindrone 0.35 mg
Monophasic low-dose estrogen oral contraceptives		
Aviane, Lessina, Levlite	Ethinyl estradiol 20 mcg	Levonorgestrel 0.1 mg
Loestrin 1/20, Loestrin Fe 1/20, Microgestin Fe 1/20	Ethinyl estradiol 20 mcg	Norethindrone 1 mg
Yasmin, Ocella, Syeda	Ethinyl estradiol 30 mcg	Drospirenone 3 mg
Levlen, Levora, Nordette, Portia	Ethinyl estradiol 30 mcg	Levonorgestrel 0.15 mg
Cryselle, Lo/Ovral, Low-Ogestrel	Ethinyl estradiol 30 mcg	Norgestrel 0.3 mg
Apri, Desogen, Ortho-Cept	Ethinyl estradiol 30 mcg	Desogestrel 0.15 mg
Ovcon-35	Ethinyl estradiol 30 mcg	Norethindrone 0.4 mg
Brevicon, Modicon, Necon 0.5/35, Nortrel 0.5/35	Ethinyl estradiol 35 mcg	Norethindrone 0.5 mg
Necon 1/35, Norinyl 1+35, Nortrel 1/35, Ortho-Novum 1/35–28	Ethinyl estradiol 35 mcg	Norethindrone 1 mg
Monophasic high-dose estrogen oral contraceptives		
Ogestrel 0.5/50–28	Ethinyl estradiol 50 mcg	Norgestrel 0.5 mg
Zovia 1/50	Ethinyl estradiol 50 mcg	Ethynodiol diacetate 1 mg
Ovcon-50	Ethinyl estradiol 50 mcg	Norethindrone 1 mg
Biphasic oral contraceptives		
Necon 10/11	Ethinyl estradiol 35 mcg	Norethindrone 0.5 mg × 10 days; 1 mg × 11 days
Mircette, Kariva	Ethinyl estradiol 20 mcg × 21 days, placebo × 2 days, then 10 mcg × 5 days	Desogestrel 0.15 mg × 21 days
Triphasic oral contraceptives		
Enpresse, Trivora, Levonest	Ethinyl estradiol 30 mcg × 6 days, 40 mcg × 5 days, 30 mcg × 10 days	Levonorgestrel 0.05 mg × 6 days; 0.075 mg × 5 days; 0.125 mg × 10 days.
Tri-Norinyl, Leena, Aranelle	Ethinyl estradiol 35 mcg × 21 days	Norethindrone 0.5 mg × 7 days, 1 mg × 9 days, 0.5 mg × 5 days
Necon 7/7/7, Ortho-Novum 7/7/7, Nortrel 7/7/7	Ethinyl estradiol 35 mcg × 21 days	Norethindrone 0.5 mg × 7 days, 0.75 mg × 7 days, 1 mg × 7 days
Cyclessa, Velivet	Ethinyl estradiol 25 mcg × 21 days	Desogestrel 0.1 mg × 7 days, 0.125 mg × 7 days, 0.15 mg × 7 days
Ortho Tri-Cyclen Lo	Ethinyl estradiol 25 mcg × 21 days	Norgestimate 0.18 mg × 7 days, 0.215 mg × 7 days, 0.25 mg × 7 days
Ortho Tri-Cyclen, Trinessa	Ethinyl estradiol 35 mcg × 21 days	Norgestimate 0.18 mg × 7 days, 0.215 mg × 7 days, 0.25 mg × 7 days
Estrostep Fe, Tilia Fe	Ethinyl estradiol 20 mcg × 5 days, 30 mcg × 7 days, 35 mcg × 9 days	Norethindrone 1 mg × 21 days
Four phasic		
Natazia	Estradiol valerate 3 mg × 2 days, then 2 mg × 22 days, then 1 mg × 2 days, then 2 day pill-free interval	Dienogest none × 2 days, then 2 mg × 5 days, then 3 mg × 17 days, then none × 4 days

Table 19-2. Prescription Contraceptive Products *(Continued)*

Product	Estrogen	Progestin
Extended-cycle oral contraceptives		
Lo Loestrin Fe, Lo Minastrin Fe chewable	Ethinyl estradiol 10 mcg × 26 days	Norethindrone 1 mg × 24 days
Minastrin 24 Fe Chewable	Ethinyl estradiol 20 mcg × 24 days	Norethindrone 1 mg × 24 days
Seasonale, Jolessa, Quasense	Ethinyl estradiol 30 mcg × 84 days	Levonorgestrel 0.15 mg × 84 days
Yaz, Beyaz, Gianvi	Ethinyl estradiol 20 mcg × 24 days	Drospirenone 3 mg × 24 days
Quartette	Ethinyl estradiol 20 mcg × 42 days, 25 mcg × 21 days, 30 mcg × 21 days, then 10 mcg × 7 days	Levonorgestrel 0.15 mg × 84 days
Continuous-cycle oral contraceptives		
Amethyst (no placebo or pill-free interval)	Ethinyl estradiol 20 mcg	Levonorgestrel 90 mcg
Transdermal contraceptive system		
Ortho Evra	Ethinyl estradiol 20 mcg per 24 hours	Norelgestromin 0.15 mg per 24 hours; applied weekly
Vaginal ring contraceptive system		
NuvaRing	Ethinyl estradiol 15 mcg per 24 hours	Etonogestrel 0.12 mg per 24 hours; insert for 3 weeks, then remove 1 week
Contraceptive implants		
Nexplanon	n.a.	Etonogestrel subdermal rod; release rate varies over time for up to 3 years
Contraceptive injection		
Depo-Provera CI	n.a.	Medroxyprogesterone acetate 150 mg intramuscular q 3 months
Depo-SubQ Provera	n.a.	Medroxyprogesterone acetate 104 mg subcutaneous q 3 months
Intrauterine contraceptive systems		
Mirena	n.a.	Levonorgestrel 20 mcg/day × 5 years

Adapted from Shrader, Ragucci, 2014; O'Mara, 2013.
n.a., not applicable.

Drospirenone

- Progestin with progestogenic, antiandrogenic, and antimineralocorticoid activity

Drug Therapy

Mechanism of action

Estrogens prevent development of a dominant follicle by suppression of follicle-stimulating hormone. They do not block ovulation.

Progestin inhibits ovulation. It contributes to the production of thick and impermeable cervical mucus. It also contributes to involution and atrophy of the endometrium.

Patient instructions and counseling

- Efficacy is high (99 %) with perfect use, but it depends on adherence. (Efficacy is 92% with typical use.)
- Oral contraceptives do not prevent the transmission of sexually transmitted diseases.

- Patients should be educated on warning signs of serious complications:
  - Severe abdominal pain
  - Severe chest pain, shortness of breath, coughing up of blood
  - Severe headache
  - Eye problems (i.e., blurred vision, flashing lights, blindness)
  - Severe leg pain in the calf or thigh
- Patients should be advised to expect changes in characteristics of the menstrual cycle.
- Use of a backup contraceptive method is advised if more than one dose is missed per cycle.

Adverse drug events

The World Health Organization (WHO) suggests refraining from prescribing COCs to women with the following diagnoses:

- Breast cancer
- Deep-vein thrombosis or pulmonary embolism
- Cerebrovascular disease or coronary artery disease
- Diabetes with nephropathy, neuropathy, retinopathy, or other vascular disease
- Migraine headaches
- Uncontrolled hypertension ($\geq$ 160/90 mm Hg)
- Breast-feeding women (< 6 weeks postpartum)
- Liver disease
- Pregnancy
- Surgery with prolonged immobilization or any surgery on the legs
- Age > 35 years and currently smoking ($\geq$ 15 cigarettes a day)
- Hypercoagulable states (e.g., factor V Leiden, protein C or S deficiency)
- Complicated valvular heart disease (pulmonary hypertension, risk of atrial fibrillation, history of endocarditis)
- Peripartum cardiomyopathy
- Migraine, with aura

For these medical conditions, use of progestin-only oral contraceptives, DMPA, or an IUD may be an appropriate contraceptive choice.

The most common adverse drug events with COCs are as follows:

- Nausea and vomiting (usually resolves within 3 months)
- Breakthrough bleeding, spotting, amenorrhea, altered menstrual flow

- Melasma (hyperpigmentation of the skin, usually on the face)
- Headache or migraine
- Weight change or edema

Serious but less common effects are venous thrombosis, pulmonary embolism, myocardial infarction, coronary thrombosis, arterial thromboembolism, and cerebral thrombosis.

Potential hormonal effects are associated with an imbalance in estrogen and progestin (Table 19-3).

Drug–drug and drug–disease interactions

Interaction with the following drugs may result in decreased pharmacologic effect of oral contraceptives:

- Ampicillin, griseofulvin, sulfonamides, and tetracycline
- Anticonvulsants (barbiturates, carbamazepine, felbamate, phenytoin, topiramate)
- Some antiretroviral medications (e.g., nevirapine, lopinavir + ritonavir)
- Rifampin

Table 19-3. Potential Hormonal Effects Associated with an Imbalance in Estrogen or Progestin

Type of imbalance	Effect
Too much estrogen	■ Breast tenderness, fullness ■ Nausea ■ Edema and bloating ■ Hypertension ■ Melasma ■ Headache
Too much progestin	■ Acne or oily scalp ■ Breast tenderness ■ Depression or irritability ■ Hypomenorrhea ■ Increased appetite and weight gain ■ Fatigue ■ Constipation
Too little estrogen	■ Breakthrough bleeding (early, days 1–9 of cycle) ■ Hypomenorrhea ■ Vasomotor symptoms
Too little progestin	■ Amenorrhea ■ Breakthrough bleeding (late, days 14–21 of cycle) ■ Hypermenorrhea

Adapted from Shrader, Ragucci, 2014; El-Ibiary, White, 2010.

Interaction with these drugs may result in increased plasma levels of oral contraceptives:

- Atorvastatin
- Vitamin C
- CYP450 3A4 inhibitors

Interaction with the following drugs may result in decreased pharmacologic effect of the interacting drug:

- Anticoagulants (estrogens have a procoagulant effect)
- Some benzodiazepines (e.g., lorazepam, oxazepam, temazepam)
- Methyldopa
- Phenytoin

Interaction with the following may result in increased pharmacologic effect of interacting drug:

- Tricyclic antidepressants
- Some benzodiazepines (other than the benzodiazepines previously listed)
- β-blockers
- Theophylline

Parameters to monitor

Patients must monitor themselves for warning signs of serious complications previously listed. Laboratory monitoring is not recommended with use of oral contraceptives.

Nondrug Therapy

Nondrug therapy includes use of the following:

- Condoms
- Diaphragms
- IUDs
- Spermicides

19-5. Osteoporosis

Osteoporosis is characterized by low bone mineral density and deterioration of bone tissue, increasing fragility of bone, and subsequent risk of fracture.

Diagnostic Criteria

Dual-energy x-ray absorptiometry scans are used to diagnose osteoporosis. T-scores are used to guide diagnosis and decision to treat osteoporosis. The WHO classification of bone mass is based on T-scores:

- *Osteopenia:* T-score −1 to −2.5 standard deviations below the young adult mean
- *Osteoporosis:* T-score *below* −2.5 standard deviations below the young adult mean

Risk factors for osteoporosis are as follows:

- Advanced age
- Amenorrhea
- Cigarette smoking
- Current low bone mass
- Late menarche or early menopause
- Ethnicity (Caucasian or Asian)
- Excessive alcohol use
- Family history of osteoporosis or history of fracture in a primary relative
- Female
- History of fracture over the age of 50
- Sedentary lifestyle
- Low lifetime calcium intake
- Low testosterone levels in men (hypogonadism)
- Thin or small frame
- Vitamin D deficiency

Medical conditions associated with increased risk of osteoporosis are as follows:

- Acquired immune deficiency syndrome (AIDS)
- Cushing's disease
- Eating disorders
- Hyperthyroidism
- Hyperparathyroidism
- Inflammatory bowel disease
- Type 1 diabetes
- Malabsorption syndromes
- Rheumatoid arthritis
- Chronic kidney disease
- Chronic obstructive pulmonary disease

The following drugs are associated with an increased risk of osteoporosis:

- Anticonvulsants (phenobarbital, phenytoin)
- Glucocorticoids
- Immunosuppressants
- Long-term heparin or low molecular weight heparin
- DMPA
- Excessive thyroid supplementation
- Tamoxifen (premenopausal)
- Aromatase inhibitors
- Antiretroviral therapy
- Protease inhibitors
- Selective serotonin reuptake inhibitors
- Thiazolidinediones
- Proton pump inhibitors

Women 65 years of age and older should be screened for osteoporosis. In addition, postmenopausal women < 65 years of age with a family history of osteoporosis or clinical risk factors and women with a history of fractures unrelated to trauma should be screened.

Clinical Presentation

- Loss of height
- Vertebra, hip, or forearm fracture
- Kyphosis
- Bone pain (especially back pain, which could indicate vertebral compression fracture)

Pathophysiology

There are two types of bone: trabecular (i.e., vertebrae, wrist and ankle, and ends of long bones, which are the most susceptible to fracture) and cortical. Osteoblasts (formation) and osteoclasts (destruction) create a constant state of bone remodeling.

Bone formation exceeds destruction during childhood. Peak bone mass is reached around age 25–35; then bone density begins to decline at a rate of 3–4% per decade in men and 8–12% per decade in women 10 years after menopause.

Following menopause (postmenopausal osteoporosis), estrogen production declines and osteoclastic activity increases.

Treatment Principles

Adequate calcium and vitamin D intake through diet or supplementation is recommended for everyone (calcium 1,000–1,200 mg daily plus 600–1,000 IU vitamin D daily) (Table 19-4).

Lifestyle modifications are recommended, including weight-bearing exercise, smoking cessation, limited alcohol intake, dietary calcium, and vitamin D.

Prescription drug therapy should be initiated on an individual basis, considering risk factors, bone mineral density, fracture history, and concomitant diseases and medications.

Initiation of Treatment

The National Osteoporosis Foundation recommends initiation of therapy in the following situations:

- History of vertebral or hip fracture
- T-score below −2.5 (osteoporosis)
- T-score −1 to −2.5 (osteopenia) with
  - Secondary causes (steroids, immobility)
  - History of other fractures

Table 19-4. Select Calcium Supplement Products

Product	Calcium (mg)
Calcium citrate (24% calcium content)	
Citracal	Tablet: 200; liquitab: 500
Citracal Calcium + D₃ Slow Release	1,200 calcium plus 1,000 IU vitamin D₃
Calcium carbonate (40% calcium content)	
Caltrate 600	600
Tums	Chewable: 200, 300, 400, 500, 1,000
Viactiv chews	500 plus 500 IU vitamin D (1 chew)
Calcium carbonate + vitamin D	
Caltrate 600 + D	600 plus 800 IU vitamin D
Os-Cal + vitamin D	500 plus 200 IU vitamin D
Os-Cal Ultra + vitamin D	600 plus 500 IU vitamin D
Os-Cal Chewable	500 plus 600 IU vitamin D
Calcium phosphate tribasic (39% calcium content)	
Posture-D	600 plus 500 IU vitamin D

- 10-year probability of hip fracture ≥ 3% or 10-year probability of any major fracture ≥ 20% based on the U.S.-adapted WHO algorithm (Fracture Risk Assessment Tool, or FRAX; www.shef.ac.uk/FRAX/index.aspx?lang=En)

Drug Therapy

Calcium and vitamin D

Mechanism of action

Calcium is necessary to improve bone mass. It is absorbed through the gastrointestinal (GI) tract, stored in the bone, and made available when calcium levels become low.

Vitamin D facilitates absorption and regulation of calcium levels.

Patient instructions and counseling

- Approximately 500 mg of calcium can be absorbed from the GI tract at a time; separate doses appropriately to achieve a dose of 1,000–1,200 mg per day.
- Calcium carbonate contains the highest level of elemental calcium; take with food to facilitate absorption.
- Calcium citrate products may be administered without regard to meals.

The National Osteoporosis Foundation (NOF) recommends vitamin D intake of 800–1,000 IU per day. The Institute of Medicine of the National Academies' Dietary Reference Intakes recommends 600 IU of vitamin D up to age 70 and 800 IU daily for adults age 71 and older. The NOF recommends that vitamin D be supplemented to achieve a serum 25-hydroxyvitamin D [25(OH)D] level of at least 30 ng/mL.

Adverse drug events
The most common adverse drug events with calcium are as follows:

- GI upset (nausea, vomiting, cramping, flatulence, especially with carbonate)
- Hypophosphatemia and hypercalcemia
- Nephrolithiasis (especially with higher doses)

Drug–drug and drug–disease interactions
Concomitant administration with calcium may decrease the bioavailability of fluoroquinolones, tetracyclines, and levothyroxine.

Parameters to monitor
Laboratory monitoring is not recommended.

Bisphosphonates

Table 19-5 provides summary information about bisphosphonates.

Mechanism of action
Bisphosphonates are incorporated into the hydroxyapatite of the bone to increase and stabilize bone mass. They inhibit osteoclasts and have a very long half-life in the bone.

Patient instructions and counseling
- Bisphosphonates must be taken with a full glass of water (8 oz) 30–60 minutes prior to the first meal of the day and 30–60 minutes before any other medications.
- Remain in an upright position for at least 30 minutes following ingestion.
- Take medication on a regularly scheduled basis.
- Adherence may be increased by extended dosing intervals (weekly, monthly, quarterly); however, the studies that demonstrated fracture risk reduction used daily dosing.
- Appropriate calcium and vitamin D intake must be assured when taking bisphosphonates.

Adverse drug events
The most common adverse drug events are GI related: abdominal pain, dyspepsia, constipation, diarrhea, flatulence, nausea, gastritis, and esophageal ulceration (if not taken appropriately). Rarely, patients experience osteonecrosis of the jaw (mostly in cancer patients on intravenous bisphosphonates), myalgia, arthralgia, or flu-like symptoms (especially with intravenous zoledronic acid). Atrial fibrillation may be associated with bisphosphonates.

Drug–drug and drug–disease interactions
Concomitant administration of bisphosphonates with calcium supplements and antacids may result in decreased pharmacologic effect of bisphosphonates.

Parameters to monitor
Laboratory monitoring is not recommended.

Estrogen therapy

ET has a beneficial effect on bone mineral density and fracture risk, but the risks of long-term therapy appear to outweigh that benefit. ET should be used at the lowest effective dose for the shortest duration in women experiencing vasomotor symptoms or vulvovaginal atrophy.

Estrogen agonist–antagonist (selective estrogen receptor modulator): Raloxifene (Evista)

Mechanism of action
Raloxifene is an estrogen receptor agonist in the bone. It decreases resorption of bone and overall bone turnover. It acts as an antagonist in breast tissue.

Patient instructions and counseling
- This medication may be taken without regard to food.
- This medication will not treat symptoms of menopause such as hot flashes and may aggravate them.
- In the event of prolonged immobilization, when possible discontinue raloxifene 3 days prior to and during the period of immobility.

Adverse drug events
The most common adverse drug events are as follows:

- **Cardiovascular:** Hot flashes, chest pain, syncope
- **GI:** Nausea, diarrhea, vomiting

Table 19-5. Antiresorptive Agents

Medication	Dosing	FDA indication and availability
Bisphosphonates		
Alendronate (Fosamax) (Binosto—effervescent tablet)	Prevention: 5 mg daily or 35 mg weekly Treatment: 10 mg daily or 70 mg weekly	Prevention and treatment of postmenopausal osteoporosis Osteoporosis in men and glucocorticoid-induced osteoporosis Avoid if CrCl < 35 mL/min.
Risedronate (Actonel)	Prevention: 5 mg daily	Prevention and treatment of postmenopausal osteoporosis. Avoid if CrCl < 30 mL/min.
(Atelvia—delayed release)	Treatment: 5 mg daily or 35 mg po weekly, 75 mg po daily × 2 consecutive days monthly, or 150 mg po monthly	Osteoporosis in men Glucocorticoid-induced osteoporosis Available as tablets and tablets plus calcium
Ibandronate (Boniva)	2.5 mg po daily, 150 mg po monthly, 3 mg IV q 3 months	Prevention and treatment of postmenopausal osteoporosis. Avoid if CrCl < 35 mL/min.
Zoledronic acid (Reclast)	5 mg IV infusion over 15 minutes once yearly	Treatment of postmenopausal osteoporosis. Avoid if CrCl < 35 mL/min.
Selective estrogen receptor modulator		
Raloxifene (Evista)	60 mg daily	Prevention and treatment of postmenopausal osteoporosis
Other agents		
Calcitonin (Miacalcin)	Intranasal: 200 IU daily, alternating nostrils Intramuscular or subcutaneous: 100 IU every other day	Treatment of postmenopausal osteoporosis in women at least 5 years postmenopause
Teriparatide (Forteo)	20 mcg subcutaneously daily	Treatment of postmenopausal women with osteoporosis who are at high risk for fractures or who have failed or are intolerant to other therapies Treatment of men with primary or hypogonadal osteoporosis who are at high risk for fractures
Denosumab (Prolia)	60 mg subcutaneously every 6 months	RANK ligand (RANKL) inhibitor indicated for: Treatment of postmenopausal women with osteoporosis at high risk for fracture Men at high risk for fracture receiving androgen deprivation therapy Women receiving aromatase inhibitor therapy who are at high risk for fracture

Adapted from O'Connell, Borchert, 2014; National Osteoporosis Foundation, www.nof.org.
IV, intravenous.

- **Musculoskeletal:** Arthralgia, myalgia, nocturnal leg cramps
- **Central nervous system (CNS):** Insomnia, neuralgia
- **Skin:** Rash, sweating
- **Thrombotic:** Deep-vein thrombosis, pulmonary embolism

Drug–drug and drug–disease interactions
- **Cholestyramine:** Absorption and entero-hepatic cycling are reduced. Do not administer together.

Parameters to monitor
Laboratory monitoring is not recommended.

Calcitonin (Miacalcin, Fortical)

Mechanism of action

Calcitonin is involved in the regulation of calcium and bone metabolism. It inhibits bone resorption by binding to osteoclast receptors.

Patient instructions and counseling

- Proper education regarding administration techniques for both the injection and the nasal spray preparation is necessary.
- If this medication is administered as a subcutaneous injection, it should be given in the upper arm, thigh, or buttocks.
- Patient should be advised that if an injection is missed, the injection should be administered as soon as possible, but not if it is almost time for the next dose.
- Store the nasal spray in the refrigerator until time for use. Warm the spray to room temperature prior to first use and then store at room temperature. Prime the pump prior to first use.

Adverse drug events

The most common adverse drug events are as follows:

- **Skin:** Facial flushing and hand flushing (most common overall)
- **GI:** Nausea, diarrhea, vomiting, abdominal pain
- **Taste disorder:** Salty taste
- **Genitourinary:** Nocturia, urinary frequency
- **Nasal (with nasal spray):** Rhinitis, nasal dryness, irritation, itching, congestion
- **Ophthalmic:** Blurred vision, abnormal lacrimation

Drug–drug and drug–disease interactions

Salmon calcitonin should be avoided in patients with a true allergy to seafood.

Parameters to monitor

Laboratory monitoring is not recommended.

Parathyroid hormone: Teriparatide (Forteo)

Mechanism of action

Teriparatide increases the rate of bone formation by stimulating osteoblasts, thereby increasing bone mass density and decreasing fracture risk.

Because of limited long-term safety data (< 2 years) and risks of osteosarcoma in animal models, this medication is recommended for use only in patients at high risk of fracture.

Patient instructions and counseling

Patients should be educated regarding appropriate use of the prefilled pen delivery device, storage (refrigerator), and adverse effects (orthostasis with first dose).

Adverse drug events

The most common adverse drug events are as follows:

- **Musculoskeletal:** Pain, arthralgia
- **CNS:** Paresthesias
- **GI:** Nausea, diarrhea, abdominal cramps
- **Taste disorder:** Metallic taste
- **Skin:** Injection pain, urticaria

Drug–drug and drug–disease interactions

No drug–drug or drug–disease interactions are known; however, teriparatide is contraindicated in patients who are at increased risk of osteosarcoma, including those who have received radiation to the bone, adolescents or young adults with open epiphyses, and individuals with Paget's disease.

Parameters to monitor

Laboratory monitoring is not recommended.

Denosumab (Prolia)

Mechanism of action

Denosumab is a monoclonal antibody that binds to RANKL (receptor activator of nuclear factor kappa-B ligand), preventing osteoclast formation and decreasing bone resorption.

Patient instructions and counseling

- Prolia is available as a refrigerated prefilled pen or a single-use vial.
- Dosage is 60 mg subcutaneously every 6 months.
- Treatment should also include supplemental calcium (at least 1,000 mg/day) and vitamin D (at least 400 IU/day).
- Prior to administration, allow to stand for 15–30 minutes at room temperature.
- It should be injected subcutaneously in the upper arm, thigh, or abdomen.

Adverse drug events

- **CNS:** Fatigue, headache
- **GI:** Nausea, diarrhea
- **Dermatologic:** Rash, dermatitis, eczema
- **Neuromuscular:** Weakness, arthralgia
- **Dental:** Osteonecrosis of the jaw
- **Infectious:** Endocarditis, upper respiratory infection

Drug–drug and drug–disease interactions

Patients who are immunocompromised or who are taking immunosuppressants may have an increased risk of infection.

Hypocalcemia should be resolved prior to initiating therapy.

Parameters to monitor

Monitor serum calcium, creatinine, phosphorus, and magnesium.

Nondrug Therapy

Nondrug therapies include the following:

- Weight-bearing and balance-improving exercises
- Smoking cessation
- Moderation of alcohol consumption
- Calcium-rich diet
- Strategies to reduce the risk of falls

19-6. Questions

1. A. J. is a 35-year-old premenopausal woman who is concerned about her family history of osteoporosis. She does not eat dairy products because she is lactose intolerant. Her recent bone mineral density screening revealed a T-score of 1. Select the appropriate therapy recommendation from the choices below.

    A. Daily estrogen replacement therapy
    B. Daily calcium and vitamin D supplementation
    C. Daily combined estrogen and progestin replacement therapy
    D. Daily teriparatide injections
    E. Daily calcitonin nasal spray

2. The pharmacist receives a prescription for Fosamax 70 mg daily for prevention of osteoporosis with instructions to the patient to take with food and remain upright for at least 30 minutes following ingestion. From the following choices, identify the errors in this prescription.

    A. The dose of Fosamax should be 35 mg weekly for prevention.
    B. Fosamax should be taken at least 30 minutes prior to a meal.
    C. Fosamax should not be taken with food.

D. Patients should lie down for 1 hour following administration of Fosamax.
E. Choices A, B, and C are correct.

3. What is the recommended dosage of daily calcium intake for a 65-year-old woman?

    A. 250 mg
    B. 500 mg
    C. 750 mg
    D. 1,000 mg
    E. 1,200 mg

4. Which of the following agents is considered first-line therapy for postmenopausal osteoporosis?

    A. Risedronate
    B. Calcitonin
    C. Prempro
    D. Denosumab
    E. Teriparatide

5. Which of the following products is available in an injectable and nasal spray dosage form?

    A. Raloxifene
    B. Alendronate
    C. Teriparatide
    D. Calcitonin
    E. Prempro

6. Which of the following drugs may increase the risk of osteoporosis?

    A. Hydrochlorothiazide
    B. Warfarin
    C. Lisinopril
    D. Oral contraceptives
    E. Depo-Provera

7. What is the recommended dose of raloxifene in the prevention and treatment of postmenopausal osteoporosis?

    A. 10 mg daily
    B. 15 mg daily
    C. 40 mg daily
    D. 60 mg daily
    E. 120 mg daily

8. S. T. is a 32-year-old woman who wants to begin using a prescription contraceptive product. She is a new mother and would like to know if any products are safe for use during breast-feeding. S. T. states that she is not

interested in using a device intravaginally and experiences irritation and inflammation with condom use. Which of the following product(s) would be an appropriate choice for S. T.?

A. Ortho Tri-Cyclen
B. Micronor
C. Depo-Provera
D. Seasonale
E. Premarin

9. T. H. is a 33-year-old woman currently taking Nordette oral contraceptive pills. She presents to your pharmacy with a prescription for oral rifampin for 6 weeks to treat prosthetic valve endocarditis. Which of the following choices describes appropriate action taken by the pharmacist?

A. Call the physician, and request a change to amoxicillin to avoid a drug interaction between Nordette and rifampin.
B. Dispense the rifampin, and counsel T. H. on the appropriate administration and duration of therapy for the antibiotic.
C. Dispense the rifampin, and counsel T. H. regarding the potential for rifampin to interfere with the efficacy of Nordette. Instruct T. H. to use a backup method of contraception throughout her course of rifampin therapy.
D. Refuse to fill the rifampin prescription, and counsel T. H. that she should never take antibiotics while she is on oral contraceptives.
E. Dispense the rifampin, and stop the patient's Nordette prescription.

10. Which of the following oral contraceptives is a biphasic product?

A. Ortho Tri-Cyclen
B. Ortho-Novum 10/11
C. Ortho-Novum 1/35
D. Yasmin
E. Amethyst

11. Which of the following products is a four-phasic oral contraceptive?

A. Nordette
B. Ortho Tri-Cyclen
C. Nor-QD
D. Natazia
E. Necon 1/35

12. A 26-year-old female who is recently initiated on a combination hormonal oral contraceptive complains of late-cycle breakthrough bleeding. Which of the following is she most likely experiencing?

A. Too much estrogen
B. Too little estrogen
C. Too much progestin
D. Too little progestin
E. Too much androgen

13. What is the highest dose of estrogen (ethinyl estradiol) offered in an oral contraceptive?

A. 25 mcg
B. 30 mcg
C. 35 mcg
D. 40 mcg
E. 50 mcg

14. A progestin-only oral contraceptive would be preferable over a combination oral contraceptive in which of the following cases?

A. A 24-year-old college student who is sexually active
B. A 48-year-old perimenopausal female with irregular menstrual cycles
C. A woman who is breast-feeding her infant
D. A 30-year-old obese patient with type 2 diabetes mellitus
E. A 52-year-old postmenopausal woman

15. R. J. is a 55-year-old woman who presents to your pharmacy with a prescription for Premarin 0.625 mg daily. She has an intact uterus and has been recently diagnosed with menopause. Which of the following statements describes the appropriate action to be taken by the pharmacist?

A. Refuse to fill the prescription, and recommend a phytoestrogen supplement.
B. Call the physician and confirm that the patient has an intact uterus, and recommend a product containing estrogen plus progestin.
C. Fill the prescription, and counsel the patient regarding administration instructions and potential adverse effects.
D. Call the physician and confirm that the patient has an intact uterus, and suggest a transdermal estrogen product.

E. Call the physician, recommend cancelling the Premarin prescription, and recommend starting a Provera prescription.

16. Which of the following factors is a contra-indication to the use of HT in postmenopausal women?

 A. Diabetes
 B. Basal cell skin cancer
 C. Thromboembolic disease
 D. Depression
 E. Obesity

17. From the following choices, select the most common side effect associated with estrogen therapy.

 A. Breast tenderness
 B. Depression
 C. Diarrhea
 D. Brittle fingernails
 E. Hair loss

18. The Women's Health Initiative study found an association between HT and all of the following conditions *except*

 A. breast cancer.
 B. stroke.
 C. cardiovascular disease.
 D. colon cancer.
 E. deep-vein thrombosis.

19. Which of the following product dosing regimens is correct?

 A. Climara Transdermal: Apply to skin once daily.
 B. Vagifem: 1 tablet vaginally once daily for 2 weeks, then 1 tablet vaginally twice weekly.
 C. Estring: Insert ring intravaginally once daily at bedtime.
 D. Premarin tablets: 0.625–2.5 mg tid.
 E. Premarin vaginal cream: 20–40 g vaginally once daily.

20. Which of the following drug interactions may result in increased pharmacologic effect of estrogen?

 A. Macrolide antibiotics
 B. Itraconazole
 C. Ketoconazole
 D. A and C
 E. A, B, and C

19-7. Answers

1. **B.** A. J. has neither osteopenia nor osteoporosis with a T-score of 1. At this point, preventive therapy is appropriate, with adequate calcium and vitamin D intake. Prescription therapy is not indicated at this time.

2. **E.** The appropriate use of Fosamax (alendronate sodium) for prevention of osteoporosis includes a 35 mg weekly or 5 mg daily dose. The 70 mg weekly dose is for treatment of osteoporosis. The medication should be taken with a full glass of water at least 30 minutes prior to ingesting food or other beverages. Patients should remain in the upright position for at least 30 minutes following ingestion of Fosamax.

3. **E.** According to the National Osteoporosis Foundation, daily calcium intake should be 1,000 mg per day for men age 50–70 and 1,200 mg per day for women age 51 and older and men age 71 and older.

4. **A.** Bisphosphonates (e.g., risedronate) are first-line therapy for osteoporosis because data demonstrate that they reduce the risk of fracture.

5. **D.** Injectable and nasal spray dosage forms of calcitonin are available. Teriparatide is available as an injection only. Prempro, raloxifene, and alendronate are available only in oral dosage forms.

6. **E.** Depo-Provera may have a negative effect on bone mineral density. Hydrochlorothiazide may actually have a beneficial effect on bone as it decreases calcium loss in the urine.

7. **D.** The approved and recommended dose of raloxifene is 60 mg once daily.

8. **E.** Micronor is a progestin-only oral contraceptive and is considered compatible with breastfeeding. Depo-Provera is an injectable progestin-only contraceptive option that is considered safe and appropriate for women who desire to breastfeed because it does not affect milk production or adversely affect infant development. Ortho Tri-Cyclen is a combined oral contraceptive that may decrease the quantity of breast milk available and may adversely affect the infant.

9. **C.** Rifampin has a pharmacokinetic inter-action with combined hormonal contraceptives. Women taking rifampin should be educated

about the possibility of oral contraceptive failure and should be encouraged to use nonhormonal contraception throughout the course of therapy.

10. **B.** Ortho-Novum 10/11 is a biphasic oral contraceptive.

11. **D.** Natazia is a four-phasic oral contraceptive.

12. **D.** Too little progestin may result in breakthrough bleeding late in the menstrual cycle. She should be changed to a product with a higher progestin content.

13. **E.** The highest dose of estrogen (ethinyl estradiol) offered in an oral contraceptive is 50 mcg.

14. **C.** Progestin-only oral contraceptives are preferred in breast-feeding women because they do not negatively affect milk supply. Perimenopausal females may take combined oral contraceptives to regulate their menstrual cycle.

15. **B.** Unopposed estrogen is not recommended in women with an intact uterus because of an increased risk of endometrial hyperplasia and endometrial cancer. Women with an intact uterus should receive a product containing estrogen plus progestin.

16. **C.** Thromboembolic disease is a definite contraindication to the use of HT therapy in postmenopausal women.

17. **A.** Breast tenderness and nausea are the most common side effects associated with estrogen therapy.

18. **D.** The WHI study demonstrated a decreased risk of colon cancer with HT.

19. **B.** Vagifem dosage is 1 tablet vaginally once daily for 2 weeks; then 1 tablet vaginally twice weekly.

20. **E.** Macrolide antibiotics, itraconazole, and ketoconazole may result in increased pharmacologic effect of estrogen by inhibiting CYP450 3A4.

19-8. References

Postmenopausal Hormone Therapy

Kalantaridou SN, Dang DK, Calis KA. Hormone therapy in women. In: Dipiro JT, Talbert RL, Yee GC, et al., eds. *Pharmacotherapy: A Pathophysiologic Approach.* 9th ed. New York, NY: McGraw-Hill; 2014:1315–36.

Hester, SA. PL Detail-Document, Postmenopausal Hormone Therapy. *Pharmacist's Letter/Prescriber's Letter.* March 2014.

North American Menopause Society. The 2012 hormone therapy position statement of the North American Menopause Society. *Menopause.* 2012; 19(3):257–71.

O'Neil CK. Health issues in older women. In: Dunsworth T, Richardson M, Chant C, et al., eds. *Pharmacotherapy Self-Assessment Program.* 6th ed. Book 7: *Women's and Men's Health.* Lenexa, KS: American College of Clinical Pharmacy, 2008; 143–57.

Contraception

Centers for Disease Control and Prevention. U.S. Medical Eligibility Criteria for Contraceptive Use, 2010. *MMWR.* 2010;59(May 28):7–33.

El-Ibiary SY, White JL. Hormonal contraception. In: Borgelt LM, O'Connell MB, Smith JA, Calis KA. *Women's Health Across the Lifespan: A Pharmacotherapeutic Approach.* Bethesda, MD: American Society of Health-System Pharmacists; 2010: 289–310.

O'Mara NB. Contraception for women with chronic medical conditions. *Pharmacist's Letter/Prescriber's Letter.* 2011;27(3):270–306.

O'Mara, NB. PL Detail-Document, Comparison of Oral Contraceptives and Non-Oral Alternatives. *Pharmacist's Letter/Prescriber's Letter.* March 2013.

Shrader SP, Ragucci KR. Contraception. In: Dipiro JT, Talbert RL, Yee GC, et al., eds. *Pharmacotherapy: A Pathophysiologic Approach.* 9th ed. New York, NY: McGraw-Hill; 2014:1271–86.

Osteoporosis

MacLaughlin EJ, Raehl CL. ASHP therapeutic position statement on the prevention and treatment of osteoporosis in adults. *Am J Health-Syst Pharm.* 2008;65:343–57.

National Osteoporosis Foundation. *Clinician's Guide to Prevention and Treatment of Osteoporosis.* Washington, DC: National Osteoporosis Foundation; 2013. http://nof.org/hcp/clinicians-guide.

O'Connell MB, Borchert JS. Osteoporosis and other metabolic bone diseases. In: Dipiro JT, Talbert RL, Yee GC, et al., eds. *Pharmacotherapy: A Pathophysiologic Approach.* 9th ed. New York, NY: McGraw-Hill; 2014:1477–504.

Kidney Disease

Joanna Q. Hudson

20-1. Key Points

Acute Kidney Injury

- Acute kidney injury (AKI) is classified on the basis of criteria for changes in serum creatinine or glomerular filtration rate (GFR) and urine output defined by the RIFLE system (risk, injury, failure, loss, and end-stage renal disease), the Acute Kidney Injury Network (AKIN) staging system (stages 1–3), and the Kidney Disease: Improving Global Outcomes (KDIGO) staging system (stages 1–3).
- The types of AKI include prerenal, intrinsic, and postrenal.
- Prevention of kidney dysfunction in high-risk patients is the most effective strategy to address AKI.
- Conditions that increase the risk of AKI include decreased perfusion of the kidney (attributable to dehydration or poor effective circulating volume such as with congestive heart failure, severe liver failure, etc.) and administration of nephrotoxic agents, particularly under conditions of decreased perfusion.
- Early recognition and treatment of AKI may prevent irreversible kidney damage.
- Goals of treatment for patients with AKI are achievement of baseline kidney function and prevention of both chronic kidney disease (CKD) and the need for chronic renal replacement therapy.
- Supportive care includes maintaining hemodynamic stability, providing nutritional support, avoiding nephrotoxic agents, and using renal replacement therapy if indicated.
- Diuretics are often used in patients with AKI to maintain fluid balance and hemodynamic stability.
- A review of medications is frequently necessary to ensure appropriate dose adjustments based on kidney function.
- Estimating equations to assess kidney function that depend on stable kidney function should not be used in patients with AKI.

Chronic Kidney Disease

- CKD is classified on the basis of the cause of kidney disease, the GFR, and the level of proteinuria.
- Screening for albuminuria and proteinuria and assessment of kidney function in individuals at high risk for kidney disease are important to identify patients with kidney disease and to monitor progression of the disease.
- Therapy to delay progression of kidney disease is based on the underlying cause, but it typically includes control of diabetes and hypertension (two leading causes of CKD in the United States); initiation of therapy with angiotensin-converting enzyme inhibitors or angiotensin receptor blockers; and protein restriction, if indicated, in more advanced disease.
- Common secondary complications of CKD include fluid and electrolyte abnormalities, anemia, CKD mineral and bone disorder (CKD-MBD), metabolic acidosis, cardiovascular complications, and malnutrition.
- Management of anemia includes administration of erythropoiesis-stimulating agents (ESAs; epoetin alfa [Epogen and Procrit], darbepoetin alfa [Aranesp]) and iron supplementation with oral

iron (multiple preparations) or intravenous iron (sodium ferric gluconate [Ferrlecit], iron sucrose [Venofer], ferumoxytol [Feraheme], ferric carboxymaltose [Injectafer], or iron dextran [INFeD and Dexferrum]) to achieve target hemoglobin, while preventing iron deficiency. Caution is warranted when using ESAs because of the increased risk of cardiovascular events and mortality in patients with CKD when ESAs are used to target a hemoglobin > 11 g/dL.

- Hyperphosphatemia associated with CKD-MBD is managed by dietary phosphorus restriction, phosphate-binding agents (calcium-containing products, lanthanum carbonate [Fosrenol], sevelamer carbonate [Renvela], sevelamer hydrochloride [Renagel], or sucroferric oxy-hydroxide [Velphoro]), and with dialysis in patients with end-stage renal disease.

- Management of secondary hyperparathyroidism associated with CKD-MBD includes control of serum calcium and phosphorus and administration of vitamin D therapy—including vitamin D precursors in early CKD based on kidney function (ergocalciferol [Drisdol and Calciferol] or cholecalciferol)—and active vitamin D therapy for more severe kidney disease (calcitriol [Calcijex and Rocaltrol], paricalcitol [Zemplar], or doxercalciferol [Hectorol]). The calcimimetic agent cinacalcet (Sensipar) is indicated for management of secondary hyperparathyroidism in patients with end-stage renal disease who are on dialysis and is used in conjunction with phosphate binders and vitamin D.

- Nutritional requirements must be reevaluated on the basis of severity of kidney disease (e.g., protein restriction to delay progression of CKD versus increased protein requirements for patients on dialysis).

20-2. Study Guide Checklist

The following topics may guide your study of AKI:

- Risk factors for AKI
- Considerations for drug dosing in AKI
- Mechanism of action of diuretics
- Diuretic resistance
- KDIGO guideline for AKI
- Indications for renal replacement therapy (e.g., dialysis)
- Drug removal by renal replacement therapy

The following topics may guide your study of CKD:

- Risk factors for CKD
- Estimating equations to assess kidney function
- American Diabetes Association guidelines for management of diabetes
- Review of antihypertensive agents
- KDIGO guidelines for CKD, CKD-MBD, and anemia
- National Kidney Foundation Kidney Disease Outcomes Quality Initiative (KDOQI) guidelines for CKD, bone metabolism and disease, and anemia

20-3. Acute Kidney Injury

Definition and Classification of Acute Kidney Injury

Acute kidney injury (AKI) is defined as rapid (hours to days) deterioration of kidney function resulting in azotemia (retention of nitrogenous waste products such as urea) and failure of the kidney to maintain fluid, electrolyte, and acid–base homeostasis.

A reduction in urine output frequently occurs, but normal urine output does not rule out AKI (i.e., reduction in urine output is not a specific marker of AKI). Urine output is classified as nonoliguric (urine output > 400 mL/day), oliguric (urine output < 400 mL/day), or anuric (urine output < 50 mL/day).

One classification system proposed to distinguish between mild or severe and early or late cases of AKI is known as RIFLE: *R*isk of kidney dysfunction, *I*njury to the kidney, *F*ailure or *L*oss of kidney function, and *E*nd-stage renal disease (ESRD):

- **Risk:** A 1.5-fold increase in the serum creatinine or a decrease in glomerular filtration rate (GFR) by 25% or urine output < 0.5 mL/kg/h for 6 hours
- **Injury:** A twofold increase in the serum creatinine or a decrease of GFR by 50% or urine output < 0.5 mL/kg/h for 12 hours
- **Failure:** A threefold increase in the serum creatinine, a decrease of GFR by 75% or urine output of < 0.3 mL/kg/h for 24 hours, or anuria for 12 hours
- **Loss:** Complete loss of kidney function (e.g., need for renal replacement therapy) for more than 4 weeks
- **ESRD:** Complete loss of kidney function (e.g., need for renal replacement therapy) for more than 3 months

A modification of RIFLE that includes slightly adapted diagnostic criteria and a staging system was proposed by the Acute Kidney Injury Network (AKIN). The classification or staging system corresponds to risk (stage 1), injury (stage 2), and failure (stage 3) of the RIFLE criteria. Because loss and ESRD were removed from the AKIN staging system and defined as outcomes, stage 3 of AKIN includes those individuals requiring renal replacement therapy.

In an effort to provide one definition of AKI, the Kidney Disease: Improving Global Outcomes (KDIGO) clinical practice guidelines for AKI were developed. KDIGO defines AKI as (1) an increase in serum creatinine by at least 0.3 mg/dL within 48 hours, (2) an increase in serum creatinine by at least 1.5 times baseline within the prior 7 days, or (3) a urine volume less than 0.5 mL/kg/h for 6 hours. The KDIGO stages of AKI are based on the following serum creatinine and urine output criteria:

- Stage 1: Increase in serum creatinine by ≥ 0.3 mg/dL or 1.5 to 1.9 times from baseline; urine output of < 0.5 mL/kg/h for 6–12 hours
- Stage 2: Increase in serum creatinine > 2–2.9 times from baseline; urine output of < 0.5 mL/kg/h for ≥ 12 hours
- Stage 3: One of the following—(1) an increase in serum creatinine of three times from baseline, (2) a serum creatinine ≥ 4 mg/dL, (3) the need for renal replacement therapy, (4) estimated GFR < 35 mL/min/1.73 m² in patients < 18 years, or (5) little to no urine output (anuria) for ≥ 12 hours.

Epidemiology

Incidence and prevalence

- Community-acquired AKI accounts for 1% of hospital admissions.
- Hospital-acquired AKI occurs in 2–20% of hospitalized patients, and the highest incidence occurs in patients in intensive care units.

Mortality

- The best prognosis is when renal replacement therapy is not required.
- The mortality rate is 15–40% for patients with hospital-acquired AKI.
- AKI that requires renal replacement therapy in critically ill patients is associated with a 40–70% mortality rate.

Types of AKI

AKI is classified according to the area of the kidney affected:

- *Prerenal AKI* is characterized by a decrease in perfusion to the kidney with or without systemic arterial hypotension. It is the most common type of AKI and is usually reversible.
- *Intrinsic or intrarenal AKI* is the result of structural damage to the parenchymal tissue of the kidney. It is divided into vascular, glomerular, interstitial, and tubular disorders (most common).
- *Postrenal AKI* is an obstruction of urine flow occurring at any level of the urinary outflow tracts.

Clinical Presentation

- Decreased urine output
- Signs of hypovolemia (prerenal causes), such as tachycardia, decreased venous and arterial pressure, and orthostasis
- Unique color and composition of urine: Cola-colored urine (suggesting bleeding) and foaming (indicating proteinuria)
- Symptoms of uremia (a clinical syndrome resulting from azotemia), including weakness, shortness of breath, fatigue, mental status changes, nausea and vomiting, bleeding, loss of appetite, and edema
- Flank pain
- Increased weight (suggesting fluid accumulation)
- Increased blood pressure (suggesting fluid accumulation)
- Signs and symptoms of electrolyte abnormalities (hyperkalemia) and metabolic acidosis (see Chapter 21 on fluids and electrolytes)
- Bladder distention or prostate enlargement (postrenal causes)
- Other findings specific to the cause of AKI (see section on pathophysiology)

Pathophysiology and Etiologies

Prerenal AKI

Prerenal AKI is caused by conditions that decrease glomerular hydrostatic pressure, leading to a decrease in GFR. Hypoperfusion leads to increased sodium and water reabsorption by the kidney and stimulates compensatory mechanisms.

The following compensatory mechanisms (also known as autoregulation) increase glomerular hydrostatic pressure and GFR:

- Vasodilation of the afferent arteriole (mediated primarily by prostaglandins)
- Vasoconstriction of the efferent arteriole (mediated primarily by angiotensin II)

Alterations in afferent and efferent arteriolar tone can affect compensatory mechanisms. Nonsteroidal anti-inflammatory drugs (NSAIDs) and cyclooxygenase-2 (COX-2) inhibitors can prevent compensatory vasodilation of the afferent arteriole. Angiotensin-converting enzyme inhibitors (ACEIs), angiotensin receptor blockers (ARBs), and renin inhibitors (aliskiren) can prevent compensatory vasoconstriction of the efferent arteriole.

Etiologies of prerenal AKI are as follows:

- Intravascular volume depletion related to excessive diuresis, vomiting, excessive gastrointestinal (GI) fluid loss, and bleeding
- Severe hypotension
- Decreased effective blood volume (volume sensed by arterial baroreceptors) as occurs with congestive heart failure, cirrhosis, nephrotic syndrome, and hepatorenal syndrome
- Systemic vasodilation as occurs with sepsis, liver failure, and anaphylaxis
- Large-vessel renal vascular disease, including renal artery thrombosis or embolism and renal artery stenosis
- Medications (see Table 20-1)

Intrinsic AKI

The primary anatomic sites of the kidney are prone to structural damage from prolonged ischemia and direct toxicity because of the high metabolic activity and concentrating ability of the kidney.

Select etiologies by anatomic site are as follows:

- ***Vascular:*** Inflammation and emboli
- ***Glomerular (glomerulonephritis):*** Systemic lupus erythematosus, immune-mediated causes, and medications (see Table 20-1)
- ***Interstitial:*** Ischemia, allergic interstitial nephritis, infections, and medications (see Table 20-1). Clinical presentation of acute allergic interstitial nephritis may include fever, rash, and eosinophilia;

Table 20-1. Drug-Induced Causes of AKI

Type of AKI	Causative drugs[a]
Prerenal AKI	ACEIs, ARBs, COX-2 inhibitors, cyclosporine, diuretics, NSAIDs, radiocontrast media, renin inhibitors, tacrolimus
Intrinsic AKI	
Vascular	*Vasculitis and thrombosis:* Bevacizumab, cisplatin, cyclosporine, hydralazine, methamphetamines, mitomycin C, propylthiouracil, tacrolimus
	Cholesterol emboli: Warfarin, thrombolytic agents
Glomerular	COX-2 inhibitors, gold, heroin, lithium, NSAIDs, pamidronate, phenytoin
Interstitial nephritis	*Allergic interstitial nephritis:* Ciprofloxacin, COX-2 inhibitors, NSAIDs, penicillins, proton pump inhibitors
	Chronic interstitial nephritis: Aristolochic acid (Chinese herbs), cyclosporine, lithium
	Papillary necrosis: Analgesic combinations
Tubular epithelial cell damage	*Acute tubular necrosis:* Adefovir, aminoglycosides, amphotericin B, carboplatin, cidofovir, cisplatin, cocaine, cyclosporine, foscarnet, ifosfamide, radiocontrast media, tacrolimus, tenofovir, zoledronate
	Osmotic nephrosis: Dextran, hydroxyethyl starch solutions, mannitol, sucrose-containing intravenous immunoglobulin
Postrenal AKI	
Obstructive	Acyclovir, foscarnet, indinavir, methotrexate, oxalate, sulfonamides
Nephrolithiasis	Allopurinol, indinavir, sulfonamides, triamterene
Nephrocalcinosis	Oral sodium phosphate solution

a. This list does not include all potential nephrotoxins.

however, these findings may be absent in patients with this type of injury.

■ *Tubular—accounts for 90% of intrinsic cases:* Intrarenal vasoconstriction, direct tubular toxicity, and intratubular obstruction; prolonged ischemia from prerenal causes; and toxins that may be endogenous or exogenous

- *Endogenous:* Myoglobin, hemoglobin, and uric acid
- *Exogenous:* Medications (see Table 20-1; aminoglycosides are common nephrotoxins leading to nonoliguric acute tubular necrosis after 5–7 days of therapy) and other exogenous substances such as ethylene glycol and pesticides

Postrenal AKI

This disease is an obstruction of urinary flow at any level from the urinary collecting system to the urethra. It must involve both kidneys (or one kidney in a patient with a single functioning kidney). Medications associated with postrenal AKI are identified in Table 20-1. Etiologies by anatomic site are as follows:

■ *Renal pelves or tubules:* Crystal deposition
■ *Ureteral:* Tumor, stricture, and stones
■ *Bladder neck obstruction:* Prostatic hypertrophy and bladder carcinoma

Diagnostic Criteria

Table 20-2 shows the diagnostic tests and the findings associated with AKI. A diagnosis requires the following:

■ *Evaluate physical findings:* Assess for signs and symptoms listed in clinical presentation.

■ *Take medication history (including over-the-counter medication and herbals):* Identify potentially nephrotoxic agents (Table 20-1). *Note:* Patients with contrast-induced nephrotoxicity (CIN) may have received the dose 24–72 hours before the time when the rise in serum creatinine is noted.

■ *Estimate GFR:* Normal is generally in the range of 90–125 mL/min/1.73 m².

- Consider limitations in using serum creatinine as a marker of kidney function (e.g., conditions of poor muscle mass) and in using equations to estimate GFR in patients with unstable kidney function. See discussion of assessment of kidney function in Section 20-4.
- Other assessment equations and methods (e.g., Jelliffe and Jelliffe equation) are available to estimate GFR in patients with unstable kidney function.

Blood tests

■ *Elevated:* Serum creatinine, blood urea nitrogen (BUN), and electrolytes (potassium and phosphorus). The BUN/serum creatinine ratio may be elevated in prerenal AKI.
■ *Decreased:* Calcium (consider albumin concentration to correct calcium), bicarbonate

Urinalysis

■ A low urine sodium and an elevated specific gravity and osmolality are indicative of prerenal causes and stimulation of sodium and water retention.

Table 20-2. Laboratory Findings to Differentiate Prerenal and Intrinsic AKI

Diagnostic test	Prerenal AKI	Intrinsic AKI
BUN:Cr ratio	> 20:1	< 15:1
Urinalysis	Normal with few cells or casts (hyaline casts normal)	Granular casts with tubular epithelial cells
Urine osmolality	> 500 mOsm/kg	≤ 300–350 mOsm/kg
Urinary Cr:Plasma Cr ratio	> 40:1	< 20:1
Specific gravity	> 1.020	< 1.015
Urine sodium	< 20 mEq/L	> 40 mEq/L
FE_{Na}	< 1%	> 2%
Urinary RBCs and WBCs	Absent	2–4+

BUN, blood urea nitrogen; Cr, creatinine; FE_{Na}, fractional excretion of sodium; RBC, red blood cell; WBC, white blood cell.

- Proteinuria includes the following:
  - Albuminuria: Microalbuminuria or moderately increased albuminuria (> 30 mg/day) and severely increased albuminuria (> 300 mg/day)
  - Proteinuria (includes albumin and other proteins): Moderately increased (> 150 mg/day) and severely increased (> 500 mg/day) proteinuria and nephrotic range proteinuria > 3.5 g/day
- Hematuria is indicated by red blood cells.
- Glucose and ketones may be present.
- Urine sediment consisting of granular casts and cellular debris suggests structural damage (hyaline casts are normal).
- White blood cells suggest inflammation.
- Eosinophils are associated with acute allergic interstitial nephritis.
- Consider whether fluids or diuretics were previously administered when interpreting urinalysis.

Urine chemistries

Evaluate urine sodium, potassium, chloride, creatinine, and urinary anion gap.

Fractional excretion of sodium (FE_{Na}) is useful to differentiate prerenal AKI from intrinsic AKI. A low value (< 1%) suggests retention of sodium and water (prerenal etiology) versus intrinsic cause.

$$FE_{Na} = \frac{U_{Na} \times P_{Cr} \times 100}{U_{Cr} \times P_{Na}}$$

where

U_{Na} = urine sodium
U_{Cr} = urine creatinine
P_{Cr} = plasma creatinine
P_{Na} = plasma sodium

Other tests

Radiographic procedures include ultrasound, plain film radiograph, radioisotope scan, and computed tomography.

Renal biopsy may be indicated for patients without cause of AKI identified by other diagnostic tests.

Treatment Principles and Goals

Prevention

Identify risk factors:

- Volume depletion
- Exposure to nephrotoxic medications
- Preexisting kidney or hepatic disease

Surgical procedures can be a risk factor. Consider baseline kidney function, age, cardiovascular status, and volume status.

Diagnostic tests requiring radiocontrast media can put patients at risk of AKI. Contrast agents are hyperosmolar compared to plasma osmolality and may cause osmotic diuresis, dehydration, and renal ischemia. Risk factors for CIN include diabetes, heart failure, age > 75, hypotension, and an estimated GFR < 60 mL/min/1.73 m². In addition to being well hydrated, usually with intravenous (IV) fluid administration, high-risk patients may benefit from oral acetylcysteine (Mucomyst) given as 4 doses of 600 mg or 1,200 mg every 12 hours with the first dose given before exposure to radiocontrast dye. Of note, in a prospective study in patients undergoing coronary and peripheral vascular angiography, acetylcysteine did not reduce the risk of CIN; therefore, this strategy is not consistently supported by available evidence. Bicarbonate may also be added to the hydration fluid.

Treatment goals

- Correct underlying causes of AKI (e.g., discontinue nephrotoxic agents, correct fluid status, treat underlying infection, address cause of urinary tract obstructions).
- Return to baseline kidney function or highest kidney function possible.
- Prevent development of chronic kidney disease and the need for chronic renal replacement therapy.
- Avoid nephrotoxic agents or take measures to reduce exposure if possible.
- Adjust doses of medications on the basis of kidney function. As kidney function recovers drug doses may need to be increased.
- Avoid agents contraindicated in patients with kidney disease, such as metformin (Glucophage) and gadolinium-based contrast dyes used for magnetic resonance imaging (MRI) procedures. Gadolinium has been shown to cause nephrogenic systemic fibrosis (NSF) in patients with preexisting kidney disease. NSF is a fibrosing disorder that involves predominantly the skin but also affects systemic organs such as the liver, heart, lungs, diaphragm, skeletal muscle, and joints.
- Address complications of AKI, such as electrolyte abnormalities (hyperkalemia), fluid overload, metabolic acidosis (see Chapter 21 on fluids and electrolytes), and hyperphosphatemia (see Section 20-4 on chronic kidney disease).

Strategies for treatment

- Address underlying cause of AKI.
- Provide supportive care with diuretic therapy (loop diuretics) and replacement fluids as needed to maintain hemodynamic stability.

Drug Therapy

Diuretics

Loop diuretics are recommended for management of fluid overload in patients with AKI (Table 20-3). They are not advocated to prevent or treat AKI and have not been shown to significantly improve outcomes of AKI.

Mechanism of action

Loop diuretics are delivered to the tubular lumen of the kidney by active secretion from the blood into the urine at the proximal tubule. Binding of the diuretic to albumin allows the drug to be confined to the plasma and minimizes glomerular filtration so the diuretic may be delivered to the organic acid secretory sites and transported into the lumen. Once at the site of action, loop diuretics cause inhibition of sodium and chloride reabsorption in the thick ascending limb of the loop of Henle to promote water excretion.

Thiazide and thiazide-like diuretics inhibit the Na^+-Cl^- cotransport in the early distal convoluted tubules. They are generally used in combination with loop diuretics for resistant edema and fluid overload, particularly metolazone (Zaroxolyn, Mykrox), which is effective at GFR < 30 mL/min. Other thiazide diuretics are generally not effective when GFR is < 30 mL/min.

Adverse drug events
Loop diuretics
Adverse drug events are as follows:

- Hypokalemia, hypomagnesemia, hyponatremia, hypovolemia, hyperuricemia, hyperglycemia
- Hypercalciuria, hypocalcemia
- Orthostatic hypotension, dehydration
- Metabolic alkalosis (partly attributable to extracellular fluid volume contraction)
- Ototoxicity
- Diarrhea, nausea

Furosemide (Lasix), bumetanide (Bumex), and torsemide (Demadex) have a sulfonamide substituent (potential for hypersensitivity reactions). Ethacrynic acid (Edecrin) is generally reserved for patients allergic to sulfa compounds.

Thiazide and thiazide-like diuretics
Adverse drug events include the following:

- Hypokalemia, hyponatremia, hypercalcemia, hyperuricemia
- Hypovolemia, orthostatic hypotension
- Hyperglycemia, hypochloremic alkalosis, hyperlipidemia
- Hypersensitivity reactions from sulfonamide substituents
- Chest pain (metolazone; more common with Mykrox, which is more rapidly and extensively absorbed than Zaroxolyn)

Drug–drug and drug–disease interactions
- Loop diuretics and aminoglycosides have an increased potential for ototoxicity.
- Diuretics and other nephrotoxins have an increased risk of nephrotoxicity if hypovolemia occurs.

Table 20-3. Loop Diuretics for Fluid Overload in AKI

Generic name	Trade name	Daily dosage range	Dosage forms	Frequency of administration[a]
Furosemide	Lasix	20–400 mg	po	q 6–12 h
		20–200 mg (up to 1–3 g/day in AKI)	IV	
Bumetanide	Bumex	0.5–10 mg	po, IV	q 12–24 h
Torsemide	Demadex	10–200 mg	po, IV	q 24 h
Ethacrynic acid	Edecrin	50–400 mg	po	q 8–12 h
		50–100 mg	IV	

a. Loop diuretics are also administered as a continuous infusion. Higher dose ranges for intermittent dosing are reserved for patients who are unresponsive to initial smaller doses.

- Diuretics and lithium (Lithane, Lithobid) used concomitantly may result in decreased renal clearance of lithium. Monitor lithium concentrations more closely.
- For diuretics and digoxin (Lanoxin, Digox), hypokalemia from diuretic use may increase risk of toxicity with digoxin. Monitor potassium and digoxin.
- Loop and thiazide diuretics may increase gout attacks because of hyperuricemia.
- For thiazide diuretics and diabetes, hyperglycemia may result from thiazides. Increase glucose monitoring.
- The following conditions decrease secretion of the diuretic to its site of action in the renal tubule:
  - Proteinuria (diuretic binds to protein and is not available at its site of action)
  - Decreased renal blood flow
  - Competitive inhibition of transport system (NSAIDs, probenecid [Probalan], cephalosporins)

Parameters to monitor
- Blood pressure (sitting and standing), pulse, urine output, fluid intake, serum creatinine, serum electrolytes, BUN, bicarbonate, calcium, glucose, uric acid

Pharmacokinetics
Loop diuretics
- ***Oral bioavailability:*** Furosemide (60%), bumetanide (85%), torsemide (85%)
- ***Oral:intravenous dose ratios:*** Furosemide (1.5), bumetanide (1), torsemide (1)
- ***Equivalent doses:*** 1 mg bumetanide = 20 mg torsemide = 40 mg furosemide
- ***Elimination route:*** Furosemide (primarily renal), bumetanide (hepatic and renal), torsemide (primarily hepatic), ethacrynic acid (hepatic and renal)

Thiazide and thiazide-like diuretics
Metolazone absorption differs between brands. Mykrox (available outside the United States) is more rapidly and extensively absorbed than Zaroxolyn.

Other factors
Patients with kidney disease generally require larger doses of diuretics to achieve adequate concentrations of the drug at the site of action in the kidney.

The brands of metolazone (Zaroxolyn and Mykrox) are not bioequivalent and should not be interchanged.

Dopamine

Low-dose dopamine is a potent vasodilator that increases renal blood flow and has been associated with an increase in urine output in AKI. Most clinical studies, however, have not shown improvement in recovery from AKI or mortality rates. KDIGO guidelines do not advocate dopamine for AKI.

Nondrug Therapy

Fluid management

Fluid intake and output should be evaluated and adjustments made to maintain hemodynamic stability (consider sensible and insensible losses).

Fluid selection (e.g., crystalloids, colloids, or normal saline) and rate of correction depend on the clinical condition of the patient. *Note:* Hetastarch should not be used in critically ill patients because of the increased risk of mortality and renal injury requiring renal replacement therapy in certain populations (e.g., patients in the intensive care unit, septic patients, patients with preexisting kidney dysfunction).

Nutritional therapy

A high-calorie diet is generally required (patient specific).

Restriction of sodium, potassium, and phosphorus should be considered.

Renal replacement therapies

Renal replacement therapies are procedures by which the blood is artificially cleared of waste and some essential metabolic products to augment the function of failed or failing kidneys. These procedures include hemodialysis and hemofiltration, in which the semipermeable membrane is a dialyzer, and peritoneal dialysis, in which the peritoneal cavity serves as this membrane. Procedures may be intermittent or continuous. Hemodialysis and hemofiltration are the modalities used for patients with AKI. Continuous renal replacement therapies (CRRTs) require lower blood and dialysate flow rates and remove fluid more gradually than intermittent procedures and are used often for patients with AKI who are hemodynamically unstable. Common terminologies used for CRRT include continuous venovenous hemofiltration, continuous venovenous hemodialysis, and continuous venovenous hemodiafiltration.

The potential for drug removal by dialysis must be considered, particularly for CRRT procedures that are performed over a prolonged period of time (e.g., > 24 hrs). Drug doses may need to be increased to account for removal by CRRT (e.g., certain antibiotics). Drug characteristics that make a drug more likely to be removed by dialysis are small molecular weight, low protein binding, and low volume of distribution.

Indications for renal replacement therapy

Any of the following refractory to more conservative measures is an indication for renal replacement therapy:

- Acidosis
- Electrolyte abnormalities (hyperkalemia)
- Intoxication (drug-induced kidney failure), if drug can be removed by dialysis
- Volume overload
- Uremia (BUN > 100 mg/dL) or uremic symptoms (pericarditis, encephalopathy, bleeding, dyscrasia, nausea, vomiting, pruritus)

20-4. Chronic Kidney Disease

Definition and Classification of Chronic Kidney Disease

Chronic kidney disease (CKD) is defined as at least a 3-month period of kidney damage with or without a decrease in GFR or a GFR < 60 mL/min/1.73 m² for greater than 3 months, with implications for health. *Kidney damage* is defined as pathologic abnormalities or markers of damage, including abnormalities in blood or urine tests or in imaging studies.

The National Kidney Foundation Kidney Disease Outcomes Quality Initiative (KDOQI) guidelines classify CKD into five stages on the basis of kidney damage and GFR (Table 20-4). ESRD occurs when patients require renal replacement therapy (either dialysis or transplantation) to sustain life. Based on the more recent recommendations from KDIGO guidelines for evaluation and management of CKD, CKD is classified by cause of kidney disease, GFR category, and albuminuria level (Table 20-5). This classification is referred to as CGA staging (Cause, GFR, Albuminuria). This section will refer to the KDOQI stage (e.g., stage 4 CKD) and corresponding KDIGO category (e.g., G4).

Table 20-4. KDOQI Stages of CKD

Stage	Description	GFR (mL/min/1.73 m²)
—	Increased risk	≥ 90 (with CKD risk factors)
1	Kidney damage with normal or increased GFR	≥ 90
2	Kidney damage with mildly decreased GFR	60–89
3	Moderately decreased GFR	30–59
4	Severely decreased GFR	15–29
5	Kidney failure (defined as ESRD if renal replacement therapy is needed)	< 15 (or need for renal replacement therapy)

Adapted from National Kidney Foundation, 2002.

Epidemiology of CKD

Incidence and prevalence

Approximately 26 million American adults have CKD. The number of patients with CKD continues to increase, with a 50% increase in the number of patients with ESRD expected by 2020. The incidence of CKD is approximately four times higher in the African American population. The incidence is greatest in individuals age 45–64.

Approximately 600,000 patients are being treated for ESRD (including patients receiving hemodialysis, peritoneal dialysis, and transplantation).

Mortality

Life expectancy is four to five times shorter in dialysis patients than in the general population. The primary causes of death in the ESRD population are cardiovascular diseases and infection. Comorbidities, estimated GFR, and albuminuria at initiation of dialysis are strong predictors of mortality in the dialysis population.

Clinical Presentation

- Changes in urine output (may not occur in earlier stages of CKD)
- Foaming of urine, which indicates proteinuria
  - Table 20-5 shows levels of albuminuria. If total protein levels are measured (including albumin and other proteins), different thresholds apply. A protein excretion ratio (PER) < 150 mg/24 h

Table 20-5. KDIGO Classification of CKD Based on GFR and Albuminuria[a]

GFR category	GFR description	GFR (mL/min/1.73 m^2)	Albuminuria category	Albuminuria description	Albumin excretion rate (mg/24 h)	Albumin to creatinine ratio (mg/g)
G1	Normal or high	≥ 90	A1	Normal to mildly increased	< 30	< 30
G2	Mildly decreased	60–89	A2	Moderately increased[b]	30–300	30–300
G3a	Mildly to moderately decreased	45–59	A3	Severely increased[c]	> 300	> 300
G3b	Moderately to severely decreased	30–44				
G4	Severely decreased	15–29				
G5	Kidney failure	< 15				

Adapted from KDIGO Chronic Kidney Disease Work Group, 2012.
a. GFR categories are similar to KDOQI stages with the exception that Stage 3 is divided into two subcategories by KDIGO (G3a and G3b).
b. Also referred to as *microalbuminuria,* although KDIGO does not advocate this terminology.
c. Also referred to as *albuminuria* (or overt *proteinuria* if proteins other than albumin are measured), although KDIGO does not advocate this terminology.

and a protein-to-creatinine ratio (PCR) of < 150 mg/g are considered normal. A PER or PCR above 150 is considered *moderately increased,* whereas levels above 500 are considered *severely increased.*

- Note: *Nephrotic syndrome* is a clinical syndrome associated with total protein in the urine in amounts > 3.5 g/day (referred to as *nephrotic range proteinuria*), hypoalbuminemia, edema, and hyperlipidemia.

▪ Increased blood pressure (hypertension is a common etiology and result of CKD)

▪ Signs and symptoms of hyperglycemia and glucosuria (diabetes is a common etiology)

▪ Signs and symptoms associated with fluid and electrolyte abnormalities (e.g., hyperkalemia, fluid overload; see Chapter 21 on fluids and electrolytes)

▪ Development of secondary complications of CKD:

- *Anemia:* Decreased hemoglobin and hematocrit, iron deficiency also common
- *CKD Mineral and Bone Disorder:* Increased serum phosphorus, decreased serum calcium (may shift to hypercalcemia as kidney disease progresses), increased intact parathyroid hormone (iPTH), vitamin D deficiency, increased fibroblast growth factor-23 (FGF-23)
- *Metabolic acidosis:* Decreased serum bicarbonate, increased anion gap

- *Malnutrition:* Decreased albumin and prealbumin (see Chapter 22 on nutrition)

▪ Signs of uremia (see Section 20-1) in later stages of CKD, that is, stage 4 CKD (G4) and stage 5 CKD (G5)

Pathophysiology of Progressive Kidney Disease and Selected Secondary Complications

Progressive kidney disease

Progressive loss of nephron function results in adaptive changes in remaining nephrons to increase single nephron glomerular filtration pressure. Over time, the compensatory increase in single nephron GFR leads to hypertrophy from sustained increases in pressure and loss of individual nephron function.

Proteinuria, one of the initial diagnostic signs, may also contribute to the progressive decline in kidney function. Loss of kidney function is usually irreversible.

Etiology of progressive kidney disease
Each of the following may result in damage to the kidney that over time leads to a decrease in functioning nephrons and in total GFR:

▪ Diabetes (accounts for primary cause in 44% of patients with ESRD)

▪ Hypertension (accounts for primary cause in 26% of patients with ESRD)

- Glomerulonephritis (multiple causes, e.g., systemic lupus erythematosus)
- Polycystic kidney disease
- HIV (human immunodeficiency virus) nephropathy
- Other contributing factors (smoking, obesity, genetic factors, gender differences)

Anemia of CKD

The primary etiology is a decrease in production of the hormone erythropoietin by the kidney as kidney disease progresses. More than 90% of erythropoietin production occurs in the kidney and approximately 10% in the liver.

CKD results in a normochromic, normocytic anemia. Red blood cell lifespan is also decreased from 120 days to approximately 60 days in patients with kidney failure. Other contributors include iron deficiency and blood loss (e.g., from uremic bleeding, dialysis).

CKD Mineral and Bone Disorder

CKD mineral and bone disorder (CKD-MBD) includes abnormalities in parathyroid hormone (PTH), calcium, phosphorus, vitamin D, FGF-23, and bone turnover. Patients with CKD-MBD are also at risk for calcifications as kidney disease progresses.

As kidney function declines, phosphorus elimination decreases. Hyperphosphatemia causes a reciprocal decrease in serum calcium concentrations (hypocalcemia). Hypocalcemia stimulates the release of PTH by the parathyroid glands. Conversion of the vitamin D precursor (25-hydroxyvitamin D) to the active form (1,25-dihydroxyvitamin D_3) occurs in the kidney. As kidney disease progresses, there is a decline in the 1α-hydroxylase enzyme that promotes the final hydroxylation step in the kidney, resulting in a deficiency in active vitamin D. Deficiencies in the precursor form of vitamin D have also been observed in CKD stage 3 (G3a and G3b) and stage 4 (G4). Active vitamin D (1,25-dihydroxyvitamin D_3) promotes increased intestinal absorption of calcium and suppresses production of parathyroid hormone by the parathyroid gland; therefore, vitamin D deficiency leads to worsening secondary hyperparathyroidism.

Increased PTH promotes the following:

- Decreased phosphorus reabsorption within the kidney
- Increased calcium reabsorption by the kidney
- Increased calcium mobilization from bone
- Stimulated production of active vitamin D

As kidney disease progresses, the following occur:

- Hyperphosphatemia and subsequent hypocalcemia progressively worsen, and secondary hyperparathyroidism becomes more severe.
- The renal effects of PTH on phosphorus and calcium are no longer maintained, and PTH predominantly stimulates calcium resorption from bone.
- Hyperphosphatemia also promotes an increase in FGF-23, produced and secreted primarily from osteocytes in bone, which reduces phosphorus by decreasing renal tubular reabsorption of phosphate and decreasing production of active vitamin D. Increases in FGF-23 are observed very early in the disease process.
- Decreased production of active vitamin D worsens hypocalcemia and secondary hyperparathyroidism.
  - In more severe CKD, stages 4 (G4) and 5 (G5), patients are prone to develop hypercalcemia, because of decreased renal elimination and use of calcium-containing phosphate binders.
  - Patients with stage 5 CKD (G5) are at risk for calcifications and calciphylaxis.
- Uncontrolled secondary hyperparathyroidism leads to hyperplasia of the parathyroid gland and renal osteodystrophy (a high bone turnover disease that results from sustained effects of PTH on bone).

Metabolic acidosis

- Decreased excretion of acid by the kidney
- Accumulation of endogenous acids attributable to impaired kidney function (e.g., phosphates, sulfates)

Diagnostic Criteria

Progressive kidney disease

There is a progressive increase in serum creatinine: > 1.1–1.2 mg/dL for females and > 1.2–1.3 mg/dL for males. Consider factors that may alter serum creatinine, such as decreased muscle mass and nutritional status.

There is a decreased GFR (see Tables 20-4 and 20-5 for CKD classifications). Consider the assessment method used to estimate creatinine clearance or GFR. The following methods are used to assess kidney function and may be used in patients with stable kidney function.

Creatinine clearance

■ Creatinine clearance (CrCl) is estimated using the Cockcroft–Gault equation (assumes stable kidney function):

$$CrCl(mL/min) = \frac{(140 - age) \times BW}{SCr \times 72}$$

where *BW* = body weight in kg and SCr = serum creatinine. Adjusted body weight is recommended if a patient's body weight is more than 30% above the ideal body weight. The result of the Cockcroft–Gault equation is multiplied by 0.85 for females.

■ CrCl is measured using urine collection methods:

$$CrCl(mL/min) = \frac{U_{Cr} \times V}{SCr \times t}$$

where
U_{Cr} = urinary creatinine concentration (mg/dL),
V = volume of urine (mL),
SCr = serum creatinine concentration (mg/dL), and
t = time period of urine collection (minutes).

Glomerular filtration rate

■ Modification of diet in renal disease (MDRD) abbreviated equation (use with nonstandardized serum creatinine):

$$GFR = 186 \times (\text{serum creatinine})^{-1.154}$$
$$\times (\text{age in years})^{-0.203}$$
$$\times 1.210 (\text{if patient is black})$$
$$\times 0.742 (\text{if patient is female})$$

■ Reexpressed MDRD abbreviated equation (use with standardized serum creatinine):

$$GFR = 175 \times (\text{serum creatinine})^{-1.154}$$
$$\times (\text{age in years})^{-0.203}$$
$$\times 1.210 (\text{if patient is black})$$
$$\times 0.742 (\text{if patient is female})$$

Note: The MDRD equation is less accurate at GFRs above 60 mL/min/1.73 m².

■ CKD-EPI (Chronic Kidney Disease Epidemiology Collaboration) equation (standardized serum creatinine should be used in this equation):

$$GFR = 141 \times \min(SCr/\kappa, 1)^{\alpha}$$
$$\times \max(SCr/\kappa, 1)^{-1.209}$$
$$\times 0.993^{Age}$$
$$\times 1.018 (\text{if patient is female})$$
$$\times 1.159 (\text{if patient is black})$$

where κ is 0.7 for females and 0.9 for males, α is −0.329 for females and −0.411 for males, *min* indicates minimum of SCr/κ or 1, and *max* indicates maximum of SCr/κ or 1. *Note:* The CKD-EPI equation can be used at all ranges of GFR. In the pediatric population, use the Schwartz equation or the Counahan–Barratt equation.

Other diagnostic criteria for CKD include the following:

■ Proteinuria as assessed by the extent of albuminuria (Table 20-5) or proteinuria
■ Abnormal serum chemistries:
  • Increased SCr and BUN
  • The following abnormalities may indicate development of secondary complications of CKD: Increased potassium, decreased serum bicarbonate, increased phosphorus, decreased calcium (may have hypercalcemia in later stages of CKD)

Anemia of CKD

Testing for anemia is recommended in all patients with CKD. Guidelines for anemia management in patients with CKD recommend further evaluation for anemia when hemoglobin is < 12 g/dL in females and < 13.5 g/dL in males.

For iron deficiency, evaluate red blood cell indices and iron indices to identify iron deficiency as a contributing factor. Iron deficiency manifests as a microcytic anemia:

■ Red blood cell count: < 4.2 × 10⁶ cells per mm²
■ Mean corpuscular volume: < 80 femtoliters
■ Serum iron: < 50 mg/dL
■ Total iron binding capacity: < 250 mg/dL
■ Transferrin saturation (TSat): < 16%
■ Serum ferritin: < 12 ng/mL

Transferrin saturation and serum ferritin should be maintained at higher values for CKD patients receiving erythropoiesis stimulating agents (TSat > 20% and serum ferritin > 100 ng/mL for CKD patients not on dialysis and for peritoneal dialysis patients, TSat > 20% and serum ferritin > 200 ng/mL for hemodialysis patients).

Evaluate for folate and vitamin B_{12} deficiencies (manifests as a macrocytic anemia), sources of blood loss (e.g., GI bleeding), and confounding disease states (e.g., cancer and HIV).

CKD-MBD

- Serum phosphorus above normal range
- Calcium abnormalities:
  - Hypocalcemia: Corrected serum calcium < 8.5 mg/dL
  - Hypercalcemia: Corrected calcium above the normal range (a concern in CKD stage 4 [G4] and stage 5 [G5]). *Note:* Corrected calcium = measured serum calcium + 0.8 × (normal serum albumin − measured serum albumin); normal serum albumin = 4 g/dL
- Elevated calcium × phosphorus product: > 55 mg^2/dL^2 (elevated product increases risk for metastatic calcifications)
- Elevated PTH: normal PTH ~ 10–60 pg/mL
- Radiographic evidence of bone abnormalities (e.g., osteitis fibrosa cystica)

Metabolic acidosis

Serum bicarbonate (HCO_3^-) < 20 mEq/L.

Typically, the anion gap is increased: anion gap = $[Na^+] − ([Cl^-] + [HCO_3^-])$.

Signs and symptoms of chronic metabolic acidosis that develop as CKD progresses are generally not of the same magnitude as those of acute metabolic acidosis (e.g., hyperventilation, cardiovascular, and central nervous system manifestations).

Treatment Principles and Goals

Progressive kidney disease

Treatment principles
- Control underlying cause of progressive CKD (e.g., hypertension and diabetes; see Chapters 12 and 17, respectively).
- Meet blood pressure goals: < 140/90 mm Hg in patients with CKD if albumin excretion rate (AER) < 30 mg/24 h or < 130/80 mm Hg for patients with CKD and AER > 30 mg/24 h.

- Prevent or minimize albuminuria or proteinuria.
- Slow the rate of progression of CKD (e.g., by achieving diabetes and hypertension goals and minimizing proteinuria).
- Prevent drug-induced causes of kidney disease:
  - Avoid chronic use of combinations of analgesics.
  - Minimize use of agents known to cause AKI, see Table 20-1. *Note:* Patients can develop an acute-on-chronic kidney disease.
- Manage secondary complications of CKD (anemia, MBD, electrolyte abnormalities).
- Control hyperlipidemia.
- Address cardiovascular risk factors (cardiovascular disease is the leading cause of death in the CKD population).
- Adjust drug doses on the basis of kidney function.
- Avoid medications contraindicated in patients with reduced kidney function. For example, metformin (Glucophage) is contraindicated in patients with elevated serum creatinine (> 1.5 mg/dL for males and > 1.4 mg/dL for females) because of the increased risk of lactic acidosis. Gadolinium-based contrast dyes used for MRI procedures should not be used in individuals with CKD stage 4 (G4) or stage 5 (G5) because of the risk of nephrogenic systemic fibrosis.
- Prepare patient for renal replacement therapy (i.e., dialysis and transplantation) as needed.
- Start dialysis if baseline GFR is less than 15 mL/min/1.73 m^2 and based on other indications (see Section 20-1 on indications for renal replacement therapy).
- Recommend smoking cessation.

Treatment strategies
- ACEIs and ARBs to delay progression of kidney disease (recommended for patients with diabetes and individuals with hypertension and an AER > 300 mg/24 h). Combination therapy with both an ACEI and an ARB is not recommended because of the risk of hyperkalemia and hypotension that outweighs any added benefit. Studies have not consistently shown that combination therapy has added benefits over use of a single agent to delay progression of CKD. The renin inhibitor aliskiren (Tekturna) also has an "unlabeled/investigational" indication for treatment of persistent proteinuria in patients with type 2 diabetes mellitus, hypertension, and nephropathy despite optimized renoprotective therapy (e.g., ARB therapy). In April 2012, the U.S. Food and Drug Administration (FDA) warned of possible risks when using aliskiren in

combination with ACEIs and ARBs in patients with diabetes or renal impairment. Recommendations being added to drug labels for aliskiren-containing products include a new contraindication against the use of aliskiren with ACEIs or ARBs in patients with diabetes because of the risk of renal impairment, hypotension, and hyperkalemia and a warning to avoid use of these combinations in patients with moderate to severe renal impairment (i.e., when GFR < 60 mL/min).

■ Diuretics for fluid balance and management of hypertension (diuretic selection based on level of kidney function)

■ Antihypertensives with diet and lifestyle modifications for control of blood pressure (see Chapter 12 on hypertension)

■ Antidiabetic agents with diet and lifestyle modifications for control of blood glucose (see Chapter 17 on diabetes)

■ Protein restriction to 0.8 g/kg/day:
  • Use only in adults with a GFR < 25 mL/min/1.73 m² because of the risk of malnutrition from prolonged protein restriction.
  • Consider for patients with > 1 g/day proteinuria despite optimal blood pressure control with a regimen that includes an ACEI or ARB.
  • Be cautious about maintaining adequate caloric intake, and avoid malnutrition.
  • Do not implement for patients < 80% of their ideal body weight or with > 10 g/day proteinuria.

■ Renal replacement therapy:
  • Consider plans for dialysis therapy (hemodialysis or peritoneal dialysis) during CKD stage 4 (G4).
  • Evaluate candidacy for kidney transplantation.

Anemia of CKD

Target hemoglobin should not exceed 11 g/dL (target hematocrit 33%) based on studies showing a greater risk for death, serious adverse cardiovascular reactions, and stroke when erythropoiesis-stimulating agents (ESAs) were used to target a hemoglobin above this threshold. *Note:* The FDA labeling for all ESAs states that initiation of therapy is recommended in patients with CKD on dialysis when the hemoglobin level is < 10 g/dL and in patients with CKD not on dialysis when the hemoglobin is < 10 g/dL and the following apply: (1) the rate of hemoglobin decline indicates the likelihood of requiring a red blood cell transfusion and (2) reducing the risk of alloimmunization and the risks of other red blood cell transfusions is a goal. A dose reduction or interruption of the ESA dose is recommended if the hemoglobin is > 11 g/dL in patients with CKD on dialysis or > 10 g/dL in CKD patients not on dialysis. This recommendation is based on safety concerns with increased hemoglobin and hematocrit targets in these patients; specifically, a greater risk for death, serious adverse cardiovascular reactions, and stroke. It is recommended to use the lowest ESA dose necessary to reduce the need for red blood cell transfusions.

Iron indices are transferrin saturation > 20% and serum ferritin > 100 ng/mL for CKD patients not on dialysis and for peritoneal dialysis patients. The goal for serum ferritin in hemodialysis patients is > 200 ng/mL. Consider the risk of iron overload if transferrin saturation and serum ferritin are elevated (e.g., transferrin saturation above 50%). *Note:* Ferritin is an acute phase reactant and may be elevated during conditions of infection or inflammation and not truly reflect iron status under these conditions.

Treatment strategies
ESAs

ESAs stimulate red blood cell production in the bone marrow. Available ESAs are listed in Table 20-6.

Table 20-6. Erythropoiesis Stimulating Agents

Generic name	Trade name	Starting dose	Route of administration	Frequency of administration
Epoetin alfa	**Epogen, Procrit**	50–100 units/kg	IV or subcutaneously	One to two doses per week
Darbepoetin alfa	**Aranesp**	0.45 mcg/kg once every 4 weeks for CKD patients not on dialysis; 0.45 mcg/kg once weekly or 0.75 mcg/kg once every 2 weeks for dialysis patients	IV or subcutaneously	Once weekly or once every other week (may prolong interval to every 3–4 weeks)

Boldface indicates one of top 100 drugs for 2012 by units sold at retail outlets, www.drugs.com/stats/top100/2012/units.

ESAs may be administered subcutaneously or intravenously (IV). Subcutaneous administration is generally preferred for patients not on hemodialysis (i.e., peritoneal dialysis, early-stage CKD patients who do not have IV access).

For epoetin alfa (Epogen and Procrit), initial doses are 50–100 units/kg IV or subcutaneously three times per week.

For darbepoetin alfa (Aranesp), initial dose is 0.45 mcg/kg administered once weekly or 0.75 mcg/kg every 2 weeks IV or subcutaneously for CKD patients on dialysis. The IV route is preferred for hemodialysis patients. For CKD patients not on dialysis, the recommended initial dose is 0.45 mcg/kg IV or subcutaneously at 4-week intervals.

Recommendations for dose conversion from epoetin alfa (units/wk) to darbepoetin alfa (mcg/wk) are provided in Table 20-7. The darbepoetin package insert states that for patients receiving epoetin alfa two to three times per week, darbepoetin alfa should be administered weekly. For patients receiving epoetin alfa once per week, darbepoetin alfa should be administered once every two weeks. In this situation, the weekly epoetin dose should be multiplied by two and that dose should be used in Table 20-7 to determine the appropriate darbepoetin dose.

For dose titration, allow at least 2–4 weeks before making a change in the ESA dose based on the change in hemoglobin or hematocrit. If a change in hemoglobin is < 1 g/dL in a 4-week period and iron stores are adequate, increase the ESA dose by 25%. If a change in hemoglobin is > 1 g/dL in a 2-week period, reduce the ESA dose by 25%.

Table 20-7. Estimated Starting Doses of Darbepoetin Alfa Based on Previous Epoetin Alfa Dose

Epoetin alfa dose (units/wk)	Darbepoetin alfa dose (mcg/wk)	
	Adult	**Pediatric**
< 1,500	6.25	—a
1,500–2,499	6.25	6.25
2,500–4,999	12.5	10
5,000–10,999	25	20
11,000–17,999	40	40
18,000–33,999	60	60
34,000–89,999	100	100
≥ 90,000	200	200

a. Insufficient data.

Iron supplementation

Iron supplementation prevents iron deficiency as a cause of resistance to therapy with ESAs. Iron deficiency should be corrected before making changes in the dose of the ESA. Common oral iron agents and all IV iron agents available in the United States are listed in Table 20-8.

Oral iron supplementation is limited by poor absorption and is often inadequate to achieve goal iron indices. It may be reasonable for patients with CKD stages 3 (G3a and G3b) and 4 (G4) and the peritoneal dialysis population (patients without IV access). The recommended dose is 200 mg elemental iron per day.

IV iron supplementation is preferred for treatment of absolute iron deficiency and in hemodialysis patients with regular IV access. A full course of iron is typically a total dose of 1 g divided over 8–10 hemodialysis sessions: 100 mg per dose for iron sucrose (Venofer) and iron dextran (INFeD, Dexferrum) or 125 mg per dose for sodium ferric gluconate (Ferrlecit). Ferumoxytol (Feraheme) may be administered as two doses to deliver 510 mg per dose and ferric carboxymaltose (Injectafer) as 750 mg per dose for two doses administered at least 7 days apart (total of 1,500 mg).

Weekly maintenances doses of iron (e.g., 25–125 mg) may be administered in hemodialysis patients to prevent absolute iron deficiency.

Approved doses for the available IV iron formulations are as follows:

- *Iron sucrose:* The 100 mg dose may be diluted in 100 mL of 0.9% NaCl (sodium chloride) administered IV over at least 15 minutes or administered undiluted over 2–5 minutes. Higher single doses are approved in nondialysis CKD patients and peritoneal dialysis patients (see below).
- *Iron dextran:* The 100 mg dose may be administered over 2 minutes IV push. Administer a 25 mg test dose because of the risk of anaphylactic reactions. Higher total dose infusions are administered in clinical practice, but the risk of reactions must be considered.
- *Sodium ferric gluconate:* The 125 mg dose may be diluted in 100 mL of 0.9% NaCl and administered IV over 1 hour or administered undiluted as an IV injection at a rate up to 12.5 mg/min. Dosing in pediatric patients is 1.5 mg/kg in 25 mL of 0.9% NaCl over 60 minutes (maximum dose 125 mg).
- *Ferumoxytol (Feraheme):* 510 mg (17 mL) as a single dose, followed by a second 510 mg dose 3–8 days after the initial dose.

Table 20-8. Iron Supplements

Generic name	Trade name[a]	Dose[b]	Dosage forms	Frequency of administration[c]
Ferrous fumarate	Femiron, Vitron-C	200 mg elemental iron per day	po	bid–tid
Ferrous gluconate	Fergon	200 mg elemental iron per day	po	bid–tid
Ferrous sulfate	Fir-In-Sol, Feosol, Slow FE	200 mg elemental iron per day	po	bid–tid
Heme iron polypeptide	Proferrin	200 mg elemental iron per day	po	tid–qid
Polysaccharide iron	Hytinic, Niferex	200 mg elemental iron per day	IV	qd–bid
Ferric carboxymaltose	Injectafer	Up to 750 mg as a single dose. Give two doses separated by at least 7 days for a total cumulative dose of 1,500 mg per treatment course.	Injection	As needed to treat iron deficiency in nondialysis CKD patients
Ferumoxytol	Feraheme	510 mg × 1 followed by second 510 mg dose 3–8 days after first dose	IV	As needed to treat iron deficiency in CKD
Iron dextran	INFeD, Dexferrum	25–1,000 mg	IV	Weekly, three times per week, or monthly[b]
Iron sucrose	Venofer	20–400 mg	IV	Weekly, three times per week, or monthly[b]
Sodium ferric gluconate	Ferrlecit	62.5–125 mg	IV	Weekly, three times per week, or monthly[c]

a. Not all trade names are included in table for oral agents.
b. Approved dosing regimens for each IV iron agent are as follows (administered IV push): iron dextran 100 mg, iron sucrose 100 mg, sodium ferric gluconate 125 mg, ferric carboxymaltose 750 mg, ferumoxytol 510 mg. If larger doses are administered, they should be infused over a prolonged period to reduce the risk of adverse events. Iron sucrose is approved at higher doses (e.g., up to 400 mg administered over 2.5 hours as part of a regimen to provide 1 g in divided doses). See product labeling for each agent.
c. For oral formulations, frequency of administration depends on the amount of elemental iron per unit; 200 mg elemental iron per day is necessary.

■ *Ferric carboxymaltose (Injectafer):* Up to 1,500 mg as a total cumulative dose administered as two 750 mg doses separated by at least 7 days. The dose may be given by either slow IV push (100 mg per minute) or infused over at least 15 minutes.

IV iron regimens may differ in peritoneal dialysis patients and patients with CKD not requiring dialysis in that typically larger doses are given at one time because these patients are not seen in a clinical environment as often as the hemodialysis population, thereby making the process of dividing doses into smaller increments less convenient. For administration of doses larger than those listed in the product labeling, the dose should be infused over a prolonged period of time to reduce the risk of adverse events.

Iron sucrose does have an approved dosing regimen in nondialysis CKD patients and peritoneal dialysis patients. The approved dosing regimen for iron sucrose

in nondialysis CKD patients is 200 mg over 2–5 minutes on five different occasions within a 14-day period. Peritoneal dialysis patients may receive 300 mg in 0.9% NaCl administered IV over 1.5 hours, followed by a second infusion of 300 mg 14 days later and then by a 400 mg dose administered over 2.5 hours 14 days later. The dose of ferumoxytol in the nondialysis CKD population is the same as in the dialysis population: 510 mg as a single dose followed by a second 510 mg dose 3–8 days later. Ferric carboxymaltose is approved in only the nondialysis CKD population, and the doses listed above and in Table 20-8 apply.

For patients with more severe anemia or when blood loss is a major contributing factor, blood transfusions may be required.

CKD-MBD

The following are goals for phosphorus, calcium, and PTH based on the KDOQI and KDIGO guidelines by stage of CKD. (KDOQI stages are listed followed by the KDIGO classification in parentheses.)

- Goal serum phosphorus:
  - KDOQI: 2.7–4.6 mg/dL for stages 3 and 4 CKD (G3a, G3b, G4) and 3.5–5.5 mg/dL for stage 5 CKD (G5) patients on dialysis
  - KDIGO: Normal range for stages 3 and 4 CKD (G3a, G3b, G4) and "toward normal" for stage 5 CKD (G5) patients on dialysis
- Goal serum calcium:
  - KDOQI: Normal range for stages 3 and 4 CKD (G3a, G3b, G4) and 8.4–9.5 mg/dL for stage 5 CKD (G5) patients on dialysis. *Note:* The lower calcium range in stage 5 CKD (G5) is recommended because of the risk of hypercalcemia and calcifications at this level of kidney function.
  - KDIGO: Normal range for stages 3–5 CKD (G3a, G3b, G4, and G5)
- Calcium × phosphorus product:
  - KDOQI: < 55 mg^2/dL^2 for all CKD stages
  - KDIGO: Specific target not recommended, but rather focuses on individual levels of each
- Goal PTH is as follows:
  - KDOQI: 35–70 pg/mL for stage 3 CKD (G3a and G3b), 70–110 pg/mL for stage 4 CKD (G4), and 150–300 pg/mL for stage 5 CKD (G5)
  - KDIGO: Upper limit of the normal range for stages 3 and 4 CKD (G3a, G3b, G4) and 2–9 times the upper limit of normal for stage 5 CKD (G5) patients on dialysis
- A 25-hydroxyvitamin D level below 30 ng/mL indicates a deficiency in the precursor form of vitamin D (25-hydroxyvitamin D is converted to the active form by the kidney). Both KDOQI and KDIGO recommend supplementation when there is a deficiency in the precursor form.

Treatment strategies

- Follow a dietary phosphorus restriction of 800–1,000 mg/day phosphorus (consult with dietitian).
- Use phosphate-binding agents—elemental (calcium, lanthanum, sucroferric oxyhydroxide) and nonelemental (sevelamer):
  - Titrate doses on the basis of phosphorus and calcium × phosphorus product.
  - Limit use of calcium-containing phosphate binders if hypercalcemia occurs.
  - Aluminum-containing agents also work to bind phosphorus, but they are not first-line agents because of the potential for aluminum

accumulation in kidney disease; prescribe only if needed for short-term use (< 30 days) to minimize the risk of accumulation.
  - Magnesium-containing agents also work to bind phosphorus, but use is limited because of GI side effects and risk of accumulation.
- Remove phosphorus by dialysis for ESRD patients. Continue phosphorus restriction and use of phosphate-binding agents with dialysis.
- Maintain goal calcium, phosphorus, and PTH.
- Provide vitamin D supplementation depending on the stage of CKD. Supplementation with the active form (calcitriol) or a vitamin D analog (doxercalciferol or paricalcitol) is necessary in more severe stages of CKD (stages 4 and 5). Supplementation with a vitamin D precursor (e.g., ergocalciferol) may be required in earlier stages, especially when 25-hydroxyvitamin D levels are below 30 ng/mL.
- Use a calcimimetic agent (cinacalcet [Sensipar]) to help control PTH in ESRD patients. Initial dose is 30 mg po daily. The dose of cinacalcet should be titrated no more frequently than every 2–4 weeks through sequential doses of 60, 90, 120, and 180 mg once daily to target goal PTH levels.
- Control metabolic acidosis (which causes bone demineralization if not controlled).

Metabolic acidosis

- Decrease in serum bicarbonate: Normal value = 22–26 mEq/L
- Decrease in blood pH: Normal value = 7.35–7.45

Treatment strategies

- Administration of sodium bicarbonate or other alkali preparation: Gradual correction (over days to weeks) is usually appropriate for asymptomatic patients with mild to moderate acidosis (serum bicarbonate 12–20 mEq/L and pH 7.2–7.4).
- Dialysis: Bicarbonate or lactate contained within the dialysate solution diffuses from dialysate to plasma and effectively treats metabolic acidosis.

Monitoring

Progressive kidney disease

- Patients at high risk for CKD (e.g., patients with diabetes or hypertension) or patients diagnosed with CKD should have the following monitored regularly:
  - ***Serum creatinine:*** Consider limitations. *Note:* Patients started on ACEIs or ARBs may have

an initial rise in serum creatinine. A 25–30% increase is generally acceptable. Increases higher than this may indicate AKI caused by the medications.

- *Estimated GFR:* Assess rate of progression (the decline in GFR in mL/min/1.73 m^2 per year).
- *Proteinuria:* Monitor annually in patients with type 1 diabetes with diabetes duration of ≥ 5 years and at diagnosis for patients with type 2 diabetes.
- *Serum electrolytes*
- *Blood pressure*
- *Blood glucose:* Assess in individuals with diabetes.
- *Medication regimens:* Evaluate and adjust on the basis of kidney function.

Anemia of CKD

- Monitor hemoglobin and hematocrit every 1–2 weeks after initiation of ESAs or following a dose change and every 2–4 weeks once a stable target hemoglobin and hematocrit are achieved.
- Monitor iron indices (transferrin saturation and serum ferritin).
- Evaluate patient for signs and symptoms of anemia.

CKD-MBD

- Phosphorus
- Calcium
- Parathyroid hormone
- Vitamin D: Measure precursor levels, 25-hydroxyvitamin D, in patients with stages 3 and 4 CKD (G3a, G3b, G4)

Metabolic acidosis

- Serum bicarbonate
- Potassium

Drug Therapy

Progressive kidney disease

- ACEIs and ARBs (see Chapter 12 on hypertension and Chapter 17 on diabetes). ACEIs and ARBs decrease intraglomerular pressure by preventing vasoconstriction of the efferent arteriole mediated by angiotensin II. This and other mechanisms independent of the effects on renal hemodynamics lead to a decrease in proteinuria and

delay progression of CKD. The renin inhibitor (aliskiren) may also be used to delay progression, but not in combination with ACEIs or ARBs.

- Antihypertensive agents (see Chapter 12 on hypertension)
- Antidiabetic agents (see Chapter 17 on diabetes)

Anemia

Anemia is treated with ESAs (Table 20-6).

Mechanism of action
These agents stimulate the division and differentiation of erythroid progenitor cells and induce the release of reticulocytes from the bone marrow into the bloodstream, where they mature into erythrocytes.

Adverse drug events
Adverse drug events include the following:

- Hypertension
- Red blood cell aplasia
- Seizures (rare)
- Polycythemia
- Thrombocytosis

Note: ESAs when dosed to achieve a higher hemoglobin (> 11 g/dL) have been shown to cause an increased risk of death, serious cardiovascular events, and stroke in patients with CKD. The package labeling for these agents contains a warning about this risk. It is recommended to use the lowest ESA dose necessary to reduce the need for red blood cell transfusions. All ESAs must be used under a risk evaluation and mitigation strategy risk management program. As part of the risk management program, a medication guide explaining the risks and benefits of ESAs must be provided to all patients receiving an ESA.

Drug–drug and drug–disease interactions
Causes of resistance to ESAs are as follows:

- Iron deficiency
- Secondary hyperparathyroidism
- Inflammatory conditions
- Aluminum accumulation
- Other disease states causing anemia (e.g., cancer, HIV)

Parameters to monitor
The following should be monitored:

- Hemoglobin and hematocrit
- Iron indices
- Blood pressure

Pharmacokinetics
Half-life:

- *Epoetin alfa:* Approximately 8.5 hours IV and 24 hours subcutaneously
- *Darbepoetin alfa:* Approximately 25 hours IV and 48 hours subcutaneously

Strengths and dosage forms
Epoetin alfa is supplied as single-dose, preservative-free solution (in vials of 2,000, 3,000, 4,000, 10,000, and 40,000 units/mL) and as a multidose, preserved solution (in vials of 10,000 and 20,000 units/mL).

Darbepoetin alfa is supplied as single-dose vials (25, 40, 60, 100, 200, and 300 mg/mL and 150 mcg/0.75 mL) and as single-dose prefilled syringes (25, 40, 60, 100, 150, 200, 300, and 500 mcg). They contain no preservatives.

Iron supplementation

Iron supplements are described in Table 20-8.

Mechanism of action
Iron supplements supply a source of elemental iron necessary for the function of hemoglobin, myoglobin, and specific enzyme systems and allow transport of oxygen via hemoglobin.

Patient instructions and counseling
- Oral iron may cause stools to be dark in color.
- Take between meals to increase absorption.
- Oral iron may be taken with food if GI upset occurs.
- Do not take with dairy products or antacids.

Adverse drug events
- Oral iron may cause stomach cramping, constipation, nausea, vomiting, and dark stools.
- In the case of IV iron, anaphylactic reactions have occurred with iron dextran (INFeD and Dexferrum); administer a 25 mg test dose before administration of the full dose. If no signs or symptoms of anaphylactic-type reactions follow the test dose, administer the full dose and continue to observe the patient.
- INFeD and Dexferrum are not identical products and differ in molecular size, which may contribute to differences in adverse effects between these two products. Iron sucrose (Venofer), ferric carboxymaltose (Injectafer), ferumoxytol (Feraheme), and sodium ferric gluconate (Ferrlecit) have less risk of hypersensitivity reactions; however, patients should be closely observed for signs of hypersensitivity during and for at least 30 minutes after administration of these agents.
- For all IV iron preparations, observe patients for diaphoresis, nausea, vomiting, lower back pain, dyspnea, and hypotension.
- Iron overload may be treated with deferoxamine (Desferal).

Drug–drug and drug–disease interactions
GI absorption of oral iron is decreased when given with antacids, quinolones, and tetracycline and increased when administered with vitamin C.

IV iron has a potential to increase risk of infection. Administration to patients with severe systemic infections is not recommended.

Ferumoxytol is a superparamagnetic iron oxide, and administration may alter MRI studies for up to 3 months following administration.

Parameters to monitor
- Ferritin and transferrin saturation
- Hemoglobin and hematocrit
- Anaphylactic or hypersensitivity reactions after IV administration

Strengths and dosage forms
- Ferric carboxymaltose (Injectafer) is supplied in single-dose vials containing 750 mg/15 mL.
- Ferumoxytol (Feraheme) is supplied in 17 mL single-dose vials containing 30 mg/mL.
- Iron dextran (INFeD and Dexferrum) is supplied in 2 mL single-dose vials containing 50 mg of elemental iron per milliliter.
- Iron sucrose (Venofer) is supplied in 50 mg/2.5 mL, 100 mg/5 mL, and 200 mg/10 mL single-use vials.
- Sodium ferric gluconate (Ferrlecit) is supplied as colorless glass ampules and in vials containing 62.5 mg elemental iron in 5 mL (12.5 mg/mL).

CKD-MBD

Phosphate-binding agents are used to treat this disorder (Table 20-9).

Mechanism of action
These agents combine with dietary phosphate in the GI tract to form an insoluble complex that is excreted in the feces.

Patient instructions and counseling
- Take with meals and snacks.
- Drug interactions (see section on drug–drug and drug–disease interactions below)

Table 20-9. Phosphate-Binding Agents[a]

Generic name	Trade name	Dosage form(s)	Starting dosage range[b]
Calcium carbonate (40% elemental calcium)	Tums, Os-Cal-500, Nephro-Calci, Caltrate 600, CalCarb HD, CaCO₃ (multiple preparations)	Multiple formulations OTC, including chewable tablet	0.8–2 g elemental calcium
Calcium acetate (25% elemental calcium)	Phos-Lo	Capsule	1,334–2,001 mg
	Phoslyra	Liquid	
	Calphron (OTC)	Tablet	
Sevelamer carbonate	Renvela	Tablet, powder	800–1,600 mg
Lanthanum carbonate	Fosrenol	Chewable tablet	250–500 mg
Sucroferric oxyhydroxide	Velphoro	Chewable tablet	500 mg
Aluminum hydroxide[c]	AlternaGel, Alu-Cap, Alu-tab, Amphojel, Basaljel	Multiple formulations OTC	300–600 mg
Magnesium carbonate[c]	Mag-Carb	Multiple formulations OTC	70 mg
Magnesium hydroxide (milk of magnesia)[c]	Various	Multiple formulations OTC	300–400 mg

OTC, over-the-counter.
a. All agents are taken orally and should be taken with meals.
b. Dose per meal.
c. Not preferred because of the risk of accumulation and adverse effects.

- Aluminum and magnesium products are not recommended because of concerns of accumulation and adverse events in patients with kidney disease.
- Lanthanum carbonate (Fosrenol) and sucroferric oxyhydroxide (Velphoro) are chewable tablets (do not swallow whole). Some forms of calcium carbonate can also be chewed.
- Sevelamer carbonate (Renvela) is available as a tablet or as a powder that should be mixed with the appropriate amount of water (1 oz for the 0.8 g packet; 2 oz for the 2.4 g packet). The powder does not dissolve and should be stirred vigorously before drinking. Drink within 30 minutes of preparation.
- Sevelamer hydrochloride [Renagel] is available as a tablet.
- Use in conjunction with dietary phosphorus restriction.

Adverse drug events
- Calcium products can result in hypercalcemia, nausea, vomiting, abdominal pain, and constipation.
- Lanthanum carbonate (Fosrenol) may cause nausea, vomiting, diarrhea, dyspepsia, abdominal pain, and constipation.
- Sevelamer carbonate (Renvela) may cause nausea, vomiting, diarrhea, dyspepsia, abdominal pain, flatulence, and constipation. Serious cases of dysphagia, bowel obstruction, and perforation have been associated with sevelamer (contraindicated in patients with bowel obstruction). *Note:* Sevelamer carbonate (Renvela) has less risk of metabolic acidosis than does sevelamer hydrochloride (Renagel).
- Sevelamer hydrochloride (Renagel) may cause metabolic acidosis, nausea, vomiting, diarrhea, dyspepsia, abdominal pain, flatulence, and constipation. Contraindicated in patients with bowel obstruction.
- Sucroferric oxyhydroxide (Velphoro) may cause discolored feces and diarrhea.
- Aluminum may cause constipation, aluminum toxicity, chalky taste, cramps, nausea, and vomiting.
- Magnesium products may cause diarrhea, hypermagnesemia, cramps, and muscle weakness.
- All products may cause hypophosphatemia.

Drug–drug and drug–disease interactions
- Drug–drug interactions: In general, to minimize the risk of the drug interactions in the follow-

ing list, administer the interacting drug at least 1–2 hours before or 3–4 hours after the phosphate binder.

- Calcium-containing binders: Oral iron salts, certain antibiotics (quinolones, tetracyclines), and mycophenolate (not inclusive of all potential drug interactions)
- Lanthanum carbonate: Certain antibiotics (quinolones, tetracyclines), cationic antacids, or levothyroxine
- Sevelamer carbonate: Quinolone antibiotics, mycophenolate, or levothyroxine (may decrease absorption of vitamin D, E, and K and folic acid)
- Sevelamer hydrochloride: Ciprofloxacin (bioavailability of ciprofloxacin may be reduced by 50%).
- Sucroferric oxyhydroxide: Alendronate, doxycycline, levothyroxine, or oral vitamin D analogs

- Sevelamer carbonate: It is associated with metabolic acidosis; however, there is less risk compared with sevelamer hydrochloride (Renagel).

Parameters to monitor
- Phosphorus, calcium, PTH, and 25-hydroxy-vitamin D levels in stages 3 and 4 CKD (G3a, G3b, G4)
- Aluminum and magnesium levels (if receiving aluminum- or magnesium-containing products)

- Serum bicarbonate with sevelamer carbonate (Renvela)

Vitamin D therapy

Vitamin D therapy is described in Table 20-10.

Mechanism of action (active vitamin D)
This therapy increases intestinal absorption of calcium, increases tubular reabsorption of calcium by the kidney (in patients with sufficient kidney function), suppresses synthesis of parathyroid hormone, and increases intestinal phosphorus absorption.

Patient instructions and counseling
- Use in conjunction with dietary phosphorus restriction and phosphate-binding agents; vitamin D therapy may need to temporarily discontinue if calcium and phosphorus are elevated.
- Notify health care provider of any of the following signs of hypercalcemia: weakness, headache, decreased appetite, and lethargy.

Adverse drug events
- *Hypercalcemia:* Decreased incidence with vitamin D analogs (paricalcitol, doxercalciferol) compared to calcitriol
- *Hyperphosphatemia:* Decreased incidence with vitamin D analogs
- *Adynamic bone disease:* Caused by over-suppression of PTH

Table 20-10. Vitamin D Therapy

Generic name	Trade name	Dosage range	Dosage forms	Frequency of administration
Vitamin D precursors				
Ergocalciferol (vitamin D$_2$ precursor)	Drisdol	400–50,000 IU	po	Daily, weekly, or monthly
Ergocalciferol	Calciferol	400–50,000 IU	po or IV	Daily, weekly, or monthly
Cholecalciferol (vitamin D$_3$ precursor)	Multiple agents	1,000 IU	po	Daily
Active vitamin D and vitamin D analogs[a]				
Calcitriol	Calcijex	0.5–5 mcg	IV	Three times per week
Calcitriol	Rocaltrol	0.25–5 mcg	po	Daily, every other day, or three times per week
Paricalcitol	Zemplar	1–4 mcg	po	Daily or three times per week
		2.5–15 mcg	IV	Three times per week
Doxercalciferol	Hectorol	5–20 mcg	po	Daily or three times per week
		2–8 mcg	IV	Three times per week

IU, international units.

a. Calcitriol is a vitamin D$_3$ agent. Paricalcitol and doxercalciferol are D$_2$ agents and are less likely to cause hypercalcemia and hyperphosphatemia.

Drug–drug and drug–disease interactions
- Cholestyramine may decrease intestinal absorption of oral products.
- Magnesium absorption may be increased with concomitant administration.

Parameters to monitor
- PTH
- Calcium
- Phosphorus
- Alkaline phosphatase
- Signs of vitamin D intoxication and hypercalcemia (e.g., weakness, headache, somnolence, nausea, vomiting, bone pain, polyuria)

Pharmacokinetics
- Calcitriol (Calcijex):
  - Half-life: 3–8 hours; protein binding 99.9%
- Paricalcitol (Zemplar):
  - Half-life: Healthy subjects 4–6 hours (oral); stages 3 and 4 CKD 17–20 hours (oral); stage 5 CKD (G5) 14–15 hours (IV)
  - Protein binding: > 99%
- Doxercalciferol (Hectorol):
  - Half-life of active metabolite: 32–37 hours

Ergocalciferol requires hydroxylation within the liver and a second hydroxylation within the kidney to form active vitamin D.

Doxercalciferol requires conversion to its active form 1α, 25-dihydroxyvitamin D_2 in the liver.

Strengths and dosage forms
- Calcitriol (Calcijex): 1 mcg/mL ampuls
- Calcitriol (Rocaltrol): 0.25 and 0.5 mcg capsules, 1 mcg/mL oral solution
- Paricalcitol (Zemplar): IV—2 and 5 mcg/mL vials; po—1, 2, 4 mcg capsules
- Doxercalciferol: IV—2 mcg/mL ampuls; po—0.5, 1, 2.5 mcg capsules

Calcimimetics: Cinacalcet (Sensipar)

Cinacalcet is approved only for patients with stage 5 CKD (G5) who are on dialysis. It is used in conjunction with phosphate binder therapy and vitamin D. The dose range is 30–180 mg/day; initial dose is 30 mg titrated every 2–4 weeks on the basis of PTH levels. Do not start therapy if corrected serum calcium is < 8.4 mg/dL.

Mechanism of action
Cinacalcet binds with the calcium-sensing receptor on the parathyroid gland and increases sensitivity of the receptor to extracellular calcium, thereby decreasing the stimulus for PTH secretion.

Patient instructions and counseling
- Cinacalcet should be taken with food or shortly after a meal.
- Tablets should be taken whole and should not be divided.

Adverse drug events
- Hypocalcemia (use with caution in patients with seizure disorder)
- Nausea, vomiting
- Diarrhea
- Myalgias

Drug–drug and drug–disease interactions
Cinacalcet is metabolized by multiple cytochrome P450 (CYP) enzymes, primarily CYP3A4, CYP2D6, and CYP1A2. Adjustments in dose may be required for patients taking agents that inhibit metabolism of cinacalcet (e.g., ketoconazole). Dose reductions of drugs with a narrow therapeutic range and with a metabolism dependent on these enzymes may also be required (e.g., tricyclic antidepressants, flecainide, thioridazine).

Parameters to monitor
Serum calcium and serum phosphorus should be measured within 1 week, and PTH should be measured 1–4 weeks after initiation or dose adjustment of cinacalcet. The dose of cinacalcet should be titrated no more frequently than every 2–4 weeks through sequential doses of 60, 90, 120, and 180 mg once daily to target the goal PTH.

Pharmacokinetics
- The maximum concentration is achieved in approximately 2–6 hours following administration and is increased with food.
- Half-life is 30–40 hours.
- Volume of distribution is approximately 1,000 L.
- Cinacalcet is approximately 93–97% bound to plasma proteins.
- Cinacalcet is metabolized primarily by CYP3A4, CYP2D6, and CYP1A2.

Strengths and dosage forms
Cinacalcet is available in 30, 60, and 90 mg tablets.

Metabolic acidosis

See Chapter 21 on critical care.

Metabolic acidosis is frequently corrected once a patient begins chronic dialysis treatments (either hemodialysis or peritoneal dialysis). If the patient required sodium bicarbonate, this medication may be discontinued once dialysis is initiated and the serum bicarbonate levels correct to the normal range.

Vitamin supplementation (specific to the dialysis population)

Water-soluble vitamins for dialysis patients are described in Table 20-11.

Mechanism of action
Vitamin supplementation replaces water-soluble vitamins lost during dialysis without providing supratherapeutic amounts of fat-soluble vitamins.

Patient instructions and counseling
- Take daily to replace water-soluble vitamins.
- Hemodialysis patients should take after dialysis.

Adverse drug events
- **General:** Nausea, headache, pruritus, flushing (depending on specific vitamin)
- **Vitamin B6 (pyridoxine):** Neuropathy, increased aspartate transaminase
- **Vitamin C (ascorbic acid):** Hyperoxaluria, dizziness, diarrhea, fatigue, nausea
- **Folic acid:** Headache, rash, pruritus

Drug–drug and drug–disease interactions
Folic acid may decrease phenytoin concentrations by increasing the metabolism.

Nondrug Therapy

- Preparation for renal replacement therapy when patients reach stage 4 CKD (G4):

Table 20-11. Water-Soluble Vitamin Supplements for Dialysis Patients[a]

Generic name	Trade name[b]
Vitamin B complex, vitamin C, and folic acid	Nephrocaps, Nephrovite, Nephrovite Rx, Rena-Vite
Vitamin B complex, vitamin C, folic acid, and iron	Nephrovite Rx + Iron
Vitamin B complex	Allbee with C

a. All these supplements are taken orally, 1 capsule or tablet once per day.
b. Not all trade names are included in table.

- Choice of chronic dialysis (hemodialysis or peritoneal dialysis) if patient is a candidate for both modalities and discussion of transplantation
- Placement of dialysis access (fistula [preferred] or graft for hemodialysis, catheter for peritoneal dialysis)
- Patient education regarding choice of renal replacement therapy and complications of CKD

Diet

- Risks and benefits of protein restriction (0.8 g/kg/day) should be considered in patients with stage 4 CKD (G4).
- Increased protein requirements should be considered for patients on dialysis (approximately 1.2 g/kg/day) and even greater requirements for peritoneal dialysis patients because of increased protein loss with the dialysis procedure.
- Nutritional supplementation should be taken as needed.
- Counseling by a renal dietitian may be beneficial to tailor a diet based on the stage of CKD.

Renal replacement therapies

Hemodialysis
The intermittent hemodialysis procedure is generally performed three times per week for 3–5 hours for patients with stage 5 (G5) kidney disease (ESRD). It requires a viable permanent access site (fistula or graft) or a temporary site for patients requiring immediate dialysis or experiencing failed permanent access sites. Fistulas are the preferred access for chronic hemodialysis.

Complications include infection, hypotension during dialysis, clotting, and dialyzer reactions. Drug removal by hemodialysis is most likely to occur for drugs with small molecular weight, low protein binding, and small volume of distribution.

Peritoneal dialysis
Peritoneal dialysis requires insertion of a catheter into the peritoneum. Types include continuous ambulatory peritoneal dialysis and automated peritoneal dialysis (which includes continuous cycling, nocturnal tidal, and nightly intermittent peritoneal dialysis).

Several complications are possible:

- Peritonitis
  - Most common Gram-positive organisms are *Staphylococcus epidermidis* and *S. aureus*.

- Most common Gram-negative organisms are *Enterobacteriaceae* and *Pseudomonas aeruginosa.*
- Empiric therapy should include Gram-positive coverage (first-generation cephalosporin or vancomycin if MRSA [methicillin-resistant *S. aureus*] is prevalent) and Gram-negative coverage (e.g., third-generation cephalosporin or aminoglycoside).
- Intraperitoneal administration of antibiotics is recommended.
- Hyperglycemia from glucose content of dialysate solution
- Malnutrition from increased protein loss

Transplantation
See Chapter 24 for information on transplantation.

20-5. Questions

Use the following case study to answer Questions 1 and 2:

A 45-year-old female is admitted to the hospital after fainting at work. Her medical history includes type 2 diabetes and rheumatoid arthritis. Her only complaint is that she has had difficulty over the past 5 days keeping down anything she eats or drinks. She has also noticed a decrease in urination over the past 24 hours. Regular medications include aspirin 325 mg daily, ibuprofen 600 mg daily for arthritis, metformin 500 mg daily, glyburide 5 mg daily, and Tylenol prn for headache. Laboratory values in the emergency department showed a serum creatinine of 2 mg/dL and BUN of 56 mg/dL, consistent with acute kidney injury. Her lab tests from 1 month ago at a regular checkup were normal.

1. The most likely etiology of this patient's acute kidney injury is
   A. dehydration from poor oral intake.
   B. age-related decreases in kidney function.
   C. kidney failure caused by diabetes.
   D. obstruction of urine outflow.

2. Which of the following medications is most likely to have contributed to her acute kidney injury?
   A. Aspirin
   B. Ibuprofen
   C. Metformin
   D. Glyburide

3. Which of the following diuretics may retain its effectiveness at a glomerular filtration rate < 30 mL/min?
   A. Hydrochlorothiazide
   B. Chlorothiazide
   C. Metolazone
   D. Spironolactone

4. Which of the following electrolyte abnormalities typically occurs in patients with severe kidney dysfunction (i.e., creatinine clearance < 15 mL/min)?
   A. Metabolic acidosis
   B. Metabolic alkalosis
   C. Hypophosphatemia
   D. Hypernatremia

5. Which set of the following laboratory values is most consistent with a diagnosis of intrinsic AKI?
   A. Urinary granular casts absent, $FE_{Na} < 1$, urinary osmolality 600 mOsm/kg
   B. Urinary granular casts absent, $FE_{Na} > 1$, urinary osmolality 600 mOsm/kg
   C. Urinary granular casts present, $FE_{Na} < 1$, urinary osmolality 300 mOsm/kg
   D. Urinary granular casts present, $FE_{Na} > 1$, urinary osmolality 300 mOsm/kg

6. Which of the following diuretics (as single-drug therapy) would be most appropriate for the initial treatment of a patient with acute kidney injury and significant volume overload?
   A. Metolazone
   B. Spironolactone
   C. Bumetanide
   D. Mannitol

7. A patient with nephrotoxicity caused by tobramycin would likely present with an increase in serum creatinine
   A. immediately after starting therapy and with nonoliguria.
   B. immediately after starting therapy and with oliguria.
   C. 5–7 days after starting therapy and with oliguria.
   D. 5–7 days after starting therapy and with nonoliguria.

8. Lisinopril may cause hemodynamically mediated acute kidney disease by preventing which of the following compensatory mechanisms by the kidney?

    A. Vasodilation of the afferent arteriole
    B. Vasoconstriction of the afferent arteriole
    C. Vasodilation of the efferent arteriole
    D. Vasoconstriction of the efferent arteriole

9. The estimated creatinine clearance for a 47-year-old male patient with an ideal body weight of 176 lb (slightly less than actual body weight) and a serum creatinine of 2.2 mg/dL is

    A. 32 mL/min.
    B. 40 mL/min.
    C. 47 mL/min.
    D. 93 mL/min.

Use the following case study to answer Questions 10 and 11:

A 53-year-old African American female (body weight = 65 kg) with hypertension and hypercholesterolemia is seen in the outpatient nephrology clinic for evaluation of kidney disease progression. Her current blood pressure is 156/82 mm Hg, SCr is 2.6 mg/dL (stable for the past 4 months), BUN is 44 mg/dL, and urinary albumin excretion rate is 600 mg/day. Her medications are enalapril 20 mg/day × 1 year and simvastatin 20 mg daily × 2 years.

10. On the basis of this patient's estimated creatinine clearance, she would be classified in which of the following KDIGO categories of chronic kidney disease?

    A. G1
    B. G2
    C. G3a
    D. G4

11. The recommended target blood pressure for this patient is

    A. < 110/70 mm Hg.
    B. < 125/90 mm Hg.
    C. < 130/80 mm Hg.
    D. < 140/90 mm Hg.

12. Which of the following is the most appropriate recommendation for a patient with stage 3 (G3b) CKD, diabetes, and an albumin-to-creatinine ratio of 200 mg/g to delay progression of CKD?

    A. Enalapril and losartan
    B. Enalapril and aliskiren
    C. Losartan and aliskiren
    D. Enalapril only

13. Epoetin alfa and darbepoetin alfa stimulate erythropoiesis by which of the following?

    A. Prevention of excessive red blood cell destruction
    B. Prevention of degradation of bone marrow stem cells
    C. Differentiation of peritubular interstitial cells of the kidney
    D. Differentiation of erythroid progenitor stem cells in the bone marrow

14. When administered intravenously, darbepoetin alfa has a terminal half-life approximately _____ that of epoetin alfa.

    A. twofold shorter than
    B. twofold longer than
    C. threefold longer than
    D. threefold shorter than

15. One of the most commonly reported adverse reactions with epoetin alfa and darbepoetin alfa is

    A. nausea.
    B. hypertension.
    C. constipation.
    D. anaphylaxis.

16. At least how much time should be allowed to lapse before a change in dose of epoetin alfa or darbepoetin alfa is made on the basis of a change in hemoglobin and hematocrit?

    A. 1 week
    B. 2–4 weeks
    C. 6–8 weeks
    D. 2 months

17. A 42-year-old male (body weight = 70 kg) on hemodialysis three times per week receives epoetin alfa for treatment of anemia. He has been stable on an epoetin dose of 4,000 units IV three times per week with an average hemoglobin of 11 g/dL (hematocrit of 33%). Over the past 3 months, his hemoglobin has

dropped to 9 g/dL. Iron indices reveal the following: serum ferritin 78 ng/mL and transferrin saturation 12%. The best initial treatment for this patient is to

A. increase the dose of epoetin alfa to maintain a hemoglobin of 11–12 g/dL (hematocrit of 33–36%).
B. administer IV iron (sodium ferric gluconate) at a maintenance dose of 125 mg/wk.
C. administer a 1 g total dose of IV iron in divided doses.
D. begin oral ferrous sulfate 325 mg tid.

18. In the gastrointestinal tract, calcitriol

A. promotes absorption of calcium and inhibits absorption of phosphorus.
B. promotes absorption of both calcium and phosphorus.
C. promotes decreased binding of calcium and phosphorus.
D. promotes increased elimination of calcium and phosphorus.

Use the following case study to answer Questions 19 and 20:

A 63-year-old female with stage 5 (G5) CKD (end-stage kidney disease) is receiving peritoneal dialysis. Her most recent laboratory analysis reveals the following: BUN 58 mg/dL, SCr 5.2 mg/dL, phosphorus 7.4 mg/dL, calcium 9 mg/dL, albumin 2.5 g/dL, and iPTH 542 pg/mL.

19. In addition to dietary restriction of phosphorus, which of the following agents is best for initial management of this patient's hyperphosphatemia?

A. Lanthanum carbonate
B. Calcium acetate
C. Aluminum hydroxide
D. Calcium carbonate

20. This patient should be instructed to take her phosphate binder

A. with meals to enhance systemic absorption of phosphorus.
B. with meals to minimize systemic absorption of phosphorus.
C. between meals to avoid food–drug interactions.
D. between meals to minimize GI side effects.

21. Which of the following agents is most appropriate for a patient with stage 5 (G5) CKD on hemodialysis, secondary hyperparathyroidism (PTH 800 pg/mL), and hypercalcemia (corrected calcium 10.5 mg/dL) who requires treatment to reduce PTH?

A. Cinacalcet
B. Paricalcitol
C. Calcitriol
D. Ergocalciferol

22. Cinacalcet is a calcimimetic that works by which of the following mechanisms?

A. It decreases the sensitivity of the calcium-sensing receptors on the parathyroid gland to calcium, which prevents secretion of PTH.
B. It increases the sensitivity of the calcium-sensing receptors on the parathyroid gland to calcium, which prevents secretion of PTH.
C. It stimulates the breakdown of PTH and prevents the effects of PTH on bone turnover.
D. It increases calcium concentrations, which suppresses secretion of PTH from the parathyroid gland.

23. A drug with which of the following characteristics is most likely to be removed by hemodialysis (Vd = volume of distribution)?

A. f_u 0.05, Vd 0.2 L/kg
B. f_u 0.05, Vd 0.6 L/kg
C. f_u 0.30, Vd 0.6 L/kg
D. f_u 0.95, Vd 0.2 L/kg

24. The best antibiotic selection for empiric treatment of peritonitis in a peritoneal dialysis patient is

A. cefazolin + vancomycin.
B. cefazolin + ceftazidime.
C. vancomycin alone.
D. gentamicin alone.

25. Which of the following supplements should be recommended daily in a patient with stage 5 (G5) CKD requiring chronic hemodialysis?

A. Multivitamin
B. Nephrocaps
C. Vitamin A
D. Nephrocaps + vitamin A

20-6. Answers

1. **A.** Dehydration is the most likely cause of AKI in this patient because she has had a decrease in oral intake over the past 5 days. Dehydration would be classified as a prerenal cause of AKI. A serum creatinine of 2 mg/dL would not be considered normal in a person age 45 years, eliminating age as a rationale for kidney disease. Diabetes would be more likely to cause a chronic decrease in her kidney function as opposed to an acute change (lab tests from 1 month ago were normal, ruling out evidence of chronic kidney disease). She has had some urine output in the past 24 hours, which rules out obstruction.

2. **B.** NSAIDs are associated with hemodynamic changes (in particular, they prevent the compensatory vasodilation of the afferent arteriole that occurs in conditions of prerenal acute kidney disease). Metformin is not a cause of AKI in this case but would need to be discontinued at this time because of the risk of lactic acidosis in a patient with decreased kidney function (serum creatinine > 1.4 mg/dL in females and > 1.5 mg/dL in males).

3. **C.** There is some evidence that metolazone is beneficial in patients with kidney disease and a GFR < 30 mL/min. This benefit is not the case with other thiazide or thiazide-like diuretics or with potassium-sparing diuretics. Metolazone is frequently used in combination with loop diuretics for this reason.

4. **D.** Metabolic acidosis is a common secondary complication of AKI. Other electrolyte abnormalities include hyperkalemia and hyperphosphatemia. Sodium disorders are usually caused by other concomitant disorders, but not by AKI alone.

5. **D.** Intrinsic AKI is generally characterized by the presence of granular casts (indicating structural damage), a fractional excretion of sodium > 1, and a urine osmolality similar to that of plasma osmolality (indicating changes in concentrating ability of the kidney).

6. **C.** A patient with AKI generally requires aggressive diuresis (while avoiding dehydration). Bumetanide is a loop diuretic that is more potent than a thiazide-like diuretic (metolazone) or a potassium-sparing diuretic (spironolactone) and would be a rational choice for initial therapy of AKI. Spironolactone may cause hyperkalemia in a patient with AKI. Mannitol is an osmotic diuretic that may cause volume depletion and requires more aggressive monitoring and is not indicated.

7. **D.** Aminoglycoside-induced nephrotoxicity is characterized by a delay in changes in serum creatinine (approximately 5–7 days) and relatively normal urine output (nonoliguria).

8. **D.** Angiotensin-converting enzyme inhibitors may contribute to development of AKI in patients with conditions resulting in prerenal kidney disease (e.g., conditions resulting in decreased perfusion of the kidney, hypovolemia, heart failure, liver disease, and so forth). ACEIs (and ARBs) prevent the compensatory vasoconstriction of the efferent arteriole mediated by angiotensin II that occurs in an attempt to increase GFR.

9. **C.** Using the Cockcroft–Gault equation to estimate creatinine clearance, one finds that this patient has an estimated creatinine clearance of 47 mL/min. For females, multiply the calculated value by 0.85.

$$CrCl = \frac{(140 - age)(BW\ in\ kg)}{72 \times SCr(mg/dL)}$$

$$BW(kg) = 176\ lbs/2.2 = 80\ kg$$

$$SCr = 2.2\ mg/dL$$

10. **D.** This patient's estimated creatinine clearance determined using the Cockcroft–Gault equation is 26 mL/min, classified as stage 4 (G4) CKD (GFR 15–29 mL/min/1.73 m²), with the result multiplied by 0.85 for a female. *Note:* The estimated GFR determined using the Modification of Diet in Renal Disease equation is 25 mL/min/1.73m².

$$CrCl = \frac{(140 - age)(BW\ in\ kg)}{72 \times SCr(mg/dL)}$$

11. **C.** The recommended blood pressure for this patient is < 130/80 mm Hg because she has stage 4 (G4) CKD and her albumin excretion ratio is > 300 mg/day.

12. **D.** A single agent (either an ACEI or an ARB) is recommended. Although ACEIs and ARBs

are advocated for patients with CKD, diabetes, and albuminuria to delay disease progression, combination therapy has not consistently shown added benefit and significantly increases the risk of hyperkalemia and hypertension. Therefore, combination therapy with ACEIs and ARBs is not recommended. A warning also exists of the possible risks when using aliskiren in combination with ACEIs and ARBs in patients with diabetes or renal impairment. The labeling for aliskiren-containing products includes a warning against the use of aliskiren with ACEIs or ARBs in patients with diabetes because of the risk of renal impairment, hypotension, and hyperkalemia and a warning to avoid use of these combinations in patients with moderate to severe renal impairment (i.e., when GFR < 60 mL/min).

13. **D.** ESAs including epoetin alfa and darbepoetin alfa work in the bone marrow to stimulate differentiation of erythroid progenitor stem cells and result in an increase in red blood cell production (increase erythrocytes).

14. **C.** The half-life of darbepoetin alfa is three times longer than that of epoetin alfa, giving this agent the added benefit of reduced frequency of administration.

15. **B.** Hypertension is the most common adverse effect in patients receiving ESAs.

16. **B.** Stimulation of erythropoiesis by epoetin alfa and darbepoetin alfa occurs immediately; however, at least 2–4 weeks will pass before substantial changes in hemoglobin and hematocrit are observed as a result of any change in dose of ESA therapy.

17. **C.** This patient is iron deficient, as indicated by his low serum ferritin (< 100 ng/mL) and transferrin saturation (< 20%). No change in epoetin alfa should be made until the iron deficiency is corrected (this is the leading cause of resistance to epoetin alfa and darbepoetin alfa therapy). This patient will require a full course of iron (1 g administered IV in divided doses with each dialysis session) as opposed to a maintenance dose, which should be administered once the patient is iron replete. Sodium ferric gluconate may be administered in doses of 125 mg per dialysis session for eight sessions to give the total 1 g dose (iron sucrose would be administered in 100 mg increments over 10 hemodialysis

sessions). Ferumoxytol would be administered as two 510 mg doses given 3–8 days apart. Absorption of oral iron is poor, making IV iron preferred in this hemodialysis patient.

18. **B.** Active vitamin D (calcitriol) promotes absorption of both calcium and phosphorus in the GI tract. This is one reason that therapy with calcitriol or a vitamin D analog may need to be withheld if the calcium × phosphorus product is elevated.

19. **A.** Lanthanum carbonate or sevelamer carbonate (Renvela) is preferred over a calcium-containing binder for initial management because this patient has a corrected calcium of 10.2 mg/dL [corrected calcium = measured serum calcium + 0.8 × (normal serum albumin − measured serum albumin)] and a calcium × phosphorus product of 75 mg^2/dL^2. This elevated product increases the risk of metastatic calcifications. She requires a phosphorus-binding agent without calcium to minimize calcium absorbed in the GI tract. Aluminum is not preferred because of the risk of accumulation and adverse effects.

20. **B.** Phosphate binders should be taken with meals to minimize systemic absorption of phosphorus from the GI tract.

21. **A.** Active vitamin D (calcitriol) and vitamin D analogs (paricalcitol and doxercalciferol) may worsen hypercalcemia in this patient through increased GI absorption and are not recommended until the calcium levels are lowered. Cinacalcet works to decrease secretion of PTH and does not cause hypercalcemia (there is a risk of hypocalcemia). This agent is approved only in patients with CKD on dialysis so would be appropriate in this case. Vitamin D should be considered when this patient's calcium levels are within the normal range. Ergocalciferol is a vitamin D precursor that requires activation by the kidney and would not be recommended as the sole vitamin D agent for a patient with stage 5 (G5) CKD without the necessary activity of the enzyme in the kidney (1α-hydroxylase) responsible for final conversion to the active form. Ergocalciferol would also carry the risk of hypercalcemia if converted to the active form.

22. **B.** The calcimimetic agent cinacalcet (Sensipar) works by binding with the calcium-sensing

receptor on the parathyroid gland and increases the sensitivity of this receptor to calcium, thereby suppressing secretion of PTH.

23. **D.** Drug characteristics that make an agent more likely to be removed by dialysis include low protein binding, small volume of distribution, and low molecular weight. Among the choices given, the agent that best meets these criteria is choice D, which has a high fraction unbound in the plasma and a low volume of distribution.

24. **B.** Empiric therapy should include antibiotics with Gram-positive and Gram-negative coverage. Choice B is most appropriate.

25. **B.** Nephrocaps include water-soluble vitamins (vitamin B complex + vitamin C + folic acid) recommended for a patient with kidney failure. Supplementation with fat-soluble vitamins is not recommended in patients with kidney failure because of toxicities associated with accumulation.

20-7. References

ACT Investigators. Acetylcysteine for prevention of renal outcomes in patients undergoing coronary and peripheral vascular angiography. *Circulation.* 2011;124:1250–59.

Cunningham J, Zehnder D. New vitamin D analogs and changing therapeutic paradigms. *Kidney Int.* 2011;79:702–7.

Dager W, Halilovic J. Acute kidney injury. In: DiPiro J, Talbert RL, Yee CG, et al., eds. *Pharmacotherapy: A Pathophysiologic Approach.* 9th ed. New York, NY: McGraw-Hill; 2014:611–32.

Eknoyan G, Levin A, Levin NW. Bone metabolism and disease in chronic kidney disease. *Am J Kidney Dis.* 2003;42(4 suppl 3):S1–201 [K/DOQI Clinical Practice Guidelines for Bone Metabolism and Disease].

Ernst ME. Use of diuretics in patients with hypertension. *N Engl J Med.* 2009;361:2153–64.

Himmelfarb J, Ikizler TA. Hemodialysis. *N Engl J Med.* 2010;363:1833–45.

Hudson JQ, Wazny LD. Chronic kidney disease. In: DiPiro JT, Talbert RL, Yee CG, et al., eds. *Pharmacotherapy: A Pathophysiologic Approach.* 9th ed. New York, NY: McGraw-Hill; 2014: 633–63.

KDIGO (Kidney Disease: Improving Global Outcomes) Chronic Kidney Disease Work Group. KDIGO 2012 clinical practice guideline for the evaluation and management of chronic kidney disease. *Kidney Int Suppl.* 2013;3:1–150.

KDIGO Acute Kidney Injury Work Group. KDIGO clinical practice guideline for acute kidney injury. *Kidney Int Suppl.* 2012;2(1):1–138.

KDIGO Chronic Kidney Disease–Mineral and Bone Disorder Work Group. KDIGO clinical practice guideline for the diagnosis, evaluation, prevention, and treatment of chronic kidney disease-mineral and bone disorder (CKD-MBD). *Kidney Int Suppl.* 2009;76(suppl 113): S1–130.

KDIGO Anemia Work Group. KDIGO clinical practice guideline for anemia in chronic kidney disease. *Kidney Int Suppl.* 2012;2(4):279–335.

Lameire NH, Bagga A, Cruz D, et al. Acute kidney injury: An increasing global concern. *Lancet.* 2013;382(9887):170–79.

Li PK, Szeto CC, Piraino B, et al. Peritoneal dialysis-related infections recommendations: 2010 update. *Perit Dial Int.* 2010;30(4):393–423.

Mannis BJ, Tonelli M. The new FDA labeling for ESA—Implications for patients and providers. *Clin J Am Soc Nephrol.* 2012;7:348–53.

National Kidney Foundation. NKF-KDOQI clinical practice guidelines for chronic kidney disease: Evaluation, classification, and stratification. *Am J Kidney Dis.* 2002;39(suppl 1):S1–266.

National Kidney Foundation. KDOQI clinical practice guidelines and clinical practice recommendations for anemia in chronic kidney disease. *Am J Kidney Dis.* 2006;47(5 suppl 3): S1–145.

National Kidney Foundation. KDOQI clinical practice guidelines for anemia of chronic kidney disease: 2007 update of hemoglobin target. *Am J Kidney Dis.* 2007;50(3):471–530.

Nolin TD, Himmelfarb J. Drug-induced kidney disease. In: DiPiro J, Talbert RL, Yee CG, et al., eds. *Pharmacotherapy: A Pathophysiologic Approach.* 9th ed. New York, NY: McGraw-Hill; 2014: 687–704.

U.S. Renal Data System. *USRDS 2013 Annual Data Report: Atlas of End-Stage Renal Disease in the United States.* Bethesda, MD: National Institutes of Health, National Institute of Diabetes and Digestive and Kidney Diseases, Bethesda, MD; 2013.

Critical Care, Fluids, and Electrolytes

G. Christopher Wood

21-1. Key Points

- Appropriate sedation and analgesia are essential because pain and agitation are common in critically ill patients. Drug selection should be based on clinical guidelines and patient parameters.
- Because benzodiazepines may be related to delirium, there is a new emphasis on avoiding benzodiazepines. Newer antipsychotics are now suggested for delirium treatment. Dexmedetomidine (Precedex) is an important new treatment option.
- Pain, agitation, and delirium should be monitored using the recommended assessment tools.
- Neuromuscular blocking (NMB) agents should be used only after sedation and analgesia have been maximized.
- NMB agents should be monitored using peripheral nerve stimulation in addition to observation of clinical signs and symptoms.
- Appropriate stress ulcer prophylaxis is recommended for patients with one or more risk factors.
- Intracranial pressure (ICP) and cerebral perfusion pressure (CPP) should be optimized using drug and nondrug therapies after severe traumatic brain injury. Phenytoin is effective at preventing early post-traumatic seizures.
- Severe sepsis and septic shock are progressions of sepsis. Therapy includes hemodynamic stabilization, appropriate antimicrobial agents, and removal of infectious foci, if possible.
- New recommendations in the Surviving Sepsis Guidelines include the selection of resuscitation fluids, amount of initial fluid therapy, selection of vasopressors, changes in suggestions for corticosteroid use, and use of serum lactate as a marker of resuscitation.
- Maintaining adequate fluid status is vital to maintaining tissue perfusion and organ function. However, many clinical factors can affect fluid and electrolyte status in critically ill patients. Finding and treating underlying causes of fluid and electrolyte abnormalities are essential.
- Fluid and electrolyte abnormalities are generally asymptomatic unless severe.
- Fluid and electrolyte therapy should be monitored closely because of patient instability and the risk of iatrogenic abnormalities (e.g., cardiac arrhythmias, fluid overload).

21-2. Study Guide Checklist

The following topics may guide your study of this subject area:

- Appropriate assessment tools for pain, agitation, and delirium
- Appropriate drug selection for pain, agitation, and delirium based on patient factors
- Treatment options for intracranial hypertension in patients with traumatic brain injury (TBI)
- Seizure prophylaxis in patients with TBI
- Risk factors for stress ulcers and appropriate prophylaxis
- Major points regarding initial therapy in severe sepsis or septic shock
- Appropriate selection of vasopressors or inotropes in severe sepsis or septic shock

- Appropriate use of corticosteroids in severe sepsis or septic shock
- Severe, life-threatening electrolyte disorders and appropriate treatments

21-3. Sedation, Analgesia, and Neuromuscular Blockade

Definition and Classifications

- *Pain:* Critically ill patients may experience acute pain, chronic pain, or both.
- *Anxiety or agitation:* Patients may experience psychophysiological response to real or imagined danger. The term *agitation* is used in this chapter.
- *ICU delirium:* Patients may experience delirium in the intensive care unit (ICU). See discussion of clinical presentation. The term *delirium* is used in this chapter.

Clinical Presentation

- The presentation of pain, agitation, or both in patients with impaired consciousness may include pulling of tubes or lines, writhing, kicking, restlessness, hypertension, tachycardia, tachypnea, diaphoresis, or moaning.
- The presentation of delirium is an acute change or fluctuation of mental status with any of the following: (1) inattention, (2) disorganized thinking, or (3) an altered level of consciousness. Patients can be hyperactive (agitated) or hypoactive (lethargic) or fluctuate between both states.

Pathophysiology

- Many states can lead to pain, agitation, or delirium including (1) injuries, (2) medical procedures and equipment (e.g., mechanical ventilation equipment or catheters), (3) mental status changes (e.g., fear, infection, hypoxia, sleep deprivation, or adverse drug effects or withdrawal), or (4) pre-existing medical conditions (e.g., chronic pain).

Diagnostic Criteria

- In patients who can communicate, pain can be self-reported. In patients who cannot communicate, pain should be assessed using the Behavioral Pain Scale (BPS) or the Critical-Care Pain Observation Tool (CPOT).
- Agitation should be assessed using the Richmond Sedation and Agitation Scale (RASS) or the Riker Sedation–Agitation Scale (SAS).
- Delirium should be assessed using the Confusion Assessment Method for the ICU (CAM-ICU) scale or the Intensive Care Delirium Screening Checklist (ICDSC).

Treatment Goals

- Treatment goals include (1) finding and removing the cause of pain, agitation, and delirium, and (2) achieving a balance between patient comfort, adverse effects, and ability to provide care. Avoiding benzodiazepines in favor of analgesia-only therapy, dexmedetomidine, or propofol may decrease the risk of delirium.
- The treatment of delirium is unclear. Formerly, haloperidol was recommended. However, the new Society of Critical Care Medicine (SCCM) guidelines suggest using newer antipsychotic agents rather than haloperidol. There are no high-quality data to guide drug selection for ICU delirium.
- Neuromuscular blocking (NMB) agents should be reserved for patients whose agitation is not controlled with maximum doses of sedation and analgesia.

Drug Therapy

Selected drug therapy is described in Table 21-1.

Mechanism of action

- *Opiates, nonsteroidal anti-inflammatory drugs (NSAIDs):* See Chapter 27 on pain management.
- *Benzodiazepines, antipsychotics:* See Chapter 29 on psychiatric disease.
- *Propofol (Diprivan):* The exact mechanism of action is unknown but may involve γ-aminobutyric acid (GABA) receptors.
- *Dexmedetomidine (Precedex):* Dexmedetomidine is a centrally acting alpha$_2$ adrenergic agonist.
- *NMB agents:* NMB agents act as cholinergic receptor antagonists; they do not provide analgesia or sedation. A recent important study suggested that 48 hours of NMB therapy was beneficial in patients with acute respiratory distress syndrome (ARDS).

Table 21-1. Selected Drug Therapy Based on Guidelines for Use in ICU Patients

Generic name	Trade name	Dosage range	Forms[a]	Schedule[b]	Notes on usage
Morphine sulfate		0.5–10 mg	IV, IM, po	Continuous; q6h	General opiate of choice
Hydromorphone	Dilaudid	0.3–1.5 mg	IV	Continuous; q6h	Used in morphine intolerance, hemodynamic instability, renal dysfunction
Fentanyl	Sublimaze	50–200 mcg/h	IV	Continuous	Used in morphine intolerance, hemodynamic instability, renal dysfunction
Acetaminophen	Ofirmev, Tylenol	Up to 4 g/day	po, PR, IV	q4–6h	NSAIDs may be added to opiates
Ibuprofen	Advil, Caldolor	100–800 mg	po, IV	q4–6h	Maximum 3,200 mg/day
Ketorolac	Toradol	10–30 mg	IV, IM, po	q6h	Maximum use 5 days
Lorazepam	Ativan	0.5–4 mg	IV, po	Continuous; q6h	Longer acting than midazolam
Midazolam	Versed	1–5 mg	IV	Continuous; q2h	Shorter acting than lorazepam
Propofol	Diprivan	1–5 mg/kg/h	IV	Continuous	Used when rapid awakening needed
Dexmedetomidine	Precedex	0.2–0.7 mcg/kg/h	IV	Continuous	Monitor for hypotension, bradycardia
Pancuronium	Pavulon	0.05–0.1 mg/kg	IV	Continuous; q2h	General NMB agent of choice (low cost); causes tachycardia, is longer acting
Vecuronium	Norcuron	0.05–0.1 mg/kg	IV	Continuous; q1h	Used in hemodynamic instability, renal dysfunction, cardiac disease
Rocuronium	Zemuron	0.6–1.2 mg/kg	IV	Continuous; q30 min	
Cisatracurium	Nimbex	0.05–0.1 mg/kg	IV	Continuous; q1h	Used in renal and hepatic dysfunction

Boldface indicates one of top 100 drugs for 2012 by units sold at retail outlets, www.drugs.com/stats/top100/2012/units.
a. Long-acting drugs and dosage forms generally are not used in ICU (e.g., fentanyl patch, controlled-release morphine, doxacurium).
b. Continuous analgesia and sedation with frequent titration (patient-controlled analgesia pump, IV infusion, or scheduled) are preferred to prn therapy alone. NMB agents used prn are preferred.

Patient instructions

When patient-controlled analgesia pumps are used, make sure the patient understands how to activate the device.

Adverse drug events

- *Opiates, NSAIDs:* See Chapter 27 on pain management.
- *Benzodiazepines, antipsychotics:* See Chapter 29 on psychiatric disease.
- *Propofol (Diprivan):* Adverse events include respiratory depression, hypotension, and hypertriglyceridemia. Propofol infusion syndrome (e.g., metabolic acidosis, rhabdomyolysis, and cardiac dysfunction) may occur at high doses (> 5 mg/kg/h for > 48 h). Thus, the maximum dose is 5 mg/kg/h.
- *Dexmedetomidine (Precedex):* The most common adverse events are hypotension and bradycardia; however, respiratory depression is less likely than with other agents.

- *NMB agents:* Adverse events include respiratory depression, prolonged weakness or paralysis after discontinuation, and tachycardia with pancuronium.

Drug interactions

- *Opiates, NSAIDs:* See Chapter 27 on pain management.
- *Benzodiazepines, antipsychotics:* See Chapter 29 on psychiatric disease.
- *Propofol (Diprivan), dexmedetomidine (Precedex):* Actions are potentiated by other sedatives.
- *NMB agents:* Actions are potentiated by corticosteroids, aminoglycosides, clindamycin, calcium channel blockers, and anesthetics; actions are inhibited by anticholinesterase inhibitors (e.g., neostigmine).

Parameters to monitor

- *Opiates, NSAIDs:* Use self-reporting if possible, or BPS or CPOT if unable to communicate. Monitor vital signs, but do not use alone for assessment. Also see Chapter 27 on pain management.

- *Sedative agents:* Use RASS or SAS. Monitor vital signs. Also see Chapter 29 on psychiatric disease. For propofol (Diprivan), also monitor serum triglycerides at baseline and one to two times per week during long-term use.
- *Antipsychotics:* Use CAM-ICU or ICDSC. Also see Chapter 29 on psychiatric disease.
- *NMB agents:* Monitor movement and breathing. Also monitor blood pressure (BP), heart rate (HR), and intracranial pressure (ICP) (acute increases may indicate suboptimal sedation or analgesia). Use peripheral nerve stimulation ("train of four" monitoring).
- *Note:* In patients with continuous sedation, a daily awakening and assessment period results in decreased sedative use and a shorter length of stay in the ICU.

Kinetics

- *Opiates, NSAIDs:* See Chapter 27 on pain management.
- *Benzodiazepines, antipsychotics:* See Chapter 29 on psychiatric disease.
- *Propofol (Diprivan):* Propofol is highly lipophilic (may accumulate over the long term), has a rapid onset (1 minute), and has a short duration (about 10 minutes). It is hepatically cleared.
- *Dexmedetomidine (Precedex):* Dexmedetomidine is hepatically cleared and has a short onset (minutes) and half-life (about 2 hours).
- *NMB agents:* Onset for all NMB agents is < 5 minutes. Duration is 60–90 minutes for pancuronium and 30–60 minutes for vecuronium and cisatracurium. Excretion of pancuronium is mostly renal; for vecuronium, it is about 50:50 (hepatic:renal). Excretion of cisatracurium is not organ dependent.

Other aspects

Propofol (Diprivan) is in a lipid vehicle that provides 1 kcal/mL. Avoid overfeeding. It should be used with caution in patients with egg allergy. It is a potential growth medium for bacteria; the maximum hang time for a bottle is 12 hours.

New IV formulations

Intravenous (IV) formulations of acetaminophen and ibuprofen are now available.

21-4. Traumatic Brain Injury

Definition

Traumatic brain injury (TBI) is defined as neurologic deficit secondary to brain trauma.

Classifications

- Severe
- Mild or moderate

Clinical Presentation

- Use the Glasgow Coma Scale (GCS) for assessment: sum of eye, motor, and verbal scores (range 3 to 15).
- TBI has a wide range of presentation from mild confusion to totally nonresponsive coma.

Pathophysiology

- TBI results from motor vehicle accidents (most common), falls and accidents, assaults, and gunshot wounds. It is most common in the 15- to 24-year-old age group. Every year in the United States, there are 375,000 TBI cases and 75,000 deaths.
- TBI consists of direct neuronal damage ± edema ± secondary ischemia-related neuronal death.

Diagnostic Criteria

- The following are used for diagnosis: (1) computed tomography (CT) scan, (2) GCS, and (3) ICP monitoring in severe patients (GCS score 3–8).

Treatment Goals

- Treatment goals include keeping ICP < 20 mm Hg and cerebral perfusion pressure (CPP) > 50 mm Hg (CPP = mean arterial pressure − ICP) and preventing seizures.

Strategies to decrease ICP

- Osmotic agents and diuretics
  - Mannitol 0.25–1 g/kg IV q4–6h
  - Hypertonic NaCl IV (e.g., 3%, 7.5%) IV q4–6h
  - Loop diuretics IV (e.g., furosemide)

- Sedation
  - Short-acting agents are preferred to allow frequent patient assessment (e.g., propofol, fentanyl).
  - Pentobarbital (1–3 mg/kg/h IV) is a long-acting agent for refractory intracranial hypertension.
- NMB agents: A short-acting agent is preferred and is used only for refractory intracranial hypertension.

Nondrug interventions

- Raising of the head of the bed (30 degrees)
- Ventricular drainage of cerebrospinal fluid via ventriculostomy
- Mild or moderate hyperventilation (pCO_2 30–35 mm Hg)
- Surgery

Strategies to increase mean arterial pressure

- Maximize fluid status. The overall goal is euvolemia.
- Vasopressors and inotropes may be used in shock after fluid status is optimized.

Seizure prevention

- Seizure prevention may be started on the basis of severity and type of injury.
- Phenytoin (Dilantin, generic) can be used: 20 mg/kg IV loading dose plus 4–8 mg/kg/day for 7 days.
  - Continue beyond 7 days if the patient has a seizure after the immediate postinjury period.
  - Alternative agents include levetiracetam (Keppra) or carbamazepine (limited data for both).
- See Chapter 28 on seizure disorders for the mechanism of action, adverse drug events, drug interactions, and kinetics.

Parameters to monitor

The overall goal is CPP > 50 mm Hg and ICP < 20 mm Hg. Drug classes are covered elsewhere.

Other Aspects

Nimodipine (Nimotop) is a calcium channel blocker given for 21 days. It is indicated for treating aneurysmal subarachnoid hemorrhage. It may also provide some benefit in traumatic subarachnoid hemorrhage.

21-5. Acute Spinal Cord Injury

Note: High-dose methylprednisolone is no longer recommended for acute spinal cord injury.

21-6. Venous Thromboembolism Prophylaxis

Note: See Chapter 41 on thromboembolic disease.

21-7. Stress Ulcer Prophylaxis

Definition

Stress ulcer prophylaxis refers to gastrointestinal (GI) mucosal damage related to metabolic stress in the ICU.

Clinical Presentation

Presentation is similar to that of peptic ulcer disease (see Chapter 25 on gastrointestinal diseases).

Pathophysiology

Shunting of blood from the GI tract to vital organs during critical illness results in breakdown of gastric mucosal defenses (e.g., bicarbonate and mucus production, epithelial cell turnover).

Risk Factors

- The primary risk factors are mechanical ventilation > 48 hours and coagulopathy.
- Other risk factors include disease states or organ dysfunction where GI perfusion may be compromised (e.g., sepsis, burns, TBI, renal failure).

Diagnostic Criteria

Diagnosis is based on signs and symptoms and can be confirmed with endoscopy.

Treatment Goals

The goal is to prevent stress ulcers.

Drug Therapy

- See Chapter 25 on gastrointestinal diseases for full drug information and treatment of ulcers that develop (stress ulcers are treated similarly to peptic ulcers). Patients in the ICU should be given stress ulcer prophylaxis if they have a risk factor listed above.

■ Proton pump inhibitors (PPIs) are a primary option. Most studies of stress ulcer prophylaxis have shown PPIs and histamine 2–receptor antagonists (H2RAs) to be equivalent; however, a recent meta-analysis suggests that PPIs are more effective. Thus, PPIs may be preferred, but this is still controversial. Another unresolved issue is concern about the association between outpatient use of PPIs with increased rates of community-acquired pneumonia and *Clostridium difficile*–associated diarrhea.

■ H2RAs are still widely considered to be a primary option. They are more effective than sucralfate for this indication and may have fewer epidemiological concerns than PPIs (see previous item).

■ Sucralfate is a secondary option that has fallen out of favor. It is less effective than H2RAs, is not available in IV form, and has significant drug-binding interactions.

■ Antacids are not recommended. They are less effective, have higher aspiration risk, and require frequent dosing.

■ Optimal duration of therapy is unknown. A reasonable approach is to discontinue prophylaxis when risk factors have resolved or upon transfer from the ICU.

21-8. Severe Sepsis and Septic Shock

Definition and Classifications

Severe sepsis is sepsis (see Chapter 33 on infectious disease) plus dysfunction of one or more major organs (e.g., hypotension responsive to fluids, oliguria, acute mental status change, lactic acidosis, respiratory insufficiency, coagulopathy).

Septic shock is severe sepsis plus hypotension that is not fully responsive to fluids (i.e., requires vasopressor therapy).

Clinical Presentation

See sepsis criteria (in Chapter 33) and the definitions of severe sepsis and septic shock.

Pathophysiology

Progression is seen in the systemic manifestations of sepsis. Imbalances in the inflammatory, immune, and coagulation systems lead to organ hypoperfusion and organ dysfunction with or without refractory hypotension. See Chapter 33 on infectious disease for typical causative organisms by site of infection.

Diagnostic Criteria

See sepsis criteria (in Chapter 33) and the definitions of severe sepsis and septic shock.

Treatment Goals

■ A primary treatment goal is to use "goal-directed therapy" to rapidly stabilize hemodynamic parameters (mean arterial pressure [MAP] > 65 mm Hg, urine output > 0.5 ml/kg/h) and reverse organ dysfunction and elevated serum lactate within 6 hours.

■ Concurrently, collect appropriate cultures based on the suspected site of infection, start appropriate antimicrobial therapy within 1 hour, and eliminate the source of infection if applicable (e.g., vascular or urinary catheter, abscess). The duration of antimicrobial therapy is typically 7–10 days depending on the site of infection and type of organism.

■ Modulate inflammatory, coagulation, and hormonal derangements if applicable.

Drug and Nondrug Therapy

See Chapter 33 on infectious disease for antimicrobial information (mechanism of action, dosing, adverse effects, etc.) and empiric antimicrobial selection. Definitive therapy should be streamlined to a narrower spectrum agent, if possible, on the basis of the final culture and sensitivity reports.

See Section 21-9 for details on fluid therapy. Initial fluid therapy for severe sepsis and septic shock should be 30 ml/kg of isotonic crystalloids (0.9% NaCl or lactated Ringer's [LR] solution). Albumin can be given as a secondary fluid in patients requiring high doses of crystalloids. Other colloids (e.g., hetastarches) are no longer recommended because of the risk of acute kidney insufficiency. Vasopressors should be used only after appropriate fluid therapy fails to adequately normalize BP (Table 21-2). Inotropes can be used if cardiac index is poor following adequate fluid resuscitation.

Table 21-2. Vasopressors[a] and Inotropes Used in Severe Sepsis and Septic Shock

Name	Dosage range	Adrenergic-receptor activity	Comments
Dopamine	< 5 mcg/kg/min	Increased renal perfusion (dopaminergic receptors)	Use of low-dose "renal tonic" dopamine is not recommended. Only use if increased β_1 activity is needed.
	5–10 mcg/kg/min	Increased cardiac output/HR (β_1) > increased BP (α_1)	
	10–20 mcg/kg/min	Increased cardiac output/HR and BP	
Norepinephrine	0.01–3 mcg/kg/min	Increased BP (α_1) > increased cardiac output/HR (β_1)	Preferred agent; fewer arrhythmias than with dopamine
Epinephrine	0.01–0.5 mcg/kg/min	Increased cardiac output/HR and BP (all receptors)	Second-line agent
Phenylephrine	0.01–5 mcg/kg/min	Increased BP only (α_1)	Use only in selected patients.
Dobutamine	5–20 mcg/kg/min	Increased cardiac output/HR (β_1)	
Vasopressin	0.01–0.04 units/min (0.03 most studied)	None; acts on vasopressin receptors	Add to catecholamine vasopressor in nonresponsive patients. Do not exceed maximum dose.

a. All catecholamine vasopressors are given as continuous IV infusions and are titrated to effect.

Mechanism of action

■ Vasopressors and inotropes are adrenergic-receptor agonists.

Adverse drug events

■ *Vasopressors and inotropes:* Adverse events include tachycardia, arrhythmias, organ and extremity ischemia, and hypertension. Norepinephrine causes fewer arrhythmias than dopamine. Thus, norepinephrine is now the preferred first-line vasopressor for most patients.

Drug–drug interactions

■ *Vasopressors and inotropes:* None

Parameters to monitor

■ *Vasopressors and inotropes:* Monitor BP, HR, cardiac output, urine output, and extremity perfusion on physical exam.

Other aspects

Hydrocortisone

Low-dose hydrocortisone (200 mg/day IV infusion × 7 days) is recommended for patients with septic shock who are not responsive to fluids and vasopressors. Patients with a poor response to cosyntropin stimulation testing (serum cortisol increase of < 9 mcg/dL) may respond better to corticosteroid supplementation. Hydrocortisone may be tapered sooner than day 7 of treatment if vasopressors are discontinued.

Vasopressin

Vasopressin infusion (0.03 units/min) may be used to increase BP in patients refractory to high doses of traditional vasopressors. Doses > 0.04 units/min are associated with severe adverse events (e.g., cardiac arrest). Patients receiving lower doses of catecholamine vasopressors (i.e., < 15 mcg/min of norepinephrine) may benefit more from vasopressin than do patients on higher doses of norepinephrine.

Prevention of ventilator-associated pneumonia

Oral chlorhexidine is suggested to reduce the risk of ventilator-associated pneumonia (VAP) in critically ill patients with severe sepsis or septic shock.

Miscellaneous therapies

The following therapies are not recommended in severe sepsis or critical illness: (1) treatment with selenium, immunoglobulins, or sodium bicarbonate (unless pH < 7.15), and (2) erythropoietin (unless already used for another indication).

21-9. Fluid and Electrolyte Abnormalities in Critically Ill Patients

See also Chapter 20 on kidney disorders (for hyperphosphatemia), Chapter 22 on nutrition, and Chapter 23 on oncology (for hypercalcemia).

Definition

Fluid and electrolyte abnormalities are pathologic alterations in fluid and electrolyte homeostasis.

Classifications

Fluid and electrolyte abnormalities are classified by electrolyte (see the discussion on clinical presentation).

Clinical Presentation

In all cases, mild to moderate abnormalities are usually asymptomatic.

Sodium (normal range: 135–145 mEq/L)

In cases of hyponatremia or hypernatremia, conditions including lethargy, nausea, headache, dry mucous membranes, poor skin turgor (depends on hydration status), and confusion may occur.

Coma, seizures, or central pontine myelinolysis may occur in severe hyponatremia or if sodium increases or decreases rapidly (> 12 mEq/L/day).

Chloride (normal range: 96–106 mEq/L)

Symptoms are related to acid–base or fluid abnormalities, not chloride itself.

Water (moves osmotically with sodium)

In cases of dehydration, conditions including dry mucous membranes, poor skin turgor, lethargy, nausea, headache, hypotension, and tachycardia occur. Seizures, coma, or death can result if dehydration is severe. Decreased urine output, metabolic acidosis, and hypotension are also found.

For edema or fluid overload, see Chapter 13 on heart failure.

Potassium (normal range: 3.5–5 mEq/L)

In cases of hypokalemia, conditions including confusion, muscle cramps, weakness, and cardiac arrhythmias occur.

In cases of hyperkalemia, conditions including muscle cramps, weakness, and cardiac arrhythmias occur.

Magnesium (normal range: 1.5–2.2 mEq/L)

With hypomagnesemia, presentation is similar to that of hypocalcemia.

In cases of hypermagnesemia, conditions including lethargy, weakness, and cardiac arrhythmias occur. Coma is possible in severe cases.

Phosphorus (normal range: 2.6–4.5 mg/dL)

In cases of hypophosphatemia, conditions including confusion, anxiety, weakness, respiratory depression, paresthesias, and lethargy occur. Seizures and coma are possible if hypophosphatemia is severe.

For hyperphosphatemia, see Chapter 20 on kidney disease.

Calcium (normal range: 8.5–10.5 mg/dL)

In cases of hypocalcemia, conditions including confusion, anxiety, paresthesias, muscle cramps, and tetany occur. Coma and cardiac arrhythmias may occur in severe cases.

For hypercalcemia, see Chapter 23 on oncology.

Pathophysiology

Normal distribution of fluids and electrolytes

- Electrolytes with high serum concentrations are primarily extracellular (Na, Cl); those with low serum concentrations are mostly intracellular or in bone (K, P, Mg, Ca).
- Total body water is approximately 60–70% of total body weight (differs by age, gender, disease states).
  - Of all water, intracellular is approximately two-thirds; extracellular is approximately one-third.
  - Of extracellular water, approximately three-fourths is interstitial; approximately one-fourth is intravascular (plasma).
- Typical fluid requirements for adults are approximately 35 mL/kg/day; they can be much higher in critical illness because of extrarenal losses (GI tract, wounds) and fluid shifts (trauma, sepsis).
- Primary hormonal controls are aldosterone (sodium retention) and antidiuretic hormone (water retention).

Hyponatremia

The first three forms of hyponatremia listed below are hypotonic:

- *Hypovolemic (sodium and water loss):* This condition is characterized by high urine osmolality. It is related to extrarenal fluid losses (GI, wounds), diuretics, and adrenal insufficiency.
- *Euvolemic (moderate water retention):* This condition occurs with syndrome of inappropriate antidiuretic hormone (SIADH) release, renal failure, carbamazepine, NSAIDs, and chlorpropamide.
- *Hypervolemic (sodium and water retention):* This condition occurs with congestive heart failure, cirrhosis, nephrotic syndrome, and glucocorticoids.
- *Hypertonic:* This condition is the dilutional effect of abnormal osmotic agents in the vasculature (severe hyperglycemia).

Hypernatremia

Hypernatremia occurs in cases of water loss or excessive sodium intake (e.g., from IV fluids). It is related to extrarenal fluid losses (GI, wounds) and diabetes insipidus.

Hypochloremia

Hypochloremia occurs with GI losses.

Hypokalemia

Hypokalemia is related to diuretics, β_2-agonists, amphotericin B, glucocorticoids, cisplatin, and GI losses.

Hyperkalemia

Hyperkalemia is related to renal dysfunction, acidosis, angiotensin-converting enzyme inhibitors, potassium-sparing diuretics, trimethoprim, orally taken salt substitutes, and adrenal insufficiency.

Hypomagnesemia

Hypomagnesemia occurs with GI losses, diuretics, amphotericin B, alcohol, and cisplatin. It should be treated prior to treating hypokalemia; Na/K-ATPase pumps require magnesium to work.

Hypermagnesemia

Hypermagnesemia is related to renal dysfunction, magnesium-containing antacids, adrenal insufficiency, and hyperparathyroidism.

Hypophosphatemia

Hypophosphatemia is related to refeeding syndrome, phosphate binders, diuretics, hypercalcemia, vitamin D deficiency, and glucocorticoids.

Hyperphosphatemia

See Chapter 20 on kidney disease for information about hyperphosphatemia.

Hypocalcemia

Hypocalcemia occurs with hypoparathyroidism, hypomagnesemia, vitamin D deficiency, and loop diuretics. Total calcium is artificially low in hypoalbuminemia (calcium is highly albumin bound).

Diagnostic Criteria

- Criteria include serum concentration, signs, and symptoms.
- Sodium analysis may use urine sodium and urine osmolality.

Treatment Goals

- Find and treat the underlying cause of abnormality.
- Treat abnormality to avoid sequelae.

Drug and Nondrug Therapy

Fluid replacement

Administer fluids as follows:

- *Crystalloids:* Salt solutions—½ or ¼ normal saline (NS) ± dextrose 5% ± KCl 20 mEq/L (approximates urine electrolytes), NS (154 mEq/L of Na), LR solution, ¼ NS, or dextrose 5%—are chosen on the basis of sodium and fluid needs. NS or LR are typically used for fluid resuscitation (sodium is the major osmotic cation in plasma).
- *Colloids:* Albumin 5–25% can be used to provide fluid resuscitation or to raise oncotic pressure (e.g., cirrhosis).
- *Vasopressors ± isotropic activity:* After fluids are optimized, vasopressors ± isotropic activity may be used (see Chapter 13 on heart failure).

Edema

Fluid restriction ± diuretics may be used. See Chapter 13 on heart failure and Chapter 20 on kidney disease.

Hyponatremia

If the case is severe, titrate 3% NaCl to maximum serum sodium increase of 12 mEq/day. Treat specific forms as follows:

- *Hypovolemic:* Replace fluid losses with IV NS (0.9% NaCl, 154 mEq/L).
- *Euvolemic (SIADH):* Use fluid restriction ± demeclocycline. Newer vasopressin antagonists conivaptan (Vaprisol) or tolvaptan (Samsca) can also be used.
- *Hypervolemic:* Use fluid restriction ± diuretics.
- *Hypertonic:* Correct hyperglycemia.

Hypernatremia

Titrate low-sodium fluids (e.g., dextrose 5%, ¼ NS) to a normal serum sodium. In cases of diabetes insipidus, use DDAVP (desmopressin).

Hyperchloremia

Give sodium acetate or LR instead of NS, especially if acidemic (acetate is converted to bicarbonate by the liver).

Hypokalemia

Administer IV (KCl) or po (KCl, K phosphate, or K acetate). Each 10 mEq dose increases serum potassium by about 0.1 mEq/L. IV administration faster than 10 mEq/h requires electrocardiogram monitoring for arrhythmias.

Hyperkalemia

Treat hyperkalemia as follows:

- *Potassium removal (slower onset of action):* Use Na polystyrene sulfonate (Kayexalate) po or PR, loop diuretics, or hemodialysis (if severe).
- *Intracellular potassium shifting (rapid onset of action):* Administer regular insulin + dextrose IV, albuterol, or Na bicarbonate.
- *Potassium antagonism of cardiac effects (rapid onset of action):* Administer IV calcium.

Hypomagnesemia

Dosages are described below. A large percentage of the dose is renally wasted. Repletion requires 3–5 days of treatment.

- *IV:* 0.5–1 mEq/kg/day (8 mEq = 1 g); administration rate = 8 mEq/h

- *IM:* Can give intramuscularly but is painful
- *po:* Magnesium-containing antacid or laxative tid–qid as tolerated or magnesium oxide 300–600 mg bid–qid

Hypermagnesemia

Treat with diuretics, IV calcium, or hemodialysis (similar to hyperkalemia).

Hypophosphatemia

If the case is severe, use IV sodium or potassium phosphate 0.16–0.64 mmol/kg at 7.5 mmol/h to avoid potassium overdose (if potassium phosphate is used), calcium precipitation, or both.

Administer po 1–2 g/day (5–60 mmol/day), for example, Neutra-Phos, Neutra-Phos-K, or Fleet Phospho-soda.

Hyperphosphatemia

See Chapter 20 on kidney disease for information about hyperphosphatemia.

Hypocalcemia

If patient is symptomatic, administer IV calcium gluconate (2–3 g) or IV calcium chloride (1 g) over 10 minutes. In addition, the following may be administered:

- IV infusion of 0.5–2 mg/kg/h of elemental calcium
- Calcium salts such as calcium carbonate (po 1–3 g elemental calcium/day ± vitamin D)

Patient counseling

In cases of po administration, advise patient about potential adverse events.

Adverse drug events

- *Sodium:* Edema or central pontine myelinolysis can occur if serum Na changes rapidly (> 12 mEq/day).
- *Crystalloids:* Vein irritation is possible with hypotonic (¼ NS, ½ NS) or hypertonic (3% NaCl) fluids. Dextrose 5% is approximately isotonic and is often added to low-sodium fluids.
- *Potassium:* Events include cardiac arrhythmias (> 10 mEq/h), vein irritation (IV), GI upset (po; worse with wax matrix controlled-release tablets), and bad taste (po liquid). With sodium

polystyrene sulfonate, constipation may occur (medication is usually mixed with sorbitol).

■ *Magnesium:* Events include diarrhea (po), flushing, sweating (IV), and vein irritation (IV).

■ *Phosphorus:* Events include diarrhea (po) and calcium phosphate precipitation (IV).

■ *Calcium:* IV calcium gluconate is less irritating than calcium chloride. Cardiac dysfunction can occur if medication is administered > 60 mg/min (elemental calcium). Events also include calcium phosphate precipitation (IV) and constipation (po).

Drug interactions

■ Hypokalemia and hypomagnesemia can predispose the patient to digoxin toxicity.

■ Binding of drugs in the GI tract by calcium or magnesium is possible (see Chapter 22 on nutrition).

Parameters to monitor

■ Serum concentrations
■ Resolution of signs and symptoms
■ With fluid replacement, normalization of the following: BP, HR, urine output (goal > 0.5 mL/kg/h), skin turgor, mucous membrane hydration, edema, cardiac output, pulmonary artery wedge pressure (see Chapter 13 on heart failure), serum lactate/base deficit

Other aspects

Glucose control in critically ill patients

Intensive glucose control (80–110 mg/dL) is not beneficial and may be harmful when compared to standard glucose control. Hypoglycemia is common with intensive glucose control. Thus, the current recommendation is to keep serum glucose < 180 mg/dL.

21-10. Questions

1. Which of the following is the most easily titratable opiate for use in the ICU?

   A. Morphine
   B. Hydromorphone
   C. Fentanyl
   D. Acetaminophen
   E. Dexmedetomidine

2. In which situations should hydromorphone or fentanyl be used for analgesia in critically ill patients?

   I. Morphine allergy
   II. Renal dysfunction
   III. Hemodynamic instability

   A. I only
   B. III only
   C. I and II only
   D. II and III only
   E. I, II, and III

3. What is the maximum duration of therapy for ketorolac?

   A. 5 days
   B. 7 days
   C. 14 days
   D. 30 days
   E. There are no restrictions on length of use.

4. Which of the following sedative agents is least likely to cause respiratory depression?

   A. Lorazepam
   B. Propofol
   C. Dexmedetomidine
   D. Midazolam
   E. Fentanyl

5. In most critically ill patients, which of the following is the NMB agent of choice?

   A. Propofol
   B. Vecuronium
   C. Cisatracurium
   D. Pancuronium
   E. Any agent may be used first line.

6. The primary advantage of cisatracurium over pancuronium and vecuronium is that

   A. elimination is not organ dependent.
   B. it has a shorter duration of action.
   C. it has a longer duration of action.
   D. it is more effective.
   E. it does not require monitoring.

7. Which of the following is preferred as a first-line sedative agent for ICP control in patients with TBI?

   A. Pentobarbital
   B. Lorazepam
   C. Propofol

D. Vecuronium

E. Sedation is not recommended for patients with TBI.

8. The regimen of choice for post-traumatic seizure prophylaxis is

   A. phenytoin indefinitely.
   B. phenytoin × 7 days.
   C. carbamazepine × 7 days.
   D. benzodiazepines prn if seizures occur.
   E. levetiracetam × 7 days.

9. Which of the following should be reserved for the treatment of intracranial hypertension that is refractory to initial treatment?

   A. Propofol
   B. Mannitol
   C. Hypertonic saline
   D. Pentobarbital
   E. Phenytoin

10. All of the following are risk factors for the development of stress ulcers *except*

   A. sepsis.
   B. coagulopathy.
   C. mechanical ventilation.
   D. age > 40 years.
   E. burns.

11. Which of the following is correct regarding stress ulcer prophylaxis?

   A. H2RAs or sucralfate are equally effective and considered drugs of choice.
   B. PPIs and H2RAs are generally considered the drugs of choice.
   C. Antacids have the most direct effect on gastric pH and are considered drugs of choice.
   D. Sucralfate is more effective than H2RAs and PPIs.
   E. All agents (H2 antagonists, sucralfate, PPIs, antacids) are equally effective.

12. Which of the following describes appropriate selection of initial resuscitation fluid in severe sepsis or septic shock?

   A. Either crystalloids or colloids are acceptable choices.
   B. Colloids are recommended as a first-line treatment because they have a lower risk of renal failure.

C. Albumin is recommended first; crystalloids may be added if refractory.

D. Crystalloids and albumin should be started together.

E. Crystalloids are recommended first; albumin may be added if refractory.

13. Which of the following describes the appropriate use of hydrocortisone in severe sepsis or septic shock?

   A. Use in all patients with severe sepsis or septic shock.
   B. Use in all patients on vasopressors (i.e., in septic shock).
   C. Use only in patients with documented adrenal insufficiency.
   D. If started, treat until the patient is discharged from the ICU.
   E. Use only if BP is refractory to fluids and vasopressors.

14. How soon after the onset of severe sepsis or septic shock should antibiotic therapy be administered?

   A. 1 hour
   B. 3 hours
   C. 4 hours
   D. 6 hours
   E. 12 hours

15. Which of the following describes appropriate use of vasopressin in septic shock?

   A. It is an option if a first-line vasopressor is failing.
   B. It is recommended as a first-line vasopressor.
   C. It should be titrated similarly to a catecholamine vasopressor.
   D. It should be used only if hydrocortisone is used.
   E. It can be used to increase cardiac output more than BP.

16. Which of the following is the general vasopressor of choice in septic shock?

   A. Dopamine
   B. Epinephrine
   C. Phenylephrine
   D. Norepinephrine
   E. Vasopressin

17. Which of the following will *not* increase BP via α_1-adrenergic activation?

    A. Phenylephrine
    B. Dopamine
    C. Epinephrine
    D. Norepinephrine
    E. Dobutamine

18. M. W. is a 25-year-old pregnant female who is admitted to the medical ICU following several days of severe nausea and vomiting. She is hypotensive, tachycardic, and confused, and her urine output is very low. Her serum sodium is 128 mEq/L. Which of the following should be given to treat her fluid and sodium abnormality?

    A. IV NS or LR solution
    B. IV 5% dextrose in water
    C. po water
    D. IV furosemide
    E. Desmopressin

19. Common fluid and electrolyte abnormalities associated with loop diuretics include all of the following *except*

    A. hypokalemia.
    B. hyperkalemia.
    C. hypomagnesemia.
    D. dehydration.
    E. hypocalcemia.

20. R. T. is a 40-year-old male admitted to the medical ICU following a severe asthma exacerbation. R. T.'s serum phosphorus is 0.9 mEq/L, and his body weight is 70 kg (100% of ideal). Which of the following acute phosphorus supplementation regimens is most appropriate?

    A. 45 mmol of sodium phosphate IV over 6 hours
    B. 45 mmol of sodium phosphate IV over 10 minutes
    C. 15 mmol of po phosphorus (e.g., Neutraphos) over the next 24 hours
    D. 15 mmol of IV sodium phosphate over 2 hours
    E. No acute phosphorus therapy is required.

21. The most common electrolyte abnormality associated with ACE inhibitors is

    A. hypomagnesemia.
    B. hypokalemia.
    C. hyperkalemia.
    D. hyperphosphatemia.
    E. hypernatremia.

22. All of the following are useful in the rapid treatment of severe hyperkalemia *except*

    A. potassium restriction.
    B. IV calcium.
    C. IV regular insulin and dextrose.
    D. IV sodium bicarbonate.
    E. oral Kayexalate.

23. Which of the following electrolyte abnormalities are most commonly associated with amphotericin?

    I. Hypokalemia
    II. Hypomagnesemia
    III. Hypocalcemia

    A. I only
    B. III only
    C. I and II only
    D. II and III only
    E. I, II, and III

24. All of the following are side effects of potassium replacement therapy *except*

    A. constipation (po).
    B. GI upset (po).
    C. cardiac arrhythmias (IV).
    D. vein irritation (IV).
    E. poor taste (po liquid).

25. Which of the following best describes GI side effects of antacids containing magnesium and calcium salts?

    A. Mg causes constipation; Ca causes diarrhea.
    B. Mg causes diarrhea; Ca causes constipation.
    C. Both cause diarrhea.
    D. Both cause constipation.
    E. Neither has GI side effects.

21-11. Answers

1. C. Fentanyl is used as a continuous infusion and is more titratable than morphine or hydromorphone. Acetaminophen and dexmedetomidine are not opiates.

2. **E.** Morphine may cause more hemodynamic instability than does hydromorphone or fentanyl because of more histamine release. In addition, morphine has a renally excreted, partially active metabolite that may accumulate in renal dysfunction. Hydromorphone and fentanyl do not have such a metabolite. The reason for using these agents in morphine allergy is self-explanatory.

3. **A.** According to the manufacturer, ketorolac should not be used longer than 5 days because of the high risk of GI bleeding with this drug.

4. **C.** Dexmedetomidine does not cause respiratory depression. All the other agents can do so.

5. **D.** Under SCCM guidelines, pancuronium is the NMB agent of choice for most critically ill patients. Pancuronium is less expensive than the other agents.

6. **A.** Cisatracurium is metabolized by nonspecific plasma esterases, whereas pancuronium and vecuronium have varying degrees of hepatic and renal elimination. Thus, SCCM guidelines recommend cisatracurium for use in patients with renal and hepatic dysfunction.

7. **C.** According to SCCM guidelines, propofol is the sedative of choice for patients who require neurologic assessment often. Patients with traumatic brain injury may require multiple neurologic assessments daily. The short duration of action of propofol allows rapid awakening.

8. **B.** According to the Brain Trauma Foundation guidelines, phenytoin for 7 days postinjury is the regimen of choice for post-traumatic seizure prophylaxis in patients requiring such therapy. There are not enough high-quality data to recommend levetiracetam (Keppra) as a first-line agent.

9. **D.** Pentobarbital should be reserved for treating refractory intracranial hypertension. Propofol, mannitol, and hypertonic saline are first-line agents. Phenytoin does not affect ICPs.

10. **D.** Increased age is not an independent risk factor for stress ulcers.

11. **B.** PPIs and H2RAs are considered by most clinicians to be the drugs of choice. PPIs have pros and cons: they may be more effective but may have other disadvantages based on outpatient use. Sucralfate is a secondary option for a number of reasons described in the text, and antacids are not used for this indication.

12. **E.** The Surviving Sepsis Guidelines recommend crystalloids first, then albumin is acceptable if the patient's hypotension is refractory. Nonalbumin colloids cause more renal dysfunction and are not recommended.

13. **E.** The Surviving Sepsis Guidelines recommend using hydrocortisone only in patients who are refractory to fluids and vasopressors. The typical duration is 7 days.

14. **A.** The Surviving Sepsis Guidelines recommend administering antibiotics within 1 hour.

15. **A.** Vasopressin is recommended in the Surviving Sepsis Guidelines for use as a second vasopressor if a first-line agent (e.g., catecholamine) is failing. It is not titrated; its use is not related to hydrocortisone use; and it improves only BP, not cardiac output.

16. **D.** Norepinephrine is the first-line vasopressor recommended in the Surviving Sepsis Guidelines.

17. **E.** Dobutamine has no α_1-adrenergic (vasoconstriction) activity.

18. **A.** M. W. is hyponatremic, and her clinical signs and symptoms indicate severe dehydration from GI losses of water and sodium. She requires rapid fluid resuscitation with a fluid that has an approximately physiologic amount of sodium (either NS 154 mEq/L or LR 130 mEq/L). This amount of sodium will increase her serum sodium into the normal range over time, and the osmotic effect will hold water in the extracellular compartment (the vasculature and interstitium) to help restore organ perfusion.

19. **B.** Loop diuretics enhance renal excretion of water, potassium, magnesium, and calcium.

20. **A.** R. T. is severely hypophosphatemic and requires high-dose IV therapy (0.64 mmol/kg × 70 kg = 44.8 mmol). The dose should be infused at 7.5 mmol/h (total time: 6 hours) to avoid precipitation with calcium.

21. **C.** ACE inhibitors cause hyperkalemia because of aldosterone inhibition.

22. **E.** Oral Kayexalate (sodium polystyrene sulfonate) does not act very quickly. It requires transit time through the intestines to bind potassium and create a gradient that pulls more potassium into the lumen of the GI tract.

23. **C.** Amphotericin B causes renal wasting of potassium and magnesium.

24. **A.** Oral potassium replacement therapy does not normally cause constipation. Cardiac arrhythmias are a concern if IV potassium is given faster than 10 mEq/h.

25. **B.** Magnesium salts (e.g., milk of magnesia) are often used as osmotic laxatives and may cause diarrhea. Calcium salts may cause constipation.

21-12. References

Allen ME, Kopp BJ, Erstad BL. Stress ulcer prophylaxis in the postoperative period. *Am J Health Syst Pharm.* 2004;61:588–96.

Alhazzani W, Alenezi F, Jaeschke RZ, et al. Proton pump inhibitors versus histamine 2–receptor antagonists for stress ulcer prophylaxis in critically ill patients: A systemic review and meta-analysis. *Crit Care Med.* 2013;41:693–705.

Barr J, Fraser GL, Puntillo K, et al. Clinical practice guidelines for the management of pain, agitation, and delirium in adult patients in the intensive care unit. *Crit Care Med.* 2013;41:263–306.

Boucher BA, Wood GC. Acute management of the brain injury patient. In: DiPiro JT, Talbert RL, Yee GC, et al., eds. *Pharmacotherapy: A Pathophysiologic Approach.* 9th ed. New York, NY: McGraw-Hill; 2014:895–910.

Brain Trauma Foundation, American Association of Neurological Surgeons, Congress of Neurological Surgeons. Guidelines for the Management of Severe Traumatic Brain Injury. *J Neurotrauma.* 2007;24:S1–S106.

Brophy DF. Disorders of potassium and magnesium homeostasis. In: DiPiro JT, Talbert RL, Yee GC, et al., eds. *Pharmacotherapy: A Pathophysiologic Approach.* 9th ed. New York, NY: McGraw-Hill; 2014:783–96.

Chessman KH, Matzke GR. Disorders of sodium and water homeostasis. In: DiPiro JT, Talbert RL, Yee GC, et al., eds. *Pharmacotherapy: A Pathophysiologic Approach.* 9th ed. New York, NY: McGraw-Hill; 2014:745–64.

Dellinger RP, Levy MM, Rhodes A, et al. Surviving Sepsis Campaign: International guidelines for management of severe sepsis and septic shock: 2012. *Crit Care Med.* 2013;41:580–637.

Hurlbert RJ, Hadley MN, Walters BC, et al. Pharmacological therapy for acute spinal cord injury. *Neurosurgery* 2013;72(suppl.):93–105.

Murray MJ, Cowen J, DeBlock H, et al. Clinical practice guidelines for sustained neuromuscular blockade in the critically ill patient. *Crit Care Med.* 2002;30:142–56.

Pai AB. Disorders of calcium and phosphorus homeostasis. In: DiPiro JT, Talbert RL, Yee GC, et al., eds. *Pharmacotherapy: A Pathophysiologic Approach.* 9th ed. New York, NY: McGraw-Hill; 2014: 765–82.

Nutrition 22

Joseph M. Swanson

22-1. Key Points

- Malnutrition can present as either undernutrition or obesity.
- The components of a nutritional assessment include a history and physical exam, anthropometric measurements, and biochemical tests.
- An increase in energy expenditure (energy needs) is defined as *hypermetabolism,* and an increase in nitrogen excretion (protein needs) is defined as *hypercatabolism.*
- Most patients receiving specialized nutrition support (parenteral or enteral nutrition) require 25–30 kcal/kg/day and 1–2 g protein/kg/day.
- Critically ill, obese patients (body mass index [BMI] > 30) should receive 11–14 kcal/kg actual body weight per day (22–25 kcal/kg/day ideal body weight) and 2 g/kg ideal body weight per day of protein if BMI = 30–40 or 2.5 g/kg ideal body weight per day if BMI > 40. This approach applies only in patients with normal renal function.
- The water requirement for most adult patients without substantial extrarenal losses is 30–40 mL/kg/day.
- Parenteral nutrition (PN) should be reserved for patients whose gastrointestinal tracts are not functional or accessible (e.g., severe acute pancreatitis, severe short bowel syndrome).

- Total nutrient admixtures (TNAs) contain dextrose, amino acids, lipid emulsion, electrolytes, vitamins, and trace elements in one container.
- The advantages of TNAs include decreased nursing administration time, decreased potential for touch contamination, and reduced expense (the patient needs only one pump and one intravenous administration set).
- The advantages of central vein PN over peripheral vein PN include the ability to concentrate the formulation, administer adequate calories and protein, and use the catheter for long-term administration.
- For PN calculations: 1 g hydrated dextrose = 3.4 kcal, 1 g amino acids = 4 kcal, and 1 g lipid = 9 kcal. (Intravenous fat emulsion actually provides 10 kcal/g because it includes calories provided as glycerol and phospholipid.)
- All PN formulations should be filtered during administration (0.22-micron filter for two-in-one PN formulations and 1.2-micron filter for TNAs).
- Enteral nutrition support is generally used in patients who cannot or will not eat but have a functional and accessible gastrointestinal tract.
- Enteral tube feeding can be provided by one of the following methods: nasogastric, nasoduodenal, nasojejunal, gastrostomy, or jejunostomy.
- Diarrhea associated with enteral tube feeding is often caused by pharmacotherapy (e.g., sorbitol in liquid drug preparations as a vehicle).
- Patients receiving phenytoin or warfarin concurrently with enteral tube feeding should have the tube feeding held at least 1 hour before and after each dose.

This chapter is based on the 10th edition chapter with the same title, written by Kevin L. Freeman.

22-2. Study Guide Checklist

The following topics may guide your study of this subject area:

■ General understanding of macronutrient and micronutrient requirements
■ Factors incorporated into a nutritional assessment
■ Determination of nutritional requirements based on patient-specific variables
■ Methods of administering nutrition support
■ Patient factors that help to choose the nutrition support route
■ Assessment of nutrition support tolerance and efficacy
■ Management of electrolytes and trace elements
■ Identification of nutrition-support complications
■ Major drug–nutrient interactions

22-3. Overview

General Nutrition

U.S. dietary guidelines (MyPlate)

■ Maintain a healthy weight.
■ Maintain a low-fat diet (< 30% of total calories).
■ Eat plenty of fruits, vegetables, and grain products.
■ Use salt, sugar, and alcohol in moderation.

Malnutrition

■ Causes of undernutrition (protein-calorie malnutrition):
  • Depressed intake of nutrients (starvation, semistarvation)
  • Alteration in nutrient metabolism (trauma, major infection)
■ Causes of obesity:
  • Excessive caloric intake (especially carbohydrate and fat)
  • Alteration in nutrient metabolism (genetic predisposition)
  • Sedentary lifestyle

Dietary reference intakes (DRIs) of selected nutrients

■ *Fiber:* 20–35 g/day (many people find this goal unpalatable)
■ *Calcium:* 1,200–1,500 mg/day in adolescents and young adults; 1,000 mg/day in men until age 65

and women until age 50; 1,200–1,500 mg/day for life thereafter (usually requires supplements)
■ *Multivitamins:* Helpful to meet daily requirements of pregnant and lactating women, elderly persons, and those who eat vegetarian or low-calorie diets

Nutritional assessment components

History and physical examination

■ Dietary intake (anorexia, bulimia, hyperphagia, taste alterations)
■ Underlying pathology affecting nutrition (cancer, burns)
■ End-organ effects (diarrhea, constipation)
■ Gastrointestinal surgery (bariatric surgery, gastrectomy, bowel resection)
■ General appearance (edema, cachexia)
■ Skin appearance (scaling skin, decubitus ulcers)
■ Musculoskeletal effects (depressed muscle mass, growth retardation)
■ Neurologic effects (depressed sensorium, encephalopathy)
■ Hepatic effects (jaundice, hepatomegaly)

Anthropometrics

■ Skinfold measurements for assessment of fat (triceps, calf)
■ Arm muscle circumference for assessment of skeletal muscle
■ Waist circumference for assessment of abdominal fat (metabolic syndrome)
■ Weight for height to determine undernutrition or obesity
  • Change in weight over time is one of the best indicators of nutritional status.
■ Head circumference in infants to document appropriate growth
■ Percentage of ideal body weight (IBW) after calculation of IBW for patient:
  • IBW of males (kg) = 50 + (2.3 × height in inches over 5 feet)
  • IBW of females (kg) = 45.5 + (2.3 × height in inches over 5 feet)
■ Body mass index (BMI) for assessment of undernutrition or obesity calculated from body weight (kg) and height (m): BMI = weight (kg)/height^2 (m^2)

Biochemical assessment
Serum albumin concentration

■ Good prognostic indicator and good for assessment of long-term nutritional status
■ Poor for repletion marker because of long half-life (21 days) and large body pool

Serum prealbumin concentration

- Good for short-term assessment of nutrition support because of short half-life (2 days) and small body pool
- Possible increase in serum prealbumin concentrations in patients with kidney disease because of impaired excretion

Serum transferrin concentration

- Good for short-term assessment of nutrition support because of short half-life (7 days) and small body pool
- Elevated in iron-deficiency anemia

Creatinine height index

- Requires 24-hour urine collection to determine levels of creatinine

Other methods of nutritional assessment

- Muscle strength testing
- Bioelectrical impedance (i.e., a low-grade electrical current runs through the body to identify body protein stores and fat stores)

Types of malnutrition

- *Starvation-related malnutrition:* Features depleted fat and muscle stores, normal biochemical measurements (e.g., classic starvation without inflammation)
- *Chronic disease-related malnutrition:* Features mild to moderate inflammation (e.g., congestive heart failure, chronic kidney disease)
- *Acute disease or injury-related malnutrition:* Features severe and acute inflammation (e.g., major infection, trauma)
- *Obesity:* Demonstrated as elevated body weight to at least 120% of IBW or BMI > 27.8 (male) or > 27.3 (female)
  - Class I obesity: BMI > 30 and < 35
  - Class II obesity: BMI > 35 and < 40
  - Class III obesity: BMI > 40

Selected definitions

- *Hypermetabolism:* An increase in energy expenditure above normal (usually > 10% above normal)
- *Hypercatabolism:* An increase in protein losses above normal (usually via urinary excretion of urea nitrogen)
- *Nutrition support therapy:* Parenteral nutrition (PN) or enteral nutrition (EN)

- *Basal energy expenditure (BEE):* A calculation of the normal energy needs of healthy adult men or women using sex, age, height, and weight
- *Harris–Benedict equations for BEE:*
  - Male (kcal/day) = 66 + 13.7 (weight in kg) + 5 (height in cm) − 6.8 (age in yr)
  - Female (kcal/day) = 655 + 9.6 (weight in kg) + 1.8 (height in cm) − 4.7 (age in yr)
- *Mifflin equations for energy expenditure:*
  - Male (kcal/day) = 10 (weight in kg) + 6.25 (height in cm) − 4.9 (age in yr) + 5
  - Female (kcal/day) = 10 (weight in kg) + 6.25 (height in cm) − 4.9 (age in yr) − 161
- *Resting energy expenditure (REE):* A measured value of energy expenditure (generally ~10% above BEE or Mifflin in health, but can be 100% above BEE in severe burns)
- *Respiratory quotient (RQ):* The value that results when carbon dioxide production (VCO_2) is divided by oxygen consumption (VO_2)
  - RQ for carbohydrate oxidation = 1
  - RQ for fat oxidation = 0.7
  - RQ for protein oxidation = 0.8
  - RQ for fat synthesis = 8
- *Indirect calorimetry:* The most accurate method to determine energy requirements. It is a noninvasive procedure that measures VO_2 and VCO_2, and resting energy requirements are then calculated using the Weir equation.
- *Body cell mass:* Lean, metabolically active tissue (skeletal muscle, body organs)
- *Lean body mass:* Body cell mass, extracellular fluid, and extracellular solids (bone, serum proteins)
- *RDI:* Recommended daily intake

22-4. Nutritional Requirements

Calorie Requirements

- Most clinicians dose nutrition support therapies in total calories (i.e., using carbohydrate, fat, and protein-calorie contributions to obtain the desired dose).
  - 25 kcal/kg/day for adults with little stress (e.g., elective surgery)
  - 30 kcal/kg/day for patients with infections and skeletal trauma
  - 35 kcal/kg/day for patients with major trauma (head injury, long-bone fractures)

- 40 kcal/kg/day for patients with major thermal injury (> 50% total body surface area burn)
- Critically ill, obese patients (BMI > 30) should receive 11–14 kcal/kg actual body weight per day (22–25 kcal/kg/day ideal body weight). This is known as hypocaloric feeding.
- Multiply BEE by the stress factor to determine calorie requirements:
  - 1 × BEE for patients with little stress
  - 1.3 × BEE for patients with infections and/or skeletal trauma
  - 1.5 × BEE for patients with major trauma
  - 2 × BEE for patients with severe thermal injury
- Measure the REE via indirect calorimetry for calorie requirements.

Caloric Contribution of the Major Macronutrients

- *Glucose:* 3.4 kcal/g because hydrated glucose is used in PN (glucose powder would be 4 kcal/g)
- *Fat:* 9 kcal/g
- *Protein:* 4 kcal/g
  - Protein requirements are usually dosed in grams per kilogram per day.
  - 0.8 g/kg/day is the adult recommended daily allowance (RDA) for protein in the United States.
  - 1 g/kg/day is the adult RDA for patients with minor stress (elective operations).
  - 1.5 g/kg/day is the adult RDA for patients with major trauma or infection.
  - 2 g/kg/day is the adult RDA for patients with severe head injury, sepsis, or severe thermal injury.
  - For critically ill, obese patients, provide 2 g/kg/day IBW when the patient's BMI = 30–40 and 2.5 g/kg/day when > 40.

Measurement of Nutritional Efficacy Using Nitrogen Balance (NB)

NB = nitrogen in – nitrogen out

- Nitrogen in (grams) is determined by dividing the grams of protein taken in on the day of balance by 6.25.
- Nitrogen out (grams) is determined by measuring the grams of urea nitrogen excreted during a 24-hour urine collection and then adding a factor of 2 or 4 g for insensible nitrogen loss or stool loss.

- Positive NB can be used to document adequacy of nutritional support:
  - In undernourished patients, +4 to +6 g/day is desired.
  - Nitrogen equilibrium (−2 to +2 g/day) is usually adequate in critically ill patients.

Other Requirements during Nutrition Support
Water

- Up to 35 mL/kg/day for average-sized adults
- 40 mL/kg/day for smaller adults and adolescents
- > 40 mL/kg/day for patients with extrarenal losses (e.g., gastrointestinal drains)

Electrolytes

- Sodium requirements:
  - 60–100 mEq/day in adults
  - 2–6 mEq/kg/day in children
- Chloride requirements:
  - 60–100 mEq/day in adults
  - 2–6 mEq/kg/day in children
- Potassium requirements:
  - 60–100 mEq/day in adults
  - 2–5 mEq/kg/day in children
- Calcium requirements:
  - 5–15 mEq/day in adults
  - 2–3 mEq/kg/day in children
- Phosphorus requirements:
  - 20–45 mmol/day in adults
  - 1–2 mmol/kg/day in children
- Magnesium requirements:
  - 10–20 mEq/day in adults
  - 0.25–1 mEq/kg/day in children

Vitamins

- Vitamins are provided daily in both PN (added) and EN (endogenous).
- Most enteral formulations provide the DRI for vitamins in a volume of 1,000–1,500 mL.
- For parenteral vitamin products:
  - Adult products contain 12 (M.V.I.-12) or 13 vitamins (Infuvite Adult, M.V.I. Adult); vitamin K is added separately when the product with 12 vitamins is used.
  - Pediatric products (M.V.I. Pediatric, Infuvite Pediatric) contain all 13 vitamins.

Trace elements

- *Zinc:* 3–5 mg/day in adults with PN; 50–250 mcg/kg/day in children with PN
- *Copper:* 0.5–1.2 mg/day in adults with PN; 20 mcg/kg/day in children with PN (maximum of 300 mcg/day)
- *Chromium:* 10–15 mcg/day in adults with PN; monitored but not given to children
- *Manganese:* 50–100 mcg/day in adults with PN; monitored but not given to children
- *Selenium:* 40–80 mcg/day in adults with PN; 1.5–3 mcg/kg/day in children with PN

22-5. Nutrition Support Therapies

Parenteral Nutrition

Indications

PN is generally used for patients who cannot be fed via the gastrointestinal tract. PN should begin after 5–7 days of lack of bowel function.

Severe acute pancreatitis
- Oral or tube feeding will usually exacerbate this condition unless given via the jejunum (e.g., nasojejunal feeding tube or jejunostomy).

Short bowel syndrome
- This condition requires PN from a few weeks to lifelong, as needed.

Ileus
- This condition is secondary to lack of bowel function (e.g., postoperative after gastrointestinal surgery).

Other indications
- Bowel obstruction
- Bowel ischemia
- Neonates who cannot eat in the first day of life
- Preoperatively for undernourished patients who are undergoing an elective operation and for whom there is no direct access to the gastrointestinal tract (e.g., partial small bowel obstruction from cancer)
- Pregnancy with severe hyperemesis gravidarum (i.e., there is an inability to tolerate oral or enteral nutrition)
- Gastrointestinal fistulae where oral or EN should be restricted

Components of parenteral nutrition

Protein
- Protein should be included in all PN formulations.
- Standard amino acids from 10%, 15%, or 20% stock solutions can be used for most patients.
- Final concentrations in the PN formulation vary from 2% to 7%.

Fat
- Fat is provided as intravenous fat emulsion either as a separate infusion or admixed with the rest of the PN formulation, making a total nutrient admixture (TNA).
- Products are manufactured as 10%, 20%, and 30% fat emulsions. (In the United States, 30% can be used only for TNAs, not for direct infusion.)
- Fat provides essential fatty acids to the patient who is most likely not eating by mouth.
- Fat provides nonprotein calories other than glucose.
- Common doses used in adults are ~1 g/kg/day (9–10 kcal/kg/day) but should not exceed 2.5 g/kg/day.
- Intravenous fat emulsions contain phospholipid to emulsify the product and glycerol to make the emulsion isotonic. (Both of these components provide modest calories that result in supplying 10 kcal/g equivalent of fat.)

Dextrose
- Common doses of dextrose in critically ill patients are 3–4 mg/kg/min (~15–20 kcal/kg/day).
- Dextrose is in all PN formulations for obligate needs (central nervous system, renal medulla, white blood cells, red blood cells, wound healing).
- PN formulations are usually made from 50% to 70% dextrose in water.
- Final concentrations in the PN formulation vary from D10W (10% dextrose in water) to D35W (35% dextrose in water).
- Dextrose should never exceed a dose of 5 mg/kg/min (~25 kcal/kg/day).

Sodium
- Sodium can be provided as chloride, acetate, or phosphate salts in PN.
- After phosphate addition, the remaining anions are added on the basis of acid–base status. They are split between chloride and acetate with a normal pH, predominantly acetate with metabolic

acidosis, and predominantly chloride with metabolic alkalosis.

- Requirements can be increased when the patient has extrarenal losses from nasogastric suction, abdominal drains, or ostomy losses.

Potassium

- Potassium can be provided as chloride, acetate, or phosphate salts in PN.
- Requirements can be increased with administration of potassium-wasting drugs (diuretics, steroids) or in severe undernutrition.
- Like sodium, the remaining potassium can be added as acetate or chloride on the basis of acid–base status after the proper dose of phosphate is determined.

Calcium

- Most practitioners add calcium as the gluconate salt.
- Higher doses of calcium (~20–25 mEq/day) are needed in patients receiving long-term PN to help prevent metabolic bone disease.
- Addition of calcium is limited in PN formulations because of the potential to precipitate with phosphate salts, which ultimately results in insoluble calcium phosphate.

Phosphate

- Phosphate is added as the sodium or potassium salt.
- Higher doses of phosphorus (e.g., 30 mmol/L) are needed to prevent refeeding syndrome in severely undernourished patients.
- Phosphorus should be decreased or removed in patients with renal failure.
- Most practitioners prefer sodium phosphate over potassium phosphate because of the higher concentration of aluminum in the latter product, especially in chronic use of PN.
- Addition of phosphorus is limited in PN formulations because of the potential to precipitate with calcium or magnesium salts to form an insoluble compound.

Magnesium

- Most practitioners add magnesium as the sulfate salt.
- Higher doses should be used in patients with alcoholism or large bowel losses or in patients receiving drugs causing renal wasting of magnesium (cisplatin, amphotericin B, aminoglycosides, loop diuretics).

- Magnesium should be restricted or deleted in patients with renal failure.

Multivitamins

- Multivitamins are given daily as part of PN.
- Parenteral multivitamin preparations contain 12 or 13 vitamins. (Vitamin K should be administered separately if the 12-vitamin preparation is used.)
- Additional thiamine and folic acid are often given to alcoholic patients who are receiving PN.
- Additional folic acid (at least 600 mcg/day) should be given to pregnant patients receiving PN.

Trace elements

- Trace elements are given daily as a cocktail of four or five trace metals.
- Extra zinc should be given in patients with ostomy or diarrhea losses.
- Copper and manganese should be reduced or eliminated in patients with cholestasis.
- Extra selenium is usually needed in homebound PN patients.

Total nutrient admixtures versus two-in-one admixtures

Advantages of TNAs

- Decreased nursing time for administration
- Potentially decreased touch contamination
- Decreased pharmacy preparation time (assuming a 24-hour hang time)
- Financial savings (use of only one pump and one intravenous administration set)

Disadvantages of TNAs

- TNAs are better media for bacterial growth than are two-in-one admixtures.
- It is impossible to visualize particulate matter.
- Filter formulation with a 0.22-micron filter is not possible.
- Some additives like calcium and phosphorus are less compatible in TNAs.

Central vein PN versus peripheral vein PN

Advantages of central vein PN

- Central vein PN can maximize caloric intake.
- Volume restriction of patients is possible.
- Long-term catheter can be maintained.

Disadvantages of central vein PN

- Mechanical complications can occur during catheter placement (e.g., pneumothorax).

- Potential hyperosmolar complications are possible (e.g., from use of hypertonic dextrose).
- Potential septic catheter complications are possible.

Advantages of peripheral vein PN

- It is easier to place the catheter (i.e., peripheral vein stick).
- Hyperosmolar complications are avoided because dilute formulations must be used.

Disadvantages of peripheral vein PN

- Incidence of thrombophlebitis is high.
- Frequent vein rotation is necessary.
- Energy intake is limited.
- Volume restriction is not possible (using dilute formulations).
- Cost is higher because more lipid calories are generally used. (Lipids are isotonic.)

Parenteral nutrition calculations

D20W (final concentration of PN formulation)

- D20W = 20% dextrose = 20 g/100 mL = 200 g/L × 3.4 kcal/g = 680 dextrose kcal/L
- 2 L/day of D20W (final concentration of PN formulation) = 1,360 dextrose kcal/day

Amino acids 5% (final concentration of PN formulation)

- 5% amino acids = 5 g/100 mL = 50 g/L × 4 kcal/g = 200 protein kcal/L
- 2 L/day of 5% amino acids = 100 g/day = 400 protein kcal/day

Lipid 2% (final concentration of TNA formulation)

- 2% lipid will deliver 200 kcal/L (includes calories from glycerol/phospholipid)
- 2 L/day of lipid 2% = 400 fat kcal/day

Lipid 20% infused at 20 mL/h × 24 h (separate infusion given with two-in-one PN formulations)

- 20% lipid = 2 kcal/mL
- 20 mL/h × 24 h = 480 mL/day
- 480 mL/day × 2 kcal/mL = 960 fat kcal/day

Example: D30W; amino acids 4%; lipid 3%; at 60 mL/h

- 60 mL/h × 24 h/day = 1,440 mL/day (1.44 L/day)
- D30W = 30% dextrose = 300 g/L × 3.4 kcal/g = 1,020 kcal/L × 1.44 L = 1,469 dextrose kcal
- 4% amino acids = 40 g/L = 160 kcal/L × 1.44 L = 230 protein kcal
- 3% lipid = 300 kcal/L × 1.44 L = 432 fat kcal
- 1,469 kcal + 230 kcal + 432 kcal = 2,131 total kcal/day from the above PN formulation

Example: dextrose 400 g; amino acids 100 g; lipids 40 g; at 85 mL/h

- Dextrose 400 g × 3.4 kcal/g = 1,360 kcal/day
- Amino acids 100 g × 4 kcal/g = 400 kcal/day
- Lipids 40 g × 10 kcal/g (includes phospholipid and glycerol) = 400 kcal/day

General principles of compounding parenteral nutrition

- Each component of the PN prescription should be reviewed to ensure a balanced PN formulation is provided.
- Each component should be assessed for dose and potential compatibility programs.
- All compounded PN formulations should be visually inspected to ensure no gross contamination or precipitation is present.
- Manufacturers of automated compounders should provide the additive sequence to ensure safety in PN preparation.

General principles of stability and compatibility of parenteral nutrition

- Parenteral multivitamins should be added shortly before dispensing and administering the PN formulation because vitamins A and C degrade fairly quickly.
- Preparation of TNAs using dual-chambered bags (lipid is kept in a separate compartment until administration) can enhance the shelf life of a PN formulation.
- Dibasic calcium phosphate can precipitate in PN formulations if the amounts of calcium gluconate and sodium or potassium phosphate are excessive.
- Generally, phosphate should be added first to the PN formulation.
- Generally, calcium should be added last to the PN formulation.
- Calcium chloride should not be used in PN because it is highly reactive with phosphate.
- Iron dextran can be added to two-in-one PN formulations but should not be added to TNAs.

Parenteral nutrition filtration

- Filters are used to prevent administration of particulate matter, microorganisms, and air.
- Use a new 0.22-micron filter each day with two-in-one PN formulations (0.22-micron filters with positive charged nylon can be used for up to 72 hours in two-in-one PN formulations).
- Use a new 1.2-micron filter each day with TNAs.

Complications of parenteral nutrition

Metabolic
Hyperglycemia
- Patients with stress of trauma or infection or those with diabetes often need regular human insulin added to the PN formulation to control hyperglycemia.
- Regular insulin continuous infusions are often needed to control hyperglycemia.

Electrolyte disorders
Hypokalemia
- Patients often require extra potassium in PN (e.g., 60 mEq/L).

Hypophosphatemia
- Patients often require extra phosphorus in PN (e.g., 30 mmol/L).

Hypomagnesemia
- Patients often require extra magnesium in PN (e.g., 16 mEq/L).

Hyponatremia
- Diagnosis of sodium disorders must include an assessment of extracellular fluid status (i.e., volume status).
  - *Volume depleted:* Add sodium and water to PN, or increase intravenous fluid administration.
  - *Volume overloaded:* Remove sodium from PN, and concentrate the formulation.
  - *Euvolemic:* Generally, water restriction is first-line therapy (concentrate the PN formula).

Acid–base disorders
- Increase acetate and decrease chloride anions if the patient has metabolic acidosis.
- Increase chloride and decrease acetate anions if the patient has metabolic alkalosis.

Essential fatty acid deficiency
- During PN, at least 4% of total calories need to be provided as intravenous lipid (easily attained when lipid is used daily as a calorie source).

Trace element disorders
- Patients with increased ostomy output or chronic diarrhea need extra zinc.
- Hold copper and manganese in patients with cholestasis.

Hepatic steatosis
- Fatty infiltration of the liver has been reported with long-term PN.
- Hepatic steatosis is thought to be primarily caused by administration of excessive dextrose calories.
- The key to prevention is through administration of an appropriate dose of dextrose (e.g., < 5 mg/kg/min).

Mechanical complications
- Pneumothorax (punctured lung) can occur during central vein cannulation.
- Subclavian artery injury can occur when the artery is cannulated instead of the vein.
- Subclavian vein thrombosis can occur with long-term central vein access. (Heparin is used in some PN patients to prevent this condition.)

Infectious complications
- Such complications are usually due to catheter-related breakdown in sterile technique.
- They are rarely solution related.

Monitoring of parenteral nutrition

Frequency and intensity of monitoring is based on the patient's condition, as assessed by

- Electrolyte balance and glucose control
- Acid–base status via arterial blood gases
- Intake and output for assessment of fluid balance
- Serum prealbumin concentrations, nitrogen balance, or both to document efficacy

Enteral Nutrition

Indications

- EN is generally used in patients who cannot or will not eat but have a functional and accessible gastrointestinal tract.
- Neonates should begin EN as early as possible, even if receiving PN.
- EN is used in elderly patients who lack the ability to ingest food orally.

Cardiac
- Cardiac patients may need fluid-restricted EN with fluid overload.

Pulmonary failure
- EN is used frequently in patients receiving mechanical ventilation.

Hepatic failure

- EN is used frequently in this population.
- In severe hepatic encephalopathy, use a formulation with high branched-chain amino acids and low aromatic amino acids.
- In the absence of encephalopathy or mild encephalopathy, use EN with standard protein.

Gastrointestinal failure

- In short bowel syndrome, EN is used to enhance small bowel hypertrophy after major bowel resection.
- In inflammatory bowel syndrome, EN is the preferred method of nutrition support.

Neurologic impairment

- EN is preferred because the patient may not be able to eat, but the gastrointestinal tract is functional and accessible.

Cancer or HIV infection

- Use EN (if possible) in these patients to prevent or treat undernutrition.

Types of enteral access

- Feeding enterostomy
  - Feeding enterostomy is used for long-term EN.
  - Gastrostomy requires a G-tube or PEG (percutaneous endoscopic gastrostomy).
  - Jejunostomy requires a laparotomy for placement.
- Oral route (by drinking supplements)
- Nasal tube feeding
  - Nasal tube feeding is usual for short-term EN.
  - Nasogastric, nasoduodenal, or nasojejunal tubes are used.

Products for enteral nutrition

- Polymeric, nutritionally complete tube feeding is used for patients with normal digestive processes (e.g., 1 kcal/mL).
- Concentrated, nutritionally complete tube feeding is used for patients who need severe fluid restriction (e.g., 2 kcal/mL).
- Polymeric, nutritionally complete, oral supplements are used to supplement an oral diet (e.g., 1 or 1.5 kcal/mL).
- Chemically defined, nutritionally complete tube feeding is used for patients with impaired digestive processes such as short bowel syndrome or pancreatic insufficiency (e.g., 1 kcal/mL).

- Fiber-containing, nutritionally complete tube feeding is beneficial in patients who receive long-term tube feeding (can prevent diarrhea and constipation; e.g., 1 or 1.2 kcal/mL).
- Concentrated, low-protein, low-electrolyte tube feeding is generally used for patients with renal failure.
- A high branched-chain amino acid, low aromatic amino acid EN formula is used for patients with liver failure and severe hepatic encephalopathy (e.g., 1 or 1.5 kcal/mL).
- High-fat, low-carbohydrate, nutritionally complete tube feeding is helpful in management of diabetic or other glucose-intolerant patients (e.g., 1 or 1.2 kcal/mL).
- Immune-enhancing formulas that contain arginine, glutamine, and omega-3 fatty acids are marketed and used in patients with high metabolic stress (e.g., severe trauma or infection; 1 or 1.3 kcal/mL).

Complications of enteral nutrition

Pulmonary (e.g., aspiration pneumonia)

- The most severe complications of EN are pulmonary.
- Pulmonary complications are caused by regurgitation of gastric contents into the lung (with or without tube feeding).
- Prevention is important.
  - Elevate the head of the bed to 30–45° if possible.
  - Frequently assess the patient's abdomen to ensure tolerance.
  - Frequently assess the placement of the feeding tube (especially nasally placed tubes).

Gastrointestinal

- Diarrhea is often associated with the administration of EN, but EN is not necessarily the cause of the diarrhea.

Increased frequency or volume of stools

- Pharmacotherapy is often the cause because of sorbitol in liquid vehicles.
- Lack of fiber and excessive infusion rate advancements can also be causes.
- Decreasing (or at least not advancing) the infusion rate is appropriate.
- Change to a fiber-containing formulation if the patient is not receiving one.
- Pseudomembranous enterocolitis can occur from antibiotic therapy.

- *Clostridium difficile* colitis can be a cause.
- Use pharmacotherapeutic treatment if the above factors are ruled out (bismuth subsalicylate, loperamide, or diphenoxylate).

Constipation (decrease in stool frequency)

- Lack of fiber can be a cause.
- Lack of water can be a cause.
- Poor mobility and drugs with anticholinergic activity can contribute.
- Keep patient well hydrated, and use a fiber-containing EN formulation.

Mechanical

- In the event of nasal necrosis, use a small-bore feeding tube and do not tape it too firmly to the nose.
- To prevent esophageal injury, use a small-bore feeding tube.
- To prevent the feeding tube from clogging, frequently flush it with warm water.
- In the event of tube displacement, discourage removing the tube; the tube may have to be anchored with a bridle.

Metabolic

Hyperglycemia

- Use regular human insulin.
- Consider a high-fat, low-carbohydrate EN formulation.
- Regular insulin continuous infusions are sometimes necessary.

Hypokalemia

- Provide additional potassium as an intravenous or per tube supplement.
- Some institutions allow the addition of potassium salts to the EN formulation.

Hypophosphatemia

- Provide additional phosphorus as an intravenous supplement (e.g., potassium phosphate).
- Some institutions allow the addition of phosphorus salts to the EN formulation (e.g., injectable sodium or potassium phosphate).

Monitoring of enteral nutrition

The intensity of monitoring will be dictated by the condition of the patient:

- Electrolyte balance and glucose control
- Acid–base status via arterial blood gases (critical care only)

- Intake and output for assessment of fluid balance
- Assessment of the patient's abdomen is required:
  - Positive bowel sounds usually should be present.
  - The abdomen should be soft, nontender, and nondistended in most cases.
  - A profoundly distended abdomen usually requires the EN to be decreased or discontinued temporarily while the etiology is investigated.
- Serum prealbumin concentrations, nitrogen balance, or both should be assessed to document efficacy.

Home Nutrition Support

Parenteral nutrition

- PN can be given from weeks to a lifetime (e.g., severe short bowel syndrome).
- PN is usually cycled at night over 10–16 hours for convenience and to decrease incidence of hepatic complications.
- Patient must be monitored closely for iron deficiency because iron supplementation is not routinely added to PN.
- Regular assessment of hemoglobin, hematocrit, and mean corpuscular volume is required.
- Serum iron, total iron-binding capacity, and ferritin are commonly used in the diagnosis of iron deficiency.
- Metabolic bone disease is another long-term complication of home PN.
  - Supplemental calcium in the PN formulation is usually required (15–25 mEq/day).
  - Adequate vitamin K for osteocalcin is important on a long-term basis.

Enteral nutrition

- EN can be given indefinitely as full nutrition support or as a supplement to an oral diet.
- Permanent feeding ostomies are used almost exclusively in home EN.
- Patients in nursing homes and extended care facilities usually receive EN as a continuous (24 hours) or intermittent (e.g., 12 hours) infusion.
- Patients who receive home EN via gastrostomy usually receive bolus feeding (e.g., two 240 mL cans tid via PEG).
- Patients who receive home EN as a supplement to oral intake are often cycled at night (e.g., 1,000 mL at 85 mL/h from 7:00 pm to 7:00 am each night).

22-6. Major Drug–Nutrient Interactions

Phenytoin and Enteral Tube Feeding

- It has been demonstrated that enteral feeding will bind to phenytoin, thus impairing the absorption dramatically, possibly because of the protein component of EN (caseinates).

Management of Phenytoin–Enteral Nutrition Interaction

- Hold the EN 2 hours before and after the daily dose of phenytoin capsules.
- Hold the EN 1 hour before and after each dose of phenytoin suspension (usually given bid or tid).
- Increase the EN infusion rate to allow the desired nutritional dose of EN to be given (i.e., to make up for the lost time while the EN is being held for drug administration).

Warfarin and Enteral Tube Feeding

- It has been reported that adequate anticoagulation with warfarin is very difficult to achieve with concurrent EN (low international normalized ratios).

Management of Warfarin–Enteral Nutrition Interaction

- Hold EN 1 hour before and after the daily warfarin dose. If this is done, the EN rate should be increased to attain the desired nutritional dose.

Management of Grapefruit Juice–Drug Interaction

- Grapefruit juice interacts with many drugs (e.g., amlodipine, carbamazepine, cyclosporine).
- Grapefruit juice from frozen concentrate has been reported to inhibit gastrointestinal cytochrome P450 3A4, resulting in enhancement of oral absorption of some drugs (toxicity).
- When taking drugs that are known to interact with grapefruit juice, patients should be advised to avoid these grapefruit products (i.e., substitute another fruit juice such as apple or orange juice).

22-7. Questions

1. What is the most appropriate calcium intake (mg/day) for adults over 65 years of age?

    A. 600–800 mg
    B. 800–1,000 mg
    C. 1,000–1,200 mg
    D. 1,200–1,500 mg
    E. 1,500–1,800 mg

Use the following case study to answer Questions 2 and 3:

A patient presents for a comprehensive nutritional assessment. She is 35 years old, is 5 feet 8 inches, and weighs 52 kg. She has a history of Crohn's disease involving both the small bowel and the colon. She has had no surgeries but has intermittent diarrhea.

Medications

- Prednisone 5 mg every other day
- Mesalamine 1 g tid
- Loperamide 2 mg q6h prn diarrhea

Measurements

- Triceps skinfold = 3 mm (normal, 10–14 mm)
- Calf skinfold = 4 mm (normal, 10–15 mm)
- Serum albumin concentration = 2.5 g/dL
- Serum prealbumin concentration = 13 mg/dL (normal, 15–45 mg/dL)

2. The triceps skinfold measurement for this patient is an anthropometric measurement for assessment of

    A. somatic protein stores.
    B. fat stores.
    C. visceral protein stores.
    D. immune competence.
    E. body cell mass.

3. What type of malnutrition does this patient have?

    A. Starvation-related
    B. Acute disease-related
    C. Obesity
    D. Chronic disease-related
    E. Injury-related

4.   A patient with a bone fracture and Gram-negative pneumonia excretes 15 g (normal, 6–8 g/day) of urea nitrogen during a 24-hour urine collection. On the basis of these data, the patient is

   A. hypercatabolic.
   B. hypermetabolic.
   C. hypocatabolic.
   D. hypometabolic.
   E. euvolemic.

5.   During nutritional assessment, the measurement of body cell mass includes

   A. bone.
   B. interstitial fluid.
   C. skeletal muscle.
   D. intravascular fluid.
   E. extracellular fluid solids.

Use the following case study to answer Questions 6–9:

   Following major gastrointestinal resection, a patient with severe short bowel syndrome is started on PN. It is anticipated that this patient may need this therapy for 6 months to 1 year. The PN prescription for this patient includes

   ▪ D20W amino acids 5% (final concentrations) at 105 mL/h (2,500 mL/day).
   ▪ Intravenous fat emulsion 20% at 10 mL/h × 24 h (240 mL/day).
   ▪ 0.45% sodium chloride injection at 50 mL/h × 24 h (1,200 mL/day).

6.   How many calories from dextrose will this patient receive each day?

   A. 1,100
   B. 1,300
   C. 1,500
   D. 1,700
   E. 1,900

7.   How many grams of protein will this patient receive each day?

   A. 25
   B. 50
   C. 75
   D. 100
   E. 125

8.   How many calories from intravenous lipid will this patient receive each day?

   A. 240
   B. 360

C. 480
D. 600
E. 720

9.   Calculate the daily nitrogen balance (grams per day) in this patient if she excretes 12 g of urea nitrogen during the urine collection and 4 g are used as insensible and stool loss each day.

   A. –4
   B. –2
   C. 0
   D. 2
   E. 4

10.   What would be an appropriate water or fluid requirement for a 60-kg patient with no extrarenal fluid losses?

   A. 800 mL
   B. 1,200 mL
   C. 2,400 mL
   D. 3,600 mL
   E. 4,800 mL

11.   Which of the following disease states or clinical conditions would usually require the administration of parenteral nutrition?

   A. Severe acute pancreatitis
   B. Motor vehicle crash resulting in femur fracture and head injury
   C. 20% body surface area burn from a house fire
   D. Laparoscopic cholecystectomy
   E. Acute exacerbation of hepatic encephalopathy

12.   What is the maximum dose (in kilocalories per kilogram per day) of dextrose in PN for adult patients?

   A. 5
   B. 10
   C. 15
   D. 20
   E. 25

13.   In a patient with metabolic acidosis, what anion salt would you use to add the majority of sodium and potassium to a PN formulation?

   A. Chloride
   B. Gluconate
   C. Phosphate
   D. Acetate
   E. Sulfate

14. If excessive amounts of calcium are added to a standard PN formulation, it will likely precipitate with

    A. phosphate.
    B. gluconate.
    C. magnesium.
    D. chloride.
    E. sodium.

15. Which vitamin should be supplemented above standard amounts during nutrition support of a pregnant patient?

    A. Cyanocobalamin
    B. Folic acid
    C. Biotin
    D. Chromium
    E. Pantothenic acid

16. Which of the following is an advantage of central vein PN over peripheral vein PN?

    A. Allows easier catheter placement
    B. Does not require a pump for administration
    C. Allows for fluid restriction
    D. Does not have to be filtered
    E. Uses dilute formulations in most cases

17. Which component of a total nutrient admixture should be added last before storing it in a refrigerator?

    A. Phosphorus
    B. Magnesium
    C. Trace elements
    D. Calcium
    E. Intravenous fat emulsion

18. Which of the following are advantages of using a 0.22-micron filter when administering a two-in-one PN formulation?

    I. Traps particulate matter
    II. Prevents precipitates from entering the patient
    III. Filters most bacteria

    A. I only
    B. III only
    C. I and II only
    D. II and III only
    E. I, II, and III

19. Which trace element should be reduced or removed in patients with cholestasis who are receiving PN?

    A. Zinc
    B. Chromium
    C. Selenium
    D. Copper
    E. Iodine

20. A 70-year-old female who has mild congestive heart failure, gastroesophageal reflux disease (GERD), type II diabetes mellitus, and rheumatoid arthritis had a recent cerebral vascular accident. She will not regain her premorbid degree of mental status, so a decision is made to give her long-term nutritional support. Which method would be most appropriate for this patient?

    A. Central parenteral nutrition
    B. Nasogastric tube feeding
    C. Peripheral parenteral nutrition
    D. Jejunostomy tube feeding
    E. Nasoduodenal tube feeding

21. A common cause of diarrhea in patients receiving EN is from the

    A. osmotic load of the EN formulation.
    B. sorbitol in drug vehicles.
    C. addition of fiber to the EN formulation.
    D. solute load from the protein component of the EN formulation.
    E. improper placement of a nasogastric feeding tube.

22. What is the drug of choice for enhancing gastric emptying in a patient receiving EN support?

    A. Bismuth subsalicylate
    B. Azithromycin
    C. Metoclopramide
    D. Loperamide
    E. Acyclovir

23. A patient is receiving phenytoin capsules 300 mg each day for seizure control. She requires tube feeding with a 1 kcal/mL formulation at 85 mL/h (2,000 mL/day). What would be the most appropriate intervention to maintain a therapeutic drug concentration and maintain the required nutrition support?

    I. Increase the dose of phenytoin to 600 mg/day.
    II. Hold the EN 2 hours before and after the dose.
    III. Increase the EN to 100 mL/h × 20 hours.

    A. I only
    B. III only
    C. I and II only
    D. II and III only
    E. I, II, and III

24. What is the mechanism for grapefruit juice to inhibit the metabolism of some drugs that can result in drug toxicity?

    A. Decreased renal excretion of drug
    B. Inhibition of gastrointestinal cytochrome P450 3A4
    C. Decreased systemic clearance of drug
    D. Inhibition of hepatic cytochrome P450 3A4
    E. Expanded apparent volume of distribution

22-8. Answers

1. **D.** Calcium requirements are 1,000 mg/day for male adults until age 65, when they increase to 1,200–1,500 mg/day. Calcium requirements are 1,000 mg/day for female adults until age 50, when they increase to 1,200–1,500 mg/day.

2. **B.** Skinfold measurements measure body fat stores, which assess the lipid component of the body. Visceral protein stores are serum proteins. Body cell mass and somatic protein stores assess skeletal muscle and visceral organs. Immune competence assessment requires a skin test with a common antigen.

3. **D.** Measurements of nutritional assessment are depressed, and the patient has a chronic disease that is contributing to inflammation (i.e., weight for height, anthropometric measurements, and biochemical serum markers of protein status).

4. **A.** Catabolism is related to loss of body protein. Because urea nitrogen output is increased, the patient would be considered hypercatabolic in this case.

5. **C.** Lean body mass includes bone, skeletal muscle, visceral organs, and extracellular solids. Body cell mass includes only the lean, metabolically active tissue such as skeletal muscle and visceral organs (e.g., liver).

6. **D.** D20W = 20 g/100 mL = 200 g/L × 2.5 L/day = 500 g/day × 3.4 kcal/g = 1,700 kcal/day.

7. **E.** 5% amino acids = 5 g/100 mL = 50 g/L × 2.5 L/day = 125 g/day.

8. **C.** Intravenous lipid emulsion 20% = 2 kcal/mL × 240 mL/day = 480 kcal/day.

9. **E.** The nitrogen intake is calculated by dividing the protein intake (125 g) by 6.25, which results in 20 g. The nitrogen output would be the sum of the urinary urea nitrogen and insen-

sible losses (12 g + 4 g = 16 g/day). Therefore, the nitrogen balance would be 20 g – 16 g = 4 g. A nitrogen balance of 4 would be suggestive of nutritional adequacy with this PN formulation.

10. **C.** Water requirements are 30–40 mL/kg/day for patients without extrarenal fluid losses: 60 kg × 40 mL/kg/day = 2,400 mL/day.

11. **A.** It is difficult to feed patients with severe pancreatitis enterally unless there is access to the small bowel (e.g., jejunostomy). The other clinical conditions, such as trauma and burns, would occur in patients in whom the gastrointestinal tract could and should be used for nutrition support. A patient receiving laparoscopic cholecystectomy would not need nutrition support. Most patients with hepatic encephalopathy can be fed enterally if they require nutrition support.

12. **E.** The dose of dextrose in PN should never exceed 5 mg/kg/min in adult patients. This dose can be converted to 25 kcal/kg/day.

13. **D.** Acetate is converted to bicarbonate in the liver and would thus help or at least not exacerbate the metabolic acidosis.

14. **A.** Calcium phosphate is a relatively insoluble compound, so manufacturer guidelines for the concentrations of these two elements must be followed closely to prevent precipitation. The order of mixing these components in the PN formulation is also important.

15. **B.** Folic acid should be given at a dose of at least 600 mcg/day during pregnancy. Many practitioners administer 1 mg/day above what the patient is eating or receiving via nutrition support. This practice has been shown to prevent neural tube defects in the newborn.

16. **C.** Hyperosmolar nutrients (dextrose, amino acids) can be used to concentrate the PN formulation, but the PN would have to be administered via a central vein.

17. **D.** If calcium is added last, the PN formulation will contain the final volume, including all other nutrients. The chance of calcium causing a precipitate will be decreased because all other components (e.g., phosphorus) are diluted in the entire volume of the PN.

18. **E.** A 0.22-micron filter will do all three. In contrast, a 1.2-micron filter (used with TNAs) will not filter most bacteria.

19. **D.** Copper is excreted via the biliary tract. Patients with severe cholestasis should have

copper removed during short-term PN. In long-term PN, copper may be required in reduced doses to prevent anemia. Serum copper concentrations should be monitored regularly in long-term patients who have cholestasis.

20. **D.** She is not a candidate for long-term PN because her gastrointestinal tract would be accessible and functional. Nasogastric and nasoduodenal methods are used only for short-term EN. A jejunostomy would be ideal because she also has GERD and perhaps gastroparesis from her diabetes.

21. **B.** Several liquid preparations for drugs contain sorbitol as a pharmaceutical vehicle. These liquid preparations are commonly used in patients with tubes because the drugs can be given easily this way, especially if the patient cannot swallow. Most EN formulations are close to being isotonic (i.e., the osmotic load or solute load is not a major factor causing diarrhea). Fiber will prevent or improve diarrhea in most cases.

22. **C.** Metoclopramide enhances gastric emptying and is commonly used in patients with gastrointestinal intolerance. This is true in both diabetics and nondiabetics.

23. **D.** Absorption of phenytoin is markedly impaired when it is given concurrently with enteral tube feeding. The enteral tube feeding should be held 2 hours before and after the daily dose of phenytoin capsules. To maintain the current dose of EN, the rate of feeding should be increased to 100 mL/h × 20 h (2,000 mL/day).

24. **B.** Drugs such as amlodipine, carbamazepine, and cyclosporine are profoundly metabolized in the gastrointestinal tract before absorption. Grapefruit juice from frozen concentrate has been shown to inhibit gastrointestinal cytochrome P450 3A4 and thus allows more of the drug to be absorbed, thereby causing drug toxicity for drugs with a narrow therapeutic index.

22-9. References

American Society for Parenteral and Enteral Nutrition Board of Directors and Clinical Guidelines Task Force. Guidelines for the use of parenteral and enteral nutrition in adult and pediatric patients. *J Parenter Enteral Nutr.* 2002;26(suppl 1):1SA–138SA.

Brown RO. Parenteral and enteral nutrition in adult patients. In: Helms RA, Quan DJ, Herfindal ET, Gourley DR, eds. *Textbook of Therapeutics: Drug and Disease Management.* 8th ed. Philadelphia, PA: Lippincott, Williams & Wilkins; 2006:749–66.

Brown RO, Dickerson RN. Drug–nutrient interactions. *Am J Managed Care.* 1999;5:345–51.

Chessman KH, Kumpf VJ. Assessment of nutrition status and nutrition requirements. In Dipiro JT, Talbert RL, Yee GC, et al., eds. *Pharmacotherapy: A Pathophysiologic Approach.* 8th ed. New York, NY: McGraw Hill; 2011. Available at: http://www.accesspharmacy.com/content.aspx?aID=8011919.

Dickerson RN, Sacks GS. Medication administration considerations with specialized nutrition support. In Dipiro JT, Talbert RL, Yee GC, et al., eds. *Pharmacotherapy: A Pathophysiologic Approach.* 8th ed. New York, NY: McGraw Hill; 2011. Available at: http://www.accesspharmacy.com/content.aspx?aID=8012240.

Hodges, BM, DeLegge M. Nutritional considerations in major organ failure. In Dipiro JT, Talbert RL, Yee GC, et al., eds. *Pharmacotherapy: A Pathophysiologic Approach.* 8th ed. New York, NY: McGraw Hill; 2011. Available at: http://www.accesspharmacy.com/content.aspx?aID=8013162.

Kumpf VJ, Chessman KH. Enteral nutrition. In Dipiro JT, Talbert RL, Yee GC, et al., eds. *Pharmacotherapy: A Pathophysiologic Approach,* 8th ed. New York, NY: McGraw Hill; 2011. Available at: http://www.accesspharmacy.com/content.aspx?aID=8012769.

Mattox TW, Crill CM. Parenteral nutrition. In Dipiro JT, Talbert RL, Yee GC, et al., eds. *Pharmacotherapy: A Pathophysiologic Approach.* 8th ed. New York, NY: McGraw Hill; 2011. Available at: http://www.accesspharmacy.com/content.aspx?iAD=8012448.

McClave SA, Martindale RG, et al. Guidelines for the provision and assessment of nutrition support therapy in the adult critically ill patient: Society of Critical Care Medicine (SCCM) and American Society for Parenteral and Enteral Nutrition (A.S.P.E.N.). *J Parenter Enteral Nutr.* 2009;33(3):277–316.

NICE-SUGAR Study Investigators. Intensive versus conventional glucose control in critically ill patients. *N Engl J Med.* 2009;360:1283–97.

Task Force for the Revision of Safe Practices for Parenteral Nutrition. Safe practices for parenteral nutrition. *J Parenter Enteral Nutr.* 2004; 28(suppl):S39–S70.

Ukleja A, Freeman KL, Gilbert K, et al. Standards for nutrition support: Adult hospitalized patients. *Nutr Clin Pract.* 2010;25:403–14.

Oncology 23

J. Aubrey Waddell

23-1. Key Points

- Oncology includes more than 100 diverse diseases that share properties of abnormal and detrimental cell growth.
- Diseases are classified on the basis of the tissue in which they originate (e.g., breast cancer metastasized to the brain is classified as breast cancer).
- Signs and symptoms of cancer often do not follow a specific pattern. A health care provider should evaluate any unusual or persistent change in body appearance or function.
- Before a diagnosis of cancer can be made and systemic treatment can begin, a positive biopsy or blood examination must confirm the presence of the disease.
- Further imaging and laboratory workup should be done to evaluate the extent of the disease (i.e., determine the stage of disease).
- Cancer therapy must be individualized to each patient on the basis of the type and severity of disease, patient characteristics, and patient and family preferences.
- Surgery, radiation, chemotherapy, and biologic therapy are all cancer treatment modalities. They are often used in combination.
- Chemotherapy is often used in combinations to take advantage of different mechanisms of action, prevent resistance, and minimize toxicities.
- Most chemotherapy is aimed at rapidly proliferating cancerous cells. However, many chemotherapy-related side effects occur in normal highly proliferative cells of the body, such as hair follicles, the gastrointestinal tract lining, and blood cells.

- Patients should be aware of expected toxicities of chemotherapy, which include alopecia, diarrhea, nausea and vomiting, infertility, myelosuppression, neurotoxicity, nephrotoxicity, hepatotoxicity, stomatitis, and pulmonary toxicity.
- All prophylactic and post-treatment medications for chemotherapy-related complications should be made available to the patient. Counsel the patient to keep a diary of events that occur prior to and after treatments. Use this record to make interventions and monitor the patient's quality of life.
- All pharmacists should be aware of the accepted cancer screening recommendations and should discuss these with patients. Many diseases can be cured if they are caught early enough.

23-2. Study Guide Checklist

The following topics may guide your study of this subject area:

- General symptoms of malignant diseases
- General goals of therapy for malignant diseases
- Definitions of the various response goals to therapy for solid tumors
- First-line antineoplastic medications for each type of cancer
- Dominant adverse reactions to the various classes of antineoplastic chemotherapy
- Medications used to prevent or treat chemotherapy-induced nausea and vomiting
- Screening recommendations for major cancer types, such as cervical, breast, colorectal, and prostate

23-3. Overview

Definition

Oncology can be defined as the science dealing with the etiology, pathogenesis, and treatment of cancers (synonymous with malignant neoplasms). It encompasses more than 100 different diseases that share characteristics of uncontrollable cell proliferation, invasion of local tissues, sustained angiogenesis, defective programmed cell death, and metastases (e.g., spread from original site).

In the United States, men have roughly a one-in-two cumulative lifetime risk of developing cancer and women have a one-in-three risk. In 2014, an estimated 1,665,540 new cases of cancer were diagnosed, and an estimated 585,720 cancer deaths occurred. The most common types of cancer are prostate, lung, and colorectal in men and breast, lung, and colorectal in women.

Classifications

Neoplastic malignancies arise from four tissue types (epithelial, connective, lymphoid, and nerve) and are classified on the basis of this origin. Table 23-1 lists the tissue origin of each type of malignancy and the corresponding medical terminology.

Table 23-1. Tissue Origin of Malignant Tumor Types

Origin	Tissue type	Malignant tumor
Epithelial	Surface epithelium	Carcinoma
	Glandular tissue	Adenocarcinoma
Connective	Fibrous	Fibrosarcoma
	Bone	Osteosarcoma
	Smooth or striated muscle	Leiomyosarcoma or rhabdomyosarcoma
	Fat	Liposarcoma
Lymphoid	Bone marrow	Leukemia
	Lymphoid	Hodgkin and non-Hodgkin lymphoma
	Plasma cell	Multiple myeloma
Neural	Glial	Glioblastoma and astrocytoma
	Nerve sheath	Neurofibrosarcoma
	Melanocytes	Malignant melanoma
Mixed	Gonadal tissue	Teratocarcinoma

Adapted from Shord, Medina, 2014.

Clinical Presentation

The first signs and symptoms of cancer (solid tumors) develop when the tumor has grown to approximately 10^9 cells (1 cm in diameter or 1 g mass). The type of cancer determines the presentation of signs and symptoms, which vary widely across tumor types.

Positive screening tests (see Table 23-11 in Section 23-5) or generalized signs of anorexia, fatigue, fever, weight loss, and anemia must also be evaluated. Box 23-1 shows the American Cancer Society's warning signs of cancer.

Pathophysiology and Etiology

The following factors promote cancer:

- *External factors:* Tobacco, chemicals, radiation, infectious organisms, and diet
- *Internal factors:* Genetics, hormones, and immune conditions

Development of cancer is genetically regulated and is a multistage process:

- *Initiation:* Normal cells are exposed to chemical, physical, or biological carcinogens. Such exposure results in irreversible damage, genetic mutations, and selective growth advantages.

Box 23-1. Warning Signs of Cancer

Unexplained weight loss

Fever

Fatigue

Pain

Skin changes

Change in bowel habits or bladder function

Sores that do not heal

White patches inside the mouth or white spots on the tongue

Unusual bleeding or discharge

Thickening or lump in the breast or other parts of the body

Indigestion or trouble swallowing

Recent change in a wart or mole or any new skin change

Nagging cough or hoarseness

American Cancer Society, 2014

- *Promotion:* Reversible environmental changes favor the growth of the mutated cells.
- *Transformation:* The cells become cancerous.
- *Progression:* Additional genetic changes occur, resulting in increased cancerous proliferation. Tumors invade local tissues, and metastasis occurs.

Genetic alterations are necessary for the development and growth of cancer. Some of the most common are the following:

- Oncogenes promote growth advantages in mutated cells and cause excessive proliferation (e.g., ras, c-myc).
- Inactivation of tumor suppressor genes (TSGs) results in inappropriate cell growth, because TSGs normally regulate the cell cycle (e.g., p53).
  - Anti-apoptotic genes are activated (e.g., bcl-2).
  - DNA (deoxyribonucleic acid) repair genes experience reduced activity.

Malignant tumor cells do not resemble their tissue of origin (in contrast to benign tumors). They are unstable and are incapable of performing normal cell functions.

Diagnostic Criteria

A sample of suspected malignant tissues or cells is needed for a definitive diagnosis. Sampling can be done with a biopsy, fine-needle aspiration, or exfoliative cytology. This tissue sample is examined by a pathologist, who assigns a stage to the cancer. This process is called *pathological staging.*

Radiation or chemotherapy should not begin without proper clinical and pathological staging. Clinical staging can be accomplished by imaging studies, which may include x-rays, computed tomography (CT), magnetic resonance imaging (MRI), positron emission tomography (PET), and bone scans. Laboratory work may include complete blood counts (CBCs), blood chemistries, and tumor markers.

If a diagnosis of cancer is made, the malignancy will need to be staged or categorized on the basis of severity of the disease and the results of the pathological staging tests. Staging guides the oncology practitioner in determining the prognosis and the treatment regimen for the patient.

The tumor, node, metastasis (TNM) staging system is the most commonly used tool for solid tumors. Tumors are scored numerically on the basis of the size of the tumor, the extent of lymph node involvement, and the presence or absence of metastases. This score allows classification of tumors by stage, from 0 to IV,

with stage IV denoting the presence of metastasis (e.g., most severe disease). A stage 0 tumor is called a carcinoma in situ, where the malignancy has not yet invaded the basement membrane of the epithelial surface.

Lymphoid tumors are staged differently and are beyond the scope of this review. Refer to Chan and Yee (2014) for more information.

Treatment Principles and Goals

Treatment regimens are based on the type of cancer, stage, age of the patient, and other prognostic factors (e.g., presence of a tumor marker, poor performance status, and ethnicity, among others).

Primary therapy is the initial and mainstay approach to treat cancer. It usually consists of removal of the tumor or debulking through surgery but may also include chemotherapy, radiation, or both.

Neoadjuvant therapy is given prior to the primary therapy. The goal is to reduce the size of the tumor, thereby increasing the efficacy of the primary treatment. Examples include chemotherapy or radiation.

Adjuvant therapy is additional therapy given after the main treatment, which is usually surgery. The goal is to ensure that all the residual disease has been eradicated. Adjuvant therapy usually consists of chemotherapy, radiation therapy, or both.

The four main cancer treatments are surgery, radiation, chemotherapy, and biologic therapy. Most regimens are a combination of these modalities:

- *Surgery* alone is reserved for solid localized tumors, where the entire cancer can be resected. It may also be combined with other modalities in later stages of the disease. It is not an option for patients with lymphoid-based disease (e.g., Hodgkin lymphoma).
- *Radiation* alone is also reserved for curing localized tumors because it treats a very focused area. It also can be combined with other treatments as neoadjuvant or adjuvant therapy to reduce disease-related symptoms or to reduce the incidence of disease recurrence.
- *Chemotherapy* is a means of systemic treatment, in contrast to the two types of local treatment just described. It can be used to treat the primary tumor as well as metastases. Chemotherapy is generally not administered to patients with local disease that can be fully resected.
- *Biologic therapy* is another systemic treatment and includes agents such as monoclonal antibodies, interferons, interleukins, and tumor vaccines. It is a relatively new type of treatment and acts by stimulating the host immune system.

The goals of cancer therapy are based on the type and stage of cancer, as well as on patient characteristics (e.g., an older patient with a short life expectancy may not be offered intense treatment that may impair quality of life). Goals may be as follows:

- *Localized or regional disease* (i.e., stages 0, I, II, and early III): Provide curative intent, and inhibit recurrence of disease. Stage 0 diseases are often not treated but monitored until clinically apparent.
- *Advanced or metastasized disease* (i.e., advanced stage III and all stage IV): Palliate symptoms, reduce tumor load, prolong survival, and increase quality of life.

Survival and response to treatment

In 2014, more than 1,600 people per day in the United States will die of a cancer-related cause, which accounts for about one in four deaths. Survival depends on patient characteristics, type of disease, stage of disease, and treatment regimen. Older patients with more severe disease, poor performance status, and faster-growing tumors have a poor prognosis.

Responses to treatment modalities for solid tumors are classified as follows:

- *Cure:* 5 years of cancer-free survival for most tumor types
- *Complete response:* Absence of all neoplastic disease for a minimum of 1 month after cessation of treatment
- *Partial response:* ≥ 50% decrease in tumor size or other disease markers for a minimum of 1 month
- *Stable disease:* No change or no meeting of criteria for partial response or progression
- *Progression:* ≥ 25% increase in tumor size or new lesion

Response to treatment for hematologic cancers is measured by the elimination of abnormal cells, a decrease in tumor markers to normal, and the improved function of affected cells.

23-4. Drug Therapy

Chemotherapy

Chemotherapeutic agents have a very narrow therapeutic index and a toxic side-effect profile. They are generally more effective in combination because of synergism through biochemical interactions. It is important to choose drugs with different mecha-nisms of action, resistance, and toxicity profiles to get the full benefit of combination therapy.

Chemotherapy has the greatest effect on rapidly dividing cells, because most of the potent chemotherapy drugs act by damaging DNA. These agents are more active in different phases of the cell cycle. A therapeutic effect is seen on cancer cells, but adverse effects are also seen on human cells that rapidly divide (e.g., hair follicles, gastrointestinal [GI] tract, and blood cells). Agents can be phase specific or phase nonspecific. Nonspecific agents are effective in all phases.

Cell Cycle Phases

- G_0 = *resting phase:* No cell division occurs, and cancer cells are generally not susceptible to chemotherapy. This lack of susceptibility is problematic for slow-growing tumors that exist primarily in this phase.
- G_1 = *postmitotic phase:* Enzymes for DNA synthesis are manufactured, lasting 18–30 hours.
- S = *DNA synthesis phase:* DNA separation and replication occur, lasting 16–20 hours.
- G_2 = *premitotic phase:* Specialized proteins and RNA (ribonucleic acid) are made, lasting 2–10 hours.
- M = *mitosis:* Actual cell division occurs, lasting 30–60 minutes.

Drug Classes

There are numerous chemotherapy agents. Drugs are grouped by class. Refer to the corresponding table for each class of drugs.

Alkylating agents

Table 23-2 provides summary information about alkylating agents.

Mechanism of action
Alkylating agents cause covalent bond formation of drugs to nucleic acids and proteins, which results in the cross-linking of one or two DNA strands and inhibition of DNA replication. These agents are not phase specific. The most commonly used agents include cyclophosphamide, ifosfamide, carmustine, dacarbazine, and temozolomide.

Patient instructions and counseling
- All drugs are carcinogenic, teratogenic, and mutagenic.
- Medications may cause sterility.

Table 23-2. Alkylating Agents

Generic name	Trade name	Dosage range	Dosage form	Frequency	Disease[a]
Nitrogen mustard					
Mechlorethamine	Mustargen	6–10 mg/m²	IV	Days 1, 8 q 4 wk	HL, NHL
Cyclophosphamide	Cytoxan, Neosar	500–2,000 mg/m², 40–100 mg/m²	IV, po	q 3 wk, daily 2–14 days	ALL, CLL, HL, NHL, myeloma, testis, neuroblastoma, breast, ovary, lung, cervix
Ifosfamide	Ifex	1.2 g/m²	IV	Daily × 5 days q 3 wk	HL, NHL, lung, bladder, sarcoma
Melphalan	Alkeran	16 mg/m², 6 mg/m²	IV, po	q 4 wk, daily 4 days q 4 wk	Myeloma, breast, ovary
Chlorambucil	Leukeran	0.1–0.2 mg/kg	po	Daily × 3–6 wk	CLL, HL, NHL
Bendamustine	Treanda	100–120 mg/m²	IV	Daily × 2 days q 21–28 days	CLL, NHL
Ethylenimines and methylmelamines					
Altretamine	Hexalen	260 mg/m²	po	Daily × 14–21 days	Ovarian
Thiotepa	Thioplex	10–20 mg/m²	IV	q 3–4 wk	Bladder, breast, ovarian, HL, NHL
Alkyl sulfonates					
Busulfan	Myleran, Busulfex	4–8 mg/kg	IV, po	Daily	CML, BMT
Nitrosureas					
Carmustine	BiCNU	150–200 mg/m²	IV	q 6 wk	HL, NHL, brain, myeloma
Streptozocin	Zanosar	500 mg/m²	IV	Daily × 5 days q 6 wk	Islet cell carcinoma
Polifeprosan 20 with carmustine implant	Gliadel	7.7 mg	Implant	n.a.	Glioblastoma multiforme

ALL, acute lymphocytic leukemia; BMT, bone marrow transplant; CLL, chronic lymphocytic leukemia; CML, chronic myelogenous leukemia; HL, Hodgkin lymphoma; n.a., not applicable; NHL, non-Hodgkin lymphoma.

a. Appearance of a disease in the list does not indicate U.S. Food and Drug Administration approval for the drug's use in treatment of that disease, but does indicate use of that drug in that disease in clinical practice.

- Let your dentist know you are on chemotherapy because of an increased risk of bleeding and infections.
- Hydration and mesna therapy are recommended for cyclophosphamide and ifosfamide.
- Let your health care provider know if you have burning when urinating.

Adverse drug events
The following adverse events may occur: myelosuppression, primarily leukopenia; mucosal ulceration; pulmonary fibrosis (carmustine) and interstitial pneumonitis; pyrexia and fatigue (bendamustine); alopecia; nausea and vomiting; amenorrhea and azoospermia; hemorrhagic cystitis (cyclophosphamide and ifosfamide); encephalopathy (ifosfamide); and seizures (polifeprosan and carmustine).

Drug interactions
Drugs with specific interactions of moderate to major severity include the following:

- *Altretamine:* Tricyclic antidepressants and monoamine oxidase inhibitors
- *Bendamustine:* Strong cytochrome P450 (CYP450) 1A2 inhibitors
- *Busulfan:* Itraconazole, phenytoin, and acetaminophen
- *Carmustine:* Cimetidine, ethyl alcohol, phenytoin, and amphotericin B

- *Cyclophosphamide:* Allopurinol, barbiturates, digoxin, phenytoin, and warfarin
- *Ifosfamide:* Allopurinol, phenytoin, and warfarin
- *Streptozocin:* Nephrotoxic agents

Monitoring parameters
Monitor pulmonary function tests, renal and hepatic tests, chest x-rays, CBC with differential (baseline and expected nadir prior to next cycle) and electro-lytes, urinalysis for red blood count detection from hemorrhagic cystitis, signs of bleeding (bruising and melena), infection (sore throat and fever), and nausea or vomiting.

Antimetabolites: S-phase specific

See Table 23-3 for general information about anti-metabolites.

Table 23-3. Antimetabolites

Generic name	Trade name	Dosage range	Dosage form	Frequency	Disease[a]
Folic acid antagonists					
Pralatrexate	Folotyn	30 mg/m^2	IV	q wk × 6 wk, then 1 wk off	Peripheral T-cell lymphoma
Pemetrexed	**Alimta**	500–600 mg/m^2	IV	q 21 days	Malignant mesothelioma
Methotrexate	Rheumatrex	10–12 mg, 1–10 g/m^2, 25 mg/m^2, 10 mg/m^2	Intrathecal, IV, IM, po	q wk, q 3 wk, q wk, q wk	NSCLC, breast, NHL, sarcoma, ALL
Pyrimidine analogs					
Azacitidine	Vidaza	75–100 mg/m^2	SC, IV	Daily × 7 days q 4 wk	Myelodysplastic syndrome
Fluorouracil, 5-FU	Adrucil	450 mg/m^2	IV	Daily × 5 days	Colorectal, breast, head, neck
Cytarabine	Cytosar-U, DepoCyt	3 g/m^2, 100–200 mg/m^2, 50 mg	IV, continuous IV, intrathecal	q 12 h days 1, 3, 5 q 6 wk, daily × 7 days q 14 days	ALL, AML, CML
Capecitabine	Xeloda	2,500 mg/m^2	po	Daily × 14 days q 3 wk	Breast, colorectal
Gemcitabine	Gemzar	1,000–1,250 mg/m^2	IV	q wk	Pancreatic, NSCLC, bladder
Decitabine	Dacogen	15 mg/m^2	IV	q 8 h × 3 days q 6 wk	Myelodysplastic syndrome
Purine analogs					
Clofarabine	Clolar	52 mg/m^2	IV	Daily × 5 days q 4 wk	ALL (pediatric)
Mercaptopurine	Purinethol	1.5–2.5 mg/kg	po	Daily	ALL
Thioguanine	Tabloid	2–3 mg/kg	po	Daily	ALL, AML
Pentostatin	Nipent	4 mg/m^2	IV	q 2 wk	CLL, hairy cell leukemia, ALL
Cladribine	Leustatin	0.09–0.1 mg/kg	IV	Daily × 7 days	NHL, hairy cell leukemia, CLL
Fludarabine	Fludara	25 mg/m^2	IV	Daily × 5 days q 4 wk	CLL, NHL
Guanosine analogs					
Nelarabine	Arranon	Children: 650 mg/m^2/day	IV	Daily × 5 days q 21 days	T-cell ALL or NHL
		Adults: 1,500 mg/m^2/day	IV	Days 1, 3, 5 q 21 days	

ALL, acute lymphocytic leukemia; AML, acute myelogenous leukemia; CLL, chronic lymphocytic leukemia; CML, chronic myelogenous leukemia; NHL, non-Hodgkin lymphoma; NSCLC, non–small cell lung cancer.
Boldface indicates one of top 100 drugs for 2012 by units sold at retail outlets, www.drugs.com/stats/top100/2012/units.
a. Appearance of a disease in the list does not indicate U.S. Food and Drug Administration approval for the drug's use in treatment of that disease, but does indicate use of that drug in that disease in clinical practice.

Mechanism of action

These agents are structural analogues of natural metabolites and act by falsely inserting themselves in place of a pyrimidine or purine ring, causing interference in nucleic acid synthesis. Phase-specific agents are most active in the S phase and in tumors with a high growth fraction. They are subdivided into three groups: folate, purine, and pyrimidine antagonists.

Patient instructions and counseling

- Avoid crowds and sick people.
- If receiving fluorouracil (5-FU), you may be asked to chew ice to reduce damage to the mucosal lining in your mouth.
- Contact your health care provider if you have uncontrollable nausea or vomiting; excessive diarrhea; or pain, swelling, or tingling in palms of hands and soles of feet (hand-foot syndrome).
- Call your health care provider if you feel dizzy or lightheaded or have trouble urinating (clofarabine).
- You should be receiving folic acid and vitamin B_{12} injections if you are receiving pemetrexed.
- Nelarabine may cause sleepiness and dizziness.

Adverse drug events

Adverse events include hand-foot syndrome and stomatitis (5-FU and capecitabine); severe diarrhea, GI mucosal damage, nausea, vomiting, fatigue, myelosuppression, alopecia, and neurotoxicity (nelarabine, cytarabine, fludarabine, and methotrexate); rash, fever, and flu-like symptoms (gemcitabine); renal toxicity and mucositis (5-FU and methotrexate); conjunctivitis (cytarabine, especially in high doses); hemolytic uremic syndrome (gemcitabine); opportunistic infections (cladribine and fludarabine); and tumor lysis syndrome, systemic inflammatory response syndrome, or capillary leak (clofarabine).

Drug interactions

Drugs with specific interactions include the following:

- **Capecitabine:** Warfarin and phenytoin
- **Cytarabine:** Digoxin
- **Fluorouracil:** Warfarin
- **Mercaptopurine:** Warfarin and allopurinol
- **Methotrexate:** Nonsteroidal anti-inflammatory drugs (NSAIDs), amiodarone, amoxicillin, sulfasalazine, doxycycline, erythromycin, hydrochlorothiazide, mercaptopurine, omeprazole, phenytoin, and folic acid
- **Pentostatin:** Cyclophosphamide and fludarabine

Monitoring parameters

Note any complaints of mucositis or mouth soreness; monitor for neurotoxicity (e.g., ask the patient to write his or her name), CBC with differential prior to each dose of drug, and hepatic and renal function; and monitor for tingling or swelling of palms of hands and soles of feet, bruising or bleeding, and international normalized ratio (capecitabine). Monitor weight, and question patient about diarrhea, jaundice, and hepatomegaly (mercaptopurine). Continuous intravenous (IV) fluids and allopurinol for prevention of tumor lysis syndrome should be administered to patients taking clofarabine, and those patients should also receive prophylactic corticosteroids for systemic inflammatory response syndrome and capillary leak. Pemetrexed toxicities are reduced by lowering plasma homocysteine levels with concomitant folic acid and vitamin B_{12}. Dexamethasone should be given to prevent cutaneous reactions caused by pemetrexed.

Antitumor antibiotics

For additional information about antitumor antibiotics, consult Table 23-4.

Mechanism of action

Anthracyclines block DNA and RNA transcription through the intercalation (insertion) of adjoining nucleic acid pairs in DNA, which results in DNA strand breakage. They also inhibit the topoisomerase II enzyme. Mitomycin is an alkylating-like agent that cross-links DNA. Dactinomycin blocks RNA synthesis. Bleomycin inhibits DNA synthesis in mitosis and G_2 stages of growth. Bleomycin is the only cell cycle–specific agent.

Patient instructions and counseling

- Contact your health care provider if you have fast, slow, or irregular heartbeats or breathing difficulties.
- Anthracyclines may cause a change of urine color or change the whites of eyes to a blue-green or orange-red color.
- Bleomycin may cause a change in skin color or nail growth.

Adverse drug events

Events include severe nausea and vomiting, alopecia, and stomatitis. Anthracyclines may cause cardiac toxicity, acute or chronic (doxorubicin = daunorubicin > idarubicin > epirubicin > mitoxantrone). All anthracyclines have limits on cumulative lifetime dosing, are vesicants, and are associated with secondary acute myelogenous leukemia (AML); avoid in patients

Table 23-4. Antitumor Antibiotics

Generic name	Trade name	Dosage range	Dosage form	Frequency	Disease[a]
Anthracyclines					
Doxorubicin	Adriamycin, Doxil (liposomal)	60–75 mg/m², 20–50 mg/m² (liposomal)	IV	q 3 wk	ALL, AML, NHL, HL, solid tumors of every major organ
Daunorubicin	Cerubidine, Daunoxome (liposomal)	45 mg/m², 40 mg/m² (liposomal)	IV	Daily × 3 days, q 2 wk	ALL, AML, NHL
Epirubicin	Ellence, Pharmarubicin	60–120 mg/m²	IV	q 3 wk	Breast, bladder, lung, ovarian, gastric
Idarubicin	Idamycin	12–13 mg/m²	IV	Daily × 3 days	AML, ALL, breast
Mitoxantrone	Novantrone	12–14 mg/m²	IV	q 3 wk	Prostate, NHL, AML, breast
Valrubicin	Valstar	800 mg	Intravesical	q wk × 6 wk	Bladder
Alkylating-like					
Mitomycin	Mutamycin	10–20 mg/m²	IV, intravesical	q 6–8 wk	Bladder, breast, NSCLC, cervix, pancreatic, colon
Chromomycin					
Dactinomycin	Cosmegen	12–15 mcg/kg	IV	Daily × 5 days	Wilms' tumor, testis, sarcoma
Miscellaneous					
Bleomycin	Blenoxane	10–20 USP units/m²/wk	IM, IV, SC	q wk	HL, NHL, testis, head, neck, lung, skin

ALL, acute lymphocytic leukemia; AML, acute myelogenous leukemia; HL, Hodgkin lymphoma; NHL, non-Hodgkin lymphoma; NSCLC, non–small cell lung cancer.

a. Appearance of a disease in the list does not indicate U.S. Food and Drug Administration approval for the drug's use in treatment of that disease, but does indicate use of that drug in that disease in clinical practice.

with a cardiac history. Myelosuppression risk exists with all agents, although mitomycin demonstrates a delayed effect. Dactinomycin may cause renal toxicity, leukopenia, and increased pigmentation of previously radiated skin. Bleomycin may cause pulmonary fibrosis and interstitial pneumonitis. Mitomycin may cause hemolytic uremic syndrome.

Drug interactions
Drugs with specific interactions include the following:

- *Bleomycin:* Phenytoin and digoxin
- *Doxorubicin:* Cisplatin, digoxin, paclitaxel, phenytoin, phenobarbital, trastuzumab, and zidovudine
- *Epirubicin:* Cimetidine and trastuzumab
- *Idarubicin:* Probenecid and trastuzumab

Monitoring parameters
Monitor hepatic and renal function, CBC with differential, and pulmonary function tests before and after treatment with bleomycin. Provide cardiac monitoring through left ventricular ejection fraction measurements for anthracyclines as well as monitoring of the cumulative lifetime dose, and be alert for extravasation and necrosis with anthracyclines. Adjust anthracycline dosing on the basis of elevated total bilirubin.

Pharmacokinetics
Anthracyclines are extensively bound in the tissue, have large volumes of distribution and long half-lives, and are excreted in the bile. Dosing adjustments are necessary in patients with hepatic impairment. Bleomycin is renally excreted and requires dosing adjustments in impaired patients.

Other factors
Lifetime doses of doxorubicin should not exceed 450–550 mg/m², taking into account other anthracycline agents received. The lifetime maximum

for epirubicin is 900 mg/m²; for idarubicin, it is 150 mg/m².

Hormones and antagonists

Table 23-5 provides information about hormones and antagonists.

Mechanism of action

This diverse group of compounds acts on hormone-dependent tumors by inhibiting or decreasing the production of the disease-causing hormone.

Patient instructions and counseling

- Avoid use in pregnant women; several agents may cause weight gain and menstrual irregularities in women.
- Be aware of leg swelling or tenderness (e.g., signs of a deep-vein thrombosis), breathing problems, and sweating.
- Transient muscle or bone pain, problems urinating, and spinal cord compression may occur initially in patients receiving luteinizing hormone–releasing hormone (LHRH) agonists.
- Take exemestane after meals.

Adverse drug events

Events include edema, menstrual disorders, hot flashes, transient muscle or bone pain, tumor flare, and transient increase in serum testosterone (LHRH agonists); thromboembolic events, gynecomastia, elevated liver enzymes, nausea and vomiting, diarrhea, erectile impotence, decreased libido, endometrial cancers with tamoxifen, and bone loss (LHRH and aromatase inhibitors); seizure (enzalutamide); and risk of ventricular arrhythmias and QT prolongation.

Drug interactions

Drugs with specific interactions include the following:

- **Aminoglutethimide:** Dexamethasone, warfarin, tamoxifen, and theophylline
- **Anastrozole:** Estrogens and antiestrogens
- **Bicalutamide:** Warfarin
- **Degarelix:** Amiodarone, procainamide, quinidine, and sotalol
- **Enzalutamide:** Strong CYP2C6 inhibitors and strong or moderate CYP3A4/2C8 inducers
- **Exemestane:** CYP3A4 inducers (such as carbamazepine and phenytoin), estrogens, and antiestrogens
- **Fluoxymesterone:** Cyclosporine, anticoagulants, and valerian
- **Flutamide:** Warfarin
- **Letrozole:** Estrogens and antiestrogens
- **Medroxyprogesterone acetate:** Aminoglutethimide and rifampin
- **Megestrol:** Dofetilide contraindication
- **Nilutamide:** Alcohol
- **Tamoxifen:** Anticoagulants and cyclophosphamide
- **Toremifene:** CYP3A4 inducers (such as carbamazepine and phenytoin)

Monitoring parameters

Check white blood counts (WBCs) with differential, platelets, liver function tests, thyroid function, and serum creatinine regularly. Note any weight changes, abnormal vaginal bleeding, body or bone pain, galactorrhea, or decreased libido. Monitor for embolic disorders and uterine cancer (in females). Check prostate-specific antigen (PSA) and testosterone levels in males. Monitor bone mineral density for LHRH agonist and aromatase inhibitors.

Pharmacokinetics

The majority of agents are available orally with longer half-lives, allowing once-daily dosing.

Other factors

Agents are often contraindicated if the patient has more than one hormone-dependent tumor. With the exception of tamoxifen, third-generation aromatase inhibitors, and LHRH agonists, the majority of agents are not indicated for first-line therapy.

Plant alkaloids

See Table 23-6 for information about plant alkaloids.

Mechanism of action

These agents inhibit the replication of cancerous cells. Taxanes and vincas interfere with microtubule assembly in the M phase. Camptothecins and epipodophyllotoxins inhibit topoisomerase I and II enzymes, respectively, causing DNA strand breaks. Topoisomerase I and II affect G_2 and S phases, respectively.

Patient instructions and counseling

- Contact your health care provider for uncontrollable diarrhea (irinotecan), nausea or vomiting, or signs and symptoms of an infection.
- Patients should receive prophylaxis for emesis and pretreatment for anaphylaxis or peripheral edema (taxanes).

Table 23-5. Hormones and Antagonists

Generic name	Trade name	Dosage range	Dosage form	Frequency	Disease[a]
Adrenocorticoids					
Aminoglutethimide	Cytadren	250 mg	po	Daily	Adrenal, breast, prostate
Progestins					
Megestrol acetate	Megace	40 mg, 40–320 mg	po	qid, daily divided	Breast, endometrial
Medroxyprogesterone	Provera, Depo-Provera	400–1,000 mg	IM	q wk	Endometrial acetate
Estrogens					
Ethinyl estradiol	Estinyl	150 mcg to 3 mg, 100 mcg to 1 mg	po	Daily	Prostate, breast
Antiestrogen					
Tamoxifen	Nolvadex	20–40 mg	po	Daily	Breast
Fulvestrant	Faslodex	500 mg	IM	q mo	Breast
Toremifene	Fareston	60 mg	po	Daily	Breast
Third-generation aromatase inhibitors					
Exemestane	Aromasin	25 mg	po	Daily	Breast
Anastrozole	Arimidex	1 mg	po	Daily	Breast
Letrozole	Femara	2.5 mg	po	Daily	Breast
Androgens					
Testosterone propionate	Delatestryl	200–400 mg	IM	Daily	Breast
Fluoxymesterone	Halotestin	10–40 mg	po	q 2–4 wk	Breast
Antiandrogens					
Flutamide	Eulexin	250 mg	po	tid	Prostate
Bicalutamide	Casodex	50 mg	po	Daily	Prostate
Nilutamide	Nilandron	300 mg, 150 mg	po	Daily × 30 days, daily	Prostate
Abiraterone acetate	Zytiga	1,000 mg	po	Daily	Prostate
Enzalutamide	Xtandi	160 mg	po	Daily	Prostate
LHRH agonists					
Triptorelin	Trelstar	3.75 mg, 11.25 mg	IM	q 28 days, q 84 days	Prostate
Leuprolide	Lupron, Eligard	7.5 mg, 22.5 mg, 30 mg, 45 mg, 65 mg	IM, SC	q mo, q 3 mo, q 4 mo, q 6 mo, q 12 mo	Prostate, breast
Goserelin	Zoladex	3.6 mg, 10.8 mg	SC	q mo, q 3 mo	Prostate, breast
GNRH antagonist					
Degarelix		240 mg, 80 mg	SC	First month, then q 28 days	Prostate

GNRH, gonadotropin-releasing hormone; LHRH, luteinizing hormone–releasing hormone.

a. Appearance of a disease in the list does not indicate U.S. Food and Drug Administration approval for the drug's use in treatment of that disease, but does indicate use of that drug in that disease in clinical practice.

Table 23-6. Plant Alkaloids

Generic name	Trade name	Dosage range	Dosage form	Frequency	Disease[a]
Taxanes					
Docetaxel	Taxotere	60–100 mg/m^2	IV	q 3 wk	NSCLC, breast, ovarian, head, neck, gastric
Paclitaxel	Taxol	135–175 mg/m^2	IV	q 3 wk	NSCLC, breast, ovarian, head
Paclitaxel (protein-bound)	Abraxane	260 mg/m^2	IV	q 3 wk	Breast
Cabazitaxel	Jevtana	25 mg/m^2	IV	q 3 wk	Prostate
Halichondrin B analog					
Eribulin	Halaven	1.4 mg/m^2	IV	q wk × 2 wk, then 1 wk off	Breast
Epothilones					
Ixabepilone	Ixempra	40 mg/m^2 (maximum 88 mg)	IV	q 3 wk	Breast
Epipodophyllotoxins					
Etoposide	VePesid	100 mg/m^2, 50 mg/m^2	IV, po	Daily × 3–5 days q 3 wk, daily × 21 days q 4 wk	SCLC, testis, NSCLC
Teniposide	Vumon	165 mg/m^2	IV	q wk × 4 doses	ALL, SCLC
Camptothecins					
Irinotecan	Camptosar	100–125 mg/m^2	IV	q wk	Colorectal, NSCLC, SCLC
Topotecan	Hycamtin	1.5 mg/m^2	IV	Daily × 5 days q 21 days	Ovarian, lung, AML, cervical
Vinca alkaloids					
Vincristine	Oncovin	1.4 mg/m^2	IV	q wk	ALL, HL, NHL, CLL
Vinblastine	Velban	6 mg/m^2	IV	q 2–3 wk	HL, NHL, testis
Vinorelbine	Navelbine	25–30 mg/m^2	IV	q wk	NSCLC, breast, ovarian

ALL, acute lymphocytic leukemia; AML, acute myelogenous leukemia; CLL, chronic lymphocytic leukemia; HL, Hodgkin lymphoma; NHL, non-Hodgkin lymphoma; NSCLC, non–small cell lung cancer; SCLC, small cell lung cancer.

a. Appearance of a disease in the list does not indicate U.S. Food and Drug Administration approval for the drug's use in treatment of that disease, but does indicate use of that drug in that disease in clinical practice.

- Patients should receive a prescription for loperamide for delayed diarrhea with irinotecan therapy.

Adverse drug events
Adverse events include myelosuppression, mucositis, nausea and vomiting, alopecia, edema, and hand-foot syndrome (docetaxel); hypotension or hypersensitivity on administration (paclitaxel); neurotoxicity (vincristine); peripheral neuropathy and myalgia or arthralgia (ixabepilone and paclitaxel); diarrhea, headache, and secondary malignancies (topoisomerase II inhibitors);

and syndrome of inappropriate antidiuretic hormone secretion (SIADH) (vinca alkaloids).

Drug interactions
Drugs with specific interactions include the following:

- ***Docetaxel:*** CYP3A4 inducers and inhibitors
- ***Etoposide:*** Cyclosporine, St. John's wort, and warfarin
- ***Irinotecan:*** St. John's wort
- ***Ixabepilone:*** CYP3A4 inducers and inhibitors
- ***Paclitaxel:*** CYP3A4 inducers and inhibitors
- ***Teniposide:*** CYP3A4 inducers and inhibitors

- *Vinblastine:* Phenytoin, erythromycin, mitomycin, and zidovudine
- *Vinca alkaloids:* CYP3A4 inhibitors, itraconazole, and voriconazole
- *Vincristine:* Phenytoin, l-asparaginase, carbamazepine, digoxin, filgrastim, nifedipine, and zidovudine

Monitoring parameters

Monitor WBCs with differential for all agents; peripheral neuropathy, liver and renal function, painful mouth sores, and blood pressure (taxanes and epipodophyllotoxins); acute and late-onset diarrhea or dyspnea on exertion (irinotecan); bilirubin elevations (taxanes and camptothecins); fluid retention (docetaxel); and neuropathy, shortness of breath, bronchospasm, and SIADH (vincas).

Pharmacokinetics

Taxanes and epipodophyllotoxins are extensively bound to plasma and tissues.

Other factors

Drug resistance may occur through p-glycoprotein pumps for all agents. Topotecan needs dose adjustments for patients with a creatinine clearance < 40 mL/min. Vincas are vesicants and need close monitoring for extravasation. Vincristine should not be administered intrathecally. In adult patients, vincristine doses are often capped at 2 mg although research to support this practice is limited.

Dose adjustments may be needed for patients with liver impairment.

Biologic Response Modifiers and Monoclonal Antibodies

Table 23-7 provides information about biologic response modifiers and monoclonal antibodies.

Mechanism of action

Biologic response modifiers activate the body's immune-mediated host defense mechanisms to malignant cells. In contrast to immunotherapy, these agents have direct biological effects on malignancies. Monoclonal antibodies bind to specific antigens and kill malignant cells through the activation of apoptosis, an antibody-mediated toxicity, or complement-mediated lysis.

Patient instructions and counseling

- Let your health care provider know if you have severe fatigue, trouble breathing, or irregular heart rhythms.
- Chills, fever, depression, and flu-like symptoms are common.
- Monoclonal antibodies can cause infusion-related reactions such as fever and chills.
- If you receive bevacizumab, you should have your blood pressure checked regularly and have tests that check for protein in your urine.
- You should wear sunscreen and avoid excessive sunlight if you are receiving cetuximab.
- You should receive medication for your thyroid if you are going to receive tositumomab.
- For both men and women, do not try to conceive until 12 months after finishing therapy.
- With thalidomide and lenalidomide, do not get pregnant. Two forms of birth control must be used both by women and by men on the drug who have sexual contact with women of childbearing age.

Adverse drug events

Events include hypotension and hypersensitivity on infusion; cardiac, pulmonary, and renal impairment; and mental status changes (e.g., depression), fever, chills, nausea, and musculoskeletal pain with all agents. Other events include tumor lysis syndrome (rituximab); bleeding, hemorrhage, hypertension, proteinuria, and skin rash (bevacizumab); cutaneous and severe infusion reactions and interstitial lung disease (cetuximab); and hypothyroidism (tositumomab). Avoid use in patients with autoimmune disorders.

Additional events include neurotoxicity (thalidomide) and neutropenia, deep-vein thrombosis, and pulmonary embolism (thalidomide and lenalidomide).

Drug interactions

Drugs with specific drug interactions include the following:

- *Aldesleukin:* Glucocorticoids, NSAIDs, and antihypertensives
- *Brentuximab vedotin:* CYP3A4 inhibitors and inducers
- *Ibritumomab:* Antiplatelets and anticoagulants
- *Interferon alfa-2b:* Zidovudine, theophylline, phenytoin, and phenobarbital
- *Tositumomab:* Antiplatelets and anticoagulants
- *Trastuzumab:* Anthracyclines, cyclophosphamide, and warfarin

Monitoring parameters

Monitor baseline and follow-up pulmonary, cardiac, and renal function tests. Check CBCs with differential, liver function tests, thyroid-stimulating hormone,

Table 23-7. Biologic Response Modifiers and Monoclonal Antibodies

Generic name	Trade name	Dosage range	Dosage form	Frequency	Disease[a]
Immune therapies					
Aldesleukin	Proleukin	600,000 units/kg	IV	q 8 h × 14 doses	Metastatic renal cell carcinoma, metastatic melanoma
Interferon alfa-2b	Intron A	20×10^6 units/m², then 10×10^6 units/m²	IV SC	Daily × 5 days per wk × 4 wk,[b] then M-W-F × 11 mo.	Malignant melanoma
		2×10^6 units/m²	SC	M-W-F × 6 mo.	Hairy cell leukemia
Peginterferon alfa-2b	PegIntron	1.5 mcg/kg	SC	q wk	Malignant melanoma
Sipuleucel-T	Provenge	Individualized	IV	q 2 wk × 3	Prostate cancer
Thalidomide	Thalomid	200 mg	po	Daily	Multiple myeloma, erythema nodosum leprosum
Lenalidomide	Revlimid	10 mg	po	Daily	Myelodysplastic syndrome
		25 mg	po	Daily days 1–21 q 28 days	Multiple myeloma
Monoclonal antibodies					
Rituximab	**Rituxan**	375 mg/m²	IV	q wk × 4–8 doses, q 3 wk	NHL, CLL
Trastuzumab	**Herceptin**	2–6 mg/kg	IV, SC	q wk	Breast
Pertuzumab	Perjeta	Initial: 840 mg	IV	Once	Breast
		420 mg	IV	q 3 wk	
Alemtuzumab	Campath	3–10 mg	IV	Daily, then 30 mg 3 × wk	B-cell CLL
Bevacizumab	**Avastin**	5–15 mg/kg	IV	q 2 wk *or* q 3 wk	Colorectal, NSCLC, breast, glioblastoma, renal cell carcinoma
Cetuximab	Erbitux	250–500 mg/m²	IV	q 1–2 wk	Colorectal, head, neck
Ofatumumab	Arzerra	300 mg, 2,000 mg	IV	Initial dose, q wk × 7 wk, then 4 wk off, then q 4 wk × 4	CLL
Ipilimumab	Yervoy	3 mg/kg	IV	q 3 wk × 4	Melanoma
Panitumumab	Vectibix	6 mg/kg	IV	q 2 wk	Colorectal
Eculizumab	Soliris	600 mg, 900 mg	IV	q wk × 4 wk, then q 2 wk	Paroxysmal nocturnal hemoglobinuria
Denileukin diftitox	Ontak	9 or 18 mcg/kg	IV	Daily × 5 days q 21 days	T-cell lymphoma
Ibritumomab tiuxetan	Zevalin[c]				NHL
Tositumomab	Bexxar[c]				NHL
Brentuximab vedotin	Adcetris	1.8 mg/kg	IV	q 3 wk	NHL

CLL, chronic lymphocytic leukemia; NHL, non-Hodgkin lymphoma; NSCLC, non–small cell lung cancer.

Boldface indicates one of top 100 drugs for 2012 by units sold at retail outlets, www.drugs.com/stats/top100/2012/units.

a. Appearance of a disease in the list does not indicate U.S. Food and Drug Administration approval for the drug's use in treatment of that disease, but does indicate use of that drug in that disease in clinical practice.

b. Induction dose.

c. See package insert for range, form, and frequency of dosing.

electrolytes, and glucose regularly. Premedicate with acetaminophen and diphenhydramine for monoclonal antibodies. Observe blood pressure during infusion (hypotension concerns) for all agents. Perform blood pressure monitoring (hypertensive concerns) and urine dipstick analysis (bevacizumab). Monitor for vital signs, itching, and swelling. Check for trouble breathing (cetuximab and ibritumomab).

Other factors

Ensure that the correct form of interferon alfa is being used (four forms). Do not administer alemtuzumab as an IV push or bolus.

Miscellaneous Agents

Miscellaneous agents are described in Table 23-8.

Platinum compounds

These compounds are alklyating-like agents that cause the inhibition of DNA synthesis. They include cisplatin, carboplatin, and oxaliplatin. Adverse effects include nephrotoxicity, peripheral neurotoxicity, myelosuppression, ototoxicity, nausea, and vomiting.

Cisplatin needs hydration therapy and premedications. It interacts with doxorubicin, rituximab, tacrolimus, topotecan, and aminoglycosides.

Carboplatin needs monitoring for thrombocytopenia. It interacts with aminoglycosides.

Oxaliplatin has unique neurotoxicities (e.g., bronchial spasms).

Sorafenib

Sorafenib inhibits multiple tyrosine kinases and is used for treatment of advanced renal cell cancer. Take tablets on an empty stomach. Sorafenib causes diarrhea, fatigue, rash, hand-foot syndrome, hypertension, nausea and vomiting, neutropenia, and alopecia. It can decrease doxorubicin and irinotecan levels.

Sunitinib

Sunitinib inhibits multiple tyrosine kinases and is used for treatment of advanced renal cell cancer and GI stromal tumors. Take it with or without food. It causes neutropenia, rash changes in skin color, fatigue, myalgia, headaches, hypertension, nausea and vomiting, diarrhea, and increased liver enzymes.

Table 23-8. Miscellaneous Agents

Generic name	Trade name	Dosage range	Dosage form	Frequency	Disease[a]
Platinum compounds					
Cisplatin	Platinol-AQ	50–100 mg/m^2	IV	q 3–4 wk	NSCLC, ovarian, testis, bladder, head, neck, lung
Carboplatin	Paraplatin	300–400 mg/m^2, AUC 6	IV	q 3–4 wk	Ovarian, testis, NSCLC, head, neck, lung
Oxaliplatin	**Eloxatin**	85–130 mg/m^2	IV	q 2 wk	Colorectal
Enzymes					
Asparaginase	Elspar	6,000 IU/m^2	IM	3 × wk	ALL
	Oncaspar	2,500 IU/m^2	IM	q 14 d	ALL
	Erwinaze	25,000 IU/m^2	IM	3 × wk	ALL
Cell-specific					
Hydroxyurea	Hydrea	20–30 mg/kg	po	Daily	CML, AML, head, neck
Histone deacetylase inhibitor					
Romidepsin	Istodax	14 mg/m^2	IV	q wk × 3 wk, then 1 wk off	Cutaneous T-cell lymphoma
mTOR inhibitors					
Temsirolimus	Torisel	25 mg	IV	q wk	Renal cell carcinoma
Everolimus	Afinitor	10 mg	po	Daily	Renal cell carcinoma, subependymal giant cell astrocytoma

Table 23-8. Miscellaneous Agents *(Continued)*

Generic name	Trade name	Dosage range	Dosage form	Frequency	Disease[a]
Unknown mechanism					
Omacetaxine	Synribo	1.25 mg/m^2	SC	Twice daily for 14 d q 28 d, after response give twice daily for 7 d q 28 d	CML
Tyrosine kinase inhibitor					
Imatinib mesylate	Gleevec	400–600 mg	po	Daily	CML, gastrointestinal stromal tumors
Erlotinib	Tarceva	150 mg	po	Daily	NSCLC
Gefitinib	Iressa	250–500 mg	po	Daily	NSCLC
Sunitinib	Sutent	50 mg	po	Daily × 28 days, then 14 days off	Kidney, gastrointestinal stromal tumors
Dasatinib	Sprycel	70 mg	po	bid	CML or AML resistant to or intolerant to imatinib
Sorafenib	Nexavar	400 mg	po	bid	Renal cell carcinoma, hepatocellular carcinoma
Lapatinib	Tykerb	1,250 mg	po	Daily × 21 days	Breast
Nilotinib	Tasigna	400 mg	po	q 12 h	CML
Pazopanib	Votrient	800 mg	po	Daily	Renal cell carcinoma
Vandetanib	Caprelsa	200–300 mg	po	Daily	Medullary thyroid cancer
Vemurafenib	Zelboraf	960 mg	po	bid	Melanoma
Crizotinib	Xalkori	250 mg	po	bid	NSCLC
Ruxolitinib	Jakafi	15–20 mg	po	bid	Myelofibrosis
Axitinib	Inlyta	5 mg	po	bid	Renal cell carcinoma
Bosutinib	Bosulif	500–600 mg	po	Daily	CML
Cabozantinib	Cometriq	140 mg	po	Daily	Medullary thyroid cancer
Ponatinib	Iclusig	45 mg	po	Daily	CML
Regorafenib	Stivarga	160 mg	po	Daily for 21 days q 28 days	Colorectal cancer
Hedgehog pathway inhibitor					
Vismodegib	Erivedge	150 mg	po	Daily	Basal cell cancer
Multiple angiogenic factor trap					
Ziv-aflibercept	Zaltrap	4 mg/kg	IV	q 2 wk	Colorectal cancer
26S Proteasome inhibitor					
Bortezomib	Velcade	1.3 mg/m^2	IV, SC	Days 1, 4, 8, 11 q 21 d	Multiple myeloma, mantle cell lymphoma
Carfilzomib	Kyprolis	27 mg/m^2 (20 mg/m^2 on 1st cycle)	IV	Days 1, 2, 8, 9, 15, 16 q 28 days	Multiple myeloma

ALL, acute lymphocytic leukemia; AML, acute myelogenous leukemia; CML, chronic myelogenous leukemia; mTOR, mammalian target of rapamycin; NSCLC, non–small cell lung cancer.

a. Appearance of a disease in the list does not indicate U.S. Food and Drug Administration approval for the drug's use in treatment of that disease, but does indicate use of that drug in that disease in clinical practice.

It is extensively metabolized by CYP3A4; CYP3A4 inhibitors may increase levels, and CYP3A4 inducers may decrease levels. Ketoconazole increases levels, and rifampin reduces levels.

Dasatinib

Dasatinib specifically targets BCR-ABL mutations (including those resistant to imatinib), thereby inhibiting leukemic cell growth. It is used for treatment of chronic myelogenous leukemia (CML) and pH+ acute lymphocytic leukemia (ALL). It causes rash neutropenia, thrombocytopenia, edema, diarrhea, nausea and vomiting, weight changes, arthralgia, myalgia, cough, shortness of breath, infection, electrolyte changes, and arrhythmias. Significant drug interactions occur with CYP3A4 inhibitors; avoid concurrent use or reduce dose. Avoid acid reduction therapies because they will reduce absorption. Avoid medications that prolong QT interval.

Lapatinib

Lapatinib inhibits multiple tyrosine kinases and is used in combination with capecitabine to treat human epidermal growth factor receptor–2 (HER2) positive breast cancer. Common adverse effects include fatigue, diarrhea, nausea, vomiting, myelosuppression, increased liver enzymes, and palmar-plantar erythrodysesthesia. Significant drug interactions occur with strong CYP3A4 inhibitors and inducers; avoid concurrent use or reduce dose. These agents should be taken by mouth, on an empty stomach, 1 hour prior to or 2 hours after a meal.

Nilotinib

Nilotinib selectively inhibits BCR-ABL kinase and is used for the treatment of pH+ CML. Adverse effects include headache, fatigue, rash, pruritus, constipation, nausea, vomiting, and diarrhea. Significant drug interactions occur with strong CYP3A4 inhibitors and inducers; avoid concurrent use or reduce dose. Capsules should be taken by mouth, on an empty stomach, and swallowed whole; do not crush or open.

Asparaginase

Asparaginase removes exogenous asparagines from leukemic cells that are required for their survival. Intradermal skin testing is needed because of severe anaphylactic reactions. Adverse effects include myelosuppression, hyperuricemia, hyperglycemia, and renal problems. Drug interactions occur with methotrexate, prednisolone, prednisone, and vincristine.

Hydroxyurea

Hydroxyurea inhibits DNA synthesis without interfering with RNA and protein synthesis. Adverse effects include myelosuppression (leukopenia), development of secondary leukemias, nausea, vomiting, diarrhea, constipation, mucositis, and rare but fatal hepatotoxicity and pancreatitis. Drug interactions occur with didanosine and stavudine.

Imatinib mesylate

Imatinib mesylate is a selective inhibitor of the Philadelphia chromosome (biomarker in CML). It causes hepatotoxicity, fluid retention (pleural effusions, weight gain), neutropenia, GI effects, muscle cramps, nausea, and vomiting. Drug interactions occur with CYP3A4 substrates (cyclosporine, simvastatin, erythromycin, itraconazole) and CYP2C9 substrates (warfarin).

Erlotinib

Erlotinib is an HER1 and epidermal growth factor receptor (EGFR) tyrosine kinase inhibitor. For oral therapy, take 1 hour before or 2 hours after meals. Erlotinib causes rash, diarrhea, anorexia, stomatitis, and interstitial lung disease. Drug interactions occur with CYP3A4 inducers and inhibitors. Monitor hepatic function.

Gefitinib

Gefitinib is an EGFR tyrosine kinase inhibitor and a third-line agent for non–small cell lung cancer (NSCLC). It causes diarrhea, rash, acne, and dry skin. Drug interactions occur with CYP3A4 inducers and inhibitors and with warfarin.

Bortezomib

Bortezomib inhibits the 26S proteasome and stabilizes regulatory proteins causing apoptosis and disrupting cell proliferation. It causes nausea, vomiting, thrombocytopenia, neuropathy, hypotension, and diarrhea.

Carfilzomib

Carfilzomib irreversibly binds to the N-terminal threonine-containing active sites of 20S proteasome. Adverse effects include fatigue, anemia, nausea, thrombocytopenia, dyspnea, diarrhea, and pyrexia.

Temsirolimus and everolimus

Temsirolimus and everolimus inhibit the mammalian target of rapamycin (mTOR) and are used for the treatment of renal cell carcinoma. Adverse effects include myelosuppression, anorexia, rash, mucositis, edema, hyperglycemia, dyslipidemia, and nausea.

Drug interactions occur with angiotensin-converting enzyme inhibitors and strong CYP3A4 inhibitors and inducers.

Axitinib

Axitinib inhibits multiple-receptor tyrosine kinases, including vascular endothelial growth factor receptors (VEGFR-1, VEGFR-2, VEGFR-3). Adverse effects include diarrhea, hypertension, fatigue, palmar-plantar erythrodysesthesia, decreased appetite and weight, nausea and vomiting, asthenia, constipation, increases in AST (aspartate aminotransferase) and ALT (alanine aminotransferase), and decreased thyroid function. Axitinib is a CYP3A4/5 substrate.

Bosutinib

Bosutinib is a tyrosine kinase inhibitor that inhibits the BCR-ABL kinase that promotes CML.

Adverse effects include diarrhea, nausea, thrombocytopenia, vomiting, abdominal pain, rash, anemia, pyrexia, and fatigue. Avoid moderate or strong CYP3A4/5 inhibitors or inducers (increased or decreased bosutinib levels), p-glycoprotein inhibitors (increased bosutinib levels), and proton pump inhibitors (decreased bosutinib levels).

Cabozantinib

Cabozantinib inhibits the tyrosine kinase activity of RET, MET, VEGFR-1, VEGFR-2, VEGFR-3, KIT, tropomyosin receptor kinase B (TRK-B), FMS-like tyrosine kinase 3 (FLT-3), AXL, and TIE-2. Adverse effects include diarrhea; stomatitis; decreased weight and appetite; nausea; fatigue; oral pain; hair color changes; dysgeusia; hypertension; palmar-planar erythrodysesthesia; constipation; increased AST, ALT, alkaline phosphatase, and bilirubin; decreased calcium and phosphorus; lymphopenia; neutropenia; and thrombocytopenia. Cabozantinib is a CYP3A4 substrate.

Ponatinib

Ponatinib is a tyrosine kinase inhibitor that inhibits the BCR-ABL kinase that promotes CML. Adverse effects include hypertension, neutropenia, leucopenia, thrombocytopenia, increased AST, increased ALT, hemorrhage, peripheral edema, cardiac failure, arterial ischemic events, pancreatitis, and venous thromboembolism. Avoid strong CYP3A CYP3A4/5 inhibitors, or reduce ponatinib dose.

Regorafenib

Regorafenib is a tyrosine kinase inhibitor that inhibits RET, VEGFR-1, VEGFR-2, VEGFR-3, KIT, plate-let derived growth factor receptor (PDGFR)-alpha, PDGFR-beta, fibroblast growth factor receptor (FGFR) 1, FGFR2, TIE-2, discoidin domain receptor (DDR) 2, TRK 2A, Ephrin (Eph) 2A, RAF-1, BRAF, BRAFV600E, SAPK2, PTK5, and ABL. Adverse effects include diarrhea; hypertension; asthenia; fatigue; decreased weight, appetite, and food intake; mucositis; palmar-plantar erythrodysesthesia; infection; and dysphonia. Regorafenib is a CYP3A4 substrate.

Vismodegib

Vismodegib is a selective Hedgehog pathway inhibitor. Adverse effects include muscle spasms, alopecia, dysgeusia, decreased appetite and weight, fatigue, diarrhea, nausea and vomiting, constipation, arthralgias, and ageusia. P-glycoprotein inhibitors may increase vismodegib concentrations. Proton pump inhibitors, H2 antagonists, and antacids may reduce drug bioavailability by increasing gastric pH. Vismodegib inhibits CYP2C8, 2C9, 2C19, and transporter breast cancer resistance protein in vitro.

Ziv-aflibercept

Ziv-aflibercept acts as a soluble receptor that binds to human VEGF-A, VEGF-B, and placental growth factor (PlGF). Adverse effects include diarrhea, neutropenia, proteinuria, thrombocytopenia, decreased weight and appetite, stomatitis, fatigue, hypertension, epistaxis, dysphonia, and increased serum creatinine.

Common Toxicities and Treatments

Common toxicities of chemotherapeutic agents are outlined in Table 23-9. They can be classified as acute, subacute, chronic, cumulative, or chronic and cumulative. Rapidly dividing cells, including mucous membranes, hair, skin, GI tract, and bone marrow, are the most common acute toxicities. Examples of delayed or cumulative toxicities include nephrotoxicity, neurotoxicity, cardiomyopathy, pulmonary fibrosis, and secondary malignancies.

The prevention and treatment of chemotherapy-induced nausea and vomiting (CINV) constitute an important area in which pharmacists may play a role in drug selection for oncology patients. The selection of antiemetic agents should be based primarily on the emetogenic potential of the drug regimen. Other factors that increase the risk of CINV include sex (female), young age, prior chemotherapy exposure, lack of chronic alcohol use, combination chemotherapy, high dosage and numerous cycles, and short infusion times. It is important that patients also receive prescriptions to prevent delayed CINV.

Table 23-9. Common Toxicities of Chemotherapeutic Agents

Toxicity	Major causative drugs[a]	Recommended therapy
Alopecia	Cyclophosphamide, doxorubicin, paclitaxel, mechlorethamine	n.a.
Cardiac toxicity	Anthracyclines, trastuzumab	Limit cumulative doses.
Diarrhea	Irinotecan, fluorouracil	Premedicate with atropine (irinotecan); treat with loperamide.
Edema	Docetaxel	Administer prophylactic dexamethasone.
Extravasation	Anthracyclines, mitomycin, vinca alkaloids, paclitaxel, mechlorethamine	Treat with heat packs for vincas and with cold compresses for all other drugs.
Hemorrhagic cystitis	Cyclophosphamide, ifosfamide	Premedicate with hydration therapy, mesna.
Hepatotoxicity	Asparaginase, cytarabine, mercaptopurine, methotrexate, imatinib, erlotinib	n.a.
Hypersensitivity	Paclitaxel, asparaginase, cisplatin, carboplatin, etoposide, teniposide	Premedicate with ranitidine or cimetidine, diphenhydramine, dexamethasone, or test dose; treat with emergency resuscitation.
Infertility	Cyclophosphamide, chlorambucil, melphalan, mechlorethamine	n.a.
Myelosuppression	Alkylating agents, fluorouracil, methotrexate, lomustine, cyclophosphamide, methotrexate	Treat with G-CSF (filgrastim, tbo-filgrastim, peg-filgrastim), platelet transfusions, red blood cell transfusions, erythropoietin-stimulating agents (unless cancer is curable).
Nausea and vomiting	Cisplatin, cyclophosphamide, cytarabine, dacarbazine, ifosfamide, melphalan, mitomycin, mechlorethamine	Premedicate with dexamethasone, phenothiazines (e.g., Compazine), 5-HT$_3$-receptor antagonists (e.g., granisetron), and neurokinin-1 antagonists.
Neurotoxicity	Paclitaxel, cisplatin, cytarabine, methotrexate, vincristine, asparaginase	Use dose reductions.
Pulmonary toxicity	Bleomycin, busulfan, carmustine, mitomycin, trastuzumab	Treat with corticosteroids.
Renal toxicity	Cisplatin, ifosfamide, methotrexate, streptozocin	Premedicate with hydration therapy.
Stomatitis	Fluorouracil, methotrexate	Have patient hold ice chips in mouth; administer palifermin.[b]

G-CSF, granulocyte colony-stimulating factor; n.a., not applicable.

a. Adverse effects are not limited to the listed drugs.

b. Use for hematologic malignancies that need myelotoxic therapy requiring hematopoietic agents only.

Table 23-10 summarizes the pertinent antiemetic drugs used in the prophylactic setting.

For highly to moderately emetogenic drug regimens, dexamethasone and 5-HT$_3$ receptor antagonists are recommended—at a minimum—for the prevention of acute CINV. Aprepitant or fosaprepitant should also be considered, especially for highly emetogenic regimens.

For low to minimally emetogenic drug regimens, dexamethasone and a phenothiazine are recommended.

For prevention of delayed CINV (> 24 hours after administration of highly emetogenic and some moderately emetogenic chemotherapy), aprepitant and dexamethasone are recommended.

All patients receiving agents with emetogenic potential should receive prophylactic therapy for CINV, with rescue medication readily available.

Miscellaneous Commonalities Across Chemotherapy Agents

■ Patients should not receive live and rotavirus vaccines during chemotherapy because of immune suppression.

Table 23-10. Pharmacologic Management for the Prevention of Acute Chemotherapy-Induced Nausea and Vomiting

Generic name	Trade name	Dosage range	Dosage form[a]	Frequency	Side effects
5-HT$_3$ receptor antagonists					
Dolasetron	Anzemet	100–200 mg	IV, po	30 min before treatment	Headache, dizziness, constipation, blurred vision, elevated liver enzymes
Granisetron	Kytril, Sancuso	1–2 mg, 34.3 mg transdermal patch	IV/po, transdermal	30 min before treatment, 24h before treatment	Headache, dizziness, constipation, blurred vision, elevated liver enzymes
Ondansetron	Zofran	8–16 mg 16–24 mg	IV po	30 min before treatment	Headache, dizziness, constipation, blurred vision, elevated liver enzymes
Palonosetron	Aloxi	0.25 mg	IV	Day 1 (not to be repeated within 7 days)	Diarrhea, headache, fatigue, insomnia, arrhythmias
Phenothiazines					
Prochlorperazine	Compazine	10–25 mg	IV, po, PR	q4h prn	Sedation, hypotension, extrapyramidal effects, lethargy
Chlorpromazine	Thorazine	25–50 mg	po	q4–6h prn	Sedation, hypotension, extrapyramidal effects, lethargy
Promethazine	Phenergan	12.5–25 mg	IV, po, PR	q4–6h prn	Sedation, hypotension, extrapyramidal effects, lethargy
Butyrophenones					
Droperidol	Inapsine	1.25–2.5 mg	IM, slow IV	q4h prn	Sedation, tachycardia, hypotension
Haloperidol	Haldol	2 mg	IV, IM, po	q4–6h prn	Sedation, tachycardia, hypotension
Corticosteroids					
Dexamethasone	Decadron	4 mg, 10–20 mg	IV, po	Varies	Anxiety, insomnia, GI upset, psychosis
Cannabinoids					
Dronabinol	Marinol	10–20 mg	po	q3–6h	Drowsiness, euphoria, dry mouth
Nabilone	Cesamet	1–2 mg	po	bid	Drowsiness, euphoria, dry mouth
Benzodiazepines					
Lorazepam	Ativan	2 mg	po	q6h	Sedation, amnesia
Benzamides					
Metoclopramide	Reglan	20 mg	po	tid–qid	Diarrhea, sedation, agitation
Neurokinin-1 antagonist					
Aprepitant	Emend	80–125 mg	po	Day 1 (125 mg); days 2–3 (80 mg daily)	Somnolence, fatigue, diarrhea
Fosaprepitant	Emend	150 mg	IV	Day 1	Somnolence, fatigue, diarrhea

a. Most agents are available in more than one dosage form. Because of space limitations, oral dosing has been given preference.

Table 23-11. American Cancer Society Screening Recommendations for Standard Risk Patients

Disease[a]	Sex	Age (years)	Procedure	Frequency
Colorectal	M and F	50+	Fecal occult blood test	Every year
	M and F	50+[b]	Flexible sigmoidoscopy, colonoscopy, double contrast barium enema, CT colonography	Every 5 years (flexible sigmoidoscopy, CT colonography, and double contrast barium enema, followed by colonoscopy if positive result), every 10 years (colonoscopy)
Breast	F	20+	Breast self-exam	Every month
	F	20–39 or 40+	Clinical breast exam	Every 3 years or every year
	F	40+	Mammography	Every year
Cervical	F	21–29[c]	Pap smear and pelvic exam	Every 3 years
		30–65	Pap smear, HPV test, and pelvic exam	Every 5 years
Prostate	M	50+	Digital rectal exam	Every 1 or 2 years
	M	50+	Prostate-specific antigen test	Every 1 or 2 years

Adapted from the American Cancer Society, 2014.
HPV, human papilloma virus.
a. No specific screening recommendations have been made for lung, skin, and testicular cancer in patients with average risk. However, after age 40, it is recommended that all men and women receive health counseling and a physical exam every year.
b. Screening should be done earlier if there is a strong family history or presence of other risk factors of cancer.
c. Screening should be done earlier if patient is sexually active.

- The majority of agents are teratogenic and mutagenic.
- Patients should avoid becoming pregnant or breast-feeding during and immediately after chemotherapy.
- Patients should have laboratory studies done on a regular basis to check for common toxicities, such as myelosuppression, renal and hepatic impairment, and electrolyte disturbances.

23-5. Nondrug Therapy

As mentioned previously, cancer treatment is generally a combination of modalities. Chemotherapy is an important component, because most patients present with advanced disease on diagnosis. Surgery plays a role in resecting primary tumors or metastases. It can also be used for diagnostic purposes to biopsy tumors or for other exploratory purposes. Radiation is used to shrink primary tumors in local disease or metastases. It can be used in neoadjuvant therapy to downsize tumors, in adjuvant therapy to eradicate residual disease, and in combination with chemotherapy as a primary treatment.

Screening is also an important part of cancer therapy, because it can allow the detection of disease in very early stages, when the survival rates are much higher. Table 23-11 refers to American Cancer Society screening recommendations for patients at average risk of developing cancer.

Tests can also be performed to screen and monitor tumor markers. They are found in the plasma, serum, or other body fluids and may be used to identify neoplastic growth. These markers are often not sensitive enough to diagnose cancer and may produce false positive results (i.e., falsely identify people with a disease that they do not have). However, they are helpful in identifying the recurrence of advanced disease in patients who had elevated levels on diagnosis.

23-6. Questions

Use Patient Profile 23-1 to answer Questions 1–5.

1. Which of the following agents that Ms. Tiny is receiving can be used to treat breast and prostate cancer?

    A. Zoladex
    B. Tamoxifen
    C. Celebrex
    D. Percocet 5/325

Patient Profile 23-1. Medication Profile: Community

Patient name:	Tina Tiny
Age:	33
Sex:	Female
Diagnosis:	1. Diagnosis on 12/01/12 of stage II right breast cancer, estrogen receptor positive and HER2 negative. Genetic testing suggests patient would not benefit from adjuvant antineoplastic chemotherapy.
	2. Right simple mastectomy with sentinel lymph node resection on 12/15/12. Sentinel lymph node was negative for breast cancer.
	3. Weight loss of 20 lb
	4. Allergies
Height:	5'8"
Weight:	150 lb
Allergies:	Sulfa, penicillin

Pharmacist notes:

Date	Note
01/01/13	Patient complained of soreness and swelling of right arm after sentinel lymph node resection.
03/01/13	Patient did not pick up allergy medication (desloratadine) last month on due date of 02/01/13. Called patient to remind her of importance of this medication with upcoming allergy season. Patient picked up refill on 02/16/13.
03/04/13	Patient is starting Zoladex 3.6 mg SC q28d at oncology clinic. Received first dose today.
03/12/13	Patient signed for pseudoephedrine 30 mg tablets.

Pharmacy medication record:

Date	Rx #	Physician	Drug and strength	Quantity	Sig	Refills
12/16/12	12345	Buford	Percocet 5/325	30	1–2 q4h prn	0
02/16/13	12346	Buford	Desloratadine 5 mg	30	1 po daily	4
03/01/13	12347	Buford	Tamoxifen 20 mg	30	1 po daily	2
03/01/13	12349	Buford	Megace 40 mg/mL	80 mg/day	—	2
03/01/13	12350	Charles	Celebrex 10 mg	30	1 po daily	2

2. When Ms. Tiny presents the tamoxifen prescription, you notice that the directions are missing. You call the health care provider to clarify the instructions for this patient. Which of the following is a correct choice?

   A. 10 mL po daily
   B. 20 mL po daily
   C. 40 mg po bid
   D. 20 mg po daily

3. Ms. Tiny presents to your pharmacy with complaints of lower leg calf pain that is tender to the touch and red. You suspect a deep-vein thrombosis. Which of the following agents is most likely to be associated with this condition?

   A. Desloratadine
   B. Pseudoephedrine
   C. Tamoxifen
   D. Percocet 5/325

4. Ms. Tiny calls you on 05/05/13. She has been experiencing frequent hot flashes and wants to know if one of her medications might be causing this adverse effect. You tell her that the hot flashes are likely caused by

   A. Tamoxifen and desloratadine.
   B. Percocet 5/325 and Zoladex.
   C. Celebrex and tamoxifen.
   D. Zoladex and tamoxifen.

5. Ms. Tiny's mother (age 59) is worried that she will develop breast cancer like her daughter. Which of the following is appropriate advice for Ms. Tiny's mother?

   A. Perform a monthly breast self-examination.
   B. Receive a clinical breast examination by a qualified health care provider once every 5 years.

C. Undergo an annual mammography and an annual clinical breast exam by a qualified health care provider.

D. Undergo annual bilateral breast biopsies.

6. Which of the following classes of agents is best known for causing infusion-related reactions, such as fever and chills?

A. Monoclonal antibodies
B. Tyrosine kinase inhibitors
C. Vinca alkaloids
D. Platinum alkylating agents

7. Your patient has just received 5-FU and irinotecan for the treatment of colorectal cancer. Before he leaves the clinic, you ensure that he has a prescription to prevent or treat which of the following side effects from irinotecan?

A. Nausea with Aloxi
B. Diarrhea with loperamide
C. Headache with aspirin
D. Delayed allergic reaction with epinephrine

8. Which of the following drugs is an oral pro-drug of 5-FU?

A. Fluorouracil
B. Xeloda
C. Fludara
D. Cytoxan

9. An elderly male patient comes to your pharmacy and is worried that he might have prostate cancer. He just had some laboratory studies done, and his health care provider told him that some level was abnormal, indicating potential prostate cancer. Which lab test might he be talking about?

A. PSA
B. Cortisol
C. ESR
D. PRR

10. *Stomatitis* is the clinical term for which of the following chemotherapy-related adverse effects?

A. Nausea, vomiting, or both
B. Inflammation of the mucosal lining of the mouth

C. Obstruction of the lower esophageal sphincter
D. Inflammation of the mucosal lining of the colon and rectum

11. Which of the following describes a known characteristic of most antineoplastic chemotherapy agents?

A. They have a narrow therapeutic index.
B. They do not interfere with DNA synthesis and replication.
C. Acute adverse effects occur primarily in slowly dividing normal cells.
D. They have only phase-specific actions.

Use Patient Profile 23-2 to answer Questions 12–17.

12. A nurse would like to know if she can administer the diphenhydramine and the ranitidine to Mr. Migash in the same IV line simultaneously. Which of the following resources will provide you with this information?

A. Wolters Kluwer Health's Facts & Comparisons
B. Trissel's *Handbook on Injectable Drugs* and *Drug Prescribing in Renal Failure*
C. Micromedex and *The Sanford Guide to Antimicrobial Therapy*
D. Trissel's *Handbook on Injectable Drugs* and Micromedex

13. Which of the following agents being taken by Mr. Migash requires the premedication regimen of dexamethasone, diphenhydramine, and ranitidine to prevent an anaphylactic reaction?

A. Taxotere
B. Taxol
C. Paraplatin
D. Cisplatin

14. On the basis of the patient's weight and height, you calculate Mr. Migash's body surface area to be 2.1 m². Paclitaxel is supplied as 6 mg/mL in 5 mL, 16.7 mL, and 50 mL vials. Your pharmacy has all quantities available. What is the best way to correctly dose this patient?

A. One 50 mL vial and one 16.7 mL vial
B. One 50 mL vial and one 5 mL vial
C. Two 16.7 mL vials
D. Two 16.7 mL vials and one 5 mL vial

Patient Profile 23-2. Medication Profile: Institution

Patient name: Cassimer Migash

Age: 60

Sex: Male

Diagnosis:
1. Diagnosis on 02/01/13 of metastatic non–small cell lung cancer
2. Chronic obstructive pulmonary disease
3. Asthma

Height: 180 cm

Weight: 200 lb

Allergies: NKDA

Lab and diagnostic tests:

Date	Test
03/01/13	WBC: 6,500/mcL
03/01/13	Absolute neutrophil count: 3,500/mcL
03/01/13	PLT: 67,000/mcL
03/01/13	Hgb: 13 g/dL
03/01/13	Hct: 39%

Medication record:

Date	Route	Drug and Strength	Sig
03/01/13	IV	Paclitaxel 175 mg/m^2	175 mg/m^2 over 3 h q 3 wk
03/01/13	IV	Carboplatin AUC 6	AUC 6 over 30 min q 3 wk
03/01/13	INH	Albuterol inhaler	2 puffs prn
03/01/13	INH	Advair inhaler	1 puff bid
03/01/13	IV	Dexamethasone 20 mg	Infuse 30 min prior to chemo
03/01/13	IV	Diphenhydramine 50 mg	Infuse 30 min prior to chemo
03/01/13	IV	Ranitidine 50 mg	Infuse 30 min prior to chemo

15. You are concerned that Mr. Migash will develop nausea and vomiting from his chemotherapy regimen. Which of the following regimens would be appropriate to prevent acute CINV?

    A. Dexamethasone, granisetron, and aprepitant
    B. Granisetron and prochlorperazine
    C. Metoclopramide, dexamethasone, and aprepitant
    D. Palonosetron and granisetron

16. On the basis of the patient's laboratory values, which of the following adverse reactions appears to have occurred as a likely result of the chemotherapy?

    A. Thrombocytopenia
    B. Anemia
    C. Neutropenia
    D. Leukocytopenia

17. The goal of Mr. Migash's treatment regimen is to

    A. cure his disease.
    B. palliate his disease-related symptoms and increase his quality of life.

    C. provide adjuvant therapy following definitive surgery.
    D. increase his survival time by several years.

18. Doxorubicin is an antineoplastic agent that

    A. is not related to epirubicin and daunorubicin.
    B. interacts with the microtubules of cells during mitosis.
    C. has an oral dosage form commercially available.
    D. causes cumulative cardiac toxicity.

19. Which of the following agents is used in cancer regimens but is *not* considered an antineoplastic agent?

    A. Methotrexate
    B. Leucovorin
    C. Doxorubicin
    D. Cyclophosphamide

20. Methotrexate (Rheumatrex) is *not* available as which of the following dosage forms?

    A. An intravenous injection
    B. An oral tablet or capsule
    C. An intrathecal injection
    D. An ointment

23-7. Answers

1. **A.** Zoladex (goserelin) is an LHRH agonist that can be used to treat both breast and prostate cancer. LHRH agonists are approved by the U.S. Food and Drug Administration for premenopausal women because they inhibit estrogen production from the ovaries.

2. **D.** The FDA-approved dose for breast cancer therapy is 20 mg po daily. The drug is not available in a liquid form.

3. **C.** Tamoxifen is well-known to increase the incidence of thromboembolic events. All patients on this medication should be counseled on the signs and symptoms of thromboembolic events.

4. **D.** Hot flashes are a common adverse effect experienced by patients taking selective estrogen receptor modifiers, such as tamoxifen, and gonadotropin-releasing hormone agonists, such as Zoladex.

5. **C.** Biopsies should never be performed as initial screening tests. However, if results from the mammography and clinical breast exam point to disease, a biopsy is needed to make a diagnosis. The American Cancer Society still recommends an annual mammography and a clinical breast exam for a woman at normal risk for breast cancer.

6. **A.** Monoclonal antibodies are commonly associated with infusion-related reactions. Patients should receive premedication, such as acetaminophen and diphenhydramine, to prevent this.

7. **B.** Diarrhea is a dose-limiting toxicity of irinotecan. Late-onset diarrhea can be life threatening. All patients should receive a prescription for loperamide to treat delayed-onset diarrhea. Patients should be instructed to take 2 mg po q2h while awake and 4 mg po q4h during the night until the diarrhea has stopped for at least 12 hours. Acute-onset diarrhea can be treated with atropine.

8. **B.** Xeloda (capecitabine) is an oral pro-drug of 5-FU. Fluorouracil is another name for 5-FU. Fludara is the brand name for fludarabine and is used to treat chronic lymphocytic leukemia and non-Hodgkin lymphoma intravenously. Cytoxan is the brand name for cyclophosphamide and is available in IV and po dosage forms.

9. **A.** PSA is a lab test that is commonly done in men over age 40. It should be performed annually in men over age 50 to check for prostate cancer.

10. **B.** *Stomatitis* is used to describe an irritation or ulceration of the mucosal lining. This side effect is common with fluorouracil and methotrexate. Having the patient hold ice chips in his or her mouth during treatment can prevent it. The cold is thought to cause vasoconstriction of the lining and prevent damage.

11. **A.** Chemotherapy agents have a very narrow therapeutic index. This is one of the main reasons these drugs have so many toxic effects. They can be phase-specific or phase-nonspecific drugs and can cause many adverse reactions to normal cells that undergo rapid proliferation.

12. **D.** Both Trissel's *Handbook on Injectable Drugs* and the Micromedex IV compatibility tool can be used to assess whether diphenhydramine and cimetidine are compatible.

13. **B.** Taxol is the brand name of paclitaxel. This agent has been shown to cause hypersensitivity reactions in patients. It is unclear if these reactions are due to the drug itself or the drug's vehicle (Cremophor). All patients receiving paclitaxel should receive a premedication regimen of dexamethasone, diphenhydramine, and ranitidine.

14. **A.** The patient requires 367.5 mg of drug. Choice A will provide 400 mg of drug, and this is the most economical way to provide the required dose.

15. **A.** This patient's regimen contains carboplatin and paclitaxel. Together these agents have a high likelihood of causing acute (and delayed) CINV. The patient should receive a corticosteroid, a 5-HT$_3$ antagonist, and a neurokinin-1 inhibitor, which makes choice B incorrect because it contains a 5-HT$_3$ antagonist and a dopamine antagonist. Aprepitant is approved in combination with a corticosteroid and a 5-HT$_3$ antagonist, which makes choice C incorrect because it adds a corticosteroid and a dopamine antagonist to the aprepitant. Choice D contains two 5-HT$_3$ antagonists. Therapy should include more than one class of agent.

16. **A.** Myelosuppression is a common adverse reaction to most chemotherapy agents. Both paclitaxel and carboplatin can cause anemia,

Solid Organ Transplantation

Benjamin Duhart, Jr.

24-1. Key Points

- The goal of solid organ transplantation is to improve patients' quality of life and survival by stabilizing or improving complications related to end-organ failure.
- The immune system is a highly intricate system with mechanisms for antigen recognition in a highly specific manner as well as in a nonspecific manner.
- Acute rejection is a normal physiologic immune response to transplantation of donor antigens.
- The incidence of acute rejection is organ specific and depends on multiple pre- and post-transplant factors.
- Selection of the post-transplant immunosuppression regimen for prevention of acute rejection should be individualized on the basis of known risk and potential toxicity.
- Adjustment in the post-transplant immunosuppression regimen should focus on the balance between acute rejection, infection, and toxicity.
- Selection of the agent to be used to treat acute rejection is organ dependent and depends on the severity of acute rejection.
- Immunosuppressive complications, both infectious and noninfectious, are an important cause of morbidity and mortality and require close management following transplantation.
- Medications commonly included in immunosuppression regimens require a clinician with expertise in immunosuppressive therapeutic drug monitoring to optimize efficacy and reduce toxicity.
- Medications commonly included in immunosuppression regimens have the potential for numerous pharmacokinetic and pharmacodynamic drug interactions.
  - Calcineurin inhibitors are considered the cornerstone of maintenance immunosuppression.
  - Use of induction therapy allows for the delay of initiation of calcineurin inhibitors.
  - Induction therapy is primarily used in patients with a high risk of rejection.
  - Immunosuppressants can increase the risk of infection and malignancies post-transplant.

24-2. Study Guide Checklist

The following topics may guide your study of this subject area:

- Factors that increase the risk for acute rejection
- Selection of immunosuppressants for induction and maintenance therapy
- Considerations for selection of immunosuppressants based on patient condition
- Actions of various categories of immunosuppressants
- Trade names and available dosage forms
- Frequency of immunosuppressive dosing regimen
- Major adverse effects specific for selected immunosuppressants
- Significant drug interactions for immunosuppressants
- Unique counseling points for selected immunosuppressants
- Selection of immunosuppressants to treat acute rejection

24-3. Organ Transplantation

Definitions

- *Acute rejection:* A systemic immunologic response to donor antigens primarily mediated by T-lymphocytes
- *Adaptive immunity:* Involves the stimulation of cells and soluble mediators in response to specific antigens with a markedly enhanced response on repeat exposure
- *Complement:* An enzyme system that is a crucial part of the basic immune response on primary exposure to an antigen and that also provides augmented signaling during memory immunity
- *Human leukocyte antigen (HLA):* Antigen-binding proteins that rescue protein fragments from intracellular catabolism (class I or II) or select antigens from the extracellular milieu that are then presented to lymphocytes (class II)
- *Induction:* Administration of short-term antibody therapy before and during the initial transplant as prophylaxis for acute rejection
- *Innate immunity:* Involves the stimulation of cells and soluble mediators that nonspecifically recognize antigens and have no ability to alter response with repeat exposure
- *Major histocompatibility complex (MHC):* A group of genes that encode for HLA class I and II
- *Opsonization:* A process by which antigens or immune complexes become coated with a molecule that facilitates binding with a phagocyte
- *Panel reactive antibody (PRA):* A test that quantifies a patient's immunologic reactivity to a given pool of antigens
- *Phagocytosis:* A process by which recognized antigens are engulfed and subsequently undergo intracellular catabolism

Basic Immunology and Acute Rejection

Fundamental types of immunity

Innate immunity
Cellular components
- *Macrophages:* Phagocytic cells found throughout the body that may function as antigen-presenting cells
- *Neutrophils:* Highly motile cells whose major physiologic role is the destruction of invading microorganisms through phagocytosis or opsonization

- *Natural killer cells:* A subset of non-B- and non-T-lymphocytes that survey for the normal biosynthesis and expression of HLA class I, making them important in immunity against viral infection and malignancy

Humoral components
- *Complement:* Activation leads to formation of lipophilic complexes, called *membrane-attack complexes,* in the cell membrane of the target cell and results in osmotic leaks.
  - *Physiologic function:* Humoral component provides a defense against pyogenic bacterial infections.
  - Bridges innate and adaptive immunity
  - Mediates disposal of immune complexes
  - Consists of acute phase proteins

Adaptive immunity
Cellular components
- *Thymus-derived lymphocytes (T-cells):* Mature T-cells become activated when they encounter an antigen-presenting cell (APC). T-cells do not recognize antigens directly.
  - CD4+ T-cells (*helper T-cells*) recognize HLA class II antigens presented via APC.
  - CD8+ T-cells (*cytotoxic T-cells*) recognize HLA class I antigens presented via APC.
- *Bone marrow–derived lymphocytes (B-cells):* B-cells encounter the antigen to which their surface immunoglobulin has specificity, through either its APC function or by interaction with an activated CD4+ T-cell. B-cell–CD4+ T-cell interaction is required for translocation into a follicle within secondary lymphoid tissue, where a germinal center forms and where high-affinity memory B-cells and plasma cells are produced and selected (somatic hypermutation).

Humoral components
- *Complement:* See the previous section on innate immunity.
- *Immunoglobulin (Ig):* This complex protein of various isotypes is formed as a consequence of B-cell activation for the purpose of binding and elimination of the activating antigen.

Acute rejection

Pathophysiology
During transplantation, the recipient is exposed to donor antigens to which he or she has no previous exposure. Although undesirable, acute rejection is

the normal physiologic response of the immune system to these donor antigens. This response can be divided into five basic phases:

1. *Recognition:* Foreign antigen is recognized via self- or nonself-recognition mediated through MHC.
2. *Presentation:* On recognition, APC presents antigens in association with native HLA class II to inactive CD4+ T-cells, also called signal 1 of T-cell-mediated rejection.
3. *Activation and proliferation:* Activation depends on antigen–HLA binding to the T-cell receptor (TCR) complex and the subsequent binding of a second signal or "co-stimulatory pathway" (also considered as signal 2 of T-cell-mediated rejection). Subsequently, the active CD4+ T-cell produces and releases various lymphokines, particularly interleukin-2 (IL-2), which is important for activation and proliferation of numerous lymphocyte lineages. The binding of IL-2 to the IL-2 receptor is commonly referred to as signal 3.
4. *Recruitment:* Recruitment is mediated through several lymphokines produced as a consequence of lymphocyte activation.
5. *Antigen and tissue destruction:* Tissue injury is mediated through induction of polyclonal immune response.

Incidence

The incidence is organ specific and depends on many pre- and post-transplant factors. Several known factors increase risk:

- Increased HLA mismatch
- Factors affecting previous sensitization (e.g., history of pregnancy, previous transplantation, previous rejection, panel reactive antibody > 20%)
- Ethnicity (i.e., African American recipients)
- Age (i.e., pediatric recipients)
- Donor source (i.e., deceased donor)
- Prolonged preservation time
- Noncompliance

Immunosuppressive Strategies

Balance of immunosuppression

Selection of an immunosuppression regimen for the prevention of acute rejection should be individualized on the basis of known risk and potential for toxicity.

Subsequent adjustment must focus on the balance of the triad: rejection, infection, and toxicity.

Phases of preventive immunosuppression

Induction

The early phase is intended to provide highly potent, multifocal suppression of the immune system for several days to a few weeks. Commonly used agents include the following:

- Corticosteroids
- Monoclonal antibody (basiliximab)
- Polyclonal antibody (antithymocyte globulin—equine or rabbit)

Maintenance

The immunosuppression regimen is designed to provide chronic, balanced immunodeficiency. Some commonly used regimens include the following:

- Double therapy:
  - Calcineurin inhibitor + steroids
  - Calcineurin inhibitor + antimetabolite
  - Calcineurin inhibitor + mTOR (mammalian target of rapamycin) inhibitor
  - mTOR inhibitor + steroids
  - mTOR inhibitor + antimetabolite
  - Antimetabolite + steroids
- Triple therapy:
  - Calcineurin inhibitor + antimetabolite + steroids
  - mTOR inhibitor + calcineurin inhibitor + steroids
  - mTOR inhibitor + antimetabolite + steroids
  - Costimulation blocker + antimetabolite + steroids

Phases of immunosuppression during treatment

Treatment

Selection of the agents is organ specific and depends on the severity of acute rejection. Commonly used agents include the following:

- Corticosteroids
- Calcineurin inhibitor
  - Tacrolimus may be used as the primary treatment of acute rejection in liver recipients.
  - Tacrolimus may also have a role as adjuvant therapy in refractory acute rejection in various other solid organ recipients.
- Monoclonal antibody (basiliximab)

■ Polyclonal antibody (antithymocyte globulin—equine or rabbit)

Maintenance reevaluation

The decision to heighten maintenance immuno-suppression depends on the cause for rejection (i.e., failure of regimen versus noncompliance).

Immunosuppressive Complications

Infectious

Infectious complications are an important cause of early morbidity and mortality. The incidence is organ specific and is closely linked to the net degree of immunodeficiency. Prevention is a key management strategy following transplantation. A list of infectious complications follows:

■ Bacterial
  • Tuberculosis: *Mycobacterium tuberculosis*
  • Nocardiosis: Various species of *Nocardia*
■ Fungal
  • Aspergillosis: Various species of *Aspergillus*
  • Blastomycosis: *Blastomyces dermatitidis*
  • Candidiasis: Various species of *Candida*
  • Coccidioidomycosis: *Coccidioides immitis*
  • Cryptococcosis: *Cryptococcus neoformans*
  • Histoplasmosis: *Histoplasma capsulatum*
  • Mucormycosis: Various species of *Mucor*
  • *Pneumocystis* pneumonia: *Pneumocystis jiroveci* (formerly known as *Pneumocystis carinii*)
■ Parasitic
  • Toxoplasmosis: *Toxoplasma gondii*
■ Viral
  • Cytomegalovirus
  • Epstein-Barr virus: including post-transplant lymphoproliferative disease
  • Herpes simplex virus
  • Varicella zoster virus
  • Human herpes viruses (i.e., HHV-6, HHV-8)
  • Parvovirus
  • Polyomavirus

Noninfectious

The noninfectious complications are specific to the agents included in the immunosuppressive regimen.

24-4. Immunosuppressants

Immunosuppressant drugs are described in Table 24-1.

Calcineurin Inhibitors

Cyclosporine

Mechanism of action

Cyclosporine inhibits calcineurin-dependent trans-location of the cytosolic subunit of NFAT (nuclear factor of activated T-cells), the promoter gene for IL-2, into the nucleus, thereby inhibiting transcription and synthesis of IL-2; thus, it inhibits IL-2-mediated monoclonal T-cell proliferation and polyclonal T-cell activation.

Administration

■ Intravenous (IV)
  • Administer 5–6 mg/kg per day divided every 12 hours or as a continuous infusion. Each milliliter of IV concentrate should be diluted in 20–100 mL of normal saline (NS) or 5% dextrose in water (D_5W) in a glass container. For bolus dosing, the dose should be infused over 2–6 hours.
■ Oral
  • *Capsules:* Administer the daily dose as two equally divided doses every 12 hours with meals.
  • *Oral solution:* Administer the daily dose as two equally divided doses every 12 hours with meals. The solution may be diluted with chocolate milk or orange juice in a glass container. Additional diluent should be used to rinse the container to ensure administration of the total dose.

Drug–drug interactions

The drug is metabolized primarily via cytochrome P450 (CYP450) 3A isoenzymes. Substances known to alter functionality of these enzymes will alter bio-availability and elimination of this drug (Table 24-2).

Drug interactions lead to altered exposure of other drugs by cyclosporine (Table 24-3).

Drug–disease interactions

■ **Altered biliary flow:** Diversion of biliary flow can significantly reduce adsorption. This more profoundly affects cyclosporine USP (United States Pharmacopeia) than it does cyclosporine USP (modified).
■ **Diabetes mellitus:** Administration worsens glycemic control in patients with preexisting diabetes.
■ *Vaccination:* In general, immunosuppressants may affect efficacy of vaccinations. The use of live vaccines should be avoided.

Table 24-1. Immunosuppressant Drugs

Generic name	Trade name	Dosage forms	Dose	Generic products
Calcineurin inhibitors				
Cyclosporine USP	Sandimmune	Injection: 50 mg/mL; oral solution: 100 mg/mL; capsules: 25, 100 mg	Intravenous: 5–6 mg/kg/day; oral: 8–14 mg/kg/day divided q12h; adjusted to desired trough concentration	Injection: 50 mg/mL; capsules: 25, 100 mg
Cyclosporine USP (modified)	Neoral	Oral solution: 100 mg/mL; capsules: 25, 100 mg	Oral: 5–10 mg/kg/day divided q12h; adjusted to desired trough concentration	Oral solution: 100 mg/mL; capsules: 25, 100 mg
Tacrolimus	Prograf	Injection: 5 mg ampules; capsules: 0.5, 1, 5 mg	Intravenous: 0.03–0.05 mg/kg/day as continuous infusion; oral: 0.1–0.2 mg/kg/day divided q12h; adjusted to desired trough concentration	Capsules: 0.5, 1, 5 mg
Tacrolimus extended release	Astagraf XL	Capsules: 0.5, 1, 5 mg	Oral: 0.1–0.2 mg/kg/day q24h; adjusted to desired trough concentration	Capsules: 0.5, 1, 5 mg
mTOR inhibitors				
Sirolimus	Rapamune	Oral solution: 1 mg/mL; tablets: 0.5, 1, 2 mg	Initial: adults: 6–15 mg po; pediatrics: $\geq$ 13 years of age and < 40 kg, 3 mg/m^2; $\geq$ 13 years of age and > 40 kg, 6 mg po Maintenance: adults: 2–5 mg po daily; adjusted to desired trough concentration; pediatrics: $\geq$ 13 years of age and < 40 kg, 1 mg/m^2; $\geq$ 13 years of age and > 40 kg, 2 mg po	Not available
Everolimus	Zortress	Tablets: 0.25, 0.5, 0.75 mg	Initial: 0.75 mg every 12 hours in combination with basiliximab induction, reduced dose cyclosporine, and corticosteroids adjusted to achieve desired trough level (3–8 ng/mL) Maintenance: Same as initial dose	Not available
T-cell co-stimulatory antagonist				
Belatacept	Nulojix	Injection: 250 mg vial	Initial: 10 mg/kg IV on day 1 (day of transplant, prior to transplantation), day 5, and end of weeks 2, 4, 8, and 12 Maintenance: 5 mg/kg end of week 16 and every 4 weeks thereafter given in combination with basiliximab induction, mycophenolate mofetil, and corticosteroids	Not available
Antiproliferative agents				
Azathioprine	Imuran	Injection: 100 mg vial; tablets: 50 mg	Initial: 3–5 mg/kg IV or po Maintenance: 1–3 mg/kg IV or po daily	Injection: 100 mg vial; tablets: 50 mg
Mycophenolate mofetil	CellCept	Injection: 500 mg vial; oral suspension: 200 mg/mL; capsules: 250 mg; tablets: 500 mg	Initial: adults: 2–3 g/day divided q8–12h IV or po; pediatrics: $\geq$ 3 months of age, 600 mg/m^2 oral suspension bid (maximum dose of 2 g/day); if BSA = 1.25–1.5 m^2, 750 mg bid; if BSA > 1.5 m^2, 1,000 mg bid Maintenance: Same as initial dose	Capsules: 250 mg; tablets: 500 mg

(continued)

Table 24-1. Immunosuppressant Drugs *(Continued)*

Generic name	Trade name	Dosage forms	Dose	Generic products
Mycophenolate sodium	Myfortic	Tablets: 180, 360 mg	Initial: adults: 720 mg po q12h; pediatrics: 400 mg/m^2 po q12h (maximum dose of 720 mg po q12h); if BSA = 1.19–1.58 m^2, 540 mg po bid (1,080 mg daily); if BSA < 1.19 m^2, cannot be accurately administered Maintenance: Same as initial dose	Not available
Monoclonal antibodies				
Basiliximab	Simulect	Injection: 10, 20 mg vials	Induction: adults and pediatrics > 35 kg: 20 mg IV on day 0 and day 4; pediatrics < 35 kg: 10 mg IV on day 0 and day 4	Not available
Polyclonal antibodies				
Antithymocyte globulin (equine)	Atgam	Injection: 50 mg vials	Induction: 10–15 mg/kg IV daily × 14 days; acute rejection: 15 mg/kg IV once daily × 14 days, then every other day if necessary for a total of 21 doses	Not available
Antithymocyte globulin (rabbit)	Thymoglobulin	Injection: 25 mg vials	Induction:[a] 1.5 mg/kg IV once daily × 3–7 days; acute rejection: 1.5 mg/kg IV once daily × 7–14 days	Not available

a. Medication is not FDA approved for induction.

Table 24-2. Drug Interactions Leading to Altered Exposure of CYP450 3A Isoenzyme Substrates

CYP450 3A4 enzyme inducers[a]	CYP450 3A4 enzyme inhibitors[b]
Anticonvulsants: phenytoin, phenobarbital, carbamazepine	Antidepressants: nefazodone
Antimicrobial agents: rifampin, rifabutin	Antiviral agents: boceprevir, delavirdine, indinavir, nelfinavir, ritonavir, saquinavir, telaprevir
Antiviral agents: nevirapine, efavirenz	Azole antifungal agents: voriconazole, posaconazole, ketoconazole, fluconazole, itraconazole, clotrimazole
Herbal products: St. John's wort	Calcium channel blockers: diltiazem, nicardipine, verapamil
	Macrolide antimicrobial agents: erythromycin, clarithromycin
	Food–drug interaction: grapefruit juice

The table shows examples only. Numerous other interactions are associated with CYP450 3A4 substrates. See current journals or drug interaction texts for a more detailed list.
a. Inducers result in increased metabolism of substrates of the same system.
b. Inhibitors result in decreased metabolism of substrates of the same system.

Table 24-3. Drug Interactions Leading to Altered Exposure of Other Drugs by Cyclosporine

Mechanism	Drug	Comment
CYP450 3A4 enzyme substrates	HMG-CoA reductase inhibitors: lovastatin, simvastatin, atorvastatin	Co-administration of these agents with CsA results in significant increases in HMG-CoA reductase inhibitor exposure and may place patients at increased risk of rhabdomyolysis.
CYP450 3A4 enzyme substrates	Sirolimus	Simultaneous administration increased C_{max} and area under the curve of sirolimus by 120–500% and 140–230%, respectively; administration 4 hours apart increased C_{max} and area under the curve of sirolimus by 30–40% and 35–80%, respectively.
Alteration in enterohepatic recycling	Mycophenolate mofetil	CsA coadministration inhibits MPAG excretion via hepatocytes, thus interfering with MPA enterohepatic recycling and leading to reduced exposure of the active metabolite, MPA.

The table shows examples only. Numerous other interactions are associated with CYP450 3A4 substrates. See current journals or drug interaction texts for a more detailed list.
CsA, cyclosporine A; HMG-CoA, 3-hydroxy-3-methyglutaryl coenzyme A; MPA, mycophenolic acid; MPAG, phenolic glucuronide of MPA.

Adverse drug reactions

■ *Central nervous system (CNS):* Seizure, hallucinations, insomnia, tremor, paresthesias
■ *Head, ears, eyes, nose, and throat (HEENT):* Gingival hyperplasia
■ *Cardiovascular (CV):* Hypertension
■ *Gastrointestinal (GI):* Hepatotoxicity
■ *Renal:* Nephrotoxicity
■ *Endocrine and metabolic:* Hyperlipidemia, hyperuricemia, hyperkalemia, hypomagnesemia, new onset diabetes after transplant
■ *Dermatologic:* Hirsutism, hypertrichosis, acne

Patient instructions

■ Keep cyclosporine stored in its original container.
■ Take the prescribed dose twice daily with meals.
■ Keep timing of dosing consistent.
■ Make sure you do not take your morning medication on the day of therapeutic drug monitoring. After the monitoring is complete, take your morning medication immediately and then return to your original medication schedule.
■ Many medications interact with this medication. Do not take anything prescribed by another physician until you verify that there are no drug interactions.

Monitoring

■ C_0 *(trough):* Goals depend on multifactorial risk assessment and assay type.
■ C_2 *(concentration 2 hours after dose):* Goals depend on multifactorial risk assessment and assay type.

Pharmacokinetics

■ *Cyclosporine USP:* Highly lipoprotein bound
  ● Bioavailability: Significant intra- and interpatient variability
  ● Mean F = 30%, range 5% to 92%
  ● Elimination: Half-life = 19 hours; range 10–28 hours (increased with hepatic dysfunction)
■ *Cyclosporine USP (modified):* Highly lipoprotein bound
  ● Bioavailability: Improved and more consistent absorption (60–70% increased C_{max})
  ● Elimination: Half-life = 8 hours; range 5–18 hours (increased with hepatic dysfunction)

Tacrolimus

Mechanism of action

Tacrolimus inhibits translocation of the cytosolic subunit of NFAT, the promoter gene for IL-2, into the nucleus via its binding with the protein FKBP-12 and a calcium-calmodulin-calcineurin complex, thereby inhibiting transcription and synthesis of IL-2. Thus, it inhibits IL-2-mediated monoclonal T-cell proliferation and polyclonal T-cell activation.

Administration

■ *Intravenous:* Dilute in NS or D_5W to a concentration between 0.004 and 0.02 mg/mL, and administer as a continuous infusion via a PVC (polyvinylchloride)–free container and tubing.

- *Oral:* Administer immediate-release product in two equally divided doses orally every 12 hours consistently, with or without food. Administer extended-release product orally once every 24 hours consistently, with or without food.

Drug–drug interactions

Because tacrolimus is metabolized primarily via CYP450 3A isoenzymes, substances known to alter functionality of these enzymes will alter bioavailability and elimination of this drug (Table 24-2).

Drug–disease interactions

- *Diabetes mellitus:* Administration worsens glycemic control in patients with preexisting diabetes.
- *Liver transplantation:* The extended-release formulation has been associated with an increased risk of mortality in female liver transplant recipients.
- *Vaccinations:* In general, immunosuppressants may affect efficacy of vaccinations. The use of live vaccines should be avoided.

Adverse drug reactions

- *CNS:* Seizure, hallucinations, insomnia, tremor, depression, psychosis, anorexia
- *HEENT:* Alopecia
- *CV:* Hypertension, QT prolongation
- *GI:* Hepatotoxicity
- *Renal:* Nephrotoxicity
- *Endocrine and metabolic:* Hyperlipidemia, hyperkalemia, hypercalcemia, hypomagnesemia, hypophosphatemia, new onset diabetes after transplant
- *Hematologic:* Anemia
- *Other:* Malignancies, infection

Patient instructions

- Take the prescribed dose at a consistent time once or twice daily (extended-release or immediate-release formulations), with or without food, but always in the same way to maintain consistency.
- Make sure you do not take your morning medication on the day of therapeutic drug monitoring. After the monitoring is complete, take your morning medication immediately and then return to your original medication schedule.
- Many medications interact with this medication. Do not take anything prescribed by another physician until you verify that there are no drug interactions.

Monitoring

Monitor C_0 (trough). Goals depend on multifactorial risk assessment (in general, 5–15 ng/mL).

Pharmacokinetics

- Highly protein bound
- Bioavailability: F = 14–32%
- Elimination: Half-life = 8 hours; range 6–11 hours (increased with hepatic dysfunction); ~ 37 hours for extended-release formulation

mTOR Inhibitors

Everolimus

Mechanism of action

Everolimus binds to FKBP-12 to form a complex that binds and inhibits activation of its target protein, mTOR, a kinase that is critical in IL-2-mediated cell-cycle progression.

Administration

- To limit variability, administer consistently with or without food.
- With tablets, administer dose po bid.

Drug–drug interactions

Because everolimus is metabolized primarily via CYP450 3A isoenzymes, substances known to alter functionality of these enzymes will alter bioavailability and elimination of this drug (Table 24-2).

Additionally, the pharmacokinetic profile of everolimus is significantly altered by concomitant cyclosporine (Table 24-3).

Drug–disease interactions

- *Kidney transplantation:* Everolimus is associated with arterial and venous thrombosis of the kidney allograft and may cause proteinuria.
- *Edema:* Everolimus has been associated with peripheral edema and pleural and pericardial effusions.
- *Infertility:* Everolimus has been associated with male infertility.
- *Hyperlipidemia:* Everolimus increases triglycerides and cholesterol.
- *Vaccinations:* In general, immunosuppressants may affect efficacy of vaccinations. The use of live vaccines should be avoided.

Adverse drug reactions

- *CNS:* Fatigue, headache
- *HEENT:* Oral ulcers
- *GI:* Anorexia, constipation, diarrhea, nausea
- *Renal:* Synergistic nephrotoxicity with calcineurin inhibitors, proteinuria
- *Endocrine and metabolic:* Hyperlipidemia, hypertension, hyperkalemia

- *Dermatologic:* Rash, acne
- *Hematologic:* Anemia, leukopenia, thrombocytopenia, pancytopenia, thrombosis
- *Other:* Lymphocele, pneumonitis

Patient instructions

- Take the prescribed dose at a consistent time twice daily, with or without food.
- Make sure you do not take your medication before therapeutic drug monitoring.
- Many medications interact with this medication. Do not take anything prescribed by another physician until you verify that there are no drug interactions.

Monitoring

Monitor C_0 (trough). Goal depends on multifactorial risk assessment and assay type (in general, 3–8 ng/mL).

Pharmacokinetics

- Bioavailability: F = 30%
- Elimination: Half-life = 30 hours (increased with hepatic dysfunction)

Sirolimus

Mechanism of action

Sirolimus binds to FKBP-12 to form a complex that binds and inhibits activation of its target protein, mTOR, a kinase that is critical in IL-2-mediated cell-cycle progression.

Administration

- To limit variability, administer consistently with or without food.
- With tablets, administer daily dose po once a day.
- With oral solution, dilute the dose in 2 oz of water or orange juice, stir vigorously, and drink at once. Then refill container with 4 oz of the chosen fluid, stir vigorously, and drink.

Drug–drug interactions

Because sirolimus is metabolized primarily via CYP450 3A isoenzymes, substances known to alter functionality of these enzymes will alter bioavailability and elimination of this drug (Table 24-2).

Additionally, the pharmacokinetic profile of sirolimus is significantly altered by concomitant cyclosporine (Table 24-3).

Drug–disease interactions

- *Edema:* Sirolimus has been associated with peripheral edema and pleural and pericardial effusions.
- *Hyperlipidemia:* Sirolimus increases levels of triglycerides and cholesterol.
- *Kidney transplantation:* Sirolimus may delay recovery of graft function post-transplant and is associated with increased urinary protein excretion after conversion from calcineurin inhibitors.
- *Liver transplantation:* Sirolimus is associated with increased incidence of mortality, graft loss, and hepatic artery thrombosis in de novo liver transplant recipients.
- *Lung transplantation:* There have been cases of fatal bronchial anastomotic dehiscence in de novo lung transplant recipients.
- *Vaccinations:* In general, immunosuppressants may affect efficacy of vaccinations. The use of live vaccines should be avoided.

Adverse drug reactions

- *CNS:* Anorexia
- *HEENT:* Oral ulcers
- *GI:* Diarrhea, esophagitis, gastritis, gastroenteritis, hepatotoxicity, hepatic artery thrombosis in de novo liver transplant recipients
- *Renal:* Synergistic nephrotoxicity with calcineurin inhibitors, proteinuria
- *Endocrine and metabolic:* Hyperlipidemia, hypertension, hyperkalemia
- *Dermatologic:* Rash, acne
- *Hematologic:* Leukopenia, thrombocytopenia, pancytopenia, thrombosis
- *Other:* Arthralgia, lymphocele, pneumonitis, bronchial anastomotic dehiscence in de novo lung transplant recipients

Patient instructions

- Take the prescribed dose at a consistent time once daily, with or without food, but in the same way to maintain consistency.
- Make sure you do not take your morning medication on the day of therapeutic drug monitoring. After the monitoring is complete, take your morning medication immediately and then return to your original medication schedule.
- Many medications interact with this medication. Do not take anything prescribed by another physician until you verify that there are no drug interactions.

Monitoring

Monitor C_0 (trough). Goal depends on multifactorial risk assessment and assay type (in general, 5–15 ng/mL).

Pharmacokinetics

- Bioavailability: F = 14%

Elimination: Half-life = 57–63 hours (increased with hepatic dysfunction)

Selective T-Cell Co-stimulation Blocker

Belatacept

Mechanism of action
Belatacept binds to co-stimulation proteins CD80 and CD86 on the APC, to prevent binding to the T-cell proteins (i.e., CD28) necessary for activation of the T-cell.

Administration
Intravenous: Reconstitute contents with 10.5 mL of sterile water for injection, NS, or D_5W. Calculate total volume of reconstituted solution necessary for prescribed dose. The reconstituted solution is diluted with NS or D_5W to a final concentration of 2–10 mg/mL. Administer peripherally or centrally over 30 minutes with a 0.1–1.2 μm low-protein-binding filter. Refer to Table 24-1 for dosing schedule.

Drug–drug interactions
No clinically significant interactions have been reported.

Drug–disease interactions
- *Liver transplantation:* In a clinical trial with more frequent administration than noted in Table 24-1, belatacept was associated with increased graft loss and mortality.
- *Post-transplant lymphoproliferative disease (PTLD):* Belatacept is associated with an increased risk of PTLD involving the central nervous system, and thus is avoided in patients that are Epstein-Barr virus seronegative or with unknown status.
- *Tuberculosis:* An increased incidence of tuberculosis has been reported with belatacept; thus patients should be evaluated for latent tuberculosis infection before administering belatacept.
- *Vaccinations:* In general, immunosuppressants may affect efficacy of vaccinations. The use of live vaccines should be avoided.

Adverse drug reactions
- *CNS:* Headache, insomnia, anxiety, PTLD
- *CV:* Hypertension
- *GI:* Diarrhea, constipation, nausea, vomiting, abdominal pain
- *Hematologic:* Anemia, leukopenia
- *Renal:* Hematuria, proteinuria, dysuria
- *Endocrine and metabolic:* Hypocalcemia, hypo- or hyperkalemia, hypophosphatemia, dyslipidemia, hyperglycemia
- *Dermatologic:* Acne
- *Other:* Urinary tract infection, peripheral edema, upper respiratory infection, progressive multifocal leukoencephalopathy, polyomavirus nephropathy

Patient instructions
Report any adverse drug reactions to your health care provider immediately.

Monitoring
Patients should be monitored closely for signs and symptoms of infection or PTLD (i.e., behavioral changes).

Pharmacokinetics
- Dosing is based on total body weight.
- Linear pharmacokinetics: First-order elimination (standard doses in Table 24-1)
- Elimination: Half-life = ~11 days

Antiproliferative Agents

Azathioprine

Mechanism of action
Azathioprine is a purine analogue pro-drug, which is cleaved to 6-mercaptopurine; 6-mercaptopurine is activated intracellularly to several active metabolites, which can be incorporated directly into DNA (deoxyribonucleic acid) as thiopurine as well as interfere with the RNA (ribonucleic acid) and DNA biosynthesis directly and via feedback inhibition.

Administration
- *Intravenous:* Dilute dose in NS or D_5W, and administer IV infusion over 5–60 minutes.
- *Oral:* Administer daily dose po once a day.

Drug–drug interactions
Xanthine oxidase is responsible for the elimination of the active metabolites of azathioprine. Concomitant use of allopurinol with azathioprine results in significantly increased azathioprine-induced toxicity. Reduce dose of azathioprine by 65–75%.

Drug–disease interactions
- *Renal insufficiency:* Bioavailability is significantly reduced in uremic patients.
- *Vaccinations:* In general, immunosuppressants may affect efficacy of vaccinations. The use of live vaccines should be avoided.

Adverse drug reactions
- *HEENT:* Retinopathy
- *GI:* Nausea, vomiting, diarrhea, anorexia, pancreatitis, hepatotoxicity
- *Dermatologic:* Rash, skin cancer
- *Hematologic:* Leukopenia, thrombocytopenia, pancytopenia

Patient instructions
- Take the prescribed dose at a consistent time once daily, with or without food, but take in the same way to maintain consistency.
- Many medications interact with this medication. Do not take anything prescribed by another physician until you verify that there are no drug interactions.

Monitoring
Pharmacokinetic monitoring is not required.

Pharmacokinetics
- Bioavailability: F = 41–47%
- Bioavailability in uremic patients: F = 17%

Mycophenolate mofetil

Mechanism of action
Mycophenolate mofetil is metabolized to mycophenolic acid (MPA), which causes noncompetitive, reversible inhibition of inosine monophosphate dehydrogenase, a critical enzyme in the de novo pathway of purine synthesis, which is crucial during lymphocyte activation and proliferation.

Administration
- *Intravenous:* Dilute in D_5W to a concentration of 6 mg/mL, and infuse over at least 2 hours.
- *Oral:* Administer as equally divided doses po every 8–12 hours consistently with or without food.

Drug–drug interactions
- *Cyclosporine:* See Table 24-3.
- *Cholestyramine:* Because of the interruption of enterohepatic recirculation, administration can decrease MPA exposure.
- *Colestipol and colesevelam:* Simultaneous administration can decrease MPA exposure.
- *Antacids:* Simultaneous administration with magnesium- or aluminum-containing antacids reduces absorption and decreases MPA exposure.

- *Note:* Efficacy of oral contraceptives may decrease with therapy. Additional birth control methods are recommended.

Drug–disease interactions
- *Severe renal impairment:* Mycophenolate mofetil reduces protein binding of MPA.
- *Vaccinations:* In general, immunosuppressants may affect efficacy of vaccinations. The use of live vaccines should be avoided.

Adverse drug reactions
- *GI:* Nausea, vomiting, diarrhea, abdominal pain
- *Hematologic:* Leukopenia, thrombocytopenia, anemia, pancytopenia

Patient instructions
- Take the prescribed dose at consistent times during the day, with or without food, but in the same way to maintain consistency.
- Make sure you do not take your medication before therapeutic drug monitoring.

Monitoring
Pharmacokinetic monitoring is not required.

Pharmacokinetics
- MPA is highly protein bound.
- Bioavailability: F = 94%
- Elimination: Half-life = 16–18 hours

Mycophenolate sodium

Mechanism of action
Delayed-release tablets deliver MPA, which causes noncompetitive, reversible inhibition of inosine monophosphate dehydrogenase, a critical enzyme in the de novo pathway of purine synthesis, which is crucial during lymphocyte activation and proliferation.

Administration
Administer as equally divided doses po every 12 hours consistently without food.

Drug–drug interactions
- *Cholestyramine:* Administration interrupts enterohepatic recirculation and decreases MPA exposure.
- *Antacids:* Simultaneous administration with magnesium- or aluminum-containing antacids reduces absorption and decreases MPA exposure.

■ *Note:* Efficacy of oral contraceptives may decrease with therapy. Additional birth control methods are recommended.

Drug–disease interactions

■ *Severe renal impairment:* Mycophenolate sodium reduces protein binding of MPA.
■ *Vaccinations:* In general, immunosuppressants may affect efficacy of vaccinations. The use of live vaccines should be avoided.

Adverse drug reactions

■ *GI:* Nausea, vomiting, diarrhea, abdominal pain
■ *Hematologic:* Leukopenia, thrombocytopenia, anemia, pancytopenia

Patient instructions

■ Take the prescribed dose at consistent times during the day, either 30 minutes before or 2 hours after meals, but take the same way each day to maintain consistency.
■ Make sure you do not take your medication before therapeutic drug monitoring.

Monitoring
Pharmacokinetic monitoring is not required.

Pharmacokinetics
■ MPA is highly protein bound.
■ Bioavailability: F = 72–92%
■ Elimination: Half-life = 8–16 hours

Corticosteroids

Selection of agent

Selection of the corticosteroid used is based on the ratio of glucocorticoid to mineralocorticoid potency.

Intravenous agents are methylprednisolone and dexamethasone. Oral agents are prednisone, prednisolone, and dexamethasone.

Mechanism of action

Corticosteroids bind to cytosolic glucocorticoid receptors, which translocate to the nucleus, where the complexes bind to regulatory DNA sequences, glucocorticoid-responsive elements (GREs) within the promoter section of various genes. Activation of these GREs modifies activities of promoter genes such as NFAT, AP-1, and NF-κB, which results in down-regulation of expression of HLA and numerous cell

adhesion molecules, as well as decreased synthesis of numerous lymphokines responsible for activation, proliferation, and migration (i.e., IL-1, IL-2, IL-6, IL-8, IFN-γ, TNF-α).

Administration

Administration depends on the individual agent.

Drug–drug interactions

Because corticosteroids are metabolized primarily via CYP450 3A isoenzymes, substances known to alter functionality of these enzymes will alter bioavailability and elimination of these drugs (Table 24-2).

Drug–disease interactions

■ *Diabetes mellitus:* Administration worsens glycemic control in patients with preexisting diabetes.
■ *Osteopenia and osteoporosis:* Administration alters calcium and phosphate absorption and excretion, as well as osteoblast activity, resulting in progression of bone loss that is common in metabolic diseases such as end-stage renal disease and liver failure.
■ *Vaccinations:* In general, immunosuppressants may affect efficacy of vaccinations. The use of live vaccines should be avoided.

Adverse drug reactions

The incidence and extent of most adverse drug reactions with corticosteroids depend on the ratio of glucocorticoid to mineralocorticoid potency. Adverse drug events include the following:

■ *CNS:* Seizure, psychosis, delirium, hallucinations, mood swings, insomnia, pseudotumor cerebri
■ *HEENT:* Cataracts, glaucoma
■ *CV:* Hypertension, cardiomyopathy
■ *GI:* Increased appetite, gastroesophageal reflux disease, peptic ulcer disease, pancreatitis
■ *Renal:* Edema, alkalosis, hyperkalemia
■ *Endocrine and metabolic:* Hyperlipidemia, hypothalamic-pituitary-adrenal axis suppression, growth suppression, new onset diabetes after transplant
■ *Dermatologic:* Hirsutism, acne, skin atrophy, impaired wound healing
■ *Hematologic:* Transient leukocytosis

■ *Musculoskeletal:* Arthralgia, myopathy, osteo-porosis, avascular necrosis

Patient instructions

■ When taking orally, take daily dose in the morning with food.
■ Many drugs interact with these agents. Do not take anything prescribed by another physician until you verify that there are no drug interactions.

Monitoring

Pharmacokinetic monitoring is not required.

Pharmacokinetics

Pharmacokinetics depend on the individual agent.

Monoclonal Antibodies

Basiliximab

Mechanism of action
Chimeric (murine and human), monoclonal IgG specifically binds to the subunit, CD25, of the human high-affinity IL-2 receptor, which is expressed only on activated lymphocytes. In this way, basiliximab competitively inhibits IL-2 and facilitates preferential elimination of activated lymphocytes.

Administration
Dilute to a concentration of 0.4 mg/mL in NS or D_5W. Administer peripherally or centrally as a bolus or continuous infusion over 20–30 minutes.

Drug–drug interactions
No clinically significant drug interactions occur.

Drug–disease interactions
In general, immunosuppressants may affect efficacy of vaccinations. The use of live vaccines should be avoided.

Adverse drug reactions
Severe acute hypersensitivity reactions, including anaphylaxis, may occur within the 24 hours following administration of the initial dose or on repeat exposure.

Patient instructions
Report any shortness of breath, palpitations, light-headedness, or itching to your health care provider immediately.

Monitoring
Pharmacokinetic monitoring is not required.

Pharmacokinetics
■ *Adults* (following a 20 mg IV infusion over 20 minutes):
  • Mean C_{max} = 7.1 ± 5.1 mg/L
  • Mean half-life = 7.2 ± 3.2 days
■ *Children:* Mean half-life = 11.5 ± 6.3 days

Pharmacodynamics
■ *Adults:* CD25 saturation is at or above serum concentration of 0.2 mcg/mL. Mean duration of saturation depends on concomitant immuno-suppressive regimen.
■ *Children:* CD25 saturation is similar to that seen in adults.

Polyclonal Antibodies

Antithymocyte globulin (equine)

Mechanism of action
This antithymocyte globulin is purified, sterile, polyclonal IgG harvested from horses immunized with human thymocytes. The preparation includes IgG directed against cell surface markers such as CD2, CD3, CD4, CD8, CD11a, and CD18. In this way, horse antithymocyte globulin targets multiple phases of immunity, including T-cell activation, homing, and cytotoxic activities.

Administration
■ Premedication:
  • *Dose 1:* Giving IV steroids, acetaminophen, and antihistamines 1 hour before the dose is strongly recommended to modify first-dose reactions.
  • *Subsequent doses:* Give acetaminophen and antihistamines 1 hour before the dose with steroids as needed for infusion reactions.
■ Dosing:
  • Dilute the dose to a concentration not to exceed 4 mg/mL in 1/2 NS or D_5W.
  • Administer centrally over 4–6 hours.

Drug–drug interactions
No clinically significant drug interactions occur.

Drug–disease interactions
In general, immunosuppressants may affect the efficacy of vaccinations. The use of live vaccines should be avoided.

Adverse drug reactions

Most adverse drug reactions with antithymocyte globulin (equine) are infusion-related reactions (i.e., fever, chills, dyspnea); leukopenia; thrombocytopenia; or rash.

Patient instructions

Report any shortness of breath, palpitations, light-headedness, tremor, fever, or itching to your health care provider immediately.

Monitoring

The goal for treatment of acute rejection is suppression of CD3 lineage to < 50 cells/mm^3.

Pharmacokinetics

Elimination: half-life = 36 hours–12 days

Antithymocyte globulin (rabbit)

Mechanism of action

This antithymocyte globulin is purified, pasteurized, polyclonal IgG harvested from pathogen-free rabbits immunized with human thymocytes. This preparation includes IgG directed against cell surface markers, such as TCRab, CD2, CD3, CD4, CD5, CD6, CD7, CD8, CD11a, CD18, CD28, CD45, CD49, CD54, CD58, CD80, CD86, HLA class I, and β_2 microglobulin. In this way, rabbit antithymocyte globulin targets multiple phases of immunity, including T-cell activation, homing, and cytotoxic activities.

Administration

- Premedication:
  - *Dose 1:* Giving IV steroids, acetaminophen, and antihistamines 1 hour before the dose is strongly recommended to modify first-dose reactions.
  - *Subsequent doses:* Give acetaminophen and antihistamines 1 hour before the dose with steroids as needed for infusion reactions.
- Dose:
  - Dilute dose to a concentration of 0.5 mg/mL in NS or D$_5$W.
  - Administer centrally over 4–6 hours through 0.22-micron in-line filter.

Drug–drug interactions

In the case of immunoglobulin, administration may decrease the degree of lymphocyte depletion achieved.

Drug–disease interactions

In general, immunosuppressants may affect efficacy of vaccinations. The use of live vaccines should be avoided.

Adverse drug reactions

Most adverse drug reactions with antithymocyte globulin (rabbit) are infusion-related reactions (i.e., fever, chills, dyspnea); leukopenia; thrombocytopenia; or rash.

Patient instructions

Report any shortness of breath, palpitations, light-headedness, tremor, fever, or itching to your health care provider immediately.

Monitoring

The goal for treatment of acute rejection is suppression of CD3 lineage to < 50 cells/mm^3.

Pharmacokinetics

A two-compartment model is used. For terminal elimination, half-life = 2–3 days for first dose; range = 14–45 days with multiple doses.

24-5. Questions

Use Patient Profile 24-1 to answer Questions 1–4.

1. Which of the following medications should be given with caution because of the patient's sulfonamide allergy?

   A. Furosemide
   B. Fluconazole
   C. Azathioprine
   D. Valganciclovir
   E. Tacrolimus

2. Which of the following combinations of drugs represents therapeutic duplication?

   A. Tacrolimus and azathioprine
   B. Azathioprine and mycophenolate mofetil
   C. Dapsone and valganciclovir
   D. Glimepiride and tacrolimus
   E. Prednisone and mycophenolate mofetil

3. Which of the following combinations of drugs interact?

   A. Fluconazole and tacrolimus
   B. Fluconazole and valganciclovir

Patient Profile 24-1. City Hospital

Patient name: John Doe

Age: 52

Gender: Male

Ethnicity: African American

Diagnoses:

h/o ESRD s/p deceased donor renal transplant 3 mo ago

DM × 20 yr

HTN × 30 yr

Drug-induced hyperkalemia

Current laboratory results:

SCr = 1.2

K = 5.3

WBC 3.8

Plt 120

Address: 101 South First Street

Height: 5′11″

Weight: 240 lb

Allergies: Sulfa

Medications prior to hospital admission:

Prograf 4 mg po bid

Amaryl 4 mg po bid

CellCept 750 mg po bid

Metoprolol 100 mg po bid

Diflucan 200 mg po daily

Dapsone 100 mg po daily

Valcyte 450 mg po daily

EC ASA 81 mg po daily

Prednisone 5 mg po daily

Additional medications prescribed during hospital course:

Lasix 40 mg po bid

Imuran 100 mg po daily

   C. Dapsone and furosemide
   D. Valcyte and prednisone
   E. Valganciclovir and ECASA

4. Mr. Doe was diagnosed with drug-induced hyperkalemia. Which medication on his profile could be responsible for this?

   A. Mycophenolate mofetil
   B. Furosemide
   C. Prednisone
   D. Tacrolimus
   E. Aspirin

5. Which of the following medications is classified as a calcineurin inhibitor?

   A. Sirolimus
   B. Everolimus
   C. Belatacept
   D. Azathioprine
   E. Cyclosporine

6. Which of the following medications causes diarrhea and myelosuppression?

   A. Sirolimus
   B. Mycophenolate mofetil
   C. Prednisone

   D. Cyclosporine
   E. Basiliximab

7. Which of the following medications require(s) bile for emulsification and absorption?

   A. Azathioprine
   B. Cyclosporine
   C. Tacrolimus
   D. Prednisone
   E. All of the above

8. All of the following are known adverse effects of cyclosporine *except*

   A. hirsutism.
   B. nephrotoxicity.
   C. oral ulceration.
   D. gingival hyperplasia.
   E. hyperlipidemia.

9. All of the following are contraindications or precautions associated with sirolimus *except*

   A. de novo lung transplant recipient.
   B. hyperlipidemia.
   C. diabetes mellitus.
   D. de novo liver transplant recipient.
   E. allergy to sirolimus.

10. What is the generic name for Imuran?

   A. Mycophenolate mofetil
   B. Azathioprine
   C. Cyclosporine
   D. Tacrolimus
   E. Prednisone

11. Which of the immunosuppressive medications listed may cause new onset diabetes after transplant?

   A. Horse antithymocyte globulin
   B. Azathioprine
   C. Mycophenolate mofetil
   D. Basiliximab
   E. Tacrolimus

12. Which of the following medications requires therapeutic drug monitoring via trough concentrations?

   A. Belatacept
   B. Tacrolimus
   C. Daclizumab
   D. Basiliximab
   E. Azathioprine

13. Which of the following medications inhibits signal 3 by binding to the CD25 subunit of the IL-2 receptor?

   A. Antithymocyte globulin (rabbit)
   B. Antithymocyte globulin (equine)
   C. Basiliximab
   D. Everolimus
   E. Belatacept

14. All of the following increase the risk of acute rejection *except*

   A. pediatric recipient.
   B. HLA mismatch.
   C. living donor.
   D. noncompliance.
   E. history of previous transplantation.

15. Which of the following medications produces a significant pharmacokinetic interaction when administered with azathioprine?

   A. Allopurinol
   B. Fluconazole
   C. Sirolimus
   D. Probenecid
   E. Tacrolimus

16. Which of the following conditions alter(s) the pharmacokinetic profile of cyclosporine?

   I. Biliary obstruction
   II. Malnutrition
   III. Hyperglycemia

   A. I only
   B. II only
   C. III only
   D. I and II only
   E. I, II, and III

17. Which of the following medications interacts with sirolimus?

   A. Erythromycin
   B. Metoprolol
   C. Furosemide
   D. Nifedipine
   E. Gentamicin

18. Which of the following immunosuppressants should *not* be administered at the same time secondary to an interaction related to timing of doses?

   A. Tacrolimus and azathioprine
   B. Sirolimus and cyclosporine
   C. Cyclosporine and azathioprine
   D. Sirolimus and tacrolimus
   E. Sirolimus and mycophenolate mofetil

19. Which type of immunity involves stimulation of cells and soluble mediators that nonspecifically recognize alloantigens with no altered response on repeat exposure?

   A. Autoimmunity
   B. Innate immunity
   C. Adaptive immunity
   D. Acute rejection
   E. Hyperacute rejection

20. Which group of genes encodes for antigens that are responsible for self- or nonself-recognition?

   A. Class I human leukocyte antigen
   B. Class II human leukocyte antigen
   C. Class III human leukocyte antigen
   D. Major histocompatibility complex
   E. Minor histocompatibility complex

21. On binding of antigen displayed by the antigen-presenting cell to the T-cell receptor

complex, what additional step is required for
T-helper-cell activation?

A. Binding of the co-stimulatory pathway
(i.e., CD58/CD2)
B. Activation of the promoter gene NFAT
C. Transcription of the IL-2 gene
D. No additional step required
E. Translation of IL-2

22. Which cytokine released by activated CD4⁺
lymphocytes plays a major role in the subsequent activation of numerous lymphocyte
lineages?

A. Interleukin-1 (IL-1)
B. Tumor necrosis factor-α (TNF-α)
C. Interleukin-2 (IL-2)
D. Interferon-γ (IFN-γ)
E. Complement

23. Which of the following medications should be
avoided in female liver transplant recipients?

A. Tacrolimus
B. Cyclosporine
C. Mycophenolate sodium
D. Azathioprine
E. Tacrolimus extended release

24. Which of the following medications is a
polyclonal antibody?

A. Belatacept
B. Basiliximab
C. Mycophenolate sodium
D. Rabbit antithymocyte globulin
E. Sirolimus

25. Which of the following medications is
a monoclonal antibody?

A. Belatacept
B. Basiliximab
C. Horse antithymocyte globulin
D. Astagraf XL
E. Zortress

24-6. Answers

1. **A.** Furosemide (Lasix) is structurally similar to
sulfonamides and would be expected to elicit a
similar allergic response.

2. **B.** Both azathioprine (Imuran) and mycophenolate mofetil (CellCept) are classified
as antiproliferative agents. Both agents
inhibit purine biosynthesis and would not act
synergistically.

3. **A.** Fluconazole (Diflucan) is an inhibitor of
cytochrome P450 3A isoenzymes, which is the
enzyme system that is responsible for metabolism of tacrolimus.

4. **D.** Hyperkalemia (incidence 20–40%) is a well-
documented adverse drug reaction with tacrolimus (Prograf).

5. **E.** Cyclosporine is a calcineurin inhibitor.

6. **B.** Mycophenolate mofetil can cause dose-
limiting diarrhea and myelosuppression.
Sirolimus (i.e., CD80/86-CD28) can cause
myelosuppression but are not commonly associated with diarrhea.

7. **B.** Cyclosporine is highly lipophilic and requires
bile for emulsification and absorption.

8. **C.** Hirsutism, nephrotoxicity, gingival hyperplasia, and hyperlipidemia are known adverse
effects of cyclosporine. Oral ulceration is not an
adverse effect of cyclosporine.

9. **C.** The use of sirolimus in de novo lung and
liver transplant recipients is contraindicated
because of an increased incidence of fatal adverse
drug reactions. Additionally, use of sirolimus
in patients with uncontrolled hyperlipidemia is
strongly discouraged because of its profound
effects on lipid biosynthesis and catabolism.

10. **B.** Azathioprine is the generic name for Imuran.

11. **E.** Tacrolimus may cause new onset diabetes
after transplant.

12. **B.** Tacrolimus requires therapeutic drug monitoring via trough concentrations to obtain desired
therapeutic effects.

13. **C.** Basiliximab selects for destruction of activated lymphocytes by binding to the CD25 subunit of the high-affinity IL-2 receptor.

14. **C.** Of the listed parameters, all are considered
to increase the risk of acute rejection *except* a
living donor as the donor source.

15. **A.** Xanthine oxidase is responsible for the
elimination of the active metabolites of azathioprine. Concomitant use of allopurinol with
azathioprine results in significantly increased

azathioprine-induced toxicity. Reduce the dose of azathioprine by 65–75%.

16. **D.** Both biliary obstruction and severe malnutrition would change the pharmacokinetic profile of cyclosporine. Cyclosporine requires bile for emulsification and absorption. If bile flow is obstructed, then the bioavailability is significantly decreased. Additionally, cyclosporine is a highly lipoprotein-bound drug. In severe malnutrition, total protein stores are depleted, thereby increasing the total free drug.

17. **A.** Erythromycin inhibits CYP450 3A isoenzymes, which is the enzyme system that is responsible for sirolimus metabolism.

18. **B.** Simultaneous administration of sirolimus and cyclosporine increases C_{max} and the area under the curve of sirolimus by 120–500% and 140–230%, respectively. Administration 4 hours apart increases C_{max} and the area under the curve of sirolimus by 30–40% and 35–80%, respectively.

19. **B.** Innate immunity is the fundamental type of immunity in which antigens are recognized in a nonspecific manner. This type of immunity is not augmented on repeat exposure.

20. **D.** Class I and II HLA are the actual antigens important for self- and nonself-recognition. The group of genes that encode for these antigens is the major histocompatibility complex.

21. **A.** Activation is dependent on antigen–HLA binding to the T-cell receptor complex and the subsequent binding of a second signal or "co-stimulatory pathway."

22. **C.** Active CD4+ T-cells produce and release various lymphokines, particularly IL-2, which is important for activation and proliferation of numerous lymphocyte lineages.

23. **E.** Tacrolimus extended release (Astagraf XL) is associated with increased mortality in female transplant recipients.

24. **D.** Rabbit antithymocyte globulin is a polyclonal antibody with an FDA indication for treatment of acute rejection.

25. **B.** Basiliximab is a monoclonal antibody with an FDA-approved indication for prevention of acute rejection.

24-7. References

Christians U, Jacobsen W, Benet LZ, et al. Mechanisms of clinically relevant drug interactions associated with tacrolimus. *Clin Pharmacokinet*. 2002;41: 813–51.

de Jonge H, Naesens M, Kuypers DR. New insights into the pharmacokinetics and pharmacodynamics of the calcineurin inhibitors and mycophenolic acid: Possible consequences for therapeutics drug monitoring in solid organ transplantation. *Ther Drug Monit*. 2009;31(4):416–35.

Delves PJ, Roitt IM. The immune system: First of two parts. *N Engl J Med*. 2000;343:37–49.

Delves PJ, Roitt IM. The immune system: Second of two parts. *N Engl J Med*. 2000;343:108–17.

Dunn CJ, Wagstaff AJ, Perry CM, et al. Cyclosporin: An updated review of the pharmacokinetic properties, clinical efficacy, and tolerability of a microemulsion-based formulation (Neoral) in organ transplantation. *Drugs*. 2001;61:1957–2016.

Garbardi S, Baroletti S. Everolimus: A proliferation signal inhibitor with clinical applications in organ transplantation, oncology, and cardiology. *Pharmacotherapy*. 2010;30(10):1044–56.

Kelly P, Kahan BD. Review: Metabolism of immunosuppressant drugs. *Curr Drug Metab*. 2002;3: 275–87.

Kirchner GI, Meier-Wiedenbach I, Manns MP. Clinical pharmacokinetics of everolimus. *Clin Pharmacokinet*. 2004;43(2):83–95.

MacDonald A, Scarola J, Burke JT, et al. Clinical pharmacokinetics and therapeutic drug monitoring of sirolimus. *Clin Ther*. 2000;22(suppl B): B101–B121.

Martin S, Tichy E, Gabardi S. Belatacept: A novel biologic for maintenance immunosuppression after renal transplantation. *Pharmacotherapy*. 2011; 31(4):394–407.

Nankivell BJ, Alexander SI. Rejection of kidney allograft. *N Engl J Med*. 2010;363:1451–62.

Newbold N, Riley B, Hardinger K. A review of enteric-coated mycophenolate sodium for renal transplant immunosuppression. *Clin Med Ther*. 2009;1:927–33.

Saad A, DePestel D, Carver P. Factors influencing the magnitude and clinical significance of drug interactions between azole antifungals and select immunosuppressants. *Pharmacotherapy*. 2006;26 (12):1730–44.

Gastrointestinal Diseases

Christa M. George

25

25-1. Key Points

Peptic Ulcer Disease

- Peptic ulcer disease (PUD) is a group of disorders of the upper gastrointestinal (GI) tract characterized by ulcerative lesions that require acid and pepsin for their formation.
- Duodenal and gastric ulcers are classified as *Helicobacter pylori* related, nonsteroidal anti-inflammatory drug (NSAID) related, or stress related.
- Epigastric pain occurring 1–3 hours after meals that is relieved by ingestion of food or antacids is the classic symptom of PUD.
- *H. pylori* is a Gram-negative microaerophilic bacterium inhabiting the area between the mucous layer and epithelial cells in the stomach. It can be found anywhere that gastric epithelium is present.
- NSAIDs are the leading cause of PUD in patients who are negative for *H. pylori* infection.
- NSAIDs are directly toxic to gastric epithelium and inhibit the synthesis of prostaglandins.
- The goals of PUD therapy are ulcer healing and elimination of the cause. Additional considerations are prevention of complications and relief of symptoms.
- Upper GI endoscopy is used to diagnose PUD. The procedure is usually reserved for patients with symptoms of PUD who are over 55 years of age or who have alarm symptoms.
- Patients with symptoms of PUD who are less than 55 years of age and have no alarm symptoms may be tested for the presence of *H. pylori* and treated with eradication therapy if results are positive.

- Histology and rapid urease testing may be performed on biopsy samples obtained during endoscopy to test for *H. pylori*.
- Serum antibody tests, urea breath tests, and fecal antibody testing do not require endoscopy to test for *H. pylori*.
- The American College of Gastroenterology treatment guidelines for *H. pylori* eradication in PUD recommend initial triple therapy with a proton pump inhibitor (PPI), clarithromycin, and either amoxicillin or metronidazole for 14 days. Amoxicillin should be used first because of low resistance rates and fewer adverse effects. Alternatively, quadruple therapy with bismuth, metronidazole, tetracycline, and either a histamine 2-receptor antagonist (H2RA) or a PPI for 10–14 days may be used.
- NSAID-related PUD treatment consists of discontinuing the offending agent and issuing antisecretory therapy for symptom relief.
- Antisecretory therapy with a PPI or an H2RA should be administered for 4 weeks to promote healing and to relieve symptoms.
- Patients with active bleeding who are hemodynamically stable should receive intravenous PPI therapy and undergo endoscopy to evaluate the risk of bleeding recurrence.
- Patients with active bleeding who are hemodynamically unstable should receive intravenous fluids and blood transfusions. They should undergo emergency endoscopy for coagulation of bleeding sites. Various modalities may be used to achieve bleeding-site coagulation.
- Surgery is reserved for patients who have refractory ulcers, recurrent bleeding, or a perforated ulcer.

- Patients should be counseled on the importance of adherence to treatment regimens, proper dosing, and the side effects of medications.
- Patients should be counseled to decrease psychological stress, discontinue drinking alcohol and smoking, stop using NSAIDs, and avoid food or beverages that exacerbate PUD symptoms.

Gastroesophageal Reflux Disease

- The American College of Gastroenterology guidelines state that gastroesophageal reflux disease (GERD) "should be defined as symptoms or complications resulting from the reflux of gastric contents into the esophagus or beyond, into the oral cavity (including larynx) or lung."
- The prevalence of GERD is highest in Western countries, with 10–20% of adults experiencing symptoms weekly.
- The manifestations of GERD are divided into esophageal and extraesophageal syndromes.
- Esophageal syndromes consist of those that are only symptomatic in nature and those that are symptomatic with esophageal injury on endoscopy. Symptomatic syndromes include the typical reflux syndrome and the reflux chest pain syndrome.
- The typical reflux syndrome is defined by the presence of troublesome heartburn or regurgitation. Patients may also have other symptoms, such as epigastric pain or sleep disturbance.
- The pathophysiology of GERD involves the prolonged contact of esophageal epithelium with refluxed gastric contents that contain acid and pepsin.
- Esophageal defenses consist of the antireflux barrier, luminal clearance mechanisms, and tissue resistance. Increased contact time of refluxate and esophageal mucosa or impaired defense mechanisms can lead to the symptoms of GERD.
- Diagnostic testing with endoscopy should be performed in patients who present with alarm symptoms and for screening patients at high risk of complications.
- Goals of therapy are to alleviate or eliminate symptoms, decrease frequency and duration of reflux, promote healing of the injured mucosa, and prevent the development of complications.
- An 8-week course of once-daily PPI therapy is the treatment of choice for symptom relief and healing of erosive esophagitis in patients with typical symptoms.

- Surgery is a treatment option for long-term therapy in GERD patients who desire to stop medical therapy, are noncompliant with medical therapy, have side effects from medical therapy, or have persistent symptoms caused by refractory GERD.
- Patients should be counseled on medication dosing and administration, side effects, drug interactions, monitoring of GERD symptoms, and lifestyle modifications.
- Weight loss should be recommended for GERD patients who are overweight or have had recent weight gain.
- Head-of-bed elevation and avoidance of meals 2 to 3 hours before bedtime should be recommended for patients with nocturnal GERD.
- The routine global elimination of food that may trigger GERD symptoms is not recommended; however, patients should avoid any food or beverage that triggers their own GERD symptoms (e.g., chocolate, caffeine, alcohol, acidic and/or spicy foods).
- GERD is considered a chronic condition, and most patients will require chronic therapy with antisecretory agents. Antisecretory therapy should be titrated to the lowest effective dose.

Inflammatory Bowel Disease

- Idiopathic inflammatory bowel disease (IBD) is divided into two major types: (1) ulcerative colitis (UC) and (2) Crohn's disease (CD).
- Ulcerative colitis is a mucosal inflammatory condition confined to the rectum and colon.
- Crohn's disease is a transmural inflammation of the GI tract that can affect any part (mouth to anus).
- The hallmark clinical symptom of ulcerative colitis is bloody diarrhea, often with rectal urgency and tenesmus.
- Clinical symptoms are categorized as mild, moderate, or severe. Endoscopic findings are categorized as distal (limited to below the splenic flexure) or extensive (extending proximal to the splenic flexure).
- Typical symptoms of Crohn's disease include chronic or nocturnal diarrhea and abdominal pain. Additional typical symptoms include weight loss, fever, and rectal bleeding.
- Symptoms differ depending on the site of inflammation and are categorized as mild, moderate, or severe.

- The etiology of IBD is unclear, but similar factors may contribute to both ulcerative colitis and Crohn's disease. The diagnosis of IBD is made on the basis of negative stool evaluation for infectious causes.
- Treatment of IBD involves medications that target inflammatory mediators and alter immuno-inflammatory processes. These medications include anti-inflammatory, antimicrobial, immunosuppressive, and biologic agents.
- Goals of therapy for ulcerative colitis and Crohn's disease include inducing and maintaining remission of symptoms, improving quality of life, resolving complications and systemic symptoms, and preventing future complications.
- Patients should be counseled on medication dosing and administration, side effects, drug interactions, monitoring of IBD symptoms, and proper nutrition.
- Patients with IBD are often malnourished because of malabsorption or maldigestion caused by chronic bowel inflammation, "short gut" syndrome from multiple bowel surgeries, or bile salt deficiency in the gut.
- Surgery may be necessary for patients with severe ulcerative colitis or Crohn's disease. Surgery (proctocolectomy) is curative for ulcerative colitis but not for Crohn's disease.

Irritable Bowel Syndrome

- Irritable bowel syndrome (IBS) is abdominal pain or discomfort that occurs in association with altered bowel habits over a period of 3 months.
- IBS is a prevalent and expensive condition. It significantly impairs health-related quality of life and leads to reduced work productivity.
- IBS is a heterogeneous disorder with various clinical presentations. Common symptoms include abdominal pain, diarrhea, and constipation.
- The pathogenesis is multifactorial, including abnormal gut sensorimotor activity, central nervous system dysfunction, psychological disturbances, genetic predisposition, enteric infection, and other luminal factors.
- No symptom-based diagnostic criteria have ideal accuracy for diagnosing IBS.
- Alarm features include rectal bleeding, weight loss, iron-deficiency anemia, nocturnal symptoms, family history of colorectal cancer, IBD, or celiac sprue. These symptoms may indicate the presence of an organic disease.

- Treatment should be offered to patients seeking medical care if the patient and physician believe that the IBS symptoms decrease the patient's quality of life.
- Goals of therapy include improving IBS symptoms and patient quality of life.
- Anticholinergic and antimuscarinic agents provide short-term relief of abdominal pain and discomfort. Psyllium has been shown to be moderately effective for IBS. Calcium polycarbophil was shown to improve symptoms in one small study. Polyethylene glycol was shown to improve stool frequency. Loperamide decreases stool frequency in patients with diarrhea-predominant IBS. Tricyclic antidepressants improve abdominal pain in IBS patients. Selective serotonin reuptake inhibitors are recommended for patients with moderate to severe abdominal pain or psychiatric comorbidities. Tegaserod improves global IBS symptoms, bloating, abdominal pain, and altered bowel habits in patients with constipation-predominant IBS. Alosetron improves global IBS symptoms, abdominal discomfort, stool consistency, and stool frequency in women with diarrhea-predominant IBS. Lubiprostone has been shown to relieve global IBS symptoms in women with constipation-predominant IBS. Linaclotide reduces abdominal pain and increases the number of spontaneous bowel movements in patients with constipation-predominant IBS.
- Patients should be counseled on medication dosing and administration, side effects, drug interactions, and monitoring of IBS symptoms.
- An effective physician–patient relationship is necessary for successful treatment.
- Education regarding disease pathophysiology and treatment and reassurance that the symptoms are real should be provided.
- Patients should be counseled to avoid foods that exacerbate symptoms.
- Cognitive behavioral therapy, dynamic psychotherapy, and hypnotherapy are more effective than usual care in relieving global symptoms of IBS.

25-2. Study Guide Checklist

The following topics may guide your study of PUD, GERD, UC, CD, and IBS:

- Definitions of PUD, GERD, UC, CD, and IBS
- Clinical signs and symptoms of PUD, GERD, UC, CD, and IBS

- Risk factors associated with NSAID-related ulcers and upper GI complications
- Drug regimens used to eradicate *H. pylori* infection
- For drugs used to treat PUD, GERD, UC, CD, and IBS:
  - Mechanism of action
  - Drug dosing frequency
  - Major adverse drug reactions
  - Clinically significant drug interactions
  - Major patient counseling points
  - Nonpharmacologic treatment of PUD, GERD, UC, CD, and IBS

25-3. Definition, Incidence, and Recognition of Peptic Ulcer Disease

Peptic ulcer disease (PUD) is a group of disorders of the upper gastrointestinal (GI) tract characterized by ulcerative lesions that depend on acid and pepsin for their formation.

Approximately 4 million individuals in the United States are affected by PUD annually. Additionally, complicated PUD leads to approximately 15,000 deaths per year.

The U.S. lifetime prevalence of PUD is approximately 12% in men and 10% in women. PUD has been estimated to cost $10 billion per year in the United States.

Classification

Ulcers are either duodenal or gastric in nature. Duodenal ulcers are more common.

The three common forms of duodenal and gastric ulcers are related to *Helicobacter pylori*, nonsteroidal anti-inflammatory drugs (NSAIDs), or stress.

Clinical Presentation

Epigastric pain occurring 1–3 hours after meals that is relieved by ingestion of food or antacids is the classic presentation of PUD. Pain typically occurs in episodes lasting weeks to months and may be followed by variable periods of spontaneous remission and recurrence.

Ten percent of patients with PUD present with complications and have no prior history of pain.

Pathophysiology

Duodenal ulcers result from the imbalance between duodenal acid load and the acid-buffering capacity of the duodenum. Duodenal ulcers are more frequently associated with an antrum-predominant gastritis.

H. pylori is a Gram-negative microaerophilic bacterium that inhabits the area between the stomach's mucosal layer and epithelial cells. The bacteria can be found anywhere gastric epithelium is present.

Over 50% of the world's population is colonized by *H. pylori*, but only 15% of colonized individuals develop clinical symptoms of PUD. The prevalence of *H. pylori* is decreasing in developed countries. It has been estimated that 30–40% of the U.S. population is infected with *H. pylori*.

H. pylori causes duodenal inflammation, increases duodenal acid load, and impairs duodenal bicarbonate secretion, which leads to duodenal ulcers. It causes inflammation of gastric epithelium, particularly in the antrum-corpus area. The inflammation disrupts mucosal defense, which also leads to gastric ulcers.

NSAIDs are the leading cause of PUD in patients negative for *H. pylori* infection. They are directly toxic to gastric epithelium and inhibit the synthesis of prostaglandins.

Inhibition of prostaglandin synthesis leads to decreased secretion of bicarbonate and mucus, decreased mucosal perfusion, decreased epithelial proliferation, and decreased mucosal resistance to injury.

NSAIDs may cause gastric or duodenal ulcers (more frequently gastric). Gastric ulcers are associated with a corpus-predominant (i.e., diffuse-predominant) gastritis. This pattern of gastritis is associated with low acid output, gastric atrophy, and adenocarcinoma.

Diagnostic Criteria

Upper GI endoscopy is used to diagnose PUD. The procedure is usually reserved for patients with symptoms of PUD who are over 55 years of age or who have alarm symptoms (bleeding, anemia, early satiety, unexplained weight loss, progressive dysphagia, odynophagia, recurrent vomiting, family history of GI cancer, previous esophagogastric cancer).

Patients with symptoms of PUD who are under 55 years of age and have no alarm symptoms may be tested for the presence of *H. pylori* and treated with eradication therapy if results are positive.

Available tests for *H. pylori* are divided into two groups: those that require endoscopy and those that do not.

Histology and rapid urease testing may be performed on biopsy samples taken during endoscopy. Rapid urease testing may be performed in patients who have *not* taken a proton pump inhibitor (PPI) within 1–2 weeks or an antibiotic or bismuth within 4 weeks of the endoscopy. Histology should be performed on patients who have recently taken PPIs, antibiotics, or bismuth.

Antibody testing, urea breath tests, and fecal antigen tests do not require endoscopy. Urea breath tests and fecal antigen tests may be used to confirm eradication of *H. pylori* no sooner than 4 weeks after completion of the treatment regimen.

25-4. Treatment Principles and Goals of PUD

The goals of PUD therapy include healing the ulcer and eliminating its cause. Additional considerations include preventing complications and relieving symptoms.

Use of PPIs is associated with faster healing rates and symptom relief than is treatment with histamine 2–receptor antagonists (H2RAs). (*Note:* H2RAs are less expensive.)

Choice of PUD therapy is based on the etiology of the case. For *H. pylori*–related PUD, antibacterial therapy is used with antisecretory therapy.

Eradication of *H. pylori* reduces the recurrence of PUD and is of prime importance.

The American College of Gastroenterology treatment guidelines for *H. pylori* eradication in PUD recommend initial triple therapy with a PPI, clarithromycin, and either amoxicillin or metronidazole for 14 days. Amoxicillin should be used first, because of low resistance rates and fewer adverse effects.

Alternatively, quadruple therapy with bismuth, metronidazole, tetracycline, and either an H2RA or a PPI for 10–14 days may be used.

Sequential therapy starting with a PPI and amoxicillin for 5 days followed by a PPI and clarithromycin for an additional 5 days requires further study.

The eradication of *H. pylori* should be confirmed with urea breath testing or fecal antigen testing no sooner than 4 weeks after completing eradication therapy.

If a patient has persistent *H. pylori* infection after the initial eradication therapy regimen, salvage therapy with bismuth quadruple therapy for 7–14 days should be administered.

Salvage therapy with a PPI, amoxicillin, and levofloxacin requires further study.

For NSAID-related PUD, discontinuation of the offending agent is imperative.

Antisecretory therapy with a PPI, H2RA, or sucralfate should be administered for 4 weeks to promote healing and to relieve symptoms.

If *H. pylori* is also present, antibacterial therapy should be initiated. Eradication of *H. pylori* does not prevent NSAID-related complications or recurrence.

PPIs, H2RAs, or misoprostol should be used to prevent PUD in patients who require chronic NSAIDs and who are at risk of developing PUD (e.g., patients who are elderly or who have concomitant cardiovascular disease, patients with a history of PUD, patients using high-dose NSAID therapy, and patients who concomitantly use corticosteroids or anticoagulants).

Sucralfate may also be used to aid in ulcer healing, but it requires multiple daily dosing and is associated with many significant drug interactions.

Non-*H. pylori*, non-NSAID-related PUD should be treated with antisecretory therapy.

Patients with GI bleeding may require hospitalization if hemodynamically unstable. Treatment of GI bleeding may include the following: fluid resuscitation, blood transfusion, endoscopic treatments (e.g., thermal therapy, sclerotherapy, epinephrine, surgical clips), and intravenous PPI therapy (with *H. pylori* eradication medications, if positive).

Drug Therapy

Mechanism of action

PPIs suppress gastric acid secretion specifically by inhibiting the H^+-K^+-ATPase enzyme system of the secretory surface of the gastric parietal cell.

H2RAs suppress gastric acid secretion by reversibly blocking histamine-2 receptors on the surface of the gastric parietal cell.

Clarithromycin, amoxicillin, metronidazole, tetracycline, bismuth subsalicylate, and furazolidone exhibit antibacterial effects against *H. pylori*.

When exposed to gastric acid, sucralfate forms a viscous adhesive that binds positively charged protein molecules in the ulcer crater, thus forming a protective barrier that protects against back-diffusion of hydrogen ions.

Misoprostol is a synthetic prostaglandin E_1 (PGE_1) analog that moderately inhibits acid secretion and enhances gastric mucosal defense.

See Table 25-1 for selected medications.

Patient counseling

Educate patients about the importance of completing the entire course of therapy to ensure the eradication of *H. pylori* and to avoid bacterial resistance.

PPIs should be taken before the first meal of the day (generally 30 to 60 minutes before). Lansoprazole and dexlansoprazole granules may be sprinkled onto applesauce for patients who have trouble swallowing pills. Lansoprazole orally disintegrating tablets should not be crushed or chewed. Omeprazole capsules should be swallowed whole. Omeprazole over-the-counter (OTC) tablets should not be crushed or chewed. Omeprazole–sodium bicarbonate capsules should be swallowed whole.

If antacids are being used to control breakthrough symptoms, the dose should be taken no less than 1–2 hours before or after an H2RA is taken. H2RAs may be taken without regard to meals.

Amoxicillin, clarithromycin, and metronidazole may be taken without regard to meals; however, taking clarithromycin and metronidazole with meals often reduces the incidence of stomach upset.

Table 25-1. Selected Medications Used in Treatment of Peptic Ulcer Disease

Generic name	Trade name	Classification	Dosage range and frequency	Dosage forms
Omeprazole	Prilosec	Proton pump inhibitor	20–40 mg daily	C, G
Omeprazole	Prilosec OTC	Proton pump inhibitor	20 mg daily × 14 days	T
Omeprazole + sodium bicarbonate	Zegerid	Proton pump inhibitor and antacid	20–40 mg daily	C, P
Omeprazole/sodium bicarbonate	Zegerid OTC	Proton pump inhibitor/ antacid	20 mg daily	C
Esomeprazole	**Nexium**	Proton pump inhibitor	20–40 mg daily	C, IV, G
Lansoprazole	Prevacid, Prevacid SoluTab	Proton pump inhibitor	15 mg daily–30 mg bid	C, ODT, L, ST
Lansoprazole	Prevacid 24 Hour	Proton pump inhibitor	15 mg daily	C
Dexlansoprazole	**Dexilant**	Proton pump inhibitor	30–60 mg daily	C
Rabeprazole	**Aciphex**	Proton pump inhibitor	10–20 mg daily	T
Pantoprazole	Protonix	Proton pump inhibitor	40–80 mg daily	T, G, IV
Cimetidine	Tagamet	H2-receptor blocker	300 mg qid–800 mg bedtime	T, L, IV
Ranitidine	Zantac	H2-receptor blocker	150 mg bid–300 mg bedtime	T, L, IV, C, EfT
Nizatidine	Axid	H2-receptor blocker	150 mg bid–300 mg bedtime	C, L, T
Famotidine	Pepcid	H2-receptor blocker	20 mg bid–40 mg bedtime	T, C, P, IV
Clarithromycin	Biaxin	Antibacterial	500 mg bid × 10–14 days	T, G
Amoxicillin	Amoxil	Antibacterial	1 g bid × 10–14 days	C, P, CT
Metronidazole	Flagyl	Antibacterial	500 mg tid × 10–14 days	T, C, IV,
Tetracycline	Various trade names	Antibacterial	500 mg qid × 10–14 days	C
Sucralfate	Carafate	Cytoprotective	1 g qid	T, L
Misoprostol	Cytotec	Prostaglandin	200 mcg qid	T

C, capsule; CT, chewable tablet; EfT, effervescent tablet; G, granules for oral suspension; IV, intravenous; L, liquid; ODT, orally disintegrating tablet; P, powder for oral suspension; ST, SoluTab; T, tablet.
Boldface indicates one of top 100 drugs for 2012 by units sold at retail outlets, www.drugs.com/stats/top100/2012/units.

Tetracycline is best taken on an empty stomach. Antacids, dairy products, or iron-containing products should be taken 2 hours before or after tetracycline.

Sucralfate should be taken 1 hour before meals and at bedtime.

Misoprostol should be taken with or after meals and at bedtime.

Adverse drug effects

- Side effects occur in 15–20% of patients, but they are usually minor.
- PPIs and H2RAs are generally well tolerated, but headache, diarrhea, and nausea have been reported.
- PPIs may increase the risk of *Clostridium difficile*-associated diarrhea. Use the lowest effective dose for the shortest treatment duration possible.
- PPIs may increase incidences of osteoporosis-related fractures of the hip in patients who have at least one additional risk factor for hip fractures. The American College of Gastroenterology Guidelines for the management of gastroesophageal reflux disease (GERD) state that patients with known osteoporosis and no other risk factors for hip fracture may remain on PPI therapy.
- PPIs may also lower magnesium levels when used chronically. Consider monitoring magnesium levels and using magnesium supplements in patients using PPIs > 3 months.
- Short-term use of PPIs may increase the risk of community-acquired pneumonia.
- Antibiotics may cause diarrhea, nausea, dysgeusia, rash, and monilial vaginitis.
- Bismuth subsalicylate may cause black, tarry stools.
- Constipation is the most common side effect of sucralfate.
- Diarrhea occurs in 10–30% of patients taking misoprostol. Abdominal cramping, nausea, flatulence, and headache may also occur.

Drug interactions

- Omeprazole inhibits the cytochrome P450 (CYP450) 2C19 enzyme, which decreases the elimination of warfarin, phenytoin, and diazepam. Some pharmacokinetic and pharmacodynamic studies show that concomitant use of omeprazole significantly reduces the ability of clopidogrel to inhibit platelet activity. This could be because clopidogrel is a pro-drug that requires the CYP450 2C19 enzyme to be converted into its active form. Since the Food and Drug Administration (FDA) issued a warning in 2009 regarding this interaction, subsequent prospective studies have shown that concomitant PPI and clopidogrel therapy does not increase the incidence of cardiovascular events. The 2013 American College of Gastroenterology Guidelines for the Management of GERD state that "PPI therapy does not need to be altered in concomitant clopidogrel users."
- Lansoprazole has been reported to increase theophylline clearance by approximately 10%.
- PPIs and H2RAs may alter the bioavailability of drugs that require an acidic environment for absorption (e.g., ketoconazole, digoxin, iron).
- Cimetidine is a potent inhibitor of the CYP450 enzyme system, which decreases the elimination of numerous drugs (e.g., warfarin, theophylline, phenytoin).
- Amoxicillin may decrease the effectiveness of oral contraceptives.
- Clarithromycin is a potent inhibitor of the CYP450 enzyme system, which decreases the elimination of warfarin, digoxin, cyclosporine, carbamazepine, theophylline, and cisapride (no longer on the market; available for restricted special use only).
- Tetracycline may decrease the effectiveness of oral contraceptives. Antacids, iron products, and dairy products bind to tetracycline, decreasing its effectiveness. Tetracycline can also increase the therapeutic effect of warfarin. Tetracycline can increase or decrease lithium serum concentrations.
- Metronidazole produces a disulfiram-like reaction when ingested with alcohol and increases the therapeutic effect of warfarin and lithium.
- Sucralfate leads to the absorption of small amounts of aluminum, which may accumulate if given to patients with renal insufficiency (especially when combined with aluminum-containing antacids).
- Sucralfate alters the absorption of numerous drugs, including warfarin, digoxin, phenytoin, ketoconazole, quinidine, and quinolones.
- Magnesium-containing antacids may increase the GI side effects of misoprostol.
- Disulfiram-like reactions have been reported with the concurrent ingestion of alcohol and furazolidone.

Monitoring parameters

Patients should monitor for the return of PUD symptoms and for the side effects of medications, as discussed in the earlier sections.

Pharmacokinetics

Several medications are substrates for or have effects on the CYP450 enzyme system in the liver, as discussed in the drug interactions section above.

Nondrug Therapy and Complications

Patients should be counseled to decrease psychological stress and to discontinue drinking alcohol and smoking, taking NSAIDs, and ingesting food or beverages that may exacerbate PUD symptoms.

Major complications (hemorrhage, perforation, penetration, obstruction) occur in approximately 25% of patients with PUD:

- Patients with active bleeding who are hemodynamically stable should receive intravenous (IV) PPI therapy and undergo endoscopy to evaluate the risk of bleeding recurrence.
- Patients with active bleeding who are hemodynamically unstable should receive IV fluids and blood transfusions. They should undergo emergency endoscopy for coagulation of bleeding sites. Various modalities may be used to achieve bleeding-site coagulation.
- As soon as patients tolerate oral intake, IV PPI therapy should be changed to oral therapy.
- Surgery is reserved for those patients who have refractory ulcers, recurrent bleeding, or a perforated ulcer.

25-5. Definition, Incidence, and Recognition of GERD

The American College of Gastroenterology guidelines state that "GERD should be defined as symptoms or complications resulting from the reflux of gastric contents into the esophagus or beyond, into the oral cavity (including larynx) or lung." It may be further classified as "the presence of symptoms without erosions on endoscopic examination (non-erosive disease/NERD) or symptoms with erosions (ERD)."

The prevalence of GERD is highest in Western countries, with 10–20% of adults experiencing symptoms weekly. It occurs equally in men and women, except that its incidence is higher in pregnant women. The incidence of GERD is higher and more frequently severe in Caucasians than in African Americans. Obesity has been strongly correlated to the incidence of GERD. GERD may also occur in children. The risk of experiencing complications from GERD increases with age.

Classification

The manifestations of GERD are divided into esophageal and extraesophageal syndromes.

Esophageal syndromes

Esophageal syndromes comprise those that are only symptomatic in nature and those that are symptomatic with esophageal injury on endoscopy. Symptomatic syndromes include the typical reflux syndrome and the reflux chest pain syndrome:

- The *typical reflux syndrome* is defined by the presence of troublesome heartburn, regurgitation, or both. Patients may have other symptoms, such as epigastric pain or sleep disturbance.
- The *reflux chest pain syndrome* occurs when GERD causes chest pain that is similar to ischemic cardiac pain. This pain can occur without concurrent heartburn or regurgitation.

Symptomatic syndromes with esophageal injury include GERD complications such as reflux esophagitis, reflux stricture, Barrett's esophagus, and esophageal adenocarcinoma.

- *Reflux esophagitis* is characterized by visible breaks in the distal esophageal mucosa.
- A *reflux stricture* is defined as a persistent luminal narrowing of the esophagus caused by GERD.
- *Barrett's esophagus* occurs when esophageal squamous epithelium from the gastroesophageal junction is replaced with metaplastic columnar epithelium. It is a risk factor for the development of *esophageal adenocarcinoma*.

Extraesophageal syndromes

Extraesophageal syndromes include those syndromes that have established associations with GERD and those with proposed associations with GERD.

Esophageal syndromes that have established associations with GERD include reflux cough syndrome, reflux laryngitis syndrome, reflux asthma syndrome, and reflux dental erosion syndrome.

Esophageal syndromes that have proposed associations with GERD include pharyngitis, sinusitis, idiopathic pulmonary fibrosis, and recurrent otitis media.

Clinical Presentation

Heartburn and regurgitation are the common characteristic symptoms of the typical reflux syndrome. *Heartburn* is defined as a burning sensation in the retrosternal area. *Regurgitation* is defined as the perception of flow of refluxed gastric content into the mouth or hypopharynx.

Symptoms usually occur shortly after having a meal, when reclining after a meal, or on lying down at bedtime. Symptoms often awaken patients from sleep.

Symptoms are exacerbated by eating a large meal (especially a high-fat meal), by bending over, and occasionally by exercising.

Symptoms suggestive of complications from GERD (i.e., alarm symptoms) include continuous pain, dysphagia, odynophagia, bleeding, unexplained weight loss, and choking.

Symptom severity does not correlate with the degree of esophagitis present on endoscopy, but severity usually does correlate with the duration of reflux.

Pathophysiology

The effortless movement of gastric contents into the esophagus is a physiologic process that occurs numerous times daily throughout life and does not produce symptoms. It occurs more frequently in patients with GERD.

The pathophysiology of GERD involves the prolonged contact of esophageal epithelium with refluxed gastric contents containing acid and pepsin. Prolonged contact between esophageal epithelium and gastric contents can overwhelm esophageal defense mechanisms and produce symptoms.

Higher-potency gastric refluxate may produce symptoms during times of esophageal contact of normal duration. The presence of refluxate in an esophagus with impaired defense mechanisms may also produce symptoms.

Esophageal defenses consist of the antireflux barrier, luminal clearance mechanisms, and tissue resistance.

- Components of the antireflux barrier are the lower esophageal sphincter (LES) and the diaphragm. The LES is a thickened ring of circular smooth muscle localized to the distal 2–3 cm of the esophagus. It is contracted at rest, thereby serving as a barrier to refluxate. The diaphragm encircles the LES and acts as a mechanical support, especially during physical exertion.
- Luminal clearance factors include gravity, esophageal peristalsis, and salivary and esophageal gland secretions (which contain acid-neutralizing bicarbonate).
- The three areas of tissue resistance are preepithelial, epithelial, and postepithelial defense. Preepithelial and epithelial tissues limit the rate of diffusion of H^+ between cell membranes. Postepithelial defense is provided by the blood supply, which removes HCl and supplies oxygen, nutrients, and bicarbonate.

Diagnostic Criteria

For patients who present with typical troublesome symptoms of GERD (e.g., heartburn, regurgitation), a trial of empiric therapy with a PPI is appropriate. A diagnosis of GERD may be assumed for patients who respond to empiric treatment. Nonresponders to PPI therapy should be referred for evaluation.

Diagnostic testing with endoscopy should be performed in patients who present with alarm symptoms and for screening patients at high risk of complications.

- Endoscopy is the preferred method for evaluating the esophageal mucosa for esophagitis and for evaluating for the presence of complications.
- Esophageal manometry is not recommended in the initial diagnosis of GERD. It should be used only to assist in the placement of transnasal pH impedance probes or before consideration of antireflux surgery to rule out conditions that would be contraindications to surgery.
- Ambulatory esophageal reflux monitoring is indicated in patients with nonerosive disease before consideration of surgery or endoscopic therapy, in patients who do not respond to PPI therapy, and in patients in whom the diagnosis of GERD is questionable.

25-6. Treatment Principles and Goals of GERD

Goals of therapy are to alleviate or eliminate symptoms, decrease frequency and duration of reflux, promote healing of the injured mucosa, and prevent the development of complications.

Therapy is aimed at increasing lower esophageal pressure, improving esophageal acid clearance and gastric emptying, protecting esophageal mucosa, decreasing the acidity of refluxate, and decreasing the amount of gastric contents being refluxed.

An 8-week course of once-daily PPI therapy is the treatment of choice for symptom relief and healing of erosive esophagitis in patients with typical symptoms. PPI therapy is associated with increased healing rates and decreased relapse rates of erosive esophagitis compared to H2RAs.

For patients who partially respond to PPI therapy, increasing the dose to twice daily or switching to a different PPI may provide additional symptom relief.

Maintenance PPI therapy should be given to patients who have symptoms when PPIs are discontinued and in patients with complications (e.g., erosive esophagitis, Barrett's esophagus) at the lowest effective dose. On-demand or intermittent therapy may also be used for maintenance.

H2RA therapy may be used as maintenance therapy in patients without erosive esophagitis if they experience symptom relief.

Bedtime therapy with H2RAs may be added to daytime PPI therapy in patients with objectively confirmed nighttime reflux, but tachyphylaxis may develop after several weeks of use.

Prokinetic therapy with metoclopramide, baclofen, or both should not be used in GERD patients without diagnostic evaluation.

Drug Therapy

Mechanism of action

For information on H2RAs and PPIs, see Section 25-3 on PUD.

Antacids neutralize gastric acid (which increases LES tone) and inhibit the conversion of pepsinogen to pepsin, thus raising the pH of gastric contents. Antacids may be useful for the self-treatment of mild, infrequent heartburn.

Alginic acid reacts with sodium bicarbonate in saliva to form sodium alginate viscous solution, which floats on the surface of gastric contents. The solution acts as a barrier to protect the esophagus from the corrosive effects of gastric reflux.

See Table 25-2 for selected medications.

Patient counseling

For information on H2RAs and PPIs, see Section 25-1 on PUD.

Antacids and alginic acid are appropriate for the initial management of symptoms of GERD that are not troublesome to the patient (e.g., mild, infrequent heartburn). Symptoms persisting longer than 2 weeks require further evaluation and treatment with prescription medications.

Refrigeration of liquid antacids may aid in palatability. Chewable tablets may be more effective than liquids because of increased adherence of antacid and saliva to the distal esophagus. Antacids must be taken at least 2 hours apart from tetracyclines, iron, and digoxin. Antacids and quinolones should be taken 4–6 hours apart.

Alginic acid is effective for the relief of GERD symptoms, but no data indicate esophageal healing on endoscopy. Alginic acid is ineffective if the patient is in the supine position and must not be taken at bedtime.

Table 25-2. Selected Antacids and Absorbents

Generic name	Trade name	Classification	Dosage range and frequency	Dosage forms
Magnesium hydroxide	Milk of magnesia	Antacid	15–30 mL prn	T, L
Aluminum hydroxide	Amphojel, ALternaGEL	Antacid	15–30 mL prn	T, L
Aluminum carbonate	Basaljel	Antacid	15–30 mL prn	T, L
Magnesium hydroxide + aluminum hydroxide	Maalox	Antacid	15–30 mL prn	T, L
Magaldrate	Riopan	Antacid	15–30 mL prn	T, L
Calcium carbonate	Tums, Titralac	Antacid	15–30 mL prn	T, L
Sodium bicarbonate	Various trade names	Antacid	15–30 mL prn	T, L
Alginic acid + aluminum hydroxide + magnesium hydroxide	Gaviscon	Absorbent + antacid	15–30 mL prn; 2 after meals	T, L

L, liquid; T, tablet.

Adverse drug effects

For information on H2RAs and PPIs, see Section 25-3 on PUD.

Magnesium-containing antacids frequently cause diarrhea. Aluminum-containing antacids frequently cause constipation and bind to phosphate in the gut, which can lead to bone demineralization. Antacids may also cause acid–base disturbances.

Magnesium and aluminum toxicity may occur when used chronically in patients with renal insufficiency. Sodium bicarbonate may cause sodium overload, particularly in patients with hypertension, congestive heart failure, and chronic renal failure. It may also lead to systemic alkalosis. It should be used on a short-term basis, if at all.

Drug interactions

For information on H2RAs and PPIs, see Section 25-3 on PUD.

When taken with antacids, the absorption and effectiveness of tetracycline, ferrous sulfate, and quinolones are reduced because the antacids form chelates with them. Antacids decrease the absorption of azoles and sucralfate by increasing gastric pH. Antacids increase urine pH, which decreases the renal clearance of quinidine. Antacids decrease the systemic absorption of digoxin and H2RAs when taken concomitantly with them. Large doses of antacid may decrease the absorption of phenytoin.

Digoxin and phenytoin serum concentrations should be monitored frequently when antacids are used concomitantly. Suspected adverse effects of antacids should be reported to a health care provider.

Monitoring parameters

Patients should monitor for the return of GERD symptoms and for the side effects of medications as discussed in the previous section.

Pharmacokinetics

Several medications are substrates for or have effects on the CYP450 enzyme system in the liver. See the discussion under drug interactions in Section 25-3.

Nondrug Therapy

- Weight loss should be recommended for GERD patients who are overweight or have had recent weight gain.

- Head-of-bed elevation and avoidance of meals 2 to 3 hours before bedtime should be recommended for patients with nocturnal GERD.
- The routine global elimination of food that may trigger GERD symptoms is not recommended; however, patients should avoid any food or beverage that triggers their own GERD symptoms (e.g., chocolate, caffeine, alcohol, acidic or spicy foods).
- Calcium channel blockers, β-blockers, nitrates, barbiturates, anticholinergics, and theophylline decrease LES pressure. Tetracyclines, NSAIDs, aspirin, bisphosphonates, iron, quinidine, and potassium chloride have direct irritant effects on the esophageal mucosa. The appropriateness of these drugs in patients with GERD should be evaluated on an individual patient basis.

Surgery is a treatment option for long-term therapy in GERD patients who desire to stop medical therapy, are noncompliant with medical therapy, have adverse effects from medical therapy, or have persistent symptoms caused by refractory GERD.

25-7. Definition, Incidence, and Recognition of Inflammatory Bowel Disease

Idiopathic inflammatory bowel disease (IBD) is divided into two major types:

- *Ulcerative colitis* is defined as a chronic mucosal inflammatory condition confined to the rectum and colon.
- *Crohn's disease* is defined as a transmural inflammation of the GI tract that can affect any part of the GI tract from mouth to anus.

The incidence of ulcerative colitis is approximately 8–12 per 100,000 persons. The prevalence of Crohn's disease is approximately 50 cases per 100,000 persons.

In the United States, approximately 500,000 persons have Crohn's disease and 500,000 persons have ulcerative colitis. Ulcerative colitis is slightly predominant in men; Crohn's disease is predominant in women. The overall incidence of IBD is similar between men and women.

North America, Northern Europe, and Great Britain have the highest incidence rates for IBD.

Ulcerative colitis typically occurs in persons between 30 and 40 years of age. Crohn's disease typically occurs between ages 20 and 30. Both may be diagnosed at any stage in life, but of all cases of IBD, 10–15% are diagnosed before adulthood.

The incidence of IBD is low for Hispanics and Asian Americans. Its incidence in African Americans has increased and is equal to that of Caucasians. In addition, its incidence rate is high among the Jewish population in North America, Europe, and Israel.

Classification

The two major types of IBD are ulcerative colitis and Crohn's disease. Clinical presentation and diagnostic tests help distinguish one form from the other.

Clinical Presentation

IBD is characterized by acute exacerbations of symptoms followed by periods of remission that are spontaneous or secondary to changes in medical therapy or concurrent illnesses.

Ulcerative colitis

The hallmark clinical symptom of ulcerative colitis is bloody diarrhea, which is often accompanied by rectal urgency and tenesmus (straining to empty an already empty bowel associated with pain and cramping).

The extent and severity of ulcerative colitis are determined by clinical and endoscopic findings. Clinical symptoms are categorized as mild, moderate, severe, and fulminant. Endoscopic findings are categorized as distal (limited to below the splenic flexure) or extensive (extending proximal to the splenic flexure).

- *Mild ulcerative colitis* is characterized by fewer than four stools per day with or without blood, without systemic disturbance, and with a normal erythrocyte sedimentation rate (ESR).
- *Moderate ulcerative colitis* is characterized by more than four stools per day with minimal signs of toxicity.
- *Severe ulcerative colitis* is characterized by more than six stools per day with blood; systemic disturbance (e.g., fever, tachycardia, anemia); and ESR greater than 30.
- *Fulminant ulcerative colitis* is characterized by more than 10 bowel movements per day, continuous bleeding, toxicity, abdominal tenderness and distension, blood transfusion requirement, and colonic dilation on abdominal plain films.

Crohn's disease

The presentation of Crohn's disease is variable, and its onset is often insidious. Typical symptoms include chronic or nocturnal diarrhea and abdominal pain. Additional typical symptoms include weight loss, fever, and rectal bleeding.

Clinical signs may include pallor, abdominal mass or tenderness, cachexia, perianal fissure, fistula, or abscess.

Extraintestinal symptoms include inflammation of the skin, joints, and eyes.

Symptoms differ depending on the site and severity of inflammation:

- *Mild to moderate Crohn's disease:* Patients are ambulatory and tolerate oral alimentation without dehydration; toxicity (fever, rigors, or prostration); abdominal tenderness; painful mass or obstruction; or weight loss > 10%.
- *Moderate to severe Crohn's disease:* Patients fail to respond to treatment for mild to moderate disease or have fever, weight loss, abdominal pain, nausea, vomiting (without obstruction), or anemia.
- *Severe to fulminant Crohn's disease:* Patients have persistent symptoms despite the use of steroids or biologic agents as outpatients, or individuals present with high fever, persistent vomiting, evidence of obstruction, rebound tenderness, cachexia, or abscess.

Symptomatic remission occurs when a patient is asymptomatic or without any symptomatic inflammatory sequelae.

The ileum and colon are the most commonly affected sites. Ileitis may mimic appendicitis. Intestinal obstruction and inflammatory masses or abscesses may also develop. Patients with colonic Crohn's disease commonly have rectal bleeding, perianal lesions, and extraintestinal manifestations (e.g., spondylarthritis, peripheral arthritis, erythema nodosum, pyoderma gangrenosum, uveitis, fatty liver, chronic active hepatitis, cirrhosis, primary sclerosing cholangitis, gallstones, cholangiocarcinoma, hypercoagulability).

Oral Crohn's disease is characterized by lesions ranging from a few aphthous ulcers to deep linear ulcers with edema and induration. Gastroduodenal involvement may mimic PUD.

Pathophysiology

The etiology of ulcerative colitis and Crohn's disease is unclear, but similar factors may contribute to both diseases. These factors include infectious agents, genetics, environmental factors, psychological factors, and immune factors. Major etiologic theories involve a combination of infectious and immunologic factors.

Ulcerative colitis is confined to the rectum and colon and affects only the mucosa and submucosa. The primary lesion of ulcerative colitis is a crypt abscess, which forms in the crypts of the mucosa. Crohn's disease most commonly affects the terminal ileum and involves extensive damage to the bowel wall.

Ulcerative colitis and Crohn's disease complications can be local or systemic. Local complications of ulcerative colitis include hemorrhoids, anal fissures, and perirectal abscesses. Toxic megacolon can lead to perforation and is a major complication that affects 1–3% of patients with ulcerative colitis or Crohn's disease. Colonic strictures and hemorrhage may also occur. Small bowel strictures, obstruction, and fistulae are common in Crohn's disease. Systemic complications (extraintestinal) can occur with ulcerative colitis and Crohn's disease.

Diagnostic Criteria

Ulcerative colitis is diagnosed on the basis of clinical symptoms, proctosigmoidoscopy or colonoscopy, tissue biopsy, and bacteria-negative stool studies. Crohn's disease is diagnosed on the basis of clinical symptoms, contrast radiography or endoscopy, tissue biopsy, and bacteria-negative stool studies. Abdominal ultrasonography, computed tomography, and magnetic resonance imaging aid in the identification of masses, abscesses, and perianal complications in ulcerative colitis and Crohn's disease.

25-8. Treatment Principles and Goals of IBD

Treatment of IBD involves medications that target inflammatory mediators and alter immuno-inflammatory processes. These medications include anti-inflammatory, antimicrobial, immunosuppressive, and biologic agents.

Nutritional considerations are also important because many patients with IBD may be malnourished.

Goals of therapy for ulcerative colitis and Crohn's disease include induction and maintenance of remission of symptoms, induction and maintenance of mucosal healing, improved quality of life, resolution of complications and systemic symptoms, and pre-

vention of future complications. For patients with Crohn's disease, remission means that patients are asymptomatic or without inflammatory sequelae, including patients who have responded to medical intervention. Patients who require steroids to maintain their condition are considered steroid dependent, not in remission.

In ulcerative colitis patients, remission is likely to last at least 1 year with medical therapy. Without medical therapy, up to two-thirds of patients will relapse within 9 months. For mild Crohn's disease, up to 40% of patients improve in 3–4 months with observation alone. Most will remain in remission for prolonged periods without medical therapy.

Mild to moderate distal colitis may be treated with oral aminosalicylates, topical mesalamine, or topical steroids; however, topical mesalamine is superior to topical steroids or oral aminosalicylates.

- Combining oral and topical aminosalicylates is more effective than using them individually.
- Patients who do not respond to oral aminosalicylates or topical corticosteroids may respond to mesalamine enemas or suppositories.
- Patients who are refractory to maximum doses of these agents or have systemic symptoms may require oral prednisone at doses up to 40–60 mg/day or infliximab with an induction regimen of 5 mg/kg at weeks 0, 2, and 6.
- For the maintenance of remission in patients with proctitis, mesalamine suppositories are effective.

For the maintenance of remission in patients with distal colitis:

- Mesalamine enemas are effective even if used only every third night. Sulfasalazine, mesalamine compounds, and balsalazide may also be used.
- The combination of oral and topical mesalamine is more effective than either one used alone.
- Topical corticosteroids are not effective for maintaining remission in distal colitis.
- In patients who do not achieve remission using the above therapies, thiopurines and infliximab may be used.

For mild to moderate extensive ulcerative colitis (acute):

- Initiate therapy with oral sulfasalazine in doses titrated up to 4–6 g/day. Alternatively, a different aminosalicylate in doses up to 4.8 g/day of the active 5–aminosalicylate moiety may be used. Combining oral and topical aminosalicylates may be of additional benefit.

- Oral steroids should be reserved for patients refractory to oral aminosalicylates in combination with topical therapy or for patients with symptoms severe enough to warrant rapid improvement.
- Thiopurines are effective for patients refractory to oral steroids with continued moderate disease who do not require acute IV therapy.
- Infliximab is effective for patients refractory to steroids, patients who are dependent on steroids despite appropriate doses of thiopurines, or patients intolerant to those medications.

For maintenance of remission in mild to moderate extensive ulcerative colitis:

- Sulfasalazine, olsalazine, mesalamine, and balsalazide are all effective.
- Chronic steroid therapy should be avoided as much as possible.
- Thiopurines may be used as steroid-sparing agents for remission not completely sustained by aminosalicylates and sometimes for patients who are steroid-dependent but not acutely ill.
- Infliximab is effective in maintaining remission in patients who respond to the infliximab induction regimen.

For severe colitis:

- If urgent hospitalization is not necessary, infliximab 5 mg/kg may be used in patients refractory to maximal oral prednisone, oral aminosalicylates, and topical medications.
- Patients with incapacitating symptoms require hospitalization and IV steroids. Patients who do not respond to IV steroids within 3 to 5 days should be treated with either IV cyclosporine or infliximab. Patients with fulminant colitis are treated similarly, except that the decision to treat with IV cyclosporine, infliximab, or surgery is made sooner.
- Adding thiopurines to maintenance therapy significantly enhances long-term remission in severe colitis.

For Crohn's disease, clinical improvement should be evident within 2–4 weeks. Maximal clinical improvement should occur within 12–16 weeks. Treatment for acute disease should be continued until remission is achieved or the patient's symptoms fail to improve.

For mild to moderate Crohn's disease localized to the ileum or right colon, controlled-release oral budesonide is appropriate initial therapy.

- Controlled-release oral budesonide is more effective than oral mesalamine and placebo. It has similar efficacy to conventional oral corticosteroids.
- Oral mesalamine has been used as first-line therapy; however, new evidence indicates that it is only minimally more effective than placebo and less effective than corticosteroids.
- Oral sulfasalazine is more effective than placebo but less effective than corticosteroids for ileocolonic and colonic Crohn's disease.
- Rectal aminosalicylates are often used to treat distal colonic Crohn's disease; however, controlled studies showing efficacy are lacking.
- Although metronidazole and ciprofloxacin are widely used in the treatment of Crohn's disease, clinical trials have not consistently demonstrated efficacy.
- No controlled data exist regarding the treatment of mild to moderate oral Crohn's disease. Lidocaine lozenges may provide symptomatic relief. Lesions will respond to systemic steroids or azathioprine in 50% of patients.
- For Crohn's disease of the stomach, esophagus, duodenum, and jejunum, PPIs, oral corticosteroids, mercaptopurine, azathioprine, methotrexate, infliximab, adalimumab, and certolizumab pegol have improved symptoms in uncontrolled trials.
- When remission is achieved, maintenance therapy should be initiated. For patients who do not respond, treatment with alternative agents for mild to moderate disease may be initiated or the treatment may be advanced to agents used for moderate to severe disease.

For patients with moderate to severe disease, oral corticosteroids are the mainstay of therapy.

- Prednisone 40–60 mg daily should be given until symptoms resolve and weight gain resumes. Steroids are not appropriate maintenance therapy.
- Infections or abscesses should be treated with appropriate antibiotics or surgical drainage.
- Azathioprine and 6-mercaptopurine may be added to oral corticosteroids to maintain a steroid-induced remission. They are also effective for steroid-dependent or steroid-refractory patients.
- Parenteral methotrexate is effective for inducing remission and allowing steroid dose reduction in patients with steroid-dependent and steroid-refractory Crohn's disease.

- Infliximab, adalimumab, and certolizumab pegol may be used in patients who do not respond to oral corticosteroids or immunosuppressive agents. They may also be used as an alternative to oral corticosteroids when the side effects of oral corticosteroids need to be avoided.
- Natalizumab may be used when patients are intolerant or unresponsive to oral corticosteroids, immunosuppressants, and biologic therapies.
- Enteral nutrition should be used to support the patient's overall nutrition status, not to induce remission of Crohn's disease.
- When remission is achieved, maintenance therapy should be initiated.

For severe to fulminant Crohn's disease, hospitalization for IV steroids and hydration is required.

- IV steroids equivalent to 40–60 mg/day of prednisone should be administered.
- Parenteral fluid and electrolyte therapy should be administered to restore hydration.
- Parenteral or enteral nutrition support should be administered after 5–7 days if the patient cannot meet adequate nutritional requirements.
- Anemic patients may require blood transfusions.
- Intestinal obstructions related to adhesions should be managed with bowel rest and nasogastric tube suctioning. Obstructions related to inflammatory strictures require antibiotic therapy and IV steroids. Surgery should be considered if obstructive symptoms do not respond to therapy.
- Abscesses should be drained and appropriate antibiotic therapy instituted.
- High-dose metronidazole or ciprofloxacin may be used in the management of fistulas. Chronic therapy may be required to prevent recurrent drainage.
- Azathioprine, 6-mercaptopurine, and infliximab may also be used in the management of fistulas.
- If patients do not respond to IV steroids after 5–7 days of therapy, cyclosporine or tacrolimus therapy may be instituted.
- When symptoms respond to initial treatment, the patient should be converted to an equivalent oral corticosteroid regimen.
- Patients who do not respond to therapy require surgical intervention.

Maintenance therapy should be initiated when remission is achieved.

- Corticosteroids should not be used as long-term maintenance therapy.
- Sulfasalazine and mesalamine have not shown consistent benefit as maintenance therapy.
- Azathioprine, 6-mercaptopurine, and methotrexate have shown benefit as maintenance therapy.
- Azathioprine may be used as maintenance therapy in steroid-naive patients who achieved remission with infliximab.
- Infliximab, adalimumab, and certolizumab pegol are effective maintenance therapies.
- Natalizumab may be used for maintenance therapy after it has been successfully used to induce remission.

Drug Therapy

See Table 25-3 for selected medications used in IBD.

Mechanism of action

Sulfasalazine is cleaved by bacteria in the gut to form sulfapyridine (excreted in the urine) and mesalamine (the active component). The sulfapyridine molecule is responsible for the many side effects associated with sulfasalazine.

Mesalamine's mechanism of action is poorly understood. Mesalamine inhibits cyclooxygenase and may also inhibit production of cyclooxygenase, thromboxane synthetase, platelet-activating factor synthetase, and interleukin-1 in macrophages. It may also act as a superoxide free-radical scavenger.

Corticosteroids have immunomodulatory effects and inhibit the production of cytokines and other inflammatory mediators.

Corticosteroids, azathioprine, 6-mercaptopurine, cyclosporine, and tacrolimus are immunosuppressive agents. For full discussion of their mechanism of action, patient counseling, side effects, drug interactions, and pharmacokinetics, see Chapter 24 on solid organ transplantation.

The exact mechanism of action of metronidazole and ciprofloxacin in IBD is not known. One theory suggests that antibacterials interrupt the role of bacteria in the inflammatory process.

Methotrexate inhibits dihydrofolate reductase and purine synthesis, reduces the production of leukotriene-B_4 and interleukin-1 and -2, and may induce T-cell apoptosis.

Infliximab is a chimeric monoclonal antibody that inhibits human tumor necrosis factor, which inhibits subsequent cytokine-triggered inflammatory processes.

Table 25-3. Selected Medications Used in Treatment of Inflammatory Bowel Disease

Generic name	Trade name	Classification	Dosage range and frequency	Dosage forms
Sulfasalazine	Azulfidine	Aminosalicylate	4–6 g/day	T
Mesalamine	Asacol	Aminosalicylate	2.4–4.8 g/day	DT
Mesalamine	Pentasa	Aminosalicylate	2–4 g/day	DC
Mesalamine	Rowasa, Salofalk, Claversal	Aminosalicylate	1–4 g/day	EN, SU
Mesalamine	Lialda	Aminosalicylate	2.4–4.8 g/day	DT
Mesalamine	Canasa	Aminosalicylate	500–1,000 mg	SU
Balsalazide	Colazal	Aminosalicylate	6.75 g/day	DC
Metronidazole	Flagyl	Antibacterial	10–20 g/day (Crohn's disease)	T, IV
Ciprofloxacin	Cipro	Antibacterial	500 mg bid (Crohn's disease)	T, IV
Prednisone	Various trade names	Corticosteroid	40–60 mg/day	T
Methylprednisolone	Solu-Medrol	Corticosteroid	60 mg/day	IV
Budesonide	Entocort EC	Corticosteroid	9 mg/day	C
Azathioprine	Imuran	Immunosuppressive	1–2.5 mg/kg/day	T, IV
6-mercaptopurine	Purinethol	Immunosuppressive	1.5 mg/kg/day	T
Methotrexate	Abitrexate	Antimetabolite	25 mg/wk	IM, subcutaneous
Infliximab	**Remicade**	Immunomodulator	Induction: 5 mg/kg at 0, 2, and 6 wks; maintenance: 5 mg/kg q 8 wks	IV
Adalimumab	**Humira**	Immunomodulator	Induction: 160 mg as 4 injections over 1–2 days, then 80 mg 2 wks later; maintenance: 40 mg q other wk starting on day 29	Subcutaneous
Certolizumab pegol	Cimzia	Immunomodulator	Induction: 400 mg (given as 2 separate doses of 200 mg each) at 0, 2, and 4 wks; maintenance: 400 mg q 4 wks	Subcutaneous
Natalizumab	Tysabri	Immunomodulator	300 mg over 1 h every 4 wks	IV
Cyclosporine	Neoral, Sandimmune	Immunosuppressive	4 mg/kg/day	IV, C, L

C, capsule; DC, delayed-release capsule; DT, delayed-release tablet; EN, enema; IM, intramuscular; IV, intravenous; L, liquid; SU, suppository; T, tablet.

Adalimumab is a recombinant monoclonal antibody that inhibits human tumor necrosis factor, which inhibits subsequent cytokine-triggered inflammatory processes.

Certolizumab pegol is a pegylated humanized antibody Fab fragment of tumor necrosis factor monoclonal antibody. It inhibits human tumor necrosis factor activity, which inhibits subsequent cytokine-triggered inflammatory processes. PEGylation delays elimination and prolongs the half-life of the drug.

Natalizumab is a monoclonal antibody against the alpha-4 subunit of integrin molecules. It blocks the association of integrin with vascular receptors, which limits adhesion and transmigration of leukocytes.

Patient counseling

Sulfasalazine should be taken after meals. Patients should avoid sun exposure while taking it. Folic acid supplementation should be given during sulfasalazine treatment to avoid anemia. Sulfasalazine may cause orange discoloration of urine and skin.

Mesalamine tablets should be swallowed whole. Suppositories should not be handled excessively, and foil wrappers should be removed before insertion. Suspension enemas should be shaken well before use.

Antacids and ciprofloxacin should be taken 4–6 hours apart. Iron- or zinc-containing products should be taken 4 hours before or 2 hours after taking ciprofloxacin. Patients should avoid excessive exposure to sunlight.

Patients taking methotrexate should avoid alcohol, salicylates, and prolonged exposure to sunlight. Female patients of childbearing age should be counseled on appropriate contraceptive measures during methotrexate therapy.

Patients receiving therapy with infliximab should be counseled on the possibility of infusion reactions, delayed hypersensitivity reactions, and increased risk of infections. Live vaccines should not be administered to patients taking infliximab.

Patients taking adalimumab should be counseled on the increased risk of infections and be instructed to report any symptoms of infection to their physician immediately. They should also be counseled on the potential for injection site reactions and be taught proper injection technique and proper sharps disposal. Live vaccines should not be administered to patients taking adalimumab.

Patients taking certolizumab pegol should be counseled on the increased risk of infections and be instructed to report any symptoms of infection to their physician immediately. They should also be counseled on the potential for injection-site reactions and be taught proper injection technique and sharps disposal. Live vaccines should not be administered to patients taking certolizumab pegol.

Patients taking natalizumab should be counseled on the risk of acute hypersensitivity infusion reactions. They should also be counseled on the increased risk of infections, particularly progressive multifocal leukoencephalopathy. Patients should report symptoms of infection to their physician immediately.

Adverse drug effects

Sulfasalazine may cause nausea, vomiting, anorexia, and headaches. The sulfapyridine moiety leads to hypersensitivity reactions (e.g., rash, fever, agranulocytosis, pancreatitis, nephritis, hepatitis) and altered spermatogenesis in males.

Mesalamine is better tolerated than sulfasalazine. Olsalazine may cause self-limited watery diarrhea. Balsalazide causes abdominal pain in 10% of patients.

Ciprofloxacin may cause nausea, diarrhea, headache, and vaginal candidiasis.

Methotrexate frequently causes nausea and leukopenia. Asymptomatic elevations in liver function tests may occur.

Infliximab may cause infusion-related reactions, upper respiratory infections, headache, rash, cough, and stomach pain. Allergic reactions have been reported. Infliximab increases the risk of serious infections (bacterial [including those caused by *Legionella* and *Listeria*], viral, and fungal infections; tuberculosis) and certain types of cancer. New onset or exacerbation of preexisting heart failure, hepatotoxicity, neuropathy, anemia, and lupus-like syndrome have also been reported.

Adalimumab may cause injection-site reactions, upper respiratory infections, headaches, rash, and nausea. Allergic reactions have been reported. Adalimumab increases the risk of serious infections (bacterial [including those caused by *Legionella* and *Listeria*], viral, and fungal infections; tuberculosis) and certain types of cancer. New onset or exacerbation of preexisting heart failure, neuropathy, anemia, and lupus-like syndrome have also been reported.

Certolizumab pegol may cause injection-site reactions, upper respiratory tract infections, rash, and urinary tract infections. Allergic reactions have been reported. Certolizumab increases the risk of serious infections (bacterial [including those caused by *Legionella* and *Listeria*], viral, and fungal infections; tuberculosis) and certain types of cancer. New onset or exacerbation of preexisting heart failure, neuropathy, anemia, and lupus-like syndrome have also been reported.

Natalizumab increases the risk of developing progressive multifocal leukoencephalopathy. Serious allergic reactions (usually within 2 hours of infusion) and hepatotoxicity have been reported. Natalizumab increases the risk of serious infections (bacterial, viral, and fungal infections; tuberculosis).

Drug interactions

Sulfasalazine may decrease the bioavailability of digoxin by inhibiting its absorption.

Azathioprine is converted into 6-mercaptopurine in vivo; 6-mercaptopurine then undergoes hepatic first-pass metabolism, which is catalyzed by xanthene oxidase. By inhibiting xanthene oxidase, allopurinol increases the bioavailability of azathioprine. The azathioprine dose should be lowered by 25–50% when the two agents are used concurrently.

Ciprofloxacin binds with antacids, zinc, and iron products. It also increases the therapeutic effects of warfarin, cyclosporine, and theophylline.

Corticosteroids should not be administered with natalizumab because of the increased risk of serious infections.

The use of methotrexate and concurrent NSAIDs has caused fatal interactions. Methotrexate may increase levels of 6-mercaptopurine.

Infliximab should not be administered with etanercept or anakinra because of the increased risk of serious infections. Live vaccines should not be administered to patients taking infliximab.

Adalimumab should not be administered with anakinra because of the increased risk of serious infections. Live vaccines should not be administered to patients taking adalimumab. Methotrexate may decrease the clearance of adalimumab; however, this effect has not been shown to be clinically significant.

Certolizumab pegol should not be administered with anakinra, abatacept, rituximab, or natalizumab because of the increased risk of serious infections. Live vaccines should not be administered to patients taking certolizumab. Certolizumab may falsely elevate the activated partial thromboplastin time and the lupus anticoagulant assays.

Natalizumab should not be administered with other immunosuppressants, such as 6-mercaptopurine, azathioprine, cyclosporine, and methotrexate, or with tumor necrosis factor inhibitors because of the increased risk of progressive multifocal leukoencephalopathy.

The dietary supplement echinacea may decrease the effectiveness of infliximab, adalimumab, certolizumab, and natalizumab.

Monitoring parameters

Serum chemistries, complete blood counts, liver function tests, blood glucose concentrations, ESR, response to therapy, and the presence of adverse effects should be monitored. Tuberculosis skin testing should be performed before administering biologic agents.

Pharmacokinetics

- Sulfasalazine is metabolized by intestinal flora to sulfapyridine and 5-aminosalicylic acid. Unchanged drug and metabolites are excreted in the urine.
- Mesalamine is metabolized in the liver and gut to 5-aminosalicylic acid. The metabolite is eliminated via the urine and feces.
- Azathioprine is thought to be hepatically metabolized to 6-mercaptopurine by glutathione S-transferase; 6-mercaptopurine is further metabolized by hypoxanthine guanine phosphoriboxyltransferase, xanthene oxidase, and thiopurine methyltransferase. Metabolites are excreted in the urine.
- Ciprofloxacin is partially metabolized in the liver. Unchanged drug and metabolites are excreted in the urine and feces.
- Metronidazole is metabolized in the liver and excreted in the urine and feces.
- Prednisone is metabolized in the liver and excreted in the urine.
- Methotrexate is primarily eliminated by the kidneys.

Nondrug Therapy

Patients with ulcerative colitis and Crohn's disease are often malnourished because of malabsorption or maldigestion caused by chronic bowel inflammation, "short gut" syndrome from multiple bowel surgeries, or bile salt deficiency in the gut. The catabolic effects of the disease process can also lead to malnutrition.

Individuals should eliminate foods that exacerbate symptoms. Patients with lactase deficiency should avoid dairy products or take lactase supplements to avoid symptoms.

Enteral or parenteral supplementation may be used in patients with severe ulcerative colitis or Crohn's disease to maintain adequate nutritional status.

Surgery may be necessary for patients with severe ulcerative colitis or Crohn's disease. Surgery involves removing diseased segments of bowel, repairing fistulas, and draining abscesses.

- In Crohn's disease, surgery is indicated for patients with severe colitis with or without toxic megacolon refractory to maximal medical therapy, less severe but intractable symptoms or intolerable medication side effects, exsanguinating hemorrhage, perforation, and documented or strongly suspected carcinoma.
- In Crohn's disease, surgery is indicated for neoplastic or preneoplastic lesions, obstructing stenoses, suppurative complications, or Crohn's disease that does not respond to pharmacotherapy. Smoking cessation should be encouraged to reduce the risk of recurrence of Crohn's disease after surgery (as well as for overall health benefits).

25-9. Definition, Incidence, and Recognition of Irritable Bowel Syndrome

Irritable bowel syndrome (IBS) is defined as abdominal pain or discomfort that occurs in association with altered bowel habits over a period of 3 months.

IBS is a prevalent and expensive condition. It significantly impairs health-related quality of life and leads to reduced work productivity.

IBS patients visit physicians more frequently, have more diagnostic tests performed, take more medications, miss more workdays, show lower work productivity, are hospitalized more frequently, and consume more direct health care costs than patients without IBS.

The prevalence of IBS is 10–15% in North America and Europe. Most cases of IBS are diagnosed before age 50. IBS affects women two times more often than men in North America. It is also more common in patients from lower socioeconomic groups.

Classifications

No symptom-based diagnostic criteria have ideal accuracy for diagnosing IBS. For this reason, two different sets of criteria are often used in combination. Once the diagnosis is made, IBS may be classified according to its predominant symptom: diarrhea predominant, constipation predominant, or mixed (symptoms may alternate). Symptoms may also be further categorized as mild, moderate, or severe.

Clinical Presentation

IBS is a heterogeneous disorder with various clinical presentations:

- Abdominal pain is generally described as crampy or achy, and the intensity and location are highly variable. Pain may be exacerbated by meals and may last from 1 to 3 hours. Stress and emotional turmoil can also exacerbate pain.
- Patients typically present with diarrhea, constipation, or alternating periods of both.
- Upper GI symptoms (heartburn, dyspepsia, early satiety, nausea) occur more frequently in patients with constipation. Women experience abdominal distention, bloating, and nausea more often than men.

- Extraintestinal symptoms are common. They include genitourinary symptoms (e.g., pelvic pain, dysmenorrhea, dyspareunia, urinary frequency, nocturia, sensation of incomplete bladder evacuation); impaired sexual function (e.g., decreased libido); and musculoskeletal complaints (e.g., lower back pain, headaches, chronic fatigue).
- Alarm features include rectal bleeding, weight loss, iron-deficiency anemia, nocturnal symptoms, family history of colorectal cancer, IBD, or celiac sprue. These symptoms may indicate the presence of an organic disease.

Pathophysiology

The pathogenesis is multifactorial and includes abnormal gut sensorimotor activity, central nervous system (CNS) dysfunction, psychological disturbances, genetic predisposition, enteric infection, and other intestinal luminal factors:

- Colonic motor abnormalities commonly occur in IBS. Patients with IBS may exhibit an exaggerated gastrocolonic response lasting up to 3 hours.
- Small intestinal motor patterns are frequently disturbed in patients with IBS. Small intestinal transit is delayed in constipation-predominant IBS and is accelerated in diarrhea-predominant IBS.
- Bloating may be the result of abnormal retrograde reflux of intestinal gas, enhanced perception of the presence of intestinal gas, or obstructive intestinal motor patterns.
- Motor dysfunction of other smooth muscles may occur in IBS. The following abnormalities may also be found: decreased LES pressures, abnormal esophageal body peristalsis, gastric slow-wave dysrhythmias, delayed gastric and gallbladder emptying, and dysfunction of the sphincter of Oddi.
- It is theorized that IBS results from sensitization of visceral afferent fibers, which causes normal physiologic events to be perceived as painful. It is unknown if sensorineural dysfunction is generalized or localized to the gut afferent fibers.
- It is unknown whether IBS is primarily a CNS disorder with centrally directed changes in gut sensorimotor function or primarily a gut disorder with inappropriate CNS input.
- Eighty percent of patients with IBS exhibit psychiatric disturbances. The onset of psychiatric disturbances usually predates or occurs

concurrently with the onset of IBS. Psychological stress triggers symptoms in many patients. IBS is also associated with a history of sexual abuse.

■ Other factors that may contribute to IBS are alterations in gut flora (controversial), antecedent GI infection, carbohydrate malabsorption, food allergies, neurohumoral disturbances, genetic factors, and abnormal stool characteristics (low concentrations of bile or short-chain fatty acids).

Relief of pain with defecation, looser stool with pain onset, more frequent stools with pain onset, and abdominal distention are significantly more common in IBS than in organic disease.

Diagnostic Criteria

■ Physical examination is usually normal.
■ Routine diagnostic testing with complete blood count, serum chemistries, thyroid function tests, stool for ova and parasites, and abdominal imaging are not recommended in patients with typical IBS symptoms and no alarm symptoms because of the low probability of diagnosing organic disease.
■ Serologic screening for celiac sprue should be pursued in patients with diarrhea-predominant or mixed-symptom IBS.
■ Lactose breath testing may be considered when lactose intolerance is suspected after dietary modification.
■ Colonoscopy should be performed in patients with IBS with alarm symptoms to rule out Crohn's disease, ulcerative colitis, and colorectal cancer.
■ Colonoscopy should be performed in patients with IBS over the age of 50 to rule out colon cancer.

25-10. Treatment Principles and Goals of IBS

Treatment should be offered to patients seeking medical care if the patient and physician believe that the IBS symptoms decrease the patient's quality of life. Goals of therapy include improving IBS symptoms and improving quality of life.

Evidence from small clinical trials is inconsistent regarding the effectiveness of anticholinergic and antimuscarinic agents (dicyclomine and hyoscyamine) in the management of IBS; however, they are often used as first-line therapy in patients with mild symptoms. They may provide short-term relief of abdominal pain and discomfort. They should be used with caution in patients with constipation.

Psyllium has been shown to be moderately effective for IBS, although the evidence is weak.

Calcium polycarbophil was shown to improve symptoms in one small study. Polyethylene glycol was shown to improve stool frequency, but not abdominal pain, in a small study of adolescents with constipation-predominant IBS. It may be used as adjunctive therapy in patients with constipation-predominant IBS.

Loperamide significantly improves stool consistency and decreases stool frequency in patients with diarrhea-predominant IBS. It has no effect on abdominal pain or global IBS symptoms.

Tegaserod improves global IBS symptoms, bloating, abdominal pain, and altered bowel habits in patients with constipation-predominant IBS. It was withdrawn from the U.S. market in March 2007 because of an increased incidence (0.11%) of cardiovascular events in patients taking the drug. It is available only through the U.S. Food and Drug Administration (FDA) under an emergency investigational drug protocol.

Tricyclic antidepressants (TCAs) improve abdominal pain in patients with IBS. They also improve global IBS symptoms in patients with diarrhea-predominant IBS but not constipation-predominant IBS.

Selective serotonin reuptake inhibitors (SSRIs) improve abdominal pain in patients with IBS and are also effective in the treatment of comorbid psychiatric disorders in patients with IBS. SSRIs are recommended for patients with moderate to severe abdominal pain or those with psychiatric comorbidities. Several types of psychological counseling and therapy are effective in some patients with IBS.

Alosetron improves global IBS symptoms, abdominal discomfort, stool consistency, and stool frequency in women with diarrhea-predominant IBS. Because of the incidence of colon ischemia and complicated constipation, alosetron is available only through a prescribing program regulated by the FDA and administered by the drug's manufacturer. It is approved for use only in women with chronic, severe, diarrhea-predominant IBS who do not respond to other therapies.

Lubiprostone has been shown to relieve global IBS symptoms in women with constipation-predominant IBS.

Linaclotide reduces abdominal pain and increases the number of spontaneous bowel movements in patients with constipation-predominant IBS.

Drug Therapy

Table 25-4 shows selected medications used to treat IBS.

Mechanism of action

The antispasmodic agent dicyclomine decreases GI motility by relaxing smooth muscle in the gut.

Hyoscyamine is an anticholinergic agent that decreases GI motility by decreasing smooth muscle tone through antimuscarinic activity in the gut.

TCAs, such as amitriptyline, delay intestinal transit and may blunt perception of visceral distention. The effect of TCAs on the cerebral processing of visceral pain is unknown.

Tegaserod maleate, a partial 5-HT$_4$ agonist that stimulates the peristaltic reflex and intestinal secretion, inhibits visceral sensitivity by binding to 5-HT$_4$ receptors in the gut.

Lactulose, milk of magnesia, and polyethylene glycol solutions are osmotic laxatives that aid in the treatment of IBS patients with constipation.

Fiber supplements (bulk laxatives) increase stool bulk and water content.

Loperamide inhibits peristalsis by directly affecting the circular and longitudinal muscles of the intestinal wall.

Diphenoxylate is a meperidine congener that directly affects the circular smooth muscle in the gut, which slows GI transit time.

Alosetron is a selective 5-HT$_3$ receptor antagonist that inhibits activation of nonselective cation channels in the gut, thereby modulating the enteric nervous system.

SSRIs inhibit the neuronal uptake of serotonin in the CNS. Citalopram has peripheral effects on colonic tone and sensitivity. Paroxetine has potent anticholinergic effects.

Lubiprostone is the only C-2 chloride channel activator available. By activating C-2 chloride channels in the gut, lubiprostone increases secretion of saltwater into the intestinal lumen. It is approved only for women with constipation-dependent IBS.

Table 25-4. Selected Medications Used in Treatment of Irritable Bowel Syndrome

Generic name	Trade name	Classification	Dosage range and frequency	Dosage forms
Dicyclomine	Bentyl	Antispasmodic, anticholinergic	10–20 mg qid prn	T, C, L
Hyoscyamine	Various trade names	Anticholinergic	0.25–0.5 mg bid–qid	T, L
Amitriptyline	Elavil	Tricyclic antidepressant	10–50 mg nightly	T
Paroxetine	Paxil	SSRI	10–60 mg/day	T, L, DT
Tegaserod	Zelnorm	Serotonin (5-HT$_4$) receptor antagonist	6 mg bid	T
Lactulose	Various trade names	Osmotic laxative	30–45 mL bid–qid prn	L
Polycarbophil	Fibercon	Bulking agent	1 g daily–qid prn	T
Polyethylene glycol	Various trade names	Osmotic laxative	250 mL q 10 min up to 4 L	L
Alosetron	Lotronex	Serotonin (5-HT$_3$) receptor antagonist	1 mg daily–bid	T
Lubiprostone	Amitiza	C-2 chloride channel activator	8 mcg bid	C
Loperamide	Imodium	Antidiarrheal	2 mg after each loose stool; maximum 16 mg/day	T, C, L
Diphenoxylate/atropine	Lomotil	Antidiarrheal	15–20 mg/day of diphenoxylate in 3–4 divided doses	T, L
Linaclotide	Linzess	Guanylate cyclase-C agonist	290 mcg once daily	C

C, capsule; DT, delayed-release tablet; L, liquid; T, tablet.

Linaclotide is a guanylate cyclase-C (GC-C) agonist. It binds to GC-C in the luminal surface of intestinal epithelium. This increases intra- and extracellular levels of cyclic guanosine monophosphate (cGMP). The increase in cGMP stimulates the secretion of chloride and bicarbonate in the intestinal lumen, causing an increase in intestinal fluid and faster transit time.

Patient counseling

Antispasmodics and anticholinergic agents are best used on an as-needed basis up to three times per day during acute attacks or before meals when postprandial symptoms are present.

Patients taking a TCA should avoid prolonged exposure to sunlight and avoid concurrent use of CNS depressants.

Tegaserod should be taken 30 minutes before meals and should not be initiated during an acute exacerbation of IBS. It is available only through an emergency investigational drug protocol from the FDA.

Osmotic laxatives should be used on an as-needed basis. Lactulose may be mixed with water or juice to increase palatability. Patients should drink plenty of water.

Patients must be enrolled in the manufacturer's prescribing program to receive alosetron. Patients should not initiate therapy with alosetron if they are currently constipated. Alosetron should be discontinued if no improvement in symptoms is seen after 4 weeks of therapy.

See Chapter 29 on psychiatric disease for a full discussion of SSRIs.

Lubiprostone should be taken with food and water. Softgel capsules should be swallowed whole.

Linaclotide should be taken on an empty stomach at least 30 minutes before breakfast. Capsules should be swallowed whole. They should not be broken or chewed.

Adverse drug effects

Dicyclomine, hyoscyamine, and TCAs may cause anticholinergic side effects (CNS depression, dry mouth, urinary retention, constipation, decreased sweating).

Tegaserod may cause diarrhea, nausea, headache, and abdominal pain. It was associated with an increased risk of cardiovascular events in clinical trials.

Osmotic laxatives may cause abdominal pain and cramping.

Alosetron may cause constipation, abdominal pain, and nausea. Intestinal obstruction, perforation, toxic megacolon, ischemic colitis, and death have occurred.

See Chapter 29 on psychiatric disease for a full discussion of SSRIs.

Lubiprostone's most common side effects are nausea, diarrhea, and headache. Allergic reactions and dyspnea within 1 hour of the first dose have also been reported. Though dyspnea may recur with repeated doses, it usually resolves within 3 hours.

Linaclotide causes diarrhea in 20% of patients. Loose stools may occur more frequently if the drug is given with a high-fat breakfast. Abdominal pain, flatulence, upper respiratory infection, abdominal distention, and sinusitis have also been reported.

Drug interactions

Anticholinergics and antispasmodics may decrease the effectiveness of antipsychotic medications. Side effects from anticholinergics are increased when they are given concurrently with a TCA.

TCA concentrations may be increased or decreased by medications that induce or inhibit the activity of the CYP450 enzyme system in the liver. TCAs should not be given concurrently with monoamine oxidase inhibitors or sympathomimetic agents.

Other medications should not be taken within 1 hour of the start of therapy with osmotic laxatives.

The levels of alosetron may be decreased by concurrent administration of rifamycin derivatives. No significant drug interactions have been reported with tegaserod, lubiprostone, or linaclotide.

Monitoring parameters

Patients should monitor for the presence of IBS symptoms and for the side effects of medications, as discussed in the section on adverse drug effects.

Pharmacokinetics

Dicyclomine, hyoscyamine, amitriptyline, paroxetine, tegaserod, alosetron, loperamide, and diphenoxylate/atropine undergo hepatic metabolism.

Lubiprostone is metabolized in the stomach and small intestine.

Linaclotide is metabolized to an active metabolite in the GI tract. It is minimally absorbed systemically. It is excreted primarily in the feces.

Nondrug Therapy

An effective physician–patient relationship is necessary for successful treatment. Education should be provided regarding disease pathophysiology and treatment, and the patient should be reassured that the symptoms are real.

Although evidence supporting exclusion diets is lacking, patients may be counseled to avoid foods that exacerbate IBS symptoms. Foods commonly implicated are fatty foods, beans, gas-producing foods, alcohol, caffeine, lactose (in lactase-deficient individuals), and occasionally excess fiber.

Cognitive behavioral therapy, dynamic psychotherapy, and hypnotherapy are more effective than usual care in relieving global symptoms of IBS. Although the quality of the evidence regarding such therapy is low, the potential benefit outweighs the potential risks.

25-11. Questions

Use the following case study to answer Questions 1 and 2:

A 59-year-old African American male was recently diagnosed with PUD on endoscopy. Tissue biopsy is positive for *H. pylori*. He has no known drug allergies.

1. Which of the following is the ideal therapeutic regimen for *H. pylori*–related PUD in this case?

   A. PPI, clarithromycin, amoxicillin
   B. PPI, bismuth, metronidazole, tetracycline
   C. Omeprazole, amoxicillin
   D. Omeprazole, bismuth, clarithromycin, furazolidone
   E. Omeprazole, sucralfate, clarithromycin, furazolidone

2. If the patient was allergic to penicillin, which treatment recommendation would you choose?

   A. PPI, clarithromycin, amoxicillin
   B. PPI, bismuth, metronidazole, tetracycline
   C. Omeprazole, metronidazole
   D. Clarithromycin, metronidazole, tetracycline
   E. Clarithromycin, metronidazole, furazolidone

3. Which of the following is the leading cause of PUD in *H. pylori*–negative patients?

   A. Mineralocorticoids
   B. NSAIDs
   C. DMARDs
   D. Antibiotics
   E. Corticosteroids

4. Which of the following are true of NSAIDs?

   I. They inhibit production of prostaglandins.
   II. They are directly toxic to gastroduodenal epithelium.
   III. They require dose adjustments in renal insufficiency.
   IV. They cause only gastric ulcers.
   V. They allow healing of PUD during continued therapy.

   A. I, II, and III only
   B. I and III only
   C. II and IV only
   D. V only
   E. All are correct.

5. Which of the following are goals of therapy for PUD?

   I. Reduce episodes of diarrhea
   II. Eliminate symptoms
   III. Reduce risk of gastric cancer
   IV. Heal ulcerations
   V. Avoid spreading *H. pylori*

   A. I, II, and III only
   B. I and III only
   C. II and IV only
   D. V only
   E. All are correct.

6. Which of the following tests do *not* require endoscopy to test for *H. pylori* infection?

   I. Serum antibody test
   II. Fecal antigen test
   III. Urea breath test
   IV. Histology test
   V. Rapid urease test

   A. I, II, and III only
   B. I and III only
   C. II and IV only
   D. V only
   E. All are correct.

Use the following case study to answer Questions 7 and 8:

A 45-year-old Caucasian female with a past medical history significant only for seizure disorder has experienced heartburn after meals intermittently for the past 2 weeks. It becomes worse when she is reclining at bedtime. Her medications include phenytoin 300 mg bedtime. She says that her symptoms are not troublesome and that she is going to self-treat with over-the-counter medications.

7. Which of the following should *not* be recommended for this patient?

    A. Aluminum hydroxide
    B. Cimetidine
    C. Famotidine
    D. Ranitidine
    E. Magnesium hydroxide

8. The patient's symptoms are not relieved after 2 weeks of OTC treatment with famotidine and lifestyle modifications. She states her symptoms are becoming "troublesome." Which of the following is the best choice?

    A. Add the prokinetic agent metoclopramide to famotidine.
    B. Endoscopy should be performed because she has symptoms suggestive of complications from GERD.
    C. Add alginic acid 2 tablets nightly to famotidine.
    D. Discontinue current therapy, and initiate therapy with omeprazole 20 mg daily.
    E. Continue famotidine for 1 more week to achieve maximum effectiveness.

9. Which of the following are the most common symptoms of the typical esophageal GERD syndrome?

    I.   Heartburn
    II. Belching
    III. Regurgitation
    IV. Hypersalivation
    V.   Hoarseness

    A. I, II, and III only
    B. I and III only
    C. II and IV only
    D. V only
    E. All are correct.

10. Which of the following diagnoses carries an increased risk for developing esophageal adenocarcinoma?

    I.   Typical reflux syndrome
    II. Reflux cough syndrome
    III. Reflux laryngitis
    IV. Nontroublesome symptoms of GERD
    V.   Barrett's esophagus

    A. I, II, and III only
    B. I and III only
    C. II and IV only
    D. V only
    E. All are correct.

11. Which of the following may exacerbate GERD symptoms by lowering the LES pressure?

    A. Quinidine
    B. Iron
    C. Potassium chloride
    D. Diltiazem
    E. Tetracycline

12. Which of the following is the best choice for the initial treatment of troublesome symptoms of the typical reflux syndrome?

    A. Nizatidine 75 mg daily
    B. Pantoprazole 40 mg daily
    C. Metoclopramide 10 mg qid
    D. A 3-month trial of lifestyle modifications
    E. Pantoprazole 40 mg daily with metoclopramide 10 mg qid

Use the following case study to answer Questions 13 and 14:

A 32-year-old Caucasian male presents with bloody diarrhea (fewer than four stools per day) for 2 days. Complete blood counts and ESR are normal. Physical exam is normal. Colonoscopy reveals distal colitis.

13. Which of the following is the best choice for initial therapy for him?

    A. Prednisone 40 mg po daily
    B. Sulfasalazine 4–6 g po daily
    C. Mesalamine 1–4 g PR nightly
    D. Mesalamine 4–6 g po daily
    E. Methylprednisolone 16 mg IV q8h

14. The patient continues to have bloody diarrhea (without systemic disturbances). Which one of the following is the best choice?

    A. Add prednisone 40 mg po daily, and discontinue enema.
    B. Add mesalamine 2–4 g po daily, and continue enema.
    C. Add methylprednisolone 16 mg IV q8h until remission is achieved.
    D. Add mesalamine 2–4 g po daily, and discontinue enema.
    E. Add azathioprine 1–2.5 mg/kg/day, and discontinue enema.

15. Which of the following is true for UC?

    I.   Aminosalicylates are the drugs of choice for maintenance therapy.
    II. Oral corticosteroids are the drugs of choice for maintenance therapy.

III. Azathioprine often allows reduction in corticosteroid dose.

IV. Topical aminosalicylates are the drugs of choice for severe or fulminant disease.

V. Ciprofloxacin is alternative first-line therapy for mild to moderate disease.

A. I, II, and III only
B. I and III only
C. II and IV only
D. V only
E. All are correct.

16. Which of the following is true for CD?

I. Infliximab is the drug of choice for mild to moderate disease.

II. Oral corticosteroids are the drugs of choice for maintenance therapy.

III. Topical aminosalicylates are the drugs of choice for mild to moderate disease.

IV. Oral cyclosporine is the drug of choice for maintenance therapy.

V. Budesonide should be used as initial therapy for CD of the ileum and right colon.

A. I, II, and III only
B. I and III only
C. II and IV only
D. V only
E. All are correct.

17. Which of the following is true for moderate to severe CD?

A. Azathioprine is the drug of choice for initial therapy.

B. Budesonide is appropriate maintenance therapy.

C. Oral corticosteroids are the drugs of choice for initial therapy.

D. Methotrexate has no role in CD therapy.

E. Topical aminosalicylates are appropriate maintenance therapy.

18. Which of the following is associated with the development of progressive multifocal leukoencephalopathy?

A. Prednisone
B. Sulfasalazine
C. Mesalamine
D. Methotrexate
E. Natalizumab

Use the following case study to answer Questions 19 and 20.

A 39-year-old female presents with mild abdominal pain and diarrhea for 12 weeks. She has no significant past medical history and occasionally misses days from her full-time job. Her symptoms are worse after meals.

19. Which of the following is the best choice for initial therapy?

I. Paroxetine 10 mg daily
II. Amitriptyline 10 mg bedtime
III. Tegaserod 6 mg bid
IV. Alosetron 1 mg daily
V. Dicyclomine 10 mg qid after meals

A. I, II, and III only
B. I and III only
C. II and IV only
D. V only
E. All are correct.

20. Her symptoms are controlled for several months until she loses her job. Her abdominal pain then returns. She has five episodes of diarrhea per day and complains of fatigue and insomnia. Which of the following are the most appropriate for this patient?

I. Initiate psychological counseling.
II. Prescribe amitriptyline 10–50 mg bedtime.
III. Add loperamide 2 mg after each loose stool (16 mg/day maximum).
IV. Add alosetron 1 mg daily.
V. Start tegaserod 6 mg bid.

A. I, II, and III only
B. I and II only
C. II and IV only
D. V only
E. All are correct.

21. Which of the following is indicated for constipation-predominant IBS?

A. Tegaserod 6 mg bid
B. Alosetron 1 mg bid
C. Loperamide 2–16 mg/day
D. Paroxetine 10–40 mg daily
E. Diphenoxylate + atropine 2 tabs qid

22. Which of the following is affected by medications that induce or inhibit the cytochrome P450 enzyme system?

A. Tegaserod
B. Alosetron

C. Fibercon
D. Polyethylene glycol
E. Amitriptyline

23. Which life-threatening complication caused the restriction of alosetron?

   A. Stevens–Johnson syndrome
   B. Toxic epidermal necrolysis
   C. Aplastic anemia
   D. Ischemic colitis
   E. Chronic diarrhea

24. Alosetron is indicated for which group of IBS patients?

   A. Women with diarrhea-predominant IBS
   B. Men with diarrhea-predominant IBS
   C. Women with constipation-predominant IBS
   D. Men with constipation-predominant IBS
   E. Children with diarrhea-predominant IBS

25-12. Answers

1. **A.** Triple-drug therapy with a PPI, clarithromycin, and amoxicillin is recommended by the American Gastroenterological Association as initial therapy for *H. pylori*. Quadruple therapy with a bismuth-based regimen is less convenient but may be used first line in patients who are penicillin allergic. Two-drug regimens are less effective and are not recommended. Furazolidone is unavailable in the United States.

2. **B.** The patient is allergic to penicillin; therefore, amoxicillin cannot be used. Two-drug regimens are less effective and not recommended. Antisecretory therapy is an integral part of *H. pylori* regimens to promote ulcer healing. Furazolidone is unavailable in the United States.

3. **B.** NSAIDs are the leading cause of PUD in patients who are negative for *H. pylori* infection.

4. **A.** NSAIDs inhibit production of prostaglandins and are directly toxic to gastroduodenal epithelium. NSAIDs require dose adjustments in renal insufficiency. NSAIDs may cause gastric or duodenal ulcers and must be discontinued to allow for ulcer healing.

5. **C.** Elimination of symptoms and healing of ulcerations are goals of therapy for PUD.

6. **A.** The serum antibody test, fecal antigen test, and urea breath test do not require endoscopy.

7. **B.** Cimetidine is a potent inhibitor of the cytochrome P450 enzyme system and will increase serum concentrations of phenytoin in this patient.

8. **D.** Prokinetic agents are useful mainly in patients with concurrent gastric motility disorders and are not routinely recommended. She does not currently exhibit symptoms of GERD complications. Alginic acid is ineffective when the patient is lying in the supine position and should not be given at bedtime. Nonprescription medications for GERD should be discontinued if symptoms are not relieved after a 2-week trial.

9. **B.** Heartburn and regurgitation are the most common symptoms of the typical reflux syndrome.

10. **D.** Patients with Barrett's esophagus have an increased risk of developing esophageal adenocarcinoma.

11. **D.** Calcium channel blockers decrease LES pressure. Quinidine, iron, potassium chloride, and tetracycline have direct irritant effects on the esophageal mucosa.

12. **B.** The correct dose of nizatidine (prescription strength) would be 150 mg bid. Metoclopramide is not routinely recommended for the treatment of the typical reflux syndrome. When patients find their symptoms "troublesome," pharmacologic therapy should be initiated.

13. **C.** Topical aminosalicylates (answer C) are more effective than oral aminosalicylates (answer B) and topical steroids for mild distal UC (although oral aminosalicylates or topical steroids may be used first line if the patient prefers). Oral and IV steroids (answers A and E, respectively) are reserved for more severe cases of UC or cases that do not respond to oral and topical aminosalicylates. The oral dose of mesalamine in answer D is incorrect.

14. **B.** Oral aminosalicylates should be added if no response is achieved with topical aminosalicylates. Oral and IV steroids are reserved for moderate to severe UC or for patients with systemic disturbances. Azathioprine may be added if UC is refractory to aminosalicylates and to allow corticosteroid dose reduction.

15. **B.** Aminosalicylates are the drugs of choice for maintenance therapy of UC, not corticosteroids. Azathioprine often allows a reduction

in dose of corticosteroids in the management of active UC. Severe or fulminant UC requires oral, not topical, therapy. Ciprofloxacin may be used as an alternative first-line therapy in the treatment of mild to moderate CD, not UC.

16. **D.** Budesonide is the treatment of choice for mild to moderate CD of the ileum and right colon. Infliximab is reserved for moderate to severe disease in patients who do not respond to oral corticosteroids or immunosuppressive agents. It may also be used in patients in whom side effects from oral corticosteroids must be avoided. Oral corticosteroids should not be used for long-term maintenance therapy. Oral budesonide is the drug of choice for mild to moderate CD, not topical corticosteroids. Oral cyclosporine has no role in CD; IV cyclosporine may be used in severe or fulminant CD that does not respond to 5–7 days of IV corticosteroids.

17. **C.** Moderate to severe disease initially requires oral corticosteroid therapy. Corticosteroids have no role in maintenance therapy. Topical aminosalicylates may be used as adjuncts in colonic CD. Methotrexate is used as maintenance therapy for moderate to severe CD.

18. **E.** Natalizumab has been associated with the development of progressive multifocal leuko-encephalopathy.

19. **D.** This patient has mild, diarrhea-predominant IBS. Symptomatic treatment with dicyclomine is appropriate initial therapy, especially because her symptoms are meal related. A TCA may be added to dicyclomine if needed. Tegaserod is indicated for constipation-predominant IBS. Alosetron is reserved for patients with severe, diarrhea-predominant disease who have failed other therapies. Paroxetine may be added if initial therapies are ineffective or if she develops severe abdominal pain or psychiatric comorbidities.

20. **A.** Alosetron is reserved for patients with severe, diarrhea-predominant disease who have failed other therapies. Several types of psychotherapy have been shown to be more effective than usual care in IBS. TCAs improve abdominal pain in IBS and may also help with insomnia. Loperamide may be used on an as-needed basis for diarrhea. Tegaserod is indicated for constipation-predominant IBS.

21. **A.** Alosetron is approved for restricted use in diarrhea-predominant IBS. Loperamide and

diphenoxylate + atropine are antidiarrheal medications that will exacerbate constipation. Paroxetine is an SSRI with potent anticholinergic effects, which could worsen constipation. Another drug should be chosen if an SSRI is needed for depression.

22. **E.** Tricyclic antidepressant serum concentrations are affected by drugs that alter cytochrome P450 activity.

23. **D.** Severe constipation, ischemic colitis, and death have been reported with alosetron.

24. **A.** Alosetron is approved for women with diarrhea-predominant IBS. It was not found to be effective in men and is not approved for use in children.

25-13. References

Peptic Ulcer Disease

Bhatt DL, Scheiman J, Abraham NS, et al. ACCF/ACG/AHA 2008 expert consensus document on reducing the gastrointestinal risks of antiplatelet therapy and NSAID use: A report of the American College of Cardiology Foundation Task Force on clinical expert consensus documents. *Am J Gastroenterol.* 2008;103:2890–907.

Chey WD, Wong BC. American College of Gastroenterology guideline on the management of *Helicobacter pylori* infection. *Am J Gastroenterol.* 2007;102:1808–25.

Del Valle, J. Peptic ulcer disease and related disorders. In: Longo DL, Fauci AS, Kasper DL, et al., eds. *Harrison's Principles of Internal Medicine.* 18th ed. New York, NY: McGraw-Hill; 2012.

Laine L, Jensen DM. American College of Gastroenterology Practice Guidelines: Management of patients with ulcer bleeding. *Am J Gastroenterol.* 2012;107:345–60.

Lanza FL, Chan FKL, Quigley EMM, et al. Guidelines for prevention of NSAID-related ulcer complications. *Am J Gastroenterol.* 2009;104:728–38.

Love BL, Thoma MN. Peptic ulcer disease. In: Dipiro JT, Talbert RL, Yee GC, et al., eds. *Pharmacotherapy: A Pathophysiologic Approach.* 9th ed. New York, NY: McGraw-Hill Education; 2014:471–95.

Malfertheiner P, Chan FKL, McColl KEL. Peptic ulcer disease. *Lancet.* 2009;374:1449–61.

Malfertheiner P, Megraud F, O'Morain C, et al. Current concepts in the management of *Helicobacter pylori* infection: The Maastricht III Consensus Report. *Gut.* 2007;56:772–81.

McColl, KEL. *Helicobacter pylori* infection. *N Engl J Med.* 2010;362:1597–604.

Rokkas T, Sechopoulos P, Robotis I, et al. Cumulative *H. pylori* eradication rates in clinical practice by adopting first- and second-line regimens proposed by the Maastrict III consensus and a third-line empirical regimen. *Am J Gastroenterol.* 2009;104:21–25.

Vakil, N. *H. pylori* treatment: New wine in old bottles? *Am J Gastroenterol.* 2009;104:26–30.

Gastroesophageal Reflux Disease

Kahrilas PJ, Hirano I. Diseases of the esophagus. In: Longo DL, Fauci AS, Kasper DL, et al., eds. *Harrison's Principles of Internal Medicine.* 18th ed. New York, NY: McGraw-Hill; 2012.

Kahrilas PJ, Shaheen NJ, Vaezi MF, et al. American Gastroenterological Association medical position statement on the management of gastroesophageal reflux disease. *Gastroenterol.* 2008;135:1383–91.

Kahrilas PJ, Shaheen NJ, Vaezi MF. American Gastroenterological Association Institute technical review on the management of gastroesophageal reflux disease. *Gastroenterol.* 2008; 135:1392–413.

Katz PO, Gerson LB, Vela MF. Guidelines for the diagnosis and management of gastroesophageal reflux disease. *Am J Gastroenterol.* 2013;108:308–28.

May DB, Rao SSC. Gastroesophageal reflux disease. In: Dipiro JT, Talbert RL, Yee GC, et al., eds. *Pharmacotherapy: A Pathophysiologic Approach.* 9th ed. New York, NY: McGraw-Hill Education; 2014:455–69.

Vakil N, van Zanten SV, Kahrilas P, et al. The Montreal definition and classification of gastroesophageal reflux disease: A global, evidence-based consensus. *Am J Gastroenterol.* 2006;101:1900–20.

Inflammatory Bowel Disease

Friedman S, Blumberg RS. Inflammatory bowel disease. In: Longo DL, Fauci AS, Kasper DL, et al., eds. *Harrison's Principles of Internal Medicine.* 18th ed. New York, NY: McGraw-Hill; 2012.

Hemstreet BA. Inflammatory bowel disease. In: Dipiro JT, Talbert RL, Yee GC, et al., eds. *Pharmacotherapy: A Pathophysiologic Approach.* 9th ed. New York, NY: McGraw-Hill Education; 2014:497–516.

Kornbluth A, Sachar DB. Ulcerative colitis practice guidelines in adults: American College of Gastroenterology, Practice Parameters Committee. *Am J Gastroenterol.* 2010;105:501–23.

Lichtenstein GR, Hanauer SB, Sandborn WJ, et al. Management of Crohn's disease in adults: American College of Gastroenterology Practice guidelines. *Am J Gastroenterol.* 2009;104:465–83.

PL detail—document, treatments for ulcerative colitis. March 2013. Pharmacist's/Prescriber's Letter Web site. http://pharmacistsletter.therapeutic research.com/pl/ArticleDD.aspx?cs=&s=PL&pt= 6&fpt=31&dd=290303&pb=PL&searchid=476 96740#dd. Accessed August 5, 2014.

Rutgeerts P, Vermeire S, Van Assche G. Biological therapies for inflammatory bowel diseases. *Gastroenterol.* 2009;136:1182–97.

Irritable Bowel Syndrome

Brandt LJ, Chey WD, Foxx-Orenstein AE, et al. An evidence-based position statement on the management of irritable bowel syndrome. *Am J Gastroenterol.* 2009;104(suppl 1):S1–S7.

Brandt LJ, Chey WD, Foxx-Orenstein AE, et al. An evidence-based systematic review on the management of irritable bowel syndrome. *Am J Gastroenterol.* 2009;104(suppl 1):S8–S35.

Drossman DA, Camilleri M, Mayer EA, et al. AGA technical review on irritable bowel syndrome. *Gastroenterol.* 2002;123:2108–31.

Fabel PH, Shealy KM. Diarrhea, constipation, and irritable bowel syndrome. In: Dipiro JT, Talbert RL, Yee GC, et al., eds. *Pharmacotherapy: A Pathophysiologic Approach.* 9th ed. New York, NY: McGraw-Hill Education; 2014: 531–47.

Longstreth G, Thompson W, Chey W, et al. Functional bowel disorders. *Gastroenterol.* 2006; 130:1480–91.

Manning A, Thompson W, Heaton K, et al. Towards positive diagnosis of the irritable bowel. *Br Med J.* 1978;2:653–54.

Owyang C. Irritable bowel syndrome. In: Longo DL, Fauci AS, Kasper DL, et al., eds. *Harrison's Principles of Internal Medicine.* 18th ed. New York, NY: McGraw-Hill; 2012.

PL detail—document, new drug: linzess (linaclotide). December 2012. Pharmacist's Letter/Prescriber's Letter Web site. http://pharmacistsletter.therapeutic research.com/pl/ArticleDD.aspx?cs=&s=PL&pt= 6&fpt=31&dd=281204&pb=PL&searchid=476 96799#dd. Accessed August 5, 2014.

Rheumatoid Arthritis, Osteoarthritis, Gout, and Lupus

Melanie P. Swims

26-1. Key Points

Rheumatoid Arthritis

- Rheumatoid arthritis (RA), a highly variable autoimmune disease characterized by symmetric, erosive synovitis, often affects extra-articular sites.
- RA usually affects diarthrodial joints, such as proximal interphalangeal joints, metacarpophalangeal joints, metatarsophalangeal joints, wrists, and ankles. Also commonly involved are the elbows, shoulders, sternoclavicular joints, temporomandibular joints, hips, and knees.
- Morning stiffness is the hallmark of RA.
- According to the American College of Rheumatology (ACR), the goals in managing RA are to prevent or control joint damage, prevent loss of function, and decrease pain.
- The ACR recommends the aggressive use of disease-modifying antirheumatic drugs (DMARDs).
- Unlike the nonsteroidal anti-inflammatory drugs (NSAIDs), DMARDs can reduce or prevent joint damage and preserve joint integrity and function. DMARDs carry the risk of various toxicities, and they must be monitored on a regular basis.

Osteoarthritis

- Osteoarthritis (OA) is the most common form of arthritis in the United States.
- Joint stiffness, a common complaint in osteoarthritis, differs from that in RA because it is relatively short in duration and resolves with movement.
- Unlike RA, pain relief is the primary treatment goal in OA. The initial drug of choice is acetaminophen.

Gout

- Gout, a systemic disease caused by the buildup of uric acid in the joints, causes inflammation, swelling, and pain.
- Primary gout is a result of an innate defect in purine metabolism or uric acid excretion.
- Patients with gout are classified as *overproducers* or *underexcreters* on the basis of 24-hour uric acid concentration levels.
- Treatment of an acute gouty arthritis attack involves the use of colchicine, NSAIDs, or glucocorticoids.
- Uricosuric agents, xanthine oxidase inhibitors, and uricase agents may be used to prevent further gout attacks. These agents should not be used during an acute gouty arthritis attack.

Systemic Lupus Erythematosus

- Systemic Lupus Erythematosus (SLE) is a chronic autoimmune inflammatory disorder that can affect any system in the body.
- Therapy for SLE is primarily driven by the clinical manifestations of the disease.

Editor's Note: This chapter is based on the 10th edition chapter written by Melanie Swims and Kevin L. Freeman.

26-2. Study Guide Checklist

The following topics may guide your study of this subject area:

- Autoimmune nature and pathophysiology of RA
- Monitoring of RA
- Mechanism of action of NSAIDs
- Adverse effects of NSAIDs
- Place in therapy of DMARDs
- Adverse effects and monitoring of DMARDs
- Pathophysiology and diagnosis of OA
- Drug therapy of OA
- Pathophysiology and diagnosis of gout
- Mechanism of action of gout drugs
- Adverse effects and monitoring of gout drugs
- Drugs for treatment of gout attacks verses prophylaxis
- Pathophysiology and diagnostic criteria of lupus
- Drugs used in lupus treatment

26-3. Rheumatoid Arthritis

Rheumatoid arthritis (RA) is a highly variable, chronic autoimmune disorder of unknown etiology characterized by symmetric, erosive synovitis. Manifestations may extend to extra-articular sites.

Incidence

RA affects 1% of the population and is two to three times more common in women than in men. Certain families, monozygotic twins, and people with specific HLA (human leukocyte antigen) genetic markers have a greater incidence of RA, which suggests a genetic predisposition.

Clinical Presentation

The onset of RA is unpredictable and varies from rapid to insidious progression.

RA usually affects diarthrodial joints such as the proximal interphalangeal (PIP) joints, metacarpophalangeal (MCP) joints, metatarsophalangeal (MTP) joints, wrists, and ankles. Also commonly involved are the elbows, shoulders, sternoclavicular joints, temporomandibular joints, hips, and knees.

The initial complaints may include generalized fatigue and multiple joint pain.

Morning stiffness is a hallmark of RA. Patients describe it as a gel-like sensation in the joints that occurs after attempting to move upon awakening.

Ulnar deviation, swan-neck deformities, boutonnière deformities, hammertoe formation, and ankylosis are common irreversible joint abnormalities that occur in RA.

The extra-articular features that occur in RA include rheumatoid nodules, vasculitis, anemia, thrombocytopenia, Felty's syndrome, and Sjögren's syndrome.

Etiology

The cause of RA remains a mystery. Factors that may be responsible are of environmental, genetic, endocrinologic, gastrointestinal, atmospheric, and infectious origin.

RA is widely held to have a strong genetic component. This assertion is supported by the fact that a greater prevalence of RA is found in patients with the major histocompatibility complex antigen HLA-DR4. This class II antigen is expressed on the surface of helper T-lymphocytes and macrophages. In combination with environmental factors, an inappropriate immune response may occur, resulting in chronic inflammation.

Pathophysiology

For unknown reasons, the body's immune system (starting with macrophages) attacks the cells within the joint capsule, thereby causing synovitis (as indicated by the warmth, swelling, redness, and pain associated with RA). Specifically, helper T-lymphocytes stimulate B-lymphocytes to attack antigen (in this case, the body's own collagen). In addition, helper T-lymphocytes release cytokines (interleukins and tumor necrosis factor), which cause further inflammation and injury in the joints. During the inflammatory process, the cells of the synovium grow and divide abnormally, causing a normally thin synovium to become thick (pannus). These abnormal synovial cells begin to invade and destroy the cartilage and bone within the joint. These effects are responsible for the pain and deformities seen in patients with RA.

Diagnostic Criteria

New classification criteria for RA were developed in 2010. To meet the diagnostic criteria, a patient must have at least one swollen joint not explained by another disease and 6 points summed from the following four factors:

1. Joint involvement in 1 large joint (shoulder, elbow, hip, knee, ankle) = 0 point; 2 to 10 large joints = 1 point; 1 to 3 small joints (metacarpophalangeal, proximal interphalangeal, metatarsophalangeal, carpal) = 2 points; 4 to 10 small joints = 3 points; or more than 10 joints (at least 1 small joint required) = 5 points.
2. Serologic studies: negative rheumatoid factor and anti–cyclic citrullinated peptide (anti-CCP) antibodies = 0 point; weakly positive rheumatoid factor or anti-CCP antibodies or both = 2 points; strong positive rheumatoid factor or anti-CCP antibodies or both = 3 points.
3. Acute-phase reactants: normal (C-reactive protein level or erythrocyte sedimentation rate or both) = 0 point; elevated = 1 point.
4. Disease duration: < 6 months = 0 point; > 6 months = 1 point.

Treatment Goals

According to the American College of Rheumatology (ACR), the goals in managing RA are to prevent or control joint damage, prevent loss of function, and decrease pain.

Monitoring

At each visit, the patient should be evaluated for subjective evidence of active disease on the basis of the following criteria:

- Degree of joint pain
- Duration of morning stiffness
- Duration of fatigue
- Presence of actively inflamed joints on examination
- Limitation of function

Periodically, the patient should be evaluated for disease activity or progression:

- Evidence of disease progression on physical examination (loss of motion, instability, malalignment, deformity)
- Erythrocyte sedimentation rate or C-reactive protein elevation
- Progression of radiographic damage of involved joints

Other parameters for assessing response to treatment (outcomes):

- Health care provider's global assessment of disease activity
- Patient's global assessment of disease activity
- Functional status or quality-of-life assessment using standardized questionnaires

The majority of clinical studies use a benchmark of 20% improvement in the preceding criteria, also known as ACR 20.

Drug Therapy

Aggressive use of disease-modifying antirheumatic drugs (DMARDs) is suggested (Table 26-1).

The ACR recommendations focus on the use of biologic and nonbiologic therapies for the treatment of RA. The use of nonmedical therapies and anti-inflammatory drugs as well as other analgesics is still a part of the optimal treatment regimen; however, it was not evaluated as part of the 2012 recommendations (Figures 26-1 and 26-2).

The 2012 ACR recommendations for the initiation or reinstitution of biologic and nonbiologic therapies depend on three factors:

- Disease duration:
  - Early (< 6 months)
  - Established RA (≥ 6 months)
- Disease activity:
  - Available indices:
    - Disease Activity Score in 28 joints
    - Simplified Disease Activity Index
    - Clinical Disease Activity Index
  - Mild disease: Typically fewer than six inflamed joints, no extra-articular disease, and no radiographic evidence of erosions
  - Severe disease: Typically more than 20 inflamed joints; elevation in C-reactive protein; and positive rheumatoid factor, extra-articular disease, or both
- Prognostic factors:
  - Physical examination, health questionnaire, and laboratory analysis
  - Poor prognosis: Functional limitation, extra-articular disease, rheumatoid factor or anti-CCP antibodies (anti-CCP antibodies may be more specific than rheumatoid factor)

Nonsteroidal anti-inflammatory drugs

Salicylates, nonsteroidal anti-inflammatory drugs (NSAIDs), and selective cyclooxygenase-2 (COX-2) inhibitors are agents with analgesic and anti-inflammatory properties useful in the management

Table 26-1. Disease-Modifying Antirheumatic Drugs

Generic name	Trade name	Dosage range	Administration schedule	Dosage forms
Nonbiologic				
Hydroxychloroquine	Plaquenil	200–400 mg	1–2 doses per day	po
Sulfasalazine	Azulfidine	1,000–3,000 mg	2–3 doses per day	po
Methotrexate	Rheumatrex	7.5–25 mg	Once weekly	po, IM, subcutaneous, IV
Gold sodium thiomalate	Myochrysine	25–50 mg	Every 2–4 weeks	IM
Auranofin	Ridaura	3–6 mg	1–2 doses per day	po
Azathioprine	Imuran	50–150 mg	1–2 doses per day	po, IV
Minocycline	Minocin	100–200 mg	2 doses per day	po
Leflunomide	Arava	10–20 mg	1–2 doses per day	po
Tofacitinib	Xeljanz	5–10 mg	Daily to bid	po
Biologic				
Certolizumab	Cimzia	200–400 mg	400 mg initially and at 2 weeks and 4 weeks, then 200 mg every other week or 400 mg every 4 weeks	Subcutaneous
Etanercept	**Enbrel**	50 mg	Once weekly	Subcutaneous
Golimumab	Simponi	50 mg	Once monthly	Subcutaneous
Infliximab	**Remicade**	3 mg/kg	Weeks 0, 2, and 6, then every 8 weeks	IV
Anakinra	Kineret	100 mg	1 dose per day	Subcutaneous
Adalimumab	**Humira**	40 mg	Every other week	Subcutaneous
Abatacept	**Orencia**	< 60 kg = 500 mg; 60–100 kg = 750 mg; > 100 kg = 1,000 mg	Weeks 0, 2, and 4, then every 4 weeks	IV
Rituximab	**Rituxan**	1,000 mg	Every 2 weeks for two doses	IV
Tocilizumab	Actemra	4 mg/kg; may be increased to 8 mg/kg on the basis of clinical response	Every 4 weeks	IV

IM, intramuscular; IV, intravenous.
Boldface indicates one of top 100 drugs for 2012 by units sold at retail outlets, www.drugs.com/stats/top100/2012/units.

of RA. These agents reduce joint pain and swelling; however, they do not inhibit joint destruction or otherwise alter the course of the disease. For this reason, they should not be considered as a sole treatment option. These agents act by inhibiting prostaglandin synthesis and release. Cyclooxygenase is present in many cells, including platelets, endothelial cells, and cells of the gastric and intestinal mucosa. The initial choice of agent is based on the efficacy, safety, cost, and convenience for any given patient. A wide range of interpatient variability exists with regard to clinical effect; several NSAIDs may need to be tried before achieving patient satisfaction. See Table 26-2.

NSAIDs

Mechanism of action
NSAIDs prevent prostaglandin formation by inhibiting the action of the enzyme cyclooxygenase. The antithrombotic effect of aspirin occurs by an irreversible inhibition of platelet cyclooxygenase. This irreversible inhibition is unique to aspirin, because the remaining NSAIDs do so in a reversible manner.

Patient instructions
NSAIDs should be taken with food or milk to decrease gastrointestinal (GI) intolerance. Patients should report any dark or black stools, abdominal pain,

Figure 26-1. 2012 American College of Rheumatology Recommendations Update for the Treatment of Early Rheumatoid Arthritis (RA), Defined as a Disease Duration < 6 Months

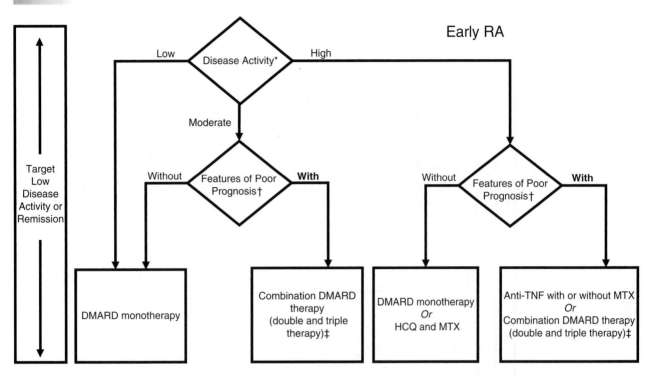

For the level of evidence supporting each recommendation, please see Supplementary Appendix 7 (available in the online version of this article at http://onlinelibrary.wiley.com/journal/10.1002/(ISSN)2151-4658). DMARD = disease-modifying antirheumatic drug (includes hydroxychloroquine [HCQ], leflunomide [LEF], methotrexate [MTX], minocycline, and sulfasalazine); anti-TNF = anti–tumor necrosis factor.
* Definitions of disease activity are discussed in Tables 2 and 3 and Supplementary Appendix 4 (available in the online version of this article at http://onlinelibrary.wiley.com/journal/10.1002/(ISSN)2151-4658) and were categorized as low, moderate, or high.
† Patients were categorized based on the presence or absence of 1 or more of the following poor prognostic features: functional limitation (e.g., Health Assessment Questionnaire score or similar valid tools), extraarticular disease (e.g., presence of rheumatoid nodules, RA vasculitis, Felty's syndrome), positive rheumatoid factor or anti–cyclic citrullinated peptide antibodies (33–37), and bony erosions by radiograph (38).
‡ Combination DMARD therapy with 2 DMARDs, which is most commonly MTX based, with some exceptions (e.g., MTX + HCQ, MTX + LEF, MTX + sulfasalazine, and sulfasalazine + HCQ), and triple therapy (MTX + HCQ + sulfasalazine) as defined in Table 2.

Reprinted with permission from the American College of Rheumatology. Singh JA, et al., 2012.

or swelling to their health care provider immediately. Studies indicate that the optimal times for taking an NSAID might be after the evening meal and immediately on awakening. Patients with a hypersensitivity to aspirin should not take NSAIDs.

Adverse drug events

Compared with patients with osteoarthritis, patients with RA on NSAID therapy are at increased risk for a serious complication.

As with aspirin, NSAIDs cause platelet dysfunction. Unlike aspirin, however, this effect is readily reversible with discontinuation of the medication.

All NSAIDs are capable of causing GI intolerance and peptic ulceration. Risk factors for the development of peptic ulcer disease include advanced age,

history of previous ulcer, concomitant use of corticosteroids or anticoagulants, higher dosage of NSAID, use of multiple NSAIDs, or serious underlying disease. Options to decrease the risk of developing GI ulceration include using a selective COX-2 inhibitor or adding a proton pump inhibitor to the patient's regimen. Misoprostol, an oral prostaglandin analog, may be added at a dose of 100–200 mcg four times daily to prevent ulceration but is not as well tolerated because of diarrhea. Misoprostol is available in combination with diclofenac and sold under the trade name Arthrotec. A 2008 joint consensus statement by the American College of Cardiology Foundation, the American Heart Association, and the American College of Gastroenterology recommends that patients with a history of ulcer disease or with risk factors for

Figure 26-2. 2012 American College of Rheumatology (ACR) Recommendations Update for the Treatment of Established Rheumatoid Arthritis (RA), Defined as a Disease Duration ≥ 6 Months or Meeting the 1987 ACR Classification Criteria

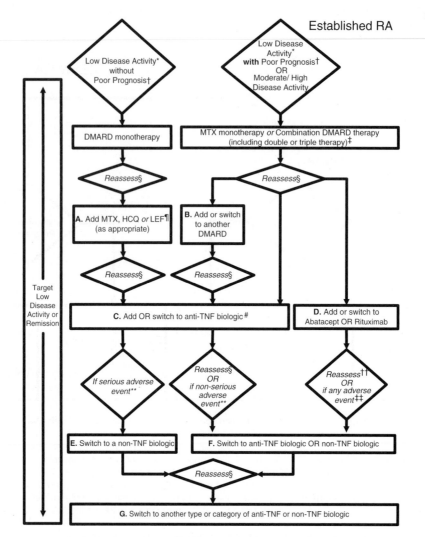

Depending on a patient's current medication regimen, the management algorithm may begin at an appropriate rectangle in the figure, rather than only at the top of the figure. Disease-modifying antirheumatic drugs (DMARDs) include hydroxychloroquine (HCQ), leflunomide (LEF), methotrexate (MTX), minocycline, and sulfasalazine (therapies are listed alphabetically; azathioprine and cyclosporine were considered but not included). DMARD monotherapy refers to treatment in most instances with HCQ, LEF, MTX, or sulfasalazine; in few instances, where appropriate, minocycline may also be used. Anti–tumor necrosis factor (anti-TNF) biologics include adalimumab, certolizumab pegol, etanercept, infliximab, and golimumab. Non-TNF biologics include abatacept, rituximab, or tocilizumab (therapies are listed alphabetically). For the level of evidence supporting each recommendation, please see Supplementary Appendix 7 (available in the online version of this article at http://onlinelibrary.wiley.com/journal/10.1002/(ISSN)2151-4658).

* Definitions of disease activity are discussed in Tables 2 and 3 and Supplementary Appendix 4 (available in the online version of this article at http://onlinelibrary.wiley.com/journal/10.1002/(ISSN)2151-4658) and were categorized as low, moderate, or high.

† Features of poor prognosis included the presence of 1 or more of the following: functional limitation (e.g., Health Assessment Questionnaire score or similar valid tools), extraarticular disease (e.g., presence of rheumatoid nodules, RA vasculitis, Felty's syndrome), positive rheumatoid factor or anti–cyclic citrullinated peptide antibodies (33–37), and bony erosions by radiograph (38).

‡ Combination DMARD therapy with 2 DMARDs, which is most commonly MTX based, with few exceptions (e.g., MTX + HCQ, MTX + LEF, MTX + sulfasalazine, sulfasalazine + HCQ), and triple therapy (MTX + HCQ + sulfasalazine).

§ Reassess after 3 months and proceed with escalating therapy if moderate or high disease activity in all instances except after treatment with a non-TNF biologic (rectangle D), where reassessment is recommended at 6 months due to a longer anticipated time for peak effect.

¶ LEF can be added in patients with low disease activity after 3–6 months of minocycline, HCQ, MTX, or sulfasalazine.

If after 3 months of intensified DMARD combination therapy or after a second DMARD has failed, the option is to add or switch to an anti-TNF biologic.

** Serious adverse events were defined per the U.S. Food and Drug Administration (FDA; see below); all other adverse events were considered nonserious adverse events.

†† Reassessment after treatment with a non-TNF biologic is recommended at 6 months due to anticipation that a longer time to peak effect is needed for non-TNF compared to anti-TNF biologics.

‡‡ Any adverse event was defined as per the U.S. FDA as any undesirable experience associated with the use of a medical product in a patient. The FDA definition of serious adverse event includes death, life-threatening event, initial or prolonged hospitalization, disability, congenital anomaly, or an adverse event requiring intervention to prevent permanent impairment or damage.

Table 26-2. Drug Therapy with Nonsteroidal Anti-Inflammatory Drugs

Generic name	Trade name	Dosage range	Administration schedule (doses/day)	Available dosage forms
Acetic acids				
Diclofenac	Voltaren	150–200 mg/day	3–4	po, ophthalmic, topical gel
	Voltaren XR	100–200 mg/day	1–2	po
Etodolac	Lodine	600–1,200 mg/day	2–4	po
	Lodine XL	400–1,000 mg/day	1	po
Indomethacin	Indocin	100–200 mg/day	2–3	po, IV, suppository
	Indocin SR	75–150 mg/day	1–2	po
Nabumetone	Relafen	1,000–2,000 mg/day	1–2	po
Tolmetin	Tolectin	600–1,800 mg/day	3	po
Sulindac	Clinoril	300–400 mg/day	2	po
Propionic acids				
Fenoprofen	Nalfon	900–3,200 mg/day	3–4	po
Flurbiprofen	Ansaid	200–300 mg/day	2–4	po
Ibuprofen	Motrin	1,200–3,200 mg/day	3–4	po
Ketoprofen	Orudis	150–300 mg/day	3–4	po
Ketoprofen SR	Oruvail	100–200 mg/day	1	po
Naproxen	Naprosyn	500–1,500 mg/day	2–3	po
Oxaprozin	Daypro	1,200–1,800 mg/day	1	po
Fenamates				
Meclofenamate	Meclomen	200–400 mg/day	3–4	po
Oxicams				
Meloxicam	Mobic	7.5–15 mg/day	1	po
Piroxicam	Feldene	10–20 mg/day	1–2	po
COX-2 selective				
Celecoxib	**Celebrex**	200–400 mg/day	1–2	po

IV, intravenous.

ulceration be treated with a proton pump inhibitor while on NSAID therapy. If the patient is taking low-dose aspirin for cardiovascular protection, a nonselective NSAID may be used in combination. However, ibuprofen should be avoided or given 2 hours later than the aspirin dose because it can render the aspirin less effective. COX-2 inhibitors should not be used in patients with cardiovascular disease.

Hepatic failure has been reported with NSAID use.

Renal blood flow can be decreased by NSAIDs, which may lead to permanent renal damage. Prostaglandins are responsible for maintaining the patency of the afferent renal tubule. Inhibition by NSAIDs decreases glomerular filtration pressure, resulting in decreased blood flow. Because of this mechanism, patients with hypertension, severe vascular disease, and kidney or liver problems and those taking diuretics must be monitored closely.

Central nervous system (CNS) side effects such as dizziness, drowsiness, and confusion may occur with all NSAIDs.

Within the class, some drug-specific adverse reactions occur. Meclofenamate, for example, has a high incidence (> 10%) of abdominal cramping and diarrhea. Paradoxically, indomethacin tends to have more severe CNS adverse effects, such as headache.

Concern exists about NSAIDs and their risk of cardiovascular events. The U.S. Food and Drug

Administration (FDA) now requires that manufacturers include a black box warning regarding the potentially serious cardiovascular and GI adverse events associated with these drugs. NSAIDs should not be used in heart failure.

Drug–drug interactions

Interactions are the same as those associated with aspirin. Ibuprofen may diminish the antiplatelet mechanism of aspirin if it is taken before aspirin or taken daily on a scheduled basis. It is recommended that aspirin be taken 2 hours before taking ibuprofen.

COX-2 inhibitors

COX-1 is the isoenzyme constitutively found in most tissues that produce the prostaglandins PGI_2 and PGE_2, which protect the gastric barrier, and thromboxane A_2, which is responsible for platelet function. COX-2 is the inducible isoenzyme present at sites of inflammation. COX-2 is also found in the brain, the kidneys, and the reproductive organs. Celecoxib (Celebrex) has been shown to have lower incidence of endoscopically demonstrated gastroduodenal lesions than do ibuprofen, naproxen, and diclofenac. The lower risk for GI complications is apparently eliminated when patients take low-dose aspirin concomitantly.

Celecoxib
Mechanism of action
Celecoxib selectively inhibits prostaglandin synthesis by specifically targeting the COX-2 isoenzyme.

Patient instructions
Patients with a history of allergic reaction to sulfonamides should avoid the use of celecoxib.

Adverse drug events
Although the rates of GI ulceration have been demonstrated to be lower with COX-2 inhibitors than with traditional NSAIDs, the risk is not completely eliminated. In addition, the risk of dyspepsia, abdominal pain, and nausea is not significantly less with COX-2 inhibitors than with traditional NSAIDs. Celecoxib now contains a black box warning regarding cardiovascular and GI risk associated with its use (as described later).

Drug–drug interactions
Interactions are the same as those associated with aspirin.

Parameters to monitor
Complete blood count (CBC) as well as creatinine should be monitored at least yearly.

Other aspects
The FDA recommended the voluntary removal of valdecoxib (Bextra) from the market in 2005 because of the lack of adequate data on the cardiovascular safety of its long-term use and the recent data demonstrating increased cardiovascular risk in short-term coronary artery bypass graft (CABG) patients. This risk is in addition to that of potentially life-threatening skin reactions. Merck removed rofecoxib (Vioxx) from the market in September 2004 because its use was shown to be associated with an increased cardiovascular risk in the VIGOR (Vioxx Gastrointestinal Outcomes Research), APPROVE (Adenomatous Polyp Prevention on Vioxx), and VICTOR (Vioxx in Colorectal Therapy, Definition of Optimal Regimen) trials. The FDA has concluded that the benefits of celecoxib outweigh the risks in properly selected and informed patients. Celecoxib contains a black box warning about cardiovascular and GI risk. Patients with a high risk of cardiovascular events should not use celecoxib, including CABG patients. Low doses of celecoxib (200 mg per day) do not seem to be associated with increased risk.

Disease-modifying antirheumatic drugs

Unlike the NSAIDs, DMARDs have the ability to reduce or prevent joint damage and preserve joint integrity and function. The ACR recommends that patients with an established diagnosis of RA be offered treatment with DMARDs. Biologic DMARDs are reserved for use after failure of nonbiologic agents, unless the patient has early disease with high activity and poor prognosis risk factors. Methotrexate is typically selected for initial therapy because of its track record to induce long-term response. Methotrexate or leflunomide may be used as monotherapy in patients with all disease durations and activity regardless of poor prognostic features. Unfortunately, all DMARDs tend to lose effectiveness over time.

Nonbiologic DMARDs

Hydroxychloroquine
Mechanism of action
Hydroxychloroquine (Plaquenil) may inhibit interleukin-1 release by monocytes, thereby decreasing macrophage chemotaxis and phagocytosis. It also inhibits the function of toll-like receptors that con-

tribute to autoimmune disease, limiting B cell and dendritic cell activation.

Patient instructions

Beneficial effect may not be seen until 1–6 months of use. Patients should report any changes in vision to their health care provider immediately.

Adverse drug events

The most serious potential adverse effect associated with hydroxychloroquine is retinal damage that can lead to vision loss. This damage is caused by the deposition of the drug in the melanin layer of the cones. A cumulative dose of 800 g and age > 70 years increase the risk. Hydroxychloroquine may also cause rash, abdominal cramping, diarrhea, myopathy, skin pigment changes, and peripheral neuropathy.

Parameters to monitor

Ophthalmic evaluations should be performed at baseline. If the patient has no risk factors (liver disease, retinal disease, age > 60) and the baseline examination is normal, the American College of Ophthalmology recommends no further testing for 5 years. High-risk patients should have annual exams.

Dose

The dose is 6–7.5 mg/kg of lean body weight daily or 200 mg bid (maximum dose).

Sulfasalazine

Mechanism of action

The intestinal flora breaks sulfasalazine (Azulfidine) down to 5-aminosalicylic acid and sulfapyridine, the active moiety in RA. Sulfapyridine likely inhibits endothelial cell proliferation, reactive oxygen species, and cytokines. In addition, it has been shown to slow radiographic progression of RA.

Patient instructions

Sulfasalazine may produce effects more quickly (within 1 month) than hydroxychloroquine. A coated tablet form may help reduce adverse GI effects.

Adverse drug events

The most common adverse reactions associated with sulfasalazine include headache, GI intolerance, dysgeusia, rash, leukopenia, and thrombocytopenia. A reversible oligozoospermia can occur in up to 33% of males and thus may impair fertility.

Drug–drug interactions

Sulfasalazine may inhibit the absorption of folic acid.

Parameters to monitor

Patient tests should include baseline CBC and liver function tests (LFTs). Patients should then have a CBC every 2–4 weeks for the first 3 months and then once every 3 months thereafter. Patients with glucose-6-phosphate dehydrogenase (G6PD) deficiency should not receive sulfasalazine.

Dose

Begin with 500 mg daily, titrated up to 1–3 g/day divided bid.

Other aspects

Patients should receive a pneumococcal vaccination before initiation.

Methotrexate

Mechanism of action

Methotrexate (Rheumatrex) inhibits dihydrofolate reductase, which reduces dihydrofolate to tetrahydrofolate. Tetrahydrofolate can be used as a carrier of single carbon units for the synthesis of nucleotides and thymidylate. Therefore, methotrexate interferes with deoxyribonucleic acid (DNA) synthesis, repair, and cellular replication.

Patient instructions

Patients should not take this medicine more than once per week. Daily dosing would be disastrous. Patients should be instructed not to drink any alcohol. Methotrexate is a teratogen and is pregnancy category X. Pregnancy and lactation should be avoided. Females should wait 3–6 months after discontinuation before conception, and males should wait 3 months before fathering a child. Doses up to 30 mg weekly do not affect female fertility but can cause a reversible male sterility.

Adverse drug events

- *Liver:* Methotrexate may cause liver damage. People with diabetes, liver problems, obesity, and psoriasis and those who are elderly or alcoholic are at higher risk. If LFTs are more than three times the upper limit of normal, methotrexate should be discontinued.
- *Bone marrow:* Leukopenia, thrombocytopenia, and pancytopenia are rare but serious adverse events associated with methotrexate therapy.
- *Lung:* Pulmonary toxicity is thought to occur in 0.1–1.2% of people who take methotrexate. Risk factors for the development of pulmonary toxicity include age; diabetes; rheumatoid involvement

of the lungs; protein in the urine; and previous use of sulfasalazine, oral gold, or penicillamine.

- *GI:* Nausea, vomiting, and stomatitis occur with an incidence of 5–30%.

Drug–drug interactions

Aspirin and other NSAIDs may increase methotrexate concentrations by as much as 30–35%. Trimethoprim-sulfamethoxazole may cause additive hematologic abnormalities because of its similar affinity for dihydrofolate reductase.

Parameters to monitor

CBC, LFTs, albumin, and creatinine should be monitored every 2–4 weeks for the first 3 months and every 8–12 weeks thereafter. Patients at risk for hepatitis B and C should be screened prior to initiation.

Other aspects

Taking folate supplements may help minimize adverse effects such as liver toxicity and should be regularly prescribed with methotrexate. Folic acid in doses up to 3 mg/day has proven effective and does not diminish methotrexate activity.

Dose

The dose is 7.5–25 mg once weekly.

Leflunomide
Mechanism of action

Leflunomide (Arava) inhibits dihydroorotate dehydrogenase (an enzyme involved in de novo pyrimidine synthesis) and has antiproliferative activity. Several in vivo and in vitro experimental models have demonstrated its anti-inflammatory effect.

Patient instructions

Leflunomide is pregnancy category X. Women taking leflunomide who wish to become pregnant should follow the drug elimination procedure outlined below under "Other aspects." Patients on leflunomide should be instructed not to drink any alcohol.

Adverse drug events

Diarrhea, elevated LFTs, alopecia, hypertension, and rash have been reported with leflunomide therapy.

Drug–drug interactions

An increased risk of liver toxicity exists when leflunomide is used in conjunction with methotrexate. Rifampin causes a 40% increase in levels of leflunomide's active metabolite, M1.

Parameters to monitor

CBC, LFTs, albumin, and creatinine should be monitored every 2–4 weeks for the first 3 months and every 8–12 weeks thereafter. If alanine aminotransferase exceeds two times the upper limit of normal, reduce the dose of leflunomide to 10 mg/day. Patients at risk for hepatitis B and C should be screened prior to initiation.

Kinetics

After absorption, 80% of the parent compound is converted to the active metabolite, M1, which is responsible for all of leflunomide's activity. Because the half-life is 2 weeks, a loading dose is necessary. In addition, M1 undergoes extensive enterohepatic recirculation.

Other aspects

Begin the following drug elimination procedure if a patient decides to become pregnant: 8 g of cholestyramine three times daily for 11 days; plasma levels of M1 < 0.02 mg/L must be verified on two separate occasions at least 14 days apart.

Many randomized controlled trials have established leflunomide as an alternative to methotrexate as monotherapy.

Dose

The dose is 100 mg daily for 3 days (loading dose), then 20 mg daily.

Gold compounds

The intramuscular (IM) gold compounds are gold sodium thiomalate (Myochrysine) and aurothioglucose (Solganal). Auranofin (Ridaura) is given orally.

Mechanism of action

The mechanism of action of gold compounds is currently unknown; they appear to suppress the synovitis seen in RA. Current research indicates that they may stimulate specific protective factors, such as interleukin-6 and interleukin-10.

Patient instructions

Patients receiving gold therapy should avoid prolonged sun exposure, which may increase the risk of serious rash.

Adverse drug events
IM gold

Patients may experience an immediate "nitroid reaction" (i.e., flushing, weakness, dizziness, sweating, syncope, hypotension). Rash is the single-largest adverse effect associated with gold therapy. The rash may range from simple erythema to exfoliative dermatitis. Gold therapy may also cause proteinuria or microscopic hematuria. Rarely, immunologic glomerulonephritis may occur, in which case gold therapy should be permanently discontinued. Leukopenia and thrombocytopenia occur with a 1–3% incidence.

Oral gold

Adverse reactions are similar to those associated with the IM formulation. However, GI complaints of nausea, diarrhea, emesis, and dysgeusia are higher.

Drug–drug interactions

Patients receiving concomitant penicillamine therapy may be subject to an increased risk of toxicity associated with gold therapy. The risk of rash is higher when gold therapy is used with hydroxychloroquine.

Parameters to monitor

At baseline, all patients should have a CBC, platelet count, creatinine profile, and urinalysis for protein. For patients receiving IM therapy, a CBC, platelet count, and urinalysis are recommended every 1–2 weeks for the first 20 weeks and then again at the time of each (or every other) injection. Those on oral therapy should have a CBC, platelet count, and urinalysis for protein every 4–12 weeks.

Other aspects

Aurothioglucose may have a lower rate of injection reactions; its sesame seed formulation slows absorption.

Dose
IM gold

A 10 mg test dose IM is followed by a 25 mg test dose on week 2 and then weekly 50 mg doses until a cumulative dose of 1 g is achieved. The maintenance regimen is 50 mg every 2 weeks for 3 months or until 1.5 g is given; then every 3 weeks; and then monthly.

Oral gold

The dose is 3 mg bid up to 3 mg tid.

Biologic DMARDs

Anti–tumor necrosis factor therapy

The drugs used in anti–tumor necrosis factor (anti-TNF) therapy are infliximab (Remicade), etanercept (Enbrel), adalimumab (Humira), golimumab (Simponi), and certolizumab (Cimzia).

Mechanism of action

Composed of human constant and murine variable regions, infliximab is an antibody that binds specifically to human tumor necrosis factor (TNF).

Similarly, by binding specifically to TNF, etanercept binds and blocks its interaction with the cell surface's TNF receptors. It is produced by recombinant technology in Chinese hamster ovaries and is not an antibody.

Adalimumab, certolizumab, and golimumab are recombinant human monoclonal antibodies that bind to TNF with high affinity. Certolizumab is unique in that it is a pegylated (polyethylene glycolated) Fab fragment derived from a high-affinity humanized anti-TNF monoclonal Ab. The Fab fragments lack the Fc portion of immunoglobulin, so the Fc responses such as complement or Ab-dependent cell-mediated cytotoxicity are not realized, which is distinct from the other anti-TNF Ab, but it still neutralizes membrane anti-TNF.

Patient instructions

Patients should not receive live vaccines during treatment. Therapy should be temporarily discontinued in the event of an acute infection.

Adverse drug events

Therapy has been associated with serious mycobacterial, fungal, and opportunistic infectious complications such as sepsis and tuberculosis, leading to requirement of an FDA black box warning to that effect in 2008. Other adverse reactions include rash, headache, nausea, and cough. Although rare, anti-TNF drugs have been associated with nerve damage that resembles the disease process in multiple sclerosis, congestive heart failure, skin cancers, and lupus-like syndromes. Lymphoma has been reported with TNF antagonists, although risk of solid tumors appears neutral. These drugs should not be used in patients with hepatitis B.

Drug–drug interactions

Live vaccines may interact with these drugs. Biologic drugs should not be used in combination because that increases the risk of infection.

Parameters to monitor

Be clinically alert for tuberculosis, histoplasmosis, and other opportunistic infections.

Other aspects

Patients should be tested for tuberculosis (skin testing, chest radiograph, or both) and hepatitis B (if risk factors are present) before initiating therapy with any biologic agent. Currently, infliximab is approved for therapy only in combination with methotrexate. Patients should receive appropriate vaccinations prior to initiation, such as pneumococcal, influenza, hepatitis B, and herpes zoster.

Dose

The dosage for infliximab is 3 mg/kg intravenous (IV) initially, at weeks 2 and 6, and then every 8 weeks in combination with methotrexate.

The dosage for etanercept is 25 mg subcutaneous twice weekly or 50 mg subcutaneous once weekly.

The dosage for adalimumab is 40 mg subcutaneous every second week.

The dosage for golimumab is 50 mg subcutaneous every 4 weeks.

The dosage for certolizumab is 400 mg subcutaneous initially and at weeks 2 and 4, followed by a dose of 200 mg every other week. Maintenance dosing up to 400 mg every 4 weeks can be considered.

Anakinra
Mechanism of action

Anakinra (Kineret) blocks the biologic activity of interleukin-1 by competitively inhibiting interleukin-1 binding to the interleukin-1 type I receptor.

Patient instructions

Kineret is supplied in a single-use, prefilled syringe that should be stored in the refrigerator. Any syringe left unrefrigerated for more than 24 hours should be discarded.

Adverse drug events

Like the anti-TNF agents, anakinra increases the risk of serious infections. Injection-site reactions are extremely common. Headache, nausea, diarrhea, sinusitis, flu-like symptoms, and abdominal pain have also been reported.

Drug–drug interactions

Live vaccines can interact with anakinra.

Parameters to monitor

Patients should have a CBC checked at baseline, then monthly for 3 months, and then once every 3 months for the first year of therapy.

Dose

The dose is 100 mg subcutaneous daily.

Abatacept
Mechanism of action

Abatacept (Orencia) selectively modulates T-cell activation causing downregulation and an anti-inflammatory effect.

Adverse drug events

Like the other biologic DMARDs, abatacept increases the risk of infections, especially upper respiratory infections. Nausea and headache are also frequently reported. In addition, patients with chronic obstructive pulmonary disease developed adverse effects more frequently than with a placebo. More cases of lung cancer were observed in patients treated with abatacept than with a placebo. The lymphoma rate was higher as well.

Drug–drug interactions

Use of abatacept is contraindicated with other biologic DMARDs because of increased risk of infection. Live vaccines are contraindicated as well.

Other aspects

Abatacept contains maltose and may falsely elevate blood glucose readings. Monitors that do not react to maltose, such as those based on glucose dehydrogenase nicotine adenine dinucleotide, glucose oxidase, or glucose hexokinase test methods, are recommended.

Dose

Dose is based on weight (< 60 kg = 500 mg; 60–100 kg = 750 mg; > 100 kg = 1,000 mg). Infusions are given over 30 minutes. After the initial dose, give at 2 and 4 weeks, followed by every 4 weeks. Alternatively, 125 mg subcutaneous weekly may be prescribed after one weight-based loading dose.

Rituximab
Mechanism of action

Rituximab (Rituxan) causes a transient depletion of B-lymphocytes by binding to the CD20 surface antigens.

Other aspects

Rituximab should be used only in patients with moderate to severe RA who have had an inadequate response or a contraindication to anti-TNF products.

Dose

Give 1,000 mg every 2 weeks for two doses; patients should be premedicated with a glucocorticoid to decrease infusion-related reactions.

Tocilizumab

Mechanism of action

Tocilizumab (Actemra) is an interleukin-6 receptor–inhibiting antibody. The FDA approved tocilizumab in 2010 for moderate to severe RA in adults who have not achieved an adequate response to one or more anti-TNF agents, with or without methotrexate. It can be used with other nonbiologic DMARDs.

Patient instructions

Side effects should be reported to the health care provider immediately.

Adverse drug events

Like the anti-TNF agents, tocilizumab increases the risk of serious infections. It also has been reported to rarely cause generalized peritonitis, diverticulitis, lower GI perforation, fistulae, and intra-abdominal abscesses. Increased transaminases, especially with methotrexate, and decreased white blood cells and platelets have also been reported, as have increased total cholesterol, LDL (low-density lipoprotein), triglycerides, and HDL (high-density lipoprotein) levels. Multiple sclerosis and chronic inflammatory demyelinating polyneuropathy cases may occur, and tocilizumab may carry a malignancy risk of 2.8%.

More common side effects include severe allergic reactions (0.2%), rash (2%), mouth ulcers (2%), abdominal pain (2%), dizziness (3%), hypertension (6%), infusion reactions (7%), headache (7%), upper respiratory infections (5–8%), and serious infections (17.5%).

Drug–drug interactions

In chronic inflammation, the formation of cytochrome P450 (CYP450) enzymes is suppressed by increased levels of cytokines such as interleukin-6. Tocilizumab could normalize the formation of CYP450 enzymes; thus, in hepatically metabolized narrow therapeutic index drugs, an increase in CYP450-mediated metabolism may lower the levels of these drugs (warfarin, theophylline, phenytoin, cyclosporine, carbamazepine, simvastatin, omeprazole, and so on).

Parameters to monitor

- Patients should have CBC and LFTs checked at baseline, then every 4–8 weeks.
- Assess lipid parameters at 4–8 weeks following initiation of therapy and every 6 months thereafter. The risk of tuberculosis is not known, but do PPD (purified protein derivative) prior to starting.

Dose

The dose is a 4 mg/kg IV infusion over 1 hour every 4 weeks. The dose may be increased to 8 mg/kg on the basis of clinical response.

Tofacitinib

Mechanism of action

Tofacitinib (Xeljanz) is a janus kinase (JAK) inhibitor. The JAK family (JAK1, JAK2, JAK3, tyrosine kinase 2 [TYK2]) are tyrosine kinase proteins that signal in pairs and facilitate the phosphorylation process of many proteins intracellularly. One such group of proteins is the signal transducers and activators of transcription (STATs). These proteins regulate the transcription of genes that control inflammatory responses. Tofacitinib affects the signaling pathway at the point of the JAK family by preventing phosphorylation and activation of STATs. Tofacitinib is approved for moderate to severe RA patients who have failed or cannot take methotrexate as monotherapy or take tofacitinib in combination with methotrexate or another nonbiologic DMARD. It cannot be combined with another biologic or immunosuppressing drug such as azathioprine or cyclosporine.

Patient instructions

Patients should not receive live vaccines during treatment. Discontinue tofacitinib during infections.

Adverse drug events

Serious infections, increased risk of malignancies, increased lipids, neutropenia, transaminases elevations, and drops in hemoglobin have been reported. One intestinal perforation was reported in clinical trials. A REMS [Risk Evaluation and Mitigation Strategy] Medication Safety Guide is available for patients.

Drug–drug interactions

Tofacitinib is metabolized by CYP3A4; therefore, drugs that inhibit or induce CYP3A4 may affect its pharmacokinetics. Drugs that inhibit CYP2C19 alone or P-glycoprotein are unlikely to affect tofacitinib.

Parameters to monitor

Patients should have baseline CBC, and then hemoglobin again at 4–8 weeks and every 3 months thereafter. Lymphocyte count should be done at baseline and every month. Lipids should be done at 4–8 weeks, and liver tests should be checked periodically. Patients should be vigilant to report any signs or symptoms of infection.

Dose

The dose is 5 mg bid or, in the following circumstances, 5 mg daily po:

- Moderate or severe renal insufficiency
- Moderate hepatic impairment
- Concomitant therapy with potential inhibitors of CYP3A4 (e.g., ketoconazole)
- Concomitant therapy with one or more drugs causing moderate inhibition of CYP3A4 and potent inhibition of CYP2C19 (e.g., fluconazole)

Other agents

Azathioprine

Azathioprine (Imuran) is a purine analogue immuno-suppressive agent that is generally reserved for refractory RA. It is associated with dose-related bone marrow suppression, stomatitis, diarrhea, rash, and liver failure. Patients must have a baseline CBC, creatinine, and liver profile. Patients should then have a CBC and platelet count every 1–2 weeks after any change in dosage and every 1–3 months thereafter. Azathioprine should not be administered with allopurinol because xanthine oxidase metabolizes 6-mercaptopurine.

Cyclosporine A

By blocking T-cell activation, cyclosporine A (Sand-immune) produces powerful immunosuppressive effects and is beneficial as monotherapy in the treatment of RA. Serious adverse effects such as hypertension, nephrotoxicity, glucose intolerance, and hepatotoxicity have limited its use.

Corticosteroids

Low-dose oral corticosteroids (< 10 mg/day of prednisone or the equivalent) and local injections of glucocorticoids are highly effective. Studies indicate that corticosteroids decrease the progression of RA. They may be useful for acute flare-ups and in patients with significant systemic manifestations of RA. RA is associated with an increased risk of osteoporosis (independent of steroid therapy), and the addition of steroidal anti-inflammatory agents increases the risk. Patients on glucocorticoids should receive 1,500 mg of elemental calcium per day and 400–800 international units (IU) of vitamin D per day.

Nondrug Therapy

Joint surgery

Patients may have arthroscopy performed to clean out the bone and cartilage fragments that cause pain

within the joint capsule. Patients may eventually require complete joint replacement surgery.

Lifestyle modifications

A mild exercise regimen can be an effective therapy.

Some evidence suggests a moderate increase in daily protein intake may be beneficial in RA.

Patients with RA benefit from a formal support group.

Rest is an important strategy as well.

26-4. Osteoarthritis

Osteoarthritis (OA), a disease that affects the weight-bearing joints of the peripheral and axial skeleton, is the most common form of arthritis in the United States. OA is also known as *degenerative joint disease*.

Incidence

Approximately 50% of people over the age of 65 have OA. Before the age of 50, men have a higher incidence primarily because of sports injuries; however, after the age of 50, women have a higher incidence.

Clinical Presentation

Pain is a common initial finding in patients with OA. This pain typically worsens with weight-bearing activity and improves with rest of the affected joint. Changes in weather and barometric pressure tend to influence the severity of pain.

Joint stiffness, including morning stiffness, is another common complaint. This stiffness differs from that of RA. It is relatively short in duration, is related to periods of inactivity, and resolves with movement.

Crepitus is common, especially when the knee joint is involved.

Joint deformities also occur in OA. Heberden's nodes, Bouchard's nodes, and osteophytes on the distal interphalangeal and proximal interphalangeal joints are commonly seen.

Pathophysiology

Although the causes of OA are not completely understood, biomechanical stresses affecting the articular cartilage and subchondral bone are thought to be the primary factors in the development of OA. In addition, inflammatory, biochemical, and immunologic components play a role. The function of the normal cartilage—that is, to dissipate the force and stress caused by normal weight-bearing activity—is impaired in OA.

- Collagen fibers are destroyed and subsequently release proteoglycans. The hydration of the cartilage increases, and the cartilage becomes thick.
- Metalloproteinases, which degrade the proteoglycans, are released to initiate the reparation process. This degradation causes an increase in chondrocyte activity.
- The resulting cartilage is thin because the chondrocyte activity cannot match the rate at which proteoglycan degradation occurs.
- With this ever-thinning layer of cartilage now exposing bone, the grinding motion stimulates osteoclast and osteoblast activity, thereby causing bone resorption and vascular changes. Ultimately, these changes lead to the formation of osteophytes.

Diagnostic Criteria

Osteoarthritis of the hip

According to the ACR classification criteria, osteoarthritis of the hip exists if the patient has hip pain and at least two of the following:

- Erythrocyte sedimentation rate < 20 mm/h
- Radiographic femoral or acetabular osteophytes
- Radiographic joint space narrowing

Other criteria include one of the following:

- Hip pain and radiographic femoral or acetabular osteophytes
- Hip pain and radiographic joint space narrowing and erythrocyte sedimentation rate < 20 mm/h

Osteoarthritis of the knee

According to ACR classification criteria, osteoarthritis of the knee exists if the patient has knee pain, radiographic osteophytes, and at least one of the following:

- Age > 50 years
- Morning stiffness ≤ 30 minutes in duration
- Crepitus on motion

Other criteria include one of the following:

- Knee pain and radiographic osteophytes
- Knee pain and age ≥ 40 years, morning stiffness ≤ 30 minutes in duration, and crepitus on motion

Treatment Principles

Treatment of patients with OA focuses on symptom control. Currently, no therapeutic options are known to change the course of the disease.

Drug Therapy

Pain relief is the primary treatment goal for patients with OA. The recommended initial drug of choice is acetaminophen. For those patients who do not respond fully, an NSAID (see discussion of this class in Section 26-3) is added. Box 26-1 outlines pharmacologic therapy for patients with osteoarthritis.

Acetaminophen

Mechanism of action
Acetaminophen centrally inhibits prostaglandin synthesis.

Patient instructions
Patients with hepatic disease or viral hepatitis are at risk of toxicity from chronic acetaminophen use.

Adverse drug events
Hepatotoxicity is the most severe side effect associated with acetaminophen therapy. For this reason, patients should not ingest more than 4 g of acetaminophen per

---

Box 26-1. Pharmacologic Therapy for Patients with Osteoarthritis

Oral

- Acetaminophen
- Oral NSAIDs, including COX-2 inhibitors
- Other pure analgesics:
  - Tramadol (Ultram) 50 mg/dose (up to 400 mg/day)
  - Ultracet 37.5 mg/dose (up to 300 mg/day)

Intra-articular (not for hand OA)

- Glucocorticoids
- Hyaluronan

Topical

- Capsaicin
- NSAIDs

Opioids

- Patients who have an inadequate response and cannot or will not have total knee or hip arthroplasty may use opioids, duloxetine, or both.

day. Long-term therapy has also been linked to renal failure.

Other aspects

Acetaminophen is generally considered the initial drug of choice; however, no clinical trials have compared its side effects, potential toxicity, or pain-relieving properties with those of NSAIDs.

Tramadol

Tramadol is a central opioid agonist that binds to mu receptors and weakly inhibits norepinephrine and serotonin reuptake.

Adverse drug events

Nausea, vomiting, constipation, and seizures are associated with tramadol use. Withdrawal symptoms may occur with abrupt discontinuation.

Drug interactions

Tramadol is contraindicated in patients taking monoamine oxidase inhibitors because of the risk of serotonin syndrome. It should be used with caution in combination with any other serotonergic drugs.

Other aspects

Tramadol is available as an immediate-release product (Ultram), as an extended-release product (Ultram ER), and in combination with acetaminophen 325 mg (Ultracet).

Topical agents

Capsaicin
Mechanism of action
Derived from the pepper plant, capsaicin works by inhibiting the release of substance P, which is responsible for transmitting pain from the peripheral to the central nervous system.

Patient instructions
Patients should avoid contact with eyes. It is important to wash hands thoroughly after use.

Adverse drug events
Patients will experience mild burning and stinging at the site of application.

Other aspects
Patients usually derive benefit after several weeks of application. Capsaicin is often used in conjunction with oral agents.

Topical NSAIDs (Diclofenac gel)
Mechanism of action
NSAIDs prevent prostaglandin formation by inhibiting the action of the enzyme cyclooxygenase.

Patient instructions
For lower extremities, apply 4 g of the 1% topical gel to the affected foot, knee, or ankle four times daily. Do not apply more than 16 g of the 1% gel to any single joint of the lower extremities. For upper extremities, apply 2 g of the 1% topical gel to the affected hand, elbow, or wrist four times daily. Gently massage the gel into the skin to ensure application to the entire affected hand (palm, back of hands, fingers), elbow, or wrist. Do not apply more than 8 g of the 1% gel to any single joint of the upper extremities.

Adverse drug events
Application site reactions may occur as well as the class effects of oral NSAIDs.

Other aspects
In persons ≥ 75 years, topical NSAIDs are preferred over oral NSAIDs.

Glucosamine sulfate and chondroitin

Mechanism of action
Glucosamine is found naturally in articular cartilage and acts as a substrate in the synthesis of proteoglycans. Chondroitin, another constituent in the cartilage, attracts and retains water, which provides shock absorption. In addition, chondroitin prevents the breakdown of cartilage and stimulates RNA (ribonucleic acid) synthesis of chondrocytes.

Patient instructions
Patients taking anticoagulants concomitantly may be at increased risk of bleeding.

Adverse drug events
Adverse events tend to be mild but include dyspepsia and euphoria.

Other aspects
This combination is available over the counter and has some clinical literature to support its use, although the American College of Rheumatology Guidelines conditionally recommend against its use in hip and knee OA.

Other agents

The FDA has approved hyaluronic acid derivatives for the treatment of pain associated with OA of the knee. These agents may be an option after all conventional therapies for OA have been exhausted. The injection of this product into the synovium appears to replenish the viscosity to the space, thus enabling normal tissue to regenerate.

Nondrug Therapy

Nondrug therapy for OA consists of the following:

- Patient education
- Self-management programs (e.g., Arthritis Foundation Self-Management Program)
- Psychosocial interventions
- Weight loss (if overweight)
- Aerobic exercise programs, tai chi
- Physical therapy
- Manual therapy, supervised exercise
- Assistive devices for ambulation
- Patellar taping, splint use
- Lateral-wedged insole for medial compartment knee OA, medially wedged insoles for lateral compartment knee OA
- Assistive devices for activities of daily living

26-5. Gout

Gout, a systemic disease caused by the buildup of uric acid in the joints, causes inflammation, swelling, and pain. *Hyperuricemia* is defined as a urate level > 7 mg/dL in men and > 6 mg/dL in women.

Incidence

Gout has been known as "the disease of kings and the king of diseases" and can be traced to the time of Hippocrates. Gout occurs in approximately 1% of the population. The vast majority of gout patients are men.

Clinical Presentation

Pain in one joint of the lower extremity is the most common first symptom of gout. The initial period of pain, usually monarticular and self-limiting, is followed by a period in which the patient is completely asymptomatic.

Termed *intercritical periods*, the time between acute gouty arthritis attacks may be 3 months to 2 years. The length of time shortens as the disease progresses.

The first attack is typically at night or in the early morning.

Gout commonly affects the ankle, heel, knee, wrist, finger, elbow, and instep. The most common site of the initial attack is the first MTP joint and is known as *podagra*.

The patient may experience fever, chills, and malaise during an acute gouty arthritis attack. Left untreated, the attack may last 1–2 weeks.

The skin over the affected joint becomes red, hot, swollen, and tender. As the patient recovers from the attack, local desquamation may occur.

Pathophysiology

Uric acid is the end product of purine metabolism (Figure 26-3). Xanthine oxidase is the rate-limiting step in the formation of uric acid. Uric acid, which serves no known biological function, has a body content of 1–1.2 g. Foods that are a source of purines (including organ meats and some seafood) and alcohol (especially beer) may need to be restricted. Intake of foods containing high fructose sweeteners should be reduced because these sweeteners increase uric acid levels.

Approximately 70% of uric acid is excreted via the kidneys. At physiologic pH, uric acid primarily exists as monosodium urate (MSU) salt.

Approximately 95% of serum uric acid is filtered across the glomerulus. Of this filtered amount, almost

Figure 26-3. Ribose–Uric Acid Pathway

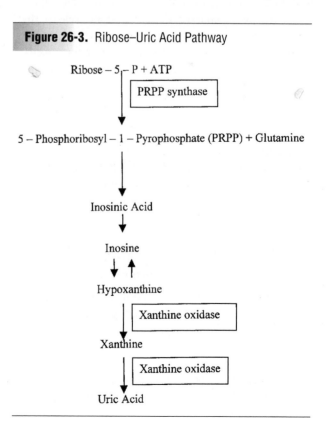

Ribose $-$ 5 $-$ P + ATP

PRPP synthase

5 – Phosphoribosyl – 1 – Pyrophosphate (PRPP) + Glutamine

Inosinic Acid

Inosine

Hypoxanthine

Xanthine oxidase

Xanthine

Xanthine oxidase

Uric Acid

100% is reabsorbed in the early part of the proximal tubule, only to be secreted back into the lumen in the more distal part of the tubule.

Primary gout is a result of an innate defect in purine metabolism or uric acid excretion. In this case, hyperuricemia may result from uric acid overproduction (in "overproducers"), impaired renal clearance of uric acid (in "underexcreters"), or a combination of both. In rare instances, enzyme defects of either hypoxanthine guanine phosphoribosyltransferase or 5-phosphoribosyl-1-pyrophosphate may cause primary gout (see Figure 26-3).

Secondary gout is associated with increased nucleic acid turnover, decreased renal function, increased purine production, or drug-induced decreased elimination of uric acid. Hematologic disorders that are lymphoproliferative and myeloproliferative in nature are known causes of secondary hyperuricemia. Salicylates such as aspirin may inhibit tubular secretion of uric acid at low doses. Diuretics, with the exception of spironolactone, may cause hyperuricemia. Ethambutol, pyrazinamide, nicotinic acid, ethanol, niacin, and cyclosporine are known to cause an increase in serum uric acid.

Acute gout attacks are caused by the deposition of MSU in the synovium of the joint. This deposition results in the stimulation of the body's inflammatory cascade. The MSU crystals undergo phagocytosis by polymorphonuclear leukocytes. These leukocytes, damaged by the sharp crystals, burst and release their contents (interleukin-1, lysosomes, prostaglandins) into the synovium, resulting in the inflammatory reaction—that is, pain, swelling, and erythema.

If left untreated, deposits of MSU crystals, also known as *tophi,* lead to joint deformity and disability. Ultimately, patients may develop one of two types of renal disease: urate nephropathy or uric acid nephropathy. Urate nephropathy results from the deposition of MSU crystals in the renal interstitium. Uric acid nephropathy results from the deposition of uric acid in the collecting tubules.

Diagnostic Criteria

The American Rheumatism Association lists the following criteria for the diagnosis of gout:

- **Definite:** Sodium urate crystals in the affected joint appear negatively birefringent when viewed through a polarized light source.
- **Suggestive:** A minimum of six of the following criteria should be met:
  - More than one attack of arthritis
  - Development of maximum inflammation within 1 day

- Oligoarthritis attack
- Redness over joint
- Painful or swollen first MTP joint
- Unilateral attack on first MTP joint
- Unilateral attack on tarsal joint
- Tophus
- Hyperuricemia
- Asymptomatic swelling within a joint

Ruling out pseudogout is also important. In pseudogout, crystals deposited into the joint synovium cause intense pain and inflammation, but the culprit is calcium pyrophosphate dihydrate, not monosodium urate.

Treatment Goals

- Relieve pain and inflammation
- Reduce serum uric acid concentration
- Prevent recurrent gout attacks

Drug Therapy

Drugs for the treatment of gout are outlined in Table 26-3.

Acute gouty arthritis attack

Three treatments are available: colchicine, NSAIDs (indomethacin in particular), and corticosteroids. Avoiding treatments that affect serum uric acid concentrations is best during an acute attack.

Colchicine
Mechanism of action
Colchicine inhibits the phagocytosis of urate crystals by leukocytes. Colchicine also inhibits the release of chemotactic factor, thus reducing the adhesion of polymorphonuclear leukocytes. The net result makes colchicine an anti-inflammatory agent without analgesic activity.

Patient instructions
Patients should immediately stop taking colchicine if abdominal cramping or diarrhea occurs. In the past, multiple doses were allowed and patients were told they should never exceed a total of 8 mg during an acute gouty arthritis attack. New recommendations state three tablets within the first day only to avoid toxicity.

Adverse drug events
Nausea, bloating, emesis, and diarrhea occur in up to 80% of patients taking colchicine. Rarely, it may cause

Table 26-3. Drugs for the Treatment of Gout

Generic name	Trade name	Classification	Normal dose	Comments	Dosage forms
Colchicine		Anti-inflammatory	1.2 mg po followed by 0.6 mg 1 hour later. Maximum dose is 1.8 mg over 1 hour.	Drug may be used for chronic suppressive therapy; dose must be adjusted for renal insufficiency.	po
Probenecid	Benemid	Uricosuric agent	250–500 mg bid	Avoid salicylates; take with plenty of water.	po
Allopurinol	Zyloprim	Xanthine oxidase inhibitor	100–300 mg daily or divided dose	Drug may cause rash; reduce dosage in renal failure.	po
Febuxostat	Uloric	Xanthine oxidase inhibitor	40 mg daily; if uric acid not less than 6 mg/dL, increase to 80 mg daily	Drug may be used in mild renal impairment.	po
Indomethacin	Indocin	NSAID	50 mg tid	Drug may cause fluid retention, GI bleeding.	po, IV, suppository

bone marrow suppression. This effect occurs with a higher incidence in those patients with underlying renal or hepatic dysfunction. When colchicine is given intravenously, possible extravasation may cause local skin necrosis. In addition, the IV route has been associated with bone marrow suppression, disseminated intravascular coagulation, seizures, and death. Thus, the IV form has now been taken off the market.

Drug–drug and drug–disease interactions

Patients with active peptic ulcer disease should not take colchicine.

Inhibitors of the CYP450 enzyme 3A4 and p-glycoproteins such as cyclosporine, ketoconazole, ritonavir, clarithromycin, azithromycin, verapamil, and diltiazem may markedly increase colchicine levels, leading to toxicity.

Parameters to monitor

With long-term therapy, patients should have a serum creatinine test, LFT, and complete white blood cell count periodically.

Dose

For the treatment of an acute gouty arthritis attack, patients should take 1.2 mg orally followed by 0.6 mg in 1 hour. Maximum dose is 1.8 mg.

Other aspects

Colchicine is most effective when initiated within 12–36 hours of the attack.

Indomethacin

Indomethacin is the most extensively studied NSAID in the treatment of an acute gouty arthritis attack. Unlike colchicine, indomethacin is effective at any point during the acute attack. For more information, see the review of NSAIDs in Section 26-3.

Corticosteroids

For the treatment of acute gout pain, corticosteroids are effective when given intra-articularly, intravenously, or orally. Their use is limited to treatment failures of colchicine and NSAIDs. Intramuscular corticotropin (adrenocorticotropic hormone) is also effective when given (40 units) to treat an acute gouty arthritis attack. The dose of prednisone for acute attacks usually is 30–60 mg prednisone equivalent once daily for 3–5 days; then taper in 5 mg decrements spread over 10–14 days until discontinuation.

Gout prophylaxis (intercritical period)

Patients with asymptomatic hyperuricemia should not be routinely treated with pharmacologic agents. These patients should undergo a workup to determine the cause of hyperuricemia. The use of low-dose (0.6–1.2 mg/day) colchicine can prevent subsequent attacks of gout. Patients in the intercritical period (after an acute gouty arthritis attack) are candidates for long-term prophylactic therapy directed at affecting serum uric acid levels if they have at least two gout attacks per year or tophi. Prophylactic treatment should be held until at least 2–4 weeks after a flare's resolution. Choice of therapy is based on the patient's pathophysiologic cause of hyperuricemia. Patients are generally classified as *overproducers* or *underexcreters*. Placing the patient on a purine-restricted diet and performing a 24-hour urine collection to measure uric acid concentration may identify overproducers of uric acid. Those patients who excrete more than 600 mg of uric acid are considered overproducers. Once this diagnosis is made, patients are treated with one of three classes of agents: xanthine oxidase inhibitors, uricosurics, and uricase agents. Uricosurics can be used in underexcreters but are less commonly used and are contraindicated in nephrolithiasis. Xanthine oxidase inhibitors should be titrated to achieve a uric acid of less than 6 mg/dL. In late 2010, the FDA announced the approval of a uricase agent, pegloticase (Krystexxa), an IV treatment for chronic gout in adults whose conditions have been refractory to conventional therapy. Pegloticase is a PEGylated uric acid–specific enzyme that lowers serum uric acid levels by catalyzing the oxidation of uric acid to allantoin, an inert and water-soluble purine metabolite that is readily eliminated, primarily by renal excretion.

Probenecid

Mechanism of action

Probenecid (Benemid) is a uricosuric agent that promotes the excretion of uric acid by blocking its reuptake at the proximal convoluted tubule.

Patient instructions

Patients should drink at least 2 liters of water per day to decrease the risk of uric acid stone formation. Patients should take probenecid with food if GI intolerance occurs.

Adverse drug events

Probenecid is generally well tolerated and is associated with very few adverse side effects. Up to 10% of patients receiving probenecid therapy develop uric acid stones. Probenecid may cause abdominal discomfort, but patients can often avoid it by taking probenecid with food.

Drug–drug interactions

Because probenecid prevents the tubular secretion of many weak organic acids, it has potential drug interactions—for example, with the penicillins, cephalosporins, nitrofurantoin, and rifampin. Although the interaction between probenecid, penicillins, and cephalosporins has been used therapeutically, the interaction with nitrofurantoin reduces nitrofurantoin's effectiveness. Using probenecid and aspirin together, even in low doses, is not advisable because aspirin blocks uric acid excretion. A crossover study in patients with gouty arthritis concluded that low-dose aspirin did not significantly interfere with the uricosuric effects of probenecid. Avoiding the combination would be reasonable, however. Additionally, the diuretic effects of furosemide and hydrochlorothiazide are magnified when probenecid is taken concomitantly. Finally, patients receiving sulfonylureas should be monitored closely for hypoglycemia when started on probenecid.

Other aspects

Patients should never begin uricosuric therapy during an acute gouty arthritis attack because of the risk of exacerbating the attack. Probenecid should not be used in patients with a creatinine clearance < 50 mL/min.

Allopurinol

Mechanism of action

Allopurinol (Zyloprim) and its metabolite, oxypurinol, inhibit xanthine oxidase formation (the rate-limiting step in uric acid synthesis), thereby facilitating the clearance of the more water-soluble precursors of uric acid, oxypurines.

Patient instructions

Patients should immediately report any signs of rash to their health care providers. Allopurinol should be taken with food to minimize GI discomfort.

Adverse drug events

Allopurinol is generally well tolerated; the overall occurrence of adverse effects is less than 1%. Patients should be advised that rash, the most common adverse effect, might occur at any time during therapy. The rash may be as simple as a maculopapular eruption or as serious as the life-threatening Stevens–Johnson syndrome (which is exfoliative and erythematous). Rarely, allopurinol may cause alopecia, neutropenia, and hepatitis.

Drug–drug interactions

The chemotherapeutic agents azathioprine and 6-mercaptopurine are metabolized via the xanthine oxidase pathway; therefore, allopurinol and its metabolite oxypurinol may increase serum levels of these agents. The concomitant administration of ampicillin or amoxicillin with allopurinol increases the risk of rash to approximately 20%.

Parameters to monitor

Patients should be encouraged to report the first signs of rash to their health care provider immediately. Patients should have serum creatinine as well as LFTs drawn periodically.

Kinetics

With a half-life of 30 hours, allopurinol is rapidly converted to its active metabolite (oxypurinol). This speed allows for once-daily dosing.

Other aspects

To reduce the risk of precipitating an acute gouty arthritis attack, allopurinol should be initiated at a dose of 100 mg/day and increased at 100 mg intervals weekly to an average dose of 300 mg/day. New guidelines suggest doses of up to 800 mg daily may be prescribed. Patients with renal insufficiency require a dose adjustment. Assuming the target dose is 300 mg/day, patients with a creatinine clearance of 10–20 mL/min should receive 200 mg/day. Those with a clearance of less than 10 mL/min should receive 100 mg/day.

Febuxostat (Uloric) was approved in February 2009 for the chronic management of hyperuricemia in patients with gout. It is also a xanthine oxidase inhibitor; however, unlike allopurinol, it is not a purine-based analog.

Febuxostat

Mechanism of action

Febuxostat (Uloric) inhibits xanthine oxidase formation (the rate-limiting step in uric acid synthesis), thereby facilitating the clearance of the more water-soluble precursors of uric acid, oxypurines.

Adverse drug events

Nausea, rash, elevated liver tests, and dizziness have been reported.

Drug–drug interactions

The chemotherapeutic agents azathioprine and 6-mercaptopurine are metabolized via the xanthine oxidase pathway; therefore, febuxostat may increase serum levels of these agents. The co-administration of theophylline and febuxostat results in higher levels of one of the metabolites of theophylline.

Parameters to monitor

Patients should have LFTs drawn at 2–4 months and then periodically thereafter.

Other aspects

Because of the risk of gout flare, prophylaxis with an NSAID medication or colchicine is recommended when febuxostat is started and may be continued for up to 6 months. Febuxostat may be used in patients with mild to moderate renal impairment.

Secondary hyperuricemia

As discussed earlier, hyperuricemia may be caused by lymphoproliferative and myeloproliferative disorders, as well as their chemotherapeutic treatments (e.g., tumor lysis syndrome). Allopurinol is commonly added to the prescribed chemotherapeutic regimen to prevent complications of hyperuricemia, for example, an acute gouty arthritis attack. Rasburicase (Elitek) is an approved therapeutic agent that is used to prevent hyperuricemia in children with leukemia, lymphoma, and solid-tumor malignancies. Rasburicase is a recombinant urate oxidase enzyme that converts uric acid to allantoin, thereby allowing it to be eliminated. Patients with G6PD deficiency should not use rasburicase.

26-6. Systemic Lupus Erythematosus

Systemic lupus erythematosus (SLE) is a chronic autoimmune inflammatory disorder that can affect any system in the body, including the skin, joints, and internal organs. Women of childbearing age are primarily affected. Fifteen-year survival rates are now approximately 76%. Lupus nephritis and infectious complications are the primary cause of mortality.

Classification

The workup of SLE must include the consideration of an alternative diagnosis. Because other autoimmune diseases have similar characteristics and because the features of SLE, RA, and scleroderma overlap, a thorough assessment is warranted. Drug-induced lupus must be ruled out as well.

Clinical Presentation

Signs and symptoms consistent with SLE include the following:

- Malar rash (a butterfly-shaped rash over the cheeks and across the bridge of the nose)
- Discoid rash (scaly, disk-shaped sores on the face, neck, or chest)
- Photosensitivity
- Oral ulcers

- Arthritis
- Serositis (inflammation of the lining around the heart, lungs, or abdomen that causes pain and shortness of breath)
- Proteinuria
- CNS problems
- Antinuclear antibodies (autoantibodies that react against the body's own cells)
- Anemia, leukopenia, lymphopenia, thrombocytopenia
- Fatigue
- Fever
- Skin rash
- Muscle aches
- Nausea
- Vomiting and diarrhea
- Anorexia
- Raynaud's phenomenon
- Weight loss

Patients typically present with chronic fatigue and depression. Dermatitis and arthritis (in multiple joints) are the most common clinical manifestations. The arthritic pain patients describe is generally out of proportion to the amount of synovitis present. Although it is rare, serious renal abnormalities can occur in patients with SLE. CNS involvement, also rare, can be serious. Lupus-related encephalopathy may occur from scarring of arterioles in the subcortical white matter. In addition, patients with SLE are at risk of stroke because of the thromboembolic nature of the antiphospholipid antibody.

Pathophysiology

The exact pathophysiology of SLE remains unknown. It is an autoimmune disease (type III hypersensitivity) in which patients have an overactivity of B-lymphocytes. The result is hypergammaglobulinemia that ultimately precipitates immune complexes on the vascular membranes, thereby causing activation of complement. Drugs, procainamide being the most predominant, may also cause SLE. Other such medications include phenytoin, chlorpromazine, hydralazine, quinidine, methyldopa, and isoniazid. Patients of the slow acetylator phenotype may have a greater risk for developing drug-induced lupus, particularly with procainamide and hydralazine. Musculoskeletal manifestations are the primary clinical manifestation of drug-induced lupus, but patients may also have fever, fatigue, pericarditis, pleurisy, and weight loss. These usually disappear with drug discontinuation. Antihistone antibodies are specific for drug-induced lupus occurring only in a small percentage of idiopathic lupus patients.

Diagnostic Criteria

Criteria for diagnosing SLE are as follows:

- Characteristic rash across the cheeks
- Discoid lesion rash
- Photosensitivity
- Oral ulcers
- Arthritis
- Inflammation of membranes in lungs, heart, or abdomen
- Evidence of kidney disease
- Evidence of severe neurologic disease
- Blood disorders, including low red blood cell, white blood cell, and platelet counts
- Immunologic abnormalities (positive for anti-double-stranded DNA antibody, anti-Smith antibody, or antiphospholipid antibody)
- Positive antinuclear antibody

A patient must experience four of the criteria before a classification of SLE can be made. These criteria, proposed by the ACR, should not be the sole characteristics for diagnosis, however.

Therapy

Therapy for each case of SLE is based on the particular symptoms of any given patient. Arthritis is commonly treated with NSAIDs or glucocorticoids. Dermatologic complications can be treated with hydroxychloroquine (see Section 26-3). Hydroxychloroquine may also be used for musculoskeletal manifestations that do not respond to NSAIDs. Thrombocytopenia generally responds to glucocorticoid therapy. Immunosuppressive agents are used in patients with lupus nephritis. Most commonly, cyclophosphamide is used, sometimes in combination with glucocorticoids, especially IV for induction therapies. Azathioprine and mycophenolate may be used as well. In early 2011, the FDA approved belimumab (Benlysta) for the treatment of adult patients with active, autoantibody-positive SLE who are receiving standard therapy. Belimumab is in the new class of drugs known as BLyS-specific inhibitors.

Belimumab

Mechanism of action
Belimumab is a monoclonal antibody that inhibits the binding of human B lymphocyte stimulator protein (BLyS) to its receptors on the B cells. Belimumab

inhibits the survival of B cells, including autoreactive B cells, and reduces the differentiation of B cells into immunoglobulin-producing plasma cells.

Adverse drug events
Migraine (5%), depression (5%), pharyngitis (5%), pain in limb (6%), insomnia (7%), bronchitis (9%) nasopharyngitis (9%), fever (10%), diarrhea (12%), and nausea (15%) have been reported.

Drug–drug interactions
None have been noted.

Parameters to monitor
Monitor for infusion reactions.

Dose
The dose is 10 mg/kg IV every 2 weeks × 3 doses, then every 4 weeks.

Other aspects
Belimumab may be helpful in more severe disease.

26-7. Questions

1. A 45-year-old man presents to his local health care provider with a complaint of extreme stiffness for the past 2 months that begins in the morning and lasts until noon on most days. He also states that he feels "drained" all the time and that both of his knees are swollen and painful. On examining the patient, the health care provider documents the presence of rheumatoid nodules. The patient's laboratory workup is significant for an elevated CRP (C-reactive protein) and ESR (erythrocyte sedimentation rate) and a positive rheumatoid factor. He states that he has been taking over-the-counter ibuprofen at a dose of 200 mg two or three times daily without relief. Which of the following represents the best drug therapy option for this patient?

   A. Increase the dose of ibuprofen to 800 mg three times daily.
   B. Increase the dose of ibuprofen, and add methotrexate 25 mg twice daily.
   C. Increase the dose of ibuprofen, and add celecoxib 100 mg twice daily.
   D. Increase the dose of ibuprofen, and add leflunomide at a dose of 100 mg daily for 3 days, followed by 20 mg daily.

2. Which of the following represents the best way to decrease potential toxicity with methotrexate while achieving optimal therapeutic benefit?

   A. Add 1–3 mg of folic acid per day to the patient's regimen.
   B. Decrease the dose of methotrexate to 25 mg once monthly.
   C. Add monthly injections of leucovorin to the patient's regimen.
   D. Add leflunomide to the patient's regimen.

3. Because combination DMARD therapy may be more efficacious in the refractory RA population, which of the following represents the *best* choice for combination therapy?

   A. Arava 20 mg once daily + Rheumatrex 5 mg once daily
   B. Remicade 3 mg/kg IV + Enbrel 50 mg once weekly
   C. Myochrysine IM weekly + Plaquenil 200 mg twice daily
   D. Remicade 3 mg/kg IV every 2 months + Rheumatrex 25 mg once weekly

4. A health care provider inquires about the recommended monitoring parameters for patients started on Ridaura. Which of the following represents the most appropriate response?

   A. Baseline ophthalmologic exam, CBC, and serum creatinine, followed by a yearly CBC, serum creatinine, and ophthalmologic exam
   B. Baseline LFTs, CBC, and albumin, followed by monthly LFTs
   C. Baseline CBC, serum creatinine, and urinalysis for protein, followed by a CBC and urinalysis for protein every 1–2 months
   D. No recommended monitoring parameters at this time

5. Which of the following represents a method to decrease the GI toxicity associated with NSAIDs?

   A. Changing patients from a COX-2 inhibitor to nonspecific NSAID
   B. Adding a proton pump inhibitor such as Prevacid to the patient's NSAID
   C. Adding glucosamine to the patient's NSAID
   D. Instructing the patient to take the NSAID at night, when acid secretion is limited

6. NSAID side effects you should counsel a patient about include

   A. category X teratogenicity.
   B. neurologic and immunologic effects.
   C. gastrointestinal and dermatologic effects.
   D. cardiovascular, renal, and gastrointestinal effects.

7. Which of the following would be a contra-indication for the use of Enbrel?

   A. Renal insufficiency
   B. Active infection
   C. Patient over the age of 65
   D. Patient with class I or II congestive heart failure

8. Regarding the biologic DMARDs, which of the following statements is correct?

   A. Kineret is unique in that it is not immunosuppressive.
   B. Patients should have a tuberculin skin test completed before initiation.
   C. FluMist is acceptable to use for influenza prevention.
   D. Patients receiving therapy are at increased risk for hepatitis.

9. The use of glucocorticoids is associated with numerous adverse effects and long-term consequences. Which of the following are initiatives to treat, prevent, or minimize these adverse effects?

   A. Instructing patients to take the glucocorti-coid in divided daily doses
   B. Instructing patients on long-term therapy to add elemental calcium and 400–800 IU of daily ergocalciferol to their regimen
   C. Adding daily chondroitin for arthritis to help offset bone effects of steroids
   D. Informing patients that stopping glucocorticoid abruptly is contraindicated

10. A young female enters your pharmacy and informs you that she plans on becoming pregnant and would like you to review her medication profile to see if any of her medications would be potentially harmful. On reviewing her profile, you notice that she is taking Arava for RA. Which is the most appropriate response?

   A. Arava is a category C drug and could potentially harm the fetus. She should discuss the risks and benefits of becoming pregnant with her health care provider first.
   B. Arava is a category X drug, and she should undergo the drug elimination procedure with cholestyramine before trying to become pregnant.
   C. Arava is a category X drug with no active metabolites and a short half-life; there-fore, she should discontinue the drug and wait 1–2 weeks before trying to become pregnant.
   D. Arava is a category B drug, and the risk of toxicity to the fetus is extremely low.

11. R. Y. is a 67-year-old man with chief com-plaints of a swollen big left toe and extreme pain. The area is erythematous and tender. Laboratory analysis reveals a uric acid level of 10 mg/dL. Review of R. Y.'s past medical his-tory reveals hypertension and congestive heart failure. A diagnosis of gout is made. Which of the following is the best choice for the treat-ment of R. Y.'s acute gouty arthritis attack?

   A. Probenecid 500 mg now, followed by 500 mg twice daily
   B. Indomethacin 50 mg now, followed by 50 mg three to four times daily
   C. Allopurinol 100 mg once daily
   D. Colchicine 1.2 mg followed by 0.6 mg in 1 hour if symptoms persist

12. Which of the following symptoms or findings is consistent with the diagnosis of gout?

   A. The presence of positively birefringent crystals in the affected synovial joint fluid
   B. The presence of calcium pyrophosphate in the affected synovial joint fluid
   C. The presence of symmetrically swollen joints
   D. The presence of hyperuricemia

13. During a routine clinic appointment, you conduct a medication review with your patient, a 35-year-old-male with RA. He states he and his wife have been trying to con-ceive for 1 year with no results. After review-ing his medication list, which drug would you most suspect as contributing to this patient's infertility issues?

A. Methotrexate
B. Hydroxychloroquine
C. Leflunomide
D. Sulfasalazine

14. Drug-induced lupus usually manifests as

    A. severe nephrotic syndrome.
    B. blood disorders including low red blood cell, white blood cell, and platelet counts.
    C. arthritis.
    D. severe neurologic disease.

15. Which of the following statements is true regarding Zyloprim?

    A. It works to decrease the formation of uric acid by inhibiting xanthine kinase.
    B. It does not require dosage adjustment in patients with renal insufficiency.
    C. Skin reactions, including Stevens–Johnson syndrome, have been reported with its use.
    D. It should be used for the treatment of an acute gouty arthritis attack.

16. Which of the following represent potentially dangerous drug interactions with Zyloprim?

    A. Amoxicillin
    B. Amoxicillin and Imuran
    C. Amoxicillin, Imuran, and aspirin
    D. Aspirin

17. Which of the following is consistent with the diagnosis of osteoarthritis?

    A. It is normally associated with elevations in C-reactive protein and ESR.
    B. A common initial finding of pain typically worsens with weight-bearing activity and subsides with rest.
    C. It commonly occurs in the wrists or the elbows.
    D. Crepitus is uncommon.

18. Which of the following medication combinations is (are) contraindicated?

    A. Tylenol and Ultram
    B. Glucosamine sulfate and chondroitin
    C. Ultram and Parnate
    D. Tylenol and glucosamine sulfate

19. Concerning treatment of osteoarthritis, which of the following statements is correct?

    A. Tylenol is generally considered the initial drug of choice.
    B. Tylenol is considered safe and effective, and it has minimal adverse effects, especially in doses greater than 4 g/day.
    C. NSAIDs may be helpful, and they have minimal side effects to consider.
    D. Hyaluronic acid derivatives have been approved by the FDA for the treatment of pain associated with osteoarthritis, and they are robustly effective.

20. Which of the following medications is considered to be a DMARD?

    A. Plaquenil
    B. Allopurinol
    C. Belimumab
    D. Nalfon

26-8. Answers

1. **D.** Although the patient currently has room to increase his dose of the NSAID, he would benefit from the addition of a DMARD. This patient has a disease duration of less than 6 months with moderate disease and poor prognostic factors. Methotrexate represents a viable option; however, the dose of 25 mg twice daily is excessive (it should be dosed once weekly). The addition of leflunomide is the best choice.

2. **A.** The addition of folic acid to the methotrexate regimen has been demonstrated to reduce the risk of liver toxicity. Lowering the dose of methotrexate is likely to decrease risk but is also likely to decrease its effectiveness. Leucovorin, an injectable formulation of folate, is normally used to reverse methotrexate toxicity.

3. **D.** Arava plus methotrexate (Rheumatrex) may be a very efficacious combination, but it increases the risk of liver toxicity significantly, and methotrexate should not be given daily. Gold therapy in combination with Plaquenil increases the risk of rash (although it may rarely be used together), and gold therapy should be given monthly. Remicade and Enbrel, two biologics, should not be used together. Remicade is approved for use in combination with Rheumatrex; this combination represents the best choice.

4. **C.** Gold therapy is associated with glomerulo-nephritis, thrombocytopenia, and leukopenia; therefore, a baseline renal evaluation and periodic testing should occur during the entire course of therapy.

5. **B.** Use a proton pump inhibitor. Glucosamine offers no GI protection. Timing the dose of NSAIDs has never been shown to change their toxicity profile. COX-2 inhibitors are less likely to cause GI damage than are nonspecific NSAIDs.

6. **D.** Cardiovascular, renal, and gastrointestinal side effects are the primary counseling points to cover.

7. **B.** Because of its effects on tumor necrosis factor, Enbrel may decrease a patient's ability to fight infection. Enbrel is contraindicated in patients with an active infection. Its use should be temporarily discontinued until the acute process has resolved.

8. **B.** Do a PPD before initiation of biologic drugs because of their immune-suppressing properties, which could cause the reactivation of a disease such as tuberculosis.

9. **D.** Because of adrenal suppression that occurs with long-term glucocorticoid therapy, patients should taper off the agent.

10. **B.** Because Arava is a teratogenic agent with an active metabolite with a long half-life, a drug elimination procedure should be performed before becoming pregnant.

11. **D.** Both probenecid and allopurinol may exacerbate an acute gouty arthritis attack and should be reserved for the prevention of further attacks only. Indomethacin is an option for the treatment of an acute gouty arthritis attack; however, because of NSAIDs' tendency to cause fluid retention in the renal tubules, it would not be the ideal agent in a patient with congestive heart failure. Colchicine represents the best option from this list.

12. **D.** The presence of calcium pyrophosphate is consistent with the diagnosis of pseudogout, not gout.

13. **D.** Sulfasalazine causes oligospermia; D is the correct answer.

14. **C.** Drug-induced lupus often manifests itself as arthritis, not the other, more severe manifestations.

15. **C.** Zyloprim's use has been associated with serious skin reactions that may occur at any point during therapy.

16. **B.** The co-administration of amoxicillin and allopurinol increases the risk of rash up to 20%. Imuran is metabolized via xanthine oxidase, whose activity is inhibited by allopurinol, thus increasing the risk of toxicity associated with Imuran.

17. **B.** RA usually exhibits elevations in ESR and C-reactive protein, unlike OA. OA typically affects the weight-bearing joints.

18. **C.** Tylenol and Ultram are marketed therapeutically as Ultracet. Glucosamine sulfate with or without chondroitin is recommended as an alternative therapy in the treatment of OA. The combination of Ultram and Parnate, a monoamine oxidase inhibitor, is contraindicated because of the risk of serotonin syndrome.

19. **A.** Tylenol is generally considered to be safe and effective, and it is considered the drug of choice initially. Doses greater than 4 g/day of Tylenol should never be used because of the risk of hepatic injury. Hyaluronidase derivatives are marginally effective. The adverse effects of NSAIDs are considerable and must always be taken into account when initiating therapy in OA.

20. **A.** Allopurinol is a xanthine oxidase inhibitor used in the treatment of gout. Nalfon is an NSAID. Belimumab is a monoclonal antibody used in the treatment of SLE.

26-9. References

Rheumatoid Arthritis

American College of Rheumatology. Recommendations for the use of nonbiologic and biologic disease-modifying antirheumatic drugs in rheumatoid arthritis. *Arthritis Rheum.* 2008;59:762–84.

Aletaha D, Neogi T, Silman, AJ, et al. Rheumatoid arthritis classification criteria: An American College of Rheumatology/European League Against Rheumatism collaborative initiative. *Ann Rheum Dis.* 2010;69:1580–88.

Bhatt DL, Scheiman J, Abraham NS, et al. ACCF/ACG/AHA 2008 expert consensus document on reducing the gastrointestinal risks of antiplatelet therapy and NSAID use. *Am J Gastroenterol.* 2008; 103:2890–907.

Boyce EG. Rheumatoid arthritis. In: Helms RA, Quan DJ, Herfindal ET, et al., eds. *Textbook of Therapeutics: Drugs and Disease Management.* 8th ed. Baltimore, MD: Lippincott Williams & Wilkins; 2006:1705–36.

Furst DE, Keyston EC, Braun J, et al. Updated consensus statement on biological agents for the treatment of rheumatic diseases. *Ann Rheum Dis.* 2011;70(suppl 1):i2–36.

Saag KG, Teng GG, Patkar NM, et al. American College of Rheumatology 2008 recommendations for the use of nonbiologic and biologic disease-modifying antirheumatic drugs in rheumatoid arthritis. *Arthritis Rheum.* 2008;59:762–84.

Singh JA, Furst DE, Bharat A, et al. Update of the 2008 American College of Rheumatology recommendations for the use of disease-modifying antirheumatic drugs and biologic agents in the treatment of rheumatoid arthritis. *Arthritis Care Res.* 2012;64(5):625–39.

Wahl K, Schuna AA. Rheumatoid arthritis. In: Dipiro JT, Talbert RL, Yee GC, et al., eds. *Pharmacotherapy: A Pathophysiologic Approach.* 9th ed. New York, NY: McGraw-Hill; 2014:1459–75.

Osteoarthritis

Buys LM, Elliott ME. Osteoarthritis. In: Dipiro JT, Talbert RL, Yee GC, et al., eds. *Pharmacotherapy: A Pathophysiologic Approach.* 9th ed. New York, NY: McGraw-Hill; 2014:1437–57.

Grosser T, Smyth EM, FitzGerald GA. Antiinflammatory, antipyretic, and analgesic agents; Pharmacotherapy of gout. In: Brunton LL, Chabner BA, Knollman BC, eds. *Goodman & Gilman's The Pharmacological Basis of Therapeutics.* 12th ed. New York, NY: McGraw-Hill; 2011:959–1004.

Hochberg MC, Altman RD, April KT, et al. American College of Rheumatology 2012 recommendations for the use of nonpharmacologic and pharmacologic therapies in osteoarthritis of the hand, hip, and knee. *Arthritis Care Res.* 2012; 64(4):455–74.

Small RE. Osteoarthritis. In: Helms RA, Quan DJ, Herfindal ET, et al., eds. *Textbook of Therapeutics: Drugs and Disease Management.* 8th ed. Baltimore, MD: Lippincott Williams & Wilkins; 2006:1737–52.

Zhang W, Nuki G, Moskowitz RW, et al. OARSI recommendations for the management of hip and knee osteoarthritis: Part III: Changes in evidence following systematic cumulative update of research published through January 2009. *Osteoarthritis Cartilage.* 2010;18(4):476–99.

Gout

Becker MA, Schumacher HR, Wortmann RL, et al. Febuxostat compared with allopurinol in patients with hyperuricemia and gout. *N Engl J Med.* 2005;353:2450–61.

Fravel MA, Ernst ME, Clark EC. Gout and hyperuricemia. In: Dipiro JT, Talbert RL, Yee GC, et al., eds. *Pharmacotherapy: A Pathophysiologic Approach.* 9th ed. New York, NY: McGraw-Hill; 2014:1505–23.

Khanna D, Fitzgerald JD, Khanna PP, et al. American College of Rheumatology guidelines for management of gout. Part 1: Systemic pharmacologic and nonpharmacologic therapeutic approaches to hyperuricemia. *Arthritis and Research.* 2012; 64(10):1431–46.

Khanna D, Khanna PP, Fitzgerald JD, et al. American College of Rheumatology guidelines for management of gout Part 2: Therapy and antiinflammatory prophylaxis of acute gouty arthritis. *Arthritis and Research.* 2012;64(10):1447–61.

McCloskey WW, Kostka-Rokosz MD. Gout and hyperuricemia. In: Helms RA, Quan DJ, Herfindal ET, et al., eds. *Textbook of Therapeutics: Drugs and Disease Management.* 8th ed. Baltimore, MD: Lippincott Williams & Wilkins; 2006:1753–66.

Neogi T. Gout. *N Eng J Med.* 2011;364:443–52.

Systemic Lupus Erythematosus

Resman-Targoff BH. Systemic lupus erythematosus. In: Dipiro JT, Talbert RL, Yee GC, et al., eds. *Pharmacotherapy: A Pathophysiologic Approach.* 9th ed. New York, NY: McGraw-Hill; 2014: 1397–411.

Krikoria S. Systemic lupus erythematosus. In: Helms RA, Quan DJ, Herfindal ET, et al., eds. *Textbook of Therapeutics: Drugs and Disease Management.* 8th ed. Baltimore, MD: Lippincott Williams & Wilkins; 2006:1767–87.

Lupus Foundation of America. Lupus. http://www.lupus.org.

Tsokos GC. Systemic lupus erythematosus. *N Engl J Med.* 2011;365(22):2110–21.

Pain Management and Migraines

Elizabeth S. Miller
Sarah T. Stapleton

27-1. Key Points

Pain Management

- Opioids relieve pain by mimicking the actions of endogenous opioid peptides at μ, δ, and κ receptors.
- Opioids fall into three categories: pure μ agonists, agonist–antagonists, and pure antagonists. Pure μ agonists are the most pharmacologically useful.
- *Addiction* is a behavior pattern involving the continued use of a substance for nonmedical reasons despite harm. *Physical dependence* is the occurrence of withdrawal syndrome after an opioid is stopped or quickly decreased without titration.
- With prolonged use, opioids produce tolerance to analgesia, euphoria, sedation, respiratory depression, and other adverse effects—but not constipation.
- Opioid overdose induces coma, respiratory depression, and pinpoint pupils. Naloxone and other pure opioid antagonists are used in cases of overdose to reverse most effects of opioids.
- Alcohol and other central nervous system (CNS) depressants can intensify opioid-induced sedation and respiratory depression. Tricyclic antidepressants and antihistamines may worsen opioid-induced constipation and urinary retention.
- Hydrocodone, codeine, fentanyl, methadone, and oxycodone are metabolized by the cytochrome P450 (CYP450) system. Thus, drug interactions through the CYP450 enzymes may exist.
- The liver extensively metabolizes opioids; dose adjustments may be required in liver dysfunction. Fentanyl, morphine, and methadone require dosing adjustments in renal dysfunction.

Migraine

- The pathogenesis of migraine is unclear and is thought to be multifactorial. The current thinking is that a primary neuronal dysfunction originates in the CNS, leading to a sequence of changes that account for the different stages of migraine.
- The goal of abortive therapy is to eliminate headache pain and associated nausea and vomiting. The goal of preventive therapy is to reduce the incidence of migraine attacks.
- Nonopioid analgesics are effective for abortive therapy of mild to moderate pain.
- Opioid analgesics are reserved for a severe migraine that has not responded to other drugs.
- Ergotamine is effective for abortive therapy but should not be used daily. Overdose with ergotamine can cause ergotism, a serious condition in which generalized constriction of peripheral arteries and arterioles causes severe tissue ischemia.
- Triptans are drugs of choice for abortive therapy of migraines. They activate 5-HT_{1B} and 5-HT_{1D} receptors, thereby causing constriction of cranial blood vessels and suppression of inflammatory neuropeptides.
- Triptans can cause coronary vasospasm and are contraindicated in patients with ischemic heart-disease, prior myocardial infarction, and uncontrolled hypertension. If a triptan is combined with another triptan or with an ergot alkaloid, excessive prolonged vasospasms could result. Because of increased triptan toxicity, triptans should not be administered concurrently with monoamine oxidase inhibitors (MAOIs) and should not be given within 2 weeks of stopping an MAOI.
- Topiramate is considered the treatment of choice. Divalproex sodium, topiramate, propranolol, and

timolol all carry U.S. Food and Drug Administration approval for use as first-line prophylaxis of migraine headaches. Amitriptyline, venlafaxine, atenolol, and nadolol are generally used as second-line treatment.

27-2. Study Guide Checklist

The following topics may guide your study of this subject area:

- Clinical presentation of various types of pain
- Considerations for selection of pain management drugs based on patient's condition and prior drug experience
- Trade names, available dosage forms, and dosing regimens of selected opioids
- Major adverse drug reactions of opioid drugs
- Significant drug disease and drug–drug interactions of opioid drugs
- Dosing of drugs to treat acute, chronic, and neuropathic pain
- Nonpharmacological treatment for pain
- Patient counseling points for specific pain management drugs

27-3. Pain

Pain is defined as real or potential tissue injury associated with any uncomfortable sensory, or emotional experience, or both. Practitioners often define pain in terms of symptoms that the patient experiences or perceives.

Currently, about 76 million Americans suffer from some form of chronic benign pain. Approximately one-third of chronic pain sufferers experience chronic pain. Billions of dollars are spent on pain treatment in the United States each year.

Types and Clinical Presentation

Pain can be classified as acute, chronic benign, or malignant.

Acute pain is caused by an injury, illness, or surgery. It responds to medications and usually resolves when the underlying cause has been treated or healed. It is often associated with physiological symptoms such as tachycardia, hypertension, diaphoresis, and mydriasis.

Chronic benign pain exists beyond an expected time for healing, typically lasting months to years. It is often associated with psychological effects, including social isolation, depression, and anxiety. Chronic pain syndromes are often not responsive to traditional analgesics and require the use of adjuvant medications.

Malignant pain may be acute, chronic, or intermittent and is often related to cancer progression or chemotherapy.

Pain is also defined by source. Such a classification divides pain into somatic, visceral, and neuropathic pain.

Somatic pain originates from the skin, muscles, tendons, ligaments, and bones. It is localized and described as sharp, stabbing, throbbing, or aching in nature. Although somatic pain can be severe, it tends to respond well to treatment with opioids.

The body's internal organs such as the liver, intestines, or stomach generate *visceral pain*. Visceral pain tends to be poorly localized and more likely to generate referred pain felt some distance away from the actual problem. Opioids are not as effective for visceral pain as they are for somatic pain.

Neuropathic pain results when the nerves themselves are damaged. It is typically burning in nature, although it may also cause numbness, aching, or a sensation like an electric shock. Opioid medications are not the most effective treatment for neuropathic pain and are recommended as second-line treatment. Specific tricyclic antidepressants, antiepileptics, and serotonin–norepinephrine reuptake inhibitors (SNRIs) are typically recommended as first-line treatment (see Table 27-1).

Pathophysiology

Nociception, the pain sensation, begins when a sensory nerve ending is stimulated and sends repetitive signals to the spinal cord along ascending nerve fibers. An individual nerve does not transmit directly to the brain but instead connects to secondary nerves in the dorsal horn of the spinal cord. The secondary nerves eventually connect to nerve cells in the brain stem.

A descending antinociceptive pathway also exists. Neurotransmitters from the descending fibers inhibit the transmission of the pain signal. Opioids chemically resemble these neurotransmitters.

Chronic pain is not a prolonged version of acute pain. As pain signals are repeatedly generated, neural pathways undergo changes that make them hypersensitive to pain signals and resistant to antinociceptive input.

Diagnostic Criteria

The individual's self-report of pain is the primary source of information in acute pain. Practitioners

Table 27-1. Prescribing Recommendations for Neuropathic Pain

Medication class and trade name	Generic name	Available strengths	Starting dosage (maximum dose)	Major adverse effects
Antidepressants				
TCAs				
Pamelor	Nortriptyline	10, 25, 50, 75 mg	25 mg daily at bedtime; 150 mg	Cardiac toxicity, anti-cholinergics SE (sedation, dry mouth, blurred vision, urinary retention)
Norpramin	Desipramine	10, 25, 50, 75, 100, 150 mg	25 mg daily bedtime; 150 mg	
SSNRIs				
Cymbalta	Duloxetine	20, 30, 60 mg	30 mg daily; 60 mg daily	Nausea
Effexor	Venlafaxine	25, 37.5, 50, 75, 100 mg	37.5 mg once or twice daily; 225 mg daily	Nausea, ↑blood pressure
Calcium channel alpha$_2$-, delta ligands[a,b]				
Neurontin	Gabapentin	100, 300, 400 mg	100–300 mg bedtime or TID; 3,600 mg daily	Dizziness, sedation, renal insufficiency
Lyrica	Pregabalin	25, 50, 75, 100, 150, 200, 225, 300 mg	50 mg TID or 75 mg BID; 600 mg daily	
Local anesthetic[a]				
Lidoderm	Lidocaine patch	5% patch	3 patches every 12 hours (starting and maximum)	Mild local reactions
Opioid agonists[c]				
MSIR, Roxicodone, Dolophine, Levo-Dromoran[b]	Morphine, oxycodone, methadone, levorphanol	Morphine 15, 30 mg; oxycodone 5, 15, 30 mg; methadone 5, 10 mg; levorphanol 2 mg	10–15 mg q4h or as needed of morphine or equianalgesic dose of other opioid analgesic, no maximum dose	Constipation, nausea, sedation
Ultram[b]	Tramadol	50 mg	50–100 mg daily or bid; 400 mg daily	Constipation, nausea, sedation, lowers the seizure threshold

Adapted from Dworkin RH, O'Connor AB, Audette J, et al., 2010; O'Connor AB, Dworkin RH, 2009.
Boldface indicates one of top 100 drugs for 2012 by units sold at retail outlets, www.drugs.com/stats/top100/2012/units.
SSNRI, selective serotonin and norepinephrine reuptake inhibitor; TCA, tricyclic antidepressant.
a. First-line treatment.
b. Consider lower starting doses and slower titration in the elderly.
c. Second-line treatment, may be appropriate as first-line treatment in certain circumstances.

often use visual analog or categorical pain scales (use of numbers or adjectives) to assess pain intensity reported by patients.

Chronic pain assessment should include a detailed history of the pain's intensity and characteristics, a physical examination emphasizing the neurological exam, and a psychosocial assessment (Figure 27-1).

The purpose of diagnostic tests, such as x-rays, computed tomography, or magnetic resonance imaging scans, or laboratory tests differs depending on the type of pain. In cancer patients, the major purpose of diagnostic testing is to visualize the disease progression. In chronic benign pain, the major purpose of diagnostic testing is to rule out the presence of any diseases for which there is a curative treatment.

Figure 27-1. Algorithm for Comprehensive Evaluation and Management of Chronic Pain

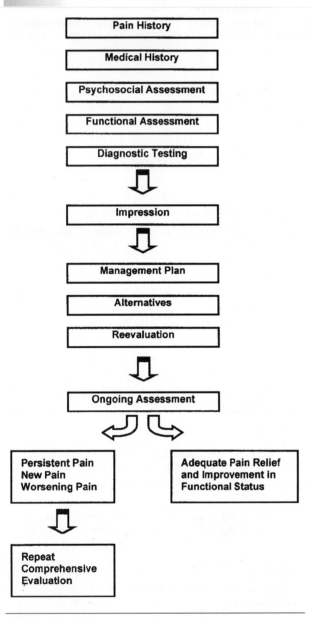

Reproduced with permission from the Pain Management Center of Paducah.

Goals of Pain Management

Acute pain

The goal in acute pain management is to provide patients with pain relief that allows them to rest comfortably and allows postsurgery or postinjury rehabilitation. This goal can be accomplished by administering short-acting medications as needed.

Malignant pain

A major goal of cancer pain management is to relieve the patient's pain without inducing disabling side effects.

The World Health Organization (WHO) has developed a three-step hierarchy for analgesic pain management in cancer pain patients (Figure 27-2). In general, this program includes using nonopioid analgesics as a baseline, supplementing with opioid analgesics as needed, and adding adjunctive medications when appropriate.

Cancer patients may suffer from constant pain that continues for months or years. For this reason, treatment with long-acting agents is more appropriate than treatment with short-acting medications. However, short-acting agents, referred to as "breakthrough" or "rescue" doses, are often available in addition to the long-acting medications.

Chronic benign pain

The goal of chronic benign pain treatment is to restore the patient to the highest degree of function possible or a decrease in pain intensity of at least 30%.

Multimodal therapy, the use of several different types of treatment, is usually required. Multi-

Figure 27-2. The WHO's Three-Step Hierarchy for Analgesic Pain Management in Cancer Patients

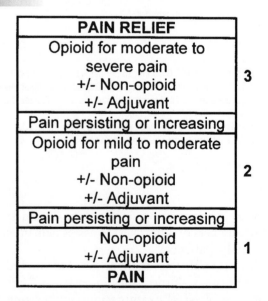

Reproduced with permission from WHO 1996.

modal therapies include nerve blocks, rehabilitation, physical therapy, pharmacotherapy, acupuncture, and psychotherapy. Basic pharmacotherapy follows the WHO guidelines for treating cancer pain (Figure 27-2).

Analgesics are categorized into nonopioid analgesics, opioid analgesics, and adjuvant analgesics. Nonopioid analgesics, such as acetaminophen and nonsteroidal anti-inflammatory drugs (NSAIDs), relieve all types of mild to moderate pain. Prescription products containing acetaminophen are limited to 325 mg per dosage unit because of the potential for severe liver failure. NSAIDs are commonly used as part of the treatment regimen for pain associated with inflammation and cancer-related bone pain. Unless contraindicated, all pain patients should first be given a trial of nonopioid analgesics. Nonopioids and opioids relieve pain via different mechanisms. Thus, combination therapy offers the potential for improved relief with decreased doses

and fewer side effects. Nonopioids do not produce tolerance, physical dependence, or addiction (see Table 27–2).

Adjuvant analgesics are drugs with a primary indication other than pain. Commonly used analgesic adjuvants include antiepileptic drugs, tricyclic antidepressants, local anesthetics, and SNRIs.

Principles of opioid use

Opioids have no ceiling effect of analgesia.

Oral medications should be used whenever possible. Intramuscular injections are painful and should be avoided.

When patients have constant or near-constant pain, analgesics should be given around the clock. Long-acting opioid analgesics are often used for this purpose.

The use of short-acting opioids as rescue medication is controversial in chronic benign pain. If allowed,

Table 27-2. Common Nonopioid Analgesics

Generic name	Common trade name and strength	Dosing interval	IV starting dose	Oral daily starting dose
Acetaminophen[a]				
Tablet	Tylenol	4–6 hours		325–600 mg (maximum 4,000 mg)
Injection	Ofirmev		650 mg	
Aspirin tablet	Ecotrin			81–325 mg (maximum 4,000 mg)
Diclofenac				
Tablet	Cataflam	8–12 hours		50–100 mg (maximum 150 mg)
Patch	Flector	Every 12 hours		
Ibuprofen				
Tablet	Motrin, Caldolor	4–6 hours		200–400 mg (maximum 3,200 mg)
Injection		6 hours	400–800 mg	
Ketoprofen tablet		6–8 hours		25–50 mg (maximum 300 mg)
Naproxen tablet	Naprosyn, Anaprox	12 hours, po		500 mg (maximum 1,000 mg)
Naproxen sodium tablet	Aleve	8–12 hours		440 mg (maximum 660 mg)
Ketorolac				
Tablet		4–6 hours po		10 mg (maximum 40 mg, 5 days)
Injection		Single dose IM, IV, or every 6 hours IV	15–30 mg (maximum 5 days)	
Celecoxib tablet	Celebrex[b]	Every 12 hours		200 mg (maximum 400 mg)

Adapted from Baumann TJ, Strickland JM, Herdon CM, et al., 2011.
a. Rare but serious skin reactions have been reported.
b. One of top 100 drugs for 2012 by units sold at retail outlets, www.drugs.com/stats/top100/2012/units.

doses of rescue medications should range from 10% to 15% of the total daily long-acting opioid dose.

Mixed agonist–antagonist opioids are not used in chronic pain. They may induce a withdrawal syndrome in patients tolerant to opioids.

Drug Therapy

Mechanism of action

Morphine and other opioid agonists are thought to produce analgesia by mimicking the action of endogenous opioid peptides that bind at opioid receptors in the antinociceptive pathway.

Opioid receptors are located in the central nervous system (CNS), pituitary gland, and gastrointestinal (GI) tract. They are abundant in the periaqueductal gray matter of the brain and the dorsal horn of the spinal cord, two areas that are very active in pain reduction.

When a drug binds to one of these receptors as an agonist, it produces analgesia. When a drug binds to one of these receptors as an antagonist, analgesia and other effects are blocked.

The three major types of opioid receptor sites involved in analgesia are mu (µ), delta (δ), and kappa (κ):

- Binding to the µ receptor produces analgesia, sedation, euphoria, respiratory depression, physical dependence, constipation, and other effects.
- Activation of δ receptors produces analgesia without many adverse events. However, there is no available δ-receptor agonist.
- Activation of the κ receptor produces analgesia and respiratory depression. In addition, psychotomimetic effects such as anxiety, strange thoughts, nightmares, and hallucinations are common.

Opioid analgesics

Opioids are classified by activity at the receptor site; that is, they are classified as pure opioid agonists, agonist–antagonists, or pure opioid antagonists.

Pure opioid agonists primarily activate µ receptors, although they may produce some κ-receptor activation (Table 27-3). Pure opioid agonists are the most clinically useful opioid analgesics.

Morphine is the prototypical pure opioid agonist. Methadone is an opioid agonist with additional antagonist activity at the NMDA (N-methyl-D-aspartate) receptor. The NMDA receptor is believed to be active primarily in chronic pain.

Mixed agonist–antagonists bind as agonists at the κ receptor, producing weak analgesia. They bind as weak antagonists at the µ receptor (Table 27-4). The result is more dysphoria and psychotomimetic effects with a lower risk of respiratory depression.

Pentazocine is the prototypical agonist–antagonist opioid. Buprenorphine is actually a partial agonist at µ and κ receptors. This opioid has limited efficacy in pain management and is primarily used in detoxification programs.

Opioid antagonists block the µ and κ receptors (Table 27-5). These drugs do not produce analgesia. They are used to reverse respiratory and CNS depression caused by overdose with opioid agonists. Naloxone and naltrexone are opioid antagonists.

Opioid analgesic adverse effects

Central nervous system

Opioids produce a number of CNS effects, including sedation, euphoria, dysphoria, changes in mood, and mental clouding. Confusion, disorientation, and cognitive impairment are also possible.

Chronic sedation can be treated with CNS stimulants such as methylphenidate or dextroamphetamine. Modafinil also promotes daytime wakefulness.

Mild to moderate muscle jerks, known as *myoclonus*, are common in patients on high doses of opioids. Myoclonus can be treated by changing the opioid dose, changing the opioid, or giving low doses of a benzodiazepine.

Neuroendocrine

Morphine acts in the hypothalamus to inhibit the release of gonadotropin-releasing hormone and corticotropin-releasing factor, thus decreasing levels of luteinizing hormone, follicle-stimulating hormone, adrenocorticotropic hormone, and β-endorphins.

Changes in hormone levels may cause decreased levels of testosterone and cortisol, disturbances in menstruation, and sexual dysfunction.

High doses of morphine and related opioids produce convulsions. Most convulsions occur at doses far in excess of those required to produce analgesia.

Respiratory

Respiratory depression is the most serious opioid-induced adverse effect. Opioids depress respiration by a direct effect on the brain-stem respiratory centers, making the brain stem less responsive to carbon dioxide.

The µ receptor is the primary receptor involved in respiratory depression, although activation of the κ receptor also contributes.

Table 27-3. Starting Doses for Strong Opioids for Severe and Moderate to Severe Pain in Adults: Mu Agonists

Generic name	Trade name and strength	Dosing interval	Equianalgesic dose		Oral/intranasal starting dose
			IV	po	
Fentanyl[a] (synthetic)					
Injection	Sublimaze 50 mcg/mL	0.5–2 hours IM or IV	0.1 mg	Not applicable	
Transdermal	Duragesic 12, 25, 50, 75, 100 mcg/h	q 2–3 days			
Transmucosal lozenge[b]	Actiq 200, 400, 600, 800, 1,200, 1,600 mcg	4 hours			200 mcg
Disintegrating tablet[b]	Fentora 100, 200, 400, 600, 800 mcg	4 hours			100 mcg
	Abstral 100, 200, 300, 400, 600, 800 mcg	2 hours			100 mcg
Nasal spray[b]	Lazanda 100 mcg/100 mcL, 400 mcg/mcL	2 hours			100 mcg/mcL
Sublingual spray[b]	Subsys 100, 200, 400, 600, 800, 1,200, 1,600 mcg	4 hours			100 mcg
Hydrocodone (semisynthetic)					
Extended-release capsules	Hydrocodone 10, 15, 20, 30, 40, 50 mg	12 hours			10 mg
Hydromorphone (semisynthetic)					
Immediate-release tablet	Dilaudid 2, 4, 8 mg	4–6 hours po; 2–3 hours IM, IV, subcutaneously	1.3–2 mg	6.5–7.5 mg	2–4 mg
Liquid	Dilaudid 1 mg/mL	3–6 hours po			2.5–10 mg
Injection	Dilaudid 1, 2, 4 mg/mL; Dilaudid HP 10 mg/mL				
Extended-release tablet	Exalgo 8, 12, 16, 32 mg	24 hours po			
Levorphanol (semisynthetic)					
Injection	Levo-Dromoran 2 mg/mL	3–6 hours IV, 6–8 hours IM, subcutaneously	2 mg	4 mg	2 mg
Tablet	Levo-Dromoran 2 mg	6–8 hours po			1 mg
Meperidine (synthetic)					
Tablet	Demerol 50, 100 mg	3–4 hours po	75 mg	300 mg	50–150 mg (not recommended)
Injection	Demerol 25, 50, 75, 100 mg/mL	3–4 hours IM or subcutaneously			
Methadone (synthetic)					
Tablet	Dolophine 5, 10 mg; Methadose 5, 10 mg; metha-dose dispersible 40 mg	8–12 hours po; 4–12 hours IM, IV, or subcutaneously	Acute: 10 mg; chronic: 2–4 mg	Acute: 20 mg; chronic: 2–4 mg	2.5–10 mg
Liquid	Methadose 10 mg/mL; meth-adone HCl 1, 2, 10 mg/mL				
Injection	Methadone HCl 10 mg/mL				

(continued)

Table 27-3. Starting Doses for Strong Opioids for Severe and Moderate to Severe Pain in Adults: Mu Agonists *(Continued)*

Generic name	Trade name and strength	Dosing interval	Equianalgesic dose		Oral/intranasal starting dose
			IV	po	
Morphine (natural)					
Immediate-release tablet	MSIR 15, 30 mg	2–4 hours po; 4 hours IM, subcutaneously, or IV; 4 hours per rectum	10 mg	30 mg	5–30 mg
Liquid	MSIR 2, 4, 20 mg/mL; morphine sulfate 2, 5 mg/mL; Roxanol 20 mg/mL				
Injection	Duramorph, Astramorph PF 0.5, 1 mg/mL; Infumorph 10, 25 mg/mL				
Controlled-release tablet	Avinza 30, 45, 60, 75, 90, 120 mg	24 hours po	Not applicable		30 mg
	Kadian 10, 20, 30, 40, 50, 60, 70, 80, 100, 130, 150, 200 mg	12–24 hours po			10–20 mg
	MS Contin 15, 30, 60, 100, 200 mg	8–12 hours po			15 mg
Oxycodone (semisynthetic)					
Tablet	Roxicodone 5, 15, 30 mg	4–6 hours po	Not applicable	20 mg	5–30 mg
	Oxecta 5, 7.5 mg	4–6 hours po			5–15 mg
Capsule	OxyIR 5 mg				
Liquid	Roxicodone 1, 20 mg/mL				
Tablet (oxycodone/ acetaminophen)	Roxicet 5/325 mg; Percocet 2.5/325, 5/325, 7.5/325, 10/325 mg				
Capsule (oxycodone/ acetaminophen)	Tylox 5/500 mg				
Liquid (oxycodone/ acetaminophen)	Roxicet 5/325 mg per 5 mL				
Tablet (oxycodone/ ibuprofen)	Combunox 5/400 mg	6 hours po			
Controlled-release tablet	**OxyContin** 10, 15, 20, 30, 40, 60, 80 mg	12 hours po		20–30 mg	10 mg
Oxymorphone (semisynthetic)					
Injection	Opana 1 mg/ml	4–6 hours po; 4 hours IM, subcutaneously, or IV	1–1.5 mg	10 mg	5–20 mg
Immediate-release tablet	Opana 5, 10 mg	4–6 hours			10–20 mg
Controlled-release tablet	Opana ER 5, 7.5, 10, 15, 20, 30, 40 mg	12 hours po	Not applicable		5 mg

a. One of top 100 drugs for 2012 by units sold at retail outlets, www.drugs.com/stats/top100/2012/units.
b. For use in breakthrough cancer pain.

Table 27-4. Opioid Dosing for Mild to Severe Pain in Adults

Generic name	Trade name and strength	Dosing interval	IV starting dose	Oral starting dose
Moderate to severe pain: Moderate-severe opioid and opioid/antagonist				
Tapentadol (synthetic)				
Immediate-release tablet	Nucynta 50, 75, 100 mg	4–6 hours po		50, 75, 100 mg; maximum 600 mg
Extended-release tablet	Nucynta ER 50, 100, 150, 200, 250 mg	12 hours po		50 mg; maximum 500 mg
Liquid	20 mg/mL	4–6 hours po		50, 75, 100 mg; maximum 600 mg
Morphine/naltrexone (natural/antagonist)				
Extended-release capsules	Embeda 20/0.8 mg, 30/1.2 mg, 50/2 mg, 60/2.4 mg, 80/3.2 mg, 100/4 mg	12–24 hours po		20/0.8 mg in opioid-naïve patients
Moderate to mild pain: Moderate-mild opioid				
Codeine (natural)				
Tablet	Codeine sulfate 15, 30, 60 mg (CII)	4 hours	30 mg	15–60 mg; maximum 360 mg
Liquid	Codeine sulfate 6 mg/mL			
Tablet (codeine/ acetaminophen)	Tylenol with Codeine, #3 (300/30 mg), #4 (300/60 mg)			
Liquid (codeine/ acetaminophen)	Tylenol with Codeine Elixir 120/12 mg per 5 mL			
Hydrocodone (semisynthetic)				
Tablet (hydrocodone/ acetaminophen[a])	Vicodin 5/300 mg; Vicodin ES 7.5/300 mg; Vicodin HP 10/300 mg; Norco 5/325, 7.5/325, 10/325 mg; Lortab 2.5/500, 5/500, 7.5/500, 10/500 mg; 10/650 mg	4–6 hours	Not applicable	2.5–10 mg
Liquid (hydrocodone/ acetaminophen[a])	Lortab Elixir 7.5/325 mg per 15 mL			
Tablet (hydrocodone/ ibuprofen)	Zydone 5/400, 7.5/400, 10/400 mg; Vicoprofen 7.5/200 mg; Reprexain 2.5/200, 5/200, 10/200 mg			
Moderate to severe pain: Agonists-antagonists				
Pentazocine				
Tablet (pentazocine/ naloxone)	50/0.5 mg	4 hours		50/0.5–100/1 mg; maximum 600 mg/day
Injection	Talwin 30 mg/mL	3–4 hours	30 mg IM, IV, or subcutaneously; maximum 360 mg/day	
Butorphanol				
Injection	Butorphanol tartrate 1, 2 mg/mL	3–4 hours	0.5–2 mg	
Nasal spray	Butorphanol tartrate 1 mg/spray			1 spray in 1 nostril

(continued)

Table 27-4. Opioid Dosing for Mild to Severe Pain in Adults *(Continued)*

Generic name	Trade name and strength	Dosing interval	IV starting dose	Oral starting dose
Buprenorphine				
Injection	Buprenex 0.3 mg/mL	6 hours	0.3–0.6 mg	
Patch	Butrans 5, 10, 15, 20 mcg/h	7 days		5 mcg/h in opioid-naïve patients; 10 mg (opioid-tolerant patients)
Miscellaneous				
Tramadol tablet	Ultram 50 mg	4–6 hours		50–100 mg; maximum 400 mg/day
Tramadol controlled-release tablet	Ultram ER 100, 200, 300 mg	24 hours		100 mg; maximum 300 mg/d
Tramadol tablet (tramadol/acetaminophen)	Ultracet 325/37.5 mg	4–6 hours		Maximum 8 tabs/day

a. One of top 100 drugs for 2012 by units sold at retail outlets, www.drugs.com/stats/top100/2012/units.

At equianalgesic doses, all pure opioid agonists depress respiration to the same degree. The agonist–antagonists have a ceiling effect (i.e., a dose beyond which no further respiratory depression or analgesia is produced), but this level is usually above recommended doses.

Opioids depress cough by inducing a direct effect on the cough reflex in the medulla.

Cardiovascular

Therapeutic doses of many opioids produce peripheral vasodilation, reduced peripheral resistance, and inhibition of the baroreceptor reflexes.

Peripheral vasodilation results primarily from opioid-induced release of histamine. Orthostatic hypotension and fainting can result. The naturally occurring and semisynthetic products are potent

Table 27-5. Opioid Antagonists

Generic name	Trade name and strength	Dosing interval	IV starting dose	Oral starting dose
Naloxone injection	Narcan (naloxone) HCl 0.4, 1 mg/mL	Every 2–3 min IM, IV, subcutaneously	Opioid overdose: 0.4–2 mg; postoperative narcotic depression: 0.1–0.2 mg (can be administered IM and subcutaneously)	
Buprenorphine/ naloxone sublingual tablet/film	Suboxone[a] tablet 2/0.5, 8/2 mg; Suboxone film 2/0.5, 4/1, 8/2, 12/3 mg	24 hours		12–16 mg/day; an alternative to methadone for opioid dependence
Naltrexone				
Tablet	Revia 50 mg; naltrexone HCl 25, 50, 100 mg	Daily, every other day, every 3 days		Alcoholism: 50 mg daily; narcotic addiction: 50 mg daily, 100 mg every other day, or 150 mg every 3 days
Injection	Vivitrol 380 mg/vial	Monthly	Alcohol and opioid dependence: 380 mg monthly	

a. One of top 100 drugs for 2012 by units sold at retail outlets, www.drugs.com/stats/top100/2012/units.

histamine releasers. Fentanyl has little propensity to release histamine.

Methadone has been associated with torsades de pointes, an atypical rapid ventricular tachycardia, at an average daily dose of 400 mg. Methadone should be used cautiously in patients on other QTc-prolonging medications. Patients should receive an electrocardiogram prior to therapy, at day 30, and once yearly while receiving methadone.

Gastrointestinal

All clinically significant μ agonists produce some degree of nausea and vomiting by direct stimulation of the chemoreceptor trigger zone in the medulla, sensitization of the vestibular system, and slowing of GI motility.

Nausea and vomiting commonly occur in ambulatory patients (28% and 15%, respectively). Both can be pretreated with an antiemetic such as promethazine or prochlorperazine.

Opioids promote constipation by delaying gastric emptying, slowing bowel motility, and decreasing peristalsis. Opioids may also reduce secretions from the colonic mucosa. At its worst, GI dysfunction results in ileus, fecal impaction, and obstruction.

Because transdermal delivery bypasses absorption from the GI tract, constipation has been reported to be less frequent with this delivery method than with other methods.

Patients on opiates do not develop tolerance to constipation. All patients taking around-the-clock opioid analgesics should be placed on prophylactic bowel regimens. Bowel regimens include increased fluid and fiber intake, daily stool softeners, and mild laxatives.

Severe constipation is managed with osmotic laxatives such as magnesium citrate and milk of magnesia.

Genitourinary

Opioids increase smooth muscle tone in the bladder and ureters and may cause bladder spasm and urgency.

An opioid-induced increase in urethral sphincter tone can make urination difficult. Urinary retention is most common in elderly men.

Biliary

Opioids increase smooth muscle tone in the biliary tract, especially in the sphincter of Oddi, which regulates the flow of bile and pancreatic fluids. This effect can result in a decrease in biliary and pancreatic secretions and a rise in the bile duct pressure. Patients may experience epigastric distress and occasionally biliary spasm.

All opioids are capable of causing constriction of the sphincter of Oddi and the biliary tract. Use caution when prescribing an opioid to a patient with biliary tract disease and pancreatitis.

Skin and eye

Therapeutic doses of morphine dilate cutaneous blood vessels, which causes flushing on the face, neck, and upper thorax. Sweating and pruritus may also occur. These changes may be caused in part by the release of histamine. Histamine release may induce or worsen asthmatic attacks in predisposed patients and can lead to wheezing, bronchoconstriction, and status asthmaticus.

Skin rash around the transdermal fentanyl patch is a common side effect caused by the patch adhesive.

Following a toxic dose of μ agonists, miosis is evident but insufficient alone to confirm a definitive diagnosis of opioid intoxication.

Overdose

Acute overdose with opioids is manifested by respiratory depression; somnolence progressing to stupor or coma; skeletal muscle flaccidity; cold, clammy skin; constricted pupils; and sometimes pulmonary edema, bradycardia, hypotension, and death.

An opioid antagonist such as naloxone may be given to block opioid receptors and reverse the effects of overdose.

Antagonist administration may cause a complete reversal of opioid effects and precipitate an acute withdrawal syndrome in persons physically dependent on opioids.

Antagonists are dosed to patient response every few minutes. If no response is observed after administration of 15 mg of naloxone, the diagnosis of opioid-induced respiratory depression should be questioned.

Tolerance and physical dependence

The use of opioids is often limited by concerns regarding tolerance, physical dependence, and addiction.

Tolerance can be defined as a state in which a larger dose is required to produce the same response that could formerly be elicited by a smaller dose. Tolerance to analgesia is demonstrated by the need for an increased dosage of a drug to produce the same level of analgesia. Tolerance is sometimes mistaken for disease progression in cancer patients.

Tolerance to adverse effects of opioids occurs after weeks of continuous administration. Tolerance to the constipating and neuroendocrine effects of opioids does not occur.

Physical dependence is the occurrence of a withdrawal syndrome after an opioid is stopped or quickly decreased without titration. Warn patients to avoid abrupt discontinuation of such drugs.

Addiction is a behavior pattern involving the continued use of a substance for nonmedical reasons despite harm. It is characterized by impaired control over drug use, compulsive use, craving, and continued use despite harm.

Pharmacokinetics of Selected Opioids

Morphine

Compared with other opioids, morphine is relatively insoluble in lipids (e.g., in adults, only small amounts of the drug cross the blood–brain barrier).

Morphine does not accumulate in tissues when given in normal doses and therefore does not cause increasing toxicity with frequent dosing.

Morphine is primarily metabolized by glucuronidation during the first pass through the liver. Approximately 50% of morphine is converted by the liver to morphine-3-glucuronide and 15% to morphine-6-glucuronide (M6G). The pharmacologic effects of morphine (both analgesia and side effects) are in part caused by M6G.

Much of an oral dose is inactivated during this first pass through the liver; consequently, oral doses need to be much larger than parenteral doses to produce the same analgesic effects.

Fentanyl

Fentanyl is highly soluble in lipids. It accumulates in skeletal muscle and fat and is released slowly into the blood. Plasma half-life is 3–4 hours after parenteral administration.

Fentanyl is rapidly metabolized, primarily by dealkylation, to inactive metabolites in the liver. This process is mediated through the cytochrome P450 (CYP450) 3A4 hepatic enzyme system. The presence of inactive metabolites makes fentanyl a preferred drug in patients with liver dysfunction.

Fentanyl is not used orally because of low oral bioavailability.

Transdermal fentanyl

The uptake of fentanyl through the skin is relatively slow and constant. The skin does not metabolize the drug, and 92% of the dose is delivered into the bloodstream as intact fentanyl.

Because of temperature-dependent increases in fentanyl release from the patch system as well as increased skin permeability, an increase in body temperature to 40°C (104°F) theoretically may increase serum fentanyl concentrations by approximately one-third.

Fentanyl is absorbed into the upper layers of the skin, forming a depot. Fentanyl then becomes available to systemic circulation. Serum fentanyl concentrations are measurable within 2 hours after application of the first patch, and analgesic effects can be observed 8–16 hours after application. Steady state is reached after several sequential patch applications.

Transmucosal fentanyl citrate lozenge

The absorption pharmacokinetics of fentanyl from the oral transmucosal dosage form is a combination of initial rapid absorption from buccal mucosa and delayed absorption of fentanyl from the GI tract. Normally 25% of the total dose is available by buccal absorption, and 25% is available from the GI tract, making the total bioavailability 50%.

Analgesia begins in 10–15 minutes, peaks in 20 minutes, and persists for 1–2 hours.

Transmucosal fentanyl is indicated only for those who are already receiving and tolerant to around-the-clock opioid therapy.

Fentanyl citrate buccal tablet

Following buccal administration, fentanyl is readily absorbed with an absolute bioavailability of 65%. Approximately 50% of the total dose administered is absorbed transmucosally and becomes systemically available. The remaining half of the total dose is swallowed and undergoes more prolonged absorption from the GI tract.

Buccal tablets are indicated only for those already receiving around-the-clock opioid therapy.

Fentanyl buccal soluble film

The pharmacokinetic absorption involves a combination of rapid absorption from the buccal mucosa and delayed absorption from the GI tract. Absorption from the buccal mucosa is 51% of the total dose, and the remaining 49% of the dose is absorbed from the GI tract. Approximately 20% of the dose absorbed from the GI tract is available for systemic absorption.

Fentanyl soluble film is indicated for breakthrough pain in cancer patients 18 years of age and older who are opioid tolerant and receiving around-the-clock opioid therapies.

Fentanyl sublingual spray

The fentanyl sublingual spray displays a mean absolute bioavailability of 76%. Its bioavailability is dependent on the amount of the dose that is absorbed through the sublingual mucosa and the amount swallowed from the gastrointestinal tract. Variable increases in fentanyl plasma concentration have occurred in patients with mucositis.

Fentanyl nasal spray

Intranasal fentanyl is absorbed from the nasal mucosa and its bioavailability is approximately 20% higher than that of transmucosal fentanyl citrate. The plasma concentration is dose dependent and increases in a linear manner across the dose range. A maximum plasma concentration is reached 15–21 minutes after a single dose.

Methadone

After therapeutic doses, about 90% of methadone is bound to plasma protein and is widely distributed in tissues. Methadone is found in low concentrations in the blood and the brain, with higher concentrations in the kidney, spleen, liver, and lung. Terminal half-life is extremely variable (15–55 hours); therefore, accumulation is possible, and dosing intervals need to be carefully monitored.

Methadone is extensively metabolized in the liver, mainly by N-demethylation. This process appears to be mediated primarily by CYP450 3A4 and to a lesser extent by CYP450 2D6. The major metabolites are excreted in the bile and urine.

Analgesic efficacy does not correspond to the half-life of the drug. Methadone may be dosed every 3 hours for pain control.

Oxycodone

Oxycodone is metabolized to noroxycodone, oxymorphone, and their glucuronides via the CYP450 enzyme system. The major circulating metabolite is noroxycodone. Noroxycodone is reported to be a weaker analgesic than oxycodone. Oxymorphone, although possessing good analgesic activity, is present in the plasma only in low concentrations. Its metabolism is mediated by CYP450 2D6.

Hydromorphone

Hydromorphone is metabolized to three major metabolites: hydromorphone 3-glucuronide, hydromorphone 3-glucoside, and dihydroisomorphine 6-glucoside. Whether hydromorphone is metabolized by the CYP450 system is not known. Hydromorphone is a poor inhibitor of CYP450 isoenzymes and is not expected to inhibit the metabolism of other drugs.

Meperidine

Normeperidine, a toxic metabolite of meperidine, produces anxiety, tremors, myoclonus, and generalized seizures when it accumulates with repetitive dosing. Patients with compromised renal function and concomitant use of benzodiazepines are particularly at risk. Naloxone does not reverse this hyperexcitability. For these reasons, meperidine should not be used for more than 48 hours in patients with renal or CNS disease or at doses greater than 600 mg every 24 hours.

Tapentadol

Tapentadol is metabolized to its major metabolite, tapentadol-O-glucuronide via glucuronidation and two minor metabolites, N-desmethyl tapentadol and hydroxy tapentadol, via the CYP450 enzyme system. The metabolism via CYP450 is not as significant as the phase 2 conjugation. Approximately 97% of the parent drug is metabolized. The major metabolic pathway is via conjugation with extensive metabolism through phase 2 pathways and minor metabolism by phase 1 oxidative pathways. The metabolites do not produce any analgesic activity. The bioavailability is approximately 32% after a single dose because of first-pass metabolism. Peak serum concentrations are typically observed 1.25 hours after a dose.

Drug Interactions and Drug–Disease Interactions

Drug interactions

All drugs with CNS-depressant actions (barbiturates, benzodiazepines, alcohol) can intensify sedation and respiratory depression caused by morphine and other opioids.

Antihistamines, tricyclic antidepressants, and atropine-like drugs can exacerbate morphine-induced constipation and urinary retention.

Antihypertensive drugs and others that lower blood pressure can exacerbate opioid-induced hypotension.

The combination of Demerol, Exalgo, Abstral, or Nucynta with a monoamine oxidase inhibitor (MAOI) may produce a syndrome characterized by excitation, delirium, hyperpyrexia, convulsions, and severe respiratory depression. Death may also occur. Although this syndrome has not been reported with other opioids, combinations containing opioids and MAOIs should be avoided. Patients should not take an opioid medication within 14 days of taking an MAOI.

Agonist–antagonists can precipitate a withdrawal syndrome if administered to an individual who is physically dependent on a pure opioid agonist.

CYP450 enzymes metabolize codeine, hydrocodone, fentanyl, methadone, and oxycodone. Although not well documented, drug interactions through this system may exist. In particular, fentanyl and oxycodone should be used with caution in a patient on a CYP450 3A4 inhibitor. The patient should be monitored over an extended period and dose adjustments made as appropriate.

Codeine, hydrocodone, and oxycodone require metabolism through CYP450 2D6 to an active drug (Table 27-6). Approximately 7% of Caucasians, 3% of African Americans, and 1% of Asians are poor metabolizers of CYP450 2D6; they produce no CYP450 2D6 or produce undetectable levels of it. Poor metabolizers may experience little or no analgesia from drugs requiring CYP450 2D6 for conversion to active metabolites.

About 5% of the patients have multiple copies of the CYP450 2D6 gene, making them ultrafast metabolizers. The clearance of some opioids may be increased, making more frequent dosing of the medications necessary.

Drug–disease interactions

In view of the extensive hepatic metabolism of opioids, their effects may be increased in patients with liver disease, particularly those with severe liver failure. Most opioids require dose reduction in severe liver disease.

Fentanyl, morphine, and methadone require dosing adjustment in renal impairment. Doses of fentanyl and morphine should be reduced 25% when creatinine clearance (CrCl) is 10–50 mL/min and by 50% when CrCl is < 10 mL/min. The dosing interval of methadone should be increased to at least every

Table 27-6. CYP450 2D6 Enzyme Activity

Substrates	Inhibitors	Inducers
Codeine	Celecoxib	Carbamazepine
Hydrocodone	Cimetidine	Ethanol
Meperidine	Citalopram	Phenobarbital
Methadone	Fluoxetine	Phenytoin
Oxycodone	Methadone	Rifampin
Tramadol	Paroxetine	
	Sertraline	

6 hours when CrCl is 10–50 mL/min and to every 8 hours when CrCl is < 10 mL/min.

Renal impairment slows the clearance of morphine conjugates, resulting in accumulation of the active metabolite M6G. For this reason, dosage reduction may be advisable in the presence of clinically significant renal impairment.

Methadone appears to be firmly bound to protein in various tissues, including the brain. After repeated administrations, methadone gradually accumulates in tissues. The risk of accumulation is greater in patients with impaired renal or hepatic function because both organs are involved in the metabolism of methadone.

Patient Counseling

Respiratory depression is increased by concurrent use of other drugs with CNS-depressant activity (e.g., alcohol, barbiturates, benzodiazepines). Outpatients should be warned against the use of alcohol with all other CNS depressants.

Constipation is commonly experienced with short- and long-term use of opioids. Suggest that patients take a stool softener and mild laxative if constipation occurs during the course of treatment. Inform patients about symptoms of hypotension (e.g., lightheadedness, dizziness). Patients should minimize hypotension by moving slowly when changing from a supine to an upright position.

Advise patients that opioids are drugs of potential abuse and should never be taken by anyone other than the person for whom they are prescribed. Patients should never adjust the dose of their medication without first consulting their health care provider.

Liquid formulations should be measured with an appropriate dose-measuring cup or spoon and not a regular teaspoon or tablespoon.

Combinations should not exceed the maximum daily dose of acetaminophen (4 g/day, no liver damage present) to prevent liver toxicity.

Women who are pregnant or planning to become pregnant should consult their health care provider before starting therapy.

Fentanyl transdermal patch

The fentanyl transdermal patch must be applied to a clean, nonhairy site on the upper torso. Only water should be used to clean the area. Soap or alcohol can increase the effects of the medication and should not be used. The patch should not be applied to oily, broken, burned, cut, or irritated skin. It must be held in place for a minimum of 30 seconds to ensure adhesion.

Each new patch should be applied to a different area of skin to avoid irritation. If a patch comes off or causes irritation, it should be removed and a new patch applied to a different site.

To dispose of the patch, fold it in half and flush down the toilet.

Do not cut or damage the patch.

Temperature-dependent increases in fentanyl release from the patch could result in an overdose. Advise patients to avoid exposing the patch to direct external heat sources such as heating pads, electric blankets, heat lamps, saunas, hot tubs, and heated waterbeds. In addition, patients who develop a high fever while wearing the patch should contact their health care provider immediately.

Long-acting opioid formulations

The long-acting formulations should be swallowed whole (i.e., not broken, chewed, or crushed).

Avinza, a long-acting morphine capsule formulation, contains fumaric acid. Doses above 1,600 mg per day contain a quantity of fumaric acid that has not been demonstrated to be safe and may result in serious renal toxicity.

Embeda (extended-release morphine sulfate and naltrexone hydrochloride) contains pellets of an extended-release oral formulation of morphine sulfate surrounding an inner core of naltrexone hydrochloride. Embeda is usually prescribed for pain when drug abuse or diversion is a concern. The capsules should be swallowed whole, or the capsule contents may be sprinkled on applesauce. Crushing, dissolving, or chewing the pellets could block the analgesic effects of morphine by causing an increased release of naltrexone and also could cause a rapid release of a potentially fatal morphine dose. Alcohol consumption may also increase the release and absorption of morphine, leading to an overdose of morphine.

Kadian and Avinza (long-acting morphine sulfate) may be opened and the beads ingested with a small amount of applesauce (sprinkle administration). In addition, Kadian is approved for sprinkle administration through a gastrostomy tube.

Patients must not consume alcoholic beverages or any medications containing alcohol while on Opana ER therapy. The co-ingestion of alcohol with Opana ER may result in increased plasma levels and a potentially fatal overdose of oxymorphone. In addition, food increases the Opana ER maximum concentration by approximately 50%. Opana ER should be ingested 1 hour before and 2 hours after a meal.

Transmucosal fentanyl citrate lozenge

The lozenge is used by placing it in the mouth between the cheek and the gum. Consumption of the lozenge should take 15 minutes. Another lozenge may be used 30 minutes after the start of the first one. Tell the patient not to bite or chew the lozenge.

To dispose of a finished lozenge, discard the handle in a place that is out of reach of children and pets. If medicine remains on the handle, place the handle under hot running tap water until the medicine is dissolved. Never leave unused or partly used lozenges where children or pets can get to them.

Fentanyl citrate buccal tablet

Once removed from the blister pack, the lozenge must be used right away. It is placed in the mouth above the back molars and between the upper cheek and gum. It is left in place until it dissolves, which may take between 14 and 25 minutes. After 30 minutes, any remaining tablet is swallowed with a glass of water.

Parameters to monitor

Evaluate for pain control 1 hour after opioid administration. If analgesia is insufficient, consider a dosage increase. Patients taking opioids chronically should be evaluated regularly for adequate doses.

Monitor the patient for respiratory depression. Higher risk for respiratory depression exists in patients who are not tolerant to opioid analgesics. Consider treatment when the respiratory rate is less than 8–12 respirations per minute for 30 minutes or longer despite stimulation or if oxygen saturation is less than 90%.

If a patient is easily arousable, he or she is unlikely to have respiratory depression.

Tramadol

Tramadol is an analog of codeine, whose mechanism of action is not completely understood. Analgesia is apparently mediated by binding of the parent molecule and the O-desmethyltramadol (M1) active metabolite to μ opioid receptors, as well as by weak inhibition of neuronal uptake of norepinephrine and serotonin. Tramadol is not a federally controlled substance; however, it is classified as a scheduled substance in some states because of the potential for abuse.

The liver extensively metabolizes tramadol. The formation of the M1 active metabolite is dependent on CYP450 2D6. M1 appears to be up to 6 times more potent than tramadol in producing analgesia and 200 times more potent in binding to μ opioid receptors. CYP450 3A4 and CYP450 2B6 also play a role in tramadol metabolism. Caution should be exercised when administering tramadol to patients on CYP450 2D6 and CYP450 3A4 inhibitors.

The most common adverse effects are sedation, dizziness, headache, dry mouth, and constipation. Respiratory depression is minimal. Seizures have been reported; avoid use of tramadol in patients with seizure disorders or recognized risk for seizure (such as head trauma, metabolic disorders, alcohol and drug withdrawal, and CNS infections) and in patients taking antidepressants and neuroleptics.

The U.S. Food and Drug Administration (FDA) requires Risk Evaluation and Mitigation Strategies (REMS) for certain medications when they are prescribed or dispensed. REMS are special requirements to ensure patient safety and may involve medication guides; training courses; and a registry for patients, prescribers, and pharmacies. REMS are required for the medications in Table 27-7.

27-4. Nonpharmacologic Treatment of Pain

General Principles of Nonpharmacologic Treatment

Nonpharmacologic strategies used in combination with appropriate drug regimens may improve pain relief by enhancing the therapeutic effects of medications and permitting use of lower doses.

Nonpharmacologic interventions should not be a substitute for analgesic use.

Physical Interventions

Physical therapy

Physical therapy is most commonly used to help restore physical strength and functioning after injury or surgery.

Physical therapy can provide pain relief for patients with musculoskeletal pain, some types of neuropathic

Table 27-7. Risk and Evaluation Mitigation Strategies (REMS)

Medication	REMS
Abstral (**fentanyl** sublingual tablet)	TIRF REMS Access program enrollment is required for prescribers (outpatient), pharmacies, and patients (outpatient).
Actiq (**fentanyl** citrate lozenge)	TIRF REMS Access program enrollment is required for prescribers (outpatient), pharmacies, and patients (outpatient).
Butrans (buprenorphine transdermal)	Prescribers must receive training.
Fentora (**fentanyl** citrate buccal tablet)	TIRF REMS Access program enrollment is required for prescribers (outpatient), pharmacies, and patients (outpatient).
Lazanda (**fentanyl** nasal spray)	TIRF REMS Access program enrollment is required for prescribers (outpatient), pharmacies, and patients (outpatient).
Methadone (40 mg tablet), indicated for detoxification and maintenance	Medication may be dispensed only in facilities that have been authorized for detoxification and maintenance treatment of patients with opioid addiction.
Opioids (extended release)	Prescriber and patient education is required.
Suboxone (sublingual buprenorphine/naloxone)	Drug Addiction Treatment Act waiver is required for prescribers. Prescribers will be issued a unique identification number (UIN) beginning with an "X," which is required to be present on the prescription.
Subsys (**fentanyl** sublingual spray)	TIRF REMS Access program enrollment is required for prescribers (outpatient), pharmacies, and patients (outpatient).
Subutex (sublingual buprenorphine)	Drug Addiction Treatment Act waiver is required for prescribers.
Vivitrol (naltrexone for extended-release injectable suspension)	Prescriber and patient education is required.

TIRF REMS, Transmucosal Immediate Release Fentanyl Risk Evaluation and Mitigation Strategy.
Boldface indicates one of top 100 drugs for 2012 by units sold at retail outlets, www.drugs.com/stats/top100/2012/units.

pain, and sympathetically mediated pain. Aquatic therapy is an alternative to land-based physical therapy for individuals who cannot perform weight-bearing exercises. Water therapy has been beneficial in improving symptoms associated with fibromyalgia in females.

Acupuncture

The National Institutes of Health recognizes the benefit of acupuncture as an adjunct treatment of painful conditions.

Transcutaneous electrical nerve stimulation

In transcutaneous electrical nerve stimulation (TENS), a controlled, low-voltage electrical current is applied through electrodes placed on the skin. Theoretically, the current will interfere with the ability of nerves to transmit pain signals to the spinal cord and brain. TENS has been used for chronic back and neck pain relief. After several decades of research, it still is not clear if TENS provides any better pain relief than placebo.

Neurostimulation

Neurostimulation involves implanting a computerized generator and electrodes near the spinal cord, near the peripheral nerves, or within the brain. Stimulators are most effective for patients with neuropathic pain and are not very beneficial in other types of pain.

Yoga

Yoga is a type of mind–body connection therapy used as adjunctive treatment for various types of chronic pain in motivated individuals. Many patients suffering from chronic pain experience a better quality of life practicing yoga by decreasing stress and anxiety and improving flexibility, strength, and mood.

Behavioral Techniques

Biofeedback

In biofeedback, electrodes connected to amplifiers are placed on the body or scalp. During biofeedback sessions, a therapist helps the patient learn to mentally control and change the signals from the electrodes, which helps the patient gain conscious control over normally unconscious functions. Biofeedback is most commonly used to relax muscles and reduce stress. Its advantages are that it is noninvasive, inexpensive, and safe.

Distraction and relaxation

Distraction and relaxation assist the patient in refocusing attention on nonpainful stimuli. Both are believed to improve mental health, which translates into improved pain control.

27-5. Migraine

Migraine is a chronic neurovascular disorder characterized by recurrent attacks of severe headache and autonomic nervous system dysfunction. Some patients also experience aura with neurologic symptoms.

Clinical Presentation and Diagnostic Criteria

Migraine headaches usually occur in the frontotemporal region. Photophobia (increased sensitivity to light) and phonophobia (increased sensitivity to sound) also are frequent complaints. A prodrome, also referred to as a premonitory phase, of mood changes, stiff neck, fatigue, or other symptoms may occur hours or days before the onset of the headache. Migraine classification is based on whether an aura of visual or sensory symptoms is present. Migraine with aura is less common than migraine without aura.

Criteria for diagnosing migraine without aura are as follows:

- The patient has at least five headaches lasting 4–72 hours each.
- The headaches have at least two of the following four characteristics:
  - Unilateral location
  - Pulsating quality
  - Moderate or severe intensity (inhibits or prohibits daily activities)
  - Aggravation with walking or similar routine physical activity
- During the headache, at least one of the following symptoms occurs:
  - Nausea or vomiting
  - Photophobia
  - Phonophobia
- Symptoms cannot be consistent with other headache types.

Criteria for diagnosis of migraine with aura are as follows:

- The patient has at least two attacks with the following criteria:
  - One or more completely reversible aura symptoms:
    - Visual
    - Sensory
    - Speech, language, or both
    - Motor
    - Brain stem
    - Retinal
  - At least two of the following characteristics:
    - At least one aura symptom develops gradually (> 5 minutes), two or more symptoms occur in succession, or both characteristics occur.
    - Each individual aura lasts 5–60 minutes.
    - At least one aura symptom is unilateral.
    - Headache follows or accompanies aura in < 1 hour.
- Symptoms cannot be consistent with other headache types, and transient ischemic attack has been ruled out.

Pathophysiology

Migraine and the brain

The pathogenesis of migraine is unclear and is thought to be multifactorial. There are a number of proposed theories to explain the vascular, electrophysical, and genetic mechanisms of migraines.

The most agreed-upon theory is that of cortical spreading depression. It suggests that a wave of depolarization spreads across the cerebral cortex from occipital to frontal regions, resulting in brain ion dysfunction and altered blood flow. These changes account for the progression and variety of symptoms that occur in patients with prodromal or aura phase.

The headache phase is probably related to inappropriate trigeminovascular activation with the release of inflammatory neuropeptides, such as substance P, neurokinin A, and calcitonin gene-related peptide.

Individuals prone to migraine may have inherited or environmentally acquired migraine thresholds that render them susceptible to a migraine attack on exposure to any of a range of patient-specific triggers. Once the threshold is exceeded, trigeminovascular activation is thought to be responsible for inducing a migraine.

Treatment Principles

Abortive therapy

The U.S. Headache Consortium identifies the following goals for successful treatment of acute attacks of migraine:

- Treat attacks rapidly and consistently, and prevent recurrence.
- Restore the patient's ability to function.
- Minimize the use of rescue medication.
- Optimize self-care, and reduce subsequent use of resources.
- Promote cost-effective therapies with minimal adverse effects.

Successful treatment of migraine depends on early intervention in relation to onset of headache and adequate dosing.

Preventive therapy

Preventive therapy should be considered in the following situations:

- Attacks unresponsive to abortive medication
- Attacks causing substantial disability
- Attacks occurring twice or more monthly
- Patient at risk for rebound headache
- Trend in increasing frequency of attacks

Two-thirds of patients taking preventive medication will have a 50% decrease in the frequency of attacks.

The minimum duration of trial for a daily preventive medication is 2–3 months. No consensus exists on the duration of the prophylaxis trial period; however, prophylaxis efficacy may continue to improve when a medication is taken continuously for months to years.

The goals of migraine preventive therapy are as follows:

- Reduce attack frequency, severity, and duration.
- Improve responsiveness to treatment of acute attacks.
- Improve function, and reduce disability.

Rebound headaches

Persons who take abortive medications daily can develop drug rebound headaches, or headaches that begin upon discontinuation of a medication. Essentially all of the medications, with the possible exception of the triptans, cause rebound headaches.

Drug Therapy

Abortive therapy: Nonprescription medications

Aspirin, acetaminophen, ibuprofen, and other aspirin-like analgesics provide adequate relief of mild to moderate migraines. Advil Migraine (ibuprofen 200 mg liquid-filled caps) and Motrin Migraine Relief (ibuprofen 200 mg) are examples of nonprescription medications indicated for migraine relief.

Combination products containing aspirin, acetaminophen, or both with caffeine are also available without a prescription. Caffeine has analgesic and possibly anti-inflammatory properties. It may also increase gastric acidity and perfusion, enhancing the absorption of aspirin. Excedrin Migraine (acetaminophen 250 mg, aspirin 250 mg, and caffeine 65 mg) is an example of an available combination nonprescription product.

Abortive therapy: Nonspecific prescription medications

Combination products containing an analgesic, caffeine, and butalbital or codeine are available. Butalbital may be useful for its sedative properties. Excessive use of these products can cause physical dependence and rebound headaches.

Opioids are well recognized as good analgesics, but strong evidence exists only for the efficacy of butorphanol nasal spray for migraine. Although opioids are commonly used, surprisingly few studies of opioid use in headache pain document whether overuse and the development of dependence are as frequent as clinically perceived.

Given intravenously, the antiemetic metoclopramide may be appropriate as monotherapy for acute attacks, particularly in patients with significant nausea. Chlorpromazine and prochlorperazine may also be considered. Serotonin receptor antagonists (5-HT_3) have not been shown to be useful migraine treatments.

Abortive therapy: Ergotamine

Mechanism of action

In cranial arteries, ergotamine acts directly to promote constriction and reduce the amplitude of pulsations. In addition, the drug can affect blood flow by depressing the vasomotor center. Antimigraine effects are possibly due to agonist activity at serotonin receptor subtypes 5-HT_{1B} and 5-HT_{1D}.

Because of the risk of dependence, ergotamine should not be taken daily on a long-term basis.

Caffeine may be added to ergotamine to enhance vasoconstriction and ergotamine absorption (Table 27-8).

Pharmacokinetics

Oral ergotamine has poor bioavailability because of extensive first-pass metabolism. Sublingual administration may not provide therapeutic blood levels.

Although the half-life of ergotamine is only 2 hours, pharmacologic effects can be seen for 24 hours after administration.

The drug is eliminated primarily by hepatic metabolism. Metabolites are excreted in the bile.

Adverse effects

Ergotamine is well tolerated at usual therapeutic doses.

Table 27-8. Ergot Alkaloids

Drug	Trade name and strengths	Maximum daily dose (weekly maximum)	Dosing instructions
Ergotamine sublingual tablet	Ergomar 2 mg	6 mg (10 mg) po	1 tablet at onset; then 1 every 30 min prn
Ergotamine/caffeine tablet	Cafergot 1/100 mg	Ergotamine 6 mg (10 mg)	2 tablets at onset; then 1 every 30 min prn
Ergotamine/caffeine suppository	Migergot 2/100 mg	Ergotamine 4 mg (10 mg)	Insert 1 at onset; repeat in 1 hour prn
Dihydroergotamine (DHE)	Injection: 1 mg/mL DHE 45	DHE 3 mL IM, 2 mL IV (6 mL IV)	0.5–1 mg IV or IM every hour as needed
	Nasal spray: Migranal 4 mg/mL	DHE 2 mg (6 mg)	Administer 1 spray (0.5 mg) in each nostril, followed in 15 min by an additional spray in each nostril

The drug can stimulate the chemoreceptor trigger zone to cause nausea and vomiting in about 10% of patients. Concurrent treatment with metoclopramide or a phenothiazine antiemetic can help suppress this response.

Other common side effects include weakness in the legs, myalgia, numbness and tingling in the periphery, angina-like pain, tachycardia, and bradycardia.

Overdose

Acute or chronic overdose can cause serious toxicity (ergotism). Symptoms include ischemia, myalgia, and paresthesia. Ischemia can progress to gangrene.

The risk of ergotism is highest in patients with sepsis, peripheral vascular disease, and renal or hepatic impairment.

Drug–drug and drug–disease interactions

Ergotamines are contraindicated with potent inhibitors of CYP450 3A4 because of the risk of cerebral or peripheral ischemia. Concomitant use with selective serotonin receptor agonists should also be avoided because of the risk of a prolonged vasospastic reaction. Separate doses of ergotamine and other migraine medications by at least 24 hours.

Ergotamine is contraindicated for patients with hepatic or renal impairment, sepsis, coronary artery disease (CAD), and peripheral vascular disease.

Patient counseling

Monitor patients to avoid overuse of the medication.

Ergotamine and its derivatives are FDA pregnancy category X. They should not be taken during pregnancy because of their ability to promote uterine contractions and cause fetal harm or abortion.

Teach patients to recognize signs of ergotism. Muscle pain, paresthesia, and cold or pale extremities should be reported immediately.

Abortive therapy: Dihydroergotamine

Mechanism of action

The action of dihydroergotamine (DHE) is similar to that of ergotamine. Like ergotamine, DHE alters transmission at serotonergic, dopaminergic, and α-adrenergic junctions.

In contrast to ergotamine, DHE causes minimal peripheral vasoconstriction, little nausea and vomiting, and no physical dependence. However, diarrhea is prominent.

Contraindications are the same as for ergotamine: CAD, peripheral vascular disease, sepsis, pregnancy, and hepatic or renal impairment.

As with ergotamine, do not administer DHE within 24 hours of a serotonin agonist.

Pharmacokinetics

DHE is not active orally because of extensive first-pass metabolism. An active metabolite, 8′-hydroxy-dihydroergotamine, contributes to its therapeutic effects. The half-life of DHE plus its active metabolite is about 21 hours.

Concomitant administration of DHE with potent CYP450 3A4 inhibitors, including protease inhibitors and macrolide antibiotics, is contraindicated. Because CYP450 3A4 inhibition elevates the serum levels of DHE, the risk for vasospasm leading to cerebral ischemia or ischemia of the extremities is increased.

Abortive therapy: Selective serotonin receptor agonists

The selective serotonin receptor agonists, also known as *triptans,* are first-line drugs for terminating a migraine attack (Table 27-9). The triptans all activate 5-HT$_{1B}$, 5-HT$_{1D}$, and, to a lesser extent, 5-HT$_{1A}$ or 5-HT$_{1F}$ receptors. Triptans have no known affinity for 5-HT$_2$ or 5-HT$_3$ and other 5-HT receptor subclasses, nor do they bind to adrenergic, dopaminergic, muscarinergic, or histaminergic receptors.

Pharmacokinetics

The pharmacokinetics of the different triptans vary somewhat. However, all are generally well tolerated and efficacious at appropriate doses.

Subcutaneous sumatriptan injection has the fastest onset of action when compared with other triptans. Sumatriptan nasal spray has a slightly slower onset than the injection.

Sumatriptan is also available through a single use, disposable, iontophoretic transdermal system (Zecuity), which delivers 6.5 mg of sumatriptan through the skin over 4 hours.

The onset of the majority of oral triptans, including the disintegrating tablets, is similar among the available agents. Rizatriptan may have a slightly faster onset of action at 30 minutes; the disintegrating tablet does not offer a faster onset.

Migraine recurrence rates may be lower with long-half-life triptans such as naratriptan and frovatriptan. However, triptans with longer half-lives tend to have a slower onset of action.

Adverse effects

Triptans are generally well tolerated. Most side effects are mild and transient. The triptans differ slightly from one another in terms of tolerability but not safety.

Table 27-9. Selective Serotonin Receptor Agonists (Triptans)

Drug	Trade name	Available strengths	Dosage (maximum daily dose)	Half-life	Onset	Metabolism
Almotriptan	Axert	Tablet: 6.25, 12.5 mg	12.5 mg; repeat in 2 hours (25 mg)	3.5 hours	60 min	CYP450; MAO
Sumatriptan	Imitrex	Tablet: 25, 50, 100 mg	50–100 mg; repeat in 2 hours (200 mg)	2.5 hours	60–120 min	MAO
		Nasal: 5, 20 mg	5 or 20 mg; repeat in 2 hours (40 mg)		15–20 min	
	Sumavel DosePro	SC injection: 4, 6 mg/0.5 mL	4 or 6 mg; repeat in 1 hour (12 mg)		10–15 min	
	Imitrex STATdose					
Eletriptan	Relpax	Tablet: 20, 40 mg	20 mg; repeat in 2 hours (80 mg)	4 hours	60 min	CYP450 3A4
Frovatriptan	Frova	Tablet: 2.5 mg	2.5 mg; repeat in 2 hours (7.5 mg)	26 hours	60–120 min	Renal 50%; CYP450 1A2
Rizatriptan	Maxalt	Tablet or wafer: 5, 10 mg	5 or 10 mg; repeat in 2 hours (30 mg)	2–3 hours	30 min	MAO
	Maxalt-MLT	Tablet SL: 5, 10 mg	10 mg (30 mg)	2–3 hours	30 min	MAO
Zolmitriptan	Zomig	Tablet: 2.5, 5 mg	2.5 or 5 mg; repeat in 2 hours (10 mg)	2.5–4 hours	45 min	CYP450; MAO
		Nasal: 5 mg	5 mg; repeat in 2 hours (10 mg)	3 hours	10–15 min	CYP450; MAO
	Zomig-ZMT	Tablet SL: 2.5, 5 mg	2.5 mg; repeat in 2 hours (10 mg)	3 hours	120 min	MAO-A
Naratriptan	Amerge	Tablet: 1, 2.5 mg	1 or 2.5 mg; repeat in 4 hours (5 mg)	6 hours	60 min	Renal 70%; CYP450
Miscellaneous agents						
Sumatriptan/naproxen	Treximet	Tablet: 85/500 mg	1 tablet; may repeat in 2 hours (2 tablets) The safety of treating more than 5 migraines in a 30-day period has not been established.	Sumatriptan 2 hours/naproxen 19 hours	60–120 min	Sumatriptan: MAO; naproxen: no significant CYP450 induction

The most frequent side effects are (1) tingling and paresthesia and (2) sensations of warmth in the head, neck, chest, and limbs. Less frequent effects are dizziness, flushing, and neck pain or stiffness.

Chest symptoms

About 50% of patients on sumatriptan experience unpleasant chest symptoms, usually described as "heavy arms" or "chest pressure" rather than pain. These symptoms are transient and not related to ischemic heart disease. Possible causes are pulmonary vasoconstriction, esophageal spasm, intercostal muscle spasm, and bronchoconstriction.

Coronary vasospasm

Rarely, sumatriptan causes angina secondary to coronary vasospasm. Electrocardiographic changes have been observed in patients with CAD or Prinzmetal's (vasospastic) angina. To reduce the risk of angina, do not give sumatriptan to patients who have risk factors for CAD. These patients include postmenopausal women; men over age 40; smokers; and patients with hypertension, hypercholesterolemia, obesity, diabetes, or a family history of CAD.

Other adverse effects

Mild reactions include vertigo, malaise, fatigue, and tingling sensations. Transient pain and redness may occur at sites of subcutaneous injection. Intranasal administration may cause irritation in the nose and throat as well as an offensive or unusual taste.

Drug–drug and drug–disease interactions

The FDA issued a warning about the combination of triptans and serotonergic drugs such as selective serotonin reuptake inhibitors (SSRIs) and serotonin–norepinephrine reuptake inhibitors (SNRIs), which can lead to the serotonin syndrome.

All triptans and ergot alkaloids cause vasoconstriction. Accordingly, if one triptan is combined with another or with an ergot alkaloid, excessive and prolonged vasospasm could result.

Do not use triptans within 24 hours of administering an ergot derivative or another triptan.

MAOIs can suppress degradation of triptans, which causes plasma levels to rise and results in toxicity. Furthermore, triptans should not be administered within 2 weeks of stopping an MAOI. Relpax is contraindicated with potent CYP450 3A4 inhibitors.

Triptans are contraindicated for patients with a history of ischemic heart disease, myocardial infarction, cerebrovascular events, uncontrolled hypertension, or other heart disease. Do not use triptans during pregnancy.

Patient counseling

Patients should be counseled to contact a health care provider if pain or tightness in the chest occurs.

Patients should not exceed daily maximum doses. If migraines occur more than three times a month, prophylactic treatment should be considered.

Migraine Prophylactic Therapy

Table 27-10 summarizes selected migraine preventive treatments.

β-adrenergic blocking agents

Propranolol is one of the drugs of choice for migraine prophylaxis. This agent can reduce the number, duration, and intensity of migraine attacks. It and timolol are the only two β-blockers that have FDA approval for migraine prophylaxis.

Not all β-blockers are active against migraines. Recommended first-line agents include metoprolol, propranolol, and timolol. Additional agents with demonstrated efficacy include atenolol, nadolol, nebivolol, and pindolol. Adverse events with these therapies include fatigue, dizziness, and hypotension. Because not all β-blockers are effective, a mechanism other than β-blockade is apparently responsible for the beneficial effects.

Anticonvulsants

Good evidence supports the efficacy of divalproex sodium and sodium valproate. Both are considered first line for prevention. Divalproex sodium carries FDA approval for migraine prophylaxis. Adverse events with these therapies include nausea, weight gain, hair loss, tremor, and teratogenic potential, such as neural tube defects. Both agents have boxed warnings for hepatotoxicity, pancreatitis, and teratogenicity. Valproate is contraindicated (pregnancy category X) for migraine prophylaxis in pregnant women because of decreased IQ scores in exposed children.

Topiramate has good scientific evidence for clinical efficacy in reducing migraine frequency, duration, and intensity. It is FDA approved for migraine prevention. In March 2014, topiramate became the first medication approved for migraine prophylaxis in adolescents ages 12 to 17. Side effects associated with use include paresthesia, fatigue, nausea, dizziness,

Table 27-10. Selected Migraine Preventive Treatments

Drug	Recommended dose/day	Selected side effects
β-adrenergic receptor antagonists		
Propranolol	80–240 mg	Reduced energy, tiredness, postural symptoms
Metoprolol	100–200 mg	
Timolol	20–30 mg	
Atenolol	100 mg	
Antidepressants		
Amitriptyline	10–150 mg	Drowsiness
Fluoxetine	10–20 mg	Headache, nausea, nervousness, insomnia, drowsiness
Calcium channel blockers		
Diltiazem	90–180 mg	Headache
Verapamil	160–320 mg	Constipation, peripheral edema, cardiac conduction disturbances
Anticonvulsants		
Divalproex	400–600 mg	Drowsiness, weight gain, tremor, hair loss, hematologic and liver abnormalities, teratogenicity
Valproate	500–1,500 mg	
Gabapentin	900–2,400 mg	Somnolence, dizziness
Topiramate	100 mg	Confusion, paresthesias, weight loss
Herbal supplements		
Petasites (butterbur)	50–75 mg bid	
MIG-99 (feverfew)	50–300 mg bid; 2.08–18.75 mg tid for MIG-99 preparation	
Magnesium	400–600 mg	Diarrhea
Coenzyme Q10	300 mg	Gastrointestinal effects
Riboflavin	400 mg	Urine discoloration (yellow)

Adapted from Goadsby P, Lipton R, Ferrari M, 2002; D'Amico D, Tepper J, 2008; Fenstermacher N, Levin M, Ward T, 2011.
Boldface indicates one of top 100 drugs for 2012 by units sold at retail outlets, www.drugs.com/stats/top100/2012/units.

and difficulty concentrating. Anorexia and weight loss may also occur.

Antidepressants

Amitriptyline has efficacy for decreasing migraine frequency. In the past, it was considered first-line prophylaxis treatment. However, as other agents moved to the forefront of migraine prophylactic therapy, its recommendation has been downgraded to second-line therapy. Somnolence, concentration difficulties, and anticholinergic symptoms are frequently reported with tricyclic antidepressants.

Venlafaxine is effective at reducing the number of migraines and their severity. It should be considered second-line therapy. Common side effects include nausea, vomiting, drowsiness, and tachycardia. SNRIs should not be used concomitantly with ergot derivatives or triptans because of increased risk of developing serotonin syndrome.

Calcium channel blockers

Calcium channel blockers were previously considered alternatives for migraine prevention. However, there is inadequate data supporting their use in improving or preventing migraines. Therefore, calcium channel blockers are no longer recommended by guidelines.

Alternative treatment

Petasites (butterbur) has been shown to be effective in reducing the frequency of migraine attacks and has the highest recommendation among herbals and nonprescription therapy for preventing migraines. MIG-99 (feverfew) leaf plays a role in migraine prevention because of the compound parthenolide, which helps relax smooth muscle spasms and release serotonin from platelets. Riboflavin (vitamin B_2) has been shown to play a role in decreasing specific cardiovascular risk (hypertension and elevated homocysteine levels) associated with migraines. Magnesium deficiency has been associated with substance P–induced neuronal inflammation. Persons who suffer from migraines have been shown to have decreased magnesium levels. Subcutaneous histamine injections (1–10 ng twice a week) showed efficacy in reducing the frequency, severity, and duration of migraine attacks. Transient itching and burning were the only reported adverse events with this therapy.

Antispasmodics

OnabotulinumtoxinA (Botox) is the first and only FDA-approved agent for prevention of chronic migraine (> 15 migraine days per month with migraines lasting at least 4 hours).

27-6. Nonpharmacologic Treatment of Migraines

General Principles of Nonpharmacologic Therapies

Nonpharmacologic approaches may be well suited to patients who have exhibited a poor tolerance or poor response to drug therapy; who have a contraindication to drug therapy; or who have a history of long-term, frequent, or excessive use of analgesics or other acute medications. Nonpharmacologic interventions may also be useful in patients who are pregnant, are planning to become pregnant, or are nursing.

Treatment Recommendations

Patients with migraine pain may experience relief by resting or sleeping in a cool, quiet, dark environment. Half of migraine patients experience considerable relief by applying a cold compress to the head.

Relaxation training, thermal biofeedback combined with relaxation training, electromyographic biofeedback, and cognitive-behavioral therapies are somewhat effective in preventing migraine.

Evidence pertaining to the treatment of migraine with acupuncture is limited, and the results are mixed. Similarly, limited evaluation has been conducted with hypnosis, TENS, cervical manipulation, and hyperbaric oxygen.

Transcutaneous Electrical Nerve Stimulation

In March 2014, the FDA approved the first TENS device, Cefaly, for migraine prophylaxis. This device is specifically labeled for use before the onset of pain in patients 18 years of age or older. It is a small, portable, battery-powered, prescription device that resembles a plastic headband worn across the forehead and atop the ears. The device applies an electric current to stimulate branches of the trigeminal nerve, which has been associated with migraine headaches. The device should be used only once per day for 20 minutes.

Trigger Management

Trigger management is important in preventing migraine attacks. Triggering factors can cause migraine. If recognized and avoided, they may impede an impending attack.

Triggers vary from person to person. Examples of triggers include changes in weather or air pressure; bright sunlight, glare, or fluorescent lights; chemical fumes; menstrual cycles; and certain foods such as processed meats, red wine, beer, dried fish, broad beans, fermented cheeses, aspartame, and monosodium glutamate.

27-7. Questions

1. Approximately how many people in the United States experience severe chronic pain?

    A. 10 million
    B. 23 million
    C. 40 million
    D. 50 million
    E. 76 million

2. Addiction is currently understood to be

    A. characterized by compulsive use of drugs.
    B. synonymous with physical dependence on a medication.
    C. the use of a substance for psychical effects.
    D. A and C
    E. A and B

3. The WHO analgesic hierarchy emphasizes

    A. concurrently using nonopioids, opioids, and adjuvant medications.
    B. avoiding opioid use.
    C. reserving opioid use only for severe pain.
    D. using single agents rather than a combination of medications.
    E. using nonopioids only for treatment of mild pain.

4. All of the following adverse effects are manifestations of μ opioid agonists *except*

    A. constipation.
    B. respiratory depression.
    C. atrial flutter.
    D. nausea.
    E. miosis.

5. The preferred route of opioid administration is

   A. oral.
   B. intravenous.
   C. subcutaneous.
   D. rectal.
   E. intramuscular.

6. Which of the following opioids has the longest duration of analgesic effect?

   A. Methadone
   B. Controlled-release morphine
   C. Hydromorphone
   D. Transdermal fentanyl
   E. Controlled-release oxycodone

7. All of the following opioids are metabolized through the cytochrome P450 hepatic enzyme system *except*

   A. hydrocodone.
   B. oxycodone.
   C. morphine.
   D. methadone.
   E. fentanyl.

8. The clearance of which of the following opioids may be increased in patients with multiple copies of the CYP450 2D6 gene?

   A. Methadone
   B. Oxycodone
   C. Fentanyl
   D. Morphine
   E. Hydromorphone

9. Which of the following statements regarding methadone pharmacokinetics is true?

   A. The half-life corresponds to analgesic efficacy.
   B. It is highly plasma protein bound and widely distributed in tissue.
   C. The clearance of methadone is rapid, resulting in frequent dosing.
   D. Methadone has low bioavailability from the GI tract and therefore is not useful when given orally.
   E. Methadone is metabolized by hepatic glucuronidation.

10. Which of the following agents can be used to reverse respiratory effects caused by opioid overdose?

    A. Naloxone
    B. Pentazocine

    C. Buprenorphine
    D. Naltrexone
    E. Tramadol

11. Which of the following opioids is not appropriate for use as an around-the-clock medication in chronic pain?

    A. Morphine
    B. Oxycodone
    C. Fentanyl
    D. Hydromorphone
    E. Methadone

12. Which of the following opioids has a toxic metabolite that can accumulate in renal dysfunction?

    A. Oxycodone
    B. Fentanyl
    C. Meperidine
    D. Hydromorphone
    E. Methadone

Use Patient Profile 27-1 to answer Questions 13 and 14.

13. Which of Mrs. Martin's medications is most likely to worsen opioid-induced constipation?

    A. Paxil
    B. Zocor
    C. Lotensin
    D. Premarin
    E. Elavil

14. The health care provider recommends changing Mrs. Martin's opioid to one that is less constipating. Which of the following medications is least likely to cause constipation?

    A. Morphine extended release
    B. Methadone
    C. Oxycodone extended release
    D. Transdermal fentanyl patch
    E. Hydromorphone

15. The rationale of adding caffeine to a simple analgesic for migraine treatment is to

    I. decrease the required dose of acetaminophen and aspirin.
    II. cause cerebral arterial vasoconstriction.

Patient name: Mary Martin	Address: 815 Elm Street	Date	Medication
Age: 65	Sex: Female	3/3	Paxil 20 mg daily
Allergies: NKDA		3/3	Zocor 40 mg daily
Diagnosis:		3/3	Lotensin 20 mg daily
Chronic low back pain		3/3	Premarin 0.625 mg
Hypertension		3/3	Morphine sulfate extended-release 60 mg bid
Hypercholesterolemia		3/3	Senokot S
Chronic constipation		3/28	Elavil 50 mg
		4/1	Milk of magnesia

III. increase gastric acidity and perfusion, enhancing aspirin absorption.

A. I only
B. III only
C. I and III only
D. II and III only
E. I, II, and III

16. Which of the following agents is a selective serotonin agonist?

A. Sumatriptan
B. Ketorolac
C. Dihydroergotamine
D. Metoclopramide
E. Caffeine

17. Which is of the following statements is true regarding the adverse effects of ergotamine?

A. Ergotamine inhibits the chemoreceptor trigger zone to minimize nausea and vomiting.
B. Ergotamine has minimal risk of dependence.
C. Muscle weakness is an uncommon side effect of ergotamine.
D. Angina-like pain reported with the triptans is not seen with ergotamine use.
E. Overuse of ergotamine can result in ischemia.

18. Which of the following statements about triptans is correct?

A. Few contraindications exist to the use of triptans.
B. Triptans are contraindicated in ischemic cardiovascular disease.

C. Triptans are preferred for migraine treatment during pregnancy.
D. Patients taking ergot alkaloids can use triptans concomitantly.
E. Triptans are strictly contraindicated in patients with hypertension.

19. Which of the following statements is true regarding the use of opioids for migraines?

A. Opioid use is not associated with rebound headaches.
B. Butorphanol nasal spray is efficacious in migraine abortive therapy.
C. Opioids in combination with butalbital and caffeine do not produce physical dependence.
D. Opioids scheduled around the clock are useful for migraine prophylaxis.
E. Opioids are not commonly prescribed for migraine treatment.

20. Which of the following statements about Treximet is correct?

I. Treximet can be used concomitantly with over-the-counter products such as Aleve.
II. Treximet dose is limited to 3 capsules per 24 hours.
III. Treximet may cause dizziness.

A. I only
B. III only
C. I and III only
D. II and III only
E. I, II, and III

Use Patient Profile 27-2 to answer Questions 23 and 24.

Patient Profile 27-2

Patient name: James Hunt

Age: 45

Allergies: NKDA

Medications:

Address: 817 Elm Street

Sex: Male

Diagnosis: Migraine with aura, controlled hypertension

Date	Drug and strength	Sig	Quantity
1/1	Sumatriptan 100 mg tablet	Oral, use as directed	#9 tabs
1/1	Lisinopril 10 mg tablet	Oral, daily	#30 tabs
2/1	Sumatriptan 100 mg tablet	Oral, use as directed	#9 tabs
2/1	Lisinopril 10 mg tablet	Oral, daily	#30 tabs
3/1	Sumatriptan 100 mg tablet	Oral, use as directed	#9 tabs
3/1	Lisinopril 10 mg tablet	Oral, daily	#30 tabs
3/9	Sumatriptan 100 mg tablet	Oral, use as directed	#9 tabs
3/14	Sumatriptan 100 mg tablet	Oral, use as directed	#9 tabs

---

21. Dihydroergotamine differs from ergotamine in which of the following ways?

    A. DHE has higher incidence of nausea and vomiting.
    B. DHE has higher incidence of physical dependence.
    C. DHE has no contraindications for ischemic cardiovascular disease.
    D. DHE has a higher incidence of diarrhea.
    E. DHE can be administered concomitantly with a triptan.

22. Which of the following statements is true regarding initiation of prophylactic migraine therapy in Mr. Hunt?

    A. Mr. Hunt is at high risk for rebound headaches caused by excessive sumatriptan use.
    B. Mr. Hunt is limiting his sumatriptan use to 3 days per week and is not a candidate for prophylactic treatment.
    C. Mr. Hunt is a candidate for prophylactic therapy because of the increasing frequency of attacks.
    D. Mr. Hunt requires prophylactic therapy because his hypertension is a contraindication to using abortive therapies.
    E. Prophylactic treatment is contraindicated in migraines with aura.

23. Which medication is appropriate to give Mr. Hunt for migraine prophylaxis?

    A. Butorphanol
    B. Propranolol
    C. Dihydroergotamine
    D. Acetaminophen
    E. Hydrocodone

27-8. Answers

1. **E.** Currently, about 76 million individuals suffer from some form of chronic benign pain.

2. **D.** Physical dependence is the occurrence of a withdrawal syndrome after an opioid is stopped or quickly decreased without titration. Addiction is the psychological dependence on the use of substances for psychical effects and is characterized by compulsive use.

3. **A.** The WHO analgesic hierarchy involves choosing among three stepped levels of treatment. Mild pain may respond to nonopioid drugs alone. Combining a low-dose opioid with a nonopioid can relieve moderate pain. More severe pain requires the addition of a higher-dose opioid preparation to the nonopioid. At any step, analgesic adjuvants may be useful.

4. **C.** Atrial flutter is not a documented adverse effect of opioids. However, therapeutic doses of many opioids produce peripheral vasodilation, reduced peripheral resistance, and inhibition of the baroreceptor reflexes. Recently, methadone has been associated with torsades de pointes, an atypical rapid ventricular tachycardia.

5. **A.** Oral medications should be used whenever possible because of convenience, flexibility, and steady serum levels.

6. **D.** Transdermal fentanyl provides analgesia for up to 72 hours. The analgesic effects of methadone do not correlate with its long half-life.

7. **C.** Morphine is metabolized by hepatic glucuronidation.

8. **B.** Oxycodone is metabolized through CYP450 2D6 to active metabolites. Fast metabolizers—those with multiple copies of the CYP450 2D6 gene—would clear oxycodone and its metabolites quickly.

9. **B.** About 90% of methadone is bound to plasma protein and is widely distributed in tissues. Methadone has a long terminal half-life, resulting in slow clearance. This half-life does not correspond to analgesic dosing. It is metabolized via the CYP450 enzyme system.

10. **A.** Naloxone is a μ antagonist useful in opioid overdose. Naltrexone is also a μ antagonist, but it is reserved for use in alcoholism and opioid addiction.

11. **D.** Hydromorphone is an opioid with a short half-life with no available long-acting formulation. Thus, it is not useful as an around-the-clock medication.

12. **C.** Normeperidine, a metabolite of meperidine, can accumulate with chronic use, with renal impairment, and when the dose exceeds 600 mg every 24 hours.

13. **E.** The anticholinergic effects of tricyclic antidepressants such as Elavil can exacerbate opioid-induced constipation and urinary retention.

14. **D.** Because transdermal delivery bypasses absorption from the GI tract, constipation has been reported to be less frequent with transdermal fentanyl than with other opioids.

15. **C.** Caffeine has analgesic and possibly anti-inflammatory properties. Therefore, reduced doses of acetaminophen and aspirin may be required. Caffeine may also increase gastric acidity and perfusion, enhancing the absorption of aspirin.

16. **A.** Sumatriptan is a selective serotonin agonist.

17. **E.** Adverse effects of ergotamine include nausea and vomiting, physical dependence, muscle weakness, and angina-like pain. Overuse of ergotamine can result in ischemia that may progress to gangrene.

18. **B.** Triptans are contraindicated in pregnancy and ischemic cardiovascular disease. They cannot be used within 24 hours of another triptan or ergot alkaloid.

19. **B.** Good evidence exists for the efficacy of butorphanol nasal spray in migraine abortive therapy. Although opioids are commonly used for abortive therapy, they may be associated with rebound headaches and physical dependence.

20. **B.** Treximet is indicated for the acute treatment of migraine attacks with or without aura in adults. This medication may cause dizziness. The dose is limited to 2 tablets per 24 hours. Because of Treximet's naproxen content, other products containing naproxen should not be used concomitantly.

21. **D.** In contrast to ergotamine, DHE causes minimal peripheral vasoconstriction, little nausea and vomiting, and no physical dependence. However, diarrhea is prominent.

22. **C.** Prophylactic therapy should be considered because his migraines occur more than twice monthly and the frequency of attacks is increasing.

23. **B.** Propranolol has been shown to be effective for migraine prophylaxis. This agent can reduce the number and intensity of attacks in about 70% of patients. Butorphanol, acetaminophen, dihydroergotamine, and hydrocodone are not approved for migraine prophylaxis.

27-9. References

Pain

American Academy of Pain Medicine. Use of opioids for the treatment of chronic pain: A statement from the American Academy of Pain Medicine. 2013. http://www.painmed.org/files/use-of-opioids

-for-the-treatment-of-chronic-pain.pdf. Accessed April 9, 2014.

American Pain Society. *Principles of Analgesic Use in the Treatment of Acute Pain and Cancer Pain.* 6th ed. Glenview, IL: American Pain Society; 2008.

American Society of Anesthesiologists Task Force on Pain Management. Practice guidelines for chronic pain management: An updated report by the American Society of Anesthesiologists Task Force on Chronic Pain Management and the American Society of Regional Anesthesia and Pain Medicine. *Anesthesiology.* 2010;112(4):810–33.

Approved Risk Evaluation and Mitigation Strategies (REMS). April 19, 2014. U.S. Food and Drug Administration Web site. www.fda.gov/drugs /drugsafety/postmarketdrugsafetyinformationfor patientsandproviders/ucm111350.htm. Accessed April 12, 2014.

Baumann TJ, Strickland JM, Herdon CM, et al. Pain management. In: DiPiro JT, Talbert RL, Yee GC, et al., eds. *Pharmacotherapy: A Pathophysiologic Approach.* 8th ed. New York, NY: McGraw-Hill; 2011:1045–59.

Bonica JJ, ed. *The Management of Pain.* 2nd ed. Philadelphia, PA: Lea & Febiger; 1990.

Boyer EW. Management of opioid analgesic overdose. *N Eng J Med.* 2012;367:146–55.

Brookoff D. Chronic pain: 1. A new disease. *Hosp Pract (Off Ed).* 2000;35:45–52, 59.

Bussing A, Ostermann T, Ludtke R, et al. Effects of yoga interventions on pain and pain-associated disability: A meta-analysis. *J of Pain.* 2012;13:1–9.

Chronic Pain Medical Treatment Guidelines: Medical Treatment Utilization Schedule. July 18, 2009. State of California Division of Workers' Compensation Web site. http://www.dir.ca.gov /dwc/DWCPropRegs/MTUS_Regulations /MTUS_Regulations.htm. Accessed March 20, 2014.

Chou R, Fanciullo GJ, Fine PG, et al. Clinical guidelines for the use of chronic opioid therapy in chronic noncancer pain. *J Pain.* 2009;10:113–30.

Duragesic [package insert]. Titusville, NJ: Janssen Pharmaceuticals; September 2013.

Dworkin RH, O'Conner AB, Audette J, et al. Recommendations for the pharmacological management of neuropathic pain: An overview and literature update. *Mayo Clin Proc.* 2010;85:S3–S14.

Embeda [package insert]. Bristol, TN: King Pharmaceuticals; June 2013.

Holdsworth M, Forman W, Killilea T, et al. Transdermal fentanyl disposition in elderly subjects. *Gerontology.* 1994;40:32–7.

Jacox A, Carr DB. *Management of Cancer Pain: Clinical Practice Guideline No. 9.* AHCPR Publication No. 94-0492. Rockville, MD: Agency for Health Care Policy and Research, U.S. Department of Health and Human Services, Public Health Service; 1994.

Joint Commission on Accreditation of Healthcare Organizations. *Pain Assessment and Management: An Organizational Approach.* Oakbrook Terrace, IL: Joint Commission on Accreditation of Healthcare Organizations; 2000.

Lazanda [package insert]. Bedminster, NJ: Archimedes Pharma US Inc.; July 2012.

Merskey H, Bogduk N, eds. *Classification of Chronic Pain: Descriptions of Chronic Pain Syndromes and Definitions of Pain Terms.* 2nd ed. Seattle, WA: IASP Press; 1994.

O'Conner AB, Dworkin RH. Treatment of neuropathic pain: An overview of recent guidelines. *Am J Med.* 2009;122(10 Suppl):S22–32.

Portenoy RK. Opioid therapy for chronic nonmalignant pain: A review of the critical issues. *J Pain Symptom Manage.* 1996;11:203–17.

Subsys [package insert]. Phoenix, AZ: Insys Therapeutics, Inc.; July 2013.

Turk DC, Melzack R, eds. *Handbook of Pain Assessment.* 2nd ed. New York, NY: Guilford Press; 2001.

World Health Organization. *Cancer Pain Relief: With a Guide to Opioid Availability.* 2nd ed. Geneva: World Health Organization; 1996.

Migraines

Anthony M, Rasmussen BK. Migraine without aura. In: Olesen J, Tfelt-Hansen P, Welch KMA, eds. *The Headaches.* New York, NY: Raven Press; 1993:255–61.

Bigal ME, Ferrari M, Silberstein SD. Migraine in the triptan era: Lessons from epidemiology, pathophysiology, and clinical science. *Headache.* 2009;49:S21–S33.

Cutrer FM. Pathophysiology of migraine. *Semin Neurol.* 2006;26:171–80.

D'Amico D, Tepper J. Prophylaxis of migraines: General principles and patient acceptance. *Neuropsychiatr Dis Treat.* 2008;4:1155–67.

DHE 45 [package insert]. Costa Mesa, CA: Valent Pharmaceuticals North America; 2002.

Diamond M. The role of concomitant headache types and non-headache comorbidities in the underdiagnosis of migraine. *Neurology.* 2002;58(suppl 6): S3–9.

FDA allows marketing of first medical device to prevent migraine headaches. FDA News Release.

March 11, 2014. U.S. Food and Drug Administration Web site. http://www.fda.gov/newsevents/newsroom/pressannouncements/ucm388765.htm. Accessed April 7, 2014.

FDA approves Topamax for migraine prevention in adolescents. FDA News Release. March 28, 2014. U.S. Food and Drug Administration Web site. http://www.fda.gov/newsevents/newsroom/pressannouncements/ucm391026.htm. Accessed April 4, 2014.

FDA Drug Podcast: Valproate anti-seizure products contraindicated for migraine prevention in pregnant women due to decreased IQ scores in exposed children. Drug Safety Podcasts. May 7, 2013. U.S. Food and Drug Administration Web site. http://www.fda.gov/drugs/drugsafety/drugsafetypodcasts/ucm351109.htm. Accessed April 4, 2014.

Fenstermacher N, Levin M, Ward T. Pharmacological prevention of migraine. *BMJ.* 2011;342:540–3.

Firnhaber J, Rickett K. What are the best prophylactic drugs for migraine? *J Pharm Pract.* 2009;58(11):608–10.

Frova [package insert]. Chadds Ford, PA: Endo Pharmaceuticals; April 2007.

Goadsby P, Lipton R, Ferrari M. Migraine: Current understanding and treatment. *N Engl J Med.* 2002;346:257–70.

Headache Classification Committee of the International Headache Society (IHS). The International Classification of Headache Disorders: 3rd edition, beta version. *Cephalalgia.* 2013;33(9):629–808.

Holland S, Silberstein SD, Freitag F, et al. Evidence-based guideline update: NSAIDs and other complementary treatments for episodic migraine prevention in adults: Report of the Quality Standards Subcommittee of the American Academy of Neurology and the American Headache Society. *Neurology.* 2012;78:1346–53.

Information for healthcare professionals: Selective serotonin reuptake inhibitors (SSRIs), selective serotonin-norepinephrine reuptake inhibitors (SNRIs), 5-hydroxytryptamine receptor agonists (triptans). Postmarket Drug Safety Information for Patients and Providers. August 14, 2013. U.S. Food and Drug Administration Web site. http://www.fda.gov/drugs/drugsafety/postmarketdrugsafetyinformationforpatientsandproviders/drugsafetyinformationforheathcareprofessionals/ucm085845.htm. Accessed April 8, 2014.

Rasmussen BK, Jensen R, Schroll M, et al. Inter-relations between migraine and tension-type headache in the general population. *Arch Neurol.* 1992;49:914–8.

Silberstein SD, Holland S, Freitag F, et al. Evidence-based guideline update: Pharmacologic treatment for episodic migraine prevention in adults: Report of the Quality Standards Subcommittee of the American Academy of Neurology and the American Headache Society. *Neurology.* 2012;78:1337–45.

Silberstein SD. Migraine. *Lancet.* 2004;363:381–91.

Silberstein SD. Practice parameter: Evidence-based guidelines for migraine headache (an evidence-based review). Report of the Quality Standards Subcommittee of the American Academy of Neurology. *Neurology.* 2000;55:754–62.

Silberstein SD. Topiramate in migraine prevention: Evidence-based medicine from clinical trials. *Arch Neurol.* 2004;61:490–5.

Spierings ELH, Ranke AH, Honkoop PC. Precipitating and aggravating factors of migraine versus tension-type headache. *Headache.* 2001;41:554–8.

Taylor FR. Nutraceuticals and headache: The biological basis. *Headache.* 2011;51(3):484–501.

Topamax [package insert]. Titusville, NJ: Ortho-McNeil Neurologics; April 2008.

Wolters Kluwer Health. Facts and comparisons online. Wolters Kluwer Health, St. Louis, MO. http://www.factsandcomparisons.com.

Seizure Disorders

28

Elizabeth L. Alford
Stephanie J. Phelps

28-1. Key Points

- Phenytoin can be mixed only with normal saline and should not be given faster than 50 mg/min.
- Gabapentin and levetiracetam are not associated with any significant drug interactions.
- As of September 2009, the following anticonvulsants carry a U.S. boxed warning: carbamazepine (aplastic anemia, dermatologic reactions); valproic acid (liver failure, teratogenicity, pancreatitis); felbamate (aplastic anemia, hepatic failure); and lamotrigine (serious rash). The U.S. Food and Drug Administration (FDA) warnings have been given for zonisamide and topiramate, which have been reported to cause oligohidrosis and hyperthermia. The FDA has found that 11 of the anticonvulsants are associated with an increased risk of suicidal behavior or ideation.
- Although absence seizures are frequently treated with ethosuximide or valproic acid (for patients ≥ 2 years of age), lamotrigine and topiramate are also used.
- Carbapenems (e.g., imipenem) and normeperidine (a metabolite of meperidine that accumulates in renal failure) may cause seizures.
- Carbamazepine undergoes autoinduction (i.e., it induces its own metabolism), and phenytoin has capacity-limited or saturable (i.e., Michaelis–Menten) pharmacokinetics.

- Because of the potential for severe life-threatening liver toxicity, valproic acid is generally not used in a patient < 2 years of age.
- There may be an association between folic acid deficiency and spina bifida; hence, all women with epilepsy who are of childbearing age should be on daily folic acid (1 mg).
- Unless a patient is experiencing a life-threatening adverse effect, an anticonvulsant should not be abruptly discontinued.
- Topiramate may cause significant weight loss, and valproic acid may cause significant weight gain.
- Topiramate and zonisamide may cause kidney stones.
- Patients with an allergy to sulfa medications should not be given zonisamide.

28-2. Study Guide Checklist

The following topics may guide your study of this subject area:

- The two main types of seizures and the differences between the two
- Drugs most often used as mono therapy in each of the two main types of seizures
- Drugs most often used as adjunctive therapy in each of the two main types of seizures
- Criteria for treatment, principles of treatment, and reasons for treatment failure of epilepsy
- FDA black box warnings and the most prevalent adverse effects for the various classes of anti-epileptic drugs (AEDs)
- Important drug–drug interactions involving AEDs
- Emergent treatment of *status epilepticus*

Editor's Note: This chapter is based on the 10th edition chapter written by Stephanie J. Phelps.

28-3. Epilepsy

Epilepsy occurs when neurons become depolarized and repetitively fire action potentials. It is involuntary and episodic. The term is applied after two unprovoked seizures. A seizure does not mean a person has epilepsy; however, epilepsy means a person has seizures. Anticonvulsants do not cure epilepsy.

Terminology

- *Aura:* A subjective sensation or motor phenomenon that marks a seizure onset and is generally associated with sensations that are localized in a particular region of the brain
- *Automatisms:* Purposeless movements seen with partial seizures
- *Postictal:* Symptoms and signs seen after a seizure

Types of Epilepsy

There are two main types of epilepsy: partial seizures and generalized seizures.

Partial seizures

Partial seizures begin in one hemisphere of the brain. They are unilateral, asymmetric movements, generally associated with an aura. Complex partial seizures are accompanied by altered consciousness.

Drugs for new-onset partial seizures
See individual drug for specific indication information.

- *Monotherapy:* Carbamazepine (drug of choice), lamotrigine, oxcarbazepine, phenobarbital, phenytoin, topiramate, valproic acid
- *Adjunctive therapy:* Eslicarbazepine, gabapentin, lacosamide, lamotrigine, levetiracetam, oxcarbazepine, perampanel, phenobarbital, phenytoin, tiagabine, topiramate, valproic acid, zonisamide

Drugs for refractory partial seizures
See individual drug for specific indication information.

- *Monotherapy:* Carbamazepine, felbamate, lamotrigine, phenytoin, phenobarbital, topiramate, valproic acid
- *Adjunctive therapy:* Eslicarbazepine, ezogabine, felbamate, gabapentin, lamotrigine, lacosamide, levetiracetam, oxcarbazepine, perampanel, phenobarbital, phenytoin, zonisamide

Generalized seizures

Generalized seizures begin simultaneously in both brain hemispheres. They are characterized by bilateral movements and have no aura.

Absence seizures
This type of generalized seizure has a sudden onset. It is brief (seconds) and characterized by a blank stare, upward rotation of the eyes, and lip smacking (confused with daydreaming). It has a three-per-second spike and wave on electroencephalography (EEG) and can be precipitated by hyperventilation.

Drugs
See individual drug for specific indication information.

Historically, ethosuximide has been the drug of choice. If a patient has both absence and generalized tonic–clonic seizures and is older than 2 years of age, many consider valproic acid to be the drug of choice. Although not labeled by the U.S. Food and Drug Administration (FDA), lamotrigine and topiramate are used.

Primary generalized tonic–clonic seizure
This type of seizure has two phases:

- *Tonic phase:* Rigid, violent, sudden muscular contractions (stiff or rigid); crying or moaning; deviation of the eyes and head to one side; rotation of the whole body and distortion of features; suppression of respiration; falling to the ground; loss of consciousness; tongue biting; involuntary urination
- *Clonic phase:* Repetitive jerks; cyanosis continues; foaming at the mouth; small grunting respirations between seizures, but deep respirations as all muscles relax at the end of the seizure

Drugs of choice
See individual drug for specific indication information.

- *Monotherapy:* Carbamazepine, phenobarbital, phenytoin, topiramate ($\geq$ 2 years of age)
- *Adjunctive therapy:* Lamotrigine, levetiracetam, topiramate, valproic acid

Juvenile myoclonic epilepsy
Juvenile myoclonic epilepsy (JME) consists of myoclonic and generalized tonic–clonic seizures. Myoclonic seizures precede generalized tonic–clonic seizures, and both seizure types generally occur on awakening. Sleep deprivation and alcohol commonly precipitate JME.

Because JME has a genetic basis, lifelong treatment is required. Although not FDA labeled for this use, valproic acid, lamotrigine, levetiracetam, topiramate, or some combination of these agents is prescribed.

Other less common seizure types

Catamenial epilepsy
Catamenial epilepsy is associated with hormonal changes during menstruation and may be treated with acetazolamide.

Infantile spasms
Infantile spasms begin in the first 6 months of life. They occur in clusters, several times a day. Parents describe symptoms that resemble colic. Infantile spasms are associated with high mortality and morbidity.

This condition is treated with adrenocorticotropic hormone (ACTH) or oral steroids, vigabatrin, or valproic acid (> 2 years). Although not FDA labeled for this purpose, topiramate and zonisamide have been used.

Lennox–Gastaut syndrome
This syndrome accounts for as few as 1–4% of childhood epilepsies, most often appears between 2–6 years of age, and is frequently accompanied by mental retardation and behavior problems. It is characterized by different types of intractable seizures.

This condition is treated with combination anticonvulsants that include clobazam (> 2 years), felbamate (> 2 years), lamotrigine (> 2 years), rufinamide (≥ 4 years), and topiramate (≥ 2 years). Although not FDA labeled for this purpose, zonisamide has been used.

Post-traumatic epilepsy
These seizures occur following head trauma and may be treated prophylactically with phenytoin or fosphenytoin for a period of 7 days. Levetiracetam is also used for this purpose. Valproic acid should not be used because it has been associated with a greater likelihood of central nervous system (CNS) bleeding and a higher mortality rate in this population. If no seizures occur within 7 days, medication should be discontinued.

Etiologies for Epilepsy

- **Mechanical:** Birth injuries, head trauma, tumors, vascular abnormalities (stroke)
- **Metabolic:** Electrolyte disturbances (low sodium, elevated calcium); glucose abnormalities (low glucose); inborn errors of metabolism
- **Genetic:** Benign familial neonatal seizures (chromosome 20), JME (chromosome 6), Baltic myoclonic (chromosome 21)
- **Other:** Fever, infection
- **Drugs:** These include, but are not limited to, the following:
  - Recreational drugs such as alcohol, cocaine and freebase cocaine, ephedra, methylphenidate, narcotics
  - Carbapenems (imipenem), lindane, local anesthetics (lidocaine), metoclopramide, theophylline, tricyclic antidepressants
  - Meperidine (the metabolite normeperidine can cause seizures in patients with renal failure who receive normal doses)
  - Anticonvulsants that are used for treatment of a nonindicated seizure type (Table 28-1)

Criteria for Treating Epilepsy

Almost no child should be treated after one seizure. Adults who have structural brain damage, a first seizure that was very severe, or an occupation that places them at risk of injury should a second seizure occur may be treated following one seizure.

Principles in the treatment of epilepsy

- **Monotherapy (one agent):** This form of treatment is always preferred.

Table 28-1. Seizures Caused by Anticonvulsants

Anticonvulsant	Absence	Seizure type Generalized tonic–clonic	Myoclonic
Carbamazepine (Tegretol, Carbitrol)	Causes	Causes	Causes
Phenytoin (Dilantin, Phenytek)	Causes		
Phenobarbital	Causes		

■ *Polytherapy (two agents):* The addition of a second anticonvulsant should not be considered until the serum concentrations (where appropriate) and doses of the first anticonvulsant have been maximized. This approach is important in a patient who has developed side effects or has not responded to the first anticonvulsant. Generally, the second anticonvulsant should work through a different mechanism of action than the first. When the patient is at full doses of the second anticonvulsant, the dose of the first drug should be slowly reduced.

■ *Polytherapy (three or more agents):* Although rarely needed, add a third anticonvulsant if (1) a combination of two anticonvulsants is tolerated and significantly reduces seizure frequency or severity, but greater control might be achieved, or (2) doses of the two anticonvulsants have been maximized. Reassess response, and slowly discontinue unnecessary anticonvulsants as soon as possible.

Reasons for Treatment Failure

■ Incorrect diagnosis
■ Wrong anticonvulsant for seizure type
■ Inappropriate dose, route, or formulation
■ Failure to recognize altered pharmacokinetics or pharmacogenomics that require a dosage alteration
■ Poor patient adherence
■ Seizures that are refractory to therapy

Patient Counseling Information Applicable to All Anticonvulsants

■ It is important that you keep a diary of your seizures and keep regular appointments with your health care provider, so that he or she can determine whether your medication is working properly and whether you are experiencing unwanted side effects.

■ The full effects of this medication may not be seen for several weeks. Continue to take the medication unless directed otherwise by your health care provider.

■ Take with food or milk if upset stomach occurs.

■ Do not drink alcohol or take CNS depressants or illegal drugs with this medication.

■ If this medication causes blurred vision or drowsiness, do not drive or operate heavy machinery while taking this medication until you have become accustomed to its effects.

■ Consult with your health care provider if you anticipate pregnancy, become pregnant, or plan to breast-feed while taking this medication.

■ Some medications decrease the effectiveness of birth control pills. You should discuss this with your health care provider or pharmacist, who may recommend that you use a backup birth control method to prevent pregnancy.

■ If you are a woman capable of having children, you should take 1 mg of folic acid a day.

■ Do not stop taking this medication unless your health care provider advises you to do so; some medicines have to be stopped slowly. Let your health care provider or pharmacist know if you stop taking this medication.

■ Check with your pharmacist or health care provider before taking or starting any new medication (prescription, over-the-counter, or herbal product).

■ If you miss a dose, take it as soon as you remember. If it is almost time for the next dose, skip the missed dose and resume your regular schedule. Do not take extra or double doses. If you miss two or more doses, contact your health care provider for further instructions.

■ Contact your health care provider immediately if skin rash occurs.

Mechanisms of Action of Anticonvulsants

Anticonvulsants work through a variety of mechanisms including the following:

■ Enhancing sodium channel inactivation
■ Reducing current through T-type calcium channels
■ Enhancing γ-aminobutyric acid (GABA) activity
■ Enhancing antiglutamate activity

28-4. Medications Used to Treat Epilepsy

Carbamazepine

Carbamazepine is the most widely used anticonvulsant in adults and children. It is the drug of choice for complex partial seizures and is indicated for use in partial seizures with complex symptomatology (psychomotor, temporal lobe), generalized tonic–clonic seizures, and mixed seizure patterns. It is ineffective in absence seizures and febrile seizures.

Pharmacokinetics

- *Bioavailability:* Good (75–85%); should be dispensed in moisture-proof containers because high humidity (as may occur in medicine cabinets) decreases bioavailability
- *Protein binding:* 75–90% bound to α-1-acid glycoprotein; the 10,11-epoxide metabolite is 50% protein bound
- *Metabolism:* Extensively hepatically metabolized to 10,11-epoxide, which is effective as an anticonvulsant and is capable of causing toxicity
- *Renal elimination:* Low (1–3%)
- *Half-life:* About one day if used as monotherapy and about 12 hours if given with more than one anticonvulsant
- *Reference range:* 4–12 mg/L (monotherapy, 8–12 mg/L; polytherapy, 4–8 mg/L)

Other aspects

Carbamazepine is one of a few drugs that induce their own metabolism. Mean time to the onset of auto-induction is 21 days (range: 17–31 days).

Side effects

Upon initiation, side effects are nausea, vomiting, drowsiness, dizziness, and neutropenia. A dose-related, transient, and reversible rash may occur, but it rarely causes the drug to be discontinued.

With chronic therapy, the following side effects may occur:

- Syndrome of inappropriate antidiuretic hormone (SIADH) causing hyponatremia and water retention
- Osteomalacia (treat with vitamin D if alkaline phosphatase is increased and 25-hydroxycholecalciferol if decreased)
- Folate deficiency causing megaloblastic anemia

Some severe or life-threatening side effects are possible:

- *FDA boxed warning:* Potentially fatal, severe dermatologic reactions (including Stevens–Johnson syndrome and toxic epidermal necrolysis) may occur. Over 90% of patients who experience these reactions do so within the first few months of treatment. Patients of Asian descent are at higher risk and should be screened for the variant HLA-B*1502 allele (genetic marker) prior to initiating therapy.
- *FDA boxed warning:* Aplastic anemia may occur. In such cases, discontinuation of carbamazepine is recommended if white blood count < 2,000–3,000 or neutrophils < 1,000–1,500.
- *FDA warning:* Direct hepatotoxicity and multi-organ hypersensitivity reactions may occur and generally present within 1 month. Carbamazepine should be discontinued if liver function tests increase more than three times above normal. Fever, rash, or fatalities may occur even if carbamazepine is stopped.
- *FDA warning:* Increased risk of suicidal behavior or ideation is possible. The FDA has analyzed suicidality reports from placebo-controlled studies involving 11 anticonvulsants (including carbamazepine) and found that patients receiving anticonvulsants had approximately twice the risk of suicidal behavior or ideation (0.43%) as patients receiving a placebo (0.22%).
- *Anticonvulsant hypersensitivity syndrome:* This syndrome is characterized by fever (90–100%), rash (90%), hepatitis (50%), and other multi-organ abnormalities (50%). Although the mechanism is unknown, patients who have experienced this syndrome should not receive anticonvulsants with an aromatic structure (i.e., hydantoin, oxcarbazepine, phenobarbital, lamotrigine).
- *Teratogenic concerns:* Carbamazepine is a pregnancy category D drug and has been associated with fetal carbamazepine syndrome (i.e., features include epicanthal folds, short nose, long philtrum, hypoplastic nails, microcephaly, developmental delay) and neural tube defects.

Drug–drug interactions

- Carbamazepine is a cytochrome (CYP) 3A4, CYP2C9, and CYP2C19 inducer.
- Erythromycin, cimetidine, and lithium increase the serum concentration of carbamazepine and may enhance the effect to cause toxicity.
- Phenobarbital, primidone, and phenytoin decrease the anticonvulsant effect of carbamazepine.
- Carbamazepine may increase the serum concentration or effect of felbamate; felbamate will increase concentrations of the 10,11-epoxide metabolite carbamazepine and cause toxicity.

Commercially available formulations

Table 28-2 shows the commercially available formulations.

Table 28-2. Dosage Forms, Normal Maintenance Doses, and Dosing Interval for Older Anticonvulsants

Generic name	Trade name	Dosage form	Adult oral maintenance dose[a]	Interval[b]
Carbamazepine	Carbatrol, Equetro	Extended-release capsule: 100, 200, 300 mg	800–1,200 mg/day	bid–tid
	Epitol	200 mg		bid–tid
	Tegretol	Suspension: 100 mg/5 mL (5, 10, 450 mL)		qid
		Chewable tablet: 100,200 mg		bid–qid
		Tablet: 100, 200, 300, 400 mg		bid
	Tegretol XR	Extended-release tablet: 100, 200, 400 mg		bid
Ethosuximide	Zarontin and generics	Capsule: 250 mg	25–1,500 mg/day	qd
		Solution: 250 mg/5 mL		bid
Fosphenytoin	Cerebyx	Injection:[c] 100 mg PE/2 mL; 500 mg PE/10 mL	NA	NA
Phenobarbital	Variety of generics	Elixir: 20 mg/5 mL (5, 7.5, 15, 480 mL)	30–120 mg/day	bid–tid
		Tablet: 15, 16.2, 30, 32.4, 60, 64.8, 97.2, 100 mg		bid-qd
		Injection: 65, 130 mg/mL (1 mL)	NA	NA
Phenytoin	Dilantin	Suspension: 125 mg/5 mL (240 mL)	100–600 mg/day	bid–tid
		Chewable tablet: 50 mg		bid–tid
		Prompt-release capsule: 30, 100 mg		bid–tid
		Extended-release capsule: 30, 100 mg		qd
		Injection: 50 mg/mL	NA	NA
	Phenytek	Extended-release capsule: 200 mg, 300 mg		qd
	Generic	Suspension: 125 mg/5 mL (240 mL)		bid–tid
		Prompt-release capsule: 100, 200, 300 mg		bid–tid
		Extended-release capsule: 100 mg		qd
		Injection: 50 mg/mL	NA	NA
Primidone	Mysoline and generics	Tablet: 50, 250 mg	250–750 mg/day	bid–qd
		Chewable tablet: 125 mg		bid–qd
Valproic acid	Depacon and generic	Injection: 100 mg/mL (5 mL)	NA	NA
	Depakene and generic	Syrup: 250 mg/5 mL (5, 10, 480 mL)	250–4,000 mg/day	bid–qid
		Gel capsule: 250 mg		bid–tid
Divalproex sodium	Stavzor	Gel capsule: 125, 250, 500 mg		bid–tid
	Depakote Sprinkles and generic	Capsule: 125 mg	30–65 mg/kg/day (max 1000 mg/day)	bid
	Depakote	Delayed-release tablet: 125, 250, 500 mg		bid
	Depakote ER and generic	Extended-release tablet: 250, 500 mg		qd

NA, not applicable; PE, phenytoin equivalent.

a. With the exception of the intravenous dosage forms, these anticonvulsants are begun at low doses and slowly titrated to a dose that will control the patient's seizures.

b. Interval may either decrease or increase in the presence of medications that induce or inhibit metabolism, respectively.

c. 150 mg of fosphenytoin = 100 mg phenytoin.

Patient counseling

See general counseling information. In addition, counsel the patient as follows:

- Shake suspension well.
- Do not store in areas of high humidity (e.g., medicine cabinets).
- Do not use with monoamine oxidase inhibitors.

Clobazam

Clobazam is a benzodiazepine indicated only for the adjunctive treatment of seizures associated with Lennox–Gaustaut syndrome in patients 2 years of age or older.

Pharmacokinetics

- *Bioavailability:* 100% for oral tablets and solution
- *Protein binding:* 80–90% for clobazam; 70% for active metabolite
- *Metabolism:* Extensively hepatic (N-demethylation by CYP3A4 mostly, some CYP2C19 and CYP2B6); N-desmethylclobazam is the active metabolite and about 20% as potent as the parent compound.
- *Renal elimination:* 82%
- *Half-life:* 36–42 hours (71–82 hours for active metabolite)

Side effects

Common side effects include constipation, somnolence or sedation, pyrexia, lethargy, and drooling.
Severe or life-threatening effects are also possible:

- *Serious dermatological reactions:* Stevens–Johnson syndrome and toxic epidermal necrolysis have been reported in children and adults during the postmarketing period. Patients should be closely monitored for signs and symptoms, especially in the first 8 weeks of treatment. Discontinuation of clobazam should be considered at the first sign of rash and alternative therapy reviewed.
- *Suicidal behavior and ideation:* Antiepileptic drugs (AEDs) may increase the risk of suicidal thoughts or behavior. Patients should be monitored for the emergence or worsening of depression, suicidal thoughts or behavior, or any unusual changes in mood or behavior.

Drug–drug interactions

Because of the metabolism of clobazam, lower doses of medications metabolized by CYP2D6 may be needed when used concomitantly with clobazam. The clobazam dose may need to be adjusted with strong or moderate CYP2C19 inhibitors. Alcohol increases levels of clobazam by approximately 50%; therefore, patients and caregivers should be cautioned against simultaneous use.

Commercially available formulations

See Table 28-3 for commercially available formulations.

Eslicarbazepine

Eslicarbazepine is the pro-drug for the major active metabolite of oxcarbazepine. It is indicated for use as adjunctive treatment of partial seizures.

Pharmacokinetics

- *Bioavailability:* Peak concentrations are obtained 1–4 hours post dose.
- *Protein binding:* Low (< 40%)
- *Metabolism:* Hydrolytic first-pass metabolism converts eslicarbazepine acetate to eslicarbazepine; minor active metabolites include (R)-licarbazepine and oxcarbazepine.
- *Renal elimination:* 100%
- *Half-life:* 13–20 hours; steady-state concentrations are attained after 4–5 days of once-daily dosing.

Side effects

Common side effects include dizziness, somnolence, nausea, headache, diplopia, vomiting, fatigue, vertigo, ataxia, blurred vision, and tremor.
Severe or life-threatening effects are also possible:

- *Suicidal behavior and ideation:* AEDs may increase the risk of suicidal thoughts or behavior. Patients should be monitored for the emergence or worsening of depression, suicidal thoughts or behavior, or any unusual changes in mood or behavior.
- *Serious dermatologic reactions:* Stevens–Johnson syndrome and toxic epidermal necrolysis have been reported with eslicarbazepine, oxcarbazepine, and carbamazepine use. Consider discontinuation of drug at the first sign of rash and alternative therapy thereafter.

Table 28-3. Dosage Forms, Normal Maintenance Doses, and Dosing Intervals for the Newer Anticonvulsants

Generic name	Trade name	Dosage form	Adult oral maintenance dose[a]	Interval[b]
Clobazam	Onfi	Suspension: 2.5 mg/mL (120 mL)	40 mg/day	bid
		Tablet: 10, 20 mg		
Eslicarbazepine	Aptiom	Tablet: 200, 400, 600, 800 mg	800–1,200 mg/day	qd
Ezogabine	Potiga	Tablet: 50, 200, 300, 400 mg	600–1,200 mg/day	tid
Felbamate	Felbatol and generics	Suspension: 600 mg/5 mL (240, 960 mL)	1,200–3,600 mg/day	tid–qid
		Tablet: 400, 600 mg		tid–qid
Gabapentin	Neurontin and generics	Capsule: 100, 300, 400 mg	900–3,600 mg/day[c]	tid
		Oral solution: 250 mg/mL (480 mL)		tid
		Tablet: 100, 300, 400, 600, 800 mg		tid
Lacosamide	Vimpat	Tablet: 50,100, 150, 200 mg	200–400 mg/day	bid
		Oral solution: 10 mg/mL		bid
		Injection: 200 mg/20 mL	NA	NA
Lamotrigine	Lamictal and generics	Chewable tablet: 2, 5, 25 mg	50–400/day	bid
		Tablet: 25, 100, 150, 200 mg		bid
	Lamictal ODT	Tablet: 25, 50, 100, 200 mg		bid
	Lamictal XR	Tablet: 25, 50, 100, 200, 250, 300 mg		qd
Levetiracetam	Keppra and generic	Tablet: 250, 500, 750, 1,000 mg	1,000–3,000 mg/day	bid
		Solution: 100 mg/mL		bid
		Injection: 500 mg/5 mL	NA	NA
	Keppra XR and generic	Extended release tablet: 500, 750 mg		qd
Oxcarbazepine	Trileptal and generics	Tablet: 150, 300, 600 mg	600–2,400 mg/day	bid
		Suspension: 300 mg/5 mL (250 mL)		bid
Perampanel	Fycompa	Tablet: 2, 4, 6, 8, 10, 12 mg	8–12 mg/day	qd
Pregabalin	**Lyrica** and generics	Capsule: 25, 50, 75, 100, 150, 200, 225, 300 mg	300–600 mg/day	bid–tid
		Solution: 20 mg/mL		bid–tid
Rufinamide	Banzel	Tablet: 200, 400 mg	45 mg/kg/day	bid
		Suspension: 40 mg/mL		bid
Tiagabine	Gabitril and generic	Tablet: 2, 4, 12, 16 mg	4–56 mg/day	bid–qid
Topiramate	Topamax and generics	Sprinkle capsule: 15, 25 mg	200–400 mg/day[d]	bid
		Tablet: 25, 50, 100, 200 mg		bid
Vigabatrin	Sabril	Capsule: 25, 50, 100, 200 mg		qd
		Tablet: 500 mg	400–600 mg/day	bid
		Powder: 500 mg		bid
Zonisamide	Zonegran and generics	Capsule: 25, 50, 100 mg	100–600 mg/day	qd

NA, not applicable.

Boldface indicates one of top 100 drugs for 2012 by units sold at retail outlets, www.drugs.com/stats/top100/2012/units.

a. With the exception of gabapentin, these anticonvulsants are begun at low doses and slowly titrated over weeks to a dose that will control the patient's seizures.

b. Interval may either decrease or increase in the presence of medications that induce or inhibit metabolism, respectively.

c. Much larger doses have been given.

d. The recommended maintenance doses for initial monotherapy and adjunctive therapy are 400 mg/day and 200–400 mg/day, respectively. Doses > 400 mg are no more effective than doses ≤ 400 mg.

■ *Drug reaction with eosinophilia and systemic symptoms:* This has been reported in patients taking eslicarbazepine. Monitor for hypersensitivity, and discontinue use if another cause cannot be established.

■ *Anaphylactic reactions and angioedema:* Rare cases of anaphylaxis and angioedema have been reported in patients taking this medication. Monitor for breathing difficulties or swelling, and discontinue if another cause cannot be established.

■ *Hyponatremia:* Significant hyponatremia (< 125 mEq/L) may occur, and thus sodium levels in patients at risk for or patients experiencing hyponatremia symptoms should be monitored.

■ *Drug-induced liver injury:* Eslicarbazepine should be discontinued in patients with jaundice or laboratory evidence of significant liver injury.

Drug–drug interactions

Several AEDs, including carbamazepine, phenobarbital, phenytoin, and primidone, can induce enzymes that metabolize eslicarbazepine and can cause decreased plasma concentrations. In addition, eslicarbazepine may decrease the effectiveness of hormonal contraceptives. Additional or alternative nonhormonal birth control should be advised. Do not use eslicarbazepine with oxcarbazepine.

Commercially available formulations

See Table 28-3 for commercially available formulations.

Ethosuximide

Indications are absence and myoclonic seizures.

Pharmacokinetics

■ *Bioavailability:* Good
■ *Protein binding:* Very low (< 10%)
■ *Metabolism:* 80% hepatically metabolized to three inactive metabolites
■ *Renal elimination:* 50% as metabolites; 10–20% as unchanged drug
■ *Half-life:* 30–60 hours
■ *Reference range:* 40–100 mg/L

Side effects

Upon initiation, side effects are nausea, vomiting, dizziness, drowsiness, lethargy, headache, rashes (including Stevens–Johnson syndrome), and urticaria.

With chronic therapy, anorexia and weight loss, as well as gum hypertrophy, could occur.

■ *Suicidal behavior and ideation:* AEDs may increase the risk of suicidal thoughts or behavior. Patients should be monitored for the emergence or worsening of depression, suicidal thoughts or behavior, or any unusual changes in mood or behavior.

Drug–drug interactions

■ Ethosuximide is a CYP3A3/4 substrate.
■ Phenytoin, carbamazepine, primidone, and phenobarbital may increase the clearance of ethosuximide.
■ Isoniazid may inhibit metabolism and increase ethosuximide serum concentrations.

Commercially available formulations

See Table 28-2 for commercially available formulations.

Ezogabine

Ezogabine is a potassium channel opener indicated for the adjunctive treatment of partial seizures in adult patients and was approved by the FDA in 2011. It should be used only in those patients with epilepsy that cannot be controlled by other agents, and the benefits versus the risks of retinal abnormalities and decline in visual acuity should be considered.

Pharmacokinetics

■ *Bioavailability:* Approximately 60%
■ *Protein binding:* Approximately 80%
■ *Metabolism:* Hepatic via extensive glucuronidation and acetylation; the N-acetyl metabolite (NAMR) is the main active metabolite with weaker antiepileptic activity.
■ *Renal elimination:* 85% renal elimination (36% unchanged drug, remainder as metabolites)
■ *Half-life:* 7–11 hours for the drug and active metabolite

Side effects

The most common adverse reactions reported are dizziness, somnolence, fatigue, confusion, vertigo, tremor, abnormal coordination, diplopia, attention disturbance, memory impairment, asthenia, blurred vision, gait disturbance, aphasia, dysarthria, and balance disorders.

Severe or life-threatening effects are also possible:

- *FDA boxed warning:* Ezogabine may cause retinal abnormalities leading to damage to the photoreceptors and vision loss. The rate of progression and reversibility is unknown. Visual acuity and dilated fundus photography is recommended at baseline and every 6 months for patients taking ezogabine. If any abnormalities are detected, the medication should be discontinued unless no other treatment options exist.
- *Urinary retention:* In placebo-controlled trials, an increased risk of urinary retention occurred while taking ezogabine. Urologic symptoms should be monitored, especially for patients with other risk factors or on concomitant medications that may affect voiding (i.e., anticholinergics).
- *Skin discoloration:* Ezogabine may cause blue, gray-blue, or brown skin discoloration that is found predominantly on or around the lips or in the nail beds. Widespread involvement to the face and legs has also been reported. This was generally reported after 2 or more years of therapy.
- *QT interval effect:* There was a mean QT prolongation in healthy volunteers of 7.7 msec that occurred within 3 hours. The QT interval should be monitored in patients using ezogabine concomitantly with medicines known to increase QT interval and in patients with known prolonged QT interval, congestive heart failure, ventricular hypertrophy, hypokalemia, or hypomagnesemia.
- *Suicidal behavior and ideation:* AEDs, including ezogabine, may increase the risk of suicidal thoughts or behavior. Patients should be monitored for the emergence or worsening of depression, suicidal thoughts or behavior, or any unusual changes in mood or behavior.

Drug–drug interactions

Concomitant administration of phenytoin or carbamazepine may reduce ezogabine plasma levels; therefore, an increased dose of ezogabine should be considered when adding either of these two drugs. The active metabolite of ezogabine may inhibit renal clearance of digoxin; thus, monitoring digoxin levels is recommended.

Commercially available formulations

See Table 28-3 for commercially available formulations.

Felbamate

Felbamate should be used only as adjunctive therapy in severe refractory partial seizures, with or without secondary generalization, in patients older than 14 years of age and in partial or generalized seizures associated with Lennox–Gastaut syndrome. It should be used only in patients with epilepsy so severe that the risk of aplastic anemia, liver failure, or both is deemed acceptable given the potential benefits of its use.

Pharmacokinetics

- *Bioavailability:* Complete (> 90%)
- *Protein binding:* Low (20–25%)
- *Metabolism:* Hepatic via hydroxylation and conjugation
- *Renal elimination:* 40–50% excreted unchanged and 40% as inactive metabolites in urine
- *Half-life:* 20–30 hours; shorter (i.e., 14 hours) with concomitant enzyme-inducing drugs; prolonged (by 9–15 hours) in renal dysfunction
- *Reference range:* Although some have proposed a therapeutic range of 30–100 mg/L, routine monitoring of serum drug concentrations is not advocated; hence, the dose should be titrated to clinical response.

Side effects

Upon initiation, nausea and vomiting, anorexia, headache, insomnia, and dizziness may occur.

With chronic therapy, weight loss significant enough to warrant discontinuing the medication is possible.

Severe or life-threatening side effects are possible:

- *FDA boxed warning:* Direct hepatotoxicity may occur at any time; however, the earliest onset of severe liver dysfunction occurred 3 weeks after starting felbamate. It is not known if dose, duration, or use of concomitant medications affects the risk. Liver enzyme and bilirubin tests should be obtained before initiation and periodically after starting felbamate, and the drug should be immediately withdrawn if liver function tests become elevated. Most cases require liver transplantation.
- *FDA boxed warning:* The risk of aplastic anemia may be 100 times greater than in the general population and can develop at any point without warning. Complete blood count with differential and platelet count should be taken before, during, and for a significant time after discontinuing

felbamate. Felbamate should be immediately withdrawn if bone marrow suppression occurs.

■ *FDA warning:* Increased risk of suicidal behavior or ideation may occur. The FDA has analyzed suicidality reports from placebo-controlled studies involving 11 anticonvulsants (including felbamate) and found that patients receiving anticonvulsants had approximately twice the risk of suicidal behavior or ideation (0.43%) as patients receiving a placebo (0.22%).

Drug–drug interactions

■ Felbamate induces CYP3A4.
■ Felbamate inhibits CYP2C19, epoxide hydroxylase, and β-oxidation.
■ Carbamazepine, phenobarbital, and phenytoin decrease the anticonvulsant effect of felbamate.
■ Phenobarbital, phenytoin, and valproic acid increase the anticonvulsant effect of felbamate.
■ Felbamate decreases carbamazepine concentrations but increases the concentration of carbamazepine 10,11-epoxide (active metabolite), which may result in toxicity.
■ Felbamate increases the serum concentrations of phenobarbital, phenytoin, and valproic acid. When felbamate is begun, a 20% reduction in phenytoin dose resulted in phenytoin concentrations comparable to those prior to initiation of felbamate.

Commercially available formulations

See Table 28-3 for commercially available formulations.

Patient counseling

See general counseling information. An information consent form is included as part of the package insert and is available from the local representative or by calling 800-526-3840. The patient or legal guardian should sign this form before receiving the medication.

Fosphenytoin

Fosphenytoin is indicated for short-term parenteral administration in treating generalized convulsive status epilepticus. The safety and effectiveness of more than 5 days' use has not been systematically evaluated.

Pharmacokinetics

■ *Bioavailability:* Time for complete conversion to phenytoin is 15 minutes and 30 minutes after intravenous (IV) and intramuscular (IM) administration, respectively.
■ *Protein binding:* Protein binding is high (95–99% primarily to albumin).
■ *Metabolism:* Each millimole of fosphenytoin is metabolized to 1 millimole of phenytoin, phosphate, and formaldehyde. Formaldehyde is then converted to formate, which is metabolized by a folate-dependent mechanism. Conversion increases the dose and infusion rate, most likely because of a decrease in fosphenytoin protein binding.
■ *Renal elimination:* None
■ *Half-life:* See the later discussion of phenytoin for the half-life of the active drug.
■ *Reference range:* 10–20 mg/L (phenytoin)

Side effects

Upon initiation, side effects include hypotension (with rapid IV administration), vasodilation, tachycardia, and bradycardia; burning, pruritus, tingling, and paresthesia (predominately in the groin area); and rash and exfoliative dermatitis. Prolonged use will result in the same side effects as those seen with phenytoin (see side effects for phenytoin).

■ *FDA warning:* The FDA is investigating the possibility of an increased risk of serious skin reactions (e.g., Stevens–Johnson syndrome, toxic epidermal necrolysis) in patients given phenytoin who have the human leukocyte antigen allele HLA-B*1502. This allele occurs almost exclusively in individuals with ancestry across broad areas of Asia, including Han Chinese, Filipinos, Malaysians, South Asian Indians, and Thais. Until the FDA evaluation is finalized, fosphenytoin should be avoided in patients who test positive for HLA-B*1502.

Drug–drug interactions

See the later discussion of phenytoin for drug–drug interactions.

Commercially available formulations

See Table 28-2 for commercially available formulations.

Gabapentin

Gabapentin is indicated as adjunctive therapy for partial seizures with and without secondary generalization in those older than 12 years of age. It is also indicated as adjunctive therapy in the treatment of partial seizures in patients 3–12 years of age.

Pharmacokinetics

- *Bioavailability:* Poor (60% with decreasing absorption as age decreases)
- *Protein binding:* Very low (< 3%)
- *Metabolism:* None
- *Renal elimination:* 100%
- *Half-life:* Short (< 12 hours); increases with decreased renal function (anuric patients: 132 hours; decreased during hemodialysis to about 4 hours)
- *Reference range:* Routine monitoring of serum concentrations not required; minimum effective concentration thought to be 2 mg/L

Side effects

Upon initiation, somnolence, dizziness, ataxia, fatigue, and nervousness may occur.

With chronic therapy, weight gain may occur. Neuropsychiatric events (i.e., emotional lability, hostility, hyperkinesias) are possible in children, especially those with mental retardation and attention deficit disorders. This problem generally resolves following a reduction in the dose.

- *FDA warning:* Increased risk of suicidal behavior or ideation is possible. The FDA has analyzed suicidality reports from placebo-controlled studies involving 11 anticonvulsants (including gabapentin) and found that patients receiving anticonvulsants had approximately twice the risk of suicidal behavior or ideation (0.43%) as patients receiving a placebo (0.22%).
- *Anticonvulsant hypersensitivity syndrome:* This syndrome is characterized by fever (90–100%), rash (90%), hepatitis (50%), and other multiorgan abnormalities (50%). Although the mechanism is unknown, patients who have experienced this syndrome should not receive anticonvulsants with an aromatic structure (i.e., hydantoin, oxcarbazepine, phenobarbitone, lamotrigine).

Drug–drug interactions

- No interactions affect metabolism; aluminum- and magnesium-containing antacids may decrease absorption.
- High protein intake can increase absorption.
- Although it is not a true drug interaction, combination with carbamazepine may cause dizziness, which will require a reduction in the dose of carbamazepine.

Commercially available formulations

See Table 28-3 for commercially available formulations.

Patient counseling

See general counseling information. In addition, the patient should be counseled as follows:

- Certain foods may decrease the extent of absorption.
- If you take antacids, wait at least 2 hours before taking gabapentin.
- Refrigerate oral solution.

Lacosamide

Lacosamide is indicated for adjunctive therapy for partial seizures in those older than 17 years of age. The injectable formulation is indicated when oral administration is temporarily not feasible.

Pharmacokinetics

- *Bioavailability:* Complete
- *Protein binding:* Very low (< 15%)
- *Metabolism:* None
- *Renal elimination:* 95% (40% as unchanged drug, 30% as inactive metabolite, 25% as uncharacterized metabolite)
- *Half-life:* About 13 hours

Side effects

Upon initiation, nausea and vomiting may occur, as well as dizziness, lack of coordination, and diplopia.

- *Suicidal behavior and ideation:* AEDs may increase the risk of suicidal thoughts or behavior. Patients should be monitored for the emergence or worsening of depression, suicidal thoughts or behavior, or any unusual changes in mood or behavior.

Commercially available formulations

See Table 28-3 for commercially available formulations.

Lamotrigine

Lamotrigine is indicated as adjunctive therapy for partial seizures (≥ 2 years), primary and secondary generalized tonic–clonic seizures (≥ 2 years), and seizures associated with Lennox–Gastaut syndrome (≥ 2 years). It is also approved for conversion to monotherapy in those ≥ 16 years of age who have been receiving monotherapy with carbamazepine, phenytoin, phenobarbital, primidone, or valproate and as adjunctive therapy for those ≥ 12 years of age. Although it is used for absence, atypical absence, atonic, and myoclonic seizures, it is not FDA labeled for these indications.

Pharmacokinetics

- *Bioavailability:* Complete
- *Protein binding:* Low (55% to albumin)
- *Metabolism:* > 75% hepatically metabolized via glucuronidation; autoinduction possible
- *Renal elimination:* 75–90% excreted as glucuronide metabolites and 10% as unchanged drug
- *Half-life:* Dependent on patient age and concomitant drug therapy
- *Reference range:* Proposed serum concentration of 1–5 mg/L, but clinical value of monitoring concentrations not established

Side effects

Upon initiation, nausea and vomiting, dizziness, sedation, somnolence, and diplopia may occur.

No additional side effects are associated with chronic therapy.

Severe or life-threatening side effects are possible:

- *FDA boxed warning:* Although rare, toxic epidermal necrolysis has been reported, and deaths have occurred. The risk of rash may be increased in those receiving valproic acid, large initial doses, or a rapid increase in dosage. The rash usually appears within 2–8 weeks of therapy initiation but has been reported after prolonged treatment (e.g., 6 months). Refer the patient to a health care provider if signs or symptoms of a rash develop. The health care provider may suggest holding a single dose until the rash is evaluated.
- *FDA warning:* Increased risk of suicidal behavior or ideation may occur. The FDA has analyzed suicidality reports from placebo-controlled studies involving 11 anticonvulsants (including lamotrigine) and found that patients receiving anticonvulsants had approximately twice the risk of suicidal behavior or ideation (0.43%) as patients receiving a placebo (0.22%).
- *Anticonvulsant hypersensitivity syndrome:* This syndrome is characterized by fever (90–100%), rash (90%), hepatitis (50%), and other multi-organ abnormalities (50%). Although the mechanism is unknown, patients who have experienced this syndrome should not receive anticonvulsants with an aromatic structure (i.e., hydantoin, oxcarbazepine, phenobarbitone, lamotrigine).

Drug–drug interactions

- Lamotrigine is a weak uridine diphosphate glucuronosyltransferase inducer.
- Valproic acid may increase the serum concentration or effect of lamotrigine.
- Carbamazepine, phenobarbital, phenytoin, primidone, and rifampin decrease the serum concentration and effect of lamotrigine.
- Estrogen-containing oral contraceptives may decrease the serum concentration of lamotrigine.
- Lamotrigine may decrease the serum concentration or effect of valproic acid.
- Although not a true drug–drug interaction, the combination with carbamazepine may cause dizziness, which requires a reduction in the dose of carbamazepine.

Commercially available formulations

See Table 28-3 for commercially available formulations.

Patient counseling

See general counseling information. In addition, patients should be counseled to notify their health care provider immediately if a skin rash occurs.

Levetiracetam

Levetiracetam is indicated as adjunctive therapy for partial onset seizures in adults and children ≥ 1 month of age; as adjunctive therapy for myoclonic seizures in adults; for JME in those ≥ 12 years of age; and as adjunctive therapy for primary generalized tonic–clonic seizures in adults and children (≥ 6 years of age) with idiopathic generalized epilepsy.

Pharmacokinetics

- *Bioavailability:* Complete
- *Protein binding:* Very low (< 10%)
- *Metabolism:* Not extensive; metabolites not active and renally eliminated
- *Renal elimination:* Undergoes glomerular filtration and subsequent partial tubular reabsorption; 66% excreted unchanged and 27% as inactive metabolites
- *Half-life:* Short (4–8 hours)
- *Reference range:* Not established; clinical value of monitoring concentrations not established

Side effects

Upon initiation, dizziness, fatigue, and sedation may occur.

No additional side effects occur with chronic therapy.

- *FDA warning:* Severe or life-threatening side effects include increased risk of suicidal behavior or ideation. The medication carries an FDA warning: The FDA has analyzed suicidality reports from placebo-controlled studies involving 11 anticonvulsants (including levetiracetam) and found that patients receiving anticonvulsants had approximately twice the risk of suicidal behavior or ideation (0.43%) as patients receiving a placebo (0.22%).

Drug–drug interactions

No significant interactions have been identified.

Commercially available formulations

See Table 28-3 for commercially available formulations.

Oxcarbazepine

Oxcarbazepine is indicated as monotherapy or adjunctive therapy in adults, as monotherapy in children 4 years of age or older, and as adjunctive therapy in children 2 years of age or older who have partial seizures.

Pharmacokinetics

- *Bioavailability:* Complete
- *Protein binding:* 67% (parent compound); 40%, monohydroxy metabolite (MHD) (primarily to albumin)
- *Metabolism:* Extensive to 10-MHD metabolite, which is active
- *Renal elimination:* > 95%
- *Half-life:* 2 hours (oxcarbazepine); 9 hours (MHD)

Side effects

Upon initiation, nausea, vomiting, drowsiness, dizziness, and neutropenia (transient) may occur. On rare instances, a dose-related, transient, and reversible rash causes the drug to be discontinued. The frequency is less than that with carbamazepine, but cross-hypersensitivity reactions with carbamazepine may occur in 25% of patients.

With chronic therapy, the following side effects are possible:

- *SIADH:* This syndrome, causing hyponatremia and water retention, is more common than with carbamazepine.
- *Anticonvulsant hypersensitivity syndrome:* This syndrome is characterized by fever (90–100%), rash (90%), hepatitis (50%), and other multi-organ abnormalities (50%). Although the mechanism is unknown, patients who have experienced this syndrome should not receive anticonvulsants that have an aromatic structure (i.e., hydantoin, carbamazepine, phenobarbitone, lamotrigine).
- *FDA warning:* Increased risk of suicidal behavior or ideation is possible. The FDA has analyzed suicidality reports from placebo-controlled studies involving 11 anticonvulsants (including oxcarbazepine) and found that patients receiving anticonvulsants had approximately twice the risk of suicidal behavior or ideation (0.43%) as patients receiving a placebo (0.22%).

Drug–drug interactions

- Oxcarbazepine is an inhibitor of CYP2C19.
- Oxcarbazepine is an inducer of CYP3A4 and CYP3A5.
- Oxcarbazepine increases serum concentrations of phenobarbital and phenytoin.
- Oxcarbazepine may decrease serum concentrations of felodipine, lamotrigine, and oral contraceptives (i.e., ethinyl estradiol, levonorgestrel).
- Carbamazepine, phenobarbital, phenytoin, and valproic acid may decrease MHD concentrations.

Commercially available formulations

See Table 28-3 for commercially available formulations.

Patient counseling

This medication decreases the effectiveness of birth control pills. Use a supplemental birth control method to prevent pregnancy while taking oxcarbazepine or contact your health care provider about a high-estrogen oral contraceptive.

Perampanel

Perampanel is a noncompetitive AMPA (α-Amino-3-hydroxy-5-methyl-4-isoxazolepropionic acid) glutamate receptor antagonist indicated for adjunctive treatment of partial seizures with or without secondary generalized seizures in patients 12 years of age and older.

Pharmacokinetics

- *Bioavailability:* Complete absorption occurs 0.5–2.5 hours after oral administration.
- *Protein binding:* High (95–96%)
- *Metabolism:* Via primary oxidation (CYP3A4, CYP3A5, or both) and sequential glucuronidation
- *Renal elimination:* 22%
- *Half-life:* 105 hours, on average

Side effects

Common side effects include dizziness, somnolence, fatigue, irritability, falls, nausea, weight gain, vertigo, ataxia, gait disturbance, and balance disorders.

Severe or life-threatening effects are also possible:

- *FDA boxed warning:* Serious or life-threatening psychiatric and behavioral adverse reactions such as aggression, hostility, irritability, anger, and homicidal ideation and threats have been reported. Monitor for these reactions as well as changes in mood, behavior, or personality, especially during the titration period and at higher doses. The perampanel dose should be reduced if these symptoms occur or discontinued immediately if these symptoms are severe or worsen.
- *Suicidal behavior and ideation:* AEDs, including perampanel, may increase the risk of suicidal thoughts or behavior. Patients should be monitored for the emergence or worsening of depression, suicidal thoughts or behavior, or any unusual changes in mood or behavior.

Drug–drug interactions

Use with contraceptives containing levonorgestrel may render them less effective; thus, additional non-hormonal forms of contraception are recommended.

The concomitant use of known CYP enzyme inducers (e.g., carbamazepine, phenytoin, or oxcarbazepine) decrease the plasma levels of perampanel by approximately 50–67%. Therefore, perampanel's starting dose should be increased when used concomitantly with enzyme-inducing AEDs. In addition, strong CYP3A inhibitors should be avoided.

Commercially available formulations

See Table 28-3 for commercially available formulations.

Phenobarbital

Phenobarbital is indicated for neonatal seizures and generalized seizures. It is ineffective in absence seizures. Other anticonvulsants are more effective in complex partial seizures.

Pharmacokinetics

- *Bioavailability:* Good (70–90%)
- *Protein binding:* Low (30–50%)
- *Metabolism:* Hepatic via hydroxylation and glucuronide conjugation
- *Renal elimination:* 20–50% unchanged in urine; increases with alkalinization of the urine
- *Half-life:* Long (20–400 hours); increasing half-life with decreasing age
- *Reference range:* 15–40 mg/L

Side effects

Upon initiation, drowsiness, dizziness, light-headedness, lack of coordination, headaches, or nervousness may occur.

With chronic therapy, the following side effects are possible:

- Hyperactivity occurs, primarily in children; however, it rarely necessitates discontinuation of therapy.
- Lower memory and concentration abilities occur. The medication slightly lowers IQ.
- Folate deficiency may cause megaloblastic anemia.
- Vitamin K–deficient hemorrhagic disease is possible. Administer vitamin K to the mother before delivery and to the newborn.

Severe or life-threatening side effects are possible:

- *Hepatic failure:* Discontinue phenobarbital if liver function tests increase to more than three times above normal.
- *Stevens–Johnson syndrome:* Refer the patient to a health care provider if a rash develops. The health care provider may suggest holding a single dose until the rash is evaluated.
- *Anticonvulsant hypersensitivity syndrome:* This syndrome is characterized by fever (90–100%), rash (90%), hepatitis (50%), and other multiorgan abnormalities (50%). Although the mechanism is unknown, patients who have experienced this syndrome should not receive anticonvulsants in the phenytoin category, carbamazepine or oxcarbazepine, barbiturates, and lamotrigine.
- *Suicidal behavior and ideation:* AEDs may increase the risk of suicidal thoughts or behavior. Patients should be monitored for the emergence or worsening of depression, suicidal thoughts or behavior, or any unusual changes in mood or behavior.
- *Teratogenic effects (phenobarbital syndrome):* Effects include developmental delay, short nose, low nasal bridge, low-set ears, wide mouth, protruding lips, and distal digital hypoplasia. The medication is pregnancy category D.

Drug–drug interactions

- Phenobarbital is an inducer of CYP1A2, CYP2B6, CYP2C8, CYP2C9, CYP2C19, CYP3A4, and uridine diphosphate glucuronosyltransferase.
- Chloramphenicol, felbamate, ketoconazole, methylphenidate, and valproic acid increase the serum concentration or effect of phenobarbital.
- Phenytoin decreases the anticonvulsant effect of phenobarbital.
- Phenobarbital may increase the serum concentration or effect of alcohol, caffeine, and monoamine oxidase inhibitors.
- Phenobarbital may decrease the serum concentration or effect of rifampin, birth control pills, corticosteroids, cyclophosphamide, cyclosporine, delavirdine, griseofulvin, haloperidol, lamotrigine, metronidazole, propranolol, quinidine, ritonavir, saquinavir, theophylline, and warfarin.

Other aspects

Phenobarbital is subject to control under the Federal Controlled Substances Act of 1970 as a schedule V (C–V) drug.

Commercially available formulations

See Table 28-2 for commercially available formulations.

Patient counseling

See general counseling information. In addition, this medication decreases the effectiveness of birth control pills. Counsel the patient to use a supplemental birth control method to prevent pregnancy while taking phenobarbital or contact a health care provider about a high-estrogen oral contraceptive.

Phenytoin

Phenytoin is indicated for all seizure types except absence and febrile seizures. It is also indicated for prevention of seizures following neurosurgery. It is frequently used to prevent post-traumatic epilepsy following head trauma but is not FDA approved for this indication.

Pharmacokinetics

- *Bioavailability:* Slow, variable, and formulation dependent; decreased in children
- *Protein binding:* Very high (90–95%); increased free fraction in neonates
- *Metabolism:* Hepatic
- *Renal elimination:* Low (< 5%)
- *Half-life:* Exhibits capacity-limited or saturable pharmacokinetics (i.e., Michaelis–Menten) and does not technically have a half-life
- *Reference range:* 10–20 mg/L (free level 1–2 mg/L)

Side effects

Upon initiation, nausea, vomiting, drowsiness, and dizziness may occur.

With chronic therapy, the following side effects are possible:

- Peripheral neuropathy may occur.
- Hydantoin facies (thickening of subcutaneous tissues, enlargement of nose and lips) is possible.
- Acne, hirsutism, and gingival hyperplasia may occur. Suggest good oral hygiene.

- Osteomalacia may occur. Treat with vitamin D if alkaline phosphatase increases and 25-hydroxycholecalciferol decreases.
- Vitamin K–deficient hemorrhagic disease is possible. Administer vitamin K to the mother before delivery and to the newborn.
- Folate deficiency may cause megaloblastic anemia.

Severe or life-threatening side effects are as follows:

- *Hepatic failure:* Discontinue if liver function tests increase more than three times above normal.
- *Stevens–Johnson syndrome:* Refer the patient to a health care provider if signs or symptoms of a rash develop. The health care provider may suggest holding a single dose until the rash is evaluated.
- *Anticonvulsant hypersensitivity syndrome:* This syndrome is characterized by fever (90–100%), rash (90%), hepatitis (50%), and other multiorgan abnormalities (50%). Although the mechanism is unknown, patients who have experienced this syndrome should not receive anticonvulsants that have an aromatic structure (e.g., hydantoin, carbamazepine or oxcarbazepine, phenobarbital, lamotrigine).
- *Suicidal behavior and ideation:* AEDs may increase the risk of suicidal thoughts or behavior. Patients should be monitored for the emergence or worsening of depression, suicidal thoughts or behavior, or any unusual changes in mood or behavior.
- *Teratogenic effects (fetal hydantoin syndrome):* Features include craniofacial anomalies, broad nasal bridges, short upturned noses, low-set and prominent ears, distal digital hypoplasia, and intrauterine growth restriction. The medication is pregnancy category D.

Drug–drug interactions

- Phenytoin induces CYP2C19, uridine 5′-diphospho-glucuronosyltransferase (UGT).
- Phenytoin inhibits CYP2C9.
- Phenytoin displaces some drugs from albumin binding sites.
- Acute alcohol use; amiodarone; chloramphenicol; chlordiazepoxide; diazepam; disulfiram; estrogens; felbamate; histamine antagonists (e.g., cimetidine); halothane; isoniazid; methylphenidate; phenothiazines; phenylbutazone; salicylates; succinimides; sulfonamides (sulfadiazine, sulfamethoxazole, sulfisoxazole); tolbutamide; trazodone; warfarin; and zidovudine increase the serum concentration or effect of phenytoin.
- Antacids, bleomycin, cisplatin, nevirapine, rifampin, ritonavir, vinblastine, zidovudine, and some herbals (i.e., shankhapushpi, kava kava, valerian) decrease the effect of phenytoin.
- Phenytoin may increase the serum concentration or effect of valproic acid.
- Phenytoin may decrease the serum concentration or effect of phenobarbital.

Drug–nutrient interactions

Patients receiving tube feedings and oral phenytoin at the same time may have a significant decrease in absorption of phenytoin. If possible, discontinue feeding 2 hours before and after a dose of phenytoin.

Commercially available formulations

See Table 28-2 for commercially available formulations.

Patient counseling

See general counseling information. In addition, counsel the patient as follows:

- Do not break, crush, or chew capsule before swallowing; swallow whole.
- Shake suspension well.
- This medication may alter your gums. Brush and floss daily, and have regular visits with your dentist.

Pregabalin

Pregabalin is indicated for adjunctive therapy in partial seizures in adults.

Side effects

Upon initiation, nausea, vomiting, dizziness, drowsiness, and lethargy may occur.

With chronic therapy, increased appetite and weight gain are possible.

Severe or life-threatening side effects may occur:

- *Angioedema:* There is some risk of angioedema (e.g., swelling of the face, tongue, lips, gums, and throat or larynx), with or without life-threatening respiratory compromise.
- *FDA warning:* Increased risk of suicidal behavior or ideation may occur. The FDA has analyzed suicidality reports from placebo-controlled

studies involving 11 anticonvulsants (including pregabalin) and found that patients receiving anticonvulsants had approximately twice the risk of suicidal behavior or ideation (0.43%) as patients receiving a placebo (0.22%).

Drug–drug interactions

No known interactions occur.

Other aspects

Pregabalin is subject to control under the Federal Controlled Substances Act of 1970 as a schedule V (C–V) drug.

Commercially available formulations

See Table 28-3 for commercially available formulations.

Primidone

Primidone is indicated for generalized tonic–clonic, complex partial, and simple partial seizures.

Pharmacokinetics

- *Bioavailability:* 60–80%
- *Protein binding:* High (99%)
- *Metabolism:* Hepatically metabolized to phenobarbital (active) and phenylethylmalonamide (PEMA)
- *Renal elimination:* Urinary excretion of active metabolites and 15–25% unchanged primidone
- *Half-life:* Primidone, 10–12 hours; PEMA, 16 hours; phenobarbital, age dependent (20–400 hours)
- *Reference range:* 5–12 mg/L for primidone; 15–45 mg/L for phenobarbital

Side effects

Upon initiation, nausea, vomiting, dizziness, drowsiness, and lethargy may occur.

With chronic therapy, malignant lymphoma-like syndrome, megaloblastic anemia, and systemic lupus-like syndrome are possible.

- *Suicidal behavior and ideation:* AEDs may increase the risk of suicidal thoughts or behavior. Patients should be monitored for the emergence or worsening of depression, suicidal thoughts or behavior, or any unusual changes in mood or behavior.

Drug–drug interactions

- Primidone is an inducer of CYP1A2, CYP2B6, CYP2C, CYP2C8, CYP3A3/4, and CYP3A5–7.
- Primidone may decrease serum concentrations of ethosuximide, valproic acid, and griseofulvin.
- Methylphenidate may increase primidone serum concentrations.
- Phenytoin may decrease primidone serum concentrations.

Commercially available formulations

See Table 28-2 for commercially available formulations.

Rufinamide

Rufinamide is indicated for adjunctive treatment of Lennox–Gastaut syndrome in children 4 years of age and older and in adults.

Pharmacokinetics

- *Bioavailability:* < 85%
- *Protein binding:* Low (34%)
- *Metabolism:* Extensively metabolized by the carboxylesterase hydrolysis (non-CYP)
- *Renal elimination:* > 85% dose excreted renally, but no change in dosage required
- *Half-life:* 6–10 hours
- *Reference range:* Not established

Side effects

Rufinamide has been reported to cause a shortening of the QT interval. Patients with familial short QT syndrome should not receive this medication.

The following side effects may occur:

- *Anticonvulsant hypersensitivity syndrome:* This syndrome is characterized by fever (90–100%), rash (90%), hepatitis (50%), and other multiorgan abnormalities (50%). Although the mechanism is unknown, patients who have experienced this syndrome should not receive anticonvulsants that have an aromatic structure (e.g., hydantoin, carbamazepine or oxcarbazepine, phenobarbitone, lamotrigine).
- *Suicidal behavior and ideation:* AEDs may increase the risk of suicidal thoughts or behavior. Patients should be monitored for the emergence or worsening of depression, suicidal thoughts or behavior, or any unusual changes in mood or behavior.

Drug–drug interactions

Patients on valproate should begin rufinamide at a lower dosage (10 mg/kg/day in children or 400 mg/day in adults).

Commercially available formulations

See Table 28-3 for commercially available formulations.

Tiagabine

Tiagabine is indicated for adjunctive therapy in the treatment of partial seizures in those ≥ 12 years of age.

Pharmacokinetics

- *Bioavailability:* Complete (> 95%)
- *Protein binding:* High (96%, mainly to albumin and alpha$_1$-acid glycoprotein)
- *Metabolism:* Hepatic via oxidation and glucuronidation; undergoes enterohepatic recirculation
- *Renal elimination:* Low (about 2% excreted unchanged in urine)
- *Half-life:* 5–10 hours
- *Reference range:* Not established

Side effects

Upon initiation, nausea and vomiting, somnolence, impaired concentration, confusion, ataxia, and speech and language problems may occur.

No additional side effects have been associated with chronic therapy to date.

- *FDA warning:* Increased risk of suicidal behavior or ideation is possible. The FDA has analyzed suicidality reports from placebo-controlled studies involving 11 anticonvulsants (including tiagabine) and found that patients receiving anticonvulsants had approximately twice the risk of suicidal behavior or ideation (0.43%) as patients receiving a placebo (0.22%).

Drug–drug interactions

- Tiagabine is a CYP3A substrate and may also be metabolized by CYP1A2, CYP2D6, or CYP2C19.
- Valproic acid may increase the serum concentration or effect of tiagabine.
- Carbamazepine, phenobarbital, primidone, and phenytoin may decrease the anticonvulsant effect of tiagabine.

- Tiagabine may decrease the serum concentration or effect of valproic acid.

Commercially available formulations

See Table 28-3 for commercially available formulations.

Topiramate

Topiramate is indicated for initial monotherapy (≥ 2 years of age) for partial onset seizures or primary generalized tonic–clonic seizures and for adjunctive therapy for patients (2–16 years of age) with partial onset seizures or primary generalized tonic–clonic seizures. It is also indicated for seizures associated with Lennox–Gastaut syndrome (≥ 2 years of age).

Pharmacokinetics

- *Bioavailability:* 80%
- *Protein binding:* 15–41%
- *Metabolism:* Minor hepatic (via hydroxylation, hydrolysis, glucuronidation)
- *Renal elimination:* 70% excreted unchanged in urine; may undergo renal tubular reabsorption
- *Half-life:* About 20 hours
- *Reference range:* Not established; clinical value of monitoring concentrations not established

Side effects

Upon initiation, drowsiness, dizziness, difficulty with concentration, loss of appetite, mood changes, and paresthesias may occur.

With chronic therapy, the following side effects are possible:

- Hyperchloremic metabolic acidosis
- Acute myopia and secondary angle closure glaucoma
- Kidney stones (caution patient that adequate hydration may reduce stone formation)
- Paresthesia
- Word-finding difficulties and decreased cognition (dose related)
- Significant weight loss

Severe or life-threatening side effects are as follows:

- *Oligohidrosis and hyperthermia:* Children taking topiramate may not adequately sweat when overheated and could develop hyperthermia and heat stroke. Caution the parent to assess the child's ability to sweat, to be cautious about the child getting overheated, and to have the child drink plenty of water.

- *FDA warning:* Increased risk of suicidal behavior or ideation may occur. The FDA has analyzed suicidality reports from placebo-controlled studies involving 11 anticonvulsants (including topiramate) and found that patients receiving anticonvulsants had approximately twice the risk of suicidal behavior or ideation (0.43%) as patients receiving a placebo (0.22%).

Drug–drug interactions

- Topiramate induces β-oxidation.
- Topiramate inhibits CYP2C19.
- CNS depressants (alcohol, morphine, codeine) and carbonic anhydrase inhibitors (acetazolamide) may increase the serum concentration or effect of topiramate.
- Phenobarbital, phenytoin, and valproic acid may decrease the anticonvulsant effect of topiramate.
- Topiramate may increase the serum concentration or effect of metformin.
- Topiramate may decrease the serum concentration or effect of oral contraceptives and valproic acid.

Commercially available formulations

See Table 28-3 for commercially available formulations.

Patient counseling

See general counseling information. In addition, counsel the patient as follows:

- If using the Topamax sprinkle capsule, sprinkle the contents on a small amount of cool, soft food (e.g., applesauce or yogurt) and swallow immediately without chewing.
- Drink plenty of fluids to avoid kidney stones.
- Confirm that children in hot climates can sweat.

Valproic Acid

Valproic acid is used as monotherapy and adjunctive therapy for all types of generalized and partial seizures; along with ethosuximide, it is the drug of choice for absence seizures. Although it is frequently used in children, it is FDA labeled for those 10 years of age or older. It is rarely used in children less than 2 years of age.

Pharmacokinetics

- *Bioavailability:* Complete
- *Protein binding:* High (80–90%; dose dependent)

- *Metabolism:* Extensive via hepatic glucuronide conjugation and oxidation
- *Renal elimination:* Low (2–3% unchanged in urine)
- *Reference range:* 50–150 mg/L (curvilinear relationship between serum concentration and protein binding)

Side effects

Upon initiation, nausea and vomiting may occur.

With chronic therapy, the following side effects are possible:

- *Weight gain:* This side effect is at times significant enough to warrant discontinuing the medication.
- *Alopecia:* Effects may be partial or total. To prevent or treat alopecia, supplement with zinc and selenium.
- *Tremor:* This effect is dose dependent. Treat it by decreasing the dose, discontinuing the drug, or adding propranolol.
- *Thrombocytopenia:* A dose-dependent decrease in platelets may occur.
- *Elevation in liver enzymes:* This side effect may be transient and responds to discontinuation of valproic acid.

Severe or life-threatening side effects are possible:

- *FDA boxed warning:* Fatal hepatotoxicity is possible. It is most common in children < 2 years of age who have severe epilepsy and are receiving multiple anticonvulsants.
- *FDA boxed warning:* Fatal hemorrhagic pancreatitis may occur.
- *FDA boxed warning:* Fetal valproate syndrome may occur. Features include craniofacial anomalies, small inverted noses, shallow philtrum, flat nasal bridge, long upper lip, congenital liver disease, and spina bifida. This medication is pregnancy category D.
- *FDA warning:* Increased risk of suicidal behavior or ideation may occur. The FDA has analyzed suicidality reports from placebo-controlled studies involving 11 anticonvulsants (including valproic acid) and found that patients receiving anticonvulsants had approximately twice the risk of suicidal behavior or ideation (0.43%) as patients receiving a placebo (0.22%).

Drug–drug interactions

- Valproic acid inhibits CYP2C9, CYP2C19, UGT, epoxide hydroxylase, and β-oxidation.
- It displaces some drugs from albumin binding sites.
- Felbamate, phenytoin, and salicylates increase the serum concentration or effect of valproic acid.
- Carbamazepine, felbamate, lamotrigine, phenytoin, phenobarbital, and primidone decrease the anticonvulsant effect of valproic acid.
- Valproic acid may increase the serum concentration or effect of amitriptyline, carbamazepine, ethosuximide, felbamate, lamotrigine, phenobarbital, primidone, and zidovudine.
- Valproic acid may decrease the serum concentration or effect of phenytoin.

Commercially available formulations

See Table 28-2 for commercially available formulations.

Patient counseling

See general counseling information. Patients should also be counseled as follows:

- You may take this medication with food or milk to reduce stomach irritation. Do not take with carbonated drinks.
- Swallow valproic acid capsules whole with water only; do not break, chew, or crush.
- Swallow divalproex sodium delayed-released capsules whole or sprinkle the contents on a small amount of cool, soft food (e.g., applesauce or pudding), and swallow without chewing immediately after preparation.
- Swallow divalproex sodium delayed-release tablets whole; do not break, chew, or crush.
- You may mix valproic acid syrup with any liquid or add it to a small amount of food.
- Report to your health care provider any sore throat, fever, fatigue, bleeding, or bruising that is severe or persists.
- Your health care provider may monitor your liver function with blood tests every 1–2 weeks initially and periodically thereafter.

Vigabatrin

Vigabatrin is indicated for infantile spasms in patients 1 month to 2 years of age.

Pharmacokinetics

- *Bioavailability:* Complete
- *Protein binding:* Low
- *Metabolism:* Minimal
- *Renal elimination:* 80% (unchanged)
- *Half-life:* 5–13 hours

Side effects

Upon initiation, fatigue, headache, drowsiness, dizziness, tremor, or agitation may occur. Hyperactivity (e.g., hyperkinesia, agitation, excitation, restlessness) has been reported in children.

With chronic therapy, permanent decrease in peripheral vision may occur. However, there is no effect on central vision or perception of color.

- *Suicidal behavior and ideation:* AEDs may increase the risk of suicidal thoughts or behavior. Patients should be monitored for the emergence or worsening of depression, suicidal thoughts or behavior, or any unusual changes in mood or behavior.
- *FDA boxed warning:* Permanent loss of peripheral vision in infants, children, and adults is possible. Due to the risk of peripheral vision loss and because vigabatrin provides an observable symptomatic benefit when it is effective, the patient who fails to show substantial benefit within a short period of time after initiation of treatment (2–4 weeks for infantile spasms; < 3 months in adults) should be withdrawn from therapy. If in the clinical judgment of the prescriber evidence of treatment failure becomes obvious earlier in treatment, vigabatrin should be discontinued at that time.

Commercially available formulations

See Table 28-3 for commercially available formulations.

Patient counseling

See general counseling information. In addition, counsel patients to notify their health care provider of any change in vision.

Zonisamide

Zonisamide is indicated for partial seizures in adults.

Pharmacokinetics

- *Bioavailability:* Complete
- *Protein binding:* Low (40%)
- *Metabolism:* Undergoes acetylation and subsequent conjugation with glucuronide in the liver
- *Renal elimination:* 62% (35% as unchanged)
- *Half-life:* 50–70 hours
- *Reference range:* proposed therapeutic range, 10–20 mg/L; concentrations > 30 mg/L associated with adverse effects

Side effects

With chronic therapy, side effects are very similar to those of topiramate:

- Kidney stones (contraindicated in patients with a history of kidney stones; should be adequately hydrated)
- Weight loss
- Reversible or irreversible psychosis (rare)

Severe or life-threatening side effects may occur:

- *FDA warning:* The medication carries an FDA warning for oligohidrosis and hyperthermia. Children taking zonisamide may not sweat as needed and could develop hyperthermia. Warn parents of the need to be aware of children getting overheated and to have them drink plenty of water.
- *FDA warning:* Zonisamide may cause a dose-dependent metabolic acidosis, which has occurred at doses as small as 25 mg/day. Metabolic acidosis is usually asymptomatic; however, chronic untreated metabolic acidosis may result in decreased growth rates in children, as well as decreased fetal growth and fetal death following exposure during pregnancy. The FDA is now recommending a serum bicarbonate level prior to initiation and periodically during therapy. If metabolic acidosis develops, consider decreasing the dose or discontinuing use with appropriate dose tapering.
- *FDA warning:* Increased risk of suicidal behavior or ideation may occur. The FDA has analyzed suicidality reports from placebo-controlled studies involving 11 anticonvulsants (including zonisamide) and found that patients receiving anticonvulsants had approximately twice the risk of suicidal behavior or ideation (0.43%) as patients receiving a placebo (0.22%).

- *Other:* Zonisamide is a sulfonamide. Life-threatening sulfonamide reactions may occur (e.g., Stevens–Johnson syndrome, toxic epidermal necrolysis, aplastic anemia, agranulocytosis, fulminant hepatic necrosis).

Drug–drug interactions

- Zonisamide is a CYP3A4 substrate.
- Carbamazepine, phenobarbital, phenytoin, and valproic acid decrease the effect of zonisamide.
- Lamotrigine may inhibit the clearance of zonisamide and increase zonisamide serum concentrations.

Commercially available formulations

See Table 28-3 for commercially available formulations.

Patient counseling

See general counseling information. In addition, counsel the patient as follows:

- Notify your pharmacist or health care provider if you are allergic to sulfa medications.
- Drink plenty of fluids to help prevent kidney stones.
- Contact your health care provider if your child is not sweating as usual.

28-5. Other Issues

Nondrug Treatment of Epilepsy

Nondrug treatments are as follows:

- Ketogenic diet
- Vagal nerve stimulator
- Surgical correction

Withdrawal of Anticonvulsants

Over half of patients who remain seizure free for 2 years can have their anticonvulsant successfully withdrawn. Most who are seizure free for 4 years can be successfully withdrawn from anticonvulsants.

Unless the patient is experiencing a severe or life-threatening adverse effect, *never* abruptly discontinue an anticonvulsant; taper slowly over 2–6 months.

Table 28-4. Treatment of Status Epilepticus

As soon as possible	▪ Assess cardiorespiratory status; insert oral airway and administer oxygen as needed.
	▪ Place secure IV, and start infusion of normal saline.
	▪ Obtain medical history; perform neurological examination.
	▪ Obtain the following tests: if the patient has been on anticonvulsants as an outpatient, obtain blood for serum drug concentrations and a chemistry panel including electrolytes, glucose, blood urea nitrogen, and urine drug screen.
	▪ Administer 25 g of glucose and 100 mg of thiamine IV.
If still seizing	▪ Administer either diazepam or lorazepam up to maximum dosage until seizure stops.
If still seizing	▪ Load with IV phenytoin (provided patient was not on phenytoin at home or has low serum concentrations), and begin maintenance doses.
	▪ Monitor blood pressure and EEG.
	▪ Load with IV phenobarbital or begin a continuous infusion of midazolam.
If still seizing	▪ Begin medically induced coma, and adjust dosage until burst suppression on EEG.
	▪ Avoid hypotension during infusion of the barbiturate.

Status Epilepticus

Status epilepticus is defined as a seizure that lasts longer than 5 minutes or two or more discrete seizures between which there is incomplete recovery of consciousness. It is a medical emergency. See Table 28-4 for suggested order of therapies.

Benzodiazepines

Benzodiazepines are first-line agents. Lorazepam is preferred.

Hydantoin (phenytoin or fosphenytoin)

Phenytoin (intravenous)
Phenytoin can be mixed only with normal saline.

If an individual is not already receiving phenytoin, give a loading dose of 15–20 mg/kg. Because phenytoin contains propylene glycol and is in itself cardiotoxic, do not infuse faster than 50 mg/min.

If the maintenance dose is to be given every 12 hours, give the first dose 12 hours after the end of the loading dose. If the maintenance dose is to be given every 24 hours, give the first dose 24 hours after the end of the loading dose.

The alkaline pH of phenytoin precludes IM administration.

Fosphenytoin
Fosphenytoin is a phenytoin pro-drug that is converted to phenytoin within minutes after infusion. It can be admixed with any IV solution.

Fosphenytoin must be dosed in PEs (phenytoin equivalents): 1 mg of phenytoin = 1.5 mg of fosphenytoin. It can be given at a rate of 150 mg/min (three times faster than phenytoin).

Phenobarbital

Phenobarbital may cause respiratory depression or arrest. The likelihood of such an effect may be increased if benzodiazepines have been given.

Phenobarbital-induced sedation may eliminate the ability to perform an accurate neurologic assessment.

Because phenobarbital contains propylene glycol and is cardiotoxic, do not infuse faster than 60 mg/min in adults and 30 mg/min in children.

Midazolam

Because of midazolam's very short half-life, the loading dose should be followed by continuous infusion.

Medically induced coma

A medically induced coma is used for severe refractory status epilepticus. It is usually achieved with pentobarbital.

Give a loading dose (20–40 mg/kg) over 1–2 hours, followed by continuous infusion (1–4 mg/kg/h).

If hypotension occurs, begin dopamine or slow the rate of infusion.

Titrate to burst suppression (isoelectric) on EEG.

Other therapies used for refractory status epilepticus

▪ Propofol
▪ Newer anticonvulsants (IV: levetiracetam, lacosamide; oral: topiramate)
▪ Magnesium
▪ Lidocaine
▪ IV immune globulin

Febrile Seizures

A febrile seizure is a benign seizure that occurs in the absence of CNS infection in a child with fever. It is the most common seizure disorder in childhood. The age of onset is 4 months to 5 years (peaks at 14–18 months).

A child is at risk if he or she has two of the following risk factors:

- A first- or second-degree relative with a history of a febrile seizure
- Developmental delay
- Delayed discharge (> 28 days) from a newborn center
- Day care attendance

Overall, the development of epilepsy in children who have experienced such seizures is rare (1–2%). However, about 15% of children who have complex febrile seizures (as defined below) will go on to develop epilepsy.

There are two types of febrile seizures:

- Simple febrile seizure:
  - Benign
  - A primary generalized seizure
  - Less than 15 minutes in duration
  - No recurrence within 24 hours
- Complex febrile seizure:
  - Focal (involves an arm, leg, or face on one side only or eye deviation toward one side)
  - Prolonged (> 15 minutes) or recurring within 24 hours of the initial seizure

Acute treatment of a simple or complex febrile seizure

Drugs of choice for prolonged febrile seizure are rectally administered benzodiazepines (rectal diazepam or lorazepam). Diastat is a commercially available gel of diazepam to be given rectally.

Prophylaxis for a simple or complex febrile seizure

If temperature is > 38°C, give the patient a nonaspirin antipyretic.

Daily anticonvulsants are not indicated for the prevention of recurrent febrile seizures.

Maintenance therapy

Maintenance therapy is not generally used. However, an anticonvulsant (i.e., phenobarbital) may be considered after a complex febrile seizure if epilepsy is suspected.

Carbamazepine and phenytoin are *not* effective in the prevention of recurrent febrile seizures.

28-6. Questions

1. Which of the following is true regarding phenytoin?

    A. The maximum rate of IV administration is 50 mg/min.
    B. If IV access cannot be established, phenytoin can be given IM.
    C. Because phenytoin contains propylene glycol, it is soluble as any IV fluid.
    D. It is an inhibitor of the cytochrome P450 system.
    E. A major limitation to the use of the product in pediatric patients is the lack of a commercially available liquid formulation.

2. A 50 kg patient with no history of epilepsy presents in status epilepticus. The patient is given an adequate dose of lorazepam and is about to be given a loading dose of IV phenytoin. Assuming a phenytoin V_d of 0.6 L/kg, what dose of phenytoin should be given to achieve a serum phenytoin concentration of ~16–18 mg/L?

    A. 18 mg/kg
    B. 500 mg
    C. 30 mg/kg
    D. 50 mg
    E. 5 g

3. Which of the following is true regarding a patient with refractory status epilepticus who is placed in a medically induced coma with a barbiturate?

    A. If the patient is mechanically ventilated, the barbiturates will induce respiratory arrest.
    B. The goal of a coma that is medically induced with a barbiturate is to induce burst suppression (isoelectric) on EEG.
    C. If hypotension develops, the patient should be given nitroprusside.
    D. The barbiturates are not associated with drug interactions.
    E. A major problem with this type of therapy is kidney failure.

4. Which of the following is associated with autoinduction?

   A. Phenobarbital
   B. Phenytoin
   C. Carbamazepine
   D. Gabapentin
   E. Levetiracetam

5. Which of these agents reduces the likelihood of congenital malformations in epileptic women receiving valproate?

   A. Folic acid
   B. Vitamin B_{12}
   C. Ginkgo biloba
   D. Iron
   E. Selenium

6. A 33-year-old woman is being started on an anticonvulsant. She is already slightly overweight and is very concerned about the effects of the various medications on her weight. Which of the following is true regarding anticonvulsants and their effect on weight?

   A. Valproic acid and phenytoin both decrease weight.
   B. Valproic acid increases weight and topiramate decreases weight.
   C. Topiramate and phenytoin both increase weight.
   D. Topiramate, valproic acid, and phenytoin cause no change in weight.
   E. Phenytoin is the only anticonvulsant known to increase weight.

7. A 24-year-old woman has complex partial seizures that are currently controlled with valproic acid, gabapentin, and topiramate. She calls your pharmacy to ask if any of her medications can cause nosebleeds because she has had one or two in the past week. You refer her to her local health care provider, where her platelet count is reported to be 95,132/mm³. Which of the following is true?

   A. None of her anticonvulsants cause thrombocytopenia.
   B. Valproate can cause a dose-related thrombocytopenia.
   C. Gabapentin has inhibited the metabolism of topiramate, and the elevated concentration of topiramate is responsible for the thrombocytopenia.

   D. Gabapentin can cause idiosyncratic thrombocytopenia.
   E. Topiramate can cause thrombocytopenia.

8. A patient has hypertension, diabetes mellitus, and chronic renal failure (SCr = 6.8) and has developed seizures. Which of the following anticonvulsants would require dosage adjustment in this patient?

   A. Gabapentin and topiramate
   B. Lamotrigine and felbamate
   C. Phenobarbital and gabapentin
   D. Phenytoin and valproic acid
   E. Phenobarbital and levetiracetam

9. Which of the following anticonvulsants is metabolized to phenobarbital?

   A. Ethosuximide
   B. Primidone
   C. Zonisamide
   D. Levetiracetam
   E. Carbamazepine

10. A 7-year-old boy on valproic acid for partial complex seizures with secondary generalization that are refractory to phenobarbital, phenytoin, carbamazepine, and gabapentin continued to have seizures and was started on lamotrigine 2 weeks ago. Today he presents with a diffuse maculopapular erythematous rash with lesions on his lips. Which of the following is correct?

    A. A rash associated with lamotrigine generally occurs within the first few days; hence, the rash is not associated with an anticonvulsant.
    B. The patient should be given diphenhydramine, and lamotrigine should be continued.
    C. Lamotrigine should be discontinued.
    D. The rash is secondary to a drug interaction between gabapentin and carbamazepine.
    E. All of the anticonvulsants are associated with a life-threatening rash. To prevent status epilepticus associated with abrupt discontinuation of the anticonvulsants, the medications should be slowly discontinued.

11. A new anticonvulsant has just been approved by the FDA. Its bioavailability is > 95%, and it is highly protein bound to α_1-acid glycoprotein. It undergoes extensive hepatic metabolism by CYP2C9. Less than 5% is excreted unchanged in the urine. It is known to inhibit CYP3A4. A patient on this anticonvulsant has developed significant depression and is being started on an antidepressant that is 93% bound to albumin and is a potent inhibitor of CYP2C19. The antidepressant is a pro-drug that is metabolized by CYP3A4 to an active metabolite that is hepatically cleared by CYP2C9. The neurologist wants to know if any drug interactions may occur that would necessitate a change in drug dosage. Which of the following is the appropriate response?

    A. No drug interactions should occur in this patient.
    B. The dose of the anticonvulsant should be reduced because of a potential protein-binding interaction that would increase the serum concentration of the anticonvulsant.
    C. The dose of the anticonvulsant should be increased.
    D. The patient may not benefit from the antidepressant, and another antidepressant that is not metabolized by CYP3A4 should be used.
    E. Because of an interaction in the gut that decreases bioavailability, the dose should be increased.

12. Which of the following AEDs is (are) *not* associated with any drug–drug interactions?

    A. Carbamazepine and gabapentin
    B. Carbamazepine and levetiracetam
    C. Gabapentin and levetiracetam
    D. Carbamazepine only
    E. Phenytoin and carbamazepine

13. A 42-year-old woman has been successfully treated with valproic acid for years, but she has experienced some undesirable side effects. She is slowly titrated onto a new anticonvulsant, and the valproic acid is gradually discontinued. She presents to the emergency department with severe flank pain and is diagnosed with a kidney stone. Which of the

following may have precipitated her current situation?

    A. Gabapentin
    B. Lamotrigine
    C. Levetiracetam
    D. Topiramate
    E. Phenytoin

14. Which of the following drugs carry an FDA boxed warning?

    A. Carbamazepine and levetiracetam
    B. Felbamate and levetiracetam
    C. Lamotrigine and clobazam
    D. Carbamazepine and felbamate
    E. Phenytoin and carbamazepine

15. Which of the following carries an FDA boxed warning for pancreatitis?

    A. Carbamazepine
    B. Felbamate
    C. Zonisamide
    D. Valproic acid
    E. Phenytoin

16. What is the drug of choice for absence seizures in a child < 2 years of age?

    A. Phenytoin
    B. Phenobarbital
    C. Ethosuximide
    D. Valproic acid
    E. Primidone

17. Diastat is given by which of the following routes?

    A. Rectally
    B. Intramuscularly
    C. Intravenously
    D. Intranasally
    E. Subcutaneously

18. Which of the following is true?

    A. Febrile seizures must be accompanied by a CNS infection.
    B. Complex febrile seizures last > 15 minutes.
    C. Most children who have a febrile seizure go on to develop epilepsy.
    D. The drug of choice for a simple febrile seizure is carbamazepine.
    E. Simple febrile seizures should never be treated.

19. Which of the following anticonvulsants is (are) available in a liquid, chewable tablet, and intravenous formulation?

    A. Phenytoin only
    B. Valproic acid and carbamazepine
    C. Carbamazepine and phenytoin
    D. Valproic acid only
    E. Primidone and valproic acid

20. Patients should be told to drink plenty of fluid when taking which of the following?

    A. Carbamazepine
    B. Topiramate
    C. Levetiracetam
    D. Gabapentin
    E. Phenytoin

21. Which of the following medications may cause seizures in an adult patient with renal failure?

    A. Meperidine
    B. Phenobarbital
    C. Carbamazepine
    D. Lamotrigine
    E. Theophylline

22. Which of the following is associated with Michaelis–Menten pharmacokinetics?

    A. Carbamazepine
    B. Valproic acid
    C. Topiramate
    D. Phenytoin
    E. Phenobarbital

23. A patient on which of the following medications should be made aware of the importance of good oral hygiene?

    A. Felbamate
    B. Phenytoin
    C. Zonisamide
    D. Phenobarbital
    E. Levetiracetam

28-7. Answers

1. **A.** Because phenytoin contains propylene glycol and is itself cardiotoxic, the IV formulation should not be infused faster than 50 mg/min. Phenytoin is extremely alkaline (pH ~13). Not only is IM administration associated with tissue damage, but also it is erratically absorbed. Phenytoin can be admixed only with normal saline, is an inducer, and is also available as a suspension and a chewable tablet.

2. **B.** The equation for calculation of a loading dose is as follows: Dose = C_p (serum concentration) desired $\times$ V_d (volume of distribution). So C_p desired is ~$17 \times (0.6 \text{ L/kg} \times 50 \text{ kg}) \approx 510$ mg.

3. **B.** The goal is to produce a "flat" EEG. If the patient is mechanically ventilated, the effect of a medication on respiration is not a factor in its administration. Although pentobarbital may cause hypotension if given too rapidly, nitroprusside is a vasodilator used to treat hypertension. The barbiturates are known inducers. A coma that is medically induced with a barbiturate does not cause kidney failure.

4. **C.** Carbamazepine induces its own metabolism, with peak effects seen about 21 days after beginning the medication or following an increase in dosage. Phenobarbital and phenytoin are inducers. Gabapentin and levetiracetam are not cleared hepatically.

5. **A.** Many of the anticonvulsants can cause folic acid deficiency. An association exists between folic acid deficiency and spina bifida; hence, all women with epilepsy who are of childbearing age should receive supplemental folic acid every day (1 mg).

6. **B.** Topiramate can cause significant weight loss, and valproate can cause significant weight gain. Phenytoin does not significantly affect weight.

7. **B.** Valproic acid can cause clinically significant thrombocytopenia. Gabapentin is not associated with any drug interaction that affects metabolism, and it does not cause a decrease in platelets. Topiramate does not cause thrombocytopenia.

8. **A.** Gabapentin and topiramate would require dosage adjustment because they are renally eliminated.

9. **B.** Primidone (Mysoline) is an active anticonvulsant, but it is also metabolized to phenobarbital.

10. **C.** Lamotrigine has an FDA boxed warning for severe rash. Because this patient has a diffuse rash and lesions on his lips, lamotrigine

should be discontinued. Because the incidence of severe rash may be higher in children than in adults, current practice would be to discontinue lamotrigine and not "treat through" the rash with diphenhydramine. Gabapentin does not interact with lamotrigine. However, the combination of valproic acid and lamotrigine is associated with a higher incidence of rash. Although abrupt discontinuation of an anticonvulsant may induce status epilepticus, an anticonvulsant may be abruptly discontinued in the face of a life-threatening event.

11. **D.** Because the new anticonvulsant inhibits CYP3A4, D is the correct answer. Because the antidepressant is a pro-drug, which must be metabolized by CYP3A4 to become active, it may not be effective. An alternative antidepressant should be considered.

12. **C.** At this time, neither gabapentin nor levetiracetam is associated with significant drug–drug interactions. The absorption of gabapentin may be reduced by concurrent administration of aluminum- or magnesium-containing antacids; hence, antacids should be given 2 hours before or after a dose of gabapentin. Carbamazepine is an inducer that is associated with numerous drug–drug interactions.

13. **D.** Both topiramate and zonisamide may cause kidney stones. Although neither agent is contraindicated in an individual with a history of kidney stones, these drugs should be used cautiously in such patients. Patients should be counseled to remain adequately hydrated because doing so may decrease the risk of stone formation.

14. **D.** Both carbamazepine and felbamate are associated with aplastic anemia and hepatic failure. Levetiracetam has no FDA boxed warning.

15. **D.** Valproic acid may cause fatal hemorrhagic pancreatitis.

16. **C.** Although valproic acid is extremely effective and is frequently used as monotherapy for absence seizures, it should not be given to a patient < 2 years of age.

17. **A.** Diastat is a commercially available gel form of diazepam that is given rectally.

18. **B.** Unlike simple febrile seizures, which last a brief period, complex febrile seizures are prolonged (> 15 minutes) or recur within 24 hours of the initial seizure. Febrile seizures must occur in the absence of CNS infection in a child with fever. Most febrile seizures are benign, and children do not go on to develop epilepsy. Carbamazepine is ineffective in febrile seizures.

19. **A.** Only phenytoin is available as a liquid (125 mg/ 5 mL), as a chewable tablet (50 mg), and in an IV dosage form. Carbamazepine is not available in an IV dosage form, and valproic acid is not available as a chewable tablet.

20. **B.** Because topiramate may cause kidney stones, patients should be encouraged to drink plenty of fluids. This would also be true for zonisamide.

21. **A.** Normeperidine, a metabolite of meperidine, can accumulate in patients with renal failure who receive normal doses and cause seizures. The other agents listed are not eliminated renally in adults.

22. **D.** Phenytoin has capacity-limited or saturable (i.e., Michaelis–Menten) pharmacokinetics.

23. **B.** Phenytoin may cause gingival hyperplasia (i.e., overgrowth of the gums). Hence, patients should be instructed to brush and floss daily and to have regular visits with the dentist.

28-8. References

Baumann RJ, Duffner PK. Treatment of children with simple febrile seizures: The AAP practice parameter. *Pediatr Neurol.* 2000;23:11–17.

Bourgeois BF. Determining the effects of antiepileptic drugs on cognitive function in pediatric patients with epilepsy. *J Child Neurol.* 2004;19(suppl 1): S15–S24.

Brophy GM, Bell R, Claassen J, et al. Guidelines for the evaluation and management of status epilepticus. *Neurocrit Care.* 2012;17(1):3–23.

Brunbech L, Sabers A. Effect of antiepileptic drugs on cognitive function in individuals with epilepsy: A comparative review of newer versus older agents. *Drugs.* 2002;62:593–604.

Deckers CL, Knoester PD, de Haan GJ, et al. Selection criteria for the clinical use of the newer antiepileptic drugs. *CNS Drugs.* 2003;17:405–21.

Hixson JD. Stopping antiepileptic drugs: When and why? *Curr Treat Options Neurol.* 2010;12(5): 434–42.

Hunter G, Young GB. Status epilepticus: A review, with emphasis on refractory cases. *Can J Neurol Sci.* 2012;39:157–69.

Italiano D, Perucca E. Clinical pharmacokinetics of new-generation antiepileptic drugs at the extremes of age: An update. *Clin Pharmacokinet.* 2013;52(8):627–45.

Johannessen SI, Battino D, Berry DJ, et al. Therapeutic drug monitoring of the newer antiepileptic drugs. *Ther Drug Monit.* 2003;25:347–463.

Krivoy N, Taer M, Neuman MG. Antiepileptic drug-induced hypersensitivity syndrome reactions. *Curr Drug Saf.* 2006;1(3):289–99.

Patsalos PN, Berry DJ, Bourgeois BFD, et al. Antiepileptic drugs—Best practice guidelines for therapeutic drug monitoring: A position paper by the subcommission on therapeutic drug monitoring, ILAE Commission on Therapeutic Strategies. *Epilepsia.* 2008;49:1239–76.

Perucca E. Clinically relevant drug interactions with antiepileptic drugs. *Br J Clin Pharmacol.* 2006; 61(3):246–55.

Steering Committee on Quality Improvement and Management, Subcommittee on Febrile Seizures. Febrile seizures: Clinical practice guideline for the long-term management of the child with simple febrile seizures. *Pediatrics.* 2008;121:1281–86.

Psychiatry 29

Jason Carter

29-1. Key Points

Schizophrenia

- Patients with schizophrenia have positive (hallucinations, delusions), negative (flat affect, avolition, anhedonia, poverty of thought), and disorganized speech and behavior symptoms. Positive symptoms usually respond to drug therapy first.
- Antipsychotics (conventional or atypical) are essential treatment for schizophrenia; atypical medications (risperidone, olanzapine, quetiapine, ziprasidone, aripiprazole, paliperidone) have been considered first-line medical treatment because they lower risk of extrapyramidal side effects (EPS) and tardive dyskinesia (TD) more than conventional medications, and they appear to be more beneficial for negative symptoms.
- Recent evidence shows that patients with schizophrenia discontinue medications frequently regardless of whether they are taking second-generation or first-generation antipsychotics. Such research questions whether the atypical antipsychotics treat negative symptoms more effectively than typical antipsychotics.
- Atypical antipsychotics (especially olanzapine) are associated with weight gain and with lipid and glucose abnormalities. (Ziprasidone and aripiprazole do not appear to have the weight gain and metabolic abnormalities.)
- Low-potency agents have more sedation, orthostatic hypotension, and anticholinergic side effects and fewer EPSs than high-potency agents. High-potency agents have more EPSs and less sedation, orthostatic hypotension, and anticholinergic effects.
- EPSs consist of dystonic reactions (to be remedied by diphenhydramine 25–50 mg intramuscular (IM) or benztropine 1–2 mg IM every 30 minutes until resolution); akathisia (to be treated with lorazepam, clonidine, or propranolol); and pseudoparkinsonism (ameliorated by amantadine or benztropine).
- Clozapine is the only agent proven effective for refractory schizophrenia.
- Consider long-acting injectable preparations in situations of poor compliance.

Bipolar Disorder

- The acute treatment for bipolar disorder focuses on slowing down the patient and reducing harm to himself or herself and others.
- Maintenance treatment focuses on preventing or reducing the number of future episodes.
- A mood stabilizer is an essential component in the treatment of bipolar disorder. First-line mood stabilizers include lithium and divalproex sodium (or valproic acid).
- The risk of lithium side effects and toxicity can be prevented by monitoring the patient for signs and symptoms of problems and by obtaining regular blood-level readings.
- Other drug therapies that may be used to treat the patient with bipolar disorder include atypical antipsychotics, gabapentin, carbamazepine, oxcarbazepine, topiramate, and lamotrigine (especially if the patient is depressed).

Major Depression

- All antidepressants are equally effective in a given population.
- Response varies from person to person. Antidepressants differ in side effect and drug-interaction profiles, and none are "speed" or "uppers."
- Choice of agent depends on the history of response of other family members to certain antidepressants (if available) and the particular side effect profile (as it relates to any given patient).
- First-line agents include selective serotonin reuptake inhibitors (SSRIs), bupropion, venlafaxine, and duloxetine; second-line agents may include mirtazapine and nefazodone; third-line agents may include tricyclic antidepressants (TCAs) and monoamine oxidase inhibitors (MAOIs).
- The goal is to reduce or eliminate target symptoms with an antidepressant; incorporating psychotherapy is optimal.
- The goal of treatment of depression is to improve the patient's ability to function and his or her quality of life.

Anxiety Disorders

- Anxiety disorders are serious, debilitating mental illnesses that have extreme anxiety as the primary mood disturbance.
- Various drug therapies include benzodiazepines, buspirone, antidepressants (especially SSRIs and venlafaxine), β-blockers, and hydroxyzine.
- Nonpharmacologic therapy of anxiety disorders is an important aspect of care (e.g., supportive therapy, cognitive behavioral therapy, relaxation techniques, and exercise and lifestyle modifications).

Eating disorders

- Anorexia nervosa is characterized by a refusal to maintain body weight (at or above a minimal normal weight for age and height), an intense fear of gaining weight, and a disturbance in self-perception of body weight.
- Bulimia nervosa is characterized by recurrent episodes of binge eating, recurrent and inappropriate compensatory behavior to prevent weight gain at least weekly for 3 months, and self-evaluation that is primarily influenced by body shape and weight.
- Eating disorders most commonly occur in young, Caucasian, middle- to upper-class females.
- Medical complications and comorbid psychiatric disorders (e.g., anxiety, depression, substance abuse) are extremely common in this population.
- Medications such as antidepressants may be helpful in treating eating disorders (especially bulimia); optimal therapy should include psychotherapy in combination with drug therapy.

29-2. Study Guide Checklist

The following topics may guide your study of this subject area:

- The *Diagnostic and Statistical Manual of Mental Disorders Text Revision* (DSM-5) of the American Psychiatric Association
- General clinical presentation and symptoms of schizophrenia, bipolar disorder, major depressive disorder, anxiety disorders, and eating disorders
- General nonpharmacologic treatment options for psychiatric illness
- Considerations for pharmacologic treatment based on patient's clinical presentation and prior drug experience
- Mechanism of action of various classes of psychotropic drugs
- Trade names and available dosage forms, particularly the "Top 100 Drugs"
- Frequency of dosing regimen, particularly long-acting injectables
- Major adverse drug reactions of psychotropic drugs
- Significant drug interactions of psychotropic drugs
- Unique patient counseling points for specific psychotropic drugs
- Monitoring of the safety and efficacy of psychotropic drugs
- Guidelines for the pharmacological treatment of schizophrenia, bipolar disorder, major depressive disorder, anxiety disorders, and eating disorders

29-3. Schizophrenia

Schizophrenia is a psychiatric disorder characterized by a profound disruption in perception, cognition, and emotion.

Epidemiology

Approximately 1% of the U.S. adult population has schizophrenia. There are 200,000 new cases reported yearly.

No gender or racial differences exist. Onset is earlier in males (average age, 18–24 years) than in females (average age, late 20s to early 40s).

Clinical Presentation

The onset of schizophrenia is typically characterized by deterioration in occupational and social situations over a period of 6 months or more.

Symptoms

Symptoms include the following:

- Hallucinations (auditory, visual, tactile, olfactory, or gustatory)
- Delusions (usually persecutory or grandiose)
- Disorganized speech
- Impaired cognition, attention, concentration, judgment, and motivation

Symptoms are commonly referred to as *positive* (hallucinations or delusions); *negative* (flat affect, avolition, anhedonia, and poverty of thought); or *disorganized* (disorganized speech or behavior).

Most patients fluctuate between acute episodes and remission, but complete remission without any symptoms is uncommon.

Associated features

Morbidity

There are many comorbid disease states (mental and medical); for example, substance abuse is found in 60–70% of persons with schizophrenia.

Mortality

Shortened life expectancy is a feature of schizophrenia. Patients with schizophrenia are at increased risk of suicide (10% commit suicide). Risk factors for suicide are as follows:

- Male
- Socially isolated
- Comorbid psychiatric disorders
- Unemployed
- < 30 years of age

Etiology

The etiology is most likely multifactorial:

- Genetic
- Neurobiologic
- Developmental (season of birth, viral illness, traumatic injury)

DSM-5 Diagnostic Criteria

Two or more of the following symptoms prevail for at least 1 month:

- Hallucinations
- Delusions
- Disorganized speech
- Grossly disorganized or catatonic behavior
- Negative symptoms
- Anhedonia
- Flat affect
- Avolition

Significant social dysfunction exists:

- Signs of the disturbance are continuous and persist for 6 months.
- Schizoaffective disorders and mood disorders, mental retardation, substance abuse, and other causative medical disorders have been ruled out.

Treatment Principles and Goals

- All antipsychotics are equally effective if used properly.
- Clozapine is the only agent proven effective in treating refractory schizophrenia.
- The basis for choosing an antipsychotic medication is the following:
  - Past history of response (patient's response or a family member's response to a medication)
  - Side effect profile of the antipsychotic
- Administer therapy with a trial of antipsychotics (at least 4–6 weeks at recommended doses).
- Do everything possible to simplify the drug regimen.
- Consider long-acting injectable preparations in situations of poor compliance.

Drug Therapy

Tables 29-1 and 29-2 provide an overview of drug therapy alternatives.

Mechanism of action

These drugs block postsynaptic dopamine-2 receptors. They share anticholinergic, antihistaminic, and α-blocking properties.

Other conventional agents

Though not commonly used, perphenazine (Trilafon), thiothixene (Navane), trifluoperazine (Stelazine), and loxapine (Loxitane) are conventional agents to treat schizophrenia. Note that loxapine has a new formulation (Adasuve) as an oral inhalation for acute treat-ment of agitation associated with schizophrenia or bipolar I disorder. Loxapine inhalation powder may be prescribed at certified facilities only, and staff training is required as part of a Risk Evaluation and Mitigation Strategies (REMS) program. Patients must be monitored at least every 15 minutes for a minimum of 1 hour following treatment with loxapine inhalation powder for signs or symptoms of bronchospasm.

Management of adverse effects

Sedation
The level of sedation depends on the drug used. Low-potency drugs in this class are more sedating than high-potency drugs.

Sedation effects are worse initially but become more tolerable over time.

Table 29-1. Typical (Conventional or Older) Antipsychotics

Drug and form	Trade name	Form	Potency	Daily dosage range	Equivalent oral dose	Clinical highlights
Chlorpromazine	Thorazine	10, 25, 50, 100, 200 mg tablets; 30, 75, 150, 200, 300 mg sustained-release capsules; 10 mg/5 mL syrup; 30 mg/mL, 100 mg/mL concentrate; 25, 100 mg rectal suppository; 25 mg/mL injection	Low	50–2,000 mg	100 mg	First antipsychotic used clinically; contributed to deinstitutionalization of many patients in the 1950s; 100 mg of chlorpromazine is equivalent to 2 mg of haloperidol
Thioridazine	Mellaril	10, 15, 25, 50, 100, 150, 200 mg tablets; 25, 100 mg/5 mL suspension; 30, 100 mg/mL concentrate	Low	50–800 mg	100 mg	Pigmentary retinopathy at daily doses > 800 mg/day; black box warning: QT prolongation
Perphenazine	Trilafon	2, 4, 8, 16 mg tablets; 5 mg/mL injection	Medium	4–64 mg in divided doses	10 mg	Moderate sedation, extra-pyramidal symptoms; low anticholinergic effect, orthostasis
Fluphenazine	Prolixin	1, 2.5, 5, 10 mg tablets; 25 mg/mL decanoate injection; 2.5 mg/mL injection; 2.5 mg/5 mL elixir; 5 mg/mL concentrate	High	1–65 mg po; 12.5–75 mg IM (decanoate) every 2 weeks	2 mg	Decanoate injection every 2 weeks; immediate-release injection, 5–10 minutes onset
Haloperidol	Haldol	0.5, 1, 2, 5, 10, 20 mg tablets; 2 mg/mL concentrate; 50, 100 mg/mL decanoate injection; 5 mg/mL injection	High	1–100 mg po; 50–300 mg IM (decanoate) every 4 weeks	2 mg	Decanoate injection every 4 weeks; immediate-release injection, 5–10 min onset

Table 29-2. Adverse Effects of Typical Antipsychotic Medications

Drug	Extrapyramidal symptoms	Sedation	Orthostasis	Weight gain	Anticholinergic effect
Chlorpromazine	+++	++++	++++	++	+++
Thioridazine	+++	++++	++++	+	++++
Perphenazine	++++	++	+	+	++
Fluphenazine	++++	+	+	+	+
Haloperidol	++++	+	+	+	+

Neuroleptic effects
Neuroleptic effects are "secondary" negative symptoms including reduced initiative, lessened interest in environment, and blunted affect.

Orthostasis
Alpha adrenergic blockade results in orthostatic hypotension. Severity depends on the drug used. Low-potency formulations promote more orthostasis than do high-potency formulations. Orthostasis is usually seen in the first few hours or days of treatment, and the patient usually develops tolerance.

This condition is especially problematic in elderly patients.

Weight gain
Weight gain is very prominent in patients taking these medications. Low doses should be used. Appropriate diet and exercise should be encouraged to offset weight gain.

Anticholinergic effect
Severity depends on the drug used. Low-potency drugs of this type are more sedating than high-potency ones.

Dry mouth, blurred vision, constipation, and urinary hesitancy may occur. Use high-potency agents in patients bothered by anticholinergic side effects.

Extrapyramidal symptoms
Extrapyramidal symptoms (EPSs) are most likely attributed to an imbalance in dopamine and acetylcholine. Antipsychotics cause a hypodopaminergic state.

Dystonic reactions
Reactions usually occur within 24–96 hours of initiating or changing the dose. They present as painful, involuntary muscle spasms in skeletal muscles (most commonly in the facial or neck muscles but sometimes in the back, arm, and leg muscles).

Treatment is benztropine (Cogentin) 1–2 mg intramuscular (IM) or diphenhydramine (Benadryl) 25–50 mg IM every 30 minutes until the reaction is relieved. Prophylaxis with oral therapy is usually initiated.

Akathisia
Akathisia usually occurs within a few weeks of initiating antipsychotic therapy. It is described as a subjective feeling of discomfort, usually seen as motor restlessness of the legs (inability to stand still or sit still).

Akathisia may be treated by decreasing the dose; changing the drug; or adding lipophilic β-blockers (e.g., propranolol), benzodiazepines, clonidine, or anticholinergic agents.

Pseudoparkinsonism
Pseudoparkinsonism usually occurs after months or years of therapy. This condition resembles Parkinson's symptoms (e.g., cogwheel rigidity, bradykinesia, tremor, shuffling gait).

It is treated with amantadine (Symmetrel) 100 mg bid or anticholinergics (including benztropine, diphenhydramine, and trihexyphenidyl).

Other adverse effects

Tardive dyskinesia
Tardive dyskinesia (TD) is an irreversible drug-induced movement disorder that occurs after years of antipsychotic therapy. It is caused by long-term suppression of dopamine.

A triad of symptoms characterize TD:

- Choreoathetosis (splayed, writhing fingers)
- Oral or buccal movements (grimacing, bruxism, lip-smacking)
- Protrusion of the tongue

The only treatment is prevention (i.e., use the lowest effective dose of antipsychotic). However, various therapies (vitamin E, lecithin, vitamin B_6) may help alleviate symptoms. Switching to clozapine may be helpful because it has not been reported to cause TD.

Monitor for TD by administering the Abnormal Involuntary Movement Scale (AIMS) to all patients taking antipsychotics.

Neuroleptic malignant syndrome

Neuroleptic malignant syndrome (NMS) has a low incidence and high mortality. It is thought to be due to dopamine blockade. Clinical presentation of NMS is as follows:

- Rapid progression (< 24 hours)
- Body temperature > 100.4°F
- Lead-pipe rigidity
- Hypertension
- Diaphoresis
- Increased heart rate
- Incontinence
- Increased liver function test (LFT), creatinine phosphokinase (CPK), and white blood count (WBC)

Treatment is as follows:

- Transport patient to an emergency room immediately.
- Discontinue antipsychotic medication.
- Administer supportive therapy (cooling blankets, hydration); the dopamine agonist bromocriptine (Parlodel); and the smooth muscle relaxant dantrolene (Dantrium).

Endocrine and metabolic effects

Such effects include amenorrhea, galactorrhea, and gynecomastia caused by hyperprolactinemia.

Dopamine regulates prolactin release. When dopamine is blocked, prolactin is elevated.

Other effects include weight gain and decreased glucose tolerance.

Dermatologic effects
(especially in long-term therapy)

Allergy to medication, photosensitivity, and pigmentation problems may occur.

Hypothalamic effects

Temperature dysregulation (i.e., sensitivity to extreme temperatures) is possible.

Cardiac effects

QT prolongation is possible. Effects are more common with thioridazine (black box warning).

The recommendation is to obtain an electrocardiogram (ECG) for all patients on antipsychotics.

Ophthalmologic effects

Pigmentary retinopathy is associated with daily thioridazine doses > 800 mg. Melanin deposits occur on the cornea and may lead to blindness.

Atypical (newer) antipsychotics

See Table 29-3 for an overview of these drugs.

Table 29-3. Atypical Antipsychotics

Drug	Trade name	Form	Usual dose	Adverse effects	Clinical highlights
Clozapine	Clozaril, FazaClo (disintegrating clozapine tablets)	25, 100 mg tablets	12.5 mg titrated up to 300–900 mg/day	Sedation, weight gain, hypersalivation; black box warning for seizure risk (> 600 mg/day), agranulocytosis, orthostasis, myocarditis, respiratory and cardiac arrest; no EPS or TD	Indicated for refractory schizophrenia only. WBC ≥ 3,500 and ANC ≥ 2,000 to initiate. Monitor weekly for 6 months, biweekly for 6 months, then every 4 weeks if no WBC ≤ 3,500 or ANC ≤ 2,000. If WBC drops to ≤ 3,500 but ≥ 3,000 or ANC > 1,500, monitor twice weekly. If WBC < 3,000, or ANC < 1,500, patient *must* discontinue medication. Black box warning for agranulocytosis, seizures, myocarditis, and other adverse cardiovascular and respiratory effects. Pregnancy category B.

Table 29-3. Atypical Antipsychotics *(Continued)*

Drug	Trade name	Form	Usual dose	Adverse effects	Clinical highlights
Risperidone	Risperdal	0.25, 0.5, 1, 2, 3, 4 mg tablets; 1 mg/mL concentrate	1 mg bid up to 4–6 mg/day; maximum dose 16 mg/day	Dose-related EPS (> 8 mg/day), +/– weight gain, +/– sedation, prolactin elevation, orthostasis	Available in concentrate; do not mix with teas or colas; used commonly in dementia (0.25–1 mg); patient must overlap Consta with oral risperidone for at least 3 weeks.
	Risperdal-M (disintegrating risperidone tablets)	0.5, 1, 2 mg			
	Risperdal Consta (long-acting injection)	25, 37.5, 50 mg			
Olanzapine	Zyprexa	2.5, 5, 7.5, 10, 15, 20 mg tablets	10–20 mg/day; higher doses have been reported	Sedation, orthostasis, weight gain	Olanzapine is also indicated for acute manic episodes of bipolar disorder; Zyprexa Zydis is useful for patients who are unable to swallow or are "cheeking" medications.
	Zyprexa Zydis (disintegrating olanzapine tablets)	5, 10, 15, 20 mg tablets			
	Zyprexa IntraMuscular	10 mg/mL injection	10 mg IM × 1; may repeat in 2 and 4h; maximum IM daily dose 30 mg	Sedation, orthostasis	
	Zyprexa Relprevv (olanzapine extended-release IM injection)	210, 300, 405 mg	Maintenance dose: 150 mg q2wk, 300 mg q2wk, or 405 mg q4wk	PIDSS (black box warning), orthostasis, weight gain, EPS, dry mouth	Patient must be observed for 3 hours in a registered facility after injection (PIDSS).
Quetiapine	Seroquel	25, 100, 200, 300, 400 mg tablets	300–800 mg/day; higher doses have been reported	Sedation, dizziness, headache	Low EPS and prolactin elevation risk; cataract risk: do lens test at baseline and every 6 months. Black box warning for suicidality in children, adolescents, and young adults.
	Seroquel XR (extended-release tablets)	50, 150, 200, 300, 400 mg			
Ziprasidone	Geodon	20, 40, 60, 80 mg capsules; 20 mg/mL injection	40–200 mg/day po; 20 mg IM × 1 dose (may repeat in 4h; maximum IM daily dose 40 mg)	+/– sedation, +/– weight gain, QT prolongation warning in package insert	Use caution with other medications that prolong QT interval.

(continued)

Table 29-3. Atypical Antipsychotics *(Continued)*

Drug	Trade name	Form	Usual dose	Adverse effects	Clinical highlights
Aripiprazole	**Abilify**	2, 5, 10, 15, 20, 30 mg tablets; 1 mg/mL concentrate; 7.5 mg/mL injection	10–30 mg/d po; 5.25–15 mg/d IM; maximum IM daily dose 30 mg	Possible insomnia, +/– weight gain	Once-daily dosing benefit; partial dopamine agonist. Black box warning for suicidality in children, adolescents, and young adults.
	Abilify Discmelt (disintegrating tablets)	10, 15 mg			
Paliperidone	Invega	3, 6, 9 mg extended-release tablets	6 mg/day; maximum dose 12 mg/day	Headache, tachycardia, somnolence, anxiety	Sustained-release tablet: do not crush or chew; tablet shell may be seen in stool.
	Invega Sustenna (paliperidone IM injectable suspension)	39, 78, 117, 156, 234 mg	234 mg day 1, 156 mg 1 wk later, then 117 mg q month; may adjust to 39–234 mg	Akathisia, somnolence, tachycardia, hyperprolactinemia	
Iloperidone	Fanapt	1, 2, 4, 6, 8, 10, 12 mg tablets 4-day titration pack	1 mg bid initial, 6–12 mg bid usual dose, maximum dose 12 mg bid; reduce dose by half with strong CYP450 2C9 and 3A4 inhibitors	Dizziness, nausea, somnolence, EPS, QT prolongation	Titrate dose to avoid significant orthostatic hypotension. If more than 3 days missed, retitrate dose.
Asenapine	Saphris	5, 10 mg sublingual tablets	5 mg bid can increase to 10 mg bid after 1 wk	EPS, insomnia, somnolence, dizziness, numbness of mouth and tongue; serious allergic reactions have been reported	Sublingual only; do not crush, chew, or swallow. Do not eat or drink for 10 minutes after dosing. Use dry hands when handling.
Lurasidone	Latuda	20, 40, 80 mg tablets	40 mg initial dose, usual dose 40–160 mg/day, maximum 80 mg/day in moderate renal/hepatic dx or moderate CYP450 3A4 inhibitors	Somnolence, nausea and vomiting, EPS (dose-related)	Take with food, at least 350 calories. Contraindicated with strong CYP450 3A4 inducers or inhibitors. Pregnancy category B.

Boldface indicates one of top 100 drugs for 2012 by units sold at retail outlets, www.drugs.com/stats/top100/2012/units.
ANC, absolute neutrophil count; PIDSS, post-injection delirium/sedation syndrome.

No universally accepted definition of *atypical* exists, but these drugs generally have the following features:

- Side effects are less severe (little or no EPS, minimal to no prolactin increase, less risk of TD).
- More weight gain, more lipid abnormalities, and a greater risk of diabetes are seen with these drugs.
- A dose-dependent increased risk of ventricular arrhythmias and sudden cardiac death is seen, possibly because of prolongation of the QT interval similar to typical antipsychotics.
- Decreased affinity for the dopamine receptor is present.
- Results from the CATIE (Clinical Antipsychotic Trials in Intervention Effectiveness) showed very high discontinuation rates for all antipsychotics secondary to inefficacy or intolerable side effects. No difference was seen between perphenazine and atypicals (except olanzapine).
- There is a black box warning for increase in mortality with atypical antipsychotics in elderly patients with dementia, and atypical antipsychotics are not approved for the treatment of patients with dementia-related psychosis.

Mechanism of action

These drugs are weak dopamine and dopamine-2 receptor blockers that block serotonin and α-adrenergic, histaminic, and muscarinic receptors in the central nervous system.

Treatment Strategies

Acute schizophrenia

- Decrease danger to self and others.
- Increase dosage of the antipsychotic until behavior improves or side effects limit the dose.
- Haloperidol or fluphenazine (immediate release) 5–10 mg IM and lorazepam 2 mg IM q4h prn may be used for psychosis or agitation. An anticholinergic may also be needed (e.g., benztropine or diphenhydramine for EPSs).
- Olanzapine 10 mg IM may be used and can be repeated in 2 hours and again 4 hours later, for a maximum of 30 mg/day for psychosis or agitation.
- Patients may use ziprasidone 10 mg IM administered every 2 hours or 20 mg IM administered every 4 hours, for a maximum of 40 mg/day for psychosis or agitation.

Maintenance

- Start an atypical antipsychotic at a recommended dose or continue a conventional agent (if it was effective for the patient before hospital admission).
- Positive symptoms will respond first.
- Monitor for side effects, and emphasize compliance.
- Lifelong therapy is usually needed.
- Use lowest effective dose to decrease risk of side effects (e.g., TD).

Recommended monitoring for patients on atypical antipsychotics

- Fasting glucose and lipids and blood pressure at baseline and at 12 weeks
- Weight (body mass index) at baseline, 4 weeks, 8 weeks, and 12 weeks, and then quarterly
- Waist circumference at baseline and then annually

Noncompliance and alternative dosing

Haloperidol decanoate (Haldol-D)

The dosage conversion from po to IM is as follows: po daily dose × 10 = IM dose every 4 weeks. For example, 20 mg daily dose × 10 = 200 mg every 4 weeks.

Steady state is reached in 8–12 weeks.

Fluphenazine decanoate (Prolixin-D)

The dosage conversion from po to IM is as follows: 1 mg po = 1.25 mg IM. For example, 20 mg daily dose × 1.25 mg = 25 mg IM every 2 weeks.

Steady state is reached in approximately 6 weeks.

Depot administration technique

Both medications are suspended in sesame seed oil. They are very viscous. Ensure that the patient has no allergy to sesame seed oil.

Administer in gluteal or deltoid muscle with a 16- or 18-gauge needle.

Risperidone long-acting injection (Risperdal Consta)

Overlap with po medication for 3 weeks.

The recommended dose is 25 mg every 2 weeks. The maximum dose is 50 mg every 2 weeks. Alternate IM administration between buttocks.

Steady state is reached in approximately 8 weeks.

Use the diluent and needle supplied in the pack to reconstitute and administer injection.

29-4. Bipolar Disorder

Bipolar disorder (manic-depressive illness) is a recurrent mood disorder with a lifetime prevalence of 0.8–1.6%. This disorder is associated with significant morbidity and mortality.

Incidence is equal in females and males. Onset is usually between ages 8 and 44. The first episode for females is usually marked by a depressive episode. For males, it is usually marked by a manic episode.

Types and Classifications

- *Bipolar I:* This type is characterized by the occurrence of manic episodes and major depressive episodes.
- *Bipolar II:* This type is characterized by the occurrence of hypomanic episodes and major depressive episodes.
- *Cyclothymia:* This type is defined as numerous episodes of hypomania and depressive episodes that cannot be classified as major depressive episodes. Diagnosis requires that cyclothymia occur for at least a 2-year period.

Clinical Presentation

See DSM-5 for complete diagnostic criteria.

Mania

Mania is characterized by heightened mood (euphoria), flight of ideas, rapid or pressured speech, grandiosity, increased energy, decreased need for sleep, irritability, and impulsivity. Judgment is significantly impaired (e.g., increased risk-taking behavior). Marked impairment also exists in social or occupational functioning.

Psychotic features are usually present. Hospitalization is needed.

Changes in sleeping patterns (especially insomnia) commonly initiate manic episodes.

Drug-induced causes include antidepressants (tricyclic antidepressants, selective serotonin reuptake inhibitors, monoamine oxidase inhibitors); bronchodilators (albuterol, salmeterol); stimulants; xanthines (caffeine, theophylline); dopamine agonists (bromocriptine, amantadine); and sympathomimetics.

Note: The STEP-BD (Systematic Treatment Enhancement Program for Bipolar Disorder) trial showed that antidepressants used in combination with mood stabilizers did not increase the risk of inducing mania in bipolar depression. However, this combination was not associated with increased efficacy.

Hypomania

Hypomania is a less severe form of mania. This disorder usually does not cause marked impairment in social or occupational functioning.

Many patients find this state highly desirable because they experience a great sense of well-being and feel productive, creative, and confident.

Mixed Features

A specifier "with mixed features" may be applied to episodes of mania or hypomania when depressive features are present.

Rapid cycling

In rapid cycling, the patient experiences more than four mood episodes in a year. Mood episodes may occur in any combination.

Rapid cycling primarily occurs in women (70–90%). The prognosis is usually poor.

Etiology

The etiology is unknown; however, the leading hypothesis supports genetic etiology. Other theories include neurotransmitter involvement, circadian rhythm, and kindling hypothesis.

Clinical Course

The mean age of onset is 21 years. The first episode for females is usually depression. For males, it is mania.

Untreated episodes may last from weeks to months. A high mortality rate exists because of suicide. Comorbid substance abuse is very common (60–70%).

Treatment Principles and Goals

Acute

In acute cases, the goal is to control the current episode (i.e., slow down the patient and reduce harm to self and others).

Maintenance

Maintenance goals are as follows:

- Prevent or minimize future episodes.
- Maintain drug therapy, and reduce adverse effects.
- Prevent drug interactions.
- Educate the patient and family about the disorder.

- Provide adequate follow-up services (including substance abuse treatment).
- Maximize the patient's functional status and quality of life.

Drug Therapy

Table 29-4 provides information about mood stabilizers.

Lithium

Indications

Lithium is indicated for acute treatment and prophylaxis of manic episodes associated with bipolar disorders. It is effective for both the manic and the depressive components.

Mechanism of action

The mechanism of action is unknown. Various theories suggest that lithium facilitates γ-aminobutyric acid (GABA) function, alters cation transport across cell membranes in nerve and muscle cells, or influences reuptake of 5-hydroxytryptamine (5-HT) or norepinephrine (NE).

Contraindications

Contraindications include renal disease, severe cardiovascular disease, history of leukemia, first trimester of pregnancy, and hypersensitivity to lithium.

Precautions

Use with caution in patients who have thyroid disease, patients who have sodium depletion, patients who are receiving diuretics, or dehydrated patients.

Monitoring (baseline and follow-up)

- **Thyroid panel:** Lithium may cause hypothyroidism. Test baseline and thyroid-stimulating hormone (TSH) every 6–12 months or as clinically indicated.

Table 29-4. Mood Stabilizers

Drug	Trade name	Form	Usual dose	Adverse effects	Clinical highlights
Lithium	Lithobid, Eskalith CR	150, 300, 600 mg caplets; 300, 450 mg CR tablets; 300 mg SR tablets; syrup, as citrate 300 mg/5 mL (Cibalith-S)	Starting: 900–1,200 mg in divided doses; titrate to desired response or level	Tremor, polydipsia or polyuria, nausea or diarrhea, weight gain, hypothyroidism, mental dulling	Many drug interactions; toxicity is a concern (pregnancy category D); monitor blood levels—acute: 0.6–1.2 mEq/L, maintenance: 0.8–1 mEq/L
Divalproex sodium	Depakote	125, 250, 500 mg DR tablets; 250, 500 mg ER tablets	Starting: 500 mg bid–tid or 15 mg/kg; maximum dose 60 mg/kg/day; ER dosed daily	GI upset, sedation, tremor, weight gain, alopecia, transient elevation in LFTs	Black box warnings: hepatotoxicity, hemorrhagic pancreatitis, teratogenicity (pregnancy category D); monitor blood levels—50–125 mcg/mL (85–125 mcg/mL for mania)
Carbamazepine	Tegretol	200 mg tablets; 100 mg chewable tablets; 100, 200, 400 mg ER tablets; 100 mg/5 mL suspension	Starting: 200 mg bid; increase to 800–1,200 mg/day (tid–qid doses); usual range 400–1,600 mg/day	Ataxia, dizziness, sedation, slurred speech, aplastic anemia	See text for contraindications; many drug interactions (pregnancy category C); monitor blood levels—4–12 mcg/mL
Lamotrigine	Lamictal	25, 100, 150, 200 mg tablets; 2, 5, 25 mg chewable tablets	Starting: 25 mg/day weeks 1 and 2; 50 mg/day weeks 3 and 4; 100 mg/day week 5; 200 mg/day week 6; 200 mg/day usual dose	Dizziness, headache, ataxia, nausea, diplopia, rash	Black box warning: severe rashes such as Stevens–Johnson syndrome; start at 25 mg and titrate to 200 mg over 6 weeks to help prevent rash

- *Serum creatinine (SCr) and blood urea nitrogen (BUN):* Lithium is 100% renally eliminated. Test baseline and every 3 months for patients with renal dysfunction and every 6–12 months otherwise or as clinically indicated.
- *Complete blood count (CBC) with differential:* Lithium may cause leukocytosis and may reactivate leukemia. Test baseline and then as clinically indicated.
- *Electrolytes:* In the event of hyponatremia, lithium toxicity may occur. Test electrolytes every 6–12 months or as clinically indicated.
- *ECG:* Lithium causes flattened or inverted T-waves. This condition is reversible. Test baseline and every 6–12 months or as clinically indicated.
- *Urinalysis:* Lithium may decrease specific gravity. Perform urinalysis every 6–12 months.
- *Pregnancy test:* Lithium may cause cardiovascular defects (e.g., Ebstein's anomaly). Perform pregnancy test every 6–12 months or as clinically indicated.
- *Lithium level:* Lithium reaches steady-state levels in 4–5 days (half-life = ~ 24 hours). Obtain the level in the morning immediately before next dose (acute: 0.6–1.2 mEq/L; maintenance: 0.8–1 mEq/L). Lithium levels should be checked after each dose increase and before the next dose increase. Steady-state levels are reached approximately 5 days after dose adjustment. Periodic monitoring of lithium levels should occur every 6 months or more frequently if clinically indicated.

Drug interactions

Table 29-5 summarizes the drug interactions associated with lithium.

In addition, several toxicity concerns are associated with the drug:

- *Mild toxicity (serum levels 1.5–2 mEq/L):* Gastrointestinal (GI) upset (nausea, vomiting, diarrhea); muscle weakness; fatigue; fine hand tremor; and difficulty with concentration and memory
- *Moderate toxicity (serum levels 2–2.5 mEq/L):* Ataxia, lethargy, nystagmus, worsening confusion, severe GI upset, coarse tremors, and increased deep tendon reflexes
- *Severe toxicity (serum levels > 3 mEq/L):* Severely impaired consciousness, coma, seizures, respiratory complications, and death

Table 29-5. Drug Interactions with Lithium

Increase level of lithium	Decrease level of lithium
Nonsteroidal anti-inflammatory drugs	Theophylline
Angiotensin-converting enzyme inhibitors	Caffeine
Angiotensin receptor blockers	Pregnancy
Fluoxetine	Osmotic diuretics (mannitol and urea)
Metronidazole	
Diuretics (e.g., thiazides)	
Sodium depletion:	
Low sodium diet	
Excessive exercise or sweating	
Vomiting or diarrhea	
Salt deficiency	

Toxicity is treated as follows:

- Discontinue lithium, and initiate gastric lavage.
- Correct electrolyte and fluid imbalances.
- Monitor neurologic changes.
- Give supportive care.
- Give dialysis if indicated.

Patient information

- Routinely monitoring serum lithium levels is important.
- Maintain a steady salt and fluid intake.
- Do not crush or chew extended- or slow-release dosage forms.

Divalproex sodium

Divalproex sodium is indicated for bipolar disorder. It is considered first-line treatment for acute manic episodes. It has unlabeled use for prophylaxis of manic episodes, is effective for rapid cyclers and patients with dysphoric mood, and is helpful in the management of agitation and aggression.

Converting from divalproex sodium delayed release to divalproex sodium extended release is not a 1:1 ratio. When converting from divalproex sodium delayed release to divalproex sodium extended release, the total daily dose must be increased by 8–20% to the nearest available dosage form.

Mechanism of action

Its mechanism of action is unknown, but divalproex sodium is thought to increase GABA or mimic its action at the postsynaptic receptor site.

Contraindications

Contraindications include the following:

- Hepatic dysfunction
- Hypersensitivity to divalproex sodium
- Patients < 2 years old
- Pregnancy

With respect to pregnancy, valproic acid (VPA) may cause neural tube defects. If the benefit outweighs the risk, supplement with 4–5 mg/day of folic acid to decrease risk of fetal damage. Perform pregnancy test every 6–12 months.

Monitoring
VPA
- VPA level reaches steady state in 5 days (half-life = 9–16 hours); 50–125 mcg/mL is optimal.
- Draw level periodically as clinically indicated.

LFT
- Test baseline, every 6–12 months, with dose changes, or as clinically indicated.
- Divalproex sodium is hepatically eliminated; it carries a black box warning for hepatotoxicity.

CBC with differential
- Test baseline, every 6–12 months, with dose changes, or as clinically indicated.
- VPA may cause thrombocytopenia.

Platelet count
- Test at baseline with dose changes, or as clinically indicated.
- Hematologic abnormalities may be seen with serum levels above 100 mcg/mL.

Serum ammonia
- Test at baseline with dose changes, or as clinically indicated.
- Divalproex may cause hyperammonemia.

Drug interactions
- Divalproex sodium is a cytochrome P450 (CYP450) 2C19 enzyme substrate, a CYP450 2C9 and 2D6 inhibitor, and a weak CYP450 3A3/4 inhibitor.
- Interactions occur with carbamazepine, lamotrigine, and phenytoin. Increased sedative effects occur with phenobarbital and benzodiazepines.

Patient information
- Take with food to avoid GI upset.
- Take a multivitamin with selenium and zinc if alopecia (hair loss) occurs.
- It is important to monitor VPA levels routinely.

Carbamazepine

Carbamazepine (CBZ) is considered second-line therapy for acute and prophylactic treatment of bipolar disorder.

Mechanism of action
The mechanism of action is unknown.

Monitoring
Monitor CBC with differential, electrolytes, LFTs, SCr or BUN, and ECG (if the patient is > 40 years old or has a preexisting heart disease).

CBZ is an autoinducer. Monitor levels routinely, especially during first few months of therapy. The optimal level is 4–12 mcg/mL.

Contraindications
Contraindications include history of previous bone marrow depression and hypersensitivity to CBZ.

Drug interactions
- CBZ is a CYP450 2C8 and 3A3/4 enzyme substrate.
- It is a CYP450 1A2, 2C, and 3A3/4 inducer.
- CBZ may induce the metabolism of benzodiazepines, clozapine, corticosteroids, oral contraceptives, VPA, warfarin, phenytoin, and tricyclic antidepressants (plus others).
- Cimetidine, clarithromycin, diltiazem, verapamil, metronidazole, and lamotrigine (plus others) inhibit CBZ.

Lamotrigine (Lamictal)

Lamotrigine is approved for maintenance treatment of bipolar I disorder. Titration of the dose is required to monitor for signs and symptoms of severe and potentially life-threatening skin rashes including Stevens–Johnson syndrome and toxic epidermal necrolysis (Table 29-6). Co-administration with VPA increases the risk.

Drug interactions and effects
- CBZ, phenytoin, oral contraceptives, rifampin, and phenobarbital decrease lamotrigine concentrations.
- VPA increases lamotrigine concentrations.
- Adverse effects include nausea, headache, tremor or anxiety, and sedation.

Other therapies

Atypical antipsychotics
These agents are approved for treatment of bipolar disorder. Olanzapine and fluoxetine (Symbyax) is

Table 29-6. Lamotrigine Dose Titration

Timing	Patients not taking carbamazepine (or other enzyme-inducing drugs) or valproate	Patients taking valproate	Patients taking carbamazepine (or other enzyme-inducing drugs) and not taking valproate
Weeks 1 and 2	25 mg daily	25 mg every other day	50 mg daily
Weeks 3 and 4	50 mg daily	25 mg daily	100 mg daily, in divided doses
Week 5	100 mg daily	50 mg daily	200 mg daily, in divided doses
Week 6	200 mg daily	100 mg daily	300 mg daily, in divided doses
Week 7	200 mg daily	100 mg daily	Up to 400 mg daily, in divided doses

indicated for the treatment of depressive episodes associated with bipolar disorder.

Gabapentin (Neurontin)

This agent may be useful as adjunctive therapy for bipolar disorder. No significant drug interactions exist. No drug serum level monitoring is required.

Gabapentin is renally eliminated. It has mild sedative effects (sedation, ataxia, fatigue).

Oxcarbazepine (Trileptal)

This agent is structurally similar to CBZ (keto-analogue of CBZ). It is sometimes used as a mood stabilizer in patients with bipolar disorder, but further studies are needed.

No autoinduction problems exist, and there are no drug serum levels to monitor. It appears to have fewer drug–drug interactions than CBZ.

Topiramate (Topamax)

This agent may be useful for treatment of bipolar disorder, but further studies are needed. Doses are usually lower than those indicated for treating seizure disorders.

Topiramate may cause weight loss, difficulties with concentration, nephrolithiasis, acute myopia, and secondary angle closure.

Calcium channel blockers

These agents are usually reserved as last-line therapy. Data in the literature are inconsistent about using verapamil for mania (other calcium channel blockers may be effective).

Although these agents are not routinely used, they could possibly be used in pregnancy.

29-5. Major Depression

Major depression is a prevalent and serious illness in the United States. It affects 10 million to 14 million people of all ages.

The condition is treatable but grossly undertreated. Most cases go unrecognized, which may be due to the social stigma surrounding depression. Several myths contribute to the problem of undertreatment (e.g., major depression is caused by personal weakness or an inability to handle life's problems).

Epidemiology

The lifetime prevalence rate is 17%. One in four females (10–24%) is affected. One in 8 males (5–12%) is affected.

Major depression is most common between the ages of 25 and 44.

Risk factors include the following:

- Family history
- Female
- Previous depressive episode
- Previous suicide attempt
- Comorbid medical or substance abuse disorder

Etiology

The etiology is unknown; however, there are many hypotheses, including the following:

- Dysregulation of neurotransmitters
- Decreased concentration of certain neurotransmitters
- Genetic basis for the disorder

- Medications that may induce or worsen depression:
  - Beta-blockers
  - Barbiturates
  - Benzodiazepines
  - Corticosteroids
  - Parkinson's agents
  - Topiramate
  - Varenicline

Clinical Presentation

Physical findings

- Fatigue
- Pain (i.e., headaches, back pain, GI upset)
- Sleep disturbances (usually insomnia)
- Appetite disturbances (usually decreased appetite)
- Psychomotor retardation or agitation

Emotional symptoms

- Anhedonia
- Depressed mood for most of the day
- Hopelessness or helplessness
- Inappropriate feelings of guilt and worthlessness
- Anxiety or worry
- Suicidal ideation

Cognitive symptoms

- Decreased ability to concentrate
- Indecisiveness

Laboratory studies

There are no diagnostic laboratory tests for depression, but the following lab work should be conducted to rule out other illnesses that may manifest as depressive symptoms:

- CBC with differential
- Thyroid function tests
- Urine drug screen

Medical conditions that may contribute to the development or worsening of depression include cancer, cerebrovascular accident, diabetes mellitus, human immunodeficiency virus, multiple sclerosis, myocardial infarction (MI), Parkinson's disease, rheumatoid arthritis, systemic lupus erythematosus, thyroid abnormalities, and vitamin deficiency. Possible drug-induced causes of depression should also be ruled out, including corticosteroids, oral contraceptives, propranolol, clonidine, and methyldopa.

Prognosis

Seventy percent of patients are responsive to antidepressant therapy. Following the first episode, 50–60% of patients will have another episode; following the second episode, 70–80% will have a third; and following the third, 90% will have another.

If untreated, an episode may resolve spontaneously within 6 to 24 months.

Approximately 15% of patients will commit suicide. Risk factors for suicide include being male, older than 50, or unemployed; having recently lost a job or spouse; being socially isolated; having access to a weapon; and experiencing comorbid substance abuse.

Males are more likely to commit suicide, but females are more likely to attempt suicide. Males commonly use more violent means of suicide (e.g., firearms and hanging) than do females (e.g., slashing of wrists and drug overdoses).

DSM-5 Diagnostic Criteria

At least five symptoms (see previous discussion of clinical presentation) must be present mostly every day for a 2-week period and represent a change from previous functioning. At least one of the symptoms must be depressed mood or anhedonia.

Treatment Principles and Goals

Goals are as follows:

- Improve patient's ability to function and quality of life.
- Reduce or eliminate target symptoms with an antidepressant.
- Optimally, incorporate psychotherapy.
- Prevent relapse.

All antidepressants are equally effective in a given population:

- Response varies from person to person.
- Each differs in side effect and drug-interaction profiles.
- None are "speed" or "uppers."

Note: The U.S. Food and Drug Administration (FDA) now requires all antidepressant drugs to include boxed warnings about increased risk of suicidal ideation and behavior in children and adolescents and in young adults (up to age 24), and a medication guide highlighting these risks is to be distributed with each new or refilled prescription for antidepressants in this population.

Basis for choosing an agent

- Past history of a patient's response or a family member's response to certain agents
- Side effect profile and the way it relates to any given patient's situation

Monitoring parameters

In the first week, the following should be noted:

- Decreased anxiety
- Trend toward normalization of appetite and sleep pattern

In the second to third week, the following should be noted:

- Increased energy
- Improved concentration and memory
- Improved somatic symptoms

Note: Risk for suicide increases at this time because the patient has the energy to carry out any ideations.
At 4–6 weeks, the following should be evident:

- Improved mood
- Decreased suicidal ideation
- Increased libido

Duration of therapy

Acute phase
The acute phase is usually 6–12 weeks or the length of time needed to stabilize depressive symptoms.

Maintenance phase
During this phase, maintain therapeutic doses of antidepressant. The duration is usually 1 year; antidepressant may be tapered for a period of time, but monitor for signs of relapse. The goal is to prevent relapse.

Prophylaxis

Chronic antidepressant therapy may be necessary for certain patients experiencing the following:

- A first-degree relative with bipolar disorder or recurrent depression
- Onset of depression before age 20 or after age 60
- Recurrence of depression within 1 year after medication discontinuation
- Severe, sudden, or life-threatening depression

Drug Therapy

Tricyclic antidepressants

Tricyclic antidepressants (TCAs) are described in Table 29-7.

Mechanism of action
TCAs increase the synaptic concentration of 5-HT or NE in the central nervous system (i.e., TCAs inhibit the presynaptic neuronal membrane's reuptake of 5-HT or NE).

Other information about TCAs
- Doses may be titrated to full dose range over 1–3 weeks.
- Many patients are dosed half-strength because of sedative effects; however, for patients with insomnia, the sedating effects may be helpful.
- These agents are deadly in overdose (blocks sinoatrial node in the heart).
- Drug serum levels are not commonly used in guiding therapy, but monitoring may be useful in patients taking amitriptyline, desipramine, imipramine, or nortriptyline.

Adverse effects
Effects include orthostatic hypotension, tachycardia, sedation, anticholinergic effects, arrhythmias (prolonged QT interval), weight gain, and sexual dysfunction.
Tertiary amines (e.g., amitriptyline, imipramine, doxepin, clomipramine) have more intense adverse effects compared to secondary amines (e.g., nortriptyline, desipramine).

Contraindications
Concomitant use of a monoamine oxidase inhibitor (MAOI) within the past 14 days, during pregnancy or lactation, and with narrow-angle glaucoma is contraindicated.

Precautions
Use with caution in patients with cardiac conduction disturbances, seizure disorders, hyperthyroidism, and renal or hepatic impairment. Avoid abrupt withdrawal in patients with prolonged use.

Drug interactions
- Increase in TCA level increases the levels of selective serotonin reuptake inhibitors (SSRIs), cimetidine, diltiazem, verapamil, labetalol,

Table 29-7. Tricyclic Antidepressants

Drug	Trade name	Form	Indications	Initial dose	Dose range
Amitriptyline	Elavil	10, 25, 50, 75, 100, 150 mg tablets; 10 mg/mL injection (pregnancy category D)	Depression, chronic and neuropathic pain, migraine prophylaxis, peripheral neuropathy	50–75 mg/day	75–300 mg
Nortriptyline	Pamelor, Aventyl	10, 25, 50, 75 mg capsules; 10 mg/5 mL injection (pregnancy category D)	Depression, chronic pain	25–50 mg/day	40–200 mg
Imipramine	Tofranil	75, 100, 125, 150 mg pamoate capsule	Depression, childhood enuresis, chronic and neuropathic pain	50–75 mg/day	75–300 mg
	Tofranil-PM	10, 25, 50 mg tablets; 12.5 mg/mL injection (pregnancy category D)			
Doxepin	Sinequan	10, 25, 50, 75, 100, 150 mg capsules; 10 mg/mL concentrate; 5% cream (pregnancy category C)	Depression; anxiety; unlabeled: chronic and neuropathic pain	75 mg/day (in divided doses)	75–300 mg
Clomipramine	Anafranil	25, 50, 75 mg (pregnancy category C)	Obsessive-compulsive disorder, depression, panic attacks, chronic pain	25–100 mg daily, titrated up for 1–2 weeks	Usual effective dose 200–250 mg/day; maximum dose 250 mg because of dose-related increased risk of seizure
Desipramine	Norpramin	10, 25, 50, 75, 100, 150 mg tablets (pregnancy category C)	Depression; chronic pain; unlabeled: peripheral neuropathy	50–75 mg/day	75–300 mg

propoxyphene, quinidine, haloperidol, and methylphenidate.

- Decrease in TCA level affects CBZ, phenytoin, and barbiturate metabolism.
- Administration with MAOIs may cause serotonin syndrome.
- Monitoring of blood pressure, pulse, ECG changes, and mental status changes is prudent; drug serum monitoring may be useful for amitriptyline, desipramine, imipramine, and nortriptyline.

Monoamine oxidase inhibitors

Table 29-8 summarizes information about MAOIs.

Mechanism of action
MAOIs increase the synaptic concentration of NE, 5-HT, and dopamine (DA) by inhibiting the breakdown enzyme—monoamine oxidase.

Note: MAOIs may be useful for patients who do not respond to other antidepressants or for treatment

Table 29-8. Monoamine Oxidase Inhibitors

Drug	Trade name	Form	Initial dose	Dose titration	Dose range
Phenelzine	Nardil	15 mg tablets	15 mg tid (> 16 years old)	Increase by 15 mg/wk	60–90 mg/day
Tranylcypromine	Parnate	10 mg tablets	30 mg/day in divided doses	Increase by 10 mg/day every 1–3 weeks	30–60 mg/day

of atypical depression; however, they are rarely used because of the need for dietary restrictions, their side effect profile, and their potentially dangerous interactions with other medications.

Adverse effects

Effects include orthostatic hypotension, weight gain, sexual dysfunction, anticholinergic effects, and hypertensive crisis.

Contraindications

Be alert for renal or hepatic dysfunction, cardiovascular disease, and concomitant sympathomimetic therapy (e.g., pseudoephedrine, ephedra).

When a patient is switched from MAOIs to SSRIs, the MAOI must be discontinued 2 weeks prior to initiation of an SSRI to prevent serotonin syndrome. When a patient is switched from SSRIs to MAOIs, the SSRI must be discontinued 2 weeks prior to initiation of MAOI, with the exception of fluoxetine, which requires 5 weeks because of its long half-life.

Precautions

Be aware of drug–food interaction with tyramine-containing foods (e.g., red wine, aged cheeses, marmite).

Drug interactions

- TCAs
- SSRIs
- Sympathomimetics
- Meperidine

Selective serotonin reuptake inhibitors

See Table 29-9 for information about SSRIs.

Mechanism of action

These agents selectively inhibit the reuptake of 5-HT.

All SSRIs should be tapered upon discontinuation of treatment (over 2–4 weeks), except fluoxetine. Side effects with abrupt withdrawal include flu-like symptoms, dizziness, nausea, tremor, anxiety, and palpitations.

Adverse effects

Effects include GI complaints, nervousness, insomnia, headache, fatigue, and sexual dysfunction, but SSRIs are safer in overdose than TCAs.

Drug interactions

Drug interactions exist with TCAs and MAOIs and among SSRIs. Interactions are variable depending on the SSRI. Reportedly there are fewer drug interactions with escitalopram and citalopram.

Serotonin–norepinephrine reuptake inhibitors

See Table 29-10 for information about serotonin–norepinephrine reuptake inhibitors (SNRIs).

Venlafaxine (Effexor, Effexor XR)
Mechanism of action

This agent inhibits the reuptake of 5-HT and NE (and also DA at higher doses). It is frequently referred to as an SNRI. Anticholinergic and antihistaminic effects are negligible. As the dose increases, NE and DA reuptake are more pronounced.

Adverse effects

Effects include GI upset, anxiety, insomnia, and headache. Elevation in blood pressure is possible; use with caution in patients with uncontrolled hypertension. An extended-release formulation is available to minimize GI upset. Other side effects are similar to those of SSRIs. Withdrawal symptoms may occur if the medication is abruptly discontinued.

Drug interactions

Cimetidine inhibits venlafaxine metabolism. Cyproheptadine induces venlafaxine metabolism. Serotonin syndrome is seen in combination with sibutramine, sumatriptan, tramadol, and trazodone. PT/INR (prothrombin time per international normalized ratio) elevations have been seen when venlafaxine is added to patients taking warfarin.

Other aspects

Venlafaxine is indicated for both generalized anxiety disorder and major depression. It is not recommended in patients with uncontrolled hypertension or recent MI or cerebrovascular disorders.

Desvenlafaxine (Pristiq)
Mechanism of action

The mechanism of action of desvenlafaxine is similar to that of venlafaxine.

Adverse effects

Common effects include GI upset, increased serum cholesterol and triglycerides, xerostomia, sleep disturbances, and erectile dysfunction. Serious effects include hypertension, hyponatremia, and abnormal bleeding.

Withdrawal symptoms may occur if the drug is abruptly discontinued.

Table 29-9. Selective Serotonin Reuptake Inhibitors

Drug	Trade name	Form	Initial dose	Usual dose	Clinical highlights
Citalopram	Celexa	10, 20, 40 mg tablets; 10 mg/5 mL syrup	10 mg	20–40 mg/day; maximum dose 40 mg/day; > 40 mg/day may cause QT prolongation. FDA issued revised recommendations for Celexa with maximum recommended dose of 20 mg for patients > 60 years old.	Used in geriatric patients; fewer drug interactions
Escitalopram	**Lexapro**	5, 10, 20 mg tablets	10 mg	10–20 mg/day	S-isomer of citalopram; 40 mg Celexa = 10 mg Lexapro
Fluvoxamine	Luvox, Luvox CR	50, 100 mg tablets; 100, 150 mg tablets	50 mg	100–300 mg/day	Available in generic; primarily used for obsessive-compulsive disorder; associated with greater amount of drug interactions relative to other SSRIs
Paroxetine	Paxil	10, 20, 30, 40 mg tablets; 10 mg/5 mL suspension	10–20 mg	10–40 mg; maximum dose 50 mg/day	Least-activating SSRI
	Paxil CR	12.5, 25, 37.5 mg tablets	12.5–25 mg	25–37.5 mg	CR formulation associated with fewer side effects; 10 mg Paxil = 12.5 mg Paxil CR
Fluoxetine	Prozac, Sarafem	10, 20, 40 mg capsules; 10, 20 mg tablets; 20 mg/5 mL syrup; 90 mg capsules	10–20 mg	20–80 mg/day	Longer half-life, so tapering unnecessary; 90 mg formulation given once weekly
Sertraline	Zoloft	25, 50, 100 mg tablets; 20 mg/mL concentrate	25–50 mg	50–100 mg/day; maximum dose 200 mg/day	Used in geriatric patients; fewer drug interactions

Boldface indicates one of top 100 drugs for 2012 by units sold at retail outlets, www.drugs.com/stats/top100/2012/units.

Drug interactions

The primary metabolic pathway is conjugation; therefore, desvenlafaxine has fewer drug interactions than venlafaxine.

Serotonin syndrome is seen in combination with MAOIs, SSRIs, sibutramine, tramadol, triptans, and linezolid.

Use in combination with unfractionated heparin, glycoprotein IIb or IIIa receptor inhibitors, warfarin, and nonsteroidal anti-inflammatory drugs may increase the risk of bleeding.

Duloxetine (Cymbalta)

Mechanism of action

The mechanism of action of duloxetine is similar to that of venlafaxine. It is a potent inhibitor of 5-HT and NE, and it has no significant affinity for dopaminergic, adrenergic, cholinergic, or histaminergic receptors.

Adverse effects

Effects include GI upset, dry mouth, dizziness, decreased appetite, elevation in blood pressure, and other side effects similar to those of SSRIs. Urinary

Table 29-10. Serotonin–Norepinephrine Reuptake Inhibitors

Drug	Trade name	Form	Initial dose	Maximum dose	Clinical highlights
Venlafaxine	Effexor	25, 37.5, 50, 75, 100 mg capsules	37.5 mg bid	375 mg/day in divided doses	Take with food; monitor blood pressure.
	Effexor XR	37.5, 75, 150, 225 mg capsules	75 mg/day	225 mg/day	Less GI upset than immediate-release formulation; monitor blood pressure.
Desvenlafaxine	Pristiq	50, 100 mg extended-release tablets	50 mg/day	50 mg/day; CrCl < 30 mL/min every other day	Fewer drug interactions due to conjugation; monitor blood pressure.
Duloxetine	**Cymbalta**	20, 30, 60 mg capsules	30 mg/day	120 mg/day	Also used for diabetic peripheral neuropathy; monitor blood pressure.

Boldface indicates one of top 100 drugs for 2012 by units sold at retail outlets, www.drugs.com/stats/top100/2012/units.
CrCl, creatinine clearance.

hesitation may occur. The patient may have withdrawal symptoms with abrupt discontinuation.

Drug interactions

CYP1A2 inhibitors (e.g., cimetidine, quinolone antibiotics) and CYP2D6 inhibitors (e.g., fluoxetine, quinidine) increase duloxetine levels. The combination of duloxetine with triptans and serotonergic drugs may cause serotonin syndrome.

Other aspects

Duloxetine is indicated for both major depression (20 or 30 mg bid or 60 mg daily) and diabetic peripheral neuropathic pain (60 mg daily). It is metabolized by CYP450 1A2 and 2D6; these inhibitors may increase plasma levels of duloxetine, causing increased side effects. Duloxetine is contraindicated in uncontrolled narrow-angle glaucoma.

Levomilnacipran (Fetzima)
Mechanism of action

The mechanism of action of levomilnacipran is similar to that of venlafaxine. Levomilnacipran is a potent inhibitor of 5-HT and NE.

Adverse effects

Effects include nausea, vomiting, constipation, increased heart rate, diaphoresis, and sexual effects.

Other aspects

Levomilnacipran is indicated for depression whereas milnacipran is indicated for fibromyalgia.

Other classes of antidepressant medication

Bupropion (Wellbutrin, Wellbutrin SR, Wellbutrin XL, and Zyban)
Mechanism of action

Bupropion, an inhibitor of NE and DA reuptake (effects on 5-HT reuptake are minimal), is a norepinephrine–dopamine reuptake inhibitor (NDRI).

Adverse effects

Effects include GI upset, insomnia, anxiety, headache, and psychosis (rare). Bupropion is less associated with sexual dysfunction than are SSRIs and other classes. It also decreases the seizure threshold.

Drug interactions

Cimetidine and ritonavir inhibit bupropion metabolism, and CBZ induces bupropion metabolism.

Other aspects

There is an increased risk of seizure with bupropion, especially in patients with a seizure disorder, eating disorder, or electrolyte imbalance. The maximum daily dose is 450 mg (400 mg SR). Titrate the dose slowly to minimize seizure risk. Bupropion is marketed as Zyban for smoking cessation.

Trazodone (Desyrel) and trazodone extended release (Oleptro)
Mechanism of action

This agent inhibits 5-HT reuptake and blocks $5-HT_{2A}$ receptors.

Adverse effects

Effects include extreme sedation, orthostatic hypotension, and priapism. There are no anticholinergic or cardiotoxic effects.

Drug interactions

Fluoxetine and ritonavir inhibit trazodone metabolism.

Other aspects

Because it causes excessive sedation, immediate-release trazodone is not clinically used as an antidepressant; rather, it is commonly used to treat insomnia (usually dosed 25–150 mg at bedtime). Extended-release trazodone is dosed 150–375 mg daily at bedtime on an empty stomach.

Nefazodone (Serzone)

Mechanism of action

This agent inhibits 5-HT and NE uptake and blocks 5-HT$_{2A}$ receptors.

Adverse effects

Effects include GI upset, sedation, dry mouth, constipation, and lightheadedness. Nefazodone is associated with minimal sexual dysfunction and orthostatic hypotension.

Drug interactions

Nefazodone is a potent inhibitor of CYP450 3A4 isoenzyme; use with caution with drugs metabolized through this enzyme (e.g., buspirone, 3-hydroxy-3-methyl-glutaryl-coenzyme A reductase inhibitors, alprazolam, triazolam, digoxin). Ritonavir inhibits nefazodone metabolism.

Other aspects

Nefazodone is usually dosed bid because of its short half-life. There is a black box warning for hepatotoxicity.

Vilazodone (Viibryd)

Mechanism of action

Vilazodone is an SSRI and 5-HT$_{1A}$ partial agonist.

Adverse effects

Effects include diarrhea, nausea and vomiting, insomnia, and decreased libido (less relative to SSRIs and SNRIs).

Other aspects

Patient starter kit is used for dosing.

Mirtazapine (Remeron and Remeron Soltab)

Mirtazapine is available in 7.5, 15, 30, and 45 mg tablets.

Mechanism of action

This agent antagonizes presynaptic α_2 autoreceptors and heteroreceptors that prevent the release of 5-HT and NE (resulting in increased 5-HT and NE in the synapses). It antagonizes 5-HT$_{2A}$ and 5-HT$_3$ receptors, thereby resulting in less GI upset and less anxiety.

Adverse effects

Effects include sedation, increased appetite, weight gain, and constipation. Elevation in LFTs and increase in triglycerides may occur. There is also a small risk of agranulocytosis or neutropenia.

Other aspects

Mirtazapine may be useful in geriatric patients because it increases appetite, is sedating, and has no significant drug interactions.

Vortioxetine (Brintellix)

Mechanism of Action

Vortioxetine inhibits reuptake of serotonin (5-HT); antagonizes 5-HT$_3$, 5-HT$_{1D}$, and 5-HT$_7$ receptors; agonizes 5-HT$_{1A}$ receptors; and is a 5-HT$_{1B}$ receptor partial agonist.

Adverse Effects

Effects include nausea, vomiting, and constipation.

Other aspects

To avoid adverse events, taper dose to 10 mg for 1 week prior to discontinuation.

Aripiprazole (Abilify), quetiapine (Seroquel), and olanzapine/fluoxetine (Symbyax)

Aripiprazole and quetiapine are approved for adjunct treatment of major depressive disorders. Olanzapine/fluoxetine is approved for treatment-resistant depression. Antipsychotic doses for the augmentation of antidepressant therapy are generally lower than doses used in the treatment of schizophrenia.

Adverse effects

See Section 29-3 on schizophrenia.

Selegiline (Emsam)

Selegiline is available in 6, 9, and 12 mg/24 hour patches.

Mechanism of action

This agent's mechanism of action is not fully understood; however, it is believed to be linked to selegiline's irreversible inhibition of monoamine oxidase.

Adverse effects

Effects include headache, insomnia, application-site reaction, diarrhea, and dry mouth.

Other aspects

There are no dietary restrictions for the 6 mg dose.

Psychostimulants

Methylphenidate has been used to treat depression (especially in the geriatric population) and has been shown to increase activity level as well as improve mood symptoms. It may cause GI upset, insomnia, and cardiovascular effects. It should be used with caution in anxious or psychotic patients. It inhibits TCA metabolism.

Nonpharmacologic Treatments

Psychotherapy

Psychotherapy is especially useful when combined with drug therapy.

Electroconvulsive therapy

Electroconvulsive therapy (ECT) is very safe and effective for treating depression. It is believed to physically "reset" receptors in the brain. ECT is usually reserved for refractory or psychotic patients.

Procedure

The patient is anesthetized and paralyzed in an outpatient setting. The patient is monitored through an electroencephalogram (EEG) during the procedure, and a seizure is induced for 30–90 seconds.

Acute and maintenance treatment

The procedure is administered every other day for 6–9 treatments. Maintenance treatment is variable for each patient, but ECT is usually administered monthly after acute treatment.

Adverse effects

Effects include short-term memory loss and confusion on the day of treatment.

Relative contraindications

ECT increases intracranial pressure and, therefore, is not recommended in patients with recent MI, intracerebral hemorrhage, or cerebral lesions.

29-6. Anxiety Disorders

Anxiety disorders are serious, debilitating mental illnesses that include a group of conditions that share extreme anxiety as the primary mood disturbance.

Epidemiology

Anxiety disorders affect approximately 19 million adults in the United States. There are no racial or cultural differences, and gender differences depend on the specific anxiety disorder.

There is significant comorbidity with other psychiatric illnesses (e.g., substance abuse).

Types and Classifications

Generalized anxiety disorder

Generalized anxiety disorder (GAD) is characterized by unprovoked excessive worry and tension. Anxiety usually consumes the patient's day, thereby affecting social and occupational functioning. Physical complaints (e.g., GI upset, headache, muscle tension, tremors, insomnia, fatigue) are common. Incidence of GAD is higher in females than in males.

Panic disorder

Panic disorder (PD) is characterized by feelings of terror that suddenly strike without warning and usually last for approximately 10–15 minutes.

Physical symptoms include increased heart rate, sweating, tremors, shortness of breath, chest pain, and dizziness. The patient feels as if death is imminent.

Obsessive-compulsive disorder

Obsessive-compulsive disorder (OCD) is characterized by intrusive, recurrent, and repetitive thoughts that severely interfere with the patient's social and occupational functioning (e.g., preoccupation with contamination, order, counting, cleanliness, safety).

Compulsions (e.g., repetitive washing of hands and checking and rechecking) are acts that must be performed in an attempt to decrease the anxiety felt about the obsessions. Prevalence of OCD is equal in males and females.

Social anxiety disorder

Social anxiety disorder is characterized by feelings of anxiety in social situations (e.g., speaking in front of others, attending social gatherings). Patients feel as though everyone is staring at and judging them. People affected by social anxiety disorder usually do not seek treatment and will, instead, self-medicate with alcohol. There is equal male and female prevalence.

Simple or specific phobias

Simple phobias are defined as specific fears (e.g., heights, dogs, mice, spiders, needles) that cause an extreme anxiety response. Affected persons usually do not seek treatment and will, instead, avoid situations that involve the phobia.

Exposure therapy to the perceived threat is common therapy. Incidence in females is greater than in males.

Post-traumatic stress disorder

Post-traumatic stress disorder (PTSD) is characterized by severe anxiety that is caused by an event outside of normal human experience (e.g., war, rape, natural disasters). Symptoms include vividly reliving the event to the extent that anxiety symptoms (i.e., flashbacks, nightmares or night terrors, extreme mood changes, feelings of fright) commonly occur. PTSD is often associated with strong guilt feelings, impaired relationships, social withdrawal, and personality changes. There is a greater prevalence in females than in males.

Anxiety due to a medical disorder

Anxiety is likely to be related to evidence of a medical condition (e.g., congestive heart failure, hyperthyroidism, chronic obstructive pulmonary disease).

Substance-induced anxiety disorder

Anxiety symptoms are likely to be a direct result of use of an agent (e.g., amphetamines, toxin, medication). Symptoms may also occur with intoxication or withdrawal.

Associated features
High comorbidity exists with other psychiatric illnesses, especially depression. High comorbidity also exists with alcohol or substance abuse.

This disorder is associated with chronic medical illnesses (e.g., chronic pain syndromes, long-term illnesses, GI distress, headaches).

Etiology
This disorder's etiology is presently unknown. Most current evidence suggests the cause is primarily biologic (imbalance of GABA, 5-HT, and NE) with genetic predisposition.

Drug Therapy

Benzodiazepines

Benzodiazepines (BZDs), the most commonly used anxiolytics, are described in Table 29-11.

Mechanism of action
BZDs potentiate the actions of GABA by increasing the influx of chloride ions into neurons. It is hypothesized that, through their effects on neurons mediated

Table 29-11. Benzodiazepines

Drug	Trade name	Time to peak plasma concentration (h)	Half-life (h)	Usual daily dose (mg/day)	Metabolic pathway
Alprazolam	Xanax, Niravam	1–2	12–15	0.5–4	Oxidation
Chlordiazepoxide	Librium	2–4	5–30	5–200	Oxidation
Clonazepam	Klonopin	1–2	18–50	1–3	Nitro reduction
Clorazepate	Tranxene	1–2	Not significant	15–60	Oxidation
Diazepam	Valium	0.5–2	20–80	2–40	Oxidation
Estazolam	ProSom	2	10–24	0.5–2	Oxidation
Flurazepam	Dalmane	0.5–2	Not significant	15–30	Oxidation
Halazepam	Paxipam	1–3	7–14	80–160	Oxidation
Lorazepam	Ativan	1–6	10–20	2–6	Conjugation
Oxazepam	Serax	2–4	5–20	30–120	Conjugation
Prazepam	Centrax	6	1.2	20–60	Oxidation
Quazepam	Doral	2	25–41	7.5–30	Oxidation
Temazepam	Restoril	2–3	10–40	15–30	Conjugation
Triazolam	Halcion	1	1.5–5	0.125–0.5	Oxidation

by receptor complexes, BZDs reduce neuronal firing and, thus, the symptoms of anxiety.

Note: The rate of absorption varies with BZDs. The more lipophilic compounds (i.e., alprazolam, diazepam, clorazepate, flurazepam) are rapidly absorbed and result in quicker onset of action. The less lipophilic BZDs are chlordiazepoxide, clonazepam, and lorazepam.

Adverse effects
Effects include sedation, dizziness, confusion, blurred vision, diplopia, syncope, residual daytime sedation, and reduced psychomotor and cognitive dysfunction.

Metabolism
Lorazepam, oxazepam, and temazepam (LOT) are conjugated and are preferred in patients with hepatic dysfunction and elderly patients.

Drug interactions
BZDs metabolized by CYP450 3A4 (e.g., alprazolam, diazepam, triazolam) have decreased clearance if taken concomitantly with CYP450 3A4 inhibitors (e.g., ketoconazole, erythromycin, nefazodone). BZDs are deadly in overdose if taken concomitantly with alcohol.

Clinical highlights
- BZDs may cause a paradoxical reaction in children, cognitively impaired elderly patients, mentally retarded patients, and post–head injury patients.
- Never abruptly discontinue BZDs because doing so may precipitate status epilepticus. Always taper the dose to avoid seizure risk and withdrawal symptoms.
- In elderly patients, the BZDs of choice are those that are conjugated (LOT). There is an increased risk of falls in this population.
- It is best to avoid use of BZDs in pregnancy (especially first trimester) because of risk of cleft palate. BZDs are also present in breast milk and should be avoided in nursing females.
- The abuse potential is great; BZDs are not recommended for patients with substance abuse issues.
- Tolerance is common, and increased doses are needed to control anxiety levels.
- Chlordiazepoxide and diazepam are also used for alcohol withdrawal treatment.
- Alprazolam extended release (Xanax XR) is dosed once daily; do not crush, chew, or break doses. It is also available as an orally disintegrating tablet (Niravam).

Buspirone (BuSpar)

Mechanism of action
The mechanism of action is poorly understood; 5-HT_{1A} is a partial agonist, and buspirone reportedly stimulates presynaptic 5-HT_{1A} receptors. In addition, the agent has a moderate affinity for D_2 receptors.

Buspirone does not interact with the BZD-GABA receptor complex.

Onset of anxiolytic effect is longer for buspirone than for BZD (2–3 weeks).

Adverse effects
Effects include GI upset, headache, and nervousness.

Benefits
Possible benefits over BZDs include the following:

- Usually less sedating than BZDs
- Little to no psychomotor or cognitive impairment
- No association with withdrawal symptoms, abuse, or physical dependence
- Not cross-tolerant with BZDs or alcohol

Antidepressants as treatment for anxiety disorders

TCAs are usually a third-line treatment because of side effects and the danger of overdose. Clomipramine is effective for OCD.

MAOIs are usually a third-line treatment because of side effects and drug–food interactions.

SSRIs and SNRIs are a first-line treatment for many anxiety disorders, especially in patients with comorbid depression and substance abuse problems.

Titrate doses of antidepressants slowly to decrease risk of initial anxiety symptoms. Ultimately, higher doses are commonly used for anxiety disorders.

Other classes of drugs used to treat anxiety disorders

β-blockers (e.g., propranolol, atenolol) ease peripheral symptoms of anxiety and may be useful for panic disorders, social anxiety disorder, and performance anxiety.

Hydroxyzine reduces anxiety and is often used in patients with substance abuse issues.

Nonpharmacologic Treatment

- Supportive psychotherapy (individual, group, family)
- Cognitive behavioral therapy
- Focus on coping with the fear of the symptoms of anxiety

- Relaxation techniques
- Exercise and lifestyle modifications (reduced caffeine and simple sugars)

29-7. Eating Disorders

Anorexia Nervosa

Characteristics

Patients suffering from anorexia nervosa refuse to maintain body weight at or above a minimal, normal weight for their age and height (85% or less of expected body weight). They experience intense fear of gaining weight or becoming fat, although they are underweight. There is a disturbance in self-perception of body weight, size, proportion, and attractiveness.

Types

- Restricting
- Binge eating and purging

Bulimia Nervosa

Characteristics

Recurrent episodes of binge eating occur (often followed by intense feelings of guilt). The patient may consume as much as 5,000–20,000 calories over 2–8 hours. Recurrent and inappropriate compensatory behavior occurs to prevent weight gain.

A person binge eats at least once weekly for 3 months. Self-evaluation is primarily influenced by body shape and weight.

Types

- Purging (vomiting, abuse of laxatives or diuretics)
- Nonpurging (excessive exercise, fasting)

Prevalence

Eating disorders are most commonly seen in Caucasian, middle- to upper-class females.

The age of onset for anorexia nervosa is 13–20 years old. The male-to-female ratio is 1:10–20. For bulimia nervosa, the age of onset is 16–18 years old, and the male-to-female ratio is 1:10.

Medical Complications and Signs of Disease

- Eating disorders produce states of semistarvation and noticeable malnutrition, especially in anorexia.

- In bulimia, patients are more difficult to identify because they are commonly of normal body weight.
- Dehydration occurs.
- There is a high incidence of comorbid anxiety, depression, OCD, and substance abuse.
- Dental caries and enamel erosion occur because of stomach acid exposure.
- Calluses on the dorsum of the hand or fingers develop because of induction of vomiting.
- Mortality rate is about 10% from starvation (primarily because of electrolyte imbalances), arrhythmia, or suicide.
- Long-term complications include endocrine or metabolic, cardiovascular, renal, gastroenterologic, hematologic, pulmonary, musculoskeletal, immunologic, and dermatologic issues.

Treatment

Psychotherapy is the mainstay of treatment. Therapy can be individual, group, family, supportive, cognitive behavioral, or insight oriented. Primary objectives are to define and examine the extent of the problem. The patient learns to accept the condition, and treatment results in a reconstruction of self-identity and self-confidence.

Dietary intake is slowly normalized with the goal of restoring normal body weight. Nutritional counseling is used. Distorted ideas about caloric intake and body shape are corrected.

Relapse prevention focuses on developing and using coping mechanisms and avoiding high-risk situations.

Drug Therapy

SSRIs are primarily used and may be more effective for patients with bulimia. Antidepressants do not appear to be beneficial in helping severely malnourished anorexia nervosa patients gain weight, but they may help patients maintain weight after it has been gained. SSRIs may decrease binge–purge behavior, anxiety, obsessions, impulsivity, and depression symptoms. Low doses of olanzapine and quetiapine may improve weight gain and psychological symptoms in anorexia nervosa. Low-dose, short-acting benzodiazepines have been shown to be beneficial in patients with severe anxiety associated with eating.

Fluoxetine (Prozac) is the only FDA-indicated medication for the treatment of bulimia nervosa. Higher doses are used; titrate to 60 mg/day every morning. Bupropion is contraindicated in bulimia nervosa because of seizure risk.

Topiramate (Topamax) and zonisamide (Zonegran) may be beneficial in binge-eating disorder and bulimia nervosa.

Ideally, treatment of eating disorders includes both psychotherapy and pharmacotherapy.

29-8. Questions

1. S. J. is a 30-year-old Caucasian female with a 10-year history of schizophrenia. Her current therapy includes haloperidol 10 mg po bid. The psychiatrist wants to convert her to haloperidol decanoate. What would be the appropriate equivalent monthly dose of haloperidol decanoate?

    A. 100 mg
    B. 10 mg
    C. 500 mg
    D. 200 mg
    E. 12.5 mg

2. B. T. reports to the nursing station with his head pulled sharply to the side and rear. He complains of severe pain in his neck and back area. The most appropriate diagnosis and treatment would be which of the following?

    A. Akathisia; propranolol 20 mg IM until resolution
    B. Dystonic reaction; diphenhydramine 50 mg IM every 30 minutes until resolution
    C. Tardive dyskinesia; physical therapy
    D. Dystonic reaction; lorazepam 2 mg IM every 30 minutes until resolution
    E. None of the above

3. A 30-year-old schizophrenic patient was receiving risperidone 3 mg bid for 12 weeks with very little response. She is currently taking quetiapine 400 mg bid for 12 weeks with little to no response. Which recommendation is the best for this patient?

    A. Increase quetiapine dose to 600 mg bid.
    B. Switch the patient to clozapine.
    C. Add risperidone 3 mg bid to quetiapine.
    D. Add fluoxetine and ECT.
    E. Continue current therapy.

4. A 48-year-old African American male arrives at the emergency department seeking his "nerve pill." He has a 27-year history of schizophrenia with multiple hospitalizations. In recent years, he has been effectively maintained on fluphenazine 10 mg po bid. He now states that he feels "really bad today." His arms and jaws are stiff, his temperature is 101°F, his blood pressure is 176/110, and his WBC is 19,000. LFTs and CPK are ordered stat. While you await the test results, you should do which of the following?

    A. Discontinue oral fluphenazine, and begin quetiapine.
    B. Discontinue oral fluphenazine.
    C. Continue oral fluphenazine, and add bromocriptine.
    D. Discontinue oral fluphenazine, and give fluphenazine decanoate 25 mg IM stat.
    E. Do nothing; labs need to be evaluated first.

Use the following case study to answer Questions 5 and 6.

A 25-year-old Caucasian male has been increasingly disruptive at home. He has been claiming that he is the president of the United States and has been staying awake all night planning bills for Congress. He has been argumentative and threatening with his friends and family. Though he appears extremely tired physically, he is constantly active.

5. The psychiatrist has decided to initiate Eskalith CR 450 mg bid in this patient. Which of the following lab tests will need to be performed for this patient before starting this drug therapy regimen?

    A. Pregnancy test
    B. LFT
    C. SCr
    D. Fasting glucose
    E. UDS

6. As the pharmacist on the treatment team, you alert the patient's family to which of the following as a common side effect of lithium:

    A. polyuria.
    B. weight loss.
    C. elevated hepatic enzymes.
    D. akathisia.
    E. euphoria.

7. Which of the following statements is (are) correct regarding the treatment of bipolar disorder?

   A. Lithium and divalproex sodium are considered first-line therapy options for mood stabilization.
   B. When treating a patient with lithium, one must monitor the WBC and ANC because of lithium's propensity to cause agranulocytosis.
   C. Patients diagnosed with bipolar I disorder exhibit intermittent cycles of mania and major depression.
   D. A and C
   E. None of the above

8. Which of the following therapies has (have) been used for the treatment of bipolar disorder?

   A. Olanzapine
   B. Topiramate
   C. Calcium channel blockers
   D. All of the above
   E. None of the above

9. Insomnia, GI upset, and headache are common side effects of which of the following antidepressants?

   A. Phenelzine
   B. Amitriptyline
   C. Fluoxetine
   D. Trazodone
   E. Both B and C

10. A 29-year-old depressed African American female has shown little improvement with fluoxetine treatment, so the psychiatrist decides to change her medication to tranylcypromine. What is your recommendation for the switch?

    A. Gradually decrease fluoxetine dosage over a 4-week period, and then start tranylcypromine.
    B. Wait 2 weeks after stopping fluoxetine, and then begin tranylcypromine.
    C. Over 6 weeks, gradually decrease fluoxetine dosage as you gradually increase the tranylcypromine dosage.
    D. Wait 5 weeks after stopping fluoxetine before initiating tranylcypromine.

    E. Maintain fluoxetine dosage, and start tranylcypromine; stop the fluoxetine when the tranylcypromine has achieved a therapeutic level.

11. Which of the following has been shown to induce or worsen depression?

    A. Oral contraceptives
    B. Amoxicillin
    C. Thiamine
    D. Methylphenidate
    E. Phenelzine

Use the following case study to answer Questions 12 and 13.

K. Y. is a 36-year-old female admitted to your mental health facility for the fifth time in the past 3 years for major depressive disorder. She presents with lack of appetite, avolition, anhedonia, and suicidal ideations with a plan. Vitals include BP 127/76, P 82, R 18, T 98.6°F. Labs include TSH 4, FBG 135, (−) UDS, and BAL 0. Her current medications are fluoxetine 40 mg daily, metformin 1,000 mg bid, and hydroxyzine 25 mg tid. K. Y. states compliance and denies side effects. Past medications include citalopram and venlafaxine.

12. What is the most likely indication for the use of hydroxyzine in this patient?

    A. Pruritus
    B. Anxiety
    C. Hypertension
    D. Appetite enhancement
    E. Diabetes

13. The psychiatrist asks for your recommendation for this patient with refractory depression. What is the best option?

    A. Discontinue fluoxetine, and initiate Pristiq.
    B. Discontinue fluoxetine, wait 2 weeks, and start Selegiline.
    C. Add Abilify to current regimen.
    D. Discontinue fluoxetine, and start Lexapro.
    E. Add Serax to current regimen.

14. Which of the following is correct regarding electroconvulsive therapy?

    A. For maximum effectiveness, seizures should last 5–10 minutes.

B. ECT is contraindicated in patients with COPD.

C. ECT is effective treatment for pregnant females with major depression.

D. Memory loss lasting 1–2 weeks is common.

E. ECT may cause amenorrhea in female patients.

15. A 33-year-old waitress is experiencing symptoms of anxiety, including night terrors and mood lability. She reports no past psychiatric history but admits that these symptoms started about 2 weeks after armed and masked gunmen robbed her restaurant. She is most likely experiencing which of the following?

A. LSD

B. PTSD

C. GAD

D. OCD

E. SAD

16. A new patient presents to your clinic. He reports that it took him 3 hours to get ready for this appointment and that he returned home several times to check to see if the door was locked. During the interview, he straightens up your desk, making sure all square items are at right angles to each other. Which medication would be most appropriate for the patient?

A. Trazodone

B. Olanzapine

C. Fluvoxamine

D. Alprazolam

E. Lithium

17. Which of the following statements regarding the use of SSRIs in anxiety disorders is most accurate?

A. SSRIs are not usually effective in the treatment of anxiety.

B. SSRI doses for anxiety should be started lower than initial doses for depression.

C. SSRIs should be used only after a failed treatment trial with benzodiazepines.

D. SSRIs may be used on a prn basis when anxiety symptoms emerge.

E. SSRIs work very rapidly to resolve symptoms of anxiety.

18. Which of the following characteristics is *not* correct regarding benzodiazepines?

A. They potentiate the effect of g-aminobutyric acid.

B. They are highly lipophilic.

C. They are cross-tolerant with alcohol.

D. Their pharmacologic action is similar to that of buspirone.

E. There is risk of seizure if they are abruptly discontinued.

For Questions 19 and 20, one or more of the answers given are correct. Answer each question as follows:

A. I only

B. II only

C. I and III only

D. II and III only

E. I, II, and III

19. Which of the following is true regarding anorexia nervosa?

I. AN is characterized by recurrent and inappropriate compensatory behavior to prevent weight gain.

II. Patients with AN generally appear to be of normal weight for age and height.

III. AN patients have an intense fear of gaining weight or becoming fat, although they are underweight.

20. Which of the following is true regarding bulimia nervosa?

I. The individual may consume 5,000–20,000 calories in a single binge episode that may last as long as 2–8 hours.

II. The two specific types of bulimic patients are the purging type and the nonpurging type.

III. There is an average of two binges per week for 3 consecutive months.

21. A 19-year-old female recently started treatment for bulimia nervosa. She is experiencing severe anxiety when eating, fearing that she will lose control. Which medication is most appropriate for her anxiety?

A. Bupropion SR 150 mg

B. Olanzapine 10 mg

C. Lithium carbonate 300 mg

D. Lorazepam 0.5 mg
E. Zonisamide 100 mg

22. Which of the following is contraindicated in anorexia nervosa and bulimia nervosa?

   A. Bupropion
   B. Sertraline
   C. Citalopram
   D. Clonazepam
   E. Fluoxetine

23. Which of the following is the most appropriate treatment for bulimia nervosa?

   A. Insight-oriented therapy
   B. Fluoxetine 20 mg daily
   C. Fluoxetine 60 mg every morning + cognitive behavioral therapy
   D. Olanzapine 10 mg at bedtime
   E. Olanzapine 20 mg at bedtime + family therapy

29-9. Answers

1. **D.** The patient is on haloperidol 10 mg bid. Therefore, to convert to the decanoate injection, the total oral daily dose is multiplied by 10. The dose would be Haldol-D 200 mg IM every 4 weeks.

2. **B.** The patient is experiencing a dystonic reaction, which can be treated with either benztropine 1–2 mg IM or diphenhydramine 25–50 mg IM every 30 minutes until resolved. The dystonic reaction is thought to occur because of an imbalance in dopamine and acetylcholine in the nigrostriatal region of the brain.

3. **B.** The only antipsychotic proven effective for refractory schizophrenia is clozapine. Because the patient has had little to no response to quetiapine, raising her quetiapine dose is inappropriate. Little evidence supports the use of multiple antipsychotics in the treatment of schizophrenia. Augmenting quetiapine therapy with fluoxetine and ECT is inappropriate because the patient has had little response to quetiapine. Guidelines for the treatment of schizophrenia recommend two adequate trials of antipsychotic monotherapy before switching the patient to clozapine, unless clozapine use is contraindicated or inappropriate for the patient.

4. **B.** The symptoms that the patient is displaying appear to be the result of neuroleptic malignant syndrome. All neuroleptics have the propensity to cause this rare but deadly adverse effect. The first steps in treating NMS are to discontinue the offending agent, offer supportive therapy, and prescribe a dopamine agonist and (commonly) a skeletal muscle relaxant.

5. **C.** Initiation of lithium requires several baseline lab tests: pregnancy test (if patient is female and of childbearing age), ECG and BP to assess cardiovascular status, thyroid function tests to rule out euthyroid goiter or hypothyroidism, SCr/BUN (lithium is 100% renally eliminated), and CBC with differential to evaluate for leukocytosis. Electrolytes should also be evaluated (decreased sodium can increase lithium levels). The pregnancy test should not be performed because the patient is male. Liver function tests must be performed prior to initiating divalproex. Baseline fasting glucose must be performed when prescribing atypical antipsychotics.

6. **A.** Common side effects that occur with the initiation of lithium include polyuria, polydipsia, tremor, and GI upset. Common side effects that may occur later in therapy include weight gain and mental dulling. Elevated hepatic enzymes and alopecia are side effects that may occur with divalproex sodium. Akathisia is an extrapyramidal side effect induced by antipsychotics.

7. **D.** Agranulocytosis is a side effect that is monitored weekly with clozapine therapy for 6 months. After 6 months, monitoring can be done every 2 weeks; after 6 more months, monitoring can be done every 4 weeks for the duration of therapy.

8. **D.** All of the therapies listed have been used for mood stabilization in bipolar disorder.

9. **C.** SSRIs commonly cause insomnia, GI upset, anxiety, headache, and sexual dysfunction. Phenelzine, amitriptyline, and trazodone cause sedative effects.

10. **D.** Because of fluoxetine's long half-life, 5 weeks should pass before initiating MAOI therapy. If fluoxetine is not cleared from the body by the time the MAOI is started, there is a risk of developing serotonin syndrome.

11. **A.** Many medications can cause or worsen depression, such as antihypertensives (reserpine, methyldopa, propranolol, clonidine);

antiparkinsonian agents (levodopa, carbidopa, amantadine); hormonal agents (estrogens, progesterone); corticosteroids; cycloserine; and the anticancer agents vinblastine and vincristine.

12. **B.** Hydroxyzine reduces anxiety and is often used in patients with substance abuse issues. Hydroxyzine is indicated for pruritus, but is likely being used for anxiety in this patient. Hydroxyzine may be confused with hydralazine, which is indicated for essential hypertension.

13. **C.** Abilify (aripiprazole) is approved as adjunctive treatment for refractory depression. The patient has already failed a trial with venlafaxine; therefore, initiating therapy with its isomer Pristiq (desvenlafaxine) may not be the best option. MAOIs are a viable fourth-line treatment option. However, you would wait 5 weeks after discontinuing fluoxetine before initiating an MAOI. Lexapro (escitalopram) is an isomer of citalopram, which the patient had already failed. Benzodiazepines are not recommended for treatment of depression.

14. **C.** ECT is a safe and effective therapy for pregnant females and patients with COPD. Relative contraindications include increased intracranial pressure, recent MI, recent intracerebral hemorrhage, and cerebral lesions. Memory loss is a common side effect, but it usually occurs only on the day of treatment and perhaps the following day. The induced seizure lasts 30–90 seconds and is monitored by an EEG. Additionally, ECT does not cause amenorrhea in female patients.

15. **B.** The patient experienced a violent and frightening episode 2 weeks before her symptoms appeared. The symptoms of reexperiencing of the event, night terrors, and mood lability are common in patients with PTSD.

16. **C.** The patient is displaying signs and symptoms of OCD (e.g., a long time is spent getting ready, and there is repeated checking behavior and preoccupation with rearranging items to 90-degree angles). These activities are time consuming and limit his social and occupational functioning. Fluvoxamine is primarily used for OCD. SSRIs are first-line agents in the treatment of OCD. Clomipramine, a tricyclic, is also FDA approved for OCD. Trazodone is an antidepressant most commonly used for insomnia.

17. **B.** Because SSRIs can be activating and may initially cause symptoms of anxiety, it is impor-

tant to "start low and go slow" with these agents when used for anxiety disorders.

18. **D.** Buspirone's mechanism of action is agonism of 5-HT_{1A} receptors. Buspirone also possesses moderate affinity for D_2 receptors. It does not interact with the BZD-GABA receptor complex like the BZDs do. The BZDs cross the blood–brain barrier and are cross-tolerant with alcohol. If BZDs are abruptly discontinued, seizures can result.

19. **C.** Patients with AN refuse to maintain body weight at or above a minimal, normal weight for age and height (less than 15% of expected body weight). Patients with AN may respond to antidepressants, but psychotherapy is usually more effective. AN is most commonly seen in Caucasian, middle- to upper-class females.

20. **E.** All of the answers are correct regarding bulimia nervosa.

21. **D.** Low-dose, short-acting benzodiazepines have shown benefit if severe anxiety associated with eating exists. Olanzapine may improve weight gain and psychological symptoms. Bupropion is contraindicated because of the risk of seizures.

22. **A.** Bupropion is contraindicated because of the risk of seizures.

23. **C.** Fluoxetine is approved for treating bulimia nervosa; 60 mg is the most common dose. A combination of psychotherapy and pharmacotherapy is preferred.

29-10. References

Adasuve (oral inhalation powder, loxapine oral inhalation powder) [product information]. Mountain View, CA: Alexza Pharmaceuticals, Inc.; 2012.

American Diabetes Association, American Psychiatric Association, American Association of Clinical Endocrinologists, North American Association for the Study of Obesity. Consensus development conference on antipsychotic drugs and obesity and diabetes. *Diabetes Care.* 2004;27:596–601.

American Psychiatric Association. *Diagnostic and Statistical Manual of Mental Disorders.* 5th ed. Text rev. Washington, DC: American Psychiatric Association; 2013.

American Psychiatric Association. Practice guideline for the treatment of patients with bipolar disorder (revision). *Am J Psychiatry.* 2002;159(suppl):1–50.

American Psychiatric Association. *Practice Guideline for the Treatment of Patients with Eating Disorders.* 3rd ed. Washington, DC: American Psychiatric Association; 2006.

American Psychiatric Association. Practice guideline for the treatment of patients with major depressive disorder. 3rd ed. *Am J Psychiatry.* 2010. http://psychiatryonline.org/content.aspx?bookid=28&sectionid=1667485.

American Psychiatric Association. Practice guideline for the treatment of patients with schizophrenia. 2nd ed. *Am J Psychiatry.* 2004. http://psychiatryonline.org/data/Books/prac/Schizophrenia2e_Inactivated_04-16-09.pdf.

Bennett JA, Dunayevich E, McElroy SL, et al. The new mood stabilizers and the treatment of bipolar disorder. *Drug Benefit Trends.* 2000;12:3–16.

Brintellix (oral tablets, vortioxetine oral tablets) [product information]. Deerfield, IL: Takeda Pharmaceuticals America, Inc.; 2013.

Canales PL, Cates M, Wells BG. Anxiety disorders. In: Herfindal ET, Gourley DR, eds. *Textbook of Therapeutics: Drug and Disease Management.* 8th ed. Philadelphia, PA: Lippincott Williams & Wilkins; 2006:1185–202.

Crismon ML, Argo TR, Buckley PF. Schizophrenia. In: DiPiro JT, Talbert RL, Yee GC, et al., eds. *Pharmacotherapy: A Pathophysiologic Approach.* 8th ed. New York, NY: McGraw-Hill; 2011: 1147–72.

DeVane CL. Keeping depression at bay. *Drug Topics.* 2001;15:49–58.

Drayton SJ. Bipolar Disorder. In: DiPiro JT, Talbert RL, Yee GC, et al., eds. *Pharmacotherapy: A Pathophysiologic Approach.* 8th ed. New York, NY: McGraw-Hill; 2011:1191–208.

Fuller MA, Sajatovic M, eds. *Drug Information for Mental Health.* 1st ed. Cleveland, OH: Lexi-Comp; 2001.

Gutierrez MA, Stimmel GL. Mood disorders. In: Helms RA, Quan DJ, Herfindal ET, et al., eds. *Textbook of Therapeutics: Drug and Disease Management.* 8th ed. Philadelphia, PA: Lippincott Williams & Wilkins; 2006:1416–31.

Gutierrez MA, Stimmel GL. Schizophrenia. In: Helms RA, Quan DJ, Herfindal ET, et al., eds. *Textbook of Therapeutics: Drug and Disease Management.* 8th ed. Philadelphia, PA: Lippincott Williams & Wilkins; 2006:1432–42.

Kane JM. Drug therapy: Schizophrenia. *N Engl J Med.* 1996;334:34–41.

Kane JM, McGlashan TH. Treatment of schizophrenia. *Lancet.* 1995;346:820–25.

Keck PE, Perlis RH, Otto MW, et al. The expert consensus guideline series: Treatment of bipolar disorder 2004. *Postgrad Med Special Report.* 2004(December):1–120.

Kirkwood CK, Melton ST. Anxiety disorders I: Generalized anxiety, panic, and social anxiety disorders. In: DiPiro JT, Talbert RL, Yee GC, et al., eds. *Pharmacotherapy: A Pathophysiologic Approach.* 8th ed. New York, NY: McGraw-Hill; 2011:1209–28.

Lieberman JA, Stroup TS, McEvoy JP, et al. Effectiveness of antipsychotic drugs in patients with chronic schizophrenia. *N Engl J Med.* 2005;353:1209–23.

Mandl DL, Iltz JL. Obesity and eating disorders. In: Herfindal ET, Gourley DR, eds. *Textbook of Therapeutics: Drug and Disease Management.* 7th ed. Philadelphia, PA: Lippincott Williams & Wilkins; 2000:1271–87.

McElroy SL, Keck PE. Pharmacologic agents for the treatment of acute bipolar mania. *Biol Psychiatry.* 2000;48:539–57.

McElroy SL, Shapira NA, Arnold LM, et al. Topiramate in the long-term treatment of binge-eating disorder associated with obesity. *J Clin Psychiatry.* 2004;65(suppl 11):1463–69.

McEvoy JP, Lieberman JA, Stroup TS, et al. Effectiveness of clozapine versus olanzapine, quetiapine, and risperidone in patients with chronic schizophrenia who did not respond to prior atypical antipsychotic treatment. *Am J Psychiatry.* 2006;163:600–10.

McEvoy JP, Scheifler PL, Frances A. The expert consensus guideline series: Treatment of schizophrenia. *J Clin Psychiatry.* 1999;60(suppl 11):3–80.

National Institute for Health Care and Excellence. Bipolar disorder: The management of bipolar disorder in adults, children and adolescents, in primary and secondary care. Clinical Guideline No 38. London, U.K.: National Institute for Health Care and Excellence; 2006.

National Institute of Mental Health. Anxiety disorders. NIH publication no. 00-3879. National Institutes of Health, Bethesda, MD; 2000.

Ray WA, Chung CP, Murray KT, et al. Atypical antipsychotic drugs and the risk of sudden cardiac death. *N Engl J Med.* 2009;360(3):225–35.

Sachs GS, Nierenberg AA, Calabrese JR, et al. Effectiveness of adjunctive antidepressant treatment for bipolar depression. *N Engl J Med.* 2007; 356:1711–22.

Sachs GS, Printz DJ, Kahn DA, et al. The expert consensus guideline series: Medication treatment of bipolar disorder 2000. *Postgrad Med.* 2000;4:1–104.

Stroup TS, Lieberman JA, McEvoy JP, et al. Effectiveness of olanzapine, quetiapine, risperidone, and ziprasidone in patients with chronic schizophrenia following discontinuation of a previous atypical antipsychotic. *Am J Psychiatry*. 2006;163:611–22.

Teter CJ, Kando JC, Wells BG. Major depressive disorder. In: DiPiro JT, Talbert RL, Yee GC, et al., eds. *Pharmacotherapy: A Pathophysiologic Approach*. 8th ed. New York, NY: McGraw-Hill; 2011; 1173–90.

Trivedi H, Rush AJ, Wisniewski SR, et al. Evaluation of outcomes with citalopram for depression using measurement-based care in STAR*D: Implications for clinical practice. *Am J Psychiatry*. 2006;163:28–40.

U.S. Food and Drug Administration. FDA drug safety communication: Revised recommendations for Celexa (citalopram hydrobromide) related to a potential risk of abnormal heart rhythms with high doses. March 28, 2012. U.S. Food and Drug Administration Web site. http://www.fda.gov /Drugs/DrugSafety/ucm297391.htm.

U.S. Food and Drug Administration. FDA proposes new warnings about suicidal thinking, behavior in young adults who take antidepressant medications. May 2, 2007. U.S. Food and Drug Administration Web site. http://www .fda.gov/NewsEvents/Newsroom/Press Announcements/2007/ucm108905.htm.

U.S. Food and Drug Administration. FDA public health advisory: Deaths with antipsychotics in elderly patients with behavioral disturbances. May 2, 2007. U.S. Food and Drug Administration Web site. http://www.fda.gov/Drugs/DrugSafety /PublicHealthAdvisories/ucm053171.htm.

U.S. Food and Drug Administration. Saphris (asenapine maleate): Drug safety communication: Serious allergic reactions. September 1, 2011. U.S. Food and Drug Administration Web site. http://www .fda.gov/Safety/MedWatch/SafetyInformation /SafetyAlertsforHumanMedicalProducts/ucm 270600.htm?utm_campaign=Google2&utm _source=fdaSearch&utm_medium=website& utm_term=saphris&utm_content=1.

Common Dermatologic Disorders

Shaunta' M. Ray

30-1. Key Points

Acne

■ Acne occurs primarily in the teenage years because of the increase of androgens during puberty that stimulates activity of the sebaceous glands.

■ Isotretinoin (Accutane) is the drug of choice for nodulocystic acne (type IV acne), which, if left untreated, will cause extensive scarring.

■ Isotretinoin is contraindicated in pregnancy because of the high incidence of serious birth defects.

■ The most common side effects of isotretinoin are cheilitis (dry, chapped lips), dry skin, and dry eyes.

Fungal Infections of the Skin

■ The most efficacious nonprescription topical antifungal is terbinafine (Lamisil).

■ Systemic antifungal therapy is required for treatment of tinea capitis (ringworm of the scalp) and tinea unguium (fungal infection of the toenails and fingernails).

Hair Loss

■ Androgenic alopecia—predominantly seen in males—is due to the conversion of testosterone to dihydrotestosterone, which binds to the hair follicles and causes progressively thinner hair.

■ In the treatment of androgenic alopecia, minoxidil (Rogaine) should be applied and left on the scalp for 4 hours for maximum benefit.

■ Finasteride (Propecia) decreases the effect of androgens on hair follicles by inhibiting 5-α-reductase, which prevents the conversion of testosterone to dihydrotestosterone.

Dry Skin

■ Dry skin occurs primarily in older adults because of decreased sebum production and decreased moisture-binding capacity of the skin.

■ Products containing urea and lactic acid improve the skin's moisture-binding capacity, thereby increasing skin hydration.

Dermatitis

■ Contact dermatitis, whether irritant or allergic, is initially treated with topical corticosteroid products.

■ The absorption and subsequent adverse systemic effects of topical corticosteroids are increased in infant skin and with occlusion, the use of high-potency agents, and long-term use.

Poison Ivy, Poison Oak, and Poison Sumac

■ Poison ivy, poison oak, and poison sumac are common causes of allergic contact dermatitis, which is the result of contact with the sap of plants of the genus *Rhus*.

■ Severe cases of poison ivy, poison oak, or poison sumac require systemic corticosteroids to relieve symptoms, decrease the severity of the rash, and shorten the course of the disorder.

Scaly Dermatoses

■ The cytostatic agents that suppress cell rate turnover—zinc pyrithione (in Head and Shoulders shampoo) and selenium sulfide (in Selsun Blue shampoo)—are the primary agents of choice for treatment of dandruff.

■ Seborrhea usually requires topical corticosteroids or the topical antifungal ketoconazole for effective treatment.

■ Psoriasis is a chronic disease characterized by inflammation and silvery scales (known as *plaques*) with sharp, delineated edges.

■ Treatment of advanced psoriasis may require systemic corticosteroids or antimetabolites in addition to topical treatments for effective management of the disease.

Pediculosis

■ Head lice (*Pediculus humanus capitis*) occur most commonly in elementary schoolchildren in the months of August and September.

■ Permethrin (Nix) is the nonprescription agent of choice for treatment of head lice because it usually does not have to be repeated in 7 to 10 days like other nonprescription pediculicidal agents (synergized pyrethrins).

Corns and Warts

■ Nonprescription products for the treatment of corns and warts contain salicylic acid.

■ Self-treatment for corns or warts with over-the-counter agents is not recommended for diabetic patients because of reduced sensation in their feet that delays awareness of possible development of infections that can lead to sepsis.

■ Warts result from an infection of the human papillomavirus and, therefore, are contagious and may spread on the body.

■ Warts may be removed by surgery, cryotherapy (freezing with liquid nitrogen), or direct application of caustics (e.g., salicylic acid, formalin, lactic acid, trichloroacetic acid, podophyllin).

30-2. Study Guide Checklist

The following topics may guide your study of this subject area:

■ Classification and clinical presentation of acne, fungal skin infections, dermatitis, *Rhus* dermatitis, psoriasis, pediculosis, warts, corns, and calluses

■ Selection of therapies for acne, fungal skin infections, dermatitis, *Rhus* dermatitis, psoriasis, pediculosis, warts, corns, and calluses based on classification

■ Selection of therapies for alopecia, dry skin, dandruff, and seborrhea

■ Important counseling points and adverse reactions for all therapies

■ Recommendations for nondrug therapies for dry skin and pediculosis

■ Options for preventive treatment for *Rhus* dermatitis

■ Actions of medications used to treat common dermatologic disorders

30-3. Acne (Acne Vulgaris)

Acne is an inflammatory disorder of the pilosebaceous glands that occurs most commonly during the teenage years, at or soon after puberty. It may reappear later or begin in adults who had clear skin in their teens, more commonly in women than in men.

Classification and Clinical Presentation

■ *Type I (comedonal):* A mild form, with primarily noninflammatory lesions (open and closed comedones), relatively few superficial inflammatory lesions, and no scarring

■ *Type II (papular):* A moderate form, with multiple papules on the face and trunk and minimal scarring

■ *Type III (pustular):* An advanced form that can lead to moderate scarring

■ *Type IV (nodulocystic):* The most severe and destructive form, with multiple deep inflammatory lesions or nodules (often called *cysts*) that lead to extensive scarring

Pathophysiology

■ Increased sebum production by androgenic hormones at the onset of puberty

■ Obstruction of hair follicle openings because of increasing adherence to and production of epithelial cells, producing closed comedones (whiteheads) that progress ultimately to open comedones (blackheads)

■ Increased growth of a primary microorganism on the skin and in the sebaceous ducts, *Propionibacterium acnes* (*P. acnes*), a Gram-positive anaerobic rod that produces enzymes (including lipases)

- Inflammation caused by the enzymatic breakdown of triglycerides into free fatty acids, which causes the influx of polymorphonuclear leukocytes, ultimately resulting in pustule formation

Treatment Principles

- *Type I (comedonal):* Topical nonprescription medications such as benzoyl peroxide, which is usually the first line of therapy
- *Type II (papular):* Topical antibiotics, topical retinoids, or both
- *Type III (pustular):* Oral antibiotics in addition to topical medications
- *Type IV (nodulocystic):* Isotretinoin

Topical Therapy

Nonprescription agents

Benzoyl peroxide is the most effective over-the-counter (OTC) agent. Examples of products containing 2.5%, 5%, and 10% benzoyl peroxide are as follows:

- Clean and Clear Gel
- Clearasil
- Clearplex
- Exact Acne Medication
- Fostex
- Neutrogena On-the-Spot Acne Treatment
- Oxy-10 Balance Spot Treatment and Face Wash
- PanOxyl Bar
- ZAPZYT Acne Treatment Gel

Mechanism of action

These agents destroy the anaerobic *P. acnes* through the release of oxygen. An exfoliant effect occurs, causing peeling of the outer layers of the skin.

P. acnes does not become resistant to benzoyl peroxide; therefore, it can be used concurrently with topical antibiotics to prevent resistance (e.g., using benzoyl peroxide for one course of therapy, alternating with a course of topical antibiotic therapy).

Patient counseling

- Use with caution with sensitive skin.
- Do not allow contact with eyes, lips, or mouth.
- Avoid unnecessary sun exposure, and use sunscreen.

Adverse effects

- These agents may cause redness, dryness, burning, itching, peeling, and swelling.
- They may bleach hair or dyed fabrics.

Other products

- **Sulfur (1–10%):** Products include Bye Bye Blemish—sulfur 10% (keratolytic and antibacterial action)
- **Salicylic acid (0.5–2%):** Products include Clearasil Ultra Rapid Action Daily Gel Wash, Neutrogena Rapid Clear Acne Defense, Noxzema, and Stridex—irritant effect, keratolytic action, and increase in turnover rate of epithelial cells
- **Resorcinol:** Keratolytic action (usually combined with sulfur)
- **Combinations such as sulfur and resorcinol:** Clearasil and Acnomel
- **Medicated soaps and cleansers:** Alcohol, acetone, and other degreasing lotions

Topical antimicrobial therapy

Topical antimicrobials are outlined in Table 30-1.

Clindamycin
Mechanism of action
Clindamycin suppresses growth of *P. acnes*. It may directly reduce free fatty acid concentrations on the skin.

Patient counseling
- Contact your health care provider if no improvement is seen within 6 weeks.
- Discontinue medication and contact your health care provider if severe diarrhea or abdominal cramps or pain develops.

Adverse effects
- Contact dermatitis or hypersensitivity
- Dry or scaly skin or peeling skin
- Rarely, pseudomembranous colitis (severe abdominal cramps, pain, bloating, severe diarrhea)

Erythromycin
Mechanism of action
Erythromycin suppresses growth of *P. acnes*.

Table 30-1. Topical Antimicrobials

Generic name	Trade name	Form
Clindamycin	Cleocin T	Liquid
Erythromycin	Theramycin Z	Liquid
	Erygel	Gel

Patient counseling

- Wait at least 1 hour before applying any other topical acne medication.
- Avoid contact with eyes, mouth, nose, and other mucous membranes.
- Although improvement is generally expected within 4 weeks, some patients do not respond for 8–12 weeks.

Adverse effects

- *More common:* Dry or scaly skin, irritation, itching
- *Less common:* Stinging sensation, peeling, redness

Retinoids

See Table 30-2 for information about retinoids.

Mechanism of action

- Retinoids are chemically related to vitamin A.
- Retinoids normalize follicular keratinization, heal comedones, decrease sebum production, and decrease inflammatory lesions.

Patient counseling

- Do not use astringents, drying agents, abrasive scrubs, or harsh soaps concurrently, and use mild soap only once or twice daily.
- Apply every other night to adjust to drying effect for the first 2 weeks.
- Apply nightly after 2 weeks.
- Expect that it may take up to 2–3 months for skin to improve.

Table 30-2. Retinoids

Generic name	Trade name	Form and strength
Tretinoin	Retin-A	0.025, 0.05, 0.1% cream; 0.01% gel
	Retin-A Micro	0.04, 0.1% gel
	Renova	0.02% cream
	Avita	0.025% cream and gel
Adapalene	Differin	0.1% cream and gel; 0.3% gel
Tazarotene	Tazorac	0.05, 0.1% cream and gel
Alitretinoin	Panretin	0.1% gel

- Use sunblock on face before sun exposure because of increased sensitivity.

Adverse drug effects

- These agents may irritate skin and cause redness, dryness, and scaling.
- Tazarotene is the most irritating retinoid.
- Adapalene appears to be least irritating and is preferred for sensitive skin.

Azelaic acid 20%

Trade names are Azelex and Finacea.

Mechanism of action

Azelaic acid 20% suppresses growth of *P. acnes*. It improves inflammatory and noninflammatory lesions. It normalizes keratinization, leading to an anticomedonal effect.

Patient counseling

- If sensitivity develops, discontinue use.
- Keep away from mouth, eyes, and mucous membranes.
- Other topical medications must be used at different times during the day.

Adverse drug effects

- Temporary dryness and skin irritation (pruritus and burning) may occur on initiation of therapy.
- Hypopigmentation may occur (caution in dark-skinned individuals).

Topical Dapsone 5%

Trade name is Aczone.

Mechanism of action

Dapsone has anti-inflammatory and antimicrobial properties and can be used to reduce the number of acne lesions in patients over 12 years old. May consider in patients unable to tolerate other topical acne medications.

Patient counseling

- If sensitivity develops, discontinue use.
- Keep away from mouth, eyes, and mucous membranes.

Adverse drug effects

- Peeling, dryness and erythema
- Phototoxicity

Systemic Therapy

Antimicrobials

Antimicrobials are useful for type II (papular) acne and type III (pustular) acne.

Dosing

See Table 30-3 for information about dosage. After 6–8 weeks, dosage may be increased if necessary. If the first antibiotic was ineffective after increasing the dosage, a second antibiotic is prescribed.

After 6 months to 1 year of therapy, the antibiotic dose may be tapered if continued at all.

Mechanism of action

Antimicrobials suppress growth of *P. acnes* in sebaceous ducts. These agents possibly have a direct anti-comedonal effect.

Patient counseling, adverse drug effects, and drug interactions

See Chapter 34 on anti-infective agents.

Isotretinoin

Isotretinoin is available in 10, 20, 30, and 40 mg capsules. Trade names are Accutane, Amnesteem, and Claravis.

Isotretinoin is for patients with severe, nodulocystic, draining acne who have not responded to systemic antibiotic therapy or who have required more than 3 years of systemic antibiotic therapy.

This agent is over 90% effective in producing an acne-free state for years following a 4- to 5-month course of therapy. Originally held in reserve for severe cases of nodulocystic acne, isotretinoin may also be indicated as first-line treatment for severe acne that results in scarring.

Table 30-3. Oral Antimicrobials

Generic name	Trade name	Dosage and form
Tetracycline	Achromycin, Sumycin	500 mg daily or bid capsules
Erythromycin	E.E.S., Erythrocin	250–500 mg daily or bid tablets
Doxycycline	Vibramycin	100 mg daily capsules or tablets
Minocycline	Minocin	50 mg bid capsules

iPLEDGE program

The U.S. Food and Drug Administration (FDA) approved an enhanced risk-management program, designed to minimize fetal exposure to isotretinoin, known as iPLEDGE. iPLEDGE requires mandatory registration of prescribers, patients, wholesalers, and pharmacies to further the public health goal of eliminating fetal exposure to isotretinoin.

Pharmacies are not able to dispense isotretinoin to people with severe acne who do not enroll in the iPLEDGE program through a health care provider who is also enrolled. After a pharmacy registers for iPLEDGE at www.ipledgeprogram.com, the "Responsible Site Pharmacist" is sent a follow-up mailing, which contains instructions on how to activate the pharmacy.

The iPLEDGE program requires that all patients meet qualification criteria and monthly program requirements. Before the patient receives his or her isotretinoin prescription each month, the prescriber must counsel the patient about the risks of isotretinoin and document it in the iPLEDGE system.

Mechanism of action

Isotretinoin reduces sebum production up to 90%. It decreases production of microcomedones, possibly by decreasing cohesiveness of follicular epithelial cells. It can have an anti-inflammatory effect.

Patient counseling

- Isotretinoin should be taken with food and is best absorbed with a fatty meal.
- Patients can take the dose divided twice daily or the entire dose with the evening meal.
- Effects are gradual, and acne may worsen during the first month of therapy. However, improvement usually begins by the sixth week of therapy.
- Use lip balm to treat cheilitis and moisturizers to treat dry skin.

Adverse drug effects

Isotretinoin is teratogenic. It is absolutely contraindicated in pregnancy because it causes significant birth defects. Females of childbearing potential must take measures to avoid pregnancy during the course of isotretinoin therapy.

Females should be tested for pregnancy before initiation of therapy and told to use two methods of contraception for at least 1 month prior to initiation of therapy and for 1 month after discontinuation of therapy.

Side effects and toxicity

- Most common (90–100%):
  - Cheilitis (chapped lips)
  - Dry mouth
  - Dry skin
  - Pruritus
- Common (30–40%):
  - Dry nose, leading to nasal crusting and epistaxis
  - Dry eyes, leading to conjunctivitis and problems with contact lenses
  - Muscular soreness or stiffness
- Less common (10–25%):
  - Headaches
  - Hyperlipidemia (primarily elevation of triglycerides, which may lead to attack of pancreatitis)
- Rare (less than 5%):
  - Decreased night vision
  - Thinning of hair
  - Easily injured skin
  - Peeling of palms and soles
  - Skin rash and skin infections
- Very rare (< 1%):
  - Acute depression (very rare, but reversible if detected early)
  - Pseudotumor cerebri (benign intracranial hypertension with visual disturbances)
- Treatment of most common side effects:
  - *Cheilitis:* Frequent use of lip balm
  - *Dry skin:* Skin lubrication with moisturizers
  - *Nosebleeds:* Lubrication of the nostrils with petrolatum
  - *Muscular soreness or stiffness:* Use of mild OTC analgesic and anti-inflammatory agents

Monitoring parameters

- Lipid panel
- Liver function tests (elevations common during initiation of therapy; usually return to normal during treatment)
- Complete blood counts
- Pregnancy testing for women prior to use of drug

Dosing

The dosage is 1 mg/kg once or twice daily with food; however, the patient may start out with 0.5 mg/kg/day for the first month before increasing. Isotretinoin is best absorbed with a fatty meal.

The goal is a total dose of 120–150 mg/kg over 4–5 months. Longer courses of 6–8 months may be required.

Other aspects

Approximately 20% of patients relapse within 1 year, and up to 40% relapse within 3 years after discontinuation of therapy. Repeat therapy for 4–6 months is acceptable and effective.

Oral corticosteroids

Oral corticosteroids are commonly known as "prom pills." These agents can temporarily suppress acne with a 7- to 10-day course of prednisone 20 mg daily. They are rapidly effective when a brief course is necessary to cause prompt improvement (e.g., important social event such as wedding, prom, and so forth).

Systemic corticosteroids used continuously may actually cause or worsen acne. Topical corticosteroids have no value in the treatment of acne, and high-potency topical corticosteroids will aggravate acne and should never be used on the faces of acne patients.

30-4. Fungal Skin Infections

Tinea are skin infections known as *dermatomycoses* caused by the fungi *Trichophyton*, *Microsporum*, and *Epidermophyton*.

Classification

- Tinea pedis (athlete's foot)
- Tinea capitis (ringworm of the scalp)
- Tinea cruris (jock itch)
- Tinea corporis (ringworm of the skin)
- Tinea unguium (onychomycosis: fungal infection of toenails and fingernails)

Pathophysiology

The fungi invade dead cells of the stratum corneum of skin, hair, and nails, digesting keratin. Unlike *Candida*, they cannot exist on unkeratinized mucous membranes.

This condition is more common in immunosuppressed patients.

Treatment Principles and Goals

- *Tinea pedis:* Self-treat topically initially; if ineffective, add oral agents.
- *Tinea capitis:* Use oral systemic therapy.
- *Tinea cruris:* Self-treat topically initially; if ineffective, add oral agents.

- *Tinea corporis:* Self-treat topically initially; if ineffective, add oral agents.
- *Tinea unguium:* Use oral systemic therapy.

Drug Therapy

OTC treatment

- Terbinafine 1% (Lamisil AT) cream, gel, and spray (most effective OTC antifungal agent)
- Miconazole 2% (Micatin, Cruex Spray powder)
- Clotrimazole 1% (Lotrimin AF lotion, solution, and cream)
- Tolnaftate 1% (Tinactin, Blis-To-Sol, Ting)
- Undecylenic acid 10–25% (Desenex)

Prescription treatment

See Table 30-4 for a description of prescription drugs.

Topical treatments
Newer antifungals are initially applied only once daily, and recurrences can be prevented by once- or twice-weekly applications.

Systemic therapy
Occasionally, topical therapy is not effective for tinea pedis, tinea cruris, and tinea corporis, and systemic antifungal therapy is required. Systemic therapy is also required for tinea capitis (ringworm of the scalp) and tinea unguium (fungal infection of the toenails and fingernails). Medications are as follows:

- Griseofulvin
- Ketoconazole
- Fluconazole
- Itraconazole
- Terbinafine

See Chapter 34 on anti-infective agents for discussion of systemic antifungals.

Table 30-4. Prescription Topical Antifungals

Generic name	Trade name
Econazole	Ecoza foam, cream
Naftifine	Naftin gel, cream
Ciclopirox	Loprox gel, cream, lotion; Penlac solution
Butenafine	Mentax cream, Lotrimin Ultra cream

30-5. Hair Loss (Alopecia)

Male pattern baldness (androgenic alopecia) is the gradual and progressive loss of hair in males as they age.

Clinical Presentation

- Onset and progression vary greatly.
- A distinct pattern of progressive hair loss develops in the frontotemporal areas and crown with sparing of the occiput.
- Hair loss is limited to the scalp.
- Miniaturization of hair is seen, where normal thick terminal hairs are converted to very fine vellus hairs.

Pathophysiology

Alopecia is primarily due to two factors:

- Heredity (genetic)
- Testosterone

Testosterone, which promotes growth of hair in the beard, axillae, pubis, and other parts of the body, does not promote the growth of scalp hair. It contributes to premature hair loss because it is converted by the enzyme 5-α-reductase to dihydrotestosterone, which binds preferentially to receptors in the hair follicles on the scalp and causes them to produce progressively thinner hair until the follicles eventually cease activity altogether.

Treatment Principles and Goals

Although androgenic alopecia has no cure, two drugs are available for its treatment:

- Minoxidil (Rogaine, available OTC)
- Finasteride (Propecia, by prescription only)

In alopecia's early stages, topical minoxidil or oral finasteride may reverse the gradually decreasing diameter of the hair shaft.

Any hair growth stimulation is temporary and lasts only as long as therapy continues. If therapy is discontinued, new hair growth is lost within 1 year.

Early hair loss occurring recently in younger men is more likely to respond to treatment than later hair loss at an older age or when hair loss is not recent.

Alopecia of the crown in males responds better to treatment than does hair loss in the frontotemporal area.

Drug Therapy

Minoxidil

OTC trade names are Rogaine 2% and Rogaine Extra Strength 5%.

Mechanism of action

Minoxidil probably increases cutaneous blood flow directly to hair follicles because of vasodilation. It possibly stimulates resting hair follicles (telogen phase) into active growth (anagen phase). It possibly stimulates hair follicle cells.

Patient counseling

- Apply 1 mL twice daily (approximately one 60 mL bottle each month).
- Minoxidil may be applied without shampooing hair.
- Use at least 4 hours before bedtime to avoid oil on pillows and bed linens.
- The drug is absorbed over a 4-hour period, so do not swim, shampoo, or walk in rain for 4 hours.
- Wash hands immediately after application to prevent unwanted absorption.
- Do not inhale mist because systemic absorption is possible.
- Do not use on infected, irritated, inflamed, or sunburned skin.
- Discontinue use immediately and contact your health care provider if chest pain, increased heart rate, faintness, dizziness, or swollen hands or feet occur.
- Women should avoid 5% strength (which has no better results than 2%); they have greater incidence of increased growth of facial hair with the 5% solution.
- Generally, treatment takes 4–6 months before any benefit occurs.
- No effects within 8 months for females and 12 months for males indicate therapeutic failure, and treatment should be discontinued.
- Patients must continue using minoxidil to maintain new hair growth.

Adverse drug effects

- Scalp dermatitis is common, producing dryness, pruritus, and flaking or scaling.
- Hypertrichosis (excessive hair growth) can occur on areas other than scalp (chest, forearms, ear rim, back, face, arms, and so forth).
- Some women report unwanted facial hair growth when minoxidil is applied to scalp, primarily with the 5% solution.

- Use may rarely produce systemic side effects (chest pain, increased heart rate, faintness, or dizziness).
- Use is contraindicated in patients less than 18 years of age.
- Use is contraindicated in women who are pregnant or breastfeeding.

Finasteride

The trade name of finasteride is Propecia 1 mg. It was originally developed for the treatment of benign prostatic hyperplasia in a 5 mg dose (Proscar). A 1 mg daily dose is approved for males only as prescription treatment for androgenic alopecia.

Over a two-year period, finasteride may halt the progressive hair loss caused by androgenic alopecia.

Mechanism of action

Finasteride inhibits the enzyme 5-α-reductase, which is responsible for the conversion of testosterone to the more powerful dihydrotestosterone—the main androgen responsible for androgenic hair loss.

Patient counseling

- Take with or without food.
- Take for at least 3 months to see if the drug is effective.
- Improvement lasts only as long as treatment continues. New hair will be lost within 1 year of stopping treatment.

Adverse drug effects

- Gynecomastia (breast enlargement and tenderness) has been reported from 2 weeks to 2 years following initial therapy, but it is usually reversible when therapy is discontinued.
- Hypersensitivity (skin rash, swelling of lips) has been reported.
- Decreased libido, erectile dysfunction, and ejaculatory dysfunction occur, which are reversible when the drug is discontinued.
- Use is contraindicated in females of childbearing age, because of abnormalities of the external genitalia in male fetuses. Finasteride is not effective in postmenopausal females.

30-6. Dry Skin

This condition refers to lack of moisture or sebum in the stratum corneum. It most commonly occurs in the winter (also known as *winter rash*). It is more commonly present in older adults.

Clinical Presentation

- Flaking and scaling
- Xerosis and roughness
- Pruritus
- Loss of skin elasticity

Pathophysiology

Dry skin is due to inadequate moisture retention in the stratum corneum, which is caused by the following factors:

- Decreased sebum production and decreasing moisture-binding capacity of skin in elderly patients
- Low humidity, which causes the skin to lose water and become dry and hardened
- Overexposure to sunlight
- Excessive cleansing and bathing, which removes lipids and other skin components
- Chronic skin diseases that impair moisture retention of skin (psoriasis, scleroderma, ichthyosis, contact dermatitis)

Treatment Principles and Goals

The goal of treatment is to increase the moisture level of the stratum corneum by increasing cell hydration and binding capacity, which improves skin permeability and restores elasticity.

Drug Therapy

Emollients and moisturizing agents

Emollients and moisturizing agents include petrolatum or mineral oil (Alpha Keri Shower and Bath Moisture Rich Oil). They increase the relative moisture content of the stratum corneum and produce a general soothing effect by reducing frictional heat and perspiration.

Humectants

Humectants include glycerin (e.g., Corn Huskers Lotion), propylene glycol, and phospholipids. They are hygroscopic agents that increase hydration of the stratum corneum.

Keratin-softening agents

Keratin-softening agents include the following:

- Urea (10–30%) (e.g., Aqua Care, Carmol)
  - Improves the skin's moisture-binding capacity
  - Provides keratolytic effect at higher concentrations
  - May cause irritation and burning
- Lactic acid (2–5%) (e.g., LactiCare)
  - Increases skin hydration by controlling the rate of keratinization
  - Is markedly hygroscopic
- Allantoin (e.g., Alphosyl, Psorex, Tegrin)
  - Relieves dry skin by disrupting keratin structure (less effective than urea)
  - Desensitizes many skin-sensitizing drugs as a protectant

Antipruritic agents

Antipruritic agents include the following:

- Camphor and menthol, which provide a cooling sensation
- Local anesthetics (e.g., benzocaine, pramoxine)
- Systemic antihistamines (H_1-receptor antagonists), which have limited effectiveness
- Colloidal oatmeal (e.g., Aveeno)

Caution: Colloidal oatmeal can cause an extremely slippery bathtub.

Hydrocortisone

Hydrocortisone reduces the inflammatory response that accompanies dry skin conditions. Although it does not directly increase skin hydration, it does prevent itching associated with dry skin and inhibits dehydration.

Ointment is better than cream for dry skin. Patients should be counseled as follows:

- Use sparingly.
- Do not use for more than 5–7 days for dry skin pruritus.

Astringents

Astringents include aluminum acetate 0.1–0.5% (e.g., Burow's solution) and Hamamelis water (witch hazel).

Protectants

Zinc oxide is a protectant.

Nondrug Recommendations and Therapy

- Bathe less frequently.
- Reduce use of soap to a minimum, and use only where necessary.

■ Lubricate skin immediately after bathing (e.g., apply bath oil after bathing and before drying).
■ Use extrafatted soaps such as Basis.

Combination products to treat dry skin

■ *Aveeno Soothing Bath Treatment:* Colloidal oatmeal and mineral oil
■ *Jergens Ultra Healing Extra Dry Skin Moisturizer:* Dimethicone, cetearyl alcohol, petrolatum, and glycerin
■ *Keri Original Dry Skin Lotion:* Mineral oil, lanolin oil, glyceryl stearate, and propylene glycol
■ *Moisturel Lotion:* Petrolatum, dimethicone, cetyl alcohol, and glycerin
■ *Neutrogena Body Oil:* Isopropyl myristate and sesame seed oil

30-7. Dermatitis

Dermatitis is a nonspecific term describing a variety of inflammatory dermatologic conditions characterized by erythema. It is a general term describing any eczematous rash of unknown etiology that cannot be classified among the major endogenous dermatoses. *Eczema* and *dermatitis* are often used interchangeably.

Types and Classification

The major classifications or types of dermatitis are as follows:

■ Atopic dermatitis (atopic eczema)
■ Chronic dermatitis (hand dermatitis)
■ Contact dermatitis (irritant and allergic)

Clinical Presentation

Atopic dermatitis (atopic eczema)

Atopic dermatitis occurs primarily in infants and children. It may disappear before adulthood. The cause is unknown but is possibly genetic.

Atopic dermatitis is usually seen on the face, knees, elbows, and neck. It is frequently seen with asthma, allergic rhinitis, and urticaria. Exacerbating factors include soaps, detergents, chemicals, temperature changes, molds, and allergens.

Chronic dermatitis (hand dermatitis or hand eczema)

Chronic dermatitis, also known as *eczema,* is a stubborn, itchy rash that occurs in certain persons with sensitive or irritable skin. The skin is very dry and easily irritated by overuse of soaps or detergents and by rough clothing.

The condition is exacerbated by very hot or very cold weather. It is probably genetically determined. No permanent cure exists.

The condition usually can be controlled by enhancing skin hydration with emollients and moisturizers and by using hydrocortisone cream to relieve itching.

Contact dermatitis

Irritant contact dermatitis (chemical contact dermatitis)
The condition is caused by exposure to irritating substances producing mechanical or chemical trauma. Examples include soap, solvents, paints, abrasive cleansers, cosmetics, lubricants, antiseptics, cacti, rose hips, thorns, peppers, and tobacco.

Irritant contact dermatitis is not a sensitization, but direct toxicity to skin tissue.

Allergic contact dermatitis
The condition is a process of sensitization with reaction on elicitation. More than 50% of all dermatitis is allergic contact dermatitis.

Examples of reactive elements include benzocaine, zinc pyrithione (ZPT), neomycin, sodium bisulfite, perfumes, many cosmetics, skin lubricants, antiseptic creams, rubber and epoxy glues, poison ivy and oak, and many other common substances.

Treatment Principles and Goals

Treat dermatitis by applying a corticosteroid, according to the following principles:

■ Ointments and creams are more lubricating than solutions, lotions, or gels.
■ Ointments should be recommended if skin is dry.
■ Lotions or gels should be recommended for a weeping, eczematous dermatitis.
■ Lotions, solutions, and gels are easier to use in hairy areas of the body.
■ Apply small amounts of corticosteroid cream or ointment, and massage in gently but thoroughly.
■ Apply the moderate- and high-strength cortisones only once daily.

- Improvement should begin within 1 week.
- Avoid excess soap, and keep skin lubricated with moisturizers.
- Treat itching with camphor, menthol, phenol, or local anesthetics.
- Occasionally with severe cases (less than 5%), patients may have to use systemic corticosteroids for 1–2 weeks.

Drug Therapy

Topical corticosteroids

See Table 30-5 for information about topical corticosteroids.

Adverse effects
- Striae may result in skin folds.
- Thinning of epidermis occurs where subcutaneous vessels become visible.

- The more potent types can cause or aggravate acne or rosacea on the face.
- Percutaneous absorption can lead to systemic effects (see Chapter 18 on endocrine drugs for complete list of systemic adverse effects) such as the following:
  - Hyperglycemia
  - Glycosuria
  - Hypothalamic–pituitary–adrenal axis suppression, which could pose a threat in case of surgery, systemic illness, trauma, or injury
- Percutaneous absorption leads to systemic effects most likely with the following:
  - Higher potency types of agents
  - Inflamed skin (also in infants and children)
  - Long-term use or use over a large area of the skin
  - *Caution:* Occlusion markedly increases absorption of topical corticosteroids and

Table 30-5. Topical Corticosteroids

Relative potency	Generic name	Trade name	Strength
Low	Hydrocortisone	Cortaid, Cortizone	1% (OTC)
		Ala-Cort, Hytone	2.5% (prescription only)
Medium	Desonide	DesOwen	0.05%
	Fluocinolone acetonide	Synalar	0.01–0.025%
	Flurandrenolide	Cordran	0.025–0.05%
	Hydrocortisone butyrate	Locoid	0.1%
	Hydrocortisone valerate	Westcort	0.2%
	Triamcinolone acetonide	Aristocort	0.025%
High	Betamethasone valerate	Valisone, Dermabet	0.1%
	Fluocinolone	Synalar, Synemol	0.025%
	Triamcinolone acetonide	Aristocort	0.1%
Very high	Desoximetasone	Topicort	0.25%
	Diflorasone diacetate	ApexiCon	0.05%
	Fluocinonide	Lidex	0.01–0.05%
	Halcinonide	Halog	0.1%
Ultra-high	Betamethasone dipropionate	Diprosone, Maxivate	0.05%
	Betamethasone dipropionate (in optimized vehicle)	Diprolene AF	0.05%
	Clobetasol propionate	Temovate	0.05%
	Diflorasone diacetate	Psorcon	0.05%
	Halobetasol propionate	Ultravate	0.05%

should therefore be used cautiously in limited areas and reserved for severe, resistant lesions.

Topical antipruritics

Topical antipruritics include the following:

- Local anesthetics (benzocaine up to 20%, pramoxine 1%)
- Benzyl alcohol
- Colloidal oatmeal (e.g., Aveeno)
- Others (camphor, menthol, phenol)

Emollients

- Petrolatum
- Lanolin
- Mineral oil

Topical immunomodulators

Topical immunomodulators are approved for atopic dermatitis. They inhibit activation of T-cells and release of certain inflammatory mediators (cytokines).

The medication is applied twice daily, with improvement in 1–3 weeks. Side effects include stinging, burning, pruritus, and rare flu-like symptoms. Patients should be cautioned to use sunscreen.

Immunomodulator products are as follows:

- Tacrolimus (Protopic) 0.03% and 0.1% ointment
- Pimecrolimus (Elidel) 1% cream

Oral corticosteroids

Corticosteroids are the only systemic anti-inflammatory agents that are effective.

Oral antihistamines

Oral antihistamines have very limited effectiveness but are possibly antipruritic.

30-8. Poison Ivy, Poison Oak, and Poison Sumac Allergy (*Rhus* Dermatitis)

Allergic reaction occurs to sap (urushiol) of some plants of the genus *Rhus* (poison ivy, poison oak, poison sumac). *Rhus* dermatitis is the most common form of allergic contact dermatitis.

Direct contact with leaves, roots, or branches is not required to get a rash. Sap can reach skin indirectly from clothing, a pet, or burning (volatilization).

A *Rhus* allergy is acquired; individuals are not born with it. Most persons are sensitized to *Rhus* because it is such a common plant; however, some people are never allergic to it. No effective way exists to desensitize a person with an allergy to *Rhus* plants.

Types and Classification

- *Mild:* Localized patches of pruritus and erythema develop, followed by appearance of vesicles and papules on the upper or lower extremities.
- *Moderate:* Extensive pruritus and irritation develop, with severe vesicles and appearance of bullae and edematous swelling.
- *Severe:* Extreme pruritus, irritation, and severe vesicle and bullae formation appear. Extensive involvement occurs, widespread over the body, face, or both. Extensive edema of the extremities or face develops. Eye, genitalia, or mucous membrane are involved.

Clinical Presentation

- *Rhus* dermatitis is not contagious.
- Fluid in blisters does not spread the rash.
- Rash appears after a latent period that varies from 4 hours to 10 days, depending on an individual's sensitivity and the amount of plant contact.
- If more rash appears after treatment has begun, these are areas with a longer latent period.
- Symptoms may last from 5 to 21 days following initial rash.
- Secondary infections can occur if scratching excoriates the skin and the abrasions become infected.

Treatment Principles and Goals

Rhus dermatitis is self-limited. Mild cases will clear without treatment within 7–14 days.

The goal of treatment is to prevent itching, excessive scratching, and possible secondary skin infections.

Treatment options

- *Mild cases:* Use topical antipruritics, such as calamine, camphor, menthol, phenol, or local anesthetics to prevent itching and topical hydrocortisone cream or ointment.

- *Moderate cases:* Use topical high-potency corticosteroids for small areas.
- *Severe cases:* Use systemic corticosteroids daily up to 2 weeks. Severe rash needs systemic corticosteroids to ease the misery and disability. Systemic corticosteroids are usually needed during early severe stages because remedies applied to skin may not penetrate deeply enough.

Therapy

OTC topical therapy

Astringents and protectants

Compresses, soaks, or wet dressings will dry the oozing, reduce the weeping, aid in removal of crusts, and soothe the skin. They include

- Aluminum acetate solution 1:40 ratio (Burow's solution)
- Aluminum sulfate (Domeboro powder)
- Calamine lotion
- Other products such as aluminum hydroxide gel, kaolin, zinc acetate, zinc carbonate, and zinc oxide

Local anesthetics

These products may contain benzocaine up to 20%, pramoxine 1%, and benzyl alcohol. They include

- *Caladryl lotion:* Calamine and pramoxine 1%
- *Rhuli calamine spray:* Calamine, benzocaine, and camphor
- *Ivarest Poison Ivy Itch Cream:* Calamine, benzyl alcohol, and diphenhydramine 2%
- *Ivy-Dry Cream:* Benzyl alcohol, camphor, menthol, and zinc acetate

Other products

Other products include

- Hydrocortisone 1% products
- Colloidal oatmeal (e.g., Aveeno) for temporary skin protection from exposures
- Ethoxylate and sodium lauroyl sarcosinate surfactants wash (Zanfel)
- Cool compresses

Prescription topical therapy

Use topical medium- to high-potency corticosteroids (see discussion on allergic contact dermatitis in Section 30-7).

Prescription systemic corticosteroid therapy

Use of systemic corticosteroids is the only therapy that will actually reduce the severity and duration of the allergic response. See the discussion on allergic contact dermatitis in Section 30-7 and the discussion on endocrine disorders in Chapter 18 for complete details.

Effects of oral corticosteroids are dramatic (patients can take up to 40–100 mg prednisone for 2 or 3 weeks if necessary); however, many cases clear up quickly with a corticosteroid dosepak (e.g., Decadron or Medrol). Extremely severe cases or large-scale rash may require a parenteral dose of corticosteroid (100 mg prednisone equivalent).

Other recommendations

Prevention

- *Avoidance:* Identify the plants—"leaves of three, let it be."
- *Removal:* Washing with soap and water within 15 minutes of exposure may reduce the extent and duration of dermatitis.
- *Use of bentoquatam 5% solution:* Marketed under the trade name IvyBlock, this lotion is an organoclay. It is the only barrier product approved by the FDA. Patient instructions are to apply the lotion 15 minutes before possible plant contact and reapply every 4 hours.

30-9. Scaly Dermatoses

The three common forms of scaly dermatoses are dandruff, seborrhea, and psoriasis.

Dandruff

Dandruff is a chronic, noninflammatory scalp condition resulting in excessive scaling of the scalp epidermis. It is a common condition affecting 20% of the population. Though not a serious disorder, dandruff can be cosmetically unsightly.

Clinical presentation

Scaling and pruritus occur, causing white flakes to accumulate on the scalp.

Pathophysiology

Increased epidermal cell turnover rate of approximately twice the normal rate (time reduced from

25–30 days to 13–15 days) prevents complete keratinization of desquamated cells caused by unknown processes. Dandruff may be related to increased *Pityrosporum ovale* (*P. ovale*), a fungal scalp organism.

Treatment

Routine shampooing with mild hypoallergenic shampoo is essential.

Cytostatic agents

Cytostatic agents suppress cell turnover. The goal is to reduce the epidermal rate of turnover of scalp cells. Agents and their mechanisms of action are as follows:

- **ZPT (0.3–2%):** Products include Denorex, Head and Shoulders, X-Seb T, and Zincon. ZPT has an antifungal effect and reduces cell turnover rate.
- **Selenium sulfide 1%:** Products include Head and Shoulders Clinical Strength Shampoo and Selsun Blue Medicated Formula. Selenium sulfide reduces the cell rate turnover and inhibits growth of *P. ovale*.
- **Coal tar:** Products include Balnetar, Denorex, DHS Tar, Ionil T, Neutrogena T, Pentrax, and Polytar. Coal tar reduces the number and size of epidermal cells.

Patients should be counseled that contact time with cytostatic agents is very important for effectiveness. Advise patients to rub shampoo in well and leave it in up to 5 minutes before rinsing it out.

Keratolytic agents

Keratolytic agents include the following:

- **Salicylic acid (1.8–3%):** Products include Ionil, Neutrogena, Scalpicin, and Sebucare. Salicylic acid can lower the pH of tissues, thereby increasing the water concentration of epidermal cells, which softens and destroys the stratum corneum. It causes the upper skin layer to become inflamed and soft, followed by desquamation. This keratolytic action removes dandruff scales.
- **Sulfur (2–5%):** Products include Sulfoam, Sul-Ray, and Exsel. Sulfur possibly exerts an antifungal effect. Sulfur is usually found in combination with salicylic acid.
- **Combination of sulfur and salicylic acid:** Products include Meted and Sebulex.

Antifungals

Antifungals include the following:

- Ketoconazole (1%) shampoo (Nizoral A-D)
- Ciclopirox 1% shampoo (Loprox)

Ciclopirox is active against *P. ovale*. Patients should be counseled to use it twice weekly or every 3 or 4 days. Stress adequate contact time for a minimum of 3 minutes. Adverse effects include itching, stinging, or irritation.

Seborrhea (Seborrheic Dermatitis)

Seborrhea is a chronic inflammatory skin disease in areas of greatest sebaceous gland activity—on the scalp and other hairy areas such as the face, trunk, armpits, and groin. Seborrhea is not contagious. It persists for life, but it can be controlled.

Clinical presentation

- Scaling rash accompanied by pruritus
- Yellowish, greasy scales unlike the dry scales of dandruff
- Inflammation, often accompanied by erythema
- Fluctuation in severity, characterized by exacerbations and remissions
- Most common on the face, eyebrows, and eyelashes, but not on the extremities
- Aggravated and worsened by nervous stress and poor health

Pathophysiology

- Accelerated cell turnover rate is approximately three times the normal rate, probably as few as 9–10 days.
- Seborrhea has a higher cell turnover rate than dandruff, but less than psoriasis.
- *P. ovale* may be causative, but this theory is not universally accepted.

Treatment

Treatment is similar to that for dandruff, but seborrhea is more difficult to treat. Overuse of selenium can make the scalp oily and actually exacerbate seborrhea.

Topical corticosteroids (e.g., Cortaid) are used to control itching and inflammation (up to 7 days). Add the topical antifungal ketoconazole 1% shampoo (Nizoral AD) or ciclopirox 1% shampoo (Loprox).

The combination is active against *P. ovale*. Patients should be counseled to use it twice weekly, every 3 or 4 days. Stress adequate contact time; leave it in for at least 3 minutes. Adverse effects include itching, stinging, or irritation.

"Cradle cap" (infantile seborrheic dermatitis)

Cradle cap is seborrhea of the scalp in newborns or infants. It is most common in the first few months of life. It is usually on top of the head and may be due to poor washing.

Cradle cap is probably not related to fungal infection. It is treated as follows:

- Massage with oils.
- Use nonmedicated shampoos.
- Use milder keratolytics (Meted and Sebulex) two or three times per week.

Psoriasis

Psoriasis is a chronic, inflammatory papulosquamous erythematous skin disease. It is marked by the presence of silvery scales with sharply delineated edges. Lesions are usually localized but can gradually grow to cover large areas.

Psoriasis can have significant physiological and psychological effects. It affects 1–3% of the population, 98% Caucasian.

Classification

- *Type I:* Characterized by early age of onset, family history, and increased frequency of human lymphocyte antigen
- *Type II:* Characterized by development later in life and no family history

Clinical presentation

- Plaque is most common and is known as *psoriasis vulgaris.*
- Plaque is known also as *scales*—silvery on top and pink to red beneath.
- Plaque may be found anywhere on the body, but more likely on the scalp, sacral area, and extensor surfaces of knees and elbows (less common on face).
- Borders of plaque are sharp with inflammation surrounding the plaque.
- Psoriasis is a chronic condition and varies from mild forms of the disease to very severe, with

such extensive coverage that it hinders social and work life.

- It is marked by spontaneous exacerbations and remissions.

Pathophysiology

A hyperproliferative skin condition results from skin cell turnover rate of approximately 10–20 times the normal rate. Skin cells of psoriatic plaque reach the outermost layer in 3–4 days.

A genetic predisposition contributes, as well as exposure of the skin to trauma or triggering factors such as stressful incidents.

Treatment

Topical treatments
Topical treatments are as follows:

- Topical corticosteroids
- Coal tar (contained in Denorex, DHS Tar, Ionil T, MG217, Neutrogena T, Polytar, Tegrin, and X-Seb T Plus)
- Keratolytics (salicylic acid, sulfur)
- Combinations of salicylic acid, sulfur, and coal tar (Sebutone)
- Retinoids (tretinoin, adapalene, tazarotene, alitretinoin)
- Anthralin (Anthraforte, Anthranol, Dritho-Scalp)
- Calcipotriene (Dovonex ointment, cream, and solution—a vitamin D_3 analog)

Caution: If used in conjugation with PUVA (psoralens with ultraviolet A light) therapy, calcipotriene should be applied after light treatment, because PUVA inactivates this product.

Systemic treatment
Systemic treatment may involve the following:

- Oral corticosteroids
- Antimetabolites, such as methotrexate and cyclosporine
- Psoralens (combined with ultraviolet light therapy)
- Immunosuppressants, such as alefacept (Amevive), etanercept (Enbrel), and ustekinumab (Stelara)
- Retinoids, such as acitretin (Soriatane)

Vitamin A analogs are reserved for severe and extensive psoriasis. Their effectiveness approaches that of methotrexate or cyclosporine when combined with ultraviolet light therapy. Adverse effects include dry lips, skin, nail changes, dry eyes, hair loss, hyperlipidemia, pancreatitis, hepatotoxicity, myalgias, and arthralgias. Such drugs are teratogenic. These adverse effects are primarily with systemic therapy; however, topical therapy may also be teratogenic.

Other therapy
Ultraviolet light therapy is also used, often following coal tar applications or concurrent with oral psoralens.

30-10. Pediculosis

Head lice are the primary or most common form of pediculosis. Lice are very common, especially in schoolchildren. They are transmitted by direct contact with the head of an infected individual or through fomites (inanimate objects capable of transmitting disease, such as shared combs, brushes, hats, or scarves). Lice are most common in August and September, after long holidays or summer camps.

Body lice are a less common form that usually occur in individuals who do not change clothing often (e.g., the homeless).

Pubic lice (crab lice) are transferred through sexual contact and are found primarily in pubic areas, but they can also affect armpits.

Classification

The three types of human pediculosis are the following:

- **Head lice:** *Pediculus humanus capitis*
- **Body lice:** *Pediculus humanus corporis* (same species as head lice)
- **Pubic lice:** *Phthirus pubis* (different species)

Clinical Presentation

- Pruritus is the most common symptom.
- Because lice are often symptomatic, diagnosis is made visually by seeing live lice.
- The flat, gray-brown adult lice are difficult to locate or visualize; the nits (larvae) firmly attached to hair shafts may be more visible.

Drug Therapy

Synergized pyrethrins (0.17–0.33%)

This drug is a natural chemical derived from chrysanthemums that is synergized by the addition of 2–4% piperonyl butoxide (petroleum derivative). Trade names include A-200, Licide, Pronto Plus, and RID.

Mechanism of action
Transmission of nerve cell impulses is blocked in lice, causing paralysis.

Patient counseling
- Wash and dry hair, and apply for 10 minutes.
- Use a lice–nit comb to remove dead lice and nits following rinsing.
- Treat all family members.
- Avoid contact with the eyes, mouth, and nose.
- Do not use on irritated or inflamed scalp.
- Repeat treatment in 1 week to 10 days.

Adverse drug effects
Adverse effects include irritation, erythema, and itching.

Permethrin 1% and 5%

Permethrin is a synthetic chemical derivative of pyrethrin. Permethrin 1% is available under the trade name Nix Cream Rinse. Permethrin 5%, at prescription-only strength, is available under the trade names Acticin and Elimite Cream.

The 1% OTC-strength treatment is approved for head lice only; however, it is effective against pubic lice. The 5% prescription-strength treatment is approved for scabies (mites) infestation.

Patients prefer these treatments because of single-application effectiveness.

Mechanism of action
Transmission of nerve cell impulses is blocked in lice, causing paralysis.

Patient information
- Apply to washed hair and scalp.
- Leave on hair for 10 minutes, and then rinse.
- After rinsing, comb hair with a lice–nit comb to remove lice and nits.
- This is a one-time treatment; do not repeat within 10 days.
- All family members should be treated.

Adverse effects
Scalp irritation, pruritus, and stinging may occur. This medication is contraindicated in patients who are allergic to chrysanthemums and in children under 2 years of age.

Lindane (Kwell shampoo, cream, and lotion; prescription only)

Formerly named gamma benzene hexachloride, lindane is effective against head lice, pubic lice, and scabies (caused by *Sarcoptes scabiei*).

Adverse effects

Lindane is absorbed significantly through the skin and has been reported to have significant neurotoxic effects, especially in infants and children. Central nervous system effects reported include convulsions, dizziness, lack of coordination, restlessness, and irritability. Other effects include rapid heartbeat, muscle cramps, and vomiting.

The OTC medications are considered much safer, especially in children.

Nondrug recommendations

- Change clothing daily.
- Treat infested clothes, and shower daily.
- All household contacts should be inspected and treated if necessary.
- All bed linens and clothes should be dry-cleaned or washed in the hot water cycle and dried on the heated-air cycle for at least 20 minutes.
- Wash hairbrushes, combs, and toys in hot water for at least 10 minutes.
- Treat surrounding environment (bedding, pillows, carpets, draperies, furniture) with A-200 Control Spray or RID Control Spray.

30-11. Warts

Warts (*verrucae*) are harmless skin growths resulting from an infectious disease caused by the human papillomavirus.

Classification

- Common warts (*verruca vulgaris*) occur on the fingers, hands, and knees.
- Common flat warts (*verruca plana*) occur on the face, hands, and legs.
- Plantar warts (*verruca plantaris*) occur on the soles of the feet.
- Anogenital warts (*verruca genitalia*) occur in the anogenital area.

Clinical Presentation

- Warts are contagious and may spread on the body.
- Warts are more common in children and immuno-compromised patients.
- Warts on the face or hands protrude.
- Warts occurring on pressure areas such as the bottom of the feet (plantar warts) grow inward from the pressure of standing and walking, are often painful, and may be confused with corns.

Treatment Principles and Goals

Warts can be eliminated by the following:

- Direct application of caustics, such as salicylic acid, formalin, lactic acid, trichloroacetic acid, and podophyllin
- Freezing (cryotherapy) with liquid nitrogen or with dimethyl ether and propane
- Surgery

OTC drug therapy

Salicylic acid

Patients should be counseled as follows:

- Use topical salicylic acid preparations on a daily basis until the wart is removed.
- Because warts are contagious, use special care in washing hands before and after treatment, and use a separate towel for drying other parts of the body.
- Do not use salicylic acid on irritated, broken, or infected skin.
- If the wart remains after 12 weeks of continuous treatment, see a dermatologist or podiatrist.

Salicylic acid products are contraindicated in patients with diabetes and other patients with poor circulation because reduced sensation in the foot delays awareness of skin breakdown, allowing possible development of infection that can lead to sepsis. Diabetic patients should see a physician or podiatrist for removal of warts.

OTC salicylic acid products are as follows:

- ***Salicylic acid 17% in flexible collodion vehicle:*** Compound W gel and liquid, Dr. Scholl's Clear Away Fast-Acting Liquid, DuoFilm
- ***Salicylic acid 40% embedded in pads or discs:*** Compound W One Step Pads, Dr. Scholl's Clear Away Medicated Discs, DuoFilm, Dr. Scholl's Clear Away Wart Remover Medicated Discs

Cryotherapy

Dimethyl ether and propane is FDA approved for OTC removal of common warts and plantar warts.

Cryotherapy irritation leads the host to produce an immune response against the causative virus (similar to liquid nitrogen, which can be administered only by a primary care provider). As a result of freezing, a blister will form under the wart. After about 10 days, the frozen skin and wart fall off, revealing newly formed skin underneath.

Cryotherapy products are as follows:

- *Dimethyl ether and propane:* Dr. Scholl's Freeze Away Wart Remover and Wartner Cryogenic Wart Removal System are approved for removal of common warts.
- *Dimethyl ether, propane, and isobutane:* Compound W Freeze Off is approved for removal of common warts and plantar warts.

Patient instructions are as follows:

- Place the applicator in the spray can, which becomes very cold (−55°C).
- After the applicator is saturated, hold it on the wart for a product-specific time period to freeze the wart (20 seconds for Wartner; 40 seconds for Compound W).
- The process may be repeated after 10 days as many as three or four times for persistent warts.
- *Caution:* Do not use in children under 4 years of age, diabetics, or pregnant or breastfeeding females; on the face, armpits, breasts, buttocks, or genitals; on irritated skin; or on mucous membranes (e.g., mouth, nose, anus).

30-12. Corns and Calluses

Corns and calluses are excessive growths of the upper keratinized layer of the skin. They are more common in women than in men.

Diabetics have an increased incidence of calluses on their feet because of the loss of sensation, preventing them from noticing the pressure that would otherwise be uncomfortable.

Classification

- *Hard corns (heloma durum):* Corns overlying a bony prominence such as the toes or bottom of the heel
- *Soft corns (heloma molle; interdigital corns):* Corns between the toes (especially the fourth and fifth)

- *Calluses (callosities):* Superficial patches of hornified epidermis; flattened, but thickened with no central core

Clinical Presentation and Pathophysiology

Corns and calluses are caused by excessive growth of the upper keratinized layer of the skin (hyperkeratosis), resulting from friction or pressure, usually from improper or tight-fitting shoes.

Treatment

The only FDA-approved OTC medication is salicylic acid formulated in flexible collodion, plasters, disks, or pads.

Mechanism of action

Salicylic acid produces a keratolytic action, which increases hydration and lowers the pH of the outer skin, initially softening and then destroying the outer layer of skin.

Patient counseling

- Do not apply to irritated, infected, or reddened skin.
- If discomfort persists after using for 14 days, see a physician or podiatrist.
- Salicylic acid products are contraindicated in diabetics.

Adverse drug effects

Salicylic acid products are contraindicated in patients with diabetes and other patients with poor circulation because reduced sensation in the foot delays awareness of skin breakdown, allowing possible development of infection that can lead to sepsis. Refer diabetics to a physician or podiatrist for removal of corns or calluses.

OTC salicylic acid (SA) corn and callus products

- Freezone Corn and Callus Remover 13.6% SA
- Freezone One Step Corn Remover 40% SA
- Curad Mediplast 40% SA plaster, cut to size
- Mosco Callus and Corn Remover 17.6% SA
- Off Ezy Corn and Callus Remover 17% SA
- One Step Callus Remover 40% SA
- Dr. Scholl's Liquid Corn/Callus Remover 12.6% SA
- Dr. Scholl's One Step Corn or Callus Remover Discs 40% SA

30-13. Questions

1. Which of the following is most appropriate for treatment of type II (papular) acne?

   A. Oral antimicrobials
   B. Isotretinoin
   C. Oral corticosteroids
   D. Topical retinoids
   E. Coal tar

2. Which of the following is the most appropriate therapy for a patient with type II acne who is unable to tolerate topical retinoids?

   A. Topical dapsone
   B. Oral clindamycin
   C. Topical tazarotene
   D. Isotretinoin
   E. Oral doxycycline

3. Which of the following is an important counseling point for patients using topical retinoids such as tretinoin (Retin-A)?

   A. Use this product twice daily for the first 2 weeks.
   B. Expect rapid improvement within 2 or 3 days of starting therapy.
   C. Astringents should be used before using this product.
   D. Use sunblock before exposure to sunlight.
   E. Product works best if followed with aggressive exfoliating scrub.

4. Which of the following is the most common side effect of isotretinoin (Accutane)?

   A. Cheilitis (dry, chapped lips)
   B. Acute depression
   C. Decreased night vision
   D. Thinning hair
   E. Insomnia

5. Which of the following is an important contraindication and precaution to the use of isotretinoin?

   A. Hypertension
   B. Migraines
   C. Allergic rhinitis
   D. Pregnancy
   E. Streptococcal infections

6. Which of the following is the most efficacious nonprescription topical antifungal?

   A. Tolnaftate (Tinactin)
   B. Terbinafine (Lamisil)
   C. Miconazole (Micatin)
   D. Undecylenic acid (Desenex)
   E. Clotrimazole (Lotrimin AF)

7. Which of the following fungal infections may be treated effectively with the use of topical antifungal agents?

   I. Tinea capitis (ringworm of the scalp)
   II. Tinea unguium (fungal infection of the toenails and fingernails)
   III. Tinea corporis (ringworm of the skin)

   A. I only
   B. II only
   C. III only
   D. I and II only
   E. I, II, and III

8. Tinea pedis is also known as

   A. athlete's foot.
   B. jock itch.
   C. onychomycosis.
   D. ringworm of the scalp.
   E. ringworm of the skin.

9. The treatment of choice for tinea unguium is

   A. clotrimazole.
   B. miconazole.
   C. undecylenic acid.
   D. griseofulvin.
   E. tolnaftate.

10. All of the following are true regarding the patient instructions for the proper use of minoxidil *except*

    A. it should be applied on the scalp and left for 4 hours for maximum effect.
    B. the patient should not swim, shampoo, or walk in rain soon after the application of minoxidil.
    C. it should not be used on infected, irritated, inflamed, or sunburned skin.
    D. the patient must continue therapy to maintain effectiveness.
    E. women with alopecia should use the 5% strength preparation of minoxidil rather than the 2% strength.

11. Which of the following is a common adverse effect of minoxidil?

    A. Dermatitis and pruritus of the scalp
    B. Hepatic damage
    C. Chest pain
    D. Dizziness
    E. Hypertension

12. The mechanism of action of finasteride (Propecia) to reduce male baldness is

    A. a direct effect on hair follicles to deepen hair roots.
    B. inhibition of the enzyme 5-a-reductase, which blocks the conversion of testosterone to dihydrotestosterone.
    C. increased cutaneous blood flow to the hair follicles on the scalp because of vasodilation.
    D. increased cutaneous blood flow to the hair follicles on the scalp because of opening the potassium channel.
    E. increased development of new hair follicles on the scalp.

13. All of the following regarding dry skin are true *except*

    A. it occurs primarily in older adults.
    B. it occurs most commonly in the summer months.
    C. it is caused by decreasing sebum production and decreased moisture-binding capacity of the skin.
    D. flaking, scaling, xerosis, and pruritus are common manifestations of dry skin.
    E. excessive cleansing and bathing removes lipids and worsens dry skin.

14. All of the following statements are true regarding the treatment of dry skin *except*

    A. hydrocortisone should be used only for short-term therapy of dry skin to relieve itching.
    B. urea-containing products improve the skin's moisture-binding capacity.
    C. lactic acid is a keratolytic agent that removes the upper epidermal skin cells and relieves the itching of dry skin.
    D. emollients and moisturizers are helpful in the treatment of dry skin, especially when applied immediately after bathing.

    E. although colloidal oatmeal may be helpful in the treatment of dry skin, patients should be cautioned about the possibility of falling because of a slippery bathtub.

15. The agents of choice for the initial treatment of contact dermatitis, whether irritant or allergic, are

    A. topical antihistamines.
    B. oral antihistamines.
    C. topical corticosteroids.
    D. local anesthetics.
    E. coal tar products.

16. An increase in topical corticosteroid systemic absorption with subsequent systemic side effects may be seen in which of the following?

    A. Occlusion
    B. Lower potency agents
    C. Use over smaller areas of skin
    D. Adults
    E. Application to the palms of hands or soles of feet

17. All of the following are true regarding poison ivy *except*

    A. it is an example of allergic contact dermatitis.
    B. it is the result of contact with the sap of plants of the genus *Rhus*.
    C. the treatment of choice is desensitization.
    D. it may be caused by direct or indirect contact (e.g., with clothing or pets).
    E. skin eruptions may occur from several hours up to 10 days following contact with the plants.

18. The treatment of choice for severe or extensive cases of poison ivy or poison oak is

    A. a local anesthetic such as benzocaine.
    B. bentoquatam (in IvyBlock).
    C. a camphor and menthol antipruritic.
    D. colloidal oatmeal.
    E. a systemic corticosteroid.

19. Which of the following agents for the treatment of dandruff is a cytostatic agent that suppresses cell rate turnover?

    A. Salicylic acid (Ionil)
    B. Sulfur (Sulfoam)
    C. Ciclopirox (Loprox)

D. Zinc pyrithione (Head and Shoulders)
E. Ketoconazole (Nizoral A–D)

20. All of the following statements are true regarding seborrhea *except*

    A. it is a chronic inflammatory skin disease seen in areas of greatest sebaceous gland activity.
    B. it fluctuates in severity and is worsened by stress and poor health.
    C. moderate to severe cases require topical corticosteroids or the topical antifungal ketoconazole for effective treatment.
    D. it is called *cradle cap* when it occurs in infants.
    E. it most commonly occurs on the legs and arms.

21. Which of the following are characteristic of psoriasis?

    I. Chronic inflammation
    II. Silvery scales (known as *plaques*) with sharply delineated edges
    III. Spontaneous exacerbations and remissions

    A. I only
    B. II only
    C. III only
    D. I and II only
    E. I, II, and III

22. Treatment of advanced psoriasis may require topical therapy combined with which of the following systemic agents?

    I. Corticosteroids
    II. Antimetabolites such as methotrexate
    III. Anthralin

    A. I only
    B. II only
    C. III only
    D. I and II only
    E. I, II, and III

23. All of the following are true statements regarding head lice (*Pediculus humanus capitis*) *except*

    A. it occurs most commonly in elementary schoolchildren.
    B. it occurs most commonly in the spring months of April and May.
    C. it is transmitted by direct contact.
    D. pruritus is the most common symptom.

    E. head lice are the most common type of pediculosis infestation.

24. All of the following statements are true regarding treatment of pediculosis with synergized pyrethrins (piperonyl butoxide and pyrethrins) *except*

    A. inspect all family contacts, and treat if necessary.
    B. apply after washing and drying the hair, and leave on overnight.
    C. remove dead lice and nits after treatment with a lice or nit comb.
    D. repeat treatment in 7–10 days.
    E. avoid contact with the eyes, nose, and mouth.

25. The most effective nonprescription agent for treatment of head lice is which of the following agents?

    A. Permethrin (Nix)
    B. Synergized pyrethrins (A-200)
    C. Lindane (Kwell)
    D. Ketoconazole
    E. Salicylic acid

26. Nonprescription products for the treatment of corns and warts contain which of the following agents?

    A. Salicylic acid
    B. Ketoconazole
    C. Lactic acid
    D. Acetylsalicylic acid
    E. Hydrocortisone

27. All of the following are true statements regarding corns *except*

    A. they are excess growths of the upper keratinized layer of skin.
    B. salicylic acid is available in pads, disks, or flexible collodion for removal of corns.
    C. self-treatment for corns or warts with OTC agents is not recommended for diabetic patients because of the reduced sensation in their feet, which delays awareness of development of infections that may lead to sepsis.
    D. they are contagious and may spread on the body.
    E. they are usually caused by pressure or friction from improper or tight-fitting shoes.

28. All of the following are true statements regarding warts *except*

    A. they result from infection with the human papillomavirus.
    B. they are contagious.
    C. they may spread on the body.
    D. plantar warts are located on the fingers, hands, and knees.
    E. they are more common in children and immunocompromised patients.

30-14. Answers

1. **D.** Topical retinoids are the agents of choice for type II acne. Oral antibiotics should be initiated in type III acne, and isotretinoin (Accutane) is reserved for nodulocystic acne (type IV acne), which, if left untreated, will lead to extensive scarring. Systemic corticosteroids should not be used continuously because they may worsen acne.

2. **A.** Topical dapsone is a good option for patients who are unable to tolerate topical retinoids because it has anti-inflammatory and antimicrobial properties. Topical tazarotene is the most irritating retinoid. Systemic therapies such as oral antibiotics or isotretinoin would not be appropriate for type II acne.

3. **D.** Topical retinoid therapy will sensitize skin to ultraviolet light rays; therefore, patients should use sunblock before sun exposure. Topical retinoids should be used every other day for the first 2 weeks, then nightly. Patients using topical retinoids should use only mild soaps for cleansing the face and avoid astringents, drying agents, and abrasive soaps. Improvement will usually occur within 2–3 weeks after initiation of therapy.

4. **A.** Cheilitis (dry, chapped lips), together with dry skin and dry eyes, are the most common side effects of isotretinoin therapy.

5. **D.** Isotretinoin is contraindicated in pregnancy because of the high incidence of serious birth defects.

6. **B.** Terbinafine (Lamisil) is the most effective nonprescription topical antifungal.

7. **C.** Topical antifungal agents are the first line of therapy against tinea corporis (ringworm of the skin). However, systemic antifungal therapy is usually required for treatment of tinea capitis (ringworm of the scalp) and tinea unguium (fungal infection of the toenails and fingernails).

8. **A.** Tinea pedis is also known as athlete's foot.

9. **D.** The treatment of choice for tinea unguium (fungal infection of the toenails and fingernails) is a systemic antifungal agent such as griseofulvin. Topical therapy is generally not effective for fungal infections of the nails.

10. **E.** Women with alopecia should use only the 2% strength preparation of minoxidil. Studies indicate that there is no greater degree of effectiveness with the 5% strength preparation, and the incidence of adverse effects (including increased growth of facial hair) is much greater in women using the 5% preparation.

11. **A.** Common adverse effects of minoxidil include hypertrichosis (increased hair growth in areas other than the scalp) and dermatitis and pruritus of the scalp. Systemic side effects such as chest pain, increased heart rate, and dizziness with topical minoxidil are rare and do not include hepatic damage.

12. **B.** The mechanism of action of finasteride to reduce male baldness is blocking of the conversion of testosterone to dihydrotestosterone by inhibiting the enzyme 5-α-reductase.

13. **B.** Dry skin occurs most commonly in the winter months and is often referred to as *winter rash*.

14. **C.** Lactic acid is used in the treatment of dry skin, not as a keratolytic agent, but as an agent that increases skin hydration.

15. **C.** Topical corticosteroids are the agents of choice for the initial treatment of irritant or allergic contact dermatitis. If the condition is severe or widespread, oral corticosteroids may be useful. Oral or topical antihistamines have minimal effect in the course of the treatment of contact dermatitis, possibly producing some antipruritic effect, but not affecting the course of the condition.

16. **A.** Topical corticosteroid systemic absorption is increased on infants' and children's skin and with occlusion, long-term use, and use of high-potency agents. Systemic corticosteroids' adverse effects may be severe and include adrenocortical suppression.

17. **C.** Desensitization has no place in the treatment of poison ivy, and most studies indicate desensitization is not an effective method to prevent poison ivy.

18. **E.** Systemic corticosteroids are the treatment of choice for severe or extensive cases of poison ivy or poison oak. Topical agents are limited in effectiveness and do not alter the course of the condition.

19. **D.** Zinc pyrithione (Head and Shoulders) and selenium sulfide (Selsun Blue) are cytostatic agents used in the treatment of dandruff that suppress cell rate turnover. Salicylic acid is a keratolytic agent. Ciclopirox is an antifungal agent.

20. **E.** Seborrhea most commonly occurs on the face, especially eyebrows and eyelashes, but not on the extremities.

21. **E.** Psoriasis is a chronic inflammatory disease marked by silvery scales (known as *plaques*) with sharp delineated edges and is characterized by spontaneous exacerbations and remissions.

22. **D.** Treatment of advanced psoriasis may require topical therapy combined with either oral corticosteroids or antimetabolites such as methotrexate.

23. **B.** Head lice occur most commonly in the months of August and September.

24. **B.** Synergized pyrethrins should be applied after washing and drying the hair and left on for 10 minutes, not overnight.

25. **A.** Permethrin (Nix) does not have to be repeated in 7–10 days as does the other available nonprescription pediculicidal agent, synergized pyrethrins (A-200). Lindane (Kwell) is not available over the counter, and significant neurologic toxicities have been reported with its use.

26. **A.** Nonprescription products for the treatment of corns and warts contain salicylic acid as the active therapeutic agent.

27. **D.** Corns are not contagious and will not spread on the body. Corns are an excess growth of the upper keratinized layer of skin, usually caused by pressure or friction from improper or tight-fitting shoes. Salicylic acid is available OTC for removal of corns in pads, disks, or flexible collodion. Self-treatment for corns or warts with OTC agents is not recommended for diabetic patients because of the reduced sensation in their feet, which delays awareness of the development of infections that could lead to sepsis.

28. **D.** Plantar warts are not located on the fingers, hands, or knees; they are located on the soles of the feet.

30-15. References

Arndt KA, Hsu J. *Manual of Dermatologic Therapeutics.* 7th ed. Philadelphia, PA: Lippincott Williams & Wilkins; 2006.

Burns T, Breathnach S, Cox N, et al., eds. *Rook's Textbook of Dermatology.* 8th ed. Oxford, UK: Wiley-Blackwell; 2010.

Covington, TR. *Nonprescription Drug Therapy: Guiding Patient Self-Care.* 6th ed. St. Louis, MO: Wolters-Kluwer/Facts & Comparisons; 2007.

DiPiro JT, Talbert RL, Yee GC, et al., eds. *Pharmacotherapy: A Pathophysiologic Approach.* 9th ed. New York, NY: McGraw-Hill Medical; 2014.

Epstein E. *Common Skin Disorders.* 6th ed. Philadelphia, PA: WB Saunders; 2001.

Fitzpatrick JE, Morelli JG. *Dermatology Secrets in Color.* 3rd ed. Philadelphia, PA: Mosby Elsevier; 2007.

Goldsmith LA, Katz S, Gilchrest B, et al., eds. *Fitzpatrick's Dermatology in General Medicine.* 8th ed. New York, NY: McGraw-Hill; 2012.

Habif TP, Campbell JL, Chapman MS, et al. *Skin Disease: Diagnosis and Treatment.* 3rd ed. Edinburgh, UK: Elsevier Saunders; 2011.

Helms RA, Quan DJ, Herfindal ET, et al., eds. *Textbook of Therapeutics.* 8th ed. Philadelphia, PA: Lippincott Williams & Wilkins; 2006.

James WD, Berger TG, Elston DM, et al., eds. *Andrew's Diseases of the Skin: Clinical Dermatology.* 11th ed. Philadelphia, PA: Saunders Elsevier; 2011.

Krinsky, DL, Berardi RR, Ferreri SP, et al., eds. *Handbook of Nonprescription Drugs.* 17th ed. Washington, DC: American Pharmacists Association; 2012.

Pray WS. *Nonprescription Product Therapeutics.* 2nd ed. Philadelphia, PA: Lippincott Williams & Wilkins; 2006.

Wolverton SE, ed. *Comprehensive Dermatologic Drug Therapy.* 3rd ed. Philadelphia, PA: Saunders Elsevier; 2012.

Nonprescription Medications

Amanda Howard-Thompson

31-1. Key Points

Cough, Cold, and Allergy

- Cough and cold products are not to be used in children < 4 years of age.
- Nonprescription drug therapy for the common cold includes symptomatic management using decongestants (nasal congestion), antihistamines (excess nasal discharge), analgesics (headache), and local anesthetic lozenges or sprays (pharyngitis).
- Nonprescription treatment of allergies includes systemic antihistamines (sedating or nonsedating), ocular antihistamines, decongestants (if nasal congestion), and intranasal steroids and cromolyn (scheduled, not as needed).
- Cough can be relieved by a product containing a cough suppressant (dextromethorphan). An expectorant (guaifenesin) should be recommended to enhance clearance of mucus.

Constipation

- Diet and lifestyle changes should always be recommended to prevent or treat constipation (exercise and an increase in fiber and fluid intake).
- Bulk-forming laxatives and stool softeners are the safest products to prevent and treat constipation and can be used chronically.
- Stimulant laxatives should be used only occasionally to prevent laxative dependence or other complications.

Diarrhea

- Loperamide or bismuth subsalicylate may be recommended to treat diarrhea.

- Maintaining adequate hydration is very important, especially in young children and elderly patients.

Nausea and Vomiting

- Nonprescription treatment options for nausea and vomiting include antihistamines (meclizine, dimenhydrinate) and phosphorated carbohydrate solution (Emetrol).
- Histamine 2–receptor antagonists (H2RAs) (cimetidine, ranitidine); antacids; or bismuth subsalicylate (Pepto-Bismol) may relieve gastric discomfort or indigestion.

Pain and Fever

- Pain and fever may be treated with aspirin and other salicylates, nonsteroidal anti-inflammatory drugs (NSAIDs), or acetaminophen.
- Aspirin and NSAIDs inhibit platelet aggregation. Nonacetylated salicylates and acetaminophen do not have antiplatelet activity.
- Salicylates and NSAIDs can cause gastropathy, including gastritis, gastric ulcers, and gastric bleeding. They may decrease the effectiveness of some antihypertensives and may have deleterious effects on kidney function.
- Acetaminophen does not have anti-inflammatory activity.

Ophthalmic Disorders

- Dry eyes can be treated with artificial tears or ocular emollients.
- Ophthalmic vasoconstrictors (ocular decongestants) cause vasoconstriction in the conjunctiva to treat redness. Naphazoline is the ocular

decongestant of choice. Ocular decongestants are contraindicated in patients with narrow-angle glaucoma because of the potential to cause rebound.

■ Ketotifen fumarate is the safest and most effective product for the treatment of allergic conjunctivitis. Twice-daily dosing and safety of this product for children ≥ 3 years of age make it the primary therapy for patients with this condition.

Otic Disorders

■ Impacted cerumen can be treated with cerumen-softening agents (carbamide peroxide in anhydrous glycerin + alcohol; hydrogen peroxide + water).
■ Water-clogged ears may be managed with the commercial preparation of isopropyl alcohol + anhydrous glycerin or with compounded acetic acid + isopropyl alcohol.

Smoking Cessation

■ First-line nonprescription agents for pharmacotherapy in smoking cessation are as follows:
  • Nicotine gum (Nicorette, generic)
  • Nicotine lozenge (Commit, generic)
  • Nicotine patch (Nicotrol, Nicoderm CQ)
■ Contraindications and precautions for nicotine replacement therapy are as follows:
  • Cardiovascular disease
    ▪ < 2 weeks postmyocardial infarction
    ▪ Serious arrhythmias
    ▪ Serious or worsening angina
  • Esophagitis and peptic ulcer disease (gum)
■ Patients should seek medical advice if pregnant or breast-feeding.
■ Patients should not smoke while using nicotine replacement therapy.

Overweight and Obese

■ The number of overweight and obese persons in the United States has reached epidemic proportions. These conditions are significant because they are associated with increased morbidity from cardiovascular disease, diabetes, gall bladder disease, osteoarthritis, respiratory problems, and several different types of cancer.
■ Orlistat (alli) is a nonprescription medication approved by the U.S. Food and Drug Administration (FDA) for the treatment of overweight patients ≥ 18 years of age. This medication has many side effects that patients may find

unpleasant, and as a result, patients should be counseled on these side effects and ways to avoid them. The use of this medication may decrease the absorption of fat-soluble vitamins from the (gastrointestinal) GI tract.

Overactive Bladder

■ Oxytrol for Women (oxybutynin) with a transdermal delivery system is indicated in women ≥ 18 years of age. The full benefit of this medication is seen in about 2 weeks. When oxybutynin is combined with daily lifestyle modifications (timed urination, pelvic floor exercises, fluid management), studies indicate a reduction of urinary accidents by 75% with Oxytrol-TDS versus 50% with a placebo. Patients must be counseled regarding anticholinergic side effects.

Home Monitoring and Testing Devices

■ When counseling patients on the use of these devices, one must ensure that they understand the directions for use (appropriate timing, causes of false-positive and false-negative results), check for expiration dates, and make certain the product is developed to give them the results they are seeking.

Natural and Herbal Products

■ Herbal products that should be stopped 7–10 days prior to surgery include ginkgo, garlic, and ginseng.
■ Note typical side effects and interactions associated with the use of the dietary supplements discussed.

31-2. Study Guide Checklist

The following topics may guide your study of this subject area:

■ Recognize conditions that are self-treatable with nonprescription drugs.
■ Assess patients' needs, risk factors, and potential for adverse events.
■ Assist patients with product selection.
■ Advise and counsel patients on therapeutic options and outcomes of therapy.
■ Monitor patients regarding their medications and related therapy.
■ Understand relevant diet, nutrition, and nondrug therapies.

31-3. Cough, Cold, and Allergy

Cough

Pathophysiology

A cough is an important defense mechanism to rid the airways of mucus and foreign bodies. A cough may be acute (< 3 weeks duration) or chronic (> 3 weeks duration).

Nonprescription treatment

Antitussives and cough suppressants
Antitussives and cough suppressants may be narcotic or nonnarcotic. Table 31-1 shows selected examples of nonprescription cough products.

Codeine
Codeine, a narcotic, is the gold standard of antitussives:

- *Availability:* Without prescription in some states
- *Mechanism of action:* Centrally mediated suppression of cough
- *Adult dose:* 10–20 mg q4–6h (120 mg/day maximum)
- *Role in therapy:* Primarily for night cough
- *Side effects:* Sedation, nausea, and constipation

Dextromethorphan
Dextromethorphan is the only category I over-the-counter (OTC) nonnarcotic antitussive:

- *Mechanism of action:* Centrally mediated suppression of cough

- *Adult dosage:* 10–30 mg q4–8h (120 mg/day maximum)
- *Role in therapy:* Nonproductive cough
- *Side effects:* Drowsiness, gastrointestinal (GI) effects
- *Drug interactions:* Monoamine oxidase (MAO) inhibitors

Diphenhydramine
Diphenhydramine is a category II antitussive:

- *Mechanism of action:* Centrally mediated suppression of cough center and anticholinergic
- *Adult dosage:* 25 mg q4h (75 mg/day maximum)

Expectorant
Guaifenesin is the only category I OTC expectorant:

- *Mechanism of action:* Thinning of mucus to enhance clearance
- *Adult dosage:*
  - Immediate-release: 200–400 mg q4h (maximum 2,400 mg/day)
  - Extended-release: 600–1,200 mg q12h (maximum 2,400 mg/day)
- *Role in therapy:* Productive cough
- *Side effects:* GI discomfort
- *Patient education:* Increase fluid intake.

Topical antitussives
Of the volatile oils, only camphor and menthol are approved by the U.S. Food and Drug Administration (FDA):

- *Mechanism of action:* Local anesthetic effect in nasal mucosa

Table 31-1. Selected Examples of Nonprescription Cough Products

Type of product	Generic name	Action	Trade name
Expectorant	Guaifenesin	Immediate release	Robitussin Chest Congestion Syrup (100 mg/5 mL)
		Extended release	Mucinex tablets (600 mg)
Cough suppressant	Dextromethorphan HBr	Immediate release	Vicks DayQuil Cough (15 mg/15 mL)
	Dextromethorphan polistirex	Extended release	Delsym suspension (30 mg/5 mL)
Combination expectorant and cough suppressant	Guaifenesin and dextromethorphan HBr		Robitussin Cough + Chest Congestion DM (100 mg/10 mg per 5 mL)
			Mucinex DM (600 mg/30 mg, 1,200 mg/60 mg tablets)
			Alka-Seltzer Plus Max Cough, Mucus, and Congestion 200 mg/10 mg capsules
Combination expectorant, cough suppressant, and decongestant	Guaifenesin, dextromethorphan HBr, and phenylephrine HCl		Robitussin Multi-Symptom Cold (100 mg/10 mg/5 mg per 5 mL)

- ■ *Product availability:* Lozenge, ointment, steam inhalation
- ■ *Patient education:* Ointment and solution are toxic if ingested.

Sore throat remedies

Sore throat remedies include the following:

- ■ Saline gargle
- ■ Sprays and lozenges:
  - • *Benzocaine:* Chloraseptic and Cepacol lozenges
  - • *Dyclonine:* Sucrets Maximum Strength lozenges
  - • *Phenol:* Chloraseptic spray
  - • *Menthol:* Vicks VapoDrops

Special populations

Pregnancy
- ■ Dextromethorphan is viewed as probably safe.

Lactation
- ■ Dextromethorphan, guaifenesin, and topical anesthetics are all low risk.
- ■ Patients may want to avoid diphenhydramine because it is excreted into breast milk and may also decrease milk production.

Common Cold

Clinical presentation

- ■ Sore throat, nasal symptoms, watery eyes, sneezing, cough, malaise, and low-grade fever occur.
- ■ There is a gradual onset with slow progression.
- ■ Duration is 1–2 weeks.

Prevention

- ■ Frequent hand cleansing
- ■ Sanitizers

Treatment

Nonpharmacologic therapy
- ■ Humidifiers
- ■ Increased fluid intake
- ■ Rest
- ■ Propping head upright
- ■ Rubber bulb nasal syringe for children < 4 years of age
- ■ Irrigation of nose with saline drops or mist

Nonprescription medication treatment (symptomatic)
- ■ Decongestants for nasal congestion
- ■ Antihistamines used in combination with a decongestant for excess nasal discharge (not effective as monotherapy for treatment of colds)

- ■ Analgesics for related pain or headaches
- ■ Local anesthetic lozenges or sprays for sore throat (pharyngitis)

Allergic Rhinitis

Clinical presentation

- ■ *Nasal:* Congestion, rhinorrhea, nasal pruritus, sneezing, postnasal drip
- ■ *Ocular:* Itching, lacrimation, redness, irritation
- ■ *General:* Headache, malaise, mood swings, irritability

Treatment

Nonpharmacologic therapy
Patients should avoid the offending allergens:

- ■ Limit outside exposure during periods of high pollen.
- ■ Avoid indoor and outdoor mold.
- ■ Avoid dust, especially in the bedroom.
- ■ Avoid pet dander, especially from cats.

Nonprescription Therapy for Treatment of the Common Cold and Allergies

Selected products for treating the common cold and allergies are shown in Tables 31-2, 31-3, and 31-4.

Antihistamines

Selected antihistamines are described in Table 31-2.

Table 31-2. Selected Nonprescription Antihistamine Products

Generic name	Trade name	Adult dosage (maximum daily dose)
Chlorpheniramine maleate	Chlor-Trimeton	4 mg q4–6h (24 mg)
Diphenhydramine HCl	Benadryl	25–50 mg q4–6h (300 mg)
Clemastine	Tavist[a]	1.34 mg q12h (2.68 mg)
Fexofenadine HCl	Allegra, Mucinex Allergy	60 mg q12h or 180 mg daily (180 mg)
Loratadine	Claritin, Alavert	10 mg daily
Cetirizine HCl	Zyrtec	10 mg daily

a. Brand name is no longer manufactured in the United States.

Table 31-3. Selected Nonprescription Oral Decongestant Products

Generic name	Products	Comments	Adult dosage (maximum daily dose)
Phenylephrine HCl	Sudafed PE	Weakest oral decongestant	10 mg q4h (60 mg)
Pseudoephedrine HCl	Sudafed	Less central nervous system stimulation	60 mg q4–6h (240 mg)

Pharmacology
- Antihistamines are H_1-receptor antagonists.
- First-generation antihistamines are nonselective and sedating.
- Second-generation antihistamines are peripherally selective and have a low incidence of sedation.

Side effects
- Sedation (primarily with first-generation antihistamines)
- Anticholinergic effects
  - Dry mouth
  - Dry eyes
  - Urinary retention
  - Constipation
- Paradoxical stimulation in some children and elderly patients

Precautions and contraindications
- Do not drive or operate heavy machinery.
- Avoid use with alcohol.
- Prostatic hyperplasia can occur.
- Narrow-angle glaucoma is possible.

Intranasal corticosteroid

Triamcinolone acetonide (Nasacort Allergy 24HR) pharmacology
- Decreases the influx of inflammatory cells and inhibits the release of cytokines, thereby reducing inflammation of the nasal mucosa

Table 31-4. Selected Nonprescription Cold, Allergy, and Sinus Combination Products

Product	Trade name	Primary ingredients
Decongestant and analgesic	Aleve-D Sinus & Cold	Pseudoephedrine 120 mg + naproxen 220 mg
	Advil Cold and Sinus	Pseudoephedrine 30 mg + ibuprofen 200 mg
	Sudafed 12 Hour Pressure + Pain	Pseudoephedrine 120 mg + naproxen 220 mg
	Sudafed PE Pressure + Pain	Phenylephrine HCl 5 mg + acetaminophen 325 mg
	Advil Congestion Relief	Phenylephrine HCl 10 mg + ibuprofen 200 mg
Antihistamine, decongestant, and analgesic	Alka-Seltzer Plus Night Severe Cold, Cough and Flu	Diphenhydramine 25 mg + phenylephrine 10 mg + acetaminophen 650 mg per packet
	Advil Allergy and Congestion Relief	Chlorpheniramine maleate 4 mg + Phenylephrine 10 mg + ibuprofen 200 mg
Antihistamine, decongestant, analgesic, and cough suppressant	Vicks Dayquil Cold and Flu LiquiCaps	Phenylephrine HCl 5 mg + acetaminophen 325 mg + dextromethorphan HBr 10 mg
	Alka-Seltzer Plus Cold and Cough Effervescent Tablets	Chlorpheniramine 4 mg + phenylephrine 15.6 mg + aspirin 650 mg + dextromethorphan 20 mg per dose
Antihistamine and decongestant	Allerest PE	Chlorpheniramine 4 mg + phenylephrine 10 mg
	Dimetapp Cold and Allergy Syrup	Brompheniramine maleate 1 mg + phenylephrine HCl 2.5 mg per 5 mL
	Zyrtec D	Cetirizine HCl 5 mg + pseudoephedrine HCl 120 mg
	Claritin-D 12 Hour	Loratadine 5 mg + pseudoephedrine 120 mg
	Claritin-D 24 Hour	Loratadine 10 mg + pseudoephedrine sulfate 240 mg
	Allegra-D 12 Hour	Fexofenadine HCl 60 mg + pseudoephedrine HCl 120 mg

- Considered first-line therapy for moderate to severe allergic rhinitis
- More effective than antihistamines, especially for treatment of late allergic rhinitis symptoms such as nasal congestion

Dosing
- Age 2–12 years: Initiate at 1 spray in each nostril daily (110 mcg/day).
  - If symptoms are not relieved:
    - Age 2–5: Refer to primary care provider (PCP).
    - Age 6–12: Increase dose to 2 sprays in each nostril daily.
- Age ≥ 12 years: Initiate at 2 sprays in each nostril daily (220 mcg/day).
  - Once symptoms are controlled, patient may be able to titrate down to 1 spray in each nostril daily.

Side effects
- Nasal discomfort
- Nasal irritation, dryness, or both
- Epistaxis
- Stinging, burning, or both
- Sneezing
- Headache
- Bitter taste
- Rhinitis medicamentosa

Precautions and contraindications
- If patient plans on using triamcinolone acetonide longer than 2 months per year, encourage patient to see PCP.
- Concerns regarding the more serious side effects:
  - Changes in vision, cataracts
  - Increased risk of infection in adults
  - Growth inhibition in children

Oral decongestants

Selected oral decongestant products are described in Table 31-3.

Pharmacology
- α-adrenergic agonists and vasoconstrictors
- Constriction of blood vessels to decrease blood supply to nasal mucosa and decrease mucosal edema
- No effect on histamine or allergy-mediated reaction

Regulation
The 2005 Combat Methamphetamine Epidemic Act has the following requirements:

- Pseudoephedrine must be kept either behind the counter or in a locked cabinet.
- Quantity is limited to 3.6 g/day and 9 g/month per patient.

Side effects
These products are relatively safe with no dependence. They can be used long term, with the most common side effects as follows:

- Nervousness
- Irritability
- Restlessness
- Insomnia

Precautions and contraindications
- **Hypertension:** These agents are generally accepted with mild or well-controlled hypertension; they should not be used with uncontrolled hypertension.
- **Heart disease (arrhythmias and ischemic heart disease):** They increase the heart rate.
- **Diabetes:** They have a minimal effect on blood sugar level.
- **Hyperthyroidism:** This condition is more sensitive to sympathomimetics.
- **Enlarged prostrate:** Benign prostatic hyperplasia (BPH) is exacerbated by constricting smooth muscle of the bladder neck.
- **Narrow-angle glaucoma:** Dilation increases intraocular pressure.
- **Blood pressure:** MAO inhibitors interact with decongestants to increase blood pressure.

Topical decongestants

Pharmacology
- α-adrenergic agonists act locally as vasoconstrictors.
- These agents constrict blood vessels, decrease blood supply to the nose, and decrease mucosal edema.
- They have no effect on histamine or allergy-mediated reaction.

Side effects
Minimal systemic absorption results in few side effects. Local effects may include burning, nasal irritation, and sneezing.

Precautions and contraindications

Rhinitis medicamentosa (rebound congestion) may occur if duration of use is > 3–5 days. The FDA recommends using these products no more than 3 days in duration.

Dosage forms of topical decongestants

Sprays

Sprays are the simplest dosage delivery. A large surface area is covered. Imprecise dosing and contamination of the bottle are possible. Products include the following:

- *Short-acting:* Phenylephrine HCl (Neo-Synephrine)
- *Longest-acting:* Oxymetazoline HCl (Afrin, Vicks Sinex)

Drops

Drops are preferred for use in small children. They cover a small surface area. They pass to the larynx, where they may be swallowed and result in systemic effects.

Nasal inhaler

A nasal inhaler requires an unobstructed airway to deliver drug to the nasal mucosa. Nasal inhalers contain sympathomimetic amines, as well as camphor and menthol. Medications lose efficacy after 2–3 months. Products include the following:

- Propylhexedrine (Benzedrex inhaler)

Nasal saline solution

This solution is very safe and is good for use in infants and children to remove dried, encrusted, or thick mucus from the nose while also moisturizing and soothing nasal passages. It can be used with oral decongestants. Products include the following:

- Saline drops (Ayr)
- Saline sprays (Ayr, Ocean Nasal Spray)
- Neti pot

Mast cell stabilizer

Cromolyn (Nasalcrom)
- *Pharmacology:* Prevention of the release of inflammatory mediators from mast cells
- *Dosage:* One spray per nostril q4–6h
- *Onset of action:* Approximately 1 week; 2–4 weeks for maximal effect

- *Efficacy:* Not efficacious if taken prn; must be taken on a scheduled basis and is more effective if started at least 1 week prior to symptom onset
- *Side effects:* Nasal irritation, nasal burning, stinging, sneezing, cough, unpleasant taste

Analgesics

Analgesics treat the pain, fever, and headaches associated with cold, flu, or allergies. Medications include the following:

- Aspirin (mostly replaced now by acetaminophen and nonsteroidal anti-inflammatory drugs [NSAIDs])
- Acetaminophen (N-acetyl-para-aminophenol, or APAP)
- NSAIDs
  - Ibuprofen (OTC not approved for children < 6 months of age)
  - Naproxen (OTC not approved for children < 12 years of age)

Special populations

Children
- Do not use cough and cold products in children < 4 years of age.
- All children < 12 years of age are excluded from self-care of allergy unless they have been diagnosed by a health care provider and are approved for nonprescription therapy.
- Second-generation antihistamines and intranasal corticosteroids can be used for self-care in children < 6 years of age (provided they have been diagnosed by a health care provider and approved for nonprescription therapy).

Pregnancy
- Avoid products containing pseudoephedrine in the first trimester.
- Oxymetazoline is the preferred topical decongestant.
- For allergy, cromolyn is considered first-line therapy, followed by the second-generation antihistamines: loratadine and cetirizine. Chlorpheniramine can also be used.

Lactation
- Avoid using the following topical decongestants: xylometazoline and naphazoline.

- All antihistamines can decrease milk production.
- For allergy, cromolyn is considered first-line therapy, followed by loratadine and chlorpheniramine.

31-4. Constipation

Clinical Presentation

- Patient has difficult or infrequent passage of stools.
- Patient may complain of abdominal or rectal fullness.

Etiology

Table 31-5 shows the common causes of constipation.

Treatment

Nonpharmacologic therapy

- Increase fluid intake.
- Increase dietary fiber.
- Exercise.
- Establish good bowel habits.

Nonprescription medication therapy

Bulk-forming laxatives

Selected bulk-forming laxative products are described in Table 31-6.

Mechanism of action

Natural or semisynthetic hydrophilic polysaccharide derivatives are present in bulk-forming laxatives. They absorb water to soften stool, increase bulk, and facilitate peristalsis and elimination. Onset of effect may not be seen for 2–3 days.

Role in therapy

Bulk-forming laxatives are the safest, most natural therapy for normal transit constipation. They are the most often recommended medication for chronic use. Use caution in patients with fluid restriction (i.e., renal dysfunction, heart failure), narcotic-associated dysmotility, and fecal impaction.

Drug interactions

- These laxatives may bind with digoxin, warfarin, and other drugs.
- Calcium complexes may bind with tetracycline, inhibiting its absorption.
- Recommend separating doses from other medications by 1–2 hours.

Side effects

- Dose should be increased gradually over several weeks to avoid bloating, flatulence, and abdominal pain.

Table 31-5. Common Causes of Constipation

Daily habits	Diseases	Medications
Inadequate fluid intake	Parkinson's disease	Antacids containing Al or Ca
Inadequate fiber intake	Multiple sclerosis	Anticholinergics
Lack of physical exercise	Cerebrovascular disease	Phenothiazines
	Irritable bowel syndrome	Tricyclic antidepressants
	Hemorrhoids	Opiates
	Polyps and tumors	Antihistamines
	Diabetes	ACE inhibitors
	Hypothyroidism	Calcium channel blockers
		Sucralfate
		Iron

ACE, angiotensin-converting enzyme.

Table 31-6. Additional Nonprescription Treatments of Constipation Not Listed in Text

Medication class	Generic name	Brand name
Bulk-forming laxatives	Psyllium seed	Metamucil, Konsyl
	Methylcellulose	Citrucel
	Calcium polycarbophil	FiberCon
Emollient laxatives	Docusate sodium	Colace
Saline laxatives	Magnesium hydroxide	Milk of Magnesia
	Magnesium citrate	Magnesium citrate
	Magnesium sulfate	Epsom salts
	Monobasic sodium phosphate	Fleets
Combination products	Senna + docusate sodium	Senokot-S

- These laxatives can cause bowel obstruction if not taken with sufficient amounts of water.
- Caution diabetics about sugar content of some products.

Emollient laxatives (stool softeners)

Emollient laxatives act as surfactants, absorbing water into the stool. Onset of effect may take 2–3 days. Emollient laxatives may cause systemic absorption of mineral oil; therefore, concurrent use is contraindicated.

Emollient laxatives are often used in combination products. They are useful in situations when straining should be avoided, such as following rectal surgery, during the postpartum time period, and following a recent myocardial infarction.

Selected emollient laxative products are described in Table 31-6.

Stimulant laxatives

Stimulant laxatives stimulate bowel motility through localized mucosal irritation. They increase secretion of fluids into the bowel. Impaired colon function occurs with chronic use.

Dangers of chronic stimulant laxative use include the following:

- Laxative habit
- Cathartic colon
- Melanosis coli
- Loss of fluids and electrolytes
- Cramping pains

Anthraquinones

Senna (Senokot and Ex-Lax) is an anthraquinone:

- **Pharmacology:** Anthraquinones are absorbed into the bloodstream with action on the large intestines. Onset of effects is 6–12 hours. This medication should be taken at bedtime.
- **Side effects:** Such effects include discoloration of urine, stimulant habituation, and melanosis coli (i.e., dark pigmentation of colonic mucosa).

Diphenylmethanes

Bisacodyl (Dulcolax tablets or suppositories) is a diphenylmethane. Minimal systemic absorption occurs with this drug. This medication is enteric coated; do not crush or take with antacids. The onset of effects varies with route of administration:

- **Oral:** 6–8 hours
- **Rectal:** 15–60 minutes

Stimulant oils

Castor oil acts on the small intestine. It is a strong cathartic and may induce fluid or electrolyte disturbances. Onset is rapid: 2–6 hours.

Hyperosmotic laxatives

Glycerin

Glycerin has an osmotic effect and is a local irritant that stimulates bowel movement. Onset of effect is usually within 30 minutes.

Products include Fleet Pedia-Lax Liquid Glycerin Suppository and Fleet Glycerin Suppository.

Polyethylene glycol 3350 (MiraLAX)

Polyethylene glycol (PEG) 3350 has a mechanism of action similar to that of glycerin. This agent is meant for short-term therapy for constipation. Onset of action is usually within 1–3 days. The adult dosage is 17 g of powder in 4–8 oz of water. Side effects are as follows:

- Bloating
- Abdominal discomfort
- Cramping
- Flatulence

Saline laxatives

With saline laxatives, nonabsorbable cations create osmotic gradient to pull water into the intestine. Onset varies depending on the route of administration:

- **Rectal:** 5–30 minutes
- **Oral:** 30 minutes to 4 hours

Twenty percent of magnesium may be absorbed systemically. Saline laxatives are contraindicated in patients with impaired renal function (magnesium- or phosphate-containing), congestive heart failure, or hypertension (sodium-containing). Selected saline laxative products are described in Table 31-6.

Enemas

Enemas include Fleet Enema (monobasic and dibasic sodium phosphates). They are typically used for acute treatment (fecal impaction), not for long-term management of constipation.

Lubricant laxatives

Selected lubricant laxative products are as follows:

- **Mineral oil:** Liquid petrolatum
- **Olive oil:** "Sweet oil"

Lubricant laxatives soften the feces by emulsifying the contents of the intestinal tract. Onset of action is 6–8 hours. Use in self-care is strongly discouraged because of high risk of adverse events in children and the elderly. Do not administer with stool softeners.

Special patient populations

Children

- Mild constipation can be treated with increases in fluids and/or fruit juices containing sorbitol, such as apple, pear, prune, apricot, nectarine, or peach juice.
- Increase dietary fiber intake.
- For children 2–6 years of age, the following products are approved for use:
  - *Rectal:* Glycerin suppositories
  - *Oral:* Docusate sodium or magnesium hydroxide
- For children 6–12 years of age, the following products are approved for use:
  - *Rectal:* Glycerin or bisacodyl suppositories
  - *Oral:* Bulk-forming laxatives, docusate, and magnesium hydroxide are preferred; oral stimulants (senna, bisacodyl) should be reserved for when preferred treatments fail.
- For patients 6–17 years of age, one could apply off-label use of PEG 3350 at doses of 1 g/kg daily (not to exceed 17 grams daily), but a health care provider must be involved with the care of this patient.
- For patients > 17 years of age, PEG 3350 is FDA approved for use.

Pregnancy

- Attempt dietary changes first by incorporating more fiber via prunes or prune juice.
- If dietary changes do not work, use bulk-forming laxatives with sufficient amounts of water.
- For complaints of primarily dry, hard stools, use docusate.
- Senna or bisacodyl can be used safely short term and have more data supporting their use than does PEG 3350, but some experts use PEG 3350 as first-line treatment.
- Avoid castor oil (causes uterine contractions) and mineral oil (impairs maternal fat-soluble vitamin absorption).

Lactation

- Senna, bisacodyl, PEG 3350, and docusate are all compatible with breast-feeding.
- Avoid castor oil and mineral oil.

31-5. Diarrhea

Clinical Presentation

Diarrhea is the abnormal increase in frequency of stools and stool looseness. It may be acute (< 14 days) or chronic (> 4 weeks).

Etiology

Common causes of diarrhea are shown in Table 31-7.

Complications

- Dehydration (especially in infants and elderly patients)
- Electrolyte abnormalities

Nonpharmacologic Treatment

- Administer oral rehydration therapy, such as Pedialyte.
- Avoid fatty and spicy foods and foods with high sugar content.

Nonprescription Medication Therapy

Loperamide HCl (Imodium AD)

Loperamide is a synthetic opioid agonist that slows GI motility. The dosage is 4 mg initially and then 2 mg after each loose stool. For OTC use, maximum dose is 8 mg/day. The pharmacist may encounter cancer patients for whom the oncologist has recommended loperamide 2 mg po q2h with a maximum dose of 16 mg/day for chemotherapy-induced diarrhea not

Table 31-7. Common Causes of Diarrhea

Infection	Medications	Diet
Viral:	Antibiotics	Allergies
Norwalk	Laxatives	Spicy foods
Rotavirus	Magnesium-containing antacids	High carbohydrate load
Bacterial:	Cytotoxic agents	Lactose intolerance
Foodborne illness		
Contaminated water		
Traveler's diarrhea		
Protozoal		

caused by irinotecan and 24 mg/day for chemotherapy-induced diarrhea caused by irinotecan, though both of these maximum doses are intended for no more than 24 hours.

The medication is well tolerated, but typical side effects are as follows:

- Constipation
- Dizziness
- Dry mouth

Precautions and contraindications are as follows:

- Loperamide is not recommended for children < 6 years of age without medical supervision.
- It should not be used if the patient has bloody or black stool; consult a health care provider before use if the patient has a fever, mucus in stool, or a history of liver disease.
- Antiperistaltic action could worsen effects of invasive or inflammatory bacterial infection.

Bismuth subsalicylate (Pepto-Bismol)

Bismuth subsalicylate reacts with stomach acid to form salicylic acid and bismuth oxychloride. It reduces frequency of diarrhea and improves stool consistency. It has a direct antimicrobial effect; therefore, it is effective in traveler's diarrhea.

Side effects include the following:

- Salicylate toxicity (tinnitus)
- Bismuth toxicity (neurotoxicity)
- Gray-black discoloration of tongue or stool

The medication is contraindicated in the following:

- Aspirin allergy
- Children and teens with viral illness (Reye's syndrome)
- Patients having a history of GI bleeding or using warfarin

31-6. Nausea and Vomiting

Physiology

Vomiting is coordinated by the vomiting center in the medulla. Stimuli from the peripheral nervous system and within the central nervous system (CNS) act on the vomiting center. Responding to these impulses, the vomiting center stimulates the abdominal muscles, stomach, and esophagus to induce vomiting.

Etiology

Common causes of nausea and vomiting are shown in Table 31-8.

Complications

- Dehydration
- Electrolyte imbalance
- Aspiration

Table 31-8. Common Causes of Nausea and Vomiting

Irritation of chemoreceptor trigger zone	Vestibular disorders	CNS disorders	GI disorders
Chemotherapy	Motion sickness	Psychogenic vomiting	Obstruction
Narcotics	Otitis interna	Migraines	Gastroparesis
Theophylline	Meniere's syndrome	Increased intracranial pressure	Gastroenteritis
Digoxin			Infection
Antibiotics			
Drug withdrawal			
Alcohol			
NSAIDs			
Antibiotics			
Ketoacidosis			
Uremia			
Pregnancy			
Electrolyte imbalances			

■ Malnutrition
■ Acid–base disturbances

Nonprescription Medication Therapy

In addition to the medications described in this section, Table 31-9 describes nonprescription drugs of choice for the nausea or vomiting associated with motion sickness.

Antihistamines

Antihistamines cross the blood-brain barrier to depress vestibular excitability.

Phosphorated carbohydrate solution (Emetrol)

This agent is a hyperosmolar solution of levulose (fructose), dextrose (glucose), and phosphoric acid. It is buffered to a pH of 1.5. It reduces gastric muscle contraction through an unknown direct effect. It must not be diluted (which raises the pH).

Bismuth subsalicylate (Pepto-Bismol)

Bismuth subsalicylate is available as nonprescription suspension, caplet, and chewable tablet. See Section 31-5 for additional information.

Histamine 2–receptor antagonists

Histamine 2–receptor antagonists (H2RAs) may provide symptomatic relief by inhibiting gastric acid secretion. Potential drug interactions occur with cimetidine.

Side effects are as follows:

■ Headache
■ Constipation
■ Diarrhea

See Section 25-4 on peptic ulcer disease in Chapter 25 for additional information on H2RAs.

Antacids

Antacids may treat nausea, dyspepsia, and stomach upset associated with excessive intake of food or drink. They are combinations of magnesium hydroxide, sodium salts, aluminum hydroxide, calcium carbonate, and magnesium carbonate. The usual adult dosage is 15 mL 30 minutes after meals and at bedtime.

Side effects include the following:

■ Constipation
■ Diarrhea
■ Sodium overload

Antacids may decrease absorption of some medications. Therefore, administer other medications 1–2 hours before or after antacids.

Special patient populations

Pregnancy
Especially during the first trimester, nonpharmacologic therapy is recommended:

■ Ensure there is fresh air in the rooms where you sleep, prepare food, and eat.
■ Eat small, frequent meals.
■ Avoid rich, fatty foods.
■ Before getting out of bed in the morning, eat several dry crackers and relax for 10–15 minutes.

Refer the patient to the health care provider if pharmacologic therapy is being considered. Once the health care provider is involved in care, the following medications are preferred for use in pregnancy:

■ Antihistamines (meclizine, cyclizine, dimenhydrinate, diphenhydramine): All have a low risk of teratogenicity but should be reserved for those

Table 31-9. Nonprescription Drugs of Choice for Prevention of Motion Sickness

| Generic name | Trade name | Adults (maximum daily dose) | Dosage | |
			Children age 6–12 (maximum daily dose)	Children age 2–6 (maximum daily dose)
Dimenhydrinate	Dramamine	50–100 mg q4–6h (400 mg)	25–50 mg q6–8h (150 mg)	12.5–25 mg q6–8h (75 mg)
Diphenhydramine	Benadryl	25–50 mg q4–6h (300 mg)	12.5–25 mg q4h (150 mg)	6.25 mg q4h (25 mg)
Cyclizine	Marezine	50 mg q4–6h (200 mg)	25 mg q6–8h (75 mg)	Not recommended
Meclizine	Bonine	25–50 mg daily (50 mg)	Not recommended	Not recommended

with severe symptoms unresponsive to non-pharmacologic measures.

- Pyridoxine (vitamin B$_6$): 10–25 mg tid–qid
- Doxylamine succinate: 12.5 mg tid–qid
- Calcium-containing antacids
- Ginger: There is evidence supporting its use in pregnancy (see Section 31-14 for herbal products).

31-7. Pain and Fever

Pathophysiology of Pain

Nociceptors are peripheral pain receptors. They send pain stimuli to the spinal cord through afferent, nociceptive nerves. Impulses then pass to the brain through dorsal root ganglia.

Pathophysiology of Fever

The core temperature is the temperature of the blood surrounding the hypothalamus. The thermoregulatory center in the anterior hypothalamus controls body temperature through physiologic and behavioral mechanisms. Pyrogens—fever-producing substances—increase the thermoregulatory set point, raising the body temperature.

Nonprescription Medication Therapy

Selected analgesic and antipyretic products are shown in Table 31-10.

Acetaminophen

Acetaminophen exerts analgesic and antipyretic activity through central inhibition of prostaglandin synthesis. It does not have peripheral anti-inflammatory activity. Acetaminophen is generally well tolerated; however, hepatotoxicity is a possible side effect. In addition, the risk for severe liver injury increases when taking multiple products that contain acetaminophen.

Drug interactions can occur as follows:

- *Alcohol:* Drinking ≥ 3 alcoholic beverages a day increases the risk of hepatotoxicity.
- *Warfarin:* Higher doses (> 1.3 grams for > 1 week) may enhance hypoprothrombinemic effect of warfarin.

Changes to McNeil (Tylenol brand) product labeling are as follows:

- Tylenol Extra Strength (500 mg tablets): Maximum dose is 3,000 mg/day or 6 tablets/day.
- Tylenol Regular Strength (325 mg tablets): Maximum dose is 3,250 mg/day or 10 tablets/day.
- These maximum doses are different than the official FDA-approved adult maximum daily dose of 4 g/day for generic acetaminophen.

Salicylates

Salicylates inhibit peripheral prostaglandin synthesis. They reduce pain, inflammation, and fever. Acetylated salicylates (e.g., aspirin) irreversibly inhibit platelet aggregation. Nonacetylated salicylates (e.g., prescription salsalate, magnesium subsalicylate) have reversible antiplatelet activity.

Side effects associated with salicylates include the following:

- Gastritis
- Gastric ulcers and bleeding
- Allergy and hypersensitivity:
  - Rare (< 1%) in the general population
  - Higher risk in individuals with asthma and nasal polyps

Table 31-10. Selected Analgesic and Antipyretic Products

Generic name	Trade name	Dosage	
		Adults (maximum daily dose)	Children (maximum daily dose)
Acetaminophen	Tylenol, FeverAll	325–1,000 mg q4–6h (4,000 mg)[a]	10–15 mg/kg q4–6h (5 doses)
Aspirin	Bayer	650–1,000 mg q4–6h (4,000 mg)	10–15 mg/kg q4–6h (80 mg/kg)
Ibuprofen	Motrin, Advil	200–400 mg q4–6h (1,200 mg OTC)	5–10 mg/kg q6–8h (40 mg/kg)
Naproxen sodium	Aleve	220 mg q8–12h (660 mg)	Not recommended < 12 years of age; ≥ 12 years of age: use adult dosage

a. FDA maximum dose. See Section 31-7 in this chapter regarding McNeil product maximum doses for acetaminophen.

- Reye's syndrome, a potentially fatal illness associated with salicylate use in children and teens with concurrent viral illness (influenza, varicella-zoster)

Drug interactions may occur with the following:

- *Alcohol:* GI toxicity is enhanced.
- *Methotrexate:* Salicylates displace methotrexate from protein-binding sites.
- *Warfarin:* Salicylates enhance hypoprothrombinemic effects of warfarin.

Patients should be aware of the following precautions and contraindications:

- Bleeding disorders
- Hemophilia
- Peptic ulcer disease
- Children or teenagers with viral illness (Reye's syndrome)
- Gout

Nonsteroidal anti-inflammatory drugs

NSAIDs provide peripheral inhibition of prostaglandin synthesis. They offer analgesic, antipyretic, and anti-inflammatory activity.
Side effects include the following:

- GI effects, including bleeding
- Rash
- Photosensitivity
- High incidence of cross-reactivity in individuals with aspirin allergy

Drug interactions may occur as follows:

- *Warfarin:* Increased bleeding risk
- *Alcohol:* Increased risk of GI bleeding
- *Methotrexate:* Decreased methotrexate clearance
- *Antihypertensives:*
  - Angiotensin-converting enzyme (ACE) inhibitors: Decreased hypotensive effects, hyperkalemia
  - β-blockers: Decreased hypotensive effects
  - Potassium-sparing diuretics: Hyperkalemia
- *Digoxin:* Decreased renal clearance, risk of digoxin toxicity

Precautions and contraindications are as follows:

- Renal impairment
- Congestive heart failure

The following patients are at increased risk of severe stomach bleed with NSAID use:

- > 60 years of age
- History of peptic ulcer disease

- Concomitant use of warfarin, other NSAIDs, or alcohol
- Duration of use longer than recommended

Special patient populations

Pregnancy and lactation
- Acetaminophen is preferred (Category B).
- Ibuprofen and naproxen are compatible with breast-feeding.
- Avoid NSAIDs in the third trimester of pregnancy (Category D).

31-8. Ophthalmic Disorders

Dry Eye

- *Definition:* Tear film instability caused by a deficiency of any component of the tear film
- *Clinical presentation:* Ocular discomfort, blurred vision, desire to rub the eyes, burning or redness

Nonpharmacologic treatment

- Avoid known irritants.
- Use a cool-mist humidifier or warm-steam vaporizer.

Nonprescription medication therapy

Table 31-11 describes the pharmacologic treatment of dry eyes.

Loose Foreign Material in the Eye

Symptoms

Symptoms include irritation, inflammation, involuntary tearing, uncontrollable blinking, and discomfort.

Nonprescription treatment

Eyewashes are isotonic, buffered solutions of sterile water. They should not be used if the patient has open wounds near the eye. Contact lens wearers should remove their lenses prior to using eyewashes. Use of eye cups should generally be avoided.

Redness Caused by Minor Irritation

Eye redness can be caused by airborne pollutants (gases or smoke), chlorinated water, infectious diseases, or glaucoma.

Table 31-11. Pharmacologic Treatment of Dry Eyes

Product	Common preparations	Comments
Artificial tears[a]		
Cellulose derivatives (carboxymethylcellulose)	Bion Tears, Refresh Celluvisc, Clear Eyes CLR	Has enhanced duration compared to other products; tends to form dry crusts, which may be easily washed off with warm water
Polyvinyl alcohol (glycerin, propylene glycol, polyethylene glycols, polysorbate 80)	Hypo Tears, Murine Tears, Oasis Tears Plus	Has shorter duration; has no crust formation
Povidone and dextran 70	AquaSite	Can cause transient stinging or burning
Ocular emollients[b]		
Lanolin, mineral oil, petrolatum, white ointment, white wax, or yellow wax	Moisture Eyes PM, Lacri-Lube SOP, Refresh PM	

a. Artificial tears act as demulcents to mimic mucin. Use twice daily as suggested.
b. Ointments have longer contact and are more likely to cause blurred vision.

Nonprescription treatment

Ophthalmic vasoconstrictors, as described in Table 31-12, are used to treat eye redness.

The medications constrict blood vessels of the conjunctiva. Instill 1–2 drops in the affected eye up to four times daily. Minimize systemic absorption by closing the eye after instillation and occluding the tear duct with a finger (punctual occlusion).

These agents are contraindicated in patients with narrow-angle glaucoma because they cause mydriasis. Contact lens wearers also should avoid ophthalmic vasoconstrictors.

A rebound hyperemia can occur, especially with overuse. If absorbed systemically, tachycardia and arrhythmias can occur.

Ocular decongestants should be avoided in patients with heart disease, high blood pressure, an enlarged prostate, or narrow-angle glaucoma.

Allergic Conjunctivitis

Symptoms

Symptoms include chronic and recurring itching. Eyes are slightly red and tear and burn, but they have little discharge.

Nonprescription treatment

Antihistamine and mast cell stabilizer
Ketotifen fumarate 0.025% (Zaditor, Alaway), an antihistamine and mast cell stabilizer, may be used to treat allergic conjunctivitis. Instill 1 drop q8–12h in the affected eye. Use in patients ≥ 3 years of age. Relief is provided within minutes, and effects may last up to 12 hours.

Combination products
The following combination products containing an ophthalmic vasoconstrictor and an ocular antihistamine may be used:

- Naphazoline + pheniramine (Naphcon A, Visine A, Opcon-A)
- Naphazoline + antazoline (Vasocon-A)

Table 31-12. Ophthalmic Vasoconstrictors

Product	Common preparations	Key points
Naphazoline	Clear Eyes, Clear Eyes Redness Relief, Allerest, All Clear, All Clear AR	Is ocular decongestant of choice
Tetrahydrozoline	Visine, Vision Clear, Visine Maximum Redness Relief, OptiClear	Is less likely to alter pupil size; may cause stinging on instillation
Oxymetazoline	Visine LR	Is relatively free of ocular or systemic side effects

Instill 1–2 drops in the affected eye up to four times daily.

Combination products containing ocular decongestants should be avoided in patients with heart disease, high blood pressure, enlarged prostate, or narrow-angle glaucoma.

Conditions Requiring Referral to a Health Care Provider or Eye Care Specialist

Corneal edema

Symptoms
Symptoms include foggy vision, haloes around lights, photophobia, irritation, sensation of a foreign body, and extreme pain.

Nonprescription treatment
After seeking medical care from a PCP, the patient can use sodium chloride (2–5%) to treat corneal edema. Instill 1–2 drops in the affected eye every 6 hours. If eye drops do not provide relief, add ointment to therapy.

Foreign body in the eye

Foreign bodies include metal shavings, wood splinters, and dust. Improper removal may lead to permanent damage.

Ocular trauma

Automobile accidents and sports injuries can result in ocular trauma.

Chemical exposure

If chemical exposure occurs, follow these steps:

- Remove contact lenses.
- Flush eye immediately with lukewarm water for at least 15 minutes.
- Do not place drops in the eyes.

31-9. Otic Disorders

Impacted Cerumen

Cerumen-softening agents

Cerumen-softening agents are used as follows:

- Instill in ear.
- Follow with warm water irrigation using otic syringe.

Various types of agents are available:

- ***Carbamide peroxide 6.5% in anhydrous glycerin:*** Products include Auro Ear Drops and Debrox Earwax Removal Aid Kit. This agent softens ear wax and facilitates its removal.
- ***Hydrogen peroxide and water:*** A 1:1 solution of warm water and 3% hydrogen peroxide is used. This mixture is not an effective drying agent.
- ***Glycerin:*** This emollient and humectant may facilitate the removal of ear wax.
- ***Olive oil:*** Sometimes called sweet oil, this agent can also be used.

Water-Clogged Ears

A solution of 95% isopropyl alcohol in 5% anhydrous glycerin (Swim Ear or Auro Dri Drops) may be used to treat water-clogged ears. This solution is the only FDA-approved ear-drying aid.

31-10. Smoking Cessation

Unless the patient has contraindications, pharmacotherapy should be offered to all patients attempting to quit smoking (Table 31-13).

First-line agents double long-term smoking abstinence rates:

- Nonprescription nicotine replacement therapy (NRT):
  - Nicotine gum (Nicorette, generic): OTC
  - Nicotine patch (Nicotrol, Nicoderm CQ, generic): OTC
  - Nicotine lozenge (Commit): OTC

Table 31-13. The "5 A's" Clinicians Should Use to Assist Patients in Smoking Cessation

Ask about tobacco use.	Identify and document tobacco use status for every patient at every visit.
Advise to quit.	In a clear, strong, and personalized manner, urge every tobacco user to quit.
Assess willingness to make a quit attempt.	Is the tobacco user willing to make a quit attempt at this time?
Assist in quit attempt.	For the patient willing to make a quit attempt, use counseling and pharmacotherapy to help him or her quit.
Arrange follow-up.	Schedule follow-up contact, preferably within the first week after the quit date.

Side Effects

NRT can have various side effects:

- Gum
  - Patients may experience an unpleasant taste, mouth irritation, jaw muscle soreness, hypersalivation, hiccups, and dyspepsia.
  - Gum can stick to dental work.
  - Warn patients against chewing the gum too fast and chewing more than one piece at a time.
  - Patients with temporomandibular joint pain may want to avoid gum.
- Lozenge
  - Mouth irritation, nausea, hiccups, cough, heartburn, headache, flatulence, and insomnia can occur.
  - Do not use more than one lozenge at a time.
- Patch
  - Local skin reactions (erythema, burning, pruritis) can occur. Treat by rotating sites or applying hydrocortisone or triamcinolone cream.
  - Vivid or abnormal dreams, insomnia, and headache can occur. These effects are more common in the 24-hour patch. Patients can minimize the effects by using the 16-hour patch or by removing the patch at night before bed.

Contraindications and precautions

Cardiovascular disease is a contraindication to the use of NRT in the following cases:

- < 2 weeks following myocardial infarction
- Serious arrhythmias
- Serious or worsening angina

NRT is also contraindicated in the following:

- Esophagitis (gum or lozenge form only)
- Peptic ulcer disease (gum or lozenge form only)

NRT patients should seek medical advice if they are pregnant or breast-feeding. Patients should attempt to stop smoking prior to starting NRT, but it is not required.

31-11. Overweight and Obese

Clinical Indicators

The definition is based on body mass index (BMI):

- Overweight = BMI 25–29.9
- Obese I = BMI 30–34.9
- Obese II = BMI 35–39.9
- Obese III = BMI ≥ 40

Waist circumference aids in assessing cardiovascular risk in anyone with a BMI of 25–34.9:

- Males with a waist circumference > 40 inches
- Females with a waist circumference > 35 inches

These persons are at increased risk of developing type 2 diabetes and cardiovascular disease.

Nonpharmacologic Therapy

Nonpharmacologic therapy involves lifestyle modification.

Caloric restriction

Usually, a reduction of 500–750 kcal/day or a 30% energy deficit is recommended. A low-calorie diet results in a typical weight loss of 1–2 lb/week. Portion control is essential. A variety of dietary approaches can be offered to an overweight or obese patient and can produce weight loss. No specific macronutrient composition has proven to be better; instead, a reduction in dietary intake is recommended. The U.S. Department of Agriculture–Department of Health and Human Services 2010 Dietary Guidelines for Americans and the 2013 AHA/ACC (American Heart Association–American College of Cardiology) Guideline on Lifestyle Management to Reduce Cardiovascular Risk recommend a diet that emphasizes the intake of vegetables, fruits, and whole grains (including low-fat dairy products, poultry, fish, legumes, nontropical vegetable oils, and nuts) while limiting the intake of sweets, sugar-sweetened beverages, and red meat.

Physical activity

The 2008 Physical Activity Guidelines for Americans by the U.S. Department of Health and Human Services recommend the following:

- *For substantial health benefits:* 150 minutes/week of moderate-intensity or 75 minutes/week of vigorous-intensity aerobic activity
- *For more extensive health benefits:* 300 minutes/week of moderate-intensity or 150 minutes/week of vigorous-intensity aerobic activity
- *Aerobic activity:* Can be broken up into 10 minute intervals
- *Additional activity:* May be required in addition to dietary caloric restriction to promote weight loss

■ *Strength training:* moderate- or high-intensity activities that involve all major muscle groups on ≥ 2 days/week

Nonprescription medication therapy

Orlistat (allī)

Orlistat decreases the absorption of dietary fats and inhibits gastric and pancreatic lipases.

Indication

This agent is used in patients ≥ 18 years of age who are overweight (BMI ≥ 25) in conjunction with lifestyle modification.

Note: According to the 2013 AHA/ACC/TOS Guideline for the Management of Overweight and Obesity in Adults, pharmacologic therapy is not recommended as an adjunct to a comprehensive lifestyle intervention unless a patient has a BMI ≥ 30 or BMI ≥ 27 in addition to one obesity-related comorbidity.

Dose

Patients should take one 60 mg capsule before meals. They do not have to take the medication if the meal does not contain fat.

Side effects

Side effects include the following:

■ Flatulence with oily spotting
■ Loose and frequent stools
■ Fatty stools
■ Fecal urgency
■ Incontinence

Decreasing the amount of ingested fat can minimize these effects. Effects generally resolve within a few weeks of initiating therapy.

Precautions

Counsel patients on the signs and symptoms associated with liver damage (anorexia, pruritis, jaundice, dark urine, light-colored stools, right upper quadrant pain).

Contraindications

Patients on cyclosporine and patients with malabsorption disorders should not use this medication. Patients with a history of thyroid disease, cholelithiasis, nephrolithiasis, or pancreatitis should consult a health care provider prior to use.

Interactions

Decreased absorption of fat-soluble vitamins (especially D and E) occurs. Take a multivitamin at bedtime or separate it from orlistat dose by at least 2 hours.

Concern exists over vitamin K absorption and possible effects on warfarin; therefore, recommend increased monitoring.

31-12. Overactive Bladder

Detrusor instability, classified as the muscle squeezing too often or without warning and causing urinary incontinence or the sudden urge to urinate, occurs.

Nonpharmacologic Treatment

■ Log consumption of food and drink.
■ Avoid foods, beverages, or both that could potentiate bladder activity.
■ Limit fluids 2–3 hours before bedtime.
■ Schedule time to use the bathroom every 2–3 hours.
■ Perform Kegel exercises.
■ Try to retrain bladder.

Nonprescription Medication Treatment

Oxytrol For Women (oxybutynin)

Transdermal delivery system (3.9 mg/day) that is indicated in women ≥ 18 years of age. Clear patch must be changed every 4 days and is applied to the abdomen, hip, or buttock. The full benefit of this medication is seen in about 2 weeks. When the agent is combined with daily lifestyle modifications (timed urination, pelvic floor exercises, fluid management), studies show a reduction of urinary accidents by 75% with Oxytrol versus 50% with placebo.

Side effects

Anticholinergic effects may occur as follows:

■ Dry mouth or eyes
■ Constipation
■ Itching, rash, or redness where patch was placed
■ Sleepiness
■ Dizziness
■ Blurry vision

Contraindications and precautions

Oxybutynin is not for use in men, women < 18 years of age, or other types of urinary incontinence.

31-13. Home Monitoring and Testing Devices

Fertility Prediction Tests

Basal thermometry

Temperatures can be taken orally, rectally, and vaginally. Temperatures are taken every morning before rising.

Resting temperatures are usually below normal for the first part of the reproductive cycle. Temperatures are closer to normal after ovulation.

Temperature results are plotted graphically against time to assess spikes (ovulation). Tests are very user dependent.

Clearblue Easy Fertility Monitor

This test for luteinizing hormone (LH) and estrone-3-glucuronide is a monitoring device with strips that are inserted into a monitor. The user tests urine daily for 10–20 consecutive days. The results are listed as low, high, and peak fertility. It can identify up to 6 fertile days; however, it is expensive in comparison to ovulation prediction kits.

OV-Watch

This device is a watch worn while sleeping that measures chloride ions in perspiration every 30 minutes. It must be worn at least 6 hours each night. This device alerts the user 4 days prior to ovulation. It is also expensive in comparison to ovulation prediction kits.

Ovulation prediction kits

This test contains antibodies that bind to the LH in urine. An LH surge is detected by a difference in color or color intensity from one day to the next.

Early morning urine collection is recommended. The user must know the length of the past three cycles before using. Testing usually begins 2–4 days prior to ovulation (based on the average of the past three cycles).

Pregnancy detection

Early testing is very important. Tests detect levels of human chorionic gonadotropin (hCG) in urine (within 1–2 weeks after conception). Antibodies designed to react with hCG form the shape of a straight line, check, or plus sign. If the user is pregnant, color is produced.

Table 31-14. Causes of Error in Home Pregnancy Testing

False positives	False negatives
Miscarriage within previous 8 weeks	Test performed first day of a missed cycle
Childbirth within previous 8 weeks	Refrigerated urine not allowed to come to room temperature
Use of fertility medications (Pergonal, Profasi)	Wax cups or household containers with soap residues used for test

Pregnancy tests are 98–100% accurate; however, human error decreases that rate to 50–75% (see Table 31-14).

Important tips for patients using pregnancy tests are as follows:

- Use of first morning urine to test is encouraged because hCG is more concentrated.
- If use of first morning urine is not possible, the patient should restrict fluids 4–6 hours before urine collection.
- Use only supplied collection devices.
- Try to test the sample immediately after collection. If this is not possible, allow refrigerated samples to come to room temperature.
- If the test is negative, wait 1 week and retest if the cycle has not yet started.
- If the test is positive, contact an obstetrician–gynecologist immediately and start prenatal vitamins.

Urinary Tract Infection Tests

AZO Test Strips are

- Tests for nitrites and leukocyte esterase
- Specific only for Gram-negative organisms

Inaccurate results are possible in the following circumstances:

- *False-negative result:* Vegetarian diet, vitamin C, or tetracycline
- *False-positive result:* Phenazopyridine

Hypertension

Mercury column devices

These devices use a blood pressure reference standard. Routine home use is discouraged because the devices are cumbersome.

Aneroid devices

Aneroid devices are light, portable, and affordable. Many come with an attached stethoscope. They require good eyesight and hearing for effective use (large-print devices are available).

Digital devices

Digital devices are less accurate than aneroid devices.

Hypercholesterolemia

Cardiocheck

Cardiocheck has the potential to test for total cholesterol (TC), high-density lipoprotein (HDL), and triglycerides (TG). Low-density lipoprotein (LDL) can be calculated or can be measured by the device, depending on the strip used. The unit stores results. It is reusable.

Fecal Occult Blood Tests

Three categories are available:

- Toilet tests (EZ-Detect Stool Blood Test), which use biodegradable paper that is placed in the toilet bowl after a bowel movement
- Stool wipes (LifeGuard)
- Manual stool application tests (Colon-Test-Sensitive)

A colorimetric assay is used for hemoglobin. A blue-green color indicates a positive test.

Tests are more likely to detect lower GI problems. False-positive tests can occur with the ingestion of red meat or vitamin C.

Human Immunodeficiency Virus (HIV)

OraQuick In-Home HIV Test screens for autoantibodies to HIV-1 and HIV-2. Patients should be aware that they need to wait for at least 3 months after exposure before testing.

An oral swab sample is obtained by the patient. Results show in the device window within 20–40 minutes. A positive result is indicated by a line present near the C and T on the device window. A negative result is indicated by a line only near the C on the device window. This test has a sensitivity of 92% and a specificity of 99.98%.

31-14. Natural and Herbal Products

Complementary and Alternative Medicine Definitions

- *Dietary supplement:* According to the Dietary Supplement and Health Education Act of 1994, "a product intended to supplement the diet that … contains one or more of the following dietary ingredients: a vitamin, mineral, herb or other botanical, amino acid; a dietary substance for use by man to supplement the diet by increasing the total daily intake; or a concentrate, metabolite, constituent, extract, or combination of these ingredients"

Regulation of Dietary Supplements

Dietary supplements are not regulated as closely as drugs. Table 31-15 provides a comparison.

The following agencies are responsible for regulation:

- *U.S. Food and Drug Administration:* Regulates labeling, safety, and manufacturing
- *U.S. Federal Trade Commission:* Regulates advertising

Herbal Products

Evening primrose oil (*Oenothera biennis*)

Common uses
Evening primrose oil is often used for the treatment of atopic dermatitis, eczema, or both.

Table 31-15. Drugs versus Dietary Supplements

Drug	Dietary supplement
Active ingredient is identified.	Active ingredient may not be identified.
Safety and efficacy are proven by manufacturer.	No proof of efficacy is required; FDA must provide proof if unsafe.
Purity and contents are regulated.	No standards exist for quality or purity.
Claims to treat, cure, or prevent disease are made.	No claims to treat, cure, or prevent specific disease are made.

Proposed mechanisms

Oil extracted from the plant seeds consists of a high amount of unsaturated fatty acids, particularly linoleic and gamma-linolenic acid (GLA), which are thought to decrease inflammation.

Side effects

Side effects include headache, nausea, diarrhea, and abdominal pain.

Contraindications and precautions

Patients on warfarin or antiplatelet agents should not use evening primrose oil because it may decrease platelet aggregation. Evening primrose oil may decrease seizure threshold, so it should be used with caution in patients with a seizure disorder. Avoid use in patients with an allergy to plants from the *Onagraceae* family. Avoid use in pregnant or lactating patients.

Asian ginseng (Panax ginseng)

Common uses

Asian ginseng is taken for enhancement of immunity and mental performance.

Proposed mechanisms

Physiologic activity is due to triterpenoid saponins and ginsenosides. This product is thought to suppress and stimulate the CNS. Corticosteroid activity and hypoglycemic activity are considered to occur.

Side effects

Side effects are insomnia, headache, blood pressure changes, anorexia, rash, mastalgia, and menstrual abnormalities. Long-term use can cause a ginseng abuse syndrome.

Contraindications

Contraindications are as follows:

- Renal failure
- Acute infection
- Pregnancy and lactation
- Active bleeding (peptic ulcer)

Precautions

Caution is warranted in the following circumstances:

- Cardiovascular disease
- Hypertension with or without medical treatment
- Diabetes (specifically with patients receiving medications that may cause hypoglycemia or having diagnosis of hypoglycemia unaware)
- History of hypotension

Interactions

- Stimulants (including caffeine)
- Antipsychotics

Coenzyme Q10 (Ubiquinone)

Common uses

Coenzyme Q10 (CoQ10) is commonly used for heart failure, hypertension, and statin-induced myopathy.

Proposed mechanisms

CoQ10 is a cofactor for many functions associated with energy production. It is a powerful antioxidant that helps in the regeneration of other antioxidants. It also stabilizes membranes and may have vasodilatory and inotropic effects.

Side effects

Side effects include nausea, GI distress, headache, irritability, and dizziness.

Interactions

- CoQ10 has a similar structure to synthetic vitamin K, which may cause a decrease in international normalized ratio (INR) levels if used concomitantly with warfarin.
- HMG-CoA (3-hydroxy-3-methylglutaryl-coenzyme A) reductase inhibitors reduce serum levels of CoQ10.

Echinacea purpurea

Common uses

Echinacea purpurea is used for the treatment of upper respiratory tract infections.

Proposed mechanisms

This product is thought to stimulate the immune system. It is believed to increase white blood cells and provide antiviral, antifungal, and anti-inflammatory action.

Dosage

Dosing should begin at the onset of viral symptoms, and treatment should continue until 24–48 hours after symptoms abate. Typical use is 14 days duration. It is not recommended for cold prevention.

Side effects

Side effects include mild GI discomfort, tingling sensation of the tongue, and headache. Allergic reactions can occur.

Contraindications

This product should not be taken by patients with severe systemic illness (HIV/AIDS, multiple sclerosis, tuberculosis) or autoimmune disorders or by patients taking immunosuppressants. Avoid in patients with an allergy to Asteraceae (daisy) family of plants and in patients with severe allergy, allergic rhinitis, or atopy.

Interactions

There are no clinical interactions of importance.

Fish oil

Common uses

Fish oil is often taken to improve cardiovascular health and by patients with coronary artery disease, hypertension, hypertriglyceridemia, or rheumatoid arthritis.

Proposed mechanisms

Fish oil provides a source of omega-3 fatty acids (docosahexaenoic acid, eicosapentaenoic acid). It is considered to increase anti-inflammatory cytokines and decrease pro-inflammatory cytokines. It is thought to decrease the intestinal absorption of cholesterol and inhibit the synthesis and degradation of very-low-density lipoprotein particles.

Dosage

- *Dosing:* Based on EPA/DHA (eicosapentaenoic acid/docosahexaenoic acid) content of capsules
- *General use:* 1–2 g daily
- *Hypertriglyceridemia:* 2–4 g daily

Side effects

Side effects include GI distress and fish burp, which may be avoided by using enteric-coated products, taking with meals, or storing the capsules in a refrigerator.

Interactions

At doses > 4 g daily, increased bleeding risk is present; therefore, patients on anticoagulation or antiplatelet therapy should be limited to 3 g daily.

Garlic (Allium sativum)

Common uses

Garlic is taken to lower cholesterol and to prevent atherosclerosis and cardiovascular disease.

Proposed mechanisms

Garlic is considered to exhibit its effects through organosulfur-containing compounds, which inhibit platelet aggregation, act as a free radical scavenger, stimulate fibrinolysis, and lower cholesterol and lipid levels by inhibition of HMG-CoA reductase.

Side effects

Side effects include malodorous breath and smell of garlic that may permeate the skin, GI discomfort, heartburn, and gas.

Contraindications

Active bleeding (peptic ulcer) can occur. Garlic should be stopped 10–14 days prior to surgery to avoid potential bleeding complications.

Interactions

- *Anticoagulants and antiplatelet agents:* Aspirin, ticlopidine, clopidogrel, dipyridamole, warfarin, ginkgo, ginseng
- *Saquinavir AUC (area under curve):* 50% decrease in healthy volunteers

Ginger

Common use

Ginger is used as an antiemetic.

Proposed mechanism

It is thought to stimulate gastric secretions and peristalsis.

Dosage

- *Pregnancy-induced nausea or vomiting:* Dried ginger 250 mg qid
- *Motion sickness:* Two 500 mg capsules taken 30 minutes prior to travel, followed by one to two more 500 mg capsules as needed every 4 hours

Side effects

Heartburn, belching, or dermatitis may occur.

Interactions

Ginger may increase the risk of hypoglycemia and alter platelet function at doses > 1 g/day. Use with caution in patients receiving antiplatelet and anticoagulation therapy.

Ginkgo biloba

Common uses

Ginkgo biloba is used to enhance memory and concentration. Credible scientific evidence supports its use in the treatment of cerebral insufficiency, dementia, generalized anxiety disorder, and schizophrenia.

Proposed mechanisms

Ginkgo biloba is thought to increase blood flow, act as an antioxidant, and inhibit platelet aggregation.

Side effects

- *Mild:* GI distress, headache, and dizziness can occur.
- *Serious:* Spontaneous bleeding has been reported (e.g., subdural hematomas, subarachnoid hemorrhage).

Interactions

This product may interact with both medications (aspirin, ticlopidine, clopidogrel, dipyridamole, warfarin) and herbs (garlic, ginseng). Interactions are due to antiplatelet or anticoagulant activity.

Contraindications

Ginkgo biloba should be stopped at least 7 days prior to surgery to avoid potential bleeding complications.

Glucosamine and chondroitin sulfate

Common uses

Glucosamine and chondroitin sulfate products are used for osteoarthritis.

Proposed mechanisms

This product serves as a precursor to glycosaminoglycans, which make up cartilage and synovial fluid. It may help regenerate cartilage and replace synovial fluid.

Dosage

Dosage is as follows:

- *Glucosamine:* 500 mg tid (with meals) glucosamine sulfate
- *Chondroitin:* 400 mg tid

These agents are often in a combination product. Full effects may not be seen for 4–6 months.

Side effects

Side effects include mild GI upset, nausea, heartburn, constipation, and diarrhea.

Contraindications

Patients with severe shellfish allergy should not take this product. Avoid in pregnancy and lactation.

Green tea

Common uses

Green tea is taken as a performance enhancer and as protection from the development of cardiovascular disease and cancer.

Proposed mechanisms

Green tea contains caffeine, which has a stimulant effect, and antioxidants (EGCG [Epigallocatechin gallate]), which protect against oxidative damage.

Side effects

GI irritation and both CNS and cardiac stimulation can occur because of caffeine content. Green tea can contain a range of 8–30 mg of caffeine per tea bag.

Drug interactions

Large doses may decrease INR levels, although brewing destroys most of the vitamin K content.

Melatonin

Common uses

Melatonin is commonly used to treat sleep disorders and to reset the sleep–wake cycle (jet lag).

Proposed mechanisms

Melatonin mimics endogenous release of melatonin from the pineal gland. Concentrations increase significantly 1–2 hours before sleep.

Dosage

Dosages are as follows:

- *Insomnia:* 0.3–5 mg 30 minutes prior to bedtime
- *Jet lag:* 2–5 mg in the evening between 5:00 pm and 10:00 pm on the day of arrival and at bedtime for 2–5 days after arrival

Long-term administration is not recommended.

Side effects

Melatonin may worsen depression. Other side effects include headache and confusion. Melatonin is possibly an immune stimulant.

Interactions

When melatonin is taken with benzodiazepines, anxiolytic effects are enhanced.

Probiotics

Common uses

Probiotics are taken for antibiotic-induced diarrhea, GI disorders, and atopic dermatitis.

Proposed mechanisms

Probiotics contain *Lactobacillus* sp, *Bifidobacterium* spp, or *Saccharomyces boulardii*. They are thought to decrease intestinal permeability, normalize gut flora, and decrease inflammatory responses. They possess immunomodulating activity.

Side effects

Bloating, flatulence, and diarrhea may occur.

Contraindications

Because of reports of systemic infection, immuno-compromised patients should avoid use. Systemic infection is more common with the use of *S. boulardii*.

Interactions

Probiotics may decrease antibiotic absorption; therefore, antimicrobial agents should be administered several hours apart from taking probiotics.

Fenugreek

Common uses

Fenugreek is often used by women to stimulate breastmilk production when lactating. It is also used for diabetes.

Proposed mechanism

Fenugreek seeds contain hormone precursors that increase milk supply. The exact mechanism is not fully understood. Fenugreek can increase a nursing mother's milk supply within 24–72 hours after first taking the herb. Once an adequate level of milk production is reached, most women can discontinue fenugreek and maintain the milk supply with adequate breast stimulation.

Dosage

The dosage is 2.5 grams orally bid.

Side effects

Urine, sweat, and breastmilk may have the odor of maple syrup.

Interactions

Use with caution in patients receiving antiplatelet and anticoagulation therapy because of possible decrease in platelet aggregation caused by fenugreek.

Contraindications and precautions

Avoid in patients with an allergy to chickpeas. Avoid in pregnancy.

Aloe Vera

Common uses

Aloe vera is commonly used topically for burns or psoriasis and systemically for constipation.

Proposed mechanisms

Aloe vera contains about 75 potentially active constituents, and multiple mechanisms of action have been proposed.

Dosage

No clear optimal topical dosage exists. It is not recommended as a first-line agent for constipation, but the dose suggested in many sources is the minimum amount to maintain a soft stool.

Side effects

Abdominal cramps and diarrhea can occur with oral use.

Interactions

Interactions do not typically occur with topical application.

Contraindications and precautions

Use caution if diabetic patients are taking aloe vera orally and are on hypoglycemic medications.

St. John's wort (Hypericum perforatum)

Common uses

St. John's wort is used to treat depression and somatoform disorders.

Proposed mechanisms

Active ingredients are hypericin and hyperforin. This product is thought to inhibit dopamine, serotonin, and norepinephrine reuptake and to decrease IL-6 (interleukin-6) concentrations.

Dosage

This product is standardized to 0.3% hypericin or 5% hyperforin. The recommended dose is 300–600 mg tid.

Side effects

The most commonly reported side effects are paresthesias, headache, nausea, dry mouth, agitation, decreased libido, and skin reactions. Photosensitivity can occur: recommend sun avoidance or sunscreen.

Interactions

Interactions are well documented and clinically significant.

Antidepressants (SSRIs [selective serotonin reuptake inhibitors] and TCAs [tricyclic antidepressants]) interact with this product because of a similar mechanism of action, which could result in serotonin syndrome.

St. John's wort is an inducer of CYP (cytochrome) 4503A4, 1A2, 2C9, 2C19, and 2E1 and P-glycoprotein, causing decreased blood levels of medications and possibly resulting in reduced therapeutic effects. Medications affected include the following:

- Cyclosporine
- Indinavir
- Digoxin
- Oral contraceptives (estradiol component)

Contraindications and precautions

Avoid in patients with schizophrenia or bipolar disorder.

31-15. Questions

1. Which of the following is the primary advantage of recommending dextromethorphan instead of codeine?

   A. It is twice as effective as codeine in suppression of cough.
   B. It has less dependence potential than codeine.
   C. It has peripheral rather than the central action of codeine.
   D. It is less expensive than codeine.
   E. It is much longer acting than codeine.

2. All of the following statements regarding guaifenesin are correct *except*

   A. it is the only OTC expectorant approved by the U.S. Food and Drug Administration.
   B. it requires large amounts of water to be effective.
   C. it is available OTC as Robitussin.
   D. it may cause a decrease in platelet aggregation and an increase in bleeding time.
   E. it is available in some prescription cough and cold formulations.

3. All of the following statements regarding diphenhydramine are true *except*

   A. it is less likely to cause drowsiness than other OTC antihistamines.
   B. it is the active ingredient in some OTC products for insomnia.
   C. it is available OTC under the trade name of Benadryl.
   D. a small percentage of children may exhibit a paradoxical CNS stimulant effect.
   E. elderly patients may experience delirium or confusion with diphenhydramine.

4. All of the following statements about the routine use of oral decongestants in treating the common cold are true *except*

   A. they cannot be used in patients on MAO inhibitor antidepressants.
   B. they are relatively safe, with no dependence.
   C. they are absolutely contraindicated in patients with controlled diabetes and mild hypertension.
   D. the most common side effects are nervousness and insomnia.
   E. their purchase is much more regulated today than in the past.

5. When should a patient using OTC Nasacort Allergy 24HR with no symptom improvement be referred for further evaluation of sinus problems?

   A. 1 week
   B. 2 weeks
   C. 1 month
   D. 2 months
   E. 6 months

6. A mother comes into the pharmacy looking for the most appropriate treatment for her 30-month-old son who has had three loose bowel movements this morning. He does not have a fever; is in good spirits; and is eating, drinking, and urinating appropriately. What should be recommended?

   A. Refer her to a primary care provider.
   B. Recommend loperamide 2 mg 2 caplets now and 1 caplet after each subsequent loose stool.
   C. Recommend loperamide (Imodium A-D) liquid for children 15 mL now and 7.5 mL after subsequent loose stools.

D. Recommend milk of magnesia 15–30 mL at bedtime.

E. Recommend oral replacement with Pedialyte; offer solution as needed after loose bowel movements depending on fluid intake.

7. Which of the following is *not* an adverse effect of Pepto-Bismol?

    A. Anticholinergic effects, dry mouth, and dry eyes
    B. Tinnitus
    C. Cross-sensitivity to aspirin allergy
    D. Grayish-black tongue
    E. Dark stools

8. Which of the following drugs exhibits analgesic and antipyretic properties, but not peripheral anti-inflammatory properties?

    A. Ibuprofen
    B. Sodium salicylate
    C. Acetaminophen
    D. Magnesium salicylate
    E. Naproxen

9. What is the maximum daily dose of Tylenol Regular Strength?

    A. 4,000 mg/day or 6 tablets per 24 hour period
    B. 3,000 mg/day or 6 tablets per 24 hour period
    C. 3,250 mg/day or 10 tablets per 24 hour period
    D. 3,000 mg/day or 10 tablets per 24 hour period
    E. 4,550 mg/day or 14 tablets per 24 hour period

10. Mary is a 32-year-old female with asthma and serious aspirin sensitivity. She comes to the pharmacist seeking assistance in selecting a nonprescription product for aches and pains. Which of the following should the pharmacist recommend for Mary?

    A. Ibuprofen
    B. Naproxen
    C. Acetaminophen
    D. Oral aloe vera
    E. Salicylate dissolvable powder

11. Nonprescription antiemetics are primarily useful for preventing which type of nausea?

    A. Nausea caused by alterations in the vestibular apparatus
    B. Nausea caused by drugs acting centrally on the chemoreceptor trigger zone
    C. Nausea caused by visceral pain
    D. Nausea caused by cortical stimulation from smells or sight
    E. Nausea caused by afferent impulses from the GI tract

12. A mother requests advice for her 6-month-old child, who has been constipated for the past 2 days after beginning cereal feedings. Which of the following agents would be the best laxative agent to recommend?

    A. Dulcolax
    B. Fletcher's Castoria
    C. Mineral oil
    D. Glycerin suppositories
    E. Milk of magnesia

13. All of the following statements about stool softeners are true *except*

    A. they are not safe to use in pregnancy.
    B. the onset of action is usually within 1–2 days.
    C. they are useful in patients with constipation who have hemorrhoids.
    D. extra water helps their effectiveness.
    E. they are often combined with mild stimulant laxatives.

14. All of the following statements about bisacodyl are true *except*

    A. it should not be taken concurrently with antacids.
    B. it can be crushed or chewed if needed.
    C. it should not be recommended in pregnancy.
    D. it is available in oral tablet and suppository dosage forms.
    E. it is the active ingredient in Dulcolax.

15. Which of the following counseling points regarding the use of Oxytrol for Women transdermal patch is the most appropriate?

    A. When used with lifestyle modifications, urinary accidents can be reduced by 10%

more than by using lifestyle modifications alone.

B. It will take up to 6 weeks to see the full benefit from the medication.

C. The best place to apply the patch is on the upper arm.

D. The patient must reapply the patch every 4 days.

E. This product should not be used by women older than 65 years of age.

Use the following case study to answer Questions 16 and 17:

Baby M is 1 year old and weighs 24 lb. He has a fever of 102°F, is irritable, seems uncomfortable, and is not sleeping well.

16. His mother is confused by the assortment of fever relief products. You recommend acetaminophen. Which product and dosage do you recommend?

A. Tylenol Infant Drops 80 mg/0.8 mL; give 1.6 mL q4–6h.

B. Tylenol Children's Liquid 160 mg/5 mL; give 2 tsp q6–8h.

C. Advil Infant Drops 50 mg/1.25 mL; give 1.25 mL q4–6h.

D. Motrin Children's Suspension 100 mg/ 5 mL; give 2.5 mL q6–8h.

E. Tylenol Infant Drops 80 mg/0.8 mL; give 3.2 mL q4–6h.

17. The next morning, baby M's mother returns to your pharmacy. Her pediatrician recommended alternating the maximum dose of ibuprofen with the acetaminophen, and she is asking for help selecting an ibuprofen product and dosage. Which do you recommend?

A. Advil Infant Drops 50 mg/1.25 mL; give 0.625 mL q8h.

B. Motrin Children's Suspension 100 mg/ 5 mL; give 2 tsp q4h.

C. Motrin Infant Drops 50 mg/1.25 mL; give 2.5 mL q6h.

D. Advil Children's Chewable Tablet 50 mg; give 1 tablet q8h.

E. Advil Children's Chewable Tablet 50 mg; give 1/2 tablet q4h.

18. A 35-year-old male requests guidance on the results of his OraQuick In-Home HIV Test. He thinks he was exposed to HIV about 1 year ago because of unprotected sex. He followed the package directions for use of the diagnostic tool correctly. The result window shows a line by the C and the T. How should this patient be counseled regarding his results?

A. The test indicates a positive result, so refer the patient to a primary care provider for confirmation.

B. The test indicates a negative result, so refer the patient to a primary care provider for confirmation.

C. The test is inconclusive because of testing too early and must be repeated.

D. The test indicates a positive result, and because of specificity of the product, confirmation is not needed.

E. The test is inaccurate when taken more than 6 months after exposure to HIV, so refer him to his primary care provider.

19. What dietary supplement can cause a user's urine and sweat to smell of maple syrup?

A. Ginseng
B. Echinacea
C. Fenugreek
D. Garlic
E. Black cohosh

20. Which of the following products should be discontinued prior to surgery?

A. Ginkgo biloba
B. Gentian root
C. Glutamine
D. Glucosamine
E. Folic acid

21. Cough and cold products are *not* to be used in children less than _____ years of age.

A. 2
B. 4
C. 6
D. 8
E. 12

22. When a patient is considering the use of nonprescription orlistat, which of the following vitamins may the patient need as additional supplementation because of decreased absorption?

    A. B$_{12}$
    B. B$_6$
    C. D
    D. C
    E. Vitamin B$_1$

31-16. Answers

1. **B.** Although there have been reports of limited recreational abuse of dextromethorphan, its potential for dependence and addiction is significantly less than that of codeine.

2. **D.** Guaifenesin does not have any effects on platelet aggregation or bleeding time. It is the only FDA-approved OTC expectorant, works better with increased fluid intake, and is included in Robitussin products.

3. **A.** Diphenhydramine, an ethanolamine, is the most sedating OTC antihistamine.

4. **C.** Systemic decongestants are not recommended in individuals with uncontrolled diabetes or hypertension because of their sympathomimetic effects. They are contraindicated with MAO inhibitors and can commonly cause nervousness or insomnia.

5. **D.** The patient will not see the full benefit of Nasacort Allergy 24HR until about 2–4 weeks of treatment. If minimal to no improvement has been seen by 2 months, the patient should seek further evaluation by a primary care provider.

6. **E.** Referring this child to a primary care provider is not needed because the child is still taking fluids and no signs and symptoms of infection are present (i.e., fever). He can be treated at home with oral rehydration solutions, such as Pedialyte. Loperamide is not for use in children < 6 years of age. Milk of magnesia would make the diarrhea worse and is not an appropriate choice of treatment for acute diarrhea.

7. **A.** Common adverse effects of Pepto-Bismol include tinnitus and grayish-black tongue or stools. Pepto-Bismol does contain a salicylate and, therefore, should not be used in individuals with aspirin allergy.

8. **C.** Acetaminophen is a centrally acting antipyretic and analgesic, but it does not exhibit peripheral anti-inflammatory activity. Salicylates and other NSAIDs do.

9. **C.** McNeil manufactures Tylenol Regular Strength (325 mg tablets). Maximum dose is 3,250 mg/day or 10 tablets/day. These maximum doses are different than the official FDA-approved adult maximum daily dose of 4 grams/day for generic acetaminophen.

10. **C.** All NSAIDs and aspirin-containing products should be avoided in individuals with aspirin sensitivity. Acetaminophen can be recommended in this setting.

11. **A.** Nonprescription antiemetics are antihistamines that exert their effect by inhibiting histamine in neural centers controlling vomiting, salivation, and vestibular excitability, making them especially well suited for motion sickness.

12. **D.** Glycerin suppositories are safe for infants. The other agents should not be used in this patient population.

13. **A.** Stool softeners are safe to use in pregnancy and usually exert their effect within 1–2 days. Stool softeners are recommended for individuals in whom hard stools or straining could cause pain or complications (e.g., hemorrhoids, postoperative or postpartum time periods, or postmyocardial infarction). Increased fluid intake enhances their effectiveness. They are frequently used in combination products containing stimulant laxatives.

14. **B.** Because bisacodyl is an enteric-coated product, it should not be taken with antacids or be crushed, chewed, or broken. It should not be used in pregnancy. It is available in both oral tablets and rectal suppositories.

15. **D.** The patient must reapply the Oxytrol for Women patch to the abdomen, hip, or buttock every 4 days. When used with lifestyle modifications, urinary accidents can be reduced by 25% more than by using lifestyle modifications alone. It will take about 2 weeks to see full benefit from this medication.

16. **A.** The pediatric dosage of acetaminophen is 10–15 mg/kg q4–6h:

$$24 \text{ lb} \times \text{kg}/2.2 \text{ lb} = 10.9 \text{ kg} \times 10\text{–}15 \text{ mg/kg}$$
$$= 109\text{–}163.5 \text{ mg}$$

Tylenol Infant Drops 80 mg/0.8 mL; 1.6 mL = 160 mg acetaminophen

17. **C.** The pediatric dosage of ibuprofen is 5–10 mg/kg q6–8h:

$$24 \text{ lb} \times \text{kg}/2.2 \text{ lb} = 10.9 \text{ kg} \times 5\text{–}10 \text{ mg/kg}$$
$$= 54.5\text{–}109 \text{ mg}$$

Motrin Infant Drops 50 mg/1.25 mL; 2.5 mL = 100 mg ibuprofen

18. **A.** OraQuick In-Home HIV Test with a line present near the C and T in the result window indicates a positive result. Exposure over 3 months allows for appropriate use of this test in this individual. This test has a specificity of 99.98%, which means 1 false-positive can occur in every 5,000 results in uninfected individuals. Therefore, a positive result does not mean that the person is definitely infected with HIV, but that additional testing by a primary care provider is required to confirm the results.

19. **C.** Fenugreek can cause the urine, sweat, and breastmilk of the user to smell of maple syrup. This supplement is typically used as a galactogogue.

20. **A.** Ginkgo biloba has antiplatelet activity and should, therefore, be withheld prior to surgical procedures.

21. **B.** The Consumer Health Care Products Association announced in October 2008 that manufacturers were voluntarily updating all cough and cold products to state "do not use" in children under 4 years of age.

22. **C.** Vitamin D is a fat-soluble vitamin that may have decreased absorption with concomitant orlistat use despite multivitamin supplementation. A multivitamin is best taken at bedtime or separate from an orlistat dose by at least 2 hours.

31-17. References

Eckel RH, Jakicic JM, Ard JD, et al. 2013 AHA/ACC Guideline on Lifestyle Management to Reduce Cardiovascular Risk: A report of the American College of Cardiology/American Heart Association Task Force on Practice Guidelines. *Circulation.* 2013:63(25).

Fiore MC, Bailey WC, Cohen SJ, et al. *Treating Tobacco Use and Dependence: Clinical Practice Guideline.* Rockville, MD: U.S. Department of Health and Human Services; 2008.

Jensen MD, Ryan DH, Apovian CM, et al. 2013 AHA/ACC/TOS guideline for the management of overweight and obesity in adults: A report of the American College of Cardiology/American Heart Association Task Force on Practice Guidelines and The Obesity Society. *J Am Coll Cardiol.* 2014;63(25):2985–3023.

Krinsky DL, ed. *Handbook of Nonprescription Drugs: An Interactive Approach to Self-Care.* 17th ed. Washington, DC: American Pharmacists Association; 2012.

Natural Standard Web site. http://naturalstandard.com/databases/herbssupplements/stjohnswort.asp?#. Accessed March 11, 2014.

OraQuick In-Home HIV Test Web site. http://www.oraquick.com/. Accessed March 11, 2014.

Oxytrol Website. http://www.oxytrolforwomen.com. Accessed March 11, 2014.

2008 Physical Activity Guidelines for Americans. Washington, DC: U.S. Department of Health and Human Services Web site. http://www.health.gov/paguidelines. Accessed May 31, 2014.

2010 Dietary Guidelines for Americans. Washington, DC: U.S. Department of Agriculture–Department of Health and Human Services Web site. http://www.cnpp.usda.gov/dietaryguidelines.htm. Accessed May 31, 2014.

Asthma and Chronic Obstructive Pulmonary Disease

Timothy H. Self

32

32-1. Key Points

Asthma

■ Asthma is primarily an inflammatory airway disease.

■ It is commonly undertreated, resulting in much unnecessary suffering and economic loss.

■ Managing patients via the principles of the National Institutes of Health (NIH) National Asthma Education and Prevention Program, Expert Panel Report 3, 2007 (EPR-3) has been clearly shown to reduce emergency department visits and hospitalizations and to improve patient quality of life.

■ Optimal long-term management includes objective assessment, environmental control, drug therapy, and patient education as a partnership.

■ Patients with persistent asthma need daily controller therapy (anti-inflammatory agents).

■ Inhaled corticosteroids are the most efficacious agents to control asthma and are the preferred first-step drug treatment for patients of all ages who have mild persistent asthma.

■ Long-acting inhaled β_2-agonists are the preferred treatment to add to inhaled corticosteroids for patients with moderate persistent or severe persistent asthma.

■ Short-acting inhaled β_2-agonists are the agents of choice for quick relief of symptoms.

■ Pharmacists should teach patients how to use inhalers (metered dose inhaler [MDI], MDI spacer, and dry powder inhaler [DPI]) by demonstrations and *observation* of the patient.

■ Pharmacists should instruct patients on how to use peak flow meters, including color-coded zone management with a written action plan. Written action plans may be based on peak flow, symptoms, or both.

■ Patients must clearly understand the purpose of daily controller or preventer medications versus quick-relief medications. Show patients airway models or colored pictures of normal versus inflamed airways.

Chronic Obstructive Pulmonary Disease

■ The overall approach to managing stable chronic obstructive pulmonary disease (COPD) should be characterized by a stepwise increase in treatment and tailored to reduce symptoms and enhance quality of life.

■ Health education can play a role in improving skills, ability to cope with COPD, and health status. It is effective in accomplishing certain goals, including smoking cessation in some patients.

■ Smoking cessation is highly important. Nicotine replacement and drug therapy improve long-term abstinence rates.

■ None of the existing medications for this disease has been shown to modify the long-term decline in pulmonary function that is the hallmark of COPD. Drug treatment for COPD is used to improve symptoms or decrease complications.

■ Bronchodilators are central to the symptomatic management of this disease. They include β_2-agonists, anticholinergics, and theophylline.

■ Inhaled therapy with long-acting agents is preferred for reasons of efficacy and convenience.

■ Combining bronchodilators may improve efficacy and decrease the risk of side effects compared with increasing the dose of a single bronchodilator.

- Inhaled corticosteroids should be added to long-acting bronchodilators in COPD patients at a high risk of exacerbations.
- Chronic treatment with systemic corticosteroids should be avoided because risks outweigh benefits.
- The long-term administration of oxygen (> 15 hours per day) to COPD patients with chronic respiratory failure has been shown to increase survival.
- Patients with COPD benefit from exercise training programs; they show improvement with respect to both exercise tolerance and symptoms of fatigue and dyspnea.
- Influenza vaccine can reduce serious illness in COPD patients. Pneumococcal polysaccharide vaccine is recommended for patients with COPD who are 65 years of age or older and for patients under 65 years of age who have a forced expiratory volume in 1 second (FEV_1) < 40% predicted.

32-2. Study Guide Checklist

The following topics may guide your study of this subject area:

- Risk factors and triggers for asthma and COPD
- Importance of environmental control
- Factors to consider when selecting drug therapy
- Actions of different classes of drugs to treat asthma and COPD
- Trade names and available dosage forms, particularly those in the "Top 100 Drugs"
- Major adverse effects and drug interactions
- Proper peak expiratory flow measurement technique and interpretation
- Considerations when choosing doses and schedules for each drug
- Importance of patient education, including correct inhaler technique
- Management of acute exacerbations
- Highly significant role of national and international evidence-based guidelines to manage asthma and COPD

32-3. Asthma

Asthma is a chronic inflammatory disorder of the airways in which many cells and cellular elements play a role, in particular mast cells, eosinophils, T-lymphocytes, neutrophils, and epithelial cells. In susceptible individuals, this inflammation causes recurrent epi-sodes of wheezing, breathlessness, chest tightness, and cough, particularly at night and in the early morning. Asthma affects about 26 million Americans and is the most common cause of missed school days for children. Morbidity and mortality caused by asthma are unacceptably high; death rates are greatest among inner-city African Americans and Hispanics.

Types and Classifications

- *Childhood-onset (atopic):* Positive family history of asthma; allergy to tree or grass pollen, house dust mites, cockroaches, household pets, and molds
- *Adult-onset:* Frequently a negative family history and negative skin tests to common aeroallergens

Classification of severity for children age 12 and over and adults is shown in Figure 32-1. This classification is extremely important in defining treatment options (see Figures 32-2 to 32-4). Classification of severity is taken from the National Institutes of Health (NIH) National Asthma Education and Prevention Program, Expert Panel Report 3, 2007 (EPR-3). See EPR-3 for classification of severity for ages 0–4 years and 5–11 years.

Clinical Presentation

- Episodic wheezing, coughing, chest tightness, and shortness of breath that is worse at night, in the early morning, and with exercise

Pathophysiology

- Asthma is an inflammatory airway disease and also a disease with bronchospasm.
- Common triggers of symptoms include aeroallergens; respiratory viral illness; exercise (especially in cold, dry air); environmental smoke; and fumes.
- Drug-induced asthma includes asthma-like symptoms caused by aspirin, nonsteroidal anti-inflammatory drugs (NSAIDs), and β-blockers. Low- to moderate-dose β_1-selective agents can be used if the patient has concurrent post myocardial infarction (atenolol or metoprolol XL) or congestive heart failure (metoprolol XL) and does not have severe asthma; cyclooxygenase-2 (COX-2) inhibitors can be used safely in many patients with aspirin-sensitive asthma. Recent research suggests that use of acetaminophen in the first year of life may be a risk factor for development of asthma in childhood, but more research is needed.

Figure 32-1. Classification of Asthma Severity (Children ≥ 12 Years of Age and Adults)

Assessing severity and initiating treatment for patients who are not currently taking long-term control medications

Components of Severity		Classification of Asthma Severity ≥12 years of age			
			Persistent		
		Intermittent	**Mild**	**Moderate**	**Severe**
Impairment **Normal FEV₁/FVC:** 8–19 yr 85% 20–39 yr 80% 40–59 yr 75% 60–80 yr 70%	Symptoms	≤2 days/week	>2 days/week but not daily	Daily	Throughout the day
	Nighttime awakenings	≤2x/month	3–4x/month	>1x/week but not nightly	Often 7x/week
	Short-acting beta₂-agonist use for symptom control (not prevention of EIB)	≤2 days/week	>2 days/week but not daily, and not more than 1x on any day	Daily	Several times per day
	Interference with normal activity	None	Minor limitation	Some limitation	Extremely limited
	Lung function	• Normal FEV₁ between exacerbations • FEV₁ >80% predicted • FEV₁/FVC normal	• FEV₁ >80% predicted • FEV₁/FVC normal	• FEV₁ >60% but <80% predicted • FEV₁/FVC reduced 5%	• FEV₁ <60% predicted • FEV₁/FVC reduced >5%
Risk	Exacerbations requiring oral systemic corticosteroids	0–1/year (see note)	≥2/year (see note) → ← Consider severity and interval since last exacerbation. → Frequency and severity may fluctuate over time for patients in any severity category. Relative annual risk of exacerbations may be related to FEV₁.		
Recommended Step for Initiating Treatment		Step 1	Step 2	Step 3	Step 4 or 5 and consider short course of oral systemic corticosteroids
		In 2–6 weeks, evaluate level of asthma control that is achieved and adjust therapy accordingly.			

Key: FEV₁, forced expiratory volume in 1 second; FVC, forced vital capacity; ICU, intensive care unit

Notes:

■ The stepwise approach is meant to assist, not replace, the clinical decisionmaking required to meet individual patient needs.

■ Level of severity is determined by assessment of both impairment and risk. Assess impairment domain by patient's/caregiver's recall of previous 2–4 weeks and spirometry. Assign severity to the most severe category in which any feature occurs.

■ At present, there are inadequate data to correspond frequencies of exacerbations with different levels of asthma severity. In general, more frequent and intense exacerbations (e.g., requiring urgent, unscheduled care, hospitalization, or ICU admission) indicate greater underlying disease severity. For treatment purposes, patients who had   2 exacerbations requiring oral systemic corticosteroids in the past year may be considered the same as patients who have persistent asthma, even in the absence of impairment levels consistent with persistent asthma.

Figure 32-2. Stepwise Approach for Managing Asthma in Infants and Young Children (0–4 Years of Age)

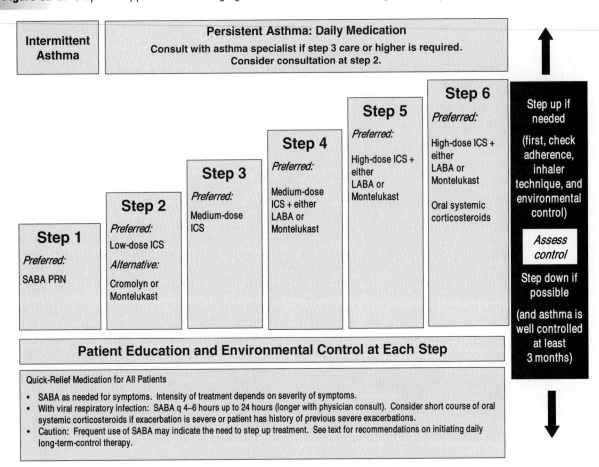

Key: **Alphabetical order is used when more than one treatment option is listed within either preferred or alternative therapy.** ICS, inhaled corticosteroid; LABA, inhaled long-acting beta$_2$-agonist; SABA, inhaled short-acting beta$_2$-agonist

Notes:

■ The stepwise approach is meant to assist, not replace, the clinical decisionmaking required to meet individual patient needs.

■ If alternative treatment is used and response is inadequate, discontinue it and use the preferred treatment before stepping up.

■ If clear benefit is not observed within 4–6 weeks and patient/family medication technique and adherence are satisfactory, consider adjusting therapy or alternative diagnosis.

■ Studies on children 0–4 years of age are limited. Step 2 preferred therapy is based on Evidence A. All other recommendations are based on expert opinion and extrapolation from studies in older children.

Figure 32-3. Stepwise Approach for Managing Asthma in Children 5–11 Years of Age: Treatment

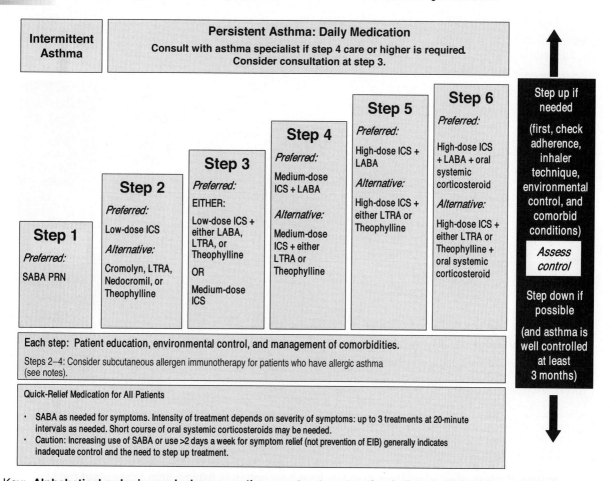

Key: **Alphabetical order is used when more than one treatment option is listed within either preferred or alternative therapy.** ICS, inhaled corticosteroid; LABA, inhaled long-acting beta₂-agonist; LTRA, leukotriene receptor antagonist; SABA, inhaled short-acting beta₂-agonist

Notes:

■ The stepwise approach is meant to assist, not replace, the clinical decisionmaking required to meet individual patient needs.

■ If alternative treatment is used and response is inadequate, discontinue it and use the preferred treatment before stepping up.

■ Theophylline is a less desirable alternative due to the need to monitor serum concentration levels.

■ Step 1 and step 2 medications are based on Evidence A. Step 3 ICS + adjunctive therapy and ICS are based on Evidence B for efficacy of each treatment and extrapolation from comparator trials in older children and adults— comparator trials are not available for this age group; steps 4–6 are based on expert opinion and extrapolation from studies in older children and adults.

■ Immunotherapy for steps 2–4 is based on Evidence B for house-dust mites, animal danders, and pollens; evidence is weak or lacking for molds and cockroaches. Evidence is strongest for immunotherapy with single allergens. The role of allergy in asthma is greater in children than in adults. Clinicians who administer immunotherapy should be prepared and equipped to identify and treat anaphylaxis that may occur.

Figure 32-4. Stepwise Approach for Managing Asthma in Children ≥ 12 Years of Age and Adults: Treatment

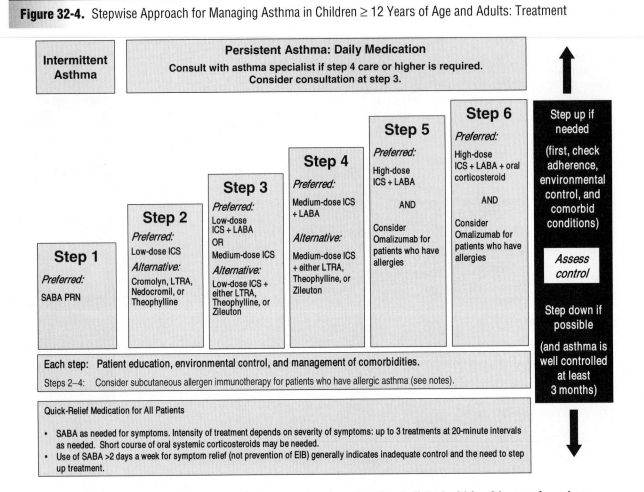

Key: **Alphabetical order is used when more than one treatment option is listed within either preferred or alternative therapy.** EIB, exercise-induced bronchospasm; ICS, inhaled corticosteroid; LABA, long-acting inhaled beta₂-agonist; LTRA, leukotriene receptor antagonist; SABA, inhaled short-acting beta₂-agonist

Notes:

■ The stepwise approach is meant to assist, not replace, the clinical decisionmaking required to meet individual patient needs.

■ If alternative treatment is used and response is inadequate, discontinue it and use the preferred treatment before stepping up.

■ Zileuton is a less desirable alternative due to limited studies as adjunctive therapy and the need to monitor liver function. Theophylline requires monitoring of serum concentration levels.

■ In step 6, before oral systemic corticosteroids are introduced, a trial of high-dose ICS + LABA + either LTRA, theophylline, or zileuton may be considered, although this approach has not been studied in clinical trials.

■ Step 1, 2, and 3 preferred therapies are based on Evidence A; step 3 alternative therapy is based on Evidence A for LTRA, Evidence B for theophylline, and Evidence D for zileuton. Step 4 preferred therapy is based on Evidence B, and alternative therapy is based on Evidence B for LTRA and theophylline and Evidence D for zileuton. Step 5 preferred therapy is based on Evidence B. Step 6 preferred therapy is based on (EPR—2 1997) and Evidence B for omalizumab.

■ Immunotherapy for steps 2–4 is based on Evidence B for house-dust mites, animal danders, and pollens; evidence is weak or lacking for molds and cockroaches. Evidence is strongest for immunotherapy with single allergens. The role of allergy in asthma is greater in children than in adults.

■ Clinicians who administer immunotherapy or omalizumab should be prepared and equipped to identify and treat anaphylaxis that may occur.

Reproduced from NIH *Expert Panel Report 3.*

- There is a complex interaction among inflammatory cells (e.g., mast cells, eosinophils, Th2-type lymphocytes); mediators (e.g., leukotrienes); and cytokines (e.g., IL-4, IL-5). The result is airway inflammation (mucus and swelling in the lining of the airways) and airway hyperreactivity.
- Early-phase response to inhaling an aeroallergen occurs immediately; late-phase response occurs 4–12 hours later.
- Asthma is worsened by poorly controlled concurrent allergic rhinitis and sinusitis. Gastroesophageal reflux disease (GERD) is common in asthma patients, but recent research revealed that although treatment with proton pump inhibitors may improve pulmonary function and asthma-related quality of life, the improvements are minor and of small clinical significance. Asthma may also worsen in the perimenstrual period.

Diagnostic Criteria

- The main basis for diagnosis is a detailed history of episodic symptoms that are typically worse at night and in the early morning and that are associated with common triggers.
- Reversible airway obstruction (improvement in pulmonary function tests [FEV_1, forced expiratory volume in 1 second] of > 12% after inhaling a short-acting β_2-agonist) is often detected.
- Alternate diagnoses (e.g., chronic obstructive pulmonary disease and vocal cord dysfunction) should be excluded.

Treatment Principles and Goals

- Optimal long-term management of asthma includes four major areas: objective assessment and monitoring, environmental control, pharmacologic therapy, and patient education as a partnership.
- Treatment goals are to achieve asthma control by *reducing impairment:*
  - Prevent chronic and troublesome symptoms (e.g., coughing or breathlessness in the daytime, during the night, or after exercise).
  - Require infrequent use (< 2 days/week) of a short-acting inhaled β_2-agonist for quick relief of symptoms.
  - Maintain (near) "normal" pulmonary function.
  - Maintain normal activity levels (including exercise and other physical activity and attendance at work or school).
  - Meet patients' and families' expectations of and satisfaction with asthma care.

- Treatment goals are to achieve asthma control by *reducing risk:*
  - Prevent recurrent exacerbations of asthma, and minimize the need for emergency department (ED) visits or hospitalization.
  - Prevent progressive loss of lung function; for children, prevent reduced lung growth.
  - Provide optimal pharmacotherapy with minimal or no adverse effects.
- A stepwise approach to managing asthma is shown in Figure 32-2 (ages 0–4), Figure 32-3 (ages 5–11), and Figure 32-4 (ages ≥ 12 and adults). These treatment guidelines are from EPR-3. See Table 32-1 for long-term control medications.
- Inhaled corticosteroids (ICSs) are the most efficacious drugs for long-term management of persistent asthma. Addition of a long-acting inhaled β_2-agonist (LABA) is recommended for patients with moderate or severe persistent asthma. Recent trials have shown that tiotropium (Spiriva) therapy added to patients inadequately controlled with ICS or ICS/LABA combination provides additional benefit.
- Omalizumab (Xolair): Anti-immunoglobulin E (IgE) therapy is primarily indicated for severe persistent asthma patients who have frequent ED visits and hospitalizations despite optimal therapy. It is given subcutaneously every 2–4 weeks.
- Drug therapy for acute exacerbations of asthma is shown in Table 32-2 (quick-relief medications) and Figure 32-5 (management of asthma exacerbations in the ED and hospital).

Monitoring

- Optimal management for the great majority of patients will result in a dramatic reduction in symptoms (including nocturnal and early morning symptoms), as well as reduced acute care visits, fewer lost work or school days, and reduced need for quick-relief medications.
- Monitoring peak expiratory flow (PEF) using a peak flow meter at home is helpful in many patients. *Green zone* is 80–100% of personal best value. *Yellow zone* is 50–79% of personal best and indicates that consultation with a health care professional is advisable. *Red zone,* or < 50% of personal best, indicates that a written action plan should be implemented, and, if there is no quick response, immediate medical attention should be sought.
- Spirometry is usually performed in the physician's office.

Table 32-1. Long-Term Asthma Control Medications[a]

Generic name	Trade name	Usual dosage range	Dosage form	Schedule[b]
Inhaled corticosteroids				
Beclomethasone HFA 40 mcg/puff; 80 mcg/puff	QVAR	80–480 mcg/day	MDI	Twice daily
Budesonide 200 mcg/inhalation	Pulmicort	1–3 inhalations/day	DPI (Flexhaler)	Twice daily
Budesonide–formoterol combination (each inhalation 4.5 mcg formoterol + budesonide 80 mcg or 160 mcg)	**Symbicort**	2 puffs	MDI	Twice daily
Budesonide 0.25 and 0.5 mg	Respules	0.5–2 mg/day	Nebulized	Twice daily
Fluticasone 44, 110, 220 mcg/puff	**Flovent HFA**	88–660 mcg/day	MDI	Twice daily
Fluticasone 50, 100, 250 mcg	Flovent Diskus	100–500 mcg/day	DPI	Twice daily
Fluticasone–salmeterol combination (each dose 50 mcg salmeterol + 100, 250, or 500 mcg fluticasone)	**Advair Diskus** (Advair 100, 250, 500)	1 inhalation	DPI (Diskus)	Twice daily
Fluticasone–salmeterol combination (each puff 21 mcg salmeterol + 45, 115, or 230 mcg fluticasone)	Advair HFA (Advair HFA 45, 115, 230)	2 inhalations/dose	MDI	Twice daily
Mometasone-formoterol combination (each puff 100 or 200 mcg mometasone + 5 mcg formoterol)	Dulera	2 inhalations	MDI	Twice daily
Mometasone 220 mcg/inhalation	Asmanex Twisthaler	1–2 inhalations daily	DPI	At bedtime
Leukotriene modifiers				
Montelukast	**Singulair**	4 mg (age 12–23 months)	Oral granules	Every night
		4 mg (age 2–5 years)	Chewable tab	Every night
		5 mg (age 6–14 years)	Chewable tab	Every night
		10 mg (adult) tablet	Tablet	Every night
Zafirlukast	Accolate	20–40 mg/day tablet	Tablet	Twice daily
Zileuton	Zyflo	600 mg/tablet	Tablet	Four times daily
	Zyflo CR	600 mg controlled release tablet (2 tablets/dose)	Controlled-release tablet	Twice daily
Long-acting inhaled β₂-agonists				
Formoterol[c]	Foradil Aerolizer	1 inhalation	DPI	Twice daily
Salmeterol[c]	Serevent Diskus	1 inhalation	DPI	Twice daily
Methylxanthines				
Theophylline (numerous products)[d]	Uniphyl	10 mg/kg/d up to 300 mg maximum in adults to start; aim for 5–15 mcg/mL steady state	Tablet	Daily; 5:00 or 6:00 pm

Boldface indicates one of top 100 drugs for 2012 by units sold at retail outlets, www.drugs.com/stats/top100/2012/units.

DPI, dry powder inhaler (breath activated); MDI, metered dose inhaler.

a. See EPR-3 and FDA-approved product literature for pediatric doses for each drug product; not a comprehensive list.

b. Usual schedule (some patients do well on once-daily dosing).

c. For asthma patients, use *only in combination product with ICS* (may use alone in COPD patients, but not asthma patients).

d. Complex, high-risk drug to dose; see references cited for details; do not use unless competent in dosing and monitoring serum theophylline concentrations. See EPR-3 for pediatric doses (< 1 year of age and > 1 year of age).

Table 32-2. Quick-Relief Asthma Medications[a]

Generic name	Trade name	Usual dosage[b]	Dosage form	Schedule
Short-acting inhaled β₂-agonists[c]				
Albuterol HFA	**Ventolin HFA,** Proventil,	2 puffs	MDI	Every 4 hours as needed
	ProAir HFA	2.5 mg	Nebulizer solution	Every 4 hours as needed
Anticholinergics				
Ipratropium	Atrovent HFA	2 puffs	MDI	Every 6 hours
		0.25 mg	Nebulizer solution	Every 6 hours
Ipratropium with albuterol	**Combivent Respimat**	1 puff	MDI	Every 6 hours
	DuoNeb	0.5 mg ipratropium plus 2.5 mg albuterol	Nebulizer solution	Every 6 hours
Systemic corticosteroids[d]				
Methylprednisolone	Medrol	1 mg/kg/day	Tablets	Daily
Prednisone		1 mg/kg/day	Tablets or liquid	Daily
Prednisolone		1 mg/kg/day	Tablets	Daily

Boldface indicates one of top 100 drugs for 2012 by units sold at retail outlets, www.drugs.com/stats/top100/2012/units.
a. See EPR-3 and FDA-approved product literature for more information, including pediatric doses for each drug product; not a comprehensive list.
b. Usual dosage for routine home use. (Dose in ED is higher and more frequent.)
c. For prevention of exercise-induced asthma, inhale 2 puffs 5–15 minutes before exercise. Increasing use indicates poor asthma control; increase anti-inflammatory therapy and reassess environmental control. (Good asthma control is indicated by infrequent need for quick-relief therapy.)
d. Short courses are used for < 2 weeks.

Mechanism of Action

For more details, see the section on mechanism of action in EPR-3.

Long-term control medications

Corticosteroids
- Corticosteroids are anti-inflammatory. They block late reaction to an allergen and reduce airway hyperresponsiveness. They inhibit cytokine production, adhesion protein activation, and inflammatory cell migration and activation.
- Corticosteroids reverse β₂-receptor down-regulation and inhibit microvascular leakage.

Long-acting β₂-agonists
- With bronchodilation, smooth muscle relaxation follows adenylate cyclase activation and an increase in cyclic adenosine monophosphate (AMP), producing functional antagonism of bronchoconstriction.

- In vitro, LABAs inhibit mast cell mediator release, decrease vascular permeability, and increase mucociliary clearance.
- Compared with a short-acting inhaled β₂-agonist, salmeterol has a slower onset of action (15–30 minutes). Formoterol has an onset of action within 3 minutes. Both LABAs have a duration of action ≥ 12 hours.

Methylxanthines
- With bronchodilation, smooth muscle relaxation results from phosphodiesterase inhibition and possibly adenosine antagonism.
- Methylxanthines may affect eosinophilic infiltration into bronchial mucosa as well as decrease T-lymphocyte numbers in epithelium.
- Methylxanthines increase diaphragm contractility and mucociliary clearance.

Leukotriene modifiers
- Leukotriene receptor antagonist; selective competitive inhibitor of CysLT₁ receptors
- 5-Lipoxygenase inhibitor

Figure 32-5. Management of Asthma Exacerbations: Emergency Department and Hospital-Based Care

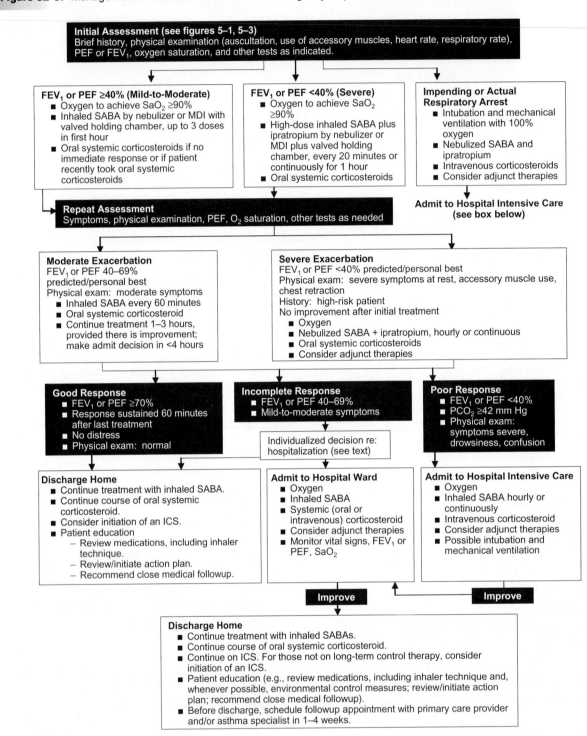

Key: FEV$_1$, forced expiratory volume in 1 second; ICS, inhaled corticosteroid; MDI, metered dose inhaler; PCO$_2$, partial pressure carbon dioxide; PEF, peak expiratory flow; SABA, short-acting beta$_2$-agonist; SaO$_2$, oxygen saturation

Reproduced from NIH *Expert Panel Report 3.*

Anti-IgE therapy
- Omalizumab (Xolair) is a humanized mono-clonal anti-IgE antibody that binds circulating IgE, thus inhibiting the allergic inflammatory cascade that results when aeroallergens bind to IgE on mast cells.

Quick-relief medications

Short-acting inhaled β₂-agonists

Short-acting inhaled β_2-agonists
- With bronchodilation, smooth muscle relaxation follows adenylate cyclase activation and an increase in cyclic AMP, producing functional antagonism of bronchoconstriction.

Anticholinergics
- With bronchodilation, there is competitive inhibition of muscarinic cholinergic receptors.
- Anticholinergics reduce intrinsic vagal tone to the airways. They may block reflex bronchoconstriction secondary to irritants or to reflux esophagus.
- Anticholinergics may decrease mucus gland secretion.

Patient Instructions and Counseling

- Patient education is absolutely essential for optimal asthma management.
- Emphasize the need to take controller–preventer medications *every day,* even when the patient feels well and is having no breathing problems.
- Instruct the patient regarding the dangers of overuse of short-acting inhaled β₂-agonists. (The patient should contact a physician if the usual dose does not give quick relief or start the written action plan given by the physician.) Patients who purchase the nonprescription racemic epinephrine inhaler (Asthmanefrin EZ Breathe Atomizer) may have persistent asthma and need daily controller medication. Even for intermittent asthma, patients need physician assessment, avoidance of asthma triggers, inhaler instruction, and written action plans. Remember that if quick-relief medication is needed more than twice weekly, the patient has persistent asthma and needs daily controller–preventer treatment.
- Demonstrate the correct use of the metered dose inhaler (MDI), the MDI plus valved holding chamber (or other "spacer"), and the dry powder inhaler (DPI), and then observe the patient using the devices. Most patients do not perform well initially; the devices can be difficult to use at first (see Figure 32-6 for MDI or MDI spacer use). For DPIs, remember to stress that inhalation must be rapid and deep.
- Demonstrate correct use of peak flow meters, and observe the patient using them (Table 32-3). Explain about the green, yellow, and red zones (including the written action plan).
- Teach the patient how to prevent exercise-induced asthma.
- Be sure patients receive an influenza vaccination every fall. For asthma patients age ≥ 19 years, also administer pneumococcal vaccine according to recent Centers for Disease Control and Prevention recommendations.

Adverse Drug Effects

For more details, see the section on adverse drug effects in EPR-3.

Long-term control medications

Inhaled corticosteroids
- Inhaled corticosteroids may cause coughing, dysphonia, and oral thrush (candidiasis).
- In high doses, systemic effects may occur, although studies are not conclusive, and the clinical significance of these effects (e.g., adrenal suppression, osteoporosis, growth suppression, skin thinning, and easy bruising) has not been established.

Long-acting inhaled β₂-agonists
- Tachycardia, skeletal muscle tremor, hypokalemia, or prolongation of QTc interval can occur in an overdose.
- Use should always be in a combination product with inhaled corticosteroid (Advair, Dulera, or Symbicort) in long-term management of asthma per EPR-3 guidelines. (Use alone could mask inflammation and increase risk of severe exacerbations.)

Methylxanthines
- Dose-related acute toxicities include tachycardia, nausea and vomiting, tachyarrhythmias (supraventricular), central nervous system stimulation, headache, seizures, hematemesis, hyperglycemia, and hypokalemia.
- Adverse effects at usual therapeutic doses include insomnia, gastric upset, aggravation of ulcer or reflux, increase in hyperactivity in some children, and difficulty in urination in elderly males with prostatism.

Figure 32-6. Steps for Using an Inhaler

Please demonstrate your inhaler technique at every visit.

1. Remove the cap and hold inhaler upright.
2. Shake the inhaler.
3. Tilt your head back slightly and breathe out slowly.
4. Position the inhaler in one of the following ways (A or B is optimal, but C is acceptable for those who have difficulty with A or B. C is required for breath-activated inhalers):

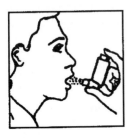
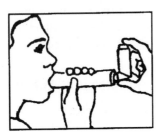
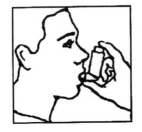
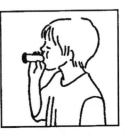

A. Open mouth with inhaler 1 to 2 inches away.

B. Use spacer/holding chamber (that is recommended especially for young children and for people using corticosteroids).

C. In the mouth. Do not use for cortico-steroids.

D. NOTE: Inhaled dry powder capsules require a different inhalation technique. To use a dry powder inhaler, it is important to close the mouth tightly around the mouthpiece of the inhaler and to inhale rapidly.

5. Press down on the inhaler to release medication as you start to breathe in slowly.
6. Breathe in slowly (3 to 5 seconds).
7. Hold your breath for 10 seconds to allow the medicine to reach deeply into your lungs.
8. Repeat puff as directed. Waiting 1 minute between puffs may permit second puff to penetrate your lungs better.
9. Spacers/holding chambers are useful for all patients. They are particularly recommended for young children and older adults and for use with inhaled corticosteroids.

Avoid common inhaler mistakes. Follow these inhaler tips:

- Breathe out *before* pressing your inhaler.
- Inhale *slowly*.
- Breathe in through your mouth, not your nose.
- Press down on your inhaler at the *start* of inhalation (or within the first second of inhalation).
- Keep inhaling as you press down on inhaler.
- Press your inhaler only *once* while you are inhaling (one breath for each puff).
- Make sure you breathe in evenly and deeply.

NOTE: Other inhalers are becoming available in addition to those illustrated above. Different types of inhalers may require different techniques.

Source: *Expert Panel Report 2: Guidelines for the Diagnosis and Management of Asthma.* National Asthma Education and Prevention Program, National Heart, Lung, and Blood Institute, 1997.

Table 32-3. Directions for Use of Peak Flow Meter

1. Stand while using the meter.
2. Position the indicator at the bottom of the scale.
3. Hold the peak flow meter so your fingers do not block the opening.
4. Inhale as deeply as possible, place the mouthpiece well into your mouth, and make sure your lips form a tight seal around it.
5. Blow out as fast and as hard as possible![a] BLAST! (Emphasize to the patient that the maneuver is highly effort dependent.)
6. Repeat steps 2–5 two more times, and record the highest of the three readings along with the date and time.

If a short-acting inhaled β_2-agonist is required in the early morning, remember to check the peak expiratory flow before using the drug and record the value; then repeat PEF testing 15 minutes later.
a. Do not accelerate air with your tongue (i.e., use a spitting motion). This incorrect maneuver will give false elevation in PEF.

Leukotriene modifiers
- Montelukast and zafirlukast are usually well tolerated.
- Zileuton can cause liver dysfunction.

Quick-relief medications

Short-acting inhaled β_2-agonists
- Tachycardia, skeletal muscle tremor, hypokalemia, increased lactic acid, headache, and rarely hyperglycemia can occur.
- In general, the inhaled route causes few systemic adverse effects; patients with preexisting cardiovascular disease, especially the elderly, may have adverse cardiovascular reactions with inhaled therapy.

Anticholinergics
- Drying of mouth and respiratory secretions; rarely, increased wheezing in some individuals; and blurred vision or acute angle-closure glaucoma can occur if aerosol inadvertently contacts eyes (e.g., ill-fitting nebulized facemask, touching of tiotropium dry powder capsule after inhalation followed by inadvertent touching of the eye).

Systemic corticosteroids
- With short-term use, reversible abnormalities in glucose metabolism, increased appetite, fluid retention, weight gain, mood alteration, hypertension, peptic ulcers, and, rarely, aseptic necrosis of the femur can occur.

- Consideration should be given to coexisting conditions that could be worsened by systemic corticosteroids, such as herpes virus infections, varicella, tuberculosis, hypertension, peptic ulcer disease, and strongyloidiasis.

Drug–Drug and Drug–Disease Interactions

- For zafirlukast, administration with meals decreases bioavailability. Patients should take at least 1 hour before or 2 hours after meals.
- Zileuton and zafirlukast may increase the effect of warfarin and increase theophylline levels.
- Well-known inducers of cytochrome P450 (carbamazepine, phenobarbital, phenytoin, and rifampin) are documented to decrease the effect of systemic corticosteroids.
- Examples of drugs that may increase the effect of systemic corticosteroids include erythromycin, clarithromycin, itraconazole, oral contraceptives, and conjugated estrogen.

Parameters to Monitor

- Refill record for daily controller–preventer medications and quick-relief medications
- Reduction in symptoms (including nocturnal and early morning symptoms)
- ED visits, hospitalizations, and unscheduled office visits
- Need for "bursts" of systemic corticosteroids
- Lost work or school days and the need for quick-relief medications
- PEF using a peak flow meter at home

In addition, if the patient also has rhinitis, monitor refills (e.g., intranasal corticosteroids) to ensure optimal control. (If rhinitis is not well controlled, asthma control will likely suffer.)

Kinetics

- Theophylline is no longer used extensively in asthma, but when it is used, knowledge of its kinetics is essential because of its high risk.
- Other drugs, disease states, smoking, age, and diet can all affect theophylline kinetics and dose requirements (see Table 32-4).
- Therapeutic serum theophylline concentrations are 5–15 mcg/mL (*not* the old recommendation of 10–20 mcg/mL; see EPR-3).
- Elimination half-life in an otherwise healthy nonsmoking adult is about 8 hours. In a smoker, it is about 4 hours, and in a small child (1 year or older), it is about 4 hours.

Table 32-4. Factors Affecting Serum Theophylline Levels

Factor	Decreases theophylline concentrations	Increases theophylline concentrations	Recommended action
Food	↓ or delays absorption of some sustained-release theophylline products	↑ rate of absorption (fatty foods) products	Select theophylline preparation that is not affected by food.
Diet	↑ metabolism (high protein)	↓ metabolism (high carbohydrate)	Inform patients that major changes in diet are not recommended while taking theophylline.
Systemic, febrile viral illness (e.g., influenza)		↓ metabolism	Decrease theophylline dose according to serum concentration level. Decrease dose by 50 percent if serum concentration measurement is not available.
Hypoxia, cor pulmonale, and decompensated congestive heart failure, cirrhosis		↓ metabolism	Decrease dose according to serum concentration level.
Age	↑ metabolism (1 to 9 years)	↓ metabolism (< 6 months, elderly)	Adjust dose according to serum concentration level.
Phenobarbital, phenytoin, carbamazepine	↑ metabolism		Increase dose according to serum concentration level.
Cimetidine		↓ metabolism	Use alternative H₂ blocker (e.g., famotidine or ranitidine).
Macrolides: TAO, erythromycin, clarithromycin		↓ metabolism	Use alternative antibiotic or adjust theophylline dose.
Quinolones: ciprofloxacin, enoxacin, pefloxacin		↓ metabolism	Use alternative antibiotic or adjust theophylline dose. Circumvent with ofloxacin if quinolone therapy is required.
Rifampin	↑ metabolism		Increase dose according to serum concentration level.
Ticlopidine		↓ metabolism	Decrease dose according to serum concentration level.
Smoking	↑ metabolism		Advise patient to stop smoking; increase dose according to serum concentration level.

Reproduced from NIH *Expert Panel Report 3*.
↓, decreases; ↑, increases; TAO, triacetyloleandomycin.
This list is not all inclusive; for discussion of other factors, see package inserts.

- Neonates have greatly prolonged elimination half-life.
- Elimination half-life in decompensated heart failure or cirrhosis is about 24 hours.
- Volume of distribution is about 0.5 L/kg.
- High-fat meals may cause "dose dumping" for some products (check product literature).

Other

- MDIs should be stored at room temperature, between 59°F and 86°F; if left in a car during freezing or near-freezing temperatures, aerosol particles will be too large to inhale into the lungs.
- MDIs should be "primed" (one dose released) only with first use or, in the case of a prn agent, used only once every 2 weeks. (Frequent priming is unnecessary and wastes expensive medications.)
- Hydrofluoroalkane (HFA) MDIs need special attention regarding weekly cleaning of the actuator (see manufacturers' instructions).
- The MDI dust cap should be left on the inhaler when not in use. Patient should check the mouthpiece for foreign objects before inhaling.

Nondrug Therapy

- An essential component of optimal asthma management is environmental control.
- Without good control of the environment at home, school, and work, drug therapy will often be inadequate.
- Have the patient identify known asthma triggers, and help the patient identify potential triggers not yet realized. (Do not forget someone smoking at home or work!)

32-4. Chronic Obstructive Pulmonary Disease (COPD)

COPD is characterized by airflow limitation that is not fully reversible. The airflow limitation is usually both progressive and associated with an abnormal inflammatory response of the lungs to noxious particles or gases. COPD is a major cause of death and suffering in the United States and around the world.

Types and Classifications

Some clinicians still refer to chronic bronchitis and emphysema in characterizing different levels of COPD (e.g., emphysema patients have destructive damage to the alveolar walls, whereas chronic bronchitis is associated with chronic productive cough). According to the Global Initiative for Chronic Obstructive Lung Disease (GOLD) 2014, COPD severity classification of airflow limitation is as follows (in patients with FEV_1/FVC [forced vital capacity] < 0.70):

- *GOLD 1. Mild:* $FEV_1 \geq 80\%$ predicted
- *GOLD 2. Moderate:* $50\% \leq FEV_1 < 80\%$ predicted
- *GOLD 3. Severe:* $30\% \leq FEV_1 < 50\%$ predicted
- *GOLD 4. Very severe:* $FEV_1 < 30\%$ predicted

In addition, examples of factors affecting the severity of COPD include frequency of exacerbations, presence of other disease states, overall health status, and severity of symptoms. GOLD 2014 includes a "Combined COPD Assessment," which includes symptomatic assessment with spirometric classification, exacerbation risk, or both. Using this assessment, 4 patient groups are summarized as follows: Group A (low risk, less symptoms), Group B (low risk, more symptoms), Group C (high risk, less symptoms), and Group D (high risk, more symptoms). These classifications are used in the initial choice for drug therapy of COPD.

Clinical Presentation

- Shortness of breath
- Cough and sputum production
- Usually, a history of cigarette smoking for several years
- In the more severe form, respiratory failure and heart failure

Pathophysiology

- COPD is usually caused by long-term smoking; it may also be caused by exposure to other noxious particles and gases.
- Chronic inflammation is found throughout the airways but via different inflammatory cells and mediators than those that cause asthma. Thus, the response to inhaled corticosteroids is much less than that seen with asthma.
- An imbalance of proteinases and antiproteinases is found in the lung.
- A rare hereditary cause of emphysema is α_1-antitrypsin deficiency.
- Pathologic changes are found in the central and peripheral airways as well as the alveoli and pulmonary vasculature.
- The following pathological changes are also found:
  - Mucus hypersecretion
  - Ciliary dysfunction
  - Airflow limitation
  - Lung hyperinflation
  - Gas exchange abnormalities
  - Secondary pulmonary hypertension
  - Cor pulmonale

Diagnostic Criteria

- History of cigarette smoking or exposure to other noxious particles or fumes
- Chronic cough and sputum production
- Spirometry (e.g., reduced FEV_1)
- Ruling out of other lung diseases

Treatment Principles and Goals

- Management of COPD includes the following principles and goals: prevent progression of disease, relieve symptoms, enhance health status, increase exercise tolerance, prevent and treat exacerbations and complications, and decrease mortality.
- Bronchodilators are central to the symptomatic treatment of COPD. These agents will increase

exercise capacity without necessarily improving FEV_1.

- Inhaled bronchodilators are preferred to oral bronchodilators for initial therapy; the specific choice of agent depends on patient response.
- Long-acting inhaled bronchodilators are more effective and convenient but more expensive. Examples of long-acting anticholinergic bronchodilators include the once-daily tiotropium (Spiriva) and twice-daily aclidinium (Tudorza Pressair). Twice-daily LABAs (formoterol and salmeterol were discussed in Section 32-3) and a once-daily LABA, indacaterol (Arcapta Neohaler) recently became available in the United States. A combination product (Breo Ellipta) with an ICS (fluticasone furoate) and LABA (vilanterol) was recently available in the United States for once-daily long-term management of COPD.
- Short-acting inhaled β_2-agonists are preferred for prn use in patients already receiving LABAs and anticholinergics.
- Inhaled corticosteroids are added to long-acting bronchodilators in COPD patients at a high risk of exacerbations.
- Theophylline is an option for maintenance therapy in patients who are not optimally controlled with β_2-agonists and anticholinergics.
- Roflumilast (Daliresp) oral tablets may decrease the frequency of exacerbations of severe COPD. This agent is a selective phosphodiesterase type-4 inhibitor.

Initial maintenance drug therapy of COPD (first choice and second choice)

For each patient group, patients should avoid risk factors (e.g., cease smoking) and receive an influenza vaccine each autumn. Also, pneumococcal vaccine should be administered per current guidelines. See the GOLD 2014 for additional second choices and alternative choice drug therapy.

- *Group A:*
  - Bronchodilator (short-acting) as needed (first choice)
  - Long-acting anticholinergic *or* LABA *or* combination of short-acting anticholinergic and short-acting β_2-agonist (second choice)
- *Group B:*
  - Long-acting anticholinergic *or* LABA (first choice)
  - Combination of long-acting inhaled bronchodilators (second choice)

- *Group C:*
  - Long-acting bronchodilator (LABA *or* long-acting anticholinergic) plus inhaled corticosteroid (first choice)
  - Combination of long-acting inhaled bronchodilators (second choice)
- *Group D:*
  - Inhaled corticosteroid plus *either* LABA *or* long-acting anticholinergic (first choice)
  - Inhaled corticosteroid plus LABA *and* long-acting anticholinergic (second choice, one option)

Drug therapy for acute exacerbations of COPD

- Inhaled albuterol with or without ipratropium
- Systemic corticosteroids (e.g., prednisone 40 mg/day for 5 days)
- Oxygen
- Antibiotics (usually oral) for purulent sputum as well as for increased sputum volume and increased dyspnea or for patients who require mechanical ventilation. The choice of antibiotic depends on local patterns of bacterial resistance. Typical initial empiric therapy is amoxicillin with or without a β-lactamase inhibitor, a macrolide, or doxycycline. For patients with frequent or severe exacerbations, appropriate cultures should be done because of the possibility of Gram-negative bacteria or microbes that are not sensitive to usual antimicrobial treatment.

Monitoring

- Spirometry: FEV_1
- Symptoms of dyspnea, cough, sputum production, and change in sputum color and volume
- PaO_2 (partial pressure of oxygen in the arterial blood)
- Exercise tolerance or fatigue

Long-term drug therapy

- See content in Table 32-1 for specific drugs.
- Tiotropium is a once-daily anticholinergic bronchodilator that is an option for step 1 treatment of moderate to severe COPD. It is administered by a DPI (HandiHaler). Each dose must be loaded, and deep inhalation does not have to be forceful but must be sufficient to hear the capsule vibrate. Another tiotropium delivery device, Respimat Soft Mist Inhaler (multidose), is available outside the United States.

Nondrug therapy

■ Smoking cessation—nicotine replacement therapy, bupropion (Zyban), varenicline (Chantix), support groups, and counseling
■ Oxygen therapy
■ Nutritional support
■ Psychosocial support
■ Pulmonary rehabilitation

Smoking cessation is the most important of these therapies.

32-5. Questions

1. In addition to airway inflammation, asthma is commonly associated with what problem?

   A. Pulmonary fibrosis
   B. Infection
   C. Interstitial lung disease
   D. Bronchospasm
   E. Granulomas

2. Which objective measure is a component of the diagnosis of asthma?

   A. PEF
   B. FEV_1
   C. FEF_{25-75}
   D. O_2 saturation
   E. PD20

3. Which device requires slow inhalation?

   A. Diskus
   B. Flexhaler
   C. Aerolizer
   D. MDI plus spacer
   E. Twisthaler

4. How many seconds is optimal for breath holding after inhaling from an MDI?

   A. 4
   B. 5
   C. 15
   D. 2
   E. 10

5. When a peak flow meter is used, what percentage of the personal best value is the green zone?

   A. > 50
   B. < 70

   C. 80–100
   D. 60–89
   E. 90–100

6. What is the trade name for mometasone + formoterol MDI?

   A. Foradil
   B. Pulmicort
   C. Combivent
   D. Symbicort
   E. Dulera

7. Which of the following disease states decrease theophylline elimination and often result in reduced dosage requirements?

   A. Hepatitis
   B. Heart failure (decompensated)
   C. Cirrhosis
   D. A and C
   E. A, B, and C

8. Which drugs are preferred for long-term treatment of moderate persistent asthma?

   A. Budesonide + formoterol
   B. Fluticasone + albuterol
   C. Beclomethasone + ipratropium
   D. A or B
   E. B or C

9. Which drug is a once-daily anticholinergic bronchodilator?

   A. Atrovent
   B. Serevent
   C. Foradil
   D. Spiriva
   E. Proventil

10. For patients with asthma or COPD exacerbations who are not responding adequately to inhaled short-acting bronchodilators, what is the agent of choice to add to manage the acute exacerbation?

    A. Fluticasone, high dose via spacer
    B. Budesonide, nebulized
    C. Montelukast, intravenously
    D. Theophylline, intravenously
    E. Prednisone, orally

11. Which drug may decrease serum theophylline concentrations?

    A. Clarithromycin
    B. Hydrochlorothiazide

C. Cimetidine

D. Rifampin

E. Losartan

12. Which side effect of inhaled corticosteroids is reduced by spacer devices?

A. Hoarseness

B. Decreased bone density

C. Thinning of skin

D. Oropharyngeal candidiasis

E. Cataracts

13. The therapeutic range for theophylline per the NIH guidelines for asthma management is

A. 5–15 mcg/mL.

B. 8–12 mcg/mL.

C. 10–20 mcg/mL.

D. 15–25 mcg/mL.

E. 10–15 mcg/mL.

14. Which asthma controller drug is preferred for mild persistent asthma in children < 12 years of age?

A. Accolate

B. Singulair

C. Xolair

D. Pulmicort

E. Medrol

15. Which disease state may worsen asthma?

A. Coronary artery disease

B. Allergic rhinitis

C. Diabetes

D. Hypertension

E. Arthritis

16. Which class of drugs is added to long-acting bronchodilators for long-term management of COPD patients who have frequent exacerbations?

A. Leukotriene receptor antagonists

B. Anticholinergics

C. Anti-IgE agent

D. Inhaled corticosteroids

E. Methylxanthines

Use Patient Profile 32-1 to answer Questions 17 and 18.

17. Which class of drugs is preferred for Mr. Johnson for optimal control of asthma?

Patient Profile 32-1 Medication Profile

Patient Name	Thomas Johnson	**Height**	5'10"
Date of birth	9-15-55	**Weight**	75 kg
Drug allergies	Aspirin sensitivity		
Allergies	NKA		

Diagnosis (1) Asthma (childhood onset, mild persistent)

(2) Allergic rhinitis

(3) Hypertension

Medications

Date	Rx #	Physician	Drug and strength	Quantity	Sig	Refills
3/16	94385	Betts	Singulair 20 mg	30	1 at bedtime	3
3/16	94386	Betts	Albuterol MDI	1	2 puffs q4h	6
3/16	94387	Betts	Fluticasone nasal spray	1	1 squirt both nostrils bid	3
3/25	95523	T. Jones	Lopressor 50 mg	60	1 bid	6
3/27	95734	Betts	Albuterol MDI	1	2 puffs q4h	5

Pharmacist notes: 3/16—discussed proper use of MDI and observed patient use. Coached Mr. Johnson to inhale slowly (he was inhaling fast); he used the MDI correctly for the other steps.

A. Anticholinergics
B. Inhaled corticosteroids
C. Methylxanthines
D. Long-acting β₂-agonists
E. Oral corticosteroids

18. What is an appropriate alternative to Lopressor for Mr. Johnson?

    A. Lisinopril
    B. Propranolol
    C. Clonidine
    D. Hydralazine
    E. Carvedilol

Use Patient Profile 32-2 to answer Questions 19 and 20.

19. What concerns regarding theophylline should the pharmacist have in the situation with Mrs. Adams?

    A. Cirrhosis is well documented to decrease elimination of theophylline.
    B. The milligrams per kilogram dose is too low.
    C. Mrs. Adams should be on a q12h product.
    D. Theophylline SR should be dosed in the morning, not evening.
    E. Long-acting inhaled β₂-agonists increase theophylline clearance.

20. Mrs. Adams has a friend who has COPD and has told her about Spiriva. Mrs. Adams asks your opinion, as her pharmacist, about her taking Spiriva.

    A. Spiriva is effective, but I am concerned about adverse effects.
    B. Spiriva is a third-line drug for COPD; I would not use it now.
    C. Spiriva is a good drug, but I want to talk to your doctor about starting a medicine called Flovent.
    D. Since you have a prescription for Atrovent, I will call your doctor and suggest changing from Atrovent to Spiriva.
    E. I think Symbicort would be better for you.

21. Which drug is best for long-term management of intermittent asthma?

    A. Albuterol, prn
    B. Montelukast
    C. Albuterol, scheduled
    D. Theophylline
    E. Budesonide

22. Which total daily dose of prednisone is best for home management of an acute exacerbation of asthma in a 20-kg child?

    A. 5 mg
    B. 60 mg

Patient Profile 32-2 Medication Profile

Patient name	Mrs. S. T. Adams	Height	5′3″
Date of birth	1-16-37	Weight	55 kg
Drug allergies	Sulfonamides		

Diagnosis	(1) COPD—53 pack/year history of smoking (quit 2 years ago); no exacerbations in 10 years
	(2) Cirrhosis

Medications

Date	Rx #	Physician	Drug and strength	Quantity	Sig	Refills
2/18	84389	Jones	Serevent Diskus	1	1 inhalation q12h	6
2/18	84390	Jones	Albuterol MDI	1	2 puffs q4h pr6	
2/18	84391	Jones	Atrovent MDI	1	2 puffs q6h	6
2/18	84392	Jones	Uniphyl 600 mg	30	1 daily 6 pm	2

Pharmacist notes: 2/18—discussed proper use of Diskus and observed patient use; taught Mrs. Adams to inhale deeply and rapidly (she was inhaling slowly for < 2 seconds). Also observed use of MDI (she forgot to exhale gently before pressing down on MDI).

C. 20 mg

D. 10 mg

E. 7.5 mg

23. Which drug is most likely to cause an asthma exacerbation in a patient sensitive to aspirin?

   A. Naproxen
   B. Acetaminophen
   C. Celecoxib
   D. Salsalate
   E. Sodium salicylate

24. Which type of inhaler does not work well in very cold temperatures?

   A. Diskus
   B. Flexhaler
   C. Aerolizer
   D. MDI
   E. Twisthaler

25. Which device requires the patient to hear the capsule vibrating?

   A. HandiHaler
   B. Twisthaler
   C. Flexhaler
   D. Diskus
   E. A and B

32-6. Answers

1. **D.** Asthma certainly does have a bronchospastic component, yet it is primarily due to inflammation, so good control of inflammation dramatically reduces bronchospasm.

2. **B.** Spirometry, primarily the FEV_1, is part of the diagnosis of asthma.

3. **D.** Dry powder inhalers for asthma therapy that are currently available require rapid inhalation. MDIs require slow inhalation to minimize impaction of aerosol in the mouth and throat.

4. **E.** Ten seconds is best; there is no need to hold longer. If 10 seconds is uncomfortable, 4–5 seconds is acceptable.

5. **C.** The green zone is 80–100%, which indicates suboptimal control. (The red zone is < 50%, which indicates that the crisis action plan should be started and medical attention should be sought.)

6. **E.** Dulera is the combination of mometasone and formoterol.

7. **E.** Hepatitis, cirrhosis, and decompensated heart failure can dramatically reduce theophylline clearance.

8. **A.** Budesonide + formoterol.

9. **D.** Spiriva (tiotropium) is inhaled once daily.

10. **E.** Prednisone or other systemic corticosteroids (e.g., methylprednisolone) are well documented to be efficacious in asthma and acute exacerbations of COPD.

11. **D.** Rifampin is well documented to decrease serum theophylline concentrations. Clarithromycin and cimetidine are well documented to increase serum concentrations. Hydrochlorothiazide and losartan do not affect serum theophylline concentrations.

12. **D.** Oropharyngeal candidiasis or thrush is correct. The other side effects are not reduced by spacers.

13. **A.** The currently accepted range for asthma is 5–15 mcg/mL (*not* the old range of 10–20 mcg/mL). There is no benefit in exceeding 15 mcg/mL, and many patients receive benefit at lower doses.

14. **D.** Pulmicort or other inhaled corticosteroid is preferred (see NIH EPR-3).

15. **B.** Allergic rhinitis that is not well controlled can worsen asthma control and outcomes.

16. **D.** This class of drugs should *not* be used routinely in COPD patients with mild disease. Inhaled corticosteroids are added to long-acting bronchodilators in COPD, especially if there are frequent exacerbations.

17. **B.** Inhaled corticosteroids are the preferred treatment (see Figures 32-2 and 32-3 for treatment choices). The pharmacist should share the NIH guidelines with Mr. Johnson's prescriber to help ensure optimal care. In addition, the pharmacist should educate the patient regarding the purpose of the medications and proper use of inhalers (e.g., the pharmacist should observe the patient using the device).

18. **A.** An ACE inhibitor, such as lisinopril, should be efficacious with few side effects (monitor for cough); β-blockers should be avoided in Mr. Johnson unless he is post myocardial infarction or had congestive heart failure (in which case, use a low dose of a β_1-selective blocker and monitor carefully).

19. **A.** Cirrhosis is well documented to decrease elimination of theophylline. Ensure a check of a steady-state theophylline level (peak), and anticipate dose reduction (usually 50% dose reduction in liver disease).

20. **D.** Because the patient has prescriptions for Atrovent and Serevent, a logical change here would be to discontinue the short-acting anticholinergic Atrovent and add the long-acting once-daily anticholinergic tiotropium (Spiriva).

21. **A.** Per EPR-3, a short-acting inhaled β_2-agonist such as albuterol is used prn for intermittent asthma (remember, if it is needed more than twice per week during the day, the patient has not intermittent but persistent asthma).

22. **C.** Twenty milligrams is an appropriate dose. If it is started as soon as the patient is in the red zone and not responding quickly to short-acting inhaled β_2-agonists, usually only a few days of treatment will be required (usually < 1 week).

23. **A.** Naproxen has the same mechanism of action as aspirin and will predictably trigger symptoms in an aspirin-sensitive patient (i.e., increased production of leukotrienes). COX-2 inhibitors are usually safe (celecoxib). Acetaminophen is the choice agent for minor pain in these patients.

24. **D.** MDIs release large aerosol particles that do not penetrate deeply into the lungs in cold temperatures. Dry powder inhalers are acceptable.

25. **A.** HandiHaler requires that the patient hear the capsule vibrating (rattling) as the medication is being inhaled.

32-7. References

Asthma

Expert Panel Report 3: Guidelines for the Diagnosis and Management of Asthma. Bethesda, MD: U.S. Department of Health and Human Services, National Heart, Lung, and Blood Institute, 2007, NIH Publication 07-4051. http://www.nhlbi.nih.gov/guidelines/asthma/asthgdln.pdf. Accessed May 16, 2014.

Kerstjens HA, Engel M, Dahl M, et al. Tiotropium in asthma poorly controlled with standard therapy. *N Engl J Med.* 2012;367:1198–207.

Kiljander TO, Junghard O, Beckman O, et al. Effect of esomeprazole 40 mg once or twice daily on asthma: A randomized, placebo-controlled study. *Am J Respir Crit Care Med.* 2010;181:1042–48.

Lemanske RF, Busse WW. The U.S. Food and Drug Administration and long-acting beta$_2$ agonists: The importance of striking the right balance between risks and benefits of therapy? *J Allergy Clin Immunol.* 2010;126:449–52.

Self TH, Wallace JL, George CM, et al. Inhalation therapy: Help patients avoid these mistakes. *J Fam Prac.* 2011;60:714–20a.

Chronic Obstructive Pulmonary Disease

Global Initiative for Chronic Obstructive Lung Disease. *Global Strategy for the Diagnosis, Management, and Prevention of Chronic Obstructive Pulmonary Disease.* Updated 2014. http://www.goldcopd.org. Accessed February 6, 2014.

Fiore MC, Schroeder SA, Baker TB. Smoke, the chief killer—strategies for targeting combustible tobacco use. *N Engl J Med.* 2014;370:297–99.

Leuppi JD, Schuetz P, Bingisser R, et al. Short-term vs. conventional glucocorticoid therapy in acute exacerbations of chronic obstructive pulmonary disease. The REDUCE randomized clinical trial. *JAMA.* 2013;309:2223–31.

Tashkin DP, Celli B, Senn S, et al. A 4-year trial of tiotropium in chronic obstructive pulmonary disease. *N Engl J Med.* 2008;359:1543–54.

Wedzicha JA, Calverley PMA, Semungal TA, et al. The prevention of chronic obstructive pulmonary disease exacerbations by salmeterol/fluticasone propionate or tiotropium bromide. *Am J Respir Crit Care Med.* 2008;177:19–26.

Wise RA, Anzueto A, Cotton D, et al. Tiotropium Respimat inhaler and the risk of death in COPD. *N Engl J Med.* 2013;369:1491–501.

Infectious Disease

W. Andrew Bell

33

33-1. Key Points

- The hallmark of empiric anti-infective therapy is to target the specific organisms associated with the disease.
- Conversely, after the identification of the organism causing the disease, anti-infective therapy should be narrowed to cover that specific organism.
- Therapy should reflect not only the best anti-infective agent for the organism but also aspects of the patient's condition (e.g., renal function, concurrent disease states).
- Combination anti-infective therapy should be reserved for infections for which there are documented clinical efficacy, therapeutic failure of monotherapy, and suspicion of multidrug-resistant pathogens.
- Clinical signs of infection should be followed to determine patient response to therapy.
- Empiric therapy of meningitis is age specific, reflecting the age-specific nature of the common pathogens. Treatment is then determined based on Gram-stain and culture results.
- Endocarditis therapy is specific to the organism isolated. The presence of a prosthetic valve generally increases the length of therapy.
- Gram-positive coverage with vancomycin is the recommended initial therapy for central line–associated blood stream infections if no additional risk factors are present.
- Monotherapy with an agent that provides Gram-positive bacteria, enteric Gram-negative bacilli,

and *Pseudomonas aeruginosa* coverage is recommended empiric therapy for febrile neutropenia.

- Many cases of bronchitis are viral in etiology, making routine antibiotic therapy controversial.
- Treatment of acute exacerbations of chronic bronchitis decreases duration of illness.
- Empiric pneumonia therapy is based on the pneumonia classification: community-acquired pneumonia (CAP), hospital-acquired pneumonia (HAP), ventilator-associated pneumonia (VAP), or health care–associated pneumonia (HCAP).
- The U.S. Centers for Disease Control and Prevention (CDC) recommends direct observed therapy for most treatment regimens for active and latent tuberculosis.
- Treatment of intra-abdominal infections is based on the severity of infection and patient risk factors.
- Diarrhea therapy should be mainly supportive, with careful use of anti-infectives and antimotility agents.
- Empiric treatment of skin and soft tissue infections (SSTIs) targets the organisms most commonly associated with the specific type of infection. The need for empiric coverage of methicillin-resistant *Staphylococcus aureus* (MRSA) is increasing.
- Diagnosis of urinary tract infections (UTIs) varies by numbers of organisms found in the urine. Higher numbers (> 105 cells/mL) are needed to diagnose UTIs in females than in males (> 103 cells/mL) because of the higher numbers of organisms able to ascend the shorter female urethra.
- Fluoroquinolones are useful in the treatment of prostatitis.

Editor's Note: This chapter is based on the 10th edition chapter written by W. Andrew Bell and Julia Underwood.

- Patients testing positive for any sexually transmitted disease should be screened for the presence of other venereal diseases.
- Patients diagnosed with syphilis should be treated appropriately to avoid progression to tertiary syphilis. Penicillin is the drug of choice for the treatment of syphilis.
- Initial therapy of sepsis should be broad in scope, covering all likely organisms, until results of cultures are obtained.
- Doxycycline is particularly useful in the treatment of tickborne systemic febrile syndromes.
- Selection of an antifungal agent is based on the suspected pathogen and severity of illness.
- Amphotericin B products are reserved for severe fungal infections because of the high incidence of toxicity.
- Chronic hepatitis B is treated with interferon alfa–based therapies or nucleos(t)ide analogue (NA) therapies.
- Treatment for chronic hepatitis C is based on genotype. Patients are treated with a combination of two or three medications: Sofosbuvir plus ribavirin is part of the preferred treatment for all genotypes, and interferon therapy is added for eligible patients with genotypes 1, 4, 5, and 6.
- Agents used for prophylaxis and treatment of influenza include oseltamivir, zanamivir, amantadine, and rimantadine.
- Acyclovir, valacyclovir, and famciclovir can be used to treat genital herpes simplex and varicella zoster infections.

33-2. Study Guide Checklist

The following topics may guide your study of this subject area:

- Signs, symptoms, and laboratory findings of common infections
- Culture and stain techniques used to identify infecting agent
- Considerations for selection of empiric anti-infective therapy based on site of infection and risk factors
- Spectrum of activity of individual anti-infective agents
- De-escalation of therapy based on culture results
- Indications for combination therapy
- Frequency and duration of anti-infective therapy

33-3. General Principles of Infectious Disease

Several infectious disease topics are addressed in other chapters of this review, including common colds in Chapter 31, human immunodeficiency virus (HIV) and acquired immune deficiency syndrome (AIDS) in Chapter 35, and otitis media in Chapter 37. For additional information about specific anti-infective agents, see Chapter 34.

Diagnosis

Diagnosis of most infectious diseases consists of isolation and identification of microorganisms, assessment of patient signs and symptoms, and analysis of other laboratory data.

Isolation of organisms

For identification of the causative agent of a disease, samples should be taken from appropriate body sites prior to the initiation of anti-infective therapy. If collection of cultures is expected to take longer than 1 hour, then antibiotic therapy should be initiated without further delay. Organisms isolated from body sites that normally are sterile (blood, urine, and spinal fluid) yield higher predictive value than do organisms isolated from body sites that are normally colonized with microorganisms (skin or fecal material).

Identification of organisms

Once a specimen is obtained, a Gram stain is performed to determine the infectious organism's cell morphology and to guide empiric therapy. The specimen is also cultured to isolate any microorganisms present. After the species of organism has been determined, it is exposed to standardized concentrations of antibiotics to determine the concentrations that inhibit its growth. The lowest concentration that prevents microbial growth is called the *minimum inhibitory concentration* (MIC). The three breakpoint concentrations of antibiotics are susceptible, intermediate, and resistant. An antibiotic's breakpoint concentration is determined by considering (1) tissue concentrations with normal dosing and (2) the organism's population distribution. The breakpoint concentration determines whether the antibiotic can be used for therapy.

Physical signs and symptoms of infection such as fever, redness, swelling, pain, and cough must be considered both for initial diagnosis and for assessment of response to antibiotic therapy.

Laboratory tests

In the initial stage of infection, the patient's neutrophil count may increase above normal, and immature neutrophil forms (bands) may appear; therefore, a white blood cell (WBC) count should be taken. The presence of greater than 10% bands, known as a left shift, is indicative of infection. Later in the course of illness, the neutrophil count may fall to below normal levels.

Inflammatory markers, such as C-reactive protein, erythrocyte sedimentation rate, and tumor necrosis factor, may increase during infection; however, they are nonspecific. Procalcitonin is an inflammatory marker that is more specific for bacterial infection.

Laboratory tests may not be reliable in patients who are elderly, malnourished, neonatal, or severely infected.

Treatment Strategies

Anti-infective agents should be used only when a significant infection has been diagnosed, when one is strongly suspected, or when prophylactic therapy is indicated.

Prophylactic anti-infective therapy is aimed at preventing infection. Prophylactic therapy commonly is used after exposure to infection (e.g., tuberculosis) or before surgical intervention in areas of high bacterial inoculum (e.g., bowel surgery).

Empiric therapy is directed toward all common pathogens associated with a disease state. Empiric therapy should be based on the organisms common to the suspected infection as well as local trends of susceptibility and prevalence.

Culture-guided therapy covers only the specific organism identified. Culture-guided therapy is preferred over empiric therapy because it is more cost-effective and it decreases bacterial resistance from unnecessary antibiotic exposure.

Choice of Anti-infective Agents

To determine optimal anti-infective therapy or to review the appropriateness of other decisions, a clinician must answer several questions:

- Is an antibiotic indicated on the basis of the clinical findings?

- Have appropriate specimens been obtained, examined, and sent for culture?
- What organisms are most likely to cause the suspected infection?
- If several antibiotics are available to treat the likely or known organism, which agent is best for the patient? (Patient allergies and concurrent disease states should be considered.)
- Is an antibiotic combination appropriate? (A combination of drugs should be given only when clinical experience has shown such therapy to be more effective than single-agent therapy in a particular setting or when there is a high suspicion for multidrug-resistant pathogens. Such multiple-agent regimens can increase the risk of toxic drug effects, and occasionally, they may result in drug antagonism and loss of effectiveness. In contrast, some combinations of anti-infective agents have demonstrated increased effectiveness that exceeds their individual effectiveness. This phenomenon is known as *synergy*. An example of synergy is the combination of an aminoglycoside, such as streptomycin or gentamicin, with a cell wall inhibitor, such as penicillin, in some Gram-positive infections.)
- What is the best route of administration? (This decision will depend on the overall plan for the patient. For example, oral therapy is preferred for outpatient therapy; many intravenous anti-infectives have oral forms with similar pharmacokinetic profiles.)
- What is the appropriate dose and dose interval? (Regimen design should take into account patient size, renal or hepatic function, the disease state being treated, and pharmacodynamics of the agents used.)
- Will initial therapy need modification after culture data are returned?
- What is the optimal duration of therapy, and is resistance during prolonged therapy likely to develop?

Lack of Therapeutic Effectiveness

When anti-infective therapy fails, careful analysis of possible causes should be made prior to changing the regimen. Factors associated with therapeutic failure include misdiagnosis of the infection, improper drug regimen, inappropriate choice of antibiotic agent, antibiotic resistance, and situations in which antibiotic therapy may not be effective without additional interventions (e.g., surgical drainage).

33-4. Common Bacterial, Fungal, and Viral Infections (Causative Agents, Clinical Presentation, Diagnostic Criteria, Treatment)

Meningitis

Meningitis, defined as inflammation of the meninges, can be caused by bacterial, fungal, or viral pathogens. This section covers treatment of bacterial meningitis.

Causative agents

A wide variety of organisms cause bacterial meningitis, including both Gram-positive and Gram-negative organisms. Patient age is one factor used to guide antibiotic selection because age is associated with specific organisms (Table 33-1).

Clinical presentation

Patients may present with a fever, headache, photophobia, nuchal rigidity, seizures, vomiting, or altered mental status. Infants may also present with a bulging anterior fontanel.

Diagnostic criteria

Blood and cerebrospinal fluid (CSF) samples should be obtained for culture if meningitis is suspected. Analysis of CSF fluid, including a Gram-stain, should also be performed. In cases of bacterial meningitis, the following abnormalities occur in the CSF: increased WBCs and protein as well as decreased glucose.

Treatment

Empiric treatment for bacterial meningitis is usually determined by patient age or comorbid neurologic conditions (Table 33-1). Because of limited antibiotic penetration by many agents, the highest safe antibiotic doses are generally used. For adults, once a Gram-stain is completed, therapy can be directed toward presumed organisms while awaiting culture results (Table 33-2). In children over 1 month of age, Vancocin (vancomycin) with either Claforan (cefotaxime) or Rocephin (ceftriaxone) is recommended until culture results are available. Additional agents may be added to the two-drug regimen based on Gram-stain. In cases of methicillin-resistant *Staphylococcus aureus* (MRSA) infections, vancomycin with the possible addition of Rifadin (rifampin) is the preferred treatment. Vancomycin loading doses of 25–30 mg/kg can be considered. Alternative treatments for MRSA meningitis include Zyvox (linezolid) or Bactrim (trimethoprim-sulfamethoxazole). Adjunctive Decadron (dexamethasone) should be considered in select patient populations based on age and presumed causative agent.

Endocarditis

Endocarditis is an infection of the endocardium, the membrane lining the heart chamber and valves. Injection drug use or heart abnormalities such as an artificial or damaged valve predispose patients to endocarditis.

Table 33-1. Empiric Therapy for Meningitis Based on Age

Age	Common organisms	Treatment
Newborn to 1 month	*Streptococcus agalactiae, Escherichia coli, Listeria monocytogenes, Klebsiella* species	Ampicillin plus either cefotaxime or an aminoglycoside
1 to 23 months	*Streptococcus pneumoniae, Neisseria meningitidis, Streptococcus agalactiae, Haemophilus influenzae, Escherichia coli*	Vancomycin plus either ceftriaxone or cefotaxime[a]
2 to 50 years	*Neisseria meningitidis, Streptococcus pneumoniae*	Vancomycin plus either ceftriaxone or cefotaxime[a]
50 years or older	*Streptococcus pneumoniae, Neisseria meningitidis, Listeria monocytogenes*, aerobic Gram-negative bacilli	Vancomycin plus ampicillin plus either ceftriaxone or cefotaxime[a]

Tunkel AR, Hartman BJ, Kaplan SL, et al. 2004.
a. Consider addition of rifampin if dexamethasone is given.

Table 33-2. Targeted Therapy for Adults with Meningitis Based on Gram-Stain

Organism	Recommended treatment	Alternative treatment
Streptococcus pneumoniae	Vancomycin plus either ceftriaxone or cefotaxime[a]	Meropenem, gatifloxacin, or moxifloxacin
Neisseria meningitidis	Ceftriaxone or cefotaxime	Penicillin G, ampicillin, chloramphenicol, fluoroquinolone, or aztreonam
Listeria monocytogenes	Ampicillin or penicillin G[b]	Trimethoprim-sulfamethoxazole or meropenem
Streptococcus agalactiae	Ampicillin or penicillin G[b]	Ceftriaxone or cefotaxime
Haemophilus influenzae	Ceftriaxone or cefotaxime	Chloramphenicol, cefepime, meropenem, or fluoroquinolone
Escherichia coli	Ceftriaxone or cefotaxime	Cefepime, meropenem, aztreonam, fluoroquinolone, trimethoprim-sulfamethoxazole

Tunkel AR, Hartman BJ, Kaplan SL, et al., 2004.
a. Consider addition of rifampin if dexamethasone is given.
b. Consider addition of an aminoglycoside to either therapy.

Causative agents

Endocarditis can result from a variety of infectious agents including fungi and bacteria. The most common bacterial organisms are *Streptococcus, Staphylococcus,* and *Enterococcus* species.

Clinical presentation

Patients may present with a low-grade fever, fatigue, weakness, new heart murmur, or petechiae.

Diagnostic criteria

Endocarditis is diagnosed on the basis of patient signs and symptoms in combination with tests such as blood cultures or an echocardiogram to visualize vegetations.

Treatment

Treatment varies depending on the causative organism, susceptibility to antibiotics, and presence or absence of prosthetic devices. Table 33-3 describes therapies for endocarditis. Published guidelines provide more specific recommendations.

Central Line–Associated Bloodstream Infections

More than 150 million vascular devices are placed in patients in the United States each year, and infections of these devices are associated with considerable morbidity, mortality, and cost. The Infectious Diseases Society of America has recently updated recommendations for the prevention and treatment of infections of intravascular catheters.

Causative agents

Like most other infections, the predominant pathogen associated with intravascular catheters varies according to the type of device, duration the device is in place, local microbiological trends, and patient-specific risk factors. In general, coagulase-negative staphylococci and *S. aureus* are the most common causes of intravascular device infections. Other commonly implicated pathogens include *Candida* species, *Enterococcus* species, *Pseudomonas aeruginosa,* and enteric Gram-negative bacilli.

Clinical presentation

The clinical presentation of intravascular catheter infections is nonspecific, consisting of fever or hypothermia, chills, tachycardia, tachypnea, hypotension, and increased or decreased WBC count. For long-term catheters, such as dialysis or tunneled catheters used for long-term intravenous (IV) therapy (chemotherapy or total parenteral nutrition), symptoms may occur when the catheter is accessed.

Diagnostic criteria

When a catheter-related infection is suspected, blood cultures should be drawn from the catheter and from a peripheral site prior to initiating antibiotics. If

Table 33-3. Treatment of Endocarditis

Organism	Native valve (duration in weeks)	Prosthetic valve (duration in weeks)
Viridans group streptococci and *Streptococcus bovis:* MIC ≤ 0.12 mcg/mL	Penicillin G (4) Ceftriaxone (4) Penicillin G (2) + gentamicin (2) Ceftriaxone (2) + gentamicin (2) Vancomycin[a] (4)	Penicillin G (6) Ceftriaxone (6) Penicillin G (6) + gentamicin (2) Ceftriaxone (6) + gentamicin (2) Vancomycin[a] (6)
Viridans group streptococci and *Streptococcus bovis:* MIC 0.12–0.5 mcg/mL	Penicillin G (4) + gentamicin (2) Ceftriaxone (4) + gentamicin (2) Vancomycin[a] (4)	Penicillin (6) + gentamicin (6) Ceftriaxone (6) + gentamicin (6) Vancomycin[a] (6)
Viridans group streptococci and *Streptococcus bovis:* MIC > 0.5 mcg/mL	Ampicillin (4–6) + gentamicin (4–6) Penicillin G (4–6) + gentamicin (4–6) Vancomycin[b] (6)	Penicillin (6) + gentamicin (6) Ceftriaxone (6) + gentamicin (6) Vancomycin[a] (6)
Oxacillin-susceptible staphylococci	Nafcillin (6) ± gentamicin (3–5 days) Oxacillin (6) ± gentamicin (3–5 days) Cefazolin[c] (6) ± gentamicin (3–5 days)	Nafcillin (≥ 6) + rifampin (≥ 6) + gentamicin (2) Oxacillin (≥ 6) + rifampin (≥ 6) + gentamicin (2) Cefazolin[c] (≥ 6) + rifampin (≥ 6) + gentamicin (2)
Oxacillin-resistant staphylococci	Vancomycin (6)	Vancomycin (≥ 6) + rifampin (≥ 6) + gentamicin (2)
Enterococci susceptible to penicillin, gentamicin, and vancomycin	Ampicillin (4–6) + gentamicin[d] (4–6) Penicillin G (4–6) + gentamicin[d] (4–6) Vancomycin[b] (6) + gentamicin[d] (6)	Ampicillin (6) + gentamicin[d] (6) Penicillin G (6) + gentamicin[d] (6) Vancomycin[b] (6) + gentamicin[d] (6)
Enterococci susceptible to aminoglycoside and vancomycin but resistant to penicillin	Ampicillin-sulbactam (6) + gentamicin (6) Vancomycin[e] (6) + gentamicin (6)	Ampicillin-sulbactam (6) + gentamicin (6) Vancomycin[e] (6) + gentamicin (6)
Enterococcus faecium resistant to penicillin, aminoglycosides, and vancomycin	Linezolid (≥ 8) Quinupristin-dalfopristin (≥ 8)	Linezolid (≥ 8) Quinupristin-dalfopristin (≥ 8)
Enterococcus faecalis resistant to penicillin, aminoglycosides, and vancomycin	Imipenem (≥ 8) + ampicillin (≥ 8) Ceftriaxone (≥ 8) + ampicillin (≥ 8)	Imipenem (≥ 8) + ampicillin (≥ 8) Ceftriaxone (≥ 8) + ampicillin (≥ 8)
HACEK Group	Ceftriaxone (4) Ampicillin-sulbactam (4) Fluoroquinolone[f] (4)	Ceftriaxone (6) Ampicillin-sulbactam (6) Fluoroquinolone[f] (6)

Baddour LM, Wilson WR, Bayer AS, et al., 2005.
HACEK = *Haemophilus, Actinobacillus, Cardiobacterium, Eikenella, Kingella.*
a. Use vancomycin only if unable to use penicillin or ceftriaxone.
b. Use vancomycin only if unable to use ampicillin or penicillin.
c. Cefazolin should be used for nonanaphylactoid penicillin-allergic patients. If the patient has an anaphylactoid allergy, use vancomycin.
d. Substitute streptomycin if patient is resistant to gentamicin.
e. Use vancomycin only if unable to use ampicillin-sulbactam or if strain has intrinsic penicillin resistance.
f. Use a fluoroquinolone only if unable to use ceftriaxone or ampicillin-sulbactam.

possible, the catheter should be removed and cultured by rolling it on a plate of agar. A definitive diagnosis is made based on the following: (1) the same organism grows from at least one bottle cultured from the catheter and one bottle cultured from the peripheral site or (2) when the same organisms grow from the blood cultured from the catheter and more than 15 colony-forming units grow from the catheter-tip culture.

Treatment

The agent selected and duration of treatment of intravascular device infections depend on the location and type of device, organism isolated, whether the device is removed, clinical response, and additional patient comorbidities. When possible, the infected device should be removed. If no specific risk factors are present, initial empiric treatment should include vancomycin to cover methicillin-resistant staphylococci (Table 33-4). If the MIC of the majority of *S. aureus* at your institution is greater than 2mg/dL, then Cubicin (daptomycin) should be used empirically. Linezolid should not be used, though, for treatment of catheter-related infections. Selection of coverage for Gram-negative organisms should be based on local susceptibility data and severity of disease. Double-coverage of Gram-negative bacteria is not recommended unless the patient has risk factors for multidrug-resistant bacteria or is extremely ill (septic shock, neutropenia). Empiric coverage of *Candida* should be given to patients with a history of femoral catheter placement, use of total parenteral nutrition, prolonged use of antibiotics, hematologic malignancy, transplant, or colonization by *Candida* species at multiple sites.

Table 33-4. Treatment of Uncomplicated Catheter-Related Infections in Patients without Malignancy or Immunosuppression

Organism	Primary treatment	Secondary treatment	Duration
Coagulase-negative Staphylococci			
Methicillin resistant	Vancomycin	Daptomycin	Remove catheter, and treat for 5–7 days.
Methicillin susceptible	Nafcillin or oxacillin	Cefazolin or vancomycin	
Staphylococcus aureus			
Methicillin resistant	Vancomycin	Daptomycin	Remove catheter, and treat for at least 14 days.
Methicillin susceptible	Nafcillin or oxacillin	Cefazolin or vancomycin	
Enterococcus			
Ampicillin susceptible	Penicillin or ampicillin	Vancomycin	Remove catheter, and treat for 7–14 days.
Vancomycin susceptible	Vancomycin +/– AMG synergy	Daptomycin	
Vancomycin resistant	Daptomycin	Linezolid or quinupristin/dalfopristin	
Gram-negative bacilli (E. coli, Klebsiella, Enterobacter, Serratia)			
ESBL negative	Third-generation cephalosporin	Ciprofloxacin or aztreonam	Remove catheter, and treat for 7–14 days.
ESBL positive	Carbapenem	Varies by susceptibility	
Pseudomonas aeruginosa	Cefepime or piperacillin/tazobactam +/– AMG	Varies by susceptibility	
Candida species			
Fluconazole susceptible	Fluconazole or echinocandin	Lipid amphotericin B preparations	Remove catheter, and treat for 14 days after first negative blood culture.
Fluconazole resistant	Echinocandin	Lipid amphotericin B preparations	

AMG = amikacin, tobramycin, or gentamicin; AMG synergy = gentamicin or streptomycin; ESBL = extended-spectrum beta-lactamase; carbapenem = doripenem, ertapenem, imipenem/cilastatin, meropenem.

Febrile Neutropenia

Patients with cancer often have marked decreases in WBCs caused by their chemotherapy regimen. *Neutropenia* is defined as an absolute neutrophil count (ANC) below 500 cells/mL [ANC = (% Bands + % Segs) × WBC]. When the ANC is less than 500 cells/mL, fever may be the only symptom of infection that the patient may display; therefore, fever in a neutropenic patient should prompt an investigation for an infection and the initiation of antibiotics.

Causative agents

Because any infection can cause fever in neutropenic patients, a wide variety of bacterial, fungal, and viral pathogens may be implicated. Site of infection, local microbiological trends, prior cultures, and current cultures all help determine the causative pathogen. The most common bacterial pathogens in neutropenic patients are coagulase-negative *Staphylococci, S. aureus, Enterococci, S. pneumoniae, S. pyogenes, E. coli, P. aeruginosa, Stenotrophomonas maltophilia, Acinetobacter, Citrobacter, Enterobacter,* and *Klebsiella* species.

Clinical presentation

Patients with febrile neutropenia can present with a range of symptoms, from fever to severe pneumonia to septic shock.

Diagnostic criteria

An ANC < 500 cells/mL with either a single oral temperature of ≥ 38.3°C or a temperature of ≥ 38°C for over 1 hour is diagnostic of febrile neutropenia. An extensive clinical evaluation to determine the cause of infection is recommended.

Treatment

Treatment is based on a severity risk assessment such as the Multinational Association for Supportive Care in Cancer (MASCC) Risk-Index score (Table 33-5). Empiric coverage should be based on suspected site of infection and risk factors for multidrug-resistant pathogens. When the site of infection is known (i.e., pneumonia, skin and soft tissue infection, catheter-related bloodstream infection), treatment should be in accordance with current guidelines. If the site of infection is not identifiable, coverage of Gram-positive bacteria, enteric Gram-negative bacilli, and *P. aeruginosa* should be provided with a single agent or combination

Table 33-5. Multinational Association for Supportive Care in Cancer Risk-Index Score

Characteristic	Weight
1. Burden of febrile neutropenia with no or mild symptoms[a]	5
2. No hypotension (systolic blood pressure > 90 mm Hg)	5
3. No chronic obstructive pulmonary disease	4
4. Solid tumor or hematologic malignancy with no previous fungal infection[b]	4
5. No dehydration requiring parenteral fluids	3
6. Burden of febrile neutropenia with moderate symptoms	3
7. Outpatient status	3
8. Age < 60 years	2

The maximum value of the score is 26.
Adapted from Klastersky J, Paesmans M, Rubenstein EB, et al., 2000.
a. Burden of febrile neutropenia refers to the general clinical status of the patient during the febrile neutropenic episode. No symptoms to mild symptoms (5); moderate symptoms (3); and severe symptoms or moribund (0). Scores of 3 and 5 are not cumulative.
b. Previous fungal infection means demonstrated fungal infection or empirically treated suspected fungal infection.

of agents. Routine coverage for MRSA, vancomycin-resistant *Enterococcus* (VRE), extended-spectrum beta-lactamase (ESBL) Gram-negatives, *Klebsiella pneumoniae* carbapenemase (KPC), and *Candida* is not recommended. In addition, double coverage of Gram-negative bacteria is not recommended. However, in select patients at risk for the previously mentioned multidrug-resistant pathogens, expanded initial coverage should be provided.

High-risk patients (MASCC score < 21) should be admitted and treated with intravenous antibiotics. Low-risk patients (MASCC score ≥ 21) may be candidates for oral antibiotic therapy or outpatient treatment. The site of infection and organism identified determines the antibiotic treatment duration. If no infectious source is identified, antibiotic treatment should be continued until the ANC is > 500 cells/mL. See Table 33-6 for treatment options.

Acute or Chronic Bronchitis

Acute bronchitis is a respiratory tract infection that typically presents with a cough as the predominant symptom with a clear chest radiograph. Chronic bron-

Table 33-6. Initial Treatment of Febrile Neutropenia

Classification	Treatment
Infection site known	Treat as immunocompromised patient and health care–associated infection in accordance with current guidelines

Infection site not known **Risk severity**	**Treatment**
Low risk	Oral ciprofloxacin + amoxicillin-clavulanate
High risk	Cefepime, piperacillin/tazobactam, or a carbapenem

High-risk patients with a past history of multidrug-resistant pathogens or in an institution with a high rate of multidrug-resistant pathogens

MRSA	Vancomycin, linezolid, or daptomycin
VRE	Daptomycin, quinupristin/dalfopristin, linezolid
ESBL	Carbapenem +/– aminoglycoside or polymyxin/colistin
KPC	Polymyxin B or colistin

Carbapenem = doripenem, imipenem/cilastatin, meropenem; aminoglycoside = amikacin, tobramycin, or gentamicin.

chitis is a disease of the bronchi that is manifested by cough and sputum expectoration occurring for at least 3 months per year for more than 2 consecutive years. Chronic bronchitis is most commonly caused by smoking or prolonged exposure to inhalation of noxious substances. When a person with chronic bronchitis experiences a worsening of symptoms, it is referred to as an acute exacerbation of chronic bronchitis.

Causative agents

The majority of acute bronchitis infections appear to be caused by respiratory viruses such as adenovirus, coronavirus, influenza A and B, parainfluenza, rhinovirus, and respiratory syncytial virus. Bacterial pathogens most commonly implicated in acute bronchitis include *Mycoplasma pneumoniae, Chlamydophila pneumoniae, Bordetella pertussis,* and *Bordetella parapertussis.* Viruses are also the most common cause of acute exacerbations of chronic bronchitis. Viral infections predispose patients to develop secondary bacterial infections. These secondary bacterial infections are often caused by *S. pneumoniae, Moraxella catarrhalis,* or *Haemophilus influenzae.*

Clinical presentation

Acute bronchitis usually presents with either productive or nonproductive cough as the predominant symptom, but fever, muscle aches, and fatigue can also be present.

Diagnostic criteria

There are no recommended diagnostic tests for acute bronchitis. Diagnosis is made by presentation with cough for less than 3 weeks with no radiological evidence of pneumonia. In addition, the common cold, asthma, and an exacerbation of chronic obstructive pulmonary disease should be ruled out.

Treatment

Acute bronchitis should not routinely be treated with antibiotics unless *B. pertussis* is suspected or known to be the causative agent (Table 33-7). However, patients with acute exacerbations of chronic bronchitis should be treated with antibiotics because treatment of exacerbations with antibiotics has been shown to decrease the duration of illness.

Pneumonia

Pneumonia is an inflammation of the lung tissue caused by bacterial, viral, or fungal infections.

Causative agents

Multiple bacterial etiologies are possible, depending on age and predisposing conditions (Table 33-8 and Table 33-9).

Table 33-7. Treatment of Acute and Chronic Bronchitis

Illness	Treatment[a]
Acute bronchitis	Antibiotics are not to be offered or given.
Acute bronchitis caused by *Bordetella pertussis*	Erythromycin, clarithromycin, azithromycin
Exacerbation of chronic bronchitis	Amoxicillin, amoxicillin-clavulanate, erythromycin, clarithromycin, azithromycin, doxycycline, minocycline

a. Usual duration is 7–10 days.

Table 33-8. Empiric Treatment of Community-Acquired Pneumonia

Treatment location	Common organisms	Treatment
Outpatient treatment	*Streptococcus pneumoniae, Mycoplasma pneumoniae, Haemophilus influenzae, Chlamydophila pneumonia*	No antimicrobials within the past 3 months: Macrolide or doxycycline
		Presence of comorbidities, immunocompromised patients, or use of antimicrobials within the past 3 months: Respiratory fluoroquinolone or combination of beta-lactam + macrolide
Inpatient treatment (non-ICU)	*Streptococcus pneumoniae, Mycoplasma pneumoniae, Chlamydophila pneumoniae, Haemophilus influenzae, Legionella* species	Respiratory fluoroquinolone or combination of beta-lactam + macrolide
Inpatient ICU treatment	*Streptococcus pneumoniae, Staphylococcus aureus, Legionella* species, Gram-negative bacilli, *Haemophilus influenzae*	Beta-lactam (cefotaxime, ceftriaxone, or ampicillin-sulbactam) + either azithromycin or respiratory fluoroquinolone (+ either vancomycin or linezolid if MRSA is suspected)
	Suspected *Pseudomonas* infection	Antipneumococcal antipseudomonal beta-lactam (piperacillin-tazobactam, cefepime, imipenem, or meropenem) + fluoroquinolone (ciprofloxacin or levofloxacin)
		Antipneumococcal antipseudomonal beta-lactam + aminoglycoside + azithromycin
		Antipneumococcal antipseudomonal beta-lactam + aminoglycoside + antipneumococcal fluoroquinolone

Mandell LA, Wunderink RG, Anzueto A, et al., 2007.
ICU = intensive care unit.

Table 33-9. Empiric Treatment of Hospital-Acquired Pneumonia, Ventilator-Associated Pneumonia, and Health Care–Associated Pneumonia

Classification	Organisms	Treatment
Early-onset HAP/VAP and no risk factors for multidrug-resistant bacteria	*Streptococcus pneumoniae, Haemophilus influenzae,* methicillin-sensitive *Staphylococcus aureus, Escherichia coli, Klebsiella pneumoniae, Enterobacter* species, *Proteus* species, *Serratia marcescens*	Ceftriaxone or fluoroquinolone (levofloxacin, moxifloxacin, or ciprofloxacin) or ampicillin-sulbactam or ertapenem
Late-onset HAP/VAP or risk factors for multidrug-resistant bacteria including HCAP	Above bacteria plus *Pseudomonas aeruginosa,* extended-spectrum beta-lactamase-positive *Klebsiella pneumoniae, Acinetobacter* species, MRSA, *Legionella pneumophila*	Antipseudomonal cephalosporin or imipenem-cilastatin, meropenem, or piperacillin-tazobactam + antipseudomonal fluoroquinolone or aminoglycoside + linezolid or vancomycin (if MRSA suspected)

American Thoracic Society Documents, 2005.

Clinical presentation

The onset of illness can be abrupt or subacute, with fever, chills, dyspnea, and productive cough predominating.

Diagnostic criteria

A diagnosis of pneumonia is based on patient signs and symptoms in combination with tests such as a chest x-ray or culture data. Blood and sputum cultures may be used to identify the causative pathogen; however, sputum cultures are often contaminated, making reliability questionable. Samples obtained by bronchoalveolar lavage (BAL) have a lower rate of contamination, but a BAL is not appropriate in all patients because it is an invasive procedure.

Treatment

Treatment decisions are based upon the pneumonia classification: community-acquired pneumonia (CAP), hospital-acquired pneumonia (HAP), ventilator-associated pneumonia (VAP), or health care–associated pneumonia (HCAP). In CAP, empiric antibiotic selection is determined by treatment location: outpatient, inpatient, or intensive care unit (Table 33-8). Recent guideline updates also advocate empiric coverage for MRSA in patients with CAP who meet one of the following criteria: intensive care unit admission, presence of necrotizing or cavitary infiltrates, or presence of empyema. In addition, factors such as alcohol abuse, travel, animal exposure, or HIV infection increase the incidence of particular pathogens, further guiding the selection of empiric antibiotics.

HAP occurs when pneumonia develops 48 hours or more after a patient is admitted to the hospital. A patient is diagnosed with VAP when pneumonia develops 48–72 hours after a patient is placed on a ventilator. Finally, HCAP refers to pneumonia that occurs in a patient exposed to a health care environment (hospitalization ≥ 2 days in the past 90 days; residence in a nursing home or other long-term care institution; IV antibiotic treatment, chemotherapy, or wound care within the past 30 days; or treatment at a hospital or hemodialysis clinic).

Treatment for HAP or VAP is based on the onset of the infection and risk factors for multidrug-resistant organisms. Patients with HAP or VAP who have been hospitalized for more than 4 days are considered to have late-onset infection and are at risk for multidrug-resistant organisms. Other risk factors for multidrug-resistant organisms include treatment with antimicrobial agents within the past 90 days, immunosuppression, or a high rate of antibiotic resistance in the community or hospital unit. Patients with HCAP are inherently at risk for multidrug-resistant organisms, and empiric antibiotics should provide appropriate coverage. Table 33-9 outlines treatment for HAP, VAP, and HCAP.

Tuberculosis

Tuberculosis is a communicable infectious disease caused by *Mycobacterium tuberculosis*. It can produce a silent, latent infection as well as an active infection. Although infection of any tissue or organ with *M. tuberculosis* is possible, the usual site of infection is pulmonary.

Clinical presentation

Tuberculosis can present with generalized symptoms of weight loss, fever, and night sweats, along with persistent cough with productive sputum. In the absence of other symptoms, latent disease is defined by a positive purified protein derivative (PPD) test or a positive interferon-gamma release assay (IGRA).

Diagnostic criteria

Diagnosis often is made by a combination of chest x-ray findings and a positive PPD skin test or IGRA. Patients with severe HIV disease may not react to the standard PPD skin test. Individuals who have been immunized with the Bacille Calmette-Guérin (BCG) vaccine may have a false positive reaction to the PPD skin test; therefore, testing with an alternative method such as an IGRA should be considered. Sputum specimens or lung tissue may be acid-fast stained to confirm the presence of *Mycobacterium* species. Mycobacterial culture can confirm speciation; however, because of the extended time needed to grow the organism, sensitivities to anti-infective agents may take weeks to months to determine.

Treatment

Tuberculosis is a very slow growing bacterium that requires prolonged treatment with multiple anti-infective agents to achieve a cure and to prevent development of resistance. To ensure compliance with therapy, the U.S. Centers for Disease Control and Prevention (CDC) recommends direct observed

Table 33-10. Treatment of Tuberculosis

Disease stage	Treatment	Duration
Latent (preferred)	Isoniazid	9 months (for children and HIV-positive patients)
	Isoniazid	6 months
	Rifampin	4 months
Latent (alternative)	Rifampin + pyrazinamide	2 months (not recommended because of hepatotoxicity)
	Isoniazid + rifapentine	3 months (not for children < 2 years of age, patients with HIV, or pregnant females)
Active disease (preferred)	Isoniazid + rifampin + pyrazinamide + ethambutol	2 months
	Followed by isoniazid + rifampin	4 months (6 months total)
Active disease (alternative)	Isoniazid + rifampin + ethambutol	2 months
	Followed by isoniazid + rifampin	7 months (9 months total)

therapy for most treatment regimens for active and latent tuberculosis.

See Table 33-10 for a summary of treatments.

Intra-abdominal Infections

Intra-abdominal infections include infections of the retroperitoneal space or the peritoneal cavity.

Causative agents

A variety of bacteria are associated with intra-abdominal infections including facultative and aerobic Gram-negative bacteria, anaerobic bacteria, and Gram-positive aerobic bacteria. Major sources of infection include *Escherichia coli* and *Bacteroides* species.

Clinical presentation

Patients may present with abdominal pain and fever. Systemic manifestation can occur in severe cases.

Diagnostic criteria

Generally, patient history and physical examination are sufficient to diagnose an intra-abdominal infection. Imaging studies or exploratory laparotomy may be necessary in select patients.

Treatment

In addition to antibiotics, fluid resuscitation may be required in cases of severe infections. Surgical procedures are essential to treatment in some patients, such as those with severe peritonitis or an abscess. Although cultures are not required in low-risk patients with a community-acquired infection, cultures of specimens obtained from the site of infection as well as susceptibility testing may prove beneficial to guiding therapy in hospital-acquired infections or higher-risk patients. Table 33-11 outlines the empiric treatment of adults with complicated intra-abdominal infections.

Infectious Diarrhea

Diarrhea is defined as an increase in frequency or liquidity of stool (or both), compared to a patient's normal stool.

Causative agents

Many disease states, drugs, and infectious organisms are associated with diarrhea.

Clinical presentation

In addition to diarrhea, the patient may present with several of the following symptoms: fever, chills, nausea, vomiting, or abdominal cramping.

Diagnostic criteria

Etiology is usually determined by patient history and physical examination. Patient history should include factors such as immune status, recent travel,

Table 33-11. Empiric Treatment of Adults with Complicated Intra-abdominal Infections

Type of infection	Treatment
Mild to moderately severe community-acquired extra-biliary infections	Single agent treatment: Cefoxitin, ertapenem, moxifloxacin, tigecycline, or ticarcillin-clavulanate
	Combination treatment: Metronidazole plus one of the following: Cefazolin, cefuroxime, ceftriaxone, cefotaxime, ciprofloxacin, or levofloxacin
Mild to moderately severe community-acquired acute cholecystitis	Cefazolin, cefuroxime, or ceftriaxone
High-risk or severe community-acquired extra-biliary infections	Single agent treatment: Imipenem, meropenem, doripenem, or piperacillin-tazobactam
	Combination treatment: Metronidazole plus one of the following: Cefepime, ceftazidime, ciprofloxacin, or levofloxacin
High-risk community-acquired acute cholecystitis	Metronidazole plus one of the following: Imipenem, meropenem, doripenem, piperacillin-tazobactam, ciprofloxacin, levofloxacin, or cefepime
Acute cholangitis after bilioenteric anastomosis	Metronidazole plus one of the following: Imipenem, meropenem, doripenem, piperacillin-tazobactam, ciprofloxacin, levofloxacin, or cefepime
Health care–associated biliary infection	Metronidazole plus vancomycin plus one of the following: Imipenem, meropenem, doripenem, piperacillin-tazobactam, ciprofloxacin, levofloxacin, or cefepime

Solomkin JS, Mazuski JE, Bradley JS, et al., 2010.

food exposure, or antibiotic use. Cultures and tests for toxins or parasites may be performed. Diagnosis of certain infectious organisms, such as those associated with foodborne illness, should be reported to appropriate agencies.

Treatment

Supportive care (hydration, electrolyte replacement, antipyretics, or antiemetics) is often the only treatment provided. Antimotility agents are usually discouraged because of the potential to cause toxic megacolon, especially in cases of bloody diarrhea, Shiga toxin–producing *Escherichia coli* (STEC) infections, or *Clostridium difficile* infections. Antibacterial therapy is reserved for severe presentations, patients with risk factors, or patients diagnosed with specific infectious causes. When indicated, patients with traveler's diarrhea can be empirically treated with fluoroquinolones in adults or Septra (trimethoprim-sulfamethoxazole) in children. Table 33-12 provides an overview of treatments for immunocompetent patients.

Skin and Soft Tissue Infections

Bacterial infections of the skin and soft tissue can result in a variety of conditions. This chapter covers the following: impetigo, erysipelas, cellulitis, necrotizing infections, and infections caused by human or animal bites.

Causative agents

Skin and soft tissue infections (SSTIs) are caused by a variety of organisms (Table 33-13).

Clinical presentation

SSTIs are usually characterized by erythema and edema of the skin. More serious infections can result in systemic symptoms, such as fever, tachycardia, or hypotension. Table 33-14 describes signs and symptoms of selected SSTIs.

Diagnostic criteria

For mild infections, diagnosis is usually made by physical examination. Blood or biopsy cultures and surgical intervention may be necessary in patients with severe infections.

Treatment

Treatment is based on the type and severity of infection. Usually treatment is empiric, targeting the organisms most commonly associated with the specific type

Table 33-12. Treatment of Infectious Diarrhea for Immunocompetent Patients

Organism	Treatment
Aeromonas, Plesiomonas	TMP-SMZ or fluoroquinolone
Campylobacter species	Erythromycin
Clostridium difficile	Initial episode or first recurrence
	Mild to moderately severe: Metronidazole (po)
	Severe: Vancomycin (po)
	Severe, complicated: Vancomycin (po) plus metronidazole (IV) (add rectal vancomycin if patient has an ileus)
	Second recurrence: Tapered or pulsed vancomycin (po)
Cryptosporidium species	Paromomycin
Cyclospora species	TMP-SMZ
Entamoeba histolytica	Metronidazole plus diiodohydroxyquin or paromomycin
Escherichia coli species	
Enterotoxigenic	TMP-SMZ or fluoroquinolone
Enteropathogenic	TMP-SMZ or fluoroquinolone
Enteroinvasive	TMP-SMZ or fluoroquinolone
Enteroaggregative	Antimicrobial treatment not defined; can consider fluoroquinolone
STEC	Avoid antimicrobials and antimotility agents
Giardia	Metronidazole
Isospora species	TMP-SMZ
Microsporidium species	Not defined
Non-*typhi* species of *Salmonella*	Generally supportive care only
	Treatment if indicated: TMP-SMZ, fluoroquinolone, or ceftriaxone
Shigella species	TMP-SMZ, fluoroquinolone, ceftriaxone, or azithromycin
Vibrio cholera	Doxycycline, tetracycline, or fluoroquinolone
Yersinia species	Generally supportive care only

Cohen SH, Gerding DN, Johnson S, et al., 2010; Guerrant RL, Van Gilder T, Steiner TS, et al., 2001.
TMP-SMZ = trimethoprim-sulfamethoxazole.

of SSTI (Table 33-13). Because of the expanding incidence of MRSA, the need for additional empiric coverage of MRSA in select SSTIs is increasing (Table 33-15). MRSA should also be considered in patients unresponsive to initial therapies lacking MRSA coverage. In patients with a necrotizing infection or in immunocompromised patients, surgical intervention may be required in combination with antibiotic therapy.

Urinary Tract Infection

Urinary tract infections (UTIs) represent a wide variety of clinical syndromes, including urethritis, cystitis, prostatitis, and pyelonephritis.

Causative agents

The most common agents are enteric Gram-negative bacilli and *Enterococcus*. Hospitalized, catheterized patients also may acquire *Pseudomonas, Morganella, Citrobacter*, and *Staphylococcus* species.

Clinical presentation

Lower urinary tract infections tend to present with dysuria, urinary urgency, polyuria, nocturia, and suprapubic heaviness or pain. Fever is rare in patients with lower urinary tract infections. Upper urinary tract infections, such as pyelonephritis, tend to present with flank pain and fever.

Table 33-13. Treatment of Skin and Soft Tissue Infections

Infection	Common organisms	Treatment
Impetigo	*Staphylococcus aureus, Streptococcus pyogenes*	Small number of lesions: Topical mupirocin
		Numerous lesions: Dicloxacillin, cephalexin, erythromycin, clindamycin, amoxicillin-clavulanate
Erysipelas	*Streptococcus* species	Penicillin
Cellulitis	*Streptococcus* species, *Staphylococcus aureus*	MSSA: Nafcillin, oxacillin, cefazolin, clindamycin, dicloxacillin, cephalexin, doxycycline, minocycline, TMP-SMZ
		MRSA: Vancomycin, linezolid, clindamycin, daptomycin, doxycycline, minocycline, TMP-SMZ
Necrotizing infections	Polymicrobial	Clindamycin + ciprofloxacin + either ampicillin-sulbactam or piperacillin-tazobactam
		Cefotaxime + either metronidazole or clindamycin
		Carbapenem (imipenem, meropenem, ertapenem)
	Streptococcus species	Penicillin + clindamycin
	Staphylococcus aureus	Nafcillin, oxacillin, cefazolin, clindamycin, vancomycin (for resistant strains)
Clostridial myonecrosis (gas gangrene)	*Clostridium* species	Clindamycin + penicillin
Animal bites	*Pasteurella* species, *Streptococcus* species, *Staphylococcus* species, *Bacteroides tectum, Fusobacterium, Capnocytophaga, Porphyromonas* species	Preferred: Amoxicillin-clavulanate
		Alternatives: Ampicillin-sulbactam, piperacillin-tazobactam, carbapenem, penicillin plus dicloxacillin, second- or third-generation cephalosporin, fluoroquinolone, doxycycline, TMP-SMZ
		Consider addition of metronidazole or clindamycin to above regimens not active against anaerobes
Human bites	Polymicrobial	Amoxicillin-clavulanate, ampicillin-sulbactam, carbapenem, cefoxitin, doxycycline, TMP-SMZ + metronidazole, clindamycin + fluoroquinolone

Lipsky BA, Berendt AR, Deery HG, et al., 2004; Stevens DL, Bisno AL, Chambers HF, et al., 2005.
MSSA = methicillin-sensitive *Staphylococcus aureus*; TMP-SMZ = trimethoprim-sulfamethoxazole.

Diagnostic criteria

Diagnosis of UTIs is based on the presence of urinary or systemic symptoms, the presence of microorganisms in significant numbers, and the presence of WBCs in the urine sample. In general, higher numbers of organisms ($> 10^5$ cells/mL) are needed to diagnose UTIs in females compared to males ($> 10^3$ cells/mL) because more organisms can ascend the shorter female urethra.

Treatment

A variety of antibacterials may be useful for the treatment of UTIs (Table 33-16), including fluoroquinolones, cephalosporins, trimethoprim-sulfamethoxazole (TMP-SMZ), and Vibramycin (doxycycline). Fluoroquinolones are especially useful for the treatment of prostatitis. Length of therapy varies according to the severity of disease.

Bacterial Venereal Diseases (Chlamydia, Gonorrhea, and Syphilis)

Venereal diseases are diseases that can be transmitted via sexual intercourse. This section covers chlamydia, gonorrhea, and syphilis. Patients testing positive for any sexually transmitted disease should be screened for the presence of other venereal diseases. In addition, all sexual partners should be screened and treated if indicated.

Table 33-14. Clinical Presentation of Selected Skin and Soft Tissue Infections

Infection	Signs and symptoms
Impetigo	Single or multiple localized, purulent lesions usually occurring on the head or extremities
Erysipelas	Raised lesions with erythema and edema; involvement limited to the upper dermis
Cellulitis	Progressive erythema and edema without raised demarcations; involvement extends into the deeper dermis and subcutaneous fat
Necrotizing infections	Rapidly progressive infection with systemic manifestations; skin necrosis and bullae may be present; involvement may extend into the fascia or muscle
Clostridial myonecrosis (gas gangrene)	Bronze or reddish purple skin with systemic manifestations; crepitant tissue resulting from gas

Stevens DL, Bisno AL, Chambers HF, et al., 2005.

Table 33-15. Empiric Treatment of MRSA Skin and Soft Tissue Infections

Infection	Signs and symptoms
Purulent cellulitis	Clindamycin, TMP-SMZ, doxycycline, minocycline, linezolid
Nonpurulent cellulitis[a]	Clindamycin, linezolid, TMP-SMZ + beta-lactam, tetracycline + beta-lactam
Complicated SSTI[b]	Vancomycin, linezolid, daptomycin, telavancin, clindamycin

Liu C, Bayer A, Cosgrove SE, et al., 2011.
a. Provide MRSA coverage if patient has a treatment failure with a beta-lactam. MRSA coverage can be considered if patient has systemic symptoms.
b. Include hospitalized patients with any of the following: deep soft tissue infections, surgical or traumatic wound infections, major abscesses, cellulitis, or infected ulcers or burns.

Table 33-16. Treatment of Urinary Tract Infections

Diagnosis	Organisms	Preferred treatments	Alternative treatment
Acute uncomplicated cystitis	*Escherichia coli, Staphylococcus saprophyticus*	TMP-SMZ × 3 days or nitrofurantoin × 5 days	Fluoroquinolone × 3 days or beta-lactam × 3–7 days
Acute pyelonephritis	*E. coli, Proteus mirabilis, Klebsiella pneumoniae, Enterococcus* species	Fluoroquinolone × 7 days or TMP-SMZ × 14 days; if severe, parenteral therapy with fluoroquinolone or broad-spectrum beta-lactam or aminoglycoside may be considered	Broad-spectrum beta-lactam plus aminoglycoside
Catheter-associated UTI	Coagulase-negative staphylococci, *E. coli, K. pneumoniae, Pseudomonas aeruginosa, Citrobacter, Enterobacter, Enterococcus, Klebsiella, Proteus, Providencia,* and *Serratia* species	Broad-spectrum beta-lactam or fluoroquinolone × 7–14 days based on resolution of symptoms / Regimen selected on the basis of severity of infection and local bacterial susceptibility	Broad-spectrum beta-lactam or fluoroquinolone plus additional Gram-positive or Gram-negative coverage if severe infection or suspicion of resistant pathogen
Prostatitis	*E. coli, Proteus* species, *K. pneumoniae*	Quinolone × 4–6 weeks or TMP-SMZ × 4–6 weeks	

Aminoglycoside = amikacin, tobramycin, or gentamicin; fluoroquinolone = ciprofloxacin, levofloxacin, ofloxacin; carbapenem = doripenem, ertapenem, imipenem/cilastatin, meropenem; beta-lactam = amoxicillin-clavulanate, cefdinir, cefaclor, cefpodoxime; broad-spectrum beta-lactam = piperacillin/tazobactam, cefepime, ceftazidime, aztreonam, or a carbapenem; Gram-positive coverage = vancomycin, daptomycin, linezolid; Gram-negative coverage = gentamicin, tobramycin, amikacin.

Chlamydia

Causative agent

Chlamydia is caused by the bacterium *Chlamydia trachomatis*.

Clinical presentation

Women with chlamydia may present with vaginal discharge, dysuria, or abdominal pain. In men, chlamydia can cause penile discharge or dysuria. The majority of patients, however, are asymptomatic, but infections can result in serious complications in women, including pelvic inflammatory disease, ectopic pregnancy, or infertility.

Diagnostic criteria

Chlamydia can be diagnosed on the basis of a swab obtained from the site of potential contact such as the endocervix, vagina, urethra, or rectum. In addition, urine tests can be used to detect urogenital infection in women or urethral infection in men.

Treatment

See Table 33-17 for treatment recommendations and alternatives for chlamydia. Additional recommendations are available for pregnant women, infants, and children.

Gonorrhea

Causative agent

Gonorrhea is caused by the Gram-negative cocci *Neisseria gonorrhoeae*.

Clinical presentation

Although patients with gonorrhea can be asymptomatic, gonorrheal infections may cause dysuria, penile discharge, or testicular pain in men. Women may experience dysuria, vaginal discharge, or vaginal bleeding. Women are also at risk of developing pelvic inflammatory disease, which can result in future infertility.

Diagnostic criteria

In symptomatic men, gonorrhea can be diagnosed by a Gram stain of a urethral swab; however, negative results in asymptomatic men are not sufficient to exclude an infection. In women and asymptomatic men, methods of diagnosis include cultures of specimen swabs and nucleic acid tests.

Treatment

N. gonorrhoeae has developed significant resistance to penicillins and fluoroquinolones; therefore, these agents are no longer recommended, leaving cephalosporins as the preferred treatment modality (Table 33-18). Because resistance to cephalosporins is anticipated to increase, vigilance is required to ensure appropriate treatment for patients with suspected cephalosporin failures or cultures demonstrating decreased susceptibilities. Because of the high rate of comorbid chlamydia infections, patients diagnosed with gonorrhea should also receive therapy against chlamydia: Zithromax (azithromycin) 1 g orally once or doxycycline 100 mg orally twice daily for 7 days. Additional recommendations are available for infants, children, and pregnant patients.

Syphilis

Causative agent

Syphilis is an infection caused by the spirochete *Treponema pallidum*.

Clinical presentation

Syphilis infections are classified into the following stages: primary, secondary, latent, and tertiary. Primary syphilis presents as a single lesion (chancre) or multiple lesions appearing at the site of infection. If not treated, primary syphilis progresses into secondary syphilis, characterized by a variety of rashes and flu-like symptoms. Untreated patients will develop latent syphilis. Patients with latent syphilis will lack signs or symptoms of syphilis, but the disease can progress further to tertiary syphilis. Symptoms of this stage include general paresis, deafness, progressive dementia, or aortic insufficiency.

Table 33-17. Treatment of Chlamydia

Treatment type	Treatment
Recommended treatments	Azithromycin 1 g orally once
	Doxycycline 100 mg orally bid × 7 days
Alternative treatments	Erythromycin base 500 mg orally qid × 7 days
	Erythromycin ethylsuccinate 800 mg orally qid × 7 days
	Levofloxacin 500 mg orally once daily × 7 days
	Ofloxacin 300 mg orally bid × 7 days

Centers for Disease Control and Prevention, 2014.

Table 33-18. Treatment of Gonorrhea

Classification	Treatment	Comments
Uncomplicated infections of the cervix, urethra, and rectum	Preferred: Ceftriaxone 250 mg IM once	
	Alternative: Cefixime 400 mg orally once or single-dose injectable cephalosporin regimen	
Uncomplicated infections of the pharynx	Ceftriaxone 250 mg IM once	
Gonococcal conjunctivitis	Ceftriaxone 1 g IM once	
Disseminated gonococcal infections	Preferred: Ceftriaxone 1 g IM or IV q24h	Continue IM or IV therapy for 24–48 hours after signs of improvement, then cefixime 400 mg orally twice daily can be used to finish at least 7 days of treatment.
	Alternative: Cefotaxime 1 g IV q8h	
Gonococcal meningitis	Ceftriaxone 1–2 g IV q12h × 10–14 days	Treat in conjunction with an infectious disease specialist.
Gonococcal endocarditis	Ceftriaxone 1–2 g IV q12h × at least 4 weeks	Treat in conjunction with an infectious disease specialist.

Centers for Disease Control and Prevention, 2014.
IM = intramuscular.

Diagnostic criteria

Darkfield tests provide a definitive diagnosis of early syphilis. A variety of serologic tests are also available to aid diagnosis; however, more than one type of serologic test should be performed because of the limitations of these tests. Patients exhibiting any signs or symptoms of neurologic or ophthalmic involvement should have additional screening including CSF analysis.

Treatment

Parenteral Pfizerpen (penicillin G) is the treatment of choice for each stage of syphilis. Table 33-19 lists the preparation, dosage, and duration of treatment based

Table 33-19. Treatment of Syphilis

Stage	Treatment	Duration
Primary	Benzathine penicillin G 2.4 million units IM	Single dose
Secondary	Benzathine penicillin G 2.4 million units IM	Single dose
Early latent syphilis (syphilis contracted within the past year)	Benzathine penicillin G 2.4 million units IM	Single dose
Late latent syphilis or latent syphilis of unknown duration	Benzathine penicillin G 2.4 million units IM weekly	Three doses
Tertiary syphilis	Benzathine penicillin G 2.4 million units IM weekly	Three doses
Neurosyphilis (syphilis with CNS manifestations)	Aqueous crystalline penicillin G 3–4 million units IV q4h or continuous infusion	10–14 days
	Alternative: Procaine penicillin 2.4 million units IM daily plus probenecid 500 mg orally four times daily	10–14 days

Centers for Disease Control and Prevention, 2014.
CNS = central nervous system; IM = intramuscular.

on the syphilis stage. Additional recommendations are available for children, patients with HIV, or pregnant patients.

Sepsis

Sepsis, as defined by the American College of Chest Physicians, is the systemic inflammatory response syndrome (SIRS) caused by a known or suspected infection. SIRS is defined as the presence of two of the following criteria: temperature > 38°C or < 36°C; heart rate > 90 bpm; respiratory rate > 20 breaths/min or $PaCo_2$ (partial pressure of carbon dioxide in the blood) < 32 mm Hg; WBC > 12,000 cells/mL or < 4,000 cells/mL; or > 10% immature form (bands).

Causative agents

The most common cause of sepsis is a bacterial infection; however, sepsis can be caused by any infectious pathogen, including aerobic and anaerobic Gram-negative or Gram-positive bacteria, atypical bacteria, fungi, parasites, and viruses.

Clinical presentation

Patients may present with any combination of symptoms, including fever or hypothermia, rigors, chills, tachycardia, tachypnea, hyperglycemia, mental status changes, tachycardia, and lethargy. As sepsis progresses to severe sepsis or septic shock, organ system failure occurs, resulting in hypoglycemia, myocardial depression, oliguria, leukopenia, coagulopathy, and pulmonary edema. This progressive deterioration can lead to multisystem organ failure and death.

Diagnostic criteria

Any suspected or confirmed infection plus the presence of two SIRS criteria are diagnostic for sepsis.

Once sepsis is suspected, an extensive clinical workup should be performed within 1 hour. Frequent monitoring of vital signs, laboratory studies, and appropriate cultures are essential to aid in selection of appropriate therapy.

Treatment

The source of the suspected infection as well as local microbiological trends and sensitivities will determine the selection of anti-infective therapy. Antibiotic therapy should be initiated within the first hour after patient presentation. Initial antibiotic therapy should comply with current guidelines once the source of infection is confirmed. In addition, empiric therapy should be broad, covering all likely pathogens. Once microbiological data are available, therapy should be de-escalated to best treat the causative pathogen.

Tickborne Systemic Febrile Syndromes (Lyme Disease, Rocky Mountain Spotted Fever, Ehrlichiosis, and Tularemia)

Tickborne illnesses are similar in transmission and natural history. The organisms responsible for these infections include *Rickettsia*, known for their intracellular growth in host cells. As such, they cannot be grown in culture media, and serologic tests are used for diagnosis. Patients present with a fever, rash, and flu-like symptoms, as well as a history of tick exposure.

Treatment

See Table 33-20 for treatment options.

Systemic Fungal Infections

Fungal infections fall into two categories: *primary* (able to cause infection in all patients) and *opportunistic*

Table 33-20. Treatment of Tickborne Systemic Febrile Syndromes

Disease	Causative agent	Primary treatment	Alternative treatment
Lyme disease	*Borrelia burgdorferi*	Amoxicillin, ceftriaxone, cefuroxime, or doxycycline	Macrolide, cefotaxime, penicillin G
Rocky Mountain spotted fever	*Rickettsia rickettsii*	Doxycycline	Chloramphenicol
Ehrlichiosis	*Ehrlichia phagocytophila*	Doxycycline	Tetracycline
Tularemia	*Francisella tularensis*	Gentamicin or streptomycin	Doxycycline, ciprofloxacin

Macrolide = azithromycin, clarithromycin, erythromycin.

(able to cause infection only in immunocompromised patients). Fungal infections affect a variety of organ systems including the skin, central nervous system, pulmonary system, and gastrointestinal tract. The incidence of fungal infection is rising as a result of increased use of antibacterial agents and the increase in the number of immunocompromised patients.

Clinical presentation

Fungal infections can present in a variety of fashions but typically have a gradual onset with general malaise, fever, and weakness that are unrelieved by antibacterial therapy. Pulmonary infections can present with pneumonia-like symptoms or with asthma-like symptoms if bronchoallergic disease is present.

Diagnostic criteria

Diagnosis is made from patient history, cultures from infected fluids or tissues, and serologic tests.

Treatment

Treatment is based on the severity of the disease and often is empiric until the organism is isolated (Table 33-21). The duration of antifungal therapy is determined by the type of fungal infection, the site and severity of infection, and the immune status of the host. Because of the relatively slow growth of most fungi and the lack of commercial testing against antifungal agents, patient response is used to determine resistance to therapy.

Viral Infections (Hepatitis, Influenza, and the Herpes Simplex Family)

Hepatitis

Hepatitis is a general term referring to a generalized inflammation of the liver.

Causative agents
Five viruses (hepatitis types A–E) have been identified as causative agents for hepatitis. Syndromes may be either acute or chronic.

Table 33-21. Treatment of Systemic Fungal Infections

Organism	Disease	Severity	Preferred treatment	Alternative treatment
Aspergillosis spp.	Invasive pulmonary disease		Voriconazole or L-AMB	AmB, itraconazole, posaconazole, caspofungin
Blastomyces dermatitidis	Cutaneous, pulmonary, or extrapulmonary disease	Severe disease	L-AMB × 1–2 weeks, then itraconazole	AmB × 1–2 weeks, then itraconazole
		Mild disease	Itraconazole	L-AMB, voriconazole, itraconazole
Candida spp.	Bloodstream infection	Severe disease	Echinocandin, fluconazole, voriconazole	Voriconazole, itraconazole
		Moderate disease	Fluconazole, echinocandin	High-dose fluconazole, L-AMB, AmB
Coccidioides immitis	Primary pulmonary disease	Severe disease	Itraconazole, fluconazole	Itraconazole, ketoconazole
Cryptococcus neoformans	Meningitis	Moderate disease	Fluconazole	AmB + fluconazole
		Immunocompromised	AmB or L-AMB + flucytosine	*or*
				fluconazole + flucytosine
		Immunocompetent	AmB or L-AMB + flucytosine	AmB or L-AMB
Histoplasma capsulatum	Pulmonary, disseminated, or localized	Severe disease	L-AMB × 2 weeks then itraconazole	AmB × 2 weeks then itraconazole
		Moderate disease	Itraconazole	Fluconazole, posaconazole, voriconazole

L-AMB = lipid amphotericin B preparations (liposomal and lipid complex); AmB = amphotericin B deoxycholate; echinocandin = anidulafungin, caspofungin, micafungin.

Clinical presentation

Patients present with a history of anorexia, nausea, fatigue, and malaise that usually progresses to fever, right-upper-quadrant pain, dark urine, light-colored stools, and worsening of systemic symptoms. Some patients have no symptoms and little hepatic damage. In addition to physical signs, laboratory tests are remarkable for elevations in AST (aspartate aminotransferase), ALT (alanine aminotransferase), and serum bilirubin.

Diagnostic criteria

Additional laboratory testing can be performed to diagnose and guide treatment of patients with hepatitis B. These tests include hepatitis B surface antigen, hepatitis B surface antibody, hepatitis B core antibody, hepatitis B deoxyribonucleic acid (DNA) levels, and genotype. There are eight hepatitis B genotypes, identified as genotypes A–H. For hepatitis C, additional tests include detection of antibodies specific to the hepatitis C virus and viral nucleic acid. Genotyping is also required to guide treatment of hepatitis C. There are six major genotypes, which are identified as genotypes 1–6.

Treatment

Treatment of hepatitis depends on the viral strain and type of presentation. The decision to initiate treatment in patients with chronic hepatitis B depends on evaluation of factors such as hepatitis B surface antigen, hepatitis B e antigen, hepatitis B DNA levels, liver function tests, patient age, and liver biopsy results. Chronic hepatitis B is treated with interferon alfa–based therapies or nucleos(t)ide analogue (NA) therapies. Agent selection and duration are based on a combination of factors, including the presence or absence of hepatitis B surface antigen, medication side effects, and the potential for the development of resistance with NAs. In general, the first-line agents are Baraclude (entecavir) or Viread (tenofovir). Peginterferon alfa is also a first-line agent in very select patient populations. Other treatments include Epivir (lamivudine), Hepsera (adefovir), Tyzeka (telbivudine), and Emtriva (emtricitabine).

For patients with acute symptomatic hepatitis B, treatment is usually not indicated unless the patient has fulminant or prolonged, severe acute hepatitis. In these patients, lamivudine or telbivudine is indicated for short-duration therapy, while entecavir is preferred for longer durations. Interferon-alfa is contraindicated in this population.

Standard therapy and duration of treatment for chronic hepatitis C is based on genotype (Table 33-22). Patients with genotype 1 are treated with a combination of three medications, peginterferon alfa with ribavirin plus Sovaldi (sofosbuvir) or Rebetol (ribavirin) plus sofosbuvir and Olysio (simeprevir). Treatment may require modifications in special patient populations, including patients with renal disease, HIV, or cirrhosis.

Acute hepatitis C can be treated with interferon-based therapy; however, the optimum duration is unclear. In addition, recommendations cannot be made concerning the benefits of combination therapy of ribavirin with interferon-based therapy in patients with acute hepatitis C.

Influenza

Influenza is an acute respiratory viral infection.

Causative agents

Three viruses, influenza A, B, and C, are responsible for most infections.

Table 33-22. Treatment of Chronic Hepatitis C

Genotype	Treatment	Standard duration
Genotype 1 treatment-naïve eligible for interferon therapy	Sofosbuvir + peginterferon alfa + ribavirin	12 weeks
Genotype 1 treatment-naïve not eligible for interferon therapy	Sofosbuvir + simeprevir + ribavirin	12 weeks
Genotypes 2 and 3 treatment-naïve	Sofosbuvir + ribavirin	Genotype 2 for 12 weeks
		Genotype 3 for 24 weeks
Genotype 4 treatment-naïve eligible for interferon therapy	Sofosbuvir + peginterferon alfa + ribavirin	12 weeks
Genotype 4 treatment-naïve not eligible for interferon therapy	Sofosbuvir + ribavirin	24 weeks
Genotype 5 or 6	Sofosbuvir + peginterferon alfa + ribavirin	12 weeks

American Association for the Study of Liver Diseases and Infectious Diseases Society of America, 2014.

Table 33-23. Treatment of Influenza

Organism	Treatment type	Treatment
Influenza A	Prophylaxis	Oseltamivir, zanamivir, amantadine, rimantadine
Influenza A	Treatment	Oseltamivir, zanamivir, amantadine, rimantadine
Influenza B	Prophylaxis	Oseltamivir, zanamivir
Influenza B	Treatment	Oseltamivir, zanamivir

Centers for Disease Control and Prevention, 2011.

Clinical presentation

Patients may present with a sudden onset of chills, fever, fatigue, headache, muscle aches, or cough. The primary viral infection may be followed by secondary bacterial infections.

Diagnostic criteria

Diagnosis is based on patient physical signs and symptoms. Rapid influenza diagnostic tests (RIDTs) are also available. RIDTs have a high specificity but low sensitivity; therefore, a negative result should not prevent treatment in patients with suspected influenza infection.

Treatment

Both prophylactic and treatment therapies are available (Table 33-23). Exact therapies are determined by the viral strain present in the community. The CDC provides yearly recommendations concerning antiviral treatments based on current circulating strains. CDC guidance should be closely monitored because resistance to antiviral treatments can develop throughout the influenza season. Therapies for the 2011–2012 influenza season included Tamiflu (oseltamivir) and Relenza (zanamivir). Recent circulating influenza A strains have demonstrated marked resistance to adamantanes; therefore, Symmetrel (amantadine) and Flumadine (rimantadine) are currently not recommended. Therapy should be initiated as soon as possible after symptoms develop, preferably within 48 hours of symptom onset.

Herpes family (herpes simplex and herpes zoster)

The herpes virus family is responsible for a variety of viral infections, including genital herpes simplex infections and varicella zoster infections (shingles).

Causative agents

A slightly different herpes virus causes each disease.

Clinical presentation

Clinical presentation varies by disease:

- *Genital herpes simplex:* Patients with an initial genital herpes infection can present with flu-like symptoms including fever, headache, malaise, and myalgias, in addition to development of painful lesions on the external genitalia. Recurrent infections may be preceded by a prodrome of tingling, dysesthesia, or numbness followed by the development of lesions. Infected patients may also be asymptomatic.
- *Varicella zoster:* Varicella zoster presents as a painful, pustular rash located on one or two dermatomes. The affected area may remain painful after the rash has resolved. Severe complications include ophthalmic manifestations and infections.

Diagnostic criteria

Diagnosis is based mostly on signs and symptoms, although additional testing may be performed.

- *Genital herpes simplex:* Virologic tests (cell culture and polymerase chain reaction [PCR]) and type-specific serologic tests for antibodies are available to diagnose genital herpes simplex and identify the type of infection. Two types of herpes simplex virus cause genital herpes: HSV-1 and HSV-2. HSV-1 is also the causative agent of oral herpes infections.
- *Varicella zoster:* Diagnosis is typically based on patient signs and symptoms, but PCR, antibody staining, and serologic tests can also be used.

Treatment

Treatment depends on the type of herpes virus and disease state.

- *Genital herpes simplex:* Zovirax (acyclovir), Famvir (famciclovir), and Valtrex (valacyclovir) are approved for the treatment of genital herpes simplex viral infections; however, antiviral treatment does not eradicate the virus. Treatment can be prescribed for initial and recurrent episodes or for suppressive therapy.
- *Varicella zoster:* Acyclovir, valacyclovir, and famciclovir can be prescribed to decrease the duration and severity of varicella zoster infections.

33-5. Questions

1. The lowest concentration of anti-infective that prevents microbial growth is called the

    A. minimum bactericidal concentration.
    B. minimum bacteriostatic concentration.
    C. minimum inhibitory concentration.
    D. minimum inhibiting concentration.
    E. minimum Schillings concentration.

2. Laboratory markers of infections, such as C-reactive protein, WBC count, and erythrocyte sedimentation rate, may not be accurate in which of the following patient populations?

    A. Elderly patients
    B. Patients with chronic obstructive pulmonary disease
    C. Malnourished patients
    D. A and C
    E. All of the above

3. The hallmark of empiric therapy is

    A. coverage of the most common pathogen associated with the infection.
    B. coverage of the common pathogens associated with the infection.
    C. coverage of all possible pathogens associated with the infection.
    D. coverage of polymicrobial pathogens associated with the infection.
    E. coverage of all viral organisms associated with the infection.

4. When two anti-infective therapies together produce a greater effect than the effects of each used alone, this phenomenon is termed

    A. commensalism.
    B. synergy.
    C. antagonism.
    D. additive.
    E. interacting.

5. Analysis of the cerebrospinal fluid may give valuable clues to the identity of the pathogen in meningitis. Given the following results, what would be indicative of a bacterial infection?

    I. Increased WBCs
    II. Increased glucose
    III. Increased protein

    A. I only
    B. II only
    C. I and III only
    D. II and III only
    E. I, II, and III

6. Empiric therapy for meningitis for patients up to 1 month of age includes

    A. vancomycin and ampicillin.
    B. aminoglycoside and ampicillin.
    C. ceftriaxone and vancomycin.
    D. vancomycin and aminoglycoside.
    E. ampicillin and ceftriaxone.

7. C. F. is a 65-year-old male diagnosed with endocarditis. Blood cultures reveal a highly sensitive strain of *Streptococcus*. Which of the following is most appropriate if C. F. has an anaphylactoid penicillin allergy?

    A. Vancomycin
    B. Gentamicin
    C. Ceftriaxone and gentamicin
    D. Meropenem
    E. Rifampin and gentamicin

8. Patients presenting with acute bronchitis without risk factors should be treated empirically with

    A. supportive care.
    B. clarithromycin.
    C. cefuroxime.
    D. ciprofloxacin.
    E. erythromycin.

9. The most common organisms associated with CAP in adults treated as outpatients are

    A. *Pseudomonas aeruginosa, Mycoplasma pneumoniae,* and *Haemophilus influenzae.*
    B. *Streptococcus pneumoniae, Haemophilus influenzae,* and *Klebsiella pneumoniae.*
    C. *Mycoplasma pneumoniae, Streptococcus pneumoniae, Haemophilus influenzae,* and *Klebsiella pneumoniae.*
    D. *Mycoplasma pneumoniae, Streptococcus pneumoniae, Haemophilus influenzae,* and *Chlamydophila pneumoniae.*
    E. *Mycoplasma pneumoniae, Streptococcus pneumoniae, Haemophilus influenzae,* and *Pseudomonas aeruginosa.*

10. Which of the following is an appropriate regimen for a patient with early-onset HAP without risk factors for multidrug-resistant pathogens?

    A. Doxycycline
    B. Azithromycin
    C. Ampicillin-sulbactam
    D. Ciprofloxacin and vancomycin
    E. Cefepime, ciprofloxacin, and vancomycin

11. Initial treatment of active tuberculosis infections in which no resistant strains of *Mycobacterium tuberculosis* are suspected should include

    A. rifabutin and pyrazinamide.
    B. rifampin and pyrazinamide.
    C. ethambutol, rifampin, isoniazid, and pyrazinamide.
    D. isoniazid, rifabutin, and pyrazinamide.
    E. ethambutol and rifampin.

12. The use of antimotility agents in a patient with suspected *Clostridium difficile* infection is

    A. discouraged because of the potential to cause toxic megacolon.
    B. encouraged because of increased cure rates.
    C. discouraged because of increased reinfections.
    D. encouraged because of decreased reinfections.
    E. discouraged because of lack of efficacy.

13. Which of the following is most likely to cause cellulitis?

    A. *Candida albicans*
    B. *Streptococcus* species
    C. *Shigella boydii*
    D. *Escherichia coli*
    E. *Klebsiella pneumoniae*

14. The best empiric regimen to treat a prostate infection is

    A. ciprofloxacin for 10 days.
    B. TMP-SMZ for 10 days.
    C. ciprofloxacin and TMP-SMZ for 10 days.
    D. ciprofloxacin for 4–6 weeks.
    E. TMP-SMZ for 4–6 weeks.

15. Tertiary syphilis in adults should be treated with

    A. benzathine penicillin G 2.4 million units for 1 day.
    B. azithromycin 1 g orally once.
    C. aqueous crystalline penicillin G 4 million units q4h for 10–14 days.
    D. benzathine penicillin G 2.4 million units once a week for 3 weeks.
    E. doxycycline 100 mg orally bid for 7 days.

16. *Candida albicans* infections of mild to moderate severity may be treated with

    A. fluconazole.
    B. amphotericin B.
    C. voriconazole.
    D. caspofungin.
    E. ketoconazole.

17. The antiviral agent(s) with the best spectrum of activity against recent influenza A strains is

    A. acyclovir.
    B. rimantadine.
    C. amantadine.
    D. oseltamivir and zanamivir.
    E. lamivudine and adefovir.

18. Which of the following agents can be used to treat genital herpes simplex infections?

    I. Acyclovir
    II. Famciclovir
    III. Valacyclovir

    A. I only
    B. III only
    C. I and II only
    D. I and III only
    E. I, II, and III

19. In the list that follows, the only organism that can be cultured easily is

    A. *Treponema pallidum.*
    B. *Mycobacterium tuberculosis.*
    C. *Rickettsia rickettsii.*
    D. *Ehrlichia phagocytophila.*
    E. *Francisella tularensis.*

20. Which of the following is the treatment of choice for an initial, mild *Clostridium difficile* infection?

    A. Metronidazole IV
    B. Metronidazole po

C. Vancomycin IV
D. Vancomycin po
E. Metronidazole IV and vancomycin po

Use the following case study to answer Questions 21 and 22:

J. B. is an 18-year-old Caucasian female diagnosed with gonorrhea.

21. What is an appropriate treatment for her uncomplicated gonorrhea infection?

A. Ceftriaxone 125 mg IM once
B. Ceftriaxone 250 mg IM once
C. Ceftriaxone 1 g IM once
D. Ceftriaxone 1g IM or IV every 24 hours until improvement, then cefixime 400 mg orally twice daily to complete a total of at least 7 days of treatment
E. Treatment is not necessary in patients with uncomplicated gonorrhea.

22. Because J. B. has gonorrhea, she should also receive treatment for

A. syphilis.
B. HIV.
C. hepatitis.
D. genital herpes.
E. chlamydia.

Use the following case study to answer Questions 23 and 24:

L. B. is a 45-year-old Caucasian female presenting to the emergency department with a fever of 103°F, flank pain, dysuria, urinary urgency, and frequency. Her laboratory tests are significant for an increased WBC count of 18,000 cells/mm^3 and 3% immature forms (bands). Her urinalysis revealed > 10^5 cells/mL of Gram-negative rods.

23. What infection does L. B. have?

A. Herpes simplex
B. Gonorrhea
C. Syphilis
D. Urinary tract infection
E. Food poisoning

24. What therapy would be useful for L. B.?

A. Oral quinolone
B. IV quinolone

C. Oral penicillin
D. IV carbapenem
E. IV vancomycin

25. R. H. is a 45-year-old male recently diagnosed with hepatitis C. Genotyping reveals R. H. is infected with hepatitis C, genotype 2. His health care provider decides to initiate treatment and asks you to select an appropriate treatment regimen. Which of the following could you recommend?

A. Peginterferon alfa for 24 weeks
B. Sofosbuvir and ribavirin for 12 weeks
C. Peginterferon alfa and ribavirin for 48 weeks
D. Boceprevir, peginterferon alfa, and ribavirin for 12 weeks followed by peginterferon alfa and ribavirin alone for 12–36 weeks
E. Telaprevir, peginterferon alfa, and ribavirin for 12 weeks followed by peginterferon alfa and ribavirin alone for 12–36 weeks

33-6. Answers

1. C. The minimum inhibitory concentration determines the level of anti-infective to which dosing regimens may be set.

2. D. Elderly and malnourished patients may not be able to respond with appropriate laboratory markers of infections because of limited reserves or deletion of inflammatory factors.

3. B. Coverage of common pathogens associated with the infection increases the probability of curing the infection without increasing anti-infective exposure to other organisms, which increases the possibility of resistance.

4. B. *Synergy* is the correct term.

5. C. Bacterial meningitis infections show an increase in WBCs and protein in the CSF, whereas CSF glucose is decreased.

6. B. This regimen covers the most likely organisms for meningitis in this age group: *Streptococcus agalactiae*, *Escherichia coli*, *Listeria monocytogenes*, and *Klebsiella* species. Ampicillin and cefotaxime would be another appropriate choice for empiric therapy in patients up to 1 month of age.

7. **A.** Vancomycin is appropriate for penicillin-allergic patients with endocarditis caused by *Streptococcus* species. Other regimens for streptococci include penicillin or ceftriaxone (with or without gentamicin), which has a potential for cross-reactivity in patients with penicillin allergies.

8. **A.** Because half of bronchitis infections are caused by a viral etiology, antibacterial therapy for low-risk patients should not be attempted, with the exception of severe presentation.

9. **D.** *Pseudomonas aeruginosa* is more likely in patients with risk factors for multidrug-resistant bacteria such as late-onset HAP or VAP. *Klebsiella pneumoniae* is also not commonly associated with CAP.

10. **C.** Empiric therapy for early-onset HAP without risk factors for multidrug-resistant pathogens is as follows: ceftriaxone, a fluoroquinolone, ampicillin-sulbactam, or ertapenem. Doxycycline or azithromycin is appropriate for outpatient treatment of CAP. Cefepime, ciprofloxacin, and vancomycin in combination are appropriate for late-onset HAP or patients with risk factors for multidrug-resistant organisms.

11. **C.** The preferred treatment for active tuberculosis infections is a four-drug regimen consisting of ethambutol, rifampin, isoniazid, and pyrazinamide for the initial 2 months, followed by rifampin with isoniazid for 4 additional months.

12. **A.** Use of antimotility agents in *Clostridium difficile* infections increases the risk of toxic megacolon.

13. **B.** Most cellulitis infections are associated with *Streptococcus* species.

14. **D.** Prostate infections are difficult to treat, requiring 4–6 weeks of therapy. Although TMP-SMZ is a reasonable choice for treating most prostate infections, ciprofloxacin is preferred because of its ability to concentrate in prostate fluid.

15. **D.** Benzathine penicillin G. 2.4 million units once a week for 3 weeks is standard therapy for either late latent syphilis or tertiary syphilis. Single-dose benzathine penicillin (2.4 million units) is appropriate for primary, secondary, or early latent syphilis. Response C is the treatment for neurosyphilis.

16. **A.** Fluconazole is the preferred treatment for mild to moderate infections caused by *Candida*

albicans. Amphotericin B, voriconazole, and caspofungin are active against *Candida* but should be reserved for more severe infections or less susceptible *Candida* species. Ketoconazole is not a preferred treatment for *Candida* infections.

17. **D.** Recent influenza A strains have demonstrated marked resistance to amantadine and rimantadine; therefore, these agents are not currently recommended. Acyclovir, lamivudine, and adefovir are not active against influenza.

18. **E.** Acyclovir, famciclovir, and valacyclovir are all approved for the treatment of genital herpes.

19. **B.** *Mycobacterium tuberculosis*, although very slow growing, can be grown on culture media. The remaining organisms cannot be grown without the use of cell culture techniques, forcing the clinician to rely on serum testing and direct staining for identification of the organism.

20. **B.** Oral metronidazole is the treatment of choice for an initial, mild-to-moderate episode of *Clostridium difficile*. An initial severe episode should be treated with vancomycin po, and an initial episode that is severe and complicated should be treated with vancomycin po and metronidazole IV. IV vancomycin is inappropriate for a *Clostridium difficile* infection.

21. **B.** Response A is no longer recommended because of decreasing cephalosporin susceptibilities and concerns about ceftriaxone treatment failures. Response C is the treatment for gonococcal conjunctivitis. Response D is the treatment for disseminated gonococcal infections.

22. **E.** Because of the high rate of comorbid chlamydia infections, patients diagnosed with gonorrhea should also receive therapy against chlamydia: azithromycin 1 g orally once or doxycycline 100 mg orally twice daily for 7 days.

23. **D.** Given the clinical presentation and laboratory test results, L. B. has a severe UTI. The presence of systemic symptoms (fever and chills) suggests an upper UTI or pyelonephritis.

24. **B.** Given the severity of disease, parenteral therapy would be reasonable for initial therapy. Because the Gram stain of the urine revealed Gram-negative rods, either a quinolone or an extended-spectrum beta-lactam would be reasonable empiric therapy until the organism is identified and sensitivities obtained. A carbapenem would be adequate but should be reserved

for infections when multidrug-resistant pathogens are suspected.

25. **B.** Response B is the recommended treatment for hepatitis C, genotype 2. Responses A, D, and E are incorrect because current guidelines do not recommend using boceprevir- or telaprevir-based regimens or interferon monotherapy to treat any hepatitis C genotype. Response C is incorrect because interferon with ribavirin is an alternate therapy for hepatitis C, genotypes 5 and 6 but not genotype 2.

33-7. References

American Association for the Study of Liver Diseases and Infectious Diseases Society of America. Recommendations for testing, managing, and treating hepatitis C. http://www.hcvguidelines.org. Accessed February 14, 2014.

American Thoracic Society Documents. Guidelines for the management of adults with hospital-acquired, ventilator-associated, and healthcare-associated pneumonia. *Am J Respir Crit Care Med.* 2005;171:388–416.

Baddour LM, Wilson WR, Bayer AS, et al. Infective endocarditis: Diagnosis, antimicrobial therapy, and management of complications: A statement for healthcare professionals from the Committee on Rheumatic Fever, Endocarditis, and Kawasaki Disease, Council on Cardiovascular Disease in the Young, and the Councils on Clinical Cardiology, Stroke, and Cardiovascular Surgery and Anesthesia, American Heart Association: Endorsed by the Infectious Diseases Society of America. *Circulation.* 2005;111:e394–433.

Braman SS. Chronic cough due to acute bronchitis: ACCP evidence-based clinical practice guidelines. *Chest.* 2006;129(suppl):95S–103S.

Braman SS. Chronic cough due to chronic bronchitis: ACCP evidence-based clinical practice guidelines. *Chest.* 2006;129(suppl):104S–115S.

Centers for Disease Control and Prevention. 2011–2012 Influenza antiviral medications: A summary for clinicians. Atlanta, GA: Centers for Disease Control and Prevention; 2011. http://www.cdc.gov/flu/pdf/professionals/antivirals/clinician-antivirals-2011.pdf. Accessed April 22, 2012.

Centers for Disease Control and Prevention. Sexually transmitted diseases. Atlanta, GA: Centers for Disease Control and Prevention; 2014. http://www.cdc.gov/std/default.htm. Accessed March 14, 2014.

Centers for Disease Control and Prevention. Treatment of tuberculosis, American Thoracic Society, CDC, and Infectious Diseases Society of America. *MMWR.* 2003;52(RR-11):1–74.

Chapman AS, Bakken JS, Folk SM, et al. Diagnosis and management of tickborne Rickettsial diseases: Rocky Mountain spotted fever, ehrlichiosis, and anaplasmosis—United States. *MMWR.* 2006;55(RR-04):1–27.

Chapman SW, Dismukes WE, Proia LA, et al. Clinical practice guidelines for the management of blastomycosis: 2008 update by the Infectious Diseases Society of America. *Clin Infect Dis.* 2008;46:1801–12.

Cohen SH, Gerding DN, Johnson S, et al. Clinical practice guidelines for *Clostridium difficile* infection in adults: 2010 update by the Society for Healthcare Epidemiology of America (SHEA) and the Infectious Diseases Society of America (IDSA). *Infect Control Hosp Epidemiol.* 2010;31(5):431–55.

Dellinger RP, Levy MM, Carlet JM, et al. Surviving Sepsis Campaign: International guidelines for management of severe sepsis and septic shock: 2008 [published correction appears in *Crit Care Med.* 2008;36:1394–96]. *Crit Care Med.* 2008;36:296–327.

Dworkin RH, Johnson RW, Breuer J, et al. Recommendations for the management of herpes zoster. *Clin Infect Dis.* 2007;1(44):S1–26.

Freifeld AG, Bow EJ, Sepkowitz KA, et al. Clinical practice guideline for the use of antimicrobial agents in neutropenic patients with cancer: 2010 update by the Infectious Diseases Society of America. *Clin Infect Dis.* 2011;52:e56–93.

Galgiani JN, Ampel NM, Blair JE, et al. Coccidioidomycosis. *Clin Infect Dis.* 2005;41:1217–23.

Ghany MG, Nelson DR, Strader DB, et al. An update on treatment of genotype 1 chronic hepatitis C virus infection: 2011 practice guideline by the American Association for the Study of Liver Diseases. *Hepatology.* 2011;54(4):1433–44.

Ghany MG, Strader DB, Thomas DL, et al. Diagnosis, management, and treatment of hepatitis C: An update. *Hepatology.* 2009;49(4):1335–74.

Global Initiative for Chronic Obstructive Lung Disease. *Global Strategy for the Diagnosis, Management, and Prevention of Chronic Obstructive Pulmonary Disease.* Updated 2014. http://www.goldcopd.org. Accessed March 19, 2014.

Guerrant RL, Van Gilder T, Steiner TS, et al. Practice guidelines for the management of infectious diarrhea. *Clin Infect Dis.* 2001;32:331–50.

Gupta K, Hooton TM, Naber KG, et al. International clinical practice guidelines for the treatment of acute uncomplicated cystitis and pyelonephritis in women: A 2010 update by the Infectious Diseases Society of America and the European Society for Microbiology and Infectious Diseases. *Clin Infect Dis.* 2011;52:e103–20.

Hooton TM, Bradley SF, Cardenas DD, et al. Diagnosis, prevention, and treatment of catheter-associated urinary tract infection in adults: 2009 international clinical practice guidelines from the Infectious Diseases Society of America. *Clin Infect Dis.* 2010;50:625–63.

Klastersky J, Paesmans M, Rubenstein EB, et al. The Multinational Association for Supportive Care in Cancer Risk Index: A multinational scoring system for identifying low-risk febrile neutropenic cancer patients. *J Clin Oncol.* 2000;18:3038–51.

Lipsky BA, Berendt AR, Deery HG, et al. Diagnosis and treatment of diabetic foot infections. *Clin Infect Dis.* 2004;39:885–910.

Liu C, Bayer A, Cosgrove SE, et al. Clinical practice guidelines by the Infectious Diseases Society of America for the treatment of methicillin-resistant *Staphylococcus aureus* infections in adults and children. *Clin Infect Dis.* 2011;52:1–38.

Lok ASF, McMahon BJ. Chronic hepatitis B: Update 2009. *Hepatology.* 2009;50(3):1–36.

Mandell LA, Wunderink RG, Anzueto A, et al. Infectious Diseases Society of America/American Thoracic Society consensus guidelines on the management of community-acquired pneumonia in adults. *Clin Infect Dis.* 2007;44:27–72.

Mermel LA, Allon M, Bouza E, et al. Clinical practice guidelines for the diagnosis and management of intravascular catheter-related infection: 2009 update by the Infectious Diseases Society of America. *Clin Infect Dis.* 2009;49:1–45.

Pappas PG, Kauffman CA, Andes D, et al. Clinical practice guidelines for the management of candidiasis: 2009 update by the Infectious Diseases Society of America. *Clin Infect Dis.* 2009;48:503–35.

Perfect JR, Dismukes WE, Dromer F, et al. Clinical practice guidelines for the management of cryptococcal disease: 2010 update by the Infectious Diseases Society of America. *Clin Infect Dis.* 2010;50:291–322.

Sexually transmitted diseases. Centers for Disease Control and Prevention Web site. http://www.cdc.gov/std/default.htm. Accessed March 14, 2014.

Shingles (herpes zoster) for healthcare professionals. Centers for Disease Control and Prevention Web site. http://www.cdc.gov/shingles/hcp/index.html. Accessed March 14, 2014.

Solomkin JS, Mazuski JE, Bradley JS, et al. Diagnosis and management of complicated intra-abdominal infection in adults and children: Guidelines by the Surgical Infection Society and the Infectious Diseases Society of America. *Clin Infect Dis.* 2010;50:133–64.

Stevens DL, Bisno AL, Chambers HF, et al. Practice guidelines for the diagnosis and management of skin and soft-tissue infections. *Clin Infect Dis.* 2005;41:1373–406.

Tunkel AR, Hartman BJ, Kaplan SL, et al. Practice guidelines for the management of bacterial meningitis. *Clin Infect Dis.* 2004;39:1267–84.

Walsh TJ, Anaissie EJ, Denning DW, et al. Treatment of aspergillosis: Clinical practice guidelines of the Infectious Diseases Society of America. *Clin Infect Dis.* 2008;46:327–60.

Wheat LJ, Freifels AG, Kleiman MB, et al. Clinical practice guidelines for the management of patients with histoplasmosis: 2007 update by the Infectious Diseases Society of America. *Clin Infect Dis.* 2007;45:807–25.

World Health Organization. *WHO Guidelines on Tularemia.* Geneva: WHO; 2007.

Wormser GP, Dattwyler RJ, Shapiro ED, et al. The clinical assessment, treatment, and prevention of Lyme disease, human granulocytic anaplasmosis, and babesiosis: Clinical practice guidelines by the Infectious Diseases Society of America. *Clin Infect Dis.* 2006;43:1089–134.

Anti-infective Agents

Anthony J. Guarascio

34-1. Key Points

Aminoglycosides

- Aminoglycoside antibiotics exhibit concentration-dependent bacterial killing.
- Aminoglycoside antibiotics are primarily used as adjunct therapy agents for severe infections or for use against multidrug-resistant bacteria.
- Aminoglycoside dosing is tailored using pharmacokinetic drug monitoring to optimize therapeutic effects and minimize toxicity.

Penicillins

- Penicillin antibiotics exhibit time-above-MIC (minimum inhibitory concentration)-dependent bacterial killing.
- All penicillins, except nafcillin and oxacillin, are renally eliminated and require dosage adjustments in patients with renal dysfunction.

Cephalosporins

- Cephalosporin antibiotics exhibit time-above-MIC-dependent bacterial killing.
- First-generation cephalosporins generally display extensive Gram-positive activity but limited Gram-negative activity.
- Second-generation cephalosporins generally have similar Gram-positive activity as first-generation agents, but more enhanced Gram-negative activity.
- Third-generation cephalosporins generally display less Gram-positive activity than that of first- and second-generation agents. However, Gram-negative activity is more extensive.
- Ceftazidime (third generation) and cefepime (fourth generation) display activity against *Pseudomonas aeruginosa*, while ceftaroline displays activity against methicillin-resistant *Staphylococcus aureus* (MRSA).

Carbapenems and Monobactam

- Carbapenem antibiotics possess a very broad spectrum of activity and should be restricted to appropriate indications to minimize development of resistance.
- The monobactam, aztreonam, is active only against aerobic Gram-negative bacteria.

Gram-Positive Antibiotics

- Daptomycin and linezolid are clinically effective against MRSA, methicillin-resistant *Staphylococcus epidermidis* (MRSE), and vancomycin-resistant *Enterococci* (VRE).
- Daptomycin is inactivated by lung surfactant and cannot be used to treat pneumonia.
- Linezolid should not be used to treat bacteremia or endovascular infections.
- Vancomycin dosing is tailored using pharmacokinetic drug monitoring to optimize therapeutic benefit and minimize toxicity.

Editor's Note: This chapter is based on the 10th edition chapter written by W. Andrew Bell.

Fluoroquinolones

■ Quinolone antibiotics exhibit concentration-dependent bacterial killing similar to that of the aminoglycosides.

■ The later-generation quinolones (levofloxacin, moxifloxacin) possess improved Gram-positive activity, particularly against beta-lactam-resistant *Streptococcus pneumoniae.*

Macrolides

■ Macrolides are a drug of choice for atypical pneumonia.

■ Macrolides are active against some Gram-positive bacteria, including streptococci.

Tetracyclines and Glycylcycline

■ Tetracyclines display activity against community-acquired MRSA strains and have reliable atypical coverage.

■ Tetracyclines are drugs of choice for Lyme disease and Rocky Mountain spotted fever.

■ The glycylcycline tigecycline displays broad-spectrum Gram-positive (including MRSA) coverage, anaerobic coverage, and Gram-negative coverage but does not cover *P. aeruginosa.*

Sulfonamides

■ Sulfamethoxazole-trimethoprim displays activity against community-acquired MRSA strains.

■ Sulfamethoxazole-trimethoprim is commonly used to treat urinary tract infections.

Miscellaneous Antibiotics

■ Clindamycin is an effective anaerobic antibiotic with activity against many community-acquired MRSA strains.

■ Metronidazole is active against many anaerobic bacteria and provides excellent *Bacteroides fragilis* coverage.

■ Fidaxomicin is an option in the treatment of *Clostridium difficile* as an alternative to metronidazole or oral vancomycin therapy.

■ The polymyxins are antibiotics reserved only for severe infections caused by multidrug-resistant Gram-negative pathogens because of a significant toxicity profile.

Antifungal Agents

■ Fluconazole is a drug of choice for *Candida albicans,* and echinocandins are drugs of choice for resistant, non–*C. albicans* species.

■ Voriconazole and amphotericin B are agents of choice for treatment of aspergillosis.

■ Imidazole and triazole antifungal antibiotics are potent inhibitors of hepatic metabolism, thereby decreasing the elimination of numerous agents.

Antitubercular Agents

■ Rifampin, isoniazid, pyrazinamide, and ethambutol (RIPE) combination therapy are agents of first choice for active tuberculosis infection.

■ Isoniazid daily therapy is the preferred regimen for latent tuberculosis infection.

34-2. Study Guide Checklist

The following topics may guide your study of this subject area:

■ General antimicrobial spectrum of anti-infective agents

■ Agents that cover the prominent bacterial pathogens MRSA and *P. aeruginosa*

■ Major toxicities associated with anti-infective agents

■ Antibiotic agents that require pharmacokinetic drug monitoring

■ Main indications for treatment with anti-infective agents

■ Drugs of choice for bacterial and fungal pathogens

■ First-line and second-line agents to treat tuberculosis

■ Important patient counseling information for anti-infective agents

34-3. Aminoglycosides

Aminoglycosides are antibiotics active against most aerobic Gram-negative bacteria and display synergistic activity for select aerobic Gram-positive bacteria. They are not effective against anaerobic bacteria. Aminoglycosides are primarily used as adjunct treatment in serious infections because of their significant toxicity. The most commonly used aminoglycosides include amikacin, gentamicin, and tobramycin.

Mechanism of Action

Aminoglycosides inhibit bacterial protein synthesis through binding to the 30S ribosomal subunit, thereby irreversibly inhibiting bacterial ribonucleic acid (RNA) synthesis. Aminoglycosides are bactericidal.

Spectrum of Activity

Amikacin is a semisynthetic parenteral aminoglycoside with the broadest antimicrobial activity of the class, and it frequently possesses activity against bacteria resistant to other aminoglycosides.

Gentamicin is a parenteral aminoglycoside that is more active against *Acinetobacter, Serratia,* and enterococci than is tobramycin.

Tobramycin is a parenteral aminoglycoside that is more active against *Pseudomonas* than is gentamicin.

Streptomycin is a parenteral aminoglycoside active against enterococci, streptococci, mycobacteria, and some Gram-negative anaerobes. Streptomycin should be administered only by intramuscular (IM) injection.

Neomycin is a minimally absorbed oral aminoglycoside used to decrease bacterial content of the bowel and is sometimes used as a preoperative bowel preparation and as an adjunct in hepatic encephalopathy.

Adverse Drug Events

Nephrotoxicity is demonstrated by an increase in blood urea nitrogen (BUN) and serum creatinine. It usually manifests as nonoliguric renal failure and may cause potassium, calcium, and magnesium wasting. Nephrotoxicity may occur in 10–25% of patients receiving aminoglycosides and is usually reversible on discontinuation of the agent. Risk factors include the following:

- Preexisting renal dysfunction
- Prolonged duration of therapy
- Concomitant use of other nephrotoxic agents
- Elevated trough concentrations:
  - Gentamicin and tobramycin > 2 mcg/mL
  - Amikacin > 8 mcg/mL

Neuromuscular blockade is an uncommon but potentially serious toxicity. Risk factors include the following:

- Concomitant use of neuromuscular blocking agents
- Myasthenia gravis
- Hypocalcemia
- Elevated peak serum concentrations

Ototoxicity is caused by eighth cranial nerve damage demonstrated by auditory and vestibular symptoms. Auditory symptoms include tinnitus and loss of high-frequency hearing. Vestibular toxicity is demonstrated by dizziness, nystagmus, vertigo, and ataxia. Ototoxicity seems to correlate with high peak concentrations. However, the true incidence is not clearly known because profound high-frequency hearing loss can occur prior to detection.

Pharmacokinetics

Aminoglycosides are renally eliminated:

- $t_{1/2}$ = 2.5–2.7 hours (normal renal function)
- $t_{1/2}$ = ~ 69 hours (anephric clearance)
- V_d = 0.27–0.3 L/kg (ideal body weight [IBW])

Dosing

Aminoglycosides are dosed on the basis of IBW unless the patient is obese (120% of IBW). For obese patients, dosing weight (DW) is adjusted. DW = IBW + 0.4 (total body weight [TBW] – IBW). Traditional and extended interval dosing parameters for aminoglycosides are described in Table 34-1.

Target serum concentrations

Traditional dosing reference levels are as follows:

- Amikacin peak = 20–30 mcg/mL
- Amikacin trough ≤ 8–10 mcg/mL
- Gentamicin and tobramycin peak = 3–10 mcg/mL
- Gentamicin and tobramycin trough ≤ 1–2 mcg/mL

Extended interval dosing

The use of extended interval dosing, dosed once daily to every other day, has been suggested to maximize efficacy and minimize nephrotoxicity of aminoglycosides. This dosing strategy is designed to yield high peak concentrations to maximize the concentration-dependent killing of bacteria and allow the trough concentrations to fall below detectable levels in the body to reduce toxicity. Aminoglycosides possess a significant postantibiotic effect, which allows them to maintain efficacy even when concentrations fall below the minimum inhibitory concentration (MIC) of the causative pathogen. Contraindications to extended interval aminoglycoside use include pregnancy, burns, ascites, and creatinine clearance < 20 mL/min. With extended interval dosing, peak and trough concentrations are not usually drawn. However, a single

Table 34-1. Aminoglycosides[a]

Generic name	Trade name	Dosage forms	Normal dose	Elimination
Amikacin	Amikin	IV, IM	Conventional dosing: 15 mg/kg daily divided q8–12h	Renal
			Extended interval: 15 mg/kg q24–48h	
Gentamicin	Garamycin	IV, IM	Conventional dosing: 3–5 mg/kg daily divided q8h	Renal
			Extended interval: 5–7 mg/kg q24–48h	
Tobramycin		IV, IM, INHL	Conventional dosing: 3–5 mg/kg daily divided q8h	Renal
			Extended interval: 5–7 mg/kg q24–48h	
			Nebulized: 300 mg q12h	
Streptomycin		IM	7.5 mg/kg IM q12h	Renal
Neomycin		po	50–100 mg/kg daily	Renal

INHL, inhaled; IV, intravenous.
a. Use ideal or adjusted body weight for all aminoglycoside dosing.

random serum level is drawn 6–14 hours after the start of the infusion and plotted on a nomogram to determine the patient-specific dosing interval (q24h, q36h, or q48h).

34-4. Penicillins

Mechanism of Action

Penicillin-binding proteins make up the bacterial cell wall. When penicillin binds to these proteins, it is able to inhibit cell wall synthesis in the bacteria, causing cell wall lysis and ultimately cell death.

Penicillins are bactericidal; they inhibit bacterial cell wall synthesis. They are known as β-lactam antibiotics because their chemical structure consists of a β-lactam ring adjoined to a thiazolidine ring.

Spectrum of Activity and Dosing

See Tables 34-2 and 34-3 for information about the spectrum of activity and dosing of penicillins, respectively.

Adverse Drug Events

Allergic or hypersensitivity reaction occurs in 3–10% of patients. Rash (4–8% of patients) or anaphylaxis (0.01–0.05% of patients) can occur within 10–20 minutes and is more common in intravenous (IV) than in oral administration.

Neurologic reactions (seizures) are seen with high doses of penicillin given to patients with renal insufficiency.

Gastrointestinal (GI) effects, including nausea and vomiting, may occur with oral use.

Hypokalemia and hypernatremia may occur, particularly with carboxypenicillins.

Penicillinase-resistant penicillins can cause interstitial nephritis and increase transaminases.

Hematologic reactions (thrombocytopenia, neutropenia, hemolytic anemia) are possible.

Drug–Drug Interactions

Probenecid competitively inhibits tubular secretion of penicillins, thus increasing plasma levels. This interaction is sometimes employed in serious central nervous system (CNS) infections to increase drug concentrations.

Concomitant use with an oral contraceptive may decrease the effectiveness of the oral contraceptive and increase incidence of breakthrough bleeding.

Other Characteristics

Nafcillin and oxacillin are eliminated primarily by biliary excretion; therefore, there is no need to adjust dosage for patients with renal dysfunction.

Penicillin G benzathine is a repository drug formulation. When it is given IM, insoluble salt allows slow drug absorption from the injection site, and therefore, it has a longer duration of action (1–4 weeks, dose-dependent).

Table 34-2. Spectrum of Activity of the Penicillins

Category	Spectrum
Natural penicillins	Natural penicillins are effective against viridans group streptococci and *Streptococcus pyogenes* and against some *S. pneumoniae,* mouth anaerobes, and *Clostridium perfringens* (gas gangrene).
	They are ineffective against *Staphylococcus aureus* because they are readily hydrolyzed by penicillinases.
Penicillinase-resistant penicillins	These agents are drugs of choice for methicillin-susceptible *Staphylococcus aureus* (MSSA). They cover some streptococci but not enterococci.
Aminopenicillins	Aminopenicillins are drugs of choice for enterococci and *Listeria monocytogenes.*
	They cover some *Streptococcus pneumoniae, Haemophilus influenzae, Escherichia coli, Klebsiella,* and *Proteus.*
Carboxypenicillins and ureidopenicillins	The spectrum is like that of aminopenicillins, but these drugs provide more Gram-negative coverage. They cover *Proteus, E. coli, Klebsiella* (not ticarcillin alone), *Enterobacter,* and *Pseudomonas.* They have in vitro activity against staphylococci, streptococci, enterococci, most *Enterobacteriaceae, Pseudomonas,* and many anaerobes, including *Bacteroides fragilis.* Ureidopenicillins possess better in vitro activity against *Pseudomonas* species than carboxypenicillins (piperacillin > ticarcillin).
β-lactamase inhibitors (clavulanic acid, sulbactam, tazobactam)	β-lactamase inhibitors are combined with penicillins to improve both Gram-negative and anaerobic activity including enhanced coverage of *H. influenzae, Moraxella catarrhalis, Bacteroides, E. coli,* and other *Enterobacteriaceae.*
Ampicillin-sulbactam and amoxicillin–clavulanic acid	This combination is active against *H. influenzae, M. catarrhalis, Proteus, E. coli, Klebsiella pneumoniae,* MSSA, and anaerobes.
Ticarcillin–clavulanic acid	This combination has activity against *Pseudomonas aeruginosa, H. influenzae, M. catarrhalis, Proteus, E. coli, K. pneumoniae,* MSSA, and anaerobes. It has enhanced activity against the nosocomial pathogen *Stenotrophomonas maltophilia* in comparison with piperacillin-tazobactam.
Piperacillin-tazobactam	This combination provides overall enhanced Gram-positive, Gram-negative (most notably *P. aeruginosa*), and anaerobic coverage compared with ticarcillin–clavulanic acid.

34-5. Cephalosporins

Cephalosporins are β-lactam antibiotics that are structurally and pharmacologically similar to penicillins.

Mechanism of Action

Cephalosporins bind to penicillin-binding proteins in a manner similar to that of other β-lactams, thereby inhibiting peptidoglycan synthesis. Cephalosporins are bactericidal agents.

Spectrum of Activity

Cephalosporins are broad-spectrum antimicrobial agents; however, the spectrum of activity varies greatly among the individual agents. Thus, cephalosporins are grouped into four broad classes, or generations,

according to their antimicrobial coverage (Table 34-4). It is important to note that no cephalosporin has clinically dependable coverage of enterococci.

First-generation agents (cefadroxil, cefazolin, cephalexin)

Gram-positive activity is extensive, including agents of choice for methicillin-susceptible *Staphylococcus aureus* (MSSA), and coverage of *Streptococcus pyogenes* (group A beta-hemolytic streptococci), *Streptococcus agalactiae* (group B streptococci), and *Streptococcus pneumoniae.* First-generation agents are inactive against methicillin-resistant staphylococci (methicillin-resistant *Staphylococcus aureus* [MRSA], methicillin-resistant *Staphylococcus epidermidis* [MRSE]), and *Listeria monocytogenes.*

Gram-negative activity is limited, although some strains of *Escherichia coli, Klebsiella pneumoniae,*

Table 34-3. Dosing of Penicillins

Type and generic name	Trade name	Elimination route	Administration route	Common doses
Natural penicillins				
Penicillin G	Pfizerpen	Renal	IV, IM, po	2 million to 4 million units IV q4h
Penicillin G procaine	Wycillin	Renal	IM	300,000–600,000 units daily
Penicillin G benzathine	Bicillin L-A	Renal	IM	Strep throat: 1.2 million units; syphilis: 2.4 million units
Penicillin V (phenoxymethyl penicillin)	Pen-Vee-K, Veetids	Renal	po	250–500 mg po bid–qid (250 mg bid for prophylaxis)
Penicillinase-resistant penicillins				
Oxacillin	Prostaphlin, Bactocill	Hepatic	po, IV, IM	1–2 g IV q4–6h
Nafcillin	Nafcil, Unipen	Hepatic	IV, IM	1–2 g IV q4–6h
Cloxacillin	Cloxapen	Renal	po	200–500 mg q6h
Dicloxacillin	Dynapen, Dycill	Renal	po	250–500 mg po q6h
Aminopenicillins				
Ampicillin	Omnipen, Principen	Renal	po, IM, IV	1–2 g IV q6h
Amoxicillin	Amoxil, Trimox, Moxatag	Renal	po	250–500 mg po q8h; 775 mg (ER) po q24h
Ureidopenicillins				
Piperacillin	Pipracil	Renal	IV, IM	3–4 g IV q4–6h
Penicillin plus β-lactamase inhibitors				
Amoxicillin–clavulanic acid	Augmentin, Augmentin XR	Renal	po	250–500 mg po tid, 500–875 mg po bid; 2,000 mg XR po q12h
Ampicillin-sulbactam	Unasyn	Renal	IV, IM	1.5 g or 3 g IV q6–8h
Piperacillin-tazobactam	Zosyn	Renal	IV	2.25 to 4.5 g IV q6h; 3.375 g IV q8h as 4-hour extended infusion
Ticarcillin–clavulanic acid	Timentin	Renal	IV	3.1 g IV q4–6h

Proteus mirabilis, and *Shigella* may display susceptibility. First-generation agents are inactive against *Haemophilus influenzae*, *Neisseria*, *Pseudomonas*, *Enterobacter*, *Citrobacter*, *Serratia*, other *Proteus* spp., and anaerobes such as *Bacteroides fragilis*.

Second-generation agents (cefaclor, cefotetan, cefoxitin, cefprozil, cefuroxime) and cephamycins (cefoxitin, cefotetan)

Gram-positive activity is similar to that of first-generation agents.

Gram-negative activity of second-generation agents is generally more extensive than that of first-

generation agents, including some strains of *E. coli*, *Klebsiella*, and *Proteus*. Second-generation agents are active against *H. influenzae*, *Neisseria*, and some (cefotetan, cefoxitin) also have anaerobic activity. Second-generation agents are inactive against *Pseudomonas*.

Third-generation agents (cefdinir, cefixime, cefotaxime, cefpodoxime, ceftazidime, ceftibuten, ceftriaxone)

In general, Gram-positive activity is reduced versus first- and second-generation agents; however, ceftriaxone displays effective *S. pneumoniae* coverage.

Table 34-4. Cephalosporins

Generic name	Trade name	Dosage forms	Dose	Elimination	Notes
First generation					More Gram-positive than Gram-negative activity
Cefadroxil	Duricef, Ultracef	po	1–2 g daily	Renal	
Cefazolin	Ancef, Kefzol	IV	250–1,000 mg q8h	Renal	
Cephalexin	Keflex	po	250–500 mg q6h	Renal	
Second generation					Enhanced Gram-negative activity versus first-generation drugs
Cefaclor	Ceclor	po	250–500 mg q8h	Renal	
Cefotetan	Cefotan	IV, IM	1–2 g q12h	Renal	Anaerobic activity, N-methylthiotetrazole side chain
Cefoxitin	Mefoxin	IV	1–2 g q6–8h	Renal	Anaerobic activity
Cefprozil	Cefzil	po	250–500 mg q12–24h	Renal	
Cefuroxime	Ceftin, Zinacef	IV, IM, po	750–1,500 mg q8h IV and IM; 250–500 mg po q12h	Renal	
Third generation					More Gram-negative than Gram-positive activity; cerebrospinal fluid penetration
Cefdinir	Omnicef	po	300 mg q12h	Renal	
Cefixime	Suprax	po	400 mg daily	Renal	
Cefotaxime	Claforan	IV	1–2 g q6–8h	Renal	
Cefpodoxime	Vantin	po	100–400 mg q12h	Renal	
Ceftazidime	Fortaz, Tazicef	IV, IM	1–2 g q8–12h	Renal	Antipseudomonal but no Gram-positive activity
Ceftibuten	Cedax	po	400 mg daily	Renal	
Ceftriaxone	Rocephin	IV, IM	1–2 q12–24h	Renal and biliary	No dosage adjustment in renal impairment
Fourth generation					Gram-positive and Gram-negative activity
Cefepime	Maxipime	IV, IM	1–2 g q8–12h	Renal	Antipseudomonal activity
Unclassified					
Ceftaroline	Teflaro	IV	600 mg q12h	Renal	MRSA, enhanced *Streptococcus pneumoniae* activity

Gram-negative activity is extensive, including *Enterobacter, Citrobacter, Serratia, Neisseria,* and *Haemophilus.* Some third-generation agents are active against *Pseudomonas* (ceftazidime).

Fourth-generation agent (cefepime)

Gram-positive activity is enhanced versus third-generation agents. Cefepime is inactive against MRSA, *Listeria,* and anaerobes.

Gram-negative activity is extensive, including enhanced activity against *Pseudomonas* and *Enterobacteriaceae* that produce inducible β-lactamases.

Unclassified agent (ceftaroline)

The spectrum of activity of ceftaroline is similar to that of the third-generation agent ceftriaxone, except ceftaroline is active against MRSA and has further enhanced *S. pneumoniae* coverage. Currently, ceftaroline is approved for the treatment of community-acquired pneumonia and skin and soft tissue infections. Ceftaroline is renally eliminated and must be dose adjusted in renal dysfunction.

Adverse Drug Events

- Hypersensitivity, including fever, rash, pruritus, urticaria, anaphylaxis, and hemolytic anemia
- GI effects, such as nausea, vomiting, and diarrhea
- Nephrotoxicity (rare)
- Seizures (potential risk with high doses in patients with renal impairment)
- *Clostridium difficile* colitis
- Bleeding or hypoprothrombinemia (cefotetan), which is attributable to the presence of an N-methylthiotetrazole (NMTT) side chain in the structure of these agents (possible prevention or reversal with administration of vitamin K)
- Blood dyscrasias (rare)

Drug–Drug Interactions

Disulfiram-like reactions have been reported with ingestion of alcohol during treatment with cephalosporin antibiotics that possess an NMTT side chain (cefotetan).

Probenecid competitively inhibits tubular secretion of cephalosporins, resulting in higher serum concentrations.

Drug–Disease Interactions

All cephalosporins (except ceftriaxone) require dosage adjustments in patients with renal insufficiency.

Monitoring Parameters

Serum concentration monitoring is not necessary. Patients should be monitored for clinical response and resolution of infection.

Patient Instructions and Counseling

Verify that the patient is not allergic to penicillins. Traditional teaching principles have noted that cross-sensitivity with penicillins has been reported in up to 10% of patients receiving cephalosporins; however, recent evidence suggests that overall cross-reactivity may be much lower (around 1–2%) and even less likely with third- and fourth-generation cephalosporins (less than 1%). Obtain a thorough history of any patient with a previous allergic reaction to a β-lactam antibiotic. Cephalosporins should be avoided in patients with a severe hypersensitivity reaction (anaphylaxis) to penicillins.

34-6. Carbapenems

Carbapenems are β-lactam-like antibiotics that are structurally and pharmacologically similar to penicillins (Table 34-5). Currently, only IV dosage forms are available for carbapenems.

Mechanism of Action

Carbapenems bind to penicillin-binding proteins in a manner similar to that of other β-lactams, thereby inhibiting peptidoglycan synthesis. Carbapenems are bactericidal in susceptible isolates.

Spectrum of Activity

Carbapenems are very broad-spectrum antibiotics with activity against most Gram-positive and Gram-negative aerobes and anaerobes, as well as activity against some *Mycobacterium* spp. They are the drugs of choice for ESBL (extended spectrum β-lactamases)–producing *Enterobacteriaceae* species. Carbapenems other than ertapenem cover *Pseudomonas* and some *Acinetobacter* spp.

Adverse Drug Events

GI adverse effects are the most common events reported with imipenem. The effects include nausea, vomiting, diarrhea (including *C. difficile* enterocolitis), gastroenteritis, and abdominal pain.

Table 34-5. Carbapenems and Monobactam

Generic name	Trade name	Dosage forms	Dose	Elimination	Notes
Carbapenems					
Imipenem-cilastatin	Primaxin	IV, IM	250–1,000 mg q6–12h, depending on the severity of infection	Renal	
Doripenem	Doribax	IV	500 mg q8h	Renal	
Meropenem	Merrem	IV	500–2,000 mg q8h	Renal	
Ertapenem	Invanz	IV, IM	1,000 mg q24h	Renal	Not for *Pseudomonas*
Monobactam					
Aztreonam	Azactam	IV, IM	1–2 g q6–12h, depending on the severity of infection	Renal	Useful in anaphylactic β-lactam allergy

Eosinophilia, leukopenia, neutropenia, agranulocytosis, hemolytic anemia, and thrombocytopenia have been reported.

Seizures have been reported in approximately 0.4% of patients receiving imipenem. Carbapenems have the highest seizure-risk profile of the β-lactams, and imipenem likely poses the greatest risk of the carbapenem class. Risk factors include the following:

- History of seizures or head trauma
- High doses
- Renal dysfunction

Imipenem-Cilastatin

Imipenem is a semisynthetic carbapenem β-lactam antibiotic. Cilastatin prevents renal metabolism of imipenem by dehydropeptidase—an enzyme present on the brush border of the proximal renal tubule—thereby increasing the concentrations of the active drug and preventing production of a nephrotoxic metabolite. Cilastatin has no antibacterial activity.

Meropenem and Doripenem

These agents are similar to imipenem with the following differences:

- Slightly lower seizure risk
- No hydrolysis by dehydropeptidases

Ertapenem

Ertapenem is dosed once daily and does not cover *Pseudomonas* spp.

34-7. Monobactam

Monobactam antibiotics are cell wall–active antibiotics like the β-lactams, but slight structural differences make them weakly immunogenic, decreasing allergic cross-reactivity with penicillins and cephalosporins (Table 34-5).

Aztreonam

Aztreonam is the only monobactam antibiotic currently available.

Mechanism of action

Monobactams bind to penicillin-binding proteins in a manner similar to that of other β-lactams, thereby inhibiting peptidoglycan synthesis. Monobactams are bactericidal in susceptible isolates.

Spectrum of activity

Aztreonam is active against many aerobic Gram-negative bacteria, but is not active against any Gram-positive or anaerobic bacteria. Though some strains of *Pseudomonas* are susceptible, resistance is increasing.

Adverse drug events

- *Hypersensitivity:* Rash, injection site reactions, eosinophilia
- *GI effects:* Nausea, vomiting, diarrhea

34-8. Gram-Positive Antibiotics

Linezolid

Linezolid is a synthetic oxazolidinone antibiotic (Table 34-6).

Mechanism of action

Linezolid binds to the 23S site of the 50S ribosomal subunit that inhibits bacterial translation and thus protein synthesis.

Spectrum of activity

Linezolid is active against *Staphylococcus* spp., including MRSA; *Enterococcus faecalis* and *E. faecium* isolates, including vancomycin-resistant enterococci (VRE); and *Streptococcus* spp., including *S. pneumoniae*. Linezolid is primarily classified as a bacteriostatic antibiotic.

Adverse drug events

Hematologic effects, including myelosuppression (primarily as thrombocytopenia, but also anemia, leukopenia, pancytopenia), have been reported. Hematologic effects are more common when therapy exceeds 14 days and appear to be reversible on discontinuation of the agent. Neurotoxicity such as peripheral neuropathy and optic neuritis has been reported with prolonged use of linezolid.

Linezolid is a weak monoamine oxidase inhibitor (MAOI), and caution should be exercised in patients receiving other serotonergic agents (MAOIs, SSRIs [selective serotonin reuptake inhibitors], TCAs [tricyclic antidepressants], meperidine, triptans) or sympathomimetics (pseudoephedrine, norepinephrine, dopaminergic agents). Serotonin syndrome has been reported, primarily in patients receiving multiple agents with serotonergic activity.

Other

Linezolid is a bacteriostatic agent that achieves higher concentrations in tissue than in plasma. Clinical data recommend against its use in bacteremia because of increased mortality.

Quinupristin-Dalfopristin

Quinupristin-dalfopristin is a semisynthetic streptogramin antibiotic. The combination acts synergistically against Gram-positive bacteria.

Mechanism of action

Quinupristin inhibits late-phase protein synthesis, while dalfopristin inhibits early-phase protein synthesis through binding to the 50S subunit of bacterial RNA.

Spectrum of activity

Quinupristin-dalfopristin is bactericidal against staphylococci (including MRSA) and streptococci and bacteriostatic against *E. faecium*, including VRE. Quinupristin-dalfopristin is not active against *E. faecalis*.

Table 34-6. Gram-Positive Antibiotics

Generic name	Trade name	Dosage forms	Dose	Elimination	Notes
Linezolid	Zyvox	IV, po	600 mg q12h	Renal	Monoamine oxidase inhibitor; no adjustment for renal dysfunction
Quinupristin-dalfopristin	Synercid	IV	7.5 mg/kg q8h	Hepatic	Infusion reactions; no adjustment for renal dysfunction
Vancomycin	Vancocin	IV, po	15–20 mg/kg IV q12h; 125–500 mg po q6h	Renal	Adjust dose per serum concentrations. Give po only for *Clostridium difficile.*
Daptomycin	Cubicin	IV	4–6 mg/kg q24h	Renal	Monitor creatine phosphokinase weekly.
Telavancin	Vibativ	IV	10 mg/kg q24h	Renal	Adjust for renal function.

Adverse drug events

Tolerability and adverse effects often preclude the use of this agent. Thrombophlebitis and severe injection site reactions are common, and the drug should be administered through a central venous catheter only.

Hyperbilirubinemia has been reported in up to 25% of patients receiving the agent.

Arthralgias and myalgias are common, some requiring discontinuation of the agent.

Other

The U.S. Food and Drug Administration (FDA) has recently repealed the VRE treatment indication for quinupristin-dalfopristin, citing the inability to verify clinical benefit.

Daptomycin

Daptomycin is a cyclic lipopeptide antibiotic.

Mechanism of action

Daptomycin binds to bacterial cell membranes, causing rapid depolarization, which results in loss of membrane potential. The loss of membrane potential inhibits protein, deoxyribonucleic acid (DNA), and RNA synthesis, resulting in cell death.

Spectrum of activity

Daptomycin is bactericidal against the Gram-positive bacteria staphylococci (including MRSA), streptococci, and enterococci (including VRE).

Adverse drug events

Dermatologic reactions include injection site reaction, rash, and pruritis. Musculoskeletal effects include increased creatine phosphokinase (CPK), which can progress to rhabdomyolysis (weekly monitoring recommended). Increased caution and CPK monitoring should be performed with concomitant use of daptomycin and statin therapy. Rarely, pulmonary eosinophilia manifesting as eosinophilic pneumonia has been reported.

Other

Daptomycin is inactivated by the surfactant in the lung and cannot be used to treat pneumonia.

Glycopeptide Antibiotics

Mechanism of action

The glycopeptides vancomycin and telavancin exhibit bactericidal killing through inhibition of peptidoglycan synthesis polymerization and cross-linking, and thus cell wall synthesis. This binding occurs at a site different from that of the penicillins.

Vancomycin

Spectrum of activity

Vancomycin is active against most Gram-positive bacteria, such as staphylococci (including MRSA), streptococci, and enterococci. It is bactericidal and acts synergistically with aminoglycosides for Gram-positive pathogens. Vancomycin is active against *C. difficile* and can be used to treat *C. difficile* infection when administered in oral dosage form.

Adverse drug events

Nephrotoxicity is manifested by an increase in serum creatinine and BUN. The incidence of nephrotoxicity is controversial but appears to be higher with concomitant nephrotoxic agents, high trough concentrations, and higher total daily doses. Renal dysfunction is normally reversible on discontinuation of the agent but may be irreversible.

Ototoxicity is induced by eighth cranial nerve damage and has been reported to cause permanent hearing loss. Vancomycin rarely causes vestibular toxicity. The incidence of ototoxicity appears to be low in the absence of concomitant ototoxic agents.

Thrombophlebitis is common and requires frequent IV site rotation.

Histamine release, or "red-man syndrome," is a reaction most commonly associated with rapid IV infusion. Histamine reactions can be minimized by slow IV infusion, not to exceed 500 mg/30 min and through the use of antihistamines such as diphenhydramine (Benadryl).

Monitoring parameters

Vancomycin trough concentrations should be monitored, whereas monitoring of vancomycin peak concentrations is not routinely required.

Pharmacokinetics

Vancomycin is renally eliminated:

- $t_{1/2} = 6$ hours (normal renal function)
- $t_{1/2} = 7$–10 days (anephric patients)
- $V_d = 0.7$ L/kg (TBW)

- Dose = 15–20 mg/kg (TBW) (Loading dose of 25–30 mg/kg may be considered.)
- Interval = q8h to intermittent dosing (based on renal function and pharmacokinetic monitoring)
- Peak concentration = 20–40 mcg/mL
- Trough concentration = 10–20 mcg/mL for pathogens with an MIC of ≤ 1 mg/dL. For serious infections (bacteremia, endocarditis, osteomyelitis, meningitis, pneumonia), trough concentrations of 15–20 mcg/mL are recommended. Lower trough concentrations of 10–15 mcg/mL are reserved for skin and soft tissue infections. An alternative Gram-positive agent should be used with an MIC ≥ 2 mg/dL to vancomycin.

Telavancin

Telavancin is a bactericidal lipoglycopeptide antibiotic that inhibits cell wall synthesis. Telavancin is available only intravenously and is currently indicated for complicated skin and soft tissue infections.

Spectrum of activity

Telavancin is active against Gram-positive bacteria such as staphylococci (including MRSA), streptococci, and vancomycin-susceptible enterococci.

Telavancin is renally eliminated, and dose and interval may be adjusted for renal dysfunction. Clinical trials have shown that efficacy may decrease with increasing age or renal dysfunction. Currently, no drug monitoring is recommended or available for telavancin.

Adverse drug events

Injection site reactions are common, including pain, pruritis, erythema, and rigor.

Nephrotoxicity is reported more often with telavancin than with vancomycin.

Neurologic effects such as dizziness, headache, and insomnia are also common.

QT prolongation can occur.

34-9. Fluoroquinolones

Quinolones are broad-spectrum antibacterial agents (Table 34-7).

Mechanism of Action

Fluoroquinolones are bactericidal agents. The mechanism of action of these agents is inhibition of topoisomerase II (DNA gyrase) and topoisomerase IV, resulting in disruption of bacterial DNA replication.

Spectrum of Activity

Gram-negative activity is extensive, including *E. coli*, *Klebsiella*, *Proteus*, *Enterobacter*, *Citrobacter*, *Salmonella*, and *Shigella*, in addition to *Moraxella catarrhalis* and *H. influenzae*. Activity against *Pseudomonas aeruginosa* varies among individual agents.

Newer fluoroquinolones (levofloxacin, moxifloxacin) demonstrate superior Gram-positive coverage versus older agents (ciprofloxacin, ofloxacin). Fluoroquinolones have limited enterococcal activity and are not recommended for the treatment of invasive staphylococcal infections or MRSA.

Moxifloxacin has some anaerobic coverage and can be used as an alternative treatment for aspiration pneumonia.

All fluoroquinolones are highly active against *Legionella* and display atypical coverage.

Table 34-7. Fluoroquinolones

Generic name	Trade name	Dosage forms	Normal dose	Elimination	Notes
Ciprofloxacin	Cipro	IV	400 mg q8–12h	Renal	Drug has enhanced antipseudomonal activity versus other fluoroquinolones.
		po	250–750 mg q12h		
Levofloxacin	Levaquin	IV, po	250–750 mg q24h	Renal	Drug covers pneumococcus and *Pseudomonas*.
Moxifloxacin	Avelox	IV, po	400 mg q24h	Hepatic	Drug does not cover *Pseudomonas* or urinary tract infection.
Ofloxacin	Floxin	po, otic, ophthalmic	100–400 mg q24h	Renal	

Adverse Drug Events

- *GI effects:* Nausea and dyspepsia
- *CNS effects:* Peripheral neuropathy, headache, dizziness, and insomnia
- *Cardiovascular effects:* QT prolongation (moxifloxacin > levofloxacin and ciprofloxacin). Avoid use in patients with preexisting QT prolongation.
- *Endocrine effects:* Hypoglycemia or hyperglycemia (reason for FDA withdrawal of gatifloxacin)
- *Other effects:* Tendinitis and tendon rupture (highest risk patients > 60 years of age, concomitant use of corticosteroids, transplant patients)
- *Rare effects:* Rash, urticaria, leukopenia, and hepatotoxicity (reason for FDA withdrawal of trovafloxacin)

Drug–Drug Interactions

Ciprofloxacin increases theophylline levels. Concomitant use should be avoided, or theophylline levels should be monitored during treatment. The risk of theophylline toxicity is lower with other fluoroquinolones.

Antacids, sucralfate, and divalent or trivalent cations (calcium, magnesium, iron) significantly decrease the absorption of fluoroquinolones. These agents should not be administered for at least 2 hours after each dose of a fluoroquinolone.

Fluoroquinolones may enhance the effects of oral anticoagulants. Monitor prothrombin time (PT) and international normalized ratio (INR) if concomitant therapy cannot be avoided.

Concomitant use of fluoroquinolones with agents that prolong the QT interval, particularly moxifloxacin, should be avoided when possible.

Drug–Disease Interactions

Dosage adjustments should be made for renally cleared fluoroquinolones based on specified CrCl except for moxifloxacin. Avoid use in myasthenia gravis.

Monitoring Parameters

Serum concentrations are not monitored. The patient should be monitored for clinical response and resolution of infection.

Patient Instructions and Counseling

- Fluoroquinolones should be avoided in children or pregnant or nursing females because of the risk of cartilage erosion in tendons and growing bone tissue.
- Do *not* take antacids; multivitamins; or other calcium, magnesium, or iron supplements for at least 2 hours after each dose.

34-10. Macrolides

Mechanism of Action

Macrolides (and ketolides) are bacteriostatic against susceptible organisms (Table 34-8). The agents bind to the 50S ribosomal subunit, thereby inhibiting RNA synthesis.

Table 34-8. Macrolides and Ketolides

Generic name	Trade name	Dosage forms	Normal dose	Elimination	Notes
Macrolides					
Azithromycin	Zithromax	po, IV	500–1,000 mg once, then 250 mg q24h, or 500 mg q24h	Hepatic	po dose = IV dose; no adjustment for renal dysfunction
Clarithromycin	Biaxin, Biaxin XL	po	250–500 mg bid or 500 mg–1 g XL q24h	Renal	XL = daily dosing
Erythromycin	Various	po	250–500 mg q6h	Hepatic	Erythromycin base, ethyl succinate, and stearate
		IV	500–1,000 mg q6h	Hepatic	Erythromycin lactobionate
Ketolides					
Telithromycin	Ketek	po	800 mg q24h	Hepatic	Use is limited because of severe hepatotoxicity reported. FDA withdrew all indications other than mild- to moderate-community-acquired pneumonia.

Spectrum of Activity

Macrolides are active against some Gram-positive organisms, including penicillin-resistant streptococci. The macrolides are also effective against *Chlamydia, Mycoplasma, Ureaplasma,* spirochetes, and mycobacteria.

Macrolides are the drugs of choice in atypical pneumonia and *Chlamydia* sexually transmitted diseases. Erythromycin is sometimes used to accelerate gastric emptying because of its stimulation of GI motility.

Adverse Drug Events

- *GI effects:* Erythromycin stimulates GI motility, leading to abdominal pain and cramping, nausea, vomiting, and diarrhea. Clarithromycin appears to be the least stimulating to the GI tract.
- *Local effects:* Erythromycin lactobionate causes venous irritation and thrombophlebitis. The agent should be diluted in at least 250 mL and infused over 30–60 minutes to decrease the venous irritation. It is not commonly used in this dosage form because of these factors.
- *Cardiac effects:* QT interval prolongation and arrhythmias have been reported. The risk of arrhythmia is highest in patients with known QT prolongation, hypokalemia, hypomagnesemia, bradycardia, and concomitant use of other antiarrhythmic agents.
- *Hepatotoxicity:* Telithromycin carries a black box warning for severe hepatotoxicity.

34-11. Tetracyclines and Glycylcyclines

Mechanism of Action

Tetracyclines and glycylcyclines are bacteriostatic. They inhibit bacterial protein synthesis by reversible binding on the 30S ribosomal subunit (Table 34-9).

Glycylcyclines (tigecycline) share the same mechanism of action as tetracyclines but have a structural modification that increases affinity and binding to the bacterial ribosome and decreases efflux from the cell.

Spectrum of Activity

Tetracyclines are used to treat the following infections:

- *Respiratory infections:* Atypical pneumonia (*Mycoplasma, Chlamydia, Legionella* spp.)
- *Genital infections:* *Chlamydia trachomatis*
- *Systemic infections:* Relapsing fever (*Borrelia* spp., including Lyme disease; *Rickettsia* spp., including Rocky Mountain spotted fever; *Vibrio* spp., including cholera)
- *Other infections:* *Pasteurella multocida, Yersinia pestis (plague),* and *Helicobacter pylori* (in combination with bismuth subsalicylate and metronidazole or clarithromycin)
- *Prophylaxis:* Mefloquine-resistant *Plasmodium falciparum* malaria

Table 34-9. Tetracyclines and Glycylcyclines

Generic name	Trade name	Dosage forms	Common doses	Primary mode of elimination
Tetracyclines				
Doxycycline	Vibramycin and others	po, IV	100 mg q12h	Renal
Minocycline	Minocin	po, IV	100–200 mg q12h	Hepatic
Tetracycline	Achromycin V, Sumycin, Tetracyn, and others	po, IV, IM	1–2 g daily	Renal
Glycylcyclines				
Tigecycline	Tygacil	IV	100 mg once, then 50 mg IV q12h	Hepatic

Doxycycline is used to treat infections caused by the following organisms:

- *Streptococcus pneumoniae* and community-acquired MRSA strains
- Adjunct therapy for nontubercular mycobacteria infections

Tetracyclines, particularly minocycline, are used in the treatment of acne (*Propionibacterium acnes*).

Tigecycline has enhanced broad-spectrum coverage including MRSA, VRE, and anaerobic coverage including *B. fragilis*. It does not cover *Pseudomonas* or *Proteus* spp. Tigecycline should not be used in bacteremia or hospital-acquired pneumonia because of increased mortality.

Patient Instructions and Counseling

Administering the drug with food can minimize GI distress.

Adverse Drug Events

Photosensitivity reactions can occur but may be less frequent with doxycycline and minocycline. Gastrointestinal intolerance includes diarrhea, nausea, vomiting, and anorexia. Tigecycline is associated with an abnormally high incidence of GI intolerance.

Tetracyclines and glycylcyclines are generally contraindicated during pregnancy and breast-feeding and in children younger than age 8 because of their association with tooth discoloration and interference with bone growth. Fanconi syndrome (kidney tubular dysfunction) can occur with outdated doxycycline.

Hepatotoxicity—specifically, acute fatty necrosis—may occur in pregnant women and in patients with renal impairment.

IV tetracyclines may cause phlebitis.

Drug–Drug and Drug–Disease Interactions

Milk, antacids, iron supplements, and probably other substances with calcium, magnesium, aluminum, and iron decrease tetracycline GI absorption considerably and should be ingested at least several hours before or after administration of tetracycline.

Anticonvulsants (e.g., barbiturates, carbamazepine, phenytoin) induce hepatic microsomal metabolism of tetracyclines and therefore decrease tetracycline serum concentrations.

Oral contraceptive efficacy may be decreased with concurrent use of tetracyclines.

Tetracyclines and glycylcyclines may potentiate warfarin-induced anticoagulation; therefore, monitor PT and INR.

Other

Tetracycline and glycylcycline doses do not have to be adjusted for renal dysfunction.

34-12. Sulfonamides

Sulfonamides are synthetic derivatives of sulfanilamide (Table 34-10).

Mechanism of Action

Sulfonamides interfere with bacterial folic acid synthesis by competitively inhibiting para aminobenzoic acid (PABA) utilization. Sulfonamides are bacteriostatic.

Spectrum of Activity

- *Gram-positive bacteria:* Staphylococci (MSSA, community-acquired MRSA strains), streptococci

Table 34-10. Sulfonamides

Generic name	Trade name	Dosage forms	Dose	Elimination	Notes
Sulfadiazine		IV, po	2–4 g daily	Renal	Used to treat toxoplasmosis in combination with pyrimethamine
Sulfamethoxazole (in combined dosage form)	Bactrim, Septra	IV, po	1–3 g daily	Renal	Combined with trimethoprim in dosage form (Bactrim, Septra)

(not enterococci), *Bacillus anthracis, Clostridium perfringens, Nocardia* spp.

- *Gram-negative bacteria: E. coli, Klebsiella, Proteus, Enterobacter, Salmonella, Shigella*
- *Other organisms: Toxoplasma gondii, Plasmodium* spp.

Adverse Drug Events

Hypersensitivity reactions appear to be cross-reactive with other sulfonamides, diuretics (including acetazolamide and thiazides), and sulfonylureas.

Dermatologic reactions include rash, urticaria, and Stevens–Johnson syndrome.

Hyperkalemia is common in trimethoprim-containing formulations (Bactrim, Septra)

34-13. Miscellaneous Antibiotics

Clindamycin

Clindamycin is a semisynthetic antibiotic derived from lincomycin (Table 34-11).

Mechanism of action

Clindamycin inhibits the 50S ribosomal subunit, thereby inhibiting RNA synthesis. Clindamycin is primarily bacteriostatic in nature.

Spectrum of activity

Clindamycin is active against aerobic Gram-positive, anaerobic Gram-positive, and some anaerobic Gram-negative bacteria. Clindamycin exhibits coverage against community-acquired MRSA strains. It has no activity against aerobic Gram-negative bacteria.

Adverse drug events

Adverse GI effects occur frequently with all forms of clindamycin, and include nausea, vomiting, diarrhea, and abdominal pain. Clindamycin has induced *C. difficile* enterocolitis because it does not cover this organism.

IV administration can lead to thrombophlebitis, erythema, and pain and swelling at the IV site. IM administration can cause pain, induration, and sterile abscesses.

Clindamycin can cause transient leukopenia, neutropenia, eosinophilia, thrombocytopenia, and agranulocytosis. These effects are usually reversible on discontinuation of the drug.

Metronidazole

Metronidazole is a nitroimidazole antibiotic that is active against anaerobic Gram-negative and Gram-positive bacteria as well as protozoa.

Table 34-11. Miscellaneous Antibiotics

Generic name	Trade name	Dosage forms	Dose	Elimination	Notes
Clindamycin	Cleocin	IV, po	600–900 mg IV q8h; 300–600 mg q6h po	Hepatic	May predispose patient to *Clostridium difficile*; no renal dose adjustment
Metronidazole	Flagyl	IV, po	250–1,000 mg tid–qid	Hepatic	Disulfiram reaction; warfarin interaction; no renal dose adjustment
Chloramphenicol	Chloromycetin	IV	12.5–25 mg/kg q6h	Hepatic	Blood dyscrasias; gray baby syndrome
Colistimethate	Coly-Mycin M	IM, IV	2.5–5 mg/kg daily divided q8–12h	Renal	Dose based on IBW and adjusted for renal function
Polymyxin B		IM, IV	15,000–25,000 units/kg daily divided q12h for IV	Renal	1 mg = 10,000 units; dose adjusted for renal function
Rifaximin	Xifaxan	po	200–400 mg tid	Fecal	For GI local use only
Fidaxomicin	Dificid	po	200 mg bid	Fecal	For *C. difficile*

Mechanism of action

Metronidazole is a pro-drug that requires metabolism by susceptible organisms for activation. Metronidazole inhibits DNA synthesis, although the complete mechanism of action is unknown.

Spectrum of activity

Metronidazole is active against many anaerobic bacteria, including being a drug of choice for *B. fragilis*. Metronidazole is also active against *Clostridium* spp., *H. pylori, Fusobacterium, Peptococcus, Peptostreptococcus,* and *Eubacterium* spp. Metronidazole is effective in the treatment of *C. difficile* infection. It is inactive against aerobic bacteria and some facultative anaerobes.

Metronidazole is active against a variety of protozoa, including *Trichomonas vaginalis, Entamoeba histolytica,* and *Giardia lamblia.*

Adverse drug events

- *GI effects:* Nausea, abdominal discomfort, taste disturbances, vomiting
- *Neurologic:* Dizziness, headache, paresthesias, peripheral neuropathy
- *Renal effect:* Dark or discolored urine, dysuria

Drug interactions

Metronidazole inhibits drug metabolism through the cytochrome P450 (CYP450) system and increases the drug level or effect of warfarin, cyclosporine, carbamazepine, ergot derivatives, fluorouracil, phenytoin, and tacrolimus. Metronidazole also produces a disulfiram-like reaction; therefore, alcohol should be avoided for at least 3 days before and after use.

Chloramphenicol

Chloramphenicol is a broad-spectrum antibiotic with life-threatening side effects; therefore, it should only be used when no safe alternative exists.

Mechanism of action

Chloramphenicol binds reversibly to the 50S ribosomal subunit, thereby inhibiting protein synthesis. Chloramphenicol is primarily bacteriostatic.

Spectrum of activity

Chloramphenicol is active against atypical pathogens and many Gram-negative and Gram-positive pathogens, including *M. catarrhalis, H. influenzae, S. pneumoniae, Streptococcus pyogenes, Neisseria gonorrhea,* and *N. meningitidis.* The broad spectrum of activity and CNS penetration of chloramphenicol make it an alternative to ceftriaxone for the treatment of meningitis in patients with life-threatening β-lactam allergy.

Adverse drug events

Chloramphenicol causes severe blood dyscrasias, and this toxicity significantly limits its use. Many of the toxicities are caused by inhibition of mammalian protein synthesis.

Black box warning: Chloramphenicol can cause life-threatening blood dyscrasias (aplastic anemia, thrombocytopenia, neutropenia)

Gray syndrome (gray baby syndrome): A fatal syndrome leading to cardiopulmonary collapse is most commonly seen in neonates that receive high doses within the first 2 days of life but has been reported in older infants or adults in overdose.

Drug interactions

Chloramphenicol is hepatically metabolized and inhibits the metabolism of cyclosporine, phenytoin, phenobarbital, tacrolimus, voriconazole, and warfarin, leading to increased concentrations and toxicity.

Drug–lab interaction: Chloramphenicol causes a false-positive urine glucose measurement.

Polymyxins

The polymyxins, polymyxin B and colistin (polymyxin E, in colistimethate dosage form), display Gram-negative spectrum with dose-limiting side effects; therefore, they should be used only when no safe alternative exists. They have reemerged in clinical practice because of an increase in multidrug-resistant *Acinetobacter* and *Pseudomonas* spp.

Mechanism of action

The polymyxins are bactericidal agents that act as anionic detergents that damage the external cell membrane of Gram-negative bacteria causing cell death.

Spectrum of activity

Polymyxins are active against many aerobic Gram-negative bacilli, including *P. aeruginosa*, *Acinetobacter*, *E. coli*, *Klebsiella*, *Enterobacter*, *Citrobacter*, and *Stenotrophomonas maltophilia*. Polymyxins are generally inactive against Gram-positive and anaerobic bacteria. Polymyxins have synergistic effect when combined with other antibiotics, most commonly β-lactams.

Adverse drug events

Nephrotoxicity and neurotoxicity are the dose-limiting side effects of the polymyxins. These toxicities limit their use:

- **Renal:** Significant incidence of renal failure (more with colistin), electrolyte abnormalities (hypocalcemia, hyponatremia, hypokalemia)
- **Neurologic:** Ataxia, dizziness, headache, myasthenia crisis, neuromuscular blockade, neurotoxicity, paresthesias, peripheral neuropathy, slurred speech, vertigo
- **Dermatologic:** Rash, urticaria, pruritis
- **Immunologic:** Anaphylaxis, fever

Drug interactions

The polymyxins have additive neurotoxic effects with neuromuscular blocking agents and aminoglycosides. They have additive nephrotoxic effects with other nephrotoxins.

Rifaximin

Rifaximin is an oral rifamycin that is not absorbed systemically and is used for enteric infections in the GI tract. Rifaximin is used for traveler's diarrhea caused by *E. coli* and for prophylaxis of hepatic encephalopathy.

Mechanism of action

Rifaximin inhibits the β-subunit of DNA-dependent RNA-polymerase, thereby inhibiting RNA synthesis.

Spectrum of activity

Rifaximin is active against Gram-negative enteric organisms and was predominantly tested against *E. coli*. As with other rifamycins, resistance to monotherapy may develop rapidly, and resistant flora was reported after 5 days of treatment in clinical trials.

Adverse drug events

Peripheral edema, nausea, dizziness, fatigue, ascites, flatulence, and headache are the most common adverse events.

Drug interactions

Currently, no drug interactions have been identified.

Fidaxomicin

Fidaxomicin is a nonabsorbable oral macrolide antibiotic used in the treatment of *C. difficile* infection.

Mechanism of action

Fidaxomicin inhibits bacterial RNA polymerases.

Spectrum of activity

Fidaxomicin is active in vitro against *Clostridium* species and has been shown clinically effective in the treatment of *C. difficile* infection.

Adverse drug events

GI events such as nausea, vomiting, pain, and bleeding are the most commonly reported side effects. Dermatologic, endocrine, and hematologic side effects have been reported, but their occurrence is less than 2%.

Drug interactions

Currently, no drug interactions have been identified.

Other

Some data suggest that *C. difficile* infection recurrence rates may be lower when fidaxomicin is used to treat nonvirulent *C. difficile* strains in comparison with metronidazole and vancomycin.

34-14. Antifungal Agents

Amphotericin B

Amphotericin B is a polyene antifungal agent used in the treatment of potentially life-threatening systemic fungal infections (Table 34-12).

Table 34-12. Antifungal Agents

Generic name	Trade name	Dosage forms	Dose	Elimination	Notes
Amphotericin B	Fungizone	IV	0.5–1 mg/kg q24h	Unknown	Dose should not exceed 1.5 mg/kg daily.
Amphotericin B (liposomal, lipid, cholesterol complex)	AmBisome, Abelcet, Amphotec	IV	3–7 mg/kg q24h	Unknown	Drug is 20–30% less nephrotoxic than conventional amphotericin B.
Caspofungin	Cancidas	IV	70 mg once and then 50 mg q24h	Hepatic	Dose adjustment is made for patients with severe hepatic dysfunction.
Micafungin	Mycamine	IV	100 mg q24h	Hepatic	
Anidulafungin	Eraxis	IV	200 mg once and then 100 mg q24h	Chemical degradation	
Fluconazole	Diflucan	IV, po	100–800 mg q24h	Renal	
Flucytosine	Ancobon	po	50–150 mg/kg daily	Renal	
Griseofulvin	Fulvicin P/G	po	500–1,000 mg daily	Hepatic	
Itraconazole	Sporanox	po	200–600 mg daily	Hepatic	Capsules require acidic environment, so solution should be taken on an empty stomach.
Ketoconazole	Nizoral	po, topical	200–400 mg bid	Hepatic	Drug requires acidic environment for dissolution and absorption.
Nystatin	Mycostatin	Topical	100,000–1,000,000 units daily to qid	Fecal	Dose, schedule, and route of administration differ by indication.
Terbinafine	Lamisil	po	250 mg daily	Hepatic	Pulse therapy is also effective.
Voriconazole	Vfend	IV, po	6 mg/kg q12h × 2 doses then 4 mg/kg IV 12h; 200 mg po q12h	Hepatic	Maximum oral dose is 800 mg per day to limit hepatotoxicity. Do *not* use IV formulation with CrCl < 50 mL/min.
Posaconazole	Noxafil	po	200–400 mg bid–qid	Hepatic	Best absorption is with high caloric, high fat meal or acidic environment.

Amphotericin B lipid formulations

Amphotericin B cholesterol sulfate complex (Amphotec), amphotericin B lipid complex (Abelcet), and amphotericin B liposomal (AmBisome) formulations are available for the treatment of severe fungal infections in patients who fail or are intolerant of conventional amphotericin B. The lipid formulations may decrease toxicity by 20–30%.

Mechanism of action

Amphotericin B is a broad-spectrum antifungal agent that binds to ergosterol in the fungal cell wall, leading to increased permeability and cell death. Amphotericin B is primarily fungicidal in nature.

Spectrum of activity

- *Aspergillus, Cryptococcus, Histoplasma, Blastomyces, Coccidioides,* and *Zygomycetes* spp.
- *Candida,* including *C. albicans, C. dubliniensis, C. glabrata, C. krusei, C. parapsilosis,* and *C. tropicalis* (*C. lusitaniae* exhibits variable sensitivity)

Adverse drug events

- ***Infusion reactions:*** Reactions can be severe to life threatening. Fever, chills, hypotension, rigors, pain, thrombophlebitis, and anaphylaxis can occur.
- ***Renal and electrolyte effects:*** Nephrotoxicity is the major dose-limiting toxicity, but significant

hypokalemia, hypocalcemia, and hypomagnesemia can occur and electrolytes should be supplemented and replaced. Lipid formulations have lower nephrotoxicity.

- *Hematologic effects:* Normocytic and normochromic anemia secondary to decreased erythropoietin production may occur.

Echinocandins

Echinocandins (caspofungin, micafungin, anidulafungin) are a class of IV antifungal agents with enhanced *Candida* spp. coverage.

Mechanism of action

Echinocandins inhibit β-(1,3) glucan synthase, thereby preventing fungi from forming an essential component of their cell wall. This loss of cell wall integrity results in cell lysis and death.

Spectrum of activity

Echinocandins are drugs of choice for most non–*Candida albicans* spp., including *C. glabrata* and *C. krusei. Candida parapsilosis* and *C. guilliermondii* have increased MICs to echinocandins, which may result in an inadequate response to treatment. Echinocandins have activity against *Aspergillus* species, but they lack activity against other molds.

Caspofungin, Micafungin, and Anidulafungin

The echinocandins are approved for the treatment of invasive *Candida* infections. They are sometimes used for treatment of aspergillosis in patients refractory to or intolerant of other therapies. Echinocandins do not require dose adjustment for renal dysfunction; however, caspofungin should be dose adjusted in severe hepatic impairment. They are generally well-tolerated agents with a mild side effect profile.

Adverse drug events

- *Hepatic effects:* Increased aspartate aminotransferase (AST) and alanine aminotransferase (ALT)
- *Sensitivity reactions:* Histamine-release reactions such as rash, pruritus, and anaphylaxis
- *Infusion reactions:* Fever, thrombophlebitis, nausea, and vomiting

Azole Antifungals

Mechanism of action

The azole antifungals appear to inhibit fungal CYP450 14-α-demethylase, thereby decreasing ergosterol concentrations in susceptible fungi.

Drug interactions

All azole antifungals are inhibitors of the CYP450 system and have many critical drug interactions attributable to decreased metabolism and, thus, toxicity.

The azole antifungals have also been shown to prolong the QT interval; thus, co-administration with other drugs that prolong the QT interval is not advised.

Fluconazole

Fluconazole is a synthetic triazole antifungal and is fungistatic.

Spectrum of activity

Fluconazole is the drug of choice for *C. albicans* infection. *Candida krusei* is inherently resistant, and *C. glabrata* most commonly displays dose-dependent susceptibility or resistance. Fluconazole also displays activity against *Cryptococcus* spp. and *Coccidioides* spp.

Adverse drug events

- *GI effects:* Nausea, vomiting, abdominal pain, and diarrhea
- *Hepatic effects:* Cholestasis and increased AST, ALT, and gamma-glutamyl transpeptidase (GGTP); hepatic necrosis; and, rarely, severe hepatic dysfunction
- *Hemolytic effects:* Eosinophilia, anemia, leukopenia, neutropenia, and thrombocytopenia

Itraconazole

Itraconazole is a synthetic triazole antifungal.

Spectrum of activity

Itraconazole is clinically used mostly for the treatment of *Histoplasma* spp. (histoplasmosis) and *Blastomyces* (blastomycosis). It also has activity against *Candida, Aspergillus,* and some *Cryptococcus* spp.

Adverse drug events

- **GI effects:** Nausea, vomiting, diarrhea, abdominal pain, dyspepsia, gastritis
- **Dermatologic and sensitivity reactions:** Rash, pruritus, urticaria, angioedema, Stevens–Johnson syndrome
- **Nervous system effects:** Headache, dizziness, tremor, neuropathy
- **Cardiovascular effects:** Congestive heart failure, peripheral edema, pulmonary edema, prolonged QT interval, ventricular dysrhythmias
- **Hepatic effects:** Increased AST and ALT
- **Electrolyte and metabolic effects:** Hypokalemia, adrenal insufficiency, gynecomastia

Patient instructions and counseling

- Capsules should be taken with food or acidic beverages to facilitate absorption.
- Oral solution should be taken on an empty stomach to help increase absorption.

Ketoconazole

Ketoconazole is a synthetic imidazole antifungal. It is no longer recommended for systemic use because of significant hepatotoxicity and adrenal insufficiency observed.

Spectrum of activity

Systemic ketoconazole activity includes candidiasis, blastomycosis, coccidioidomycosis, and histoplasmosis. Because of toxicity, it is currently used for tinea infections (dermatophytes) and for local treatment (cream, shampoo) of dermal fungal infections.

Voriconazole

Voriconazole is a synthetic triazole antifungal.

Spectrum of activity

Voriconazole is a drug of choice for aspergillosis. It displays coverage of non–*C. albicans* species as well as activity against *Histoplasma* and *Blastomyces* spp.

Adverse drug events

- Hepatic effects such as hepatitis, cholestasis, and fulminant hepatic failure (mostly with the oral formulation at high doses)
- Visual disturbances and hallucinations
- Dermatologic and sensitivity reactions, including anaphylactoid reactions, pruritus, rash, Stevens–Johnson syndrome, and photosensitivity

Other

- IV formulation should be avoided in patients with a CrCl < 50mL/min because of accumulation of the potentially toxic cyclodextrin vehicle component

Posaconazole

Posaconazole is a synthetic triazole antifungal.

Spectrum of activity

Posaconazole is primarily used for prophylaxis of invasive fungal infection in immunocompromised patients because of its coverage of *Aspergillus* and *Candida* spp. It can also be used for treatment of esophageal candidiasis. It has a broad in vitro spectrum of activity and has been effective against rare fungi such as *Zygomycetes* spp.

Adverse drug events

- **GI effects:** Nausea, vomiting, diarrhea, abdominal pain
- **Dermatologic and sensitivity reactions:** Rash, pruritus
- **Nervous system effects:** Headache, dizziness, confusion
- **Cardiovascular effects:** Hypertension, hypotension, edema, prolonged QT interval, ventricular dysrhythmias
- **Hepatic effects:** Cholestasis, increased AST and ALT

Patient instructions and counseling

Posaconazole should be taken with food (ideally high fat, caloric content) or acidic beverages to facilitate absorption. Proton pump inhibitors should be avoided because they can significantly reduce posaconazole absorption.

Flucytosine
Mechanism of action

Flucytosine enters fungal cells and is converted to 5-fluorouracil, causing cell death.

Spectrum of activity

Flucytosine is active against most strains of *Cryptococcus* and *Candida*. It is commonly combined with amphotericin B for the treatment of cryptococcal meningitis.

Adverse drug events

- *GI effects:* GI hemorrhage, ulcerative colitis caused by the antiproliferative effects, anorexia, abdominal pain, nausea, vomiting, diarrhea
- *Renal effects:* Increased serum creatinine, BUN, and crystalluria; use caution in renal impairment
- *Nervous system effects:* Confusion, hallucinations, psychosis, headache, parkinsonism, paresthesias, peripheral neuropathy, hearing loss, vertigo
- *Sensitivity reactions:* Erythema, pruritus, urticaria, rash, toxic epidermal necrolysis

Griseofulvin

Mechanism of action

Griseofulvin disrupts the fungal cell's mitotic spindle structure, thereby inhibiting the metaphase of cell division. Griseofulvin is fungistatic and should be used only for noninvasive dermatophyte infection.

Spectrum of activity

The spectrum of activity includes *Trichophyton, Microsporum,* and *Epidermophyton* (dermatomycoses). Griseofulvin does not have any *Candida* spp. activity and has been largely replaced by other antifungals for dermatophyte infections.

Adverse drug events

- *Nervous system effects:* Headache, fatigue, dizziness, paresthesias of the hands and feet after prolonged therapy
- *GI effects:* Epigastric pain, nausea, vomiting, flatulence, diarrhea
- *Renal effects:* Proteinuria, nephrosis
- *Sensitivity reactions:* Rash, urticaria, erythema multiforme, angioedema, serum sickness, photosensitivity, lupus-like reactions

Nystatin

Mechanism of action

Nystatin binds to fungal sterols. It is fungistatic.

Spectrum of activity

The spectrum of activity includes cutaneous and mucocutaneous candidiasis.

Adverse drug events

Mild nausea and diarrhea may occur.

Terbinafine

Terbinafine is a synthetic allylamine antifungal.

Mechanism of action

Terbinafine interferes with sterol biosynthesis.

Spectrum of activity

The spectrum of activity includes *Trichophyton, Microsporum, Epidermophyton,* and yeasts. Terbinafine is primarily used systemically for the treatment of onychomycosis and locally for various types of tinea infections (dermatophytes).

Adverse drug events

- *Hepatic effects:* Hepatitis, hepatic failure
- *Dermatologic and sensitivity reactions:* Anaphylactic reactions, Stevens–Johnson syndrome, erythema multiforme

34-15. Antitubercular Agents

First-Line Agents (RIPE Therapy)

For active tuberculosis (TB) infection, rifampin, isoniazid, pyrazinamide, and ethambutol (RIPE) are usually initiated for an 8-week period, then rifampin and isoniazid are continued for an additional 18 weeks (26 weeks total therapy). Various alternative regimens have been described.

Rifampin

Mechanism of action
Rifampin inhibits RNA synthesis in susceptible isolates.

Spectrum of activity
Rifampin is active against the following *Mycobacterium* species: *M. tuberculosis, M. bovis, M. kansasii,*

and some *M. avium* isolates. Rifampin also has activity against many Gram-positive and Gram-negative organisms.

Adverse drug events
- **GI effects:** Nausea, vomiting, diarrhea, and abdominal pain may require discontinuation of the agent.
- **CNS effects:** Headache, dizziness, mental confusion, and psychosis have been reported.
- **Hepatic effects:** Increased bilirubin, AST, and ALT are common; fulminant hepatotoxicity has been reported.

Patient instructions and counseling
Rifampin can cause the discoloration of body fluids such as tears, sweat, and saliva.

Other
Rifampin is a potent inducer of CYP450 enzymes.

Isoniazid

Mechanism of action
Isoniazid (INH) appears to inhibit the bacterial cell wall of susceptible isolates and, therefore, is active against actively dividing cells only.

Spectrum of activity
INH is active against the following *Mycobacterium* species: *M. tuberculosis*, *M. bovis*, and some strains of *M. kansasii*.

Adverse drug events
- **CNS effects:** Peripheral neuropathy and rarely seizures, encephalopathy, and psychosis have been reported.
- **Hepatic effects:** Increases in bilirubin, AST, and ALT are noted in up to 20% of patients receiving this agent. INH has led to fulminant hepatitis and death.
- **Hematologic effects:** Agranulocytosis, eosinophilia, thrombocytopenia, and hemolytic anemia have been reported.

Other
- INH is the drug of choice for latent TB infection (monotherapy treatment for 9 months).
- Supplement with pyridoxine (25mg daily) to decrease chances of neuropathy.
- Concomitant use with alcohol will increase risk of liver damage.

Pyrazinamide

Mechanism of action
Mycobacterium tuberculosis converts pyrazinamide (PZA) to pyrazinoic acid, which possesses antitubercular activity.

Spectrum of activity
PZA is active against *M. tuberculosis* only.

Adverse drug events
- **Hepatic effects:** Increased liver enzymes are common, and fulminant hepatitis has been reported.
- **Pain and gout:** PZA inhibits renal excretion of uric acid and may induce or worsen gout. PZA can cause polyarthralgia.

Ethambutol

Mechanism of action
Ethambutol appears to inhibit bacterial cellular metabolism and is bacteriostatic.

Spectrum of activity
Ethambutol is active against the following *Mycobacterium* species: *M. tuberculosis*, *M. bovis*, and some isolates of *M. kansasii* and *M. avium*.

Adverse drug events
Ocular effects may occur. Optic neuritis with decreased visual acuity, central and peripheral scotomas, and loss of red–green color discrimination have been noted. Peripheral neuropathy is also a common adverse effect.

Second-Line Agents

Aminosalicylic Acid

Mechanism of action
Aminosalicylic acid (para aminosalicylate, or PAS) inhibits folic acid synthesis in a manner similar to that of sulfonamides and is bacteriostatic (Table 34-13).

Spectrum of activity
Aminosalicylic acid is active against *M. tuberculosis* only.

Table 34-13. Antitubercular Agents

Generic name	Trade name	Dosage forms	Normal dose	Elimination	Notes
First-line agents					
Rifampin	Various	po, IV	10–20 mg/kg daily	Hepatic	Maximum dose: 900 mg daily
Isoniazid	Various	po	5–10 mg/kg daily	Hepatic	Maximum dose: 300 mg daily
Pyrazinamide	Various	po	15–30 mg/kg daily	Hepatic	Maximum dose: 2 g daily
Ethambutol	Myambutol	po	15–25 mg/kg daily	Hepatic	
Second-line agents					
Aminosalicylic acid	Paser	po	150 mg/kg daily	Renal	Maximum dose: 12 g daily
Capreomycin	Capastat	IM	15 mg/kg daily	Renal	Maximum dose: 1 g daily
Cycloserine	Seromycin	po	15–20 mg/kg daily	Renal	Maximum dose: 1 g daily
Ethionamide	Trecator-SC	po	500–1,000 mg daily	Hepatic	

Adverse drug events
- **GI effects:** Severe nausea, vomiting, abdominal pain, diarrhea, and anorexia can occur.
- **Vitamin and mineral absorption:** Vitamin B_{12}, folic acid, and iron malabsorption are possible.
- **Hypersensitivity reactions:** Fever, skin eruptions, joint pain, and leukopenia can occur.
- **Endocrine effects:** Hypothyroidism; check thyroid function tests

Capreomycin

Mechanism of action
The exact mechanism of action of capreomycin is unknown. The agent is bacteriostatic against susceptible isolates.

Spectrum of activity
Capreomycin is active against the following *Mycobacterium* species: *M. tuberculosis*, *M. bovis*, *M. kansasii*, and *M. avium*.

Adverse drug events
- **Renal effects:** Nephrotoxicity is exhibited in up to 30% of patients receiving the agent. It manifests as reversible acute tubular necrosis.
- **Ototoxicity:** This problem is experienced by up to 30% of patients and is caused by eighth cranial nerve damage, which can produce irreversible hearing loss.

Other
- Avoid use in pregnancy.

Cycloserine

Mechanism of action
Cycloserine is structurally similar to D-alanine and inhibits cell wall synthesis by competing for incorporation into the bacterial cell wall.

Spectrum of activity
Cycloserine is active against the following *Mycobacterium* species: *M. tuberculosis*, *M. bovis*, *M. avium*, and some *M. kansasii* isolates.

Adverse drug events
CNS effects may occur, including headache, vertigo, confusion, psychosis, and seizures.

Other
- Use with high-dose pyridoxine to help prevent neurotoxicity and seizures.

Ethionamide

Mechanism of action
Ethionamide appears to inhibit cell wall synthesis by an unidentified mechanism. It is bactericidal or bacteriostatic, depending on tissue concentrations of the agent.

Spectrum of activity
Ethionamide is active against the following *Mycobacterium* species: *M. tuberculosis*, *M. bovis*, *M. kansasii*, and some *M. avium* isolates.

Adverse drug events

Gastrointestinal adverse effects, metallic taste, peripheral and optic neuritis, hypothyroidism, gynecomastia, alopecia, impotence and, rarely, hepatitis are observed.

34-16. Questions

1. Which of the following is an antibiotic that exhibits concentration-dependent bacterial killing?

   A. Penicillin G
   B. Ceftriaxone
   C. Gentamicin
   D. Aztreonam

2. Which of the following most accurately characterizes aminoglycoside toxicity?

   A. Thrombocytopenia and neutropenia
   B. CPK elevations and myalgias
   C. QT prolongation and risk of arrhythmia
   D. Nephrotoxicity and ototoxicity

3. Which of the following β-lactam antibiotics displays the best activity against enterococci?

   A. Ampicillin
   B. Cefepime
   C. Meropenem
   D. Aztreonam

4. Which of the following β-lactam antibiotics displays activity against MRSA?

   A. Piperacillin-tazobactam
   B. Ceftaroline
   C. Imipenem-cilastatin
   D. Aztreonam

5. Which of the following penicillins does not have to be dose adjusted for renal insufficiency, yet can cause interstitial nephritis?

   A. Nafcillin
   B. Amoxicillin
   C. Ticarcillin-clavulanic acid
   D. Penicillin G

6. Which of the following cephalosporins is classified as a first-generation agent with enhanced Gram-positive activity?

   A. Cefuroxime
   B. Ceftazidime
   C. Cefepime
   D. Cefazolin

7. Which carbapenem antibiotic displays broad-spectrum antibiotic activity yet does not cover *Pseudomonas aeruginosa*?

   A. Imipenem-cilastatin
   B. Doripenem
   C. Meropenem
   D. Ertapenem

8. Which β-lactam antibiotic would be most appropriate to treat Gram-negative pathogens in a patient with a serious, anaphylactic penicillin allergy?

   A. Oxacillin
   B. Aztreonam
   C. Cephalexin
   D. Penicillin V

9. Which of the following reversible adverse effects is associated with rapid infusion time of vancomycin?

   A. Nephrotoxicity
   B. Ototoxicity
   C. Red-man syndrome
   D. Neurologic toxicity

10. Which of the following can be used as an oral formulation to treat infections caused by MRSA?

    A. Linezolid
    B. Daptomycin
    C. Vancomycin
    D. Ceftaroline

11. For which of the following antibiotics should weekly CPK levels be drawn?

    A. Vancomycin
    B. Linezolid
    C. Quinupristin-dalfopristin
    D. Daptomycin

12. Which of the following trough concentrations should be targeted for a patient receiving vancomycin for the treatment of MRSA pneumonia?

    A. 5–10 mcg/mL
    B. 10–15 mcg/mL
    C. 15–20 mcg/mL
    D. Trough monitoring is not necessary

13. Which of the following fluoroquinolones covers both *S. pneumoniae* and *P. aeruginosa*?

    A. Moxifloxacin
    B. Levofloxacin
    C. Ciprofloxacin
    D. Ofloxacin

14. Which of the following is an important patient counseling point for a patient receiving a fluoroquinolone antibiotic?

    A. Avoid antacids or calcium-containing substances within 2 hours of administration.
    B. Take only on an empty stomach.
    C. Take only with a high fat meal or an acidic beverage.
    D. Avoid proton-pump inhibitors with use.

15. Which of the following macrolide antibiotics is used primarily to accelerate gastric emptying?

    A. Azithromycin
    B. Clarithromycin
    C. Erythromycin
    D. Telithromycin

16. Which of the following is a drug of choice for *Rickettsia* infections such as Rocky Mountain spotted fever?

    A. Clindamycin
    B. Doxycycline
    C. Azithromycin
    D. Rifaximin

17. Which of the following drugs could adequately treat a skin and soft tissue infection caused by community-acquired MRSA?

    A. Metronidazole
    B. Fidaxomicin
    C. Colistimethate
    D. Sulfamethoxazole-trimethoprim

18. Which of the following antibiotics may have a higher incidence of predisposing a patient for a *Clostridium difficile* infection?

    A. Clindamycin
    B. Fidaxomicin
    C. Metronidazole
    D. Oral vancomycin

19. Which of the following agents has the best activity against the Gram-negative anaerobe *Bacteroides fragilis*?

    A. Clindamycin
    B. Colistin

    C. Fidaxomicin
    D. Metronidazole

20. Which of the following drugs is used only for severe infections caused by multidrug-resistant Gram-negative pathogens due to a significant risk of nephrotoxicity?

    A. Rifaximin
    B. Colistin
    C. Clindamycin
    D. Fidaxomicin

21. Which of the following antifungal agents is the drug of choice for infection caused by *Candida albicans*?

    A. Terbinafine
    B. Fluconazole
    C. Flucytosine
    D. Griseofulvin

22. Which of the following well-tolerated antifungal agents is commonly used to treat disseminated candidiasis caused by *Candida krusei*?

    A. Caspofungin
    B. Amphotericin B
    C. Posaconazole
    D. Fluconazole

23. Which of the following oral antifungal medications is commonly used to treat onychomycosis?

    A. Amphotericin B
    B. Caspofungin
    C. Posaconazole
    D. Terbinafine

24. Which of the following antitubercular agents is the drug of choice for latent TB infection?

    A. Isoniazid
    B. Cycloserine
    C. Ethambutol
    D. Capreomycin

25. Which of the following agents can cause red-colored staining of body fluids?

    A. Rifampin
    B. Isoniazid
    C. Pyrazinamide
    D. Ethambutol

34-17. Answers

1. **C.** Aminoglycoside antibiotics exhibit concentration-dependent bacterial killing while β-lactam antibiotics display time-dependent bacterial killing.

2. **D.** Aminoglycosides cause both nephrotoxicity and ototoxicity. Nephrotoxicity is exhibited as an acute tubular necrosis that is usually reversible and seldom requires dialysis. Ototoxicity is due to eighth cranial nerve damage and may be irreversible.

3. **A.** Ampicillin is a drug of choice for enterococci that are susceptible. No cephalosporins display reliable activity against enterococci.

4. **B.** Ceftaroline is currently the only β-lactam antibiotic that displays activity against MRSA.

5. **A.** Nafcillin is a member of the penicillinase-resistant penicillin class that does not have to be dose adjusted for renal insufficiency. However, this class of medications can cause interstitial nephritis. The first medication in this class, methicillin, was removed from the market because of a high incidence of interstitial nephritis.

6. **D.** Cefazolin is an intravenous, first-generation cephalosporin with extensive Gram-positive antibacterial activity. It is considered an agent of choice for MSSA along with the penicillinase-resistant penicillins.

7. **D.** Ertapenem is the only carbapenem that does not exhibit coverage against *P. aeruginosa*. It is also the only carbapenem that is administered once daily.

8. **B.** Aztreonam displays a purely Gram-negative spectrum of activity and tends to have the lowest allergic cross-reactivity in patients with anaphylactic penicillin allergies.

9. **C.** Red-man syndrome is a histamine-related adverse reaction that occurs when vancomycin is administered rapidly. It is important to note that this is not a true drug allergy. Red-man syndrome can be minimized by slowing the infusion time and administering antihistamines such as diphenhydramine prior to infusion.

10. **A.** Linezolid is the only Gram-positive antibiotic agent (covering MRSA) listed with an oral formulation. This can be helpful when a patient is in the outpatient setting or transitioning to outpatient care.

11. **D.** Weekly CPK levels should be drawn when patients are initiated on daptomycin therapy. Daptomycin therapy should be discontinued when CPK levels reach five times the upper limit of normal when patients are symptomatic (commonly myalgias), or 10 times the upper limit of normal when asymptomatic. Monitoring should be performed closely when patients are on concomitant statin therapy.

12. **C.** Vancomycin trough concentration targets of 15–20 mcg/mL are now recommended for the majority of vancomycin treatment indications with the exception of skin and soft tissue infections, which requires lower targets (10–15 mcg/mL).

13. **B.** Levofloxacin displays broad-spectrum activity against both pneumococci and *P. aeruginosa*. In contrast, ciprofloxacin does not display reliable activity against pneumococci, and moxifloxacin does not display reliable activity against *P. aeruginosa*.

14. **A.** Absorption and drug concentrations can be greatly reduced by the concomitant administration of cations that can bind fluoroquinolone antibiotics. This is an important patient counseling point to explain to patients to reduce the chances of treatment failure.

15. **C.** With the emergence of newer macrolide antibiotics with enhanced activity, erythromycin is now used more commonly for its adverse effect of enhancing gastric motility than for its antibacterial action.

16. **B.** Doxycycline is a drug of choice for tick-borne illnesses such as Lyme disease and Rocky Mountain spotted fever.

17. **D.** The three antibiotics commonly used to treat community-acquired MRSA skin and soft tissue infections include doxycycline, clindamycin, and sulfamethoxazole-trimethoprim.

18. **A.** Although all antibiotics can cause *C. difficile* infection, clindamycin's spectrum of activity covers many anaerobes except for *C. difficile*. For this reason, it is commonly implicated as a predisposition for *C. difficile* infection.

19. **D.** Metronidazole displays a purely anaerobic spectrum of activity and is a drug of choice for one of the main Gram-negative anaerobes *B. fragilis* typically located in the lower gastrointestinal tract.

20. **B.** Colistin is a polymyxin antibiotic that can be used for multidrug resistant Gram-negative pathogens such as *P. aeruginosa* and *Acinetobacter* spp. Its main limiting side effect is significant nephrotoxicity, and it should be reserved for severe or multidrug resistant infections.

21. **B.** Fluconazole is a drug of choice for *C. albicans*, yet it does not effectively cover some non–*Candida albicans* species including *C. glabrata* or *C. krusei*. Although fluconazole can display dose-dependent susceptibility for some *C. glabrata*, it is inherently resistant to *C. krusei*.

22. **A.** Echinocandins are drugs of choice for disseminated candidiasis caused by non-*albicans* or fluconazole-resistant *Candida* species. Echinocandins are often initiated as empiric therapy for disseminated candidiasis until the fungal species is known by culture.

23. **D.** Terbinafine is an oral antifungal agent that is commonly used to treat dermatophytes that cause onychomycosis (fungal infection of the nail, most commonly toe nails).

24. **A.** Isoniazid daily therapy is the preferred regimen for latent TB infection. Patients should be supplemented with pyridoxine and should avoid alcoholic beverages while taking isoniazid.

25. **A.** An important patient counseling point for patients being administered rifampin is to be aware of discoloration of body fluids such as tears, sweat, and saliva. Patients who wear contact lenses, for example, should be notified that the lenses may be permanently discolored.

34-18. References

Alvarez-Elcoro S, Enzler MJ. The macrolides: Erythromycin, clarithromycin, and azithromycin. *Mayo Clin Proc.* 1999;74:613–34.

Coly-Mycin M (colistimethate IV and IM injection) [product information]. Rochester, MI: JHP Pharmaceuticals; 2007.

Cubicin (daptomycin for injection) [product information]. Lexington, MA: Cubist Pharmaceuticals; 2013.

Dificid (fidaxomicin oral tablets) [product information]. San Diego, CA: Optimer Pharmaceuticals; 2011.

Doribax (doripenem IV injection) [product information]. Raritan, NJ: Ortho-McNeil; 2009.

Edson RS, Terrell CL. The aminoglycosides. *Mayo Clin Proc.* 1999;74:519–28.

Hellinger WC, Brewer NS. Carbapenems and monobactams: Imipenem, meropenem, and aztreonam. *Mayo Clin Proc.* 1999;74:420–34.

Lewis RE. Current concepts in antifungal pharmacology. *Mayo Clin Proc.* 2011;86(8):805–17.

Liu C, Bayer A, Cosgrove SE, et al. Clinical practice guidelines by the Infectious Diseases Society of America for the treatment of methicillin-resistant *Staphylococcus aureus* infection in adults and children. *Clin Infect Dis.* 2011;52:1–38.

Louie TJ, Miller MA, Mullane KM, et al. Fidaxomicin versus vancomycin for *Clostridium difficile* infection. *N Engl J Med.* 2011;364(5):422–31.

Mandell GL, Bennett JE, Dolin R, eds. *Principles and Practice of Infectious Diseases.* 7th ed. Philadelphia, PA: Churchill Livingstone; 2010.

Marshall WF, Blair JE. The cephalosporins. *Mayo Clin Proc.* 1999;74:187–95.

Polymyxin B sulfate powder for injection solution [product information]. Schaumberg, IL: Sagent Pharmaceuticals; 2013.

Sia IG, Wieland ML. Current concepts in the management of tuberculosis. *Mayo Clin Proc.* 2011;86(4):348–61.

Smilack JD. The tetracyclines. *Mayo Clin Proc.* 1999;74:727–30.

Smilack JD. Trimethoprim-sulfamethoxazole. *Mayo Clin Proc.* 1999;74:730–34.

Teflaro (ceftaroline fosamil IV injection) [prescribing information]. St. Louis, MO: Forest Pharmaceutical; 2011.

Vibativ (telavancin IV injection) [prescribing information]. South San Francisco, CA: Theravance; 2009.

Wright AJ. The penicillins. *Mayo Clin Proc.* 1999;74:290–308.

Human Immunodeficiency Virus and the Acquired Immune Deficiency Syndrome

35

Camille W. Thornton

35-1. Key Points

- *Human immunodeficiency virus* (HIV) is a virus that destroys the immune system.
- *Acquired immune deficiency syndrome* (AIDS) is caused by HIV and is defined as a CD4 cell count less than 200/mm^3 or the presence of an opportunistic infection.
- Acute retroviral syndrome occurs in 50–90% of patients within the first 2–4 weeks of infection with HIV.
- The viral load indicates the amount of virus in the body and is an indication of how well anti-retroviral medications are working.
- The CD4 cell count refers to the status of the immune system and how much a patient is at risk for developing an opportunistic infection.
- Nucleoside reverse transcriptase inhibitors (NRTIs), non-nucleoside reverse transcriptase inhibitors (NNRTIs), protease inhibitors (PIs), entry inhibitors (fusion inhibitors, CCR5 antagonists), and integrase inhibitors are the currently available classes of medications used to treat HIV.
- Vertical transmission is prevented by treating the mother with combination antiretroviral regimens.
- *Pneumocystis jiroveci* pneumonia requires primary prophylaxis at CD4 cell count < 200/mm^3. Trimethoprim-sulfamethoxazole (TMP-SMX) is the preferred treatment.
- *Mycobacterium avium* complex requires primary prophylaxis at CD4 cell count < 50/mm^3. Azithromycin is the preferred drug.
- All other opportunistic infections require treatment followed by secondary prophylaxis.

35-2. Study Guide Checklist

The following topics may guide your study of this subject area:

- Class side effects of NRTIs, NNRTIs, PIs
- Medications that contain sulfa
- Medications that need normal gastric pH for absorption
- Medications that are contraindicated with PIs and NNRTIs
- Medications that inhibit CYP3A
- When HIV medication should be started
- Preferred treatment regimens for HIV-naïve patients
- Opportunistic infections that require primary prophylaxis
- Preferred treatments for most common opportunistic infections
- When to start postexposure prophylaxis (PEP) for occupational and nonoccupational exposures
- Preferred regimen for PEP for occupational and nonoccupational exposures
- Preferred regimens to prevent mother-to-child transmission

35-3. Overview

Human immunodeficiency virus (HIV) is a retrovirus that depletes the helper T-lymphocytes (CD4 cells), resulting in continued destruction of the immune system and subsequent gradual development of opportunistic infections and malignancies.

Acquired immune deficiency syndrome (AIDS) is HIV with a CD4 cell count lower than 200 cells/mm^3 or a history of opportunistic infection (e.g., unexplained fever for more than 2 weeks, thrush, *Pneumocystis jiroveci* pneumonia, toxoplasmosis, cryptococcal meningitis, histoplasmosis, *Mycobacterium avium*).

Clinical Presentation

- Patient has an opportunistic infection.
- Patient is not ill but has tested positive for HIV.
- Patient has acute retroviral syndrome:
  - Of patients acutely infected with HIV, 50–90% experience some of the symptoms.
  - Symptoms generally appear 2–4 weeks after virus exposure.
  - Duration of the clinical syndrome is about 14 days (the range is a few days to > 10 weeks).
  - The disease is not readily recognized in the primary care setting because its symptoms are similar to those of the flu, mononucleosis, and other common illnesses.

Testing Recommendations

The U.S. Centers for Disease Control and Prevention recommend the following HIV testing in health care settings:

- Routine, voluntary, opt-out HIV screening for all persons 13–64 years of age in health care settings. Testing is not based on risk factors.
- HIV screening of pregnant women as part of the routine panel of prenatal screening tests. Testing is not based on risk factors.
- Repeat HIV screening of persons with known risk at least annually:
  - Injection drug users and their sex partners
  - Persons who exchange sex for money or drugs
  - Sex partners of HIV-infected persons
  - Men who have sex with men
  - Heterosexual persons who themselves or whose sex partners have had more than one sex partner since their most recent HIV test

Transmission

Transmission is through infected blood or hazardous body fluids, which can occur during the following activities:

- Unprotected sexual contact with an infected person
  - Multiple partners increase risk.
  - Ongoing or past medical history of sexually transmitted disease increases risk.
- Sharing of needles or syringes with an infected person
- Transfusions of infected blood or blood clotting factors (the United States began screening the blood supply in 1985)
- Vertical transmission (infected mother to infant)
- Breast-feeding

Occupational exposure and household contact are rare.

Monitoring Tools

Viral load

Viral load testing measures the amount of virus in blood. It can assess disease progression and evaluate the efficacy of antiretroviral therapy (ART). The goal of HIV treatment is to achieve and maintain an undetectable viral load. This is considered to be a viral load < 200 copies/mL, although some ultrasensitive assays have a lower limit of detection of < 20 copies/mL.

Acute illness and immunizations can cause increases in viral load for 2–4 weeks. Testing should not be performed during this time.

Monitoring of viral load in patients not on ART should occur every 3–4 months. Monitoring of viral load in patients starting a new regimen should occur 2–8 weeks after treatment initiation and then every 3–4 months.

CD4 cell count

CD4 cell count indicates the extent of immune system damage and the risk of developing opportunistic infections. Normal CD4 cell count is 800–1,200 cells/mm^3.

CD4 cell count should be measured every 3–6 months in patients on or off ART. In clinically stable patients with suppressed viral load, CD4 cell count can be monitored every 6–12 months.

Resistance testing

Genotypes should be performed to determine if resistance to medications is present. Testing should be done on all patients before starting the first treatment regimen and whenever viral loads are persistently > 500–1,000 copies/mL and the patient is currently on medications for HIV or has taken them in the past 4 weeks prior to testing.

Treatment Principles and Goals

Goals of therapy

Therapy has the following goals:

- Maximal and durable suppression of viral load
- Restoration or preservation of immunologic function

- Improvement in quality of life
- Reduction of HIV-related morbidity and mortality
- Prevention of HIV transmission

Factors involved in achieving goals of therapy are as follows:

- Adherence to the antiretroviral regimen
- Performance of pretreatment drug resistance testing
- Selection of individualized initial combination regimen

See Box 35-1 for indications for the initiation of ART in the chronically HIV-1 infected patient.

Guidelines for prevention and treatment and medications used for the treatment of HIV can be located as a living document at www.aidsinfo.nih.gov, which is updated regularly.

Box 35-1. Indications for the Initiation of ART in the Chronically HIV-1 Infected Patient

ART is recommended for all HIV-infected individuals. The strength of this recommendation varies depending on the pretreatment CD4 cell count:

- CD4 cell count < 350 cells/mm^3 (AI)
- CD4 cell count 350–500 cells/mm^3 (AII)
- CD4 cell count > 500 cells/mm^3 (BIII)

Regardless of CD4 cell count, initiation of ART is strongly recommended for individuals with the following conditions:

- Pregnancy (AI)
- History of an AIDS-defining illness (AI)
- HIV-associated nephropathy (HIVAN) (AII)
- HIV/hepatitis B virus (HBV) co-infection (AII)

Effective ART also has been shown to prevent transmission of HIV from an infected individual to a sexual partner; therefore, ART should be offered to patients who are at risk of transmitting HIV to sexual partners (AI: heterosexual transmission; AIII: other transmission risk groups)

Patients starting ART should be willing and able to commit to treatment and should understand the benefits and risks of therapy and the importance of adherence (AIII). Patients may choose to postpone therapy, and providers, on a case-by-case basis, may elect to defer therapy on the basis of clinical and/or psychosocial factors.

Rating of recommendations: A = strong; B = moderate; C = optional.

Rating of evidence: I = data from randomized controlled trials; II = data from well-designed nonrandomized trials or observational cohort studies with long-term clinical outcomes; III = expert opinion.

35-4. Drug Therapy

See Table 35-1 for antiretroviral agents recommended by the U.S. Department of Health and Human Services for initial treatment of established HIV infection.

Nucleoside Reverse Transcriptase Inhibitors

Nucleoside reverse transcriptase inhibitors (NRTIs) are described in Table 35-2. The mechanism of action of NRTIs is to interfere with HIV viral RNA (ribonucleic acid)-dependent deoxyribonucleic acid (DNA) polymerase, resulting in chain termination and inhibition of viral replication.

Didanosine (ddI), stavudine (d4T), and lamivudine (3TC) are dosed on the basis of weight. Most NRTIs are not affected by food (except didanosine). NRTIs have a low pill burden as a class and few drug interactions. All are pro-drugs requiring two or three phosphorylations for activation.

Four combination products are available:

- Combivir (zidovudine 300 mg + lamivudine 150 mg) every 12 hours
- Trizivir (zidovudine 300 mg + lamivudine 150 mg + abacavir 300 mg) every 12 hours
- Truvada (tenofovir 300 mg + emtricitabine 200 mg) every 24 hours
- Epzicom (lamivudine 300 mg + abacavir 600 mg) every 24 hours

No special storage requirements are necessary for drugs in this class.

Usually, two NRTIs are used in combination with one non-nucleoside reverse transcriptase inhibitor (NNRTI), one protease inhibitor (PI), or one integrase strand transfer inhibitor (INSTI).

All NRTIs have a boxed warning concerning the following class toxicities:

- Lactic acidosis
- Severe hepatomegaly with steatosis

The following precautions should be kept in mind regarding NRTIs:

- Most patients should be dose adjusted for renal impairment (exception: abacavir).
- Lamivudine and emtricitabine are chemically similar and should not be used in the same regimen.
- Do not use zidovudine with stavudine because of antagonism (both require thymidine for activation).

Table 35-1. Antiretroviral Regimens for Treatment of HIV Infection in Antiretroviral-Naïve Patients

Preferred Regimens (regimens with optimal and durable efficacy, favorable tolerability and toxicity profile, and ease of use)

Selection of a regimen should be individualized on the basis of virologic efficacy, toxicity, pill burden, dosing frequency, drug–drug interaction potential, resistance testing results, and comorbid conditions.

Regimen	Comments
NNRTI-based regimen • Efavirenz/tenofovir/emtricitabine[a,c]	Efavirenz should not be used during the first trimester of pregnancy or in women of childbearing potential who are trying to conceive or not using effective and consistent contraception.
PI-based regimen Atazanavir + ritonavir + tenofovir/emtricitabine[c] Darunavir + ritonavir + tenofovir/emtricitabine[c]	Tenofovir should be used with caution in patients with renal insufficiency. Atazanavir/ritonavir should not be used in patients who require > 20 mg omeprazole equivalent per day.

INSTI-based regimen
Raltegravir + tenofovir/emtricitabine[c]
Elvitegravir/cobicistat/tenofovir/emtricitabine[c]
Dolutegravir + abacavir/lamivudine[c]
Dolutegravir + tenofovir/emtricitabine[c]
	Elvitegravir/cobicistat/tenofovir/emtricitabine[c] should not be started in patients with CrCl less than 70 mL/min.
	
	1 Boosted PI:
	    Atazanavir + ritonavir
	    Lopinavir/ritonavir[c]

Preferred regimen for pregnant women[b] 2 NRTIs: Abacavir/lamivudine[c] Tenofovir/emtricitabine[c] Tenofovir + lamivudine Zidovudine/lamivudine[c]	*Or* 1 NNRTI: Efavirenz (start after 8 weeks of pregnancy)

Alternative Regimens (regimens that are effective and tolerable but have potential disadvantages compared with preferred regimens)

These regimens are based on individual patient characteristics and needs. In some instances, an alternative regimen may actually be a preferred regimen for a patient.

Regimen	Comments
NNRTI-based regimen Efavirenz + abacavir/lamivudine[c] Rilpivirine/tenofovir/emtricitabine[c] Rilpivirine + abacavir/lamivudine[c]	Rilpivirine is not recommended in patients with pretreatment viral loads > 100,000 copies/mL and should be used with caution in patients with CD4 cell count < 200 cells/mm^3. Use of PPIs with rilpivirine is contraindicated.
PI-based regimen Atazanavir + ritonavir + abacavir/lamivudine[c] Darunavir + ritonavir + abacavir/lamivudine[c] Fosamprenavir + ritonavir + abacavir/lamivudine[c] or tenofovir/emtricitabine[c] Lopinavir/ritonavir[c] + abacavir/lamivudine[c] or tenofovir/emtricitabine[c]	Abacavir should not be used in patients who test positive for HLA-B*5701. Use abacavir with caution in patients with known high risk of cardiovascular disease or with pretreatment viral loads > 100,000 copies/mL. Once-daily lopinavir/ritonavir is not recommended for use in pregnant women.
INSTI-based regimen Raltegravir + abacavir/lamivudine[c]	

INSTI, integrase strand transfer inhibitor; PPI, proton pump inhibitor.

a. Lamivudine may be substituted for emtricitabine or vice versa.

b. Refer to the perinatal guidelines for more detailed recommendations (http://aidsinfo.nih.gov/guidelines).

c. The following are available as coformulated fixed-dose combinations: efavirenz/tenofovir/emtricitabine (Atripla), tenofovir/emtricitabine (Truvada), lopinavir/ritonavir (Kaletra), zidovudine/lamivudine (Combivir), abacavir/lamivudine (Epzicom), rilpivirine/tenofovir/emtricitabine (Complera), elvitegravir/cobicistat/tenofovir/emtricitabine (Stribild).

Table 35-2. Nucleoside Reverse Transcriptase Inhibitors

	Zidovudine (AZT, ZDV)	Lamivudine (3TC)	Abacavir (ABC)	Didanosine (ddl)	Stavudine (d4T)	Tenofovir (TDF)	Emtricitabine (FTC)
Trade name	Retrovir	Epivir	Ziagen	Videx EC, Videx	Zerit	Viread	Emtriva
Form	100 mg capsules; 300 mg tablets; 10 mg/mL IV solution; 10 mg/mL oral solution; generic: 300 mg tablets; 10 mg/mL oral solution	150, 300 mg tablets; 10 mg/mL oral solution; generic; 150 mg tablets	300 mg tablets; 20 mg/mL oral solution	Videx EC capsules: 125, 200, 250, 400 mg; available as generic didanosine DR: 125, 200, 250, 400 mg capsules and 10 mg/mL oral solution	15, 20, 30, 40 mg capsules; 1 mg/mL oral solution; available as generic, same doses	150, 200, 250, 300 mg tablets; 40 mg/g oral powder	200 mg tablets; 10 mg/mL oral solution
	Combinations: Trizivir (abacavir 300 mg/lamivudine 150 mg/zidovudine 300 mg)	Combinations: Epzicom (abacavir 600 mg/lamivudine 300 mg); Combivir (lamivudine 150 mg/zidovudine 300 mg), and as generic; Trizivir (abacavir 300 mg/lamivudine 150 mg/zidovudine 300 mg)	Combinations: Epzicom (abacavir 600 mg/lamivudine 300 mg); Trizivir (abacavir 300 mg/lamivudine 150 mg/zidovudine 300 mg)			Combinations: **Truvada** (tenofovir 300 mg/emtricitabine 200 mg); **Atripla** (tenofovir 300 mg/emtricitabine 200 mg/efavirenz 600 mg); Complera (tenofovir 300 mg/emtricitabine 200 mg/rilpivirine 25 mg)	Combinations: **Truvada** (tenofovir 300 mg/emtricitabine 200 mg); **Atripla** (tenofovir 300 mg/emtricitabine 200 mg/efavirenz 600 mg); Complera (tenofovir 300 mg/emtricitabine 200 mg/rilpivirine 25 mg)
	Combivir (lamivudine 150 mg/zidovudine 300 mg), and as generic						
Dosing	300 mg twice daily; 200 mg three times daily; Combivir: twice daily; Trizivir: twice daily	150 mg twice daily or 300 mg daily; Epzicom: daily; Combivir: twice daily; Trizivir: twice daily	300 mg twice daily; 600 mg daily; Epzicom: daily; Trizivir: twice daily	> 60 kg: 400 mg daily; with tenofovir ↓ddl to 250 mg daily; < 60 kg: 250 mg daily; with tenofovir ↓ddl to 200 mg daily[b]	> 60 kg: 40 mg twice daily; < 60 kg: 30 mg twice daily[c]	Tablets: 300 mg once daily; powder: 7.5 scoops once daily. Mix oral powder with 2–4 oz of food not requiring chewing. Do not mix with liquid.	Capsules: 200 mg once daily; oral solution: 240 mg (24 mL) daily; **Truvada**: daily; **Atripla**: daily at bedtime; Complera: daily with a meal

(continued)

Table 35-2. Nucleoside Reverse Transcriptase Inhibitors *(Continued)*

	Zidovudine (AZT, ZDV)	Lamivudine (3TC)	Abacavir (ABC)	Didanosine (ddI)	Stavudine (d4T)	Tenofovir (TDF)	Emtricitabine (FTC)
						Truvada: daily; **Atripla:** daily at bedtime; Complera: daily with a meal	
Food effect	Take without regard to meals.	Take without regard to meals.	Take without regard to meals.	Take ½ hour before or 2 hours after meals.	Take without regard to meals.	Take without regard to meals except for Complera.	Take without regard to meals except for Complera.
Adverse events	Bone marrow suppression (macrocytic anemia or neutropenia), gastrointestinal intolerance, headache, insomnia, asthenia, nail pigmentation, hyperlipidemia, insulin resistance or diabetes mellitus, lipoatrophy, myopathy	Minimal toxicity; severe acute exacerbation of hepatitis may occur in HBV–co-infected patients who discontinue lamivudine.	Hypersensitivity reaction testing for HLA-B*5701 should be done before start to evaluate patient risk for hypersensitivity; only negative patients should start abacavir. Hypersensitivity symptoms include rash, fever, nausea and vomiting, malaise or fatigue, loss of appetite; respiratory symptoms include sore throat, cough, shortness of breath.	Pancreatitis, peripheral neuropathy, retinal changes, optic neuritis, nausea, vomiting, potential association with noncirrhotic portal hypertension; in some cases, patients presented with esophageal varices; insulin resistance or diabetes mellitus.	Pancreatitis; peripheral neuropathy; lipoatrophy; hyperlipidemia; insulin resistance or diabetes mellitus; rapidly progressive ascending neuromuscular weakness (rare)	Renal insufficiency, Fanconi syndrome, osteomalacia, decrease in bone mineral density, potential decrease in bone mineral density, asthenia, headache, diarrhea, nausea, vomiting, flatulence; severe acute exacerbation of hepatitis may occur in HBV–co-infected patients who discontinue TDF.	Minimal toxicity; hyperpigmentation or skin discoloration; severe acute exacerbation of hepatitis may occur in HBV–co-infected patients who discontinue FTC.

Drug interactions	Ribavirin, stavudine, methadone; with high dose: ganciclovir, TMP-SMX, other medications that can cause bone marrow suppression	Some cohort studies suggest increased risk of myocardial infarction (MI) with recent or current use of ABC, but this risk is not substantiated in other studies. Alcohol increases abacavir levels by 41%.	No clinically significant drug interactions	One cohort study suggested increased risk of MI with recent or current use of ddl, but this risk is not substantiated in other studies. Methadone, ribavirin, tenofovir, allopurinol, stavudine, alcohol; use caution with other medications that can cause peripheral neuropathy. Separate from medications that need to be taken with food.	Didanosine; use with caution with other medications that can cause peripheral neuropathy.	Didanosine, atazanavir, cidofovir, ganciclovir, valganciclovir, telaprevir	No clinically significant drug interactions
Monitoring[a]	Complete blood count, liver function tests	Signs and symptoms of hypersensitivity reaction	None necessary	Complete blood count, liver function tests; amylase, uric acid; signs and symptoms of above side effects	Signs and symptoms of above side effects	Renal function	None necessary

HBV, hepatitis B virus.

Boldface indicates one of top 100 drugs for 2012 by units sold at retail outlets, www.drugs.com/stats/top100/2012/units.

a. Monitor all for signs and symptoms of NRTI class toxicities, lactic acidosis, and hepatic steatosis; incidence is higher with stavudine than with other NRTIs.

b. Preferred dosing with oral solution is divided into two doses.

c. The World Health Organization recommends 30 mg twice daily regardless of body weight.

- Do not use didanosine with stavudine during pregnancy because of increased risk of lactic acidosis and liver damage.
- Tenofovir increases didanosine levels and decreases atazanavir levels. Dosage adjustments are required.
- Patients should be tested for HLA-B*5701 to determine risk for hypersensitivity reaction to abacavir. Only patients testing negative should start abacavir.
- The "D" drugs (ddI and d4T) can cause pancreatitis and peripheral neuropathy; when used together, this effect can be additive.
- The "D" drugs are more closely associated with lactic acidosis.

Non-nucleoside Reverse Transcriptase Inhibitors

NNRTIs are described in Table 35-3. Their mechanism of action is to competitively inhibit reverse transcriptase, thereby resulting in inhibition of HIV replication.

One-step mutation (K103N) confers resistance to first-generation NNRTIs (efavirenz, nevirapine, delavirdine) but not to the second-generation NNRTI etravirine (and rilpivirine in vitro). All should be dose adjusted for hepatic impairment.

Efavirenz should be taken on an empty stomach. Rilpivirine should be taken with the largest meal of the day. Efavirenz is contraindicated in pregnancy (pregnancy category D: risk of neural tube defects in first trimester).

Usually, one NNRTI is used in combination with two NRTIs. Two single-tablet regimens (STRs) include medications from this class:

- Atripla (tenofovir 300 mg + emtricitabine 200 mg + efavirenz 600 mg) every 24 hours
- Complera (tenofovir 300 mg + emtricitabine 200 mg + rilpivirine 25 mg) every 24 hours

No special storage requirements are necessary for drugs in this class. Class toxicities include rash and hepatic toxicity.

Drug interactions can occur (see Tables 35-4 and 35-5). All are cytochrome P450 (CYP) 3A4 inducers or inhibitors. Rilpivirine requires normal acid levels in the stomach for absorption. Class side effects include rash and elevations in liver enzymes.

Protease Inhibitors

Protease inhibitors are described in Table 35-6. Their mechanism of action is to inhibit protease, which then prevents the cleavage of HIV polyproteins and subsequently induces the formation of immature noninfectious viral particles.

Table 35-3. Non-nucleoside Reverse Transcriptase Inhibitors

	Efavirenz (EFV)	Nevirapine (NVP)	Rilpivirine (RPV)	Etravirine (ETR)
Trade name	Sustiva	Viramune	Edurant	Intelence
Form	50, 200 mg capsules; 600 mg tablets	200 mg tablets; 400 mg XR tablets; 10 mg/mL oral suspension	25 mg tablets	100, 200 mg tablets
	Combination: **Atripla** (efavirenz 600 mg/emtricitabine 200 mg/tenofovir 300 mg)		Combination: Complera (rilpivirine 25 mg/ tenofovir 300 mg/ emtricitabine 200 mg)	
Dosing recommendations	600 mg at or before bedtime; **Atripla** at or before bedtime	200 mg daily × 14 days, then 200 mg twice or 400 mg XR daily; use only in women with starting CD4 cell count > 250 cells/mm³ and men with CD4 cell count > 400 cells/mm³ to decrease incidence of side effects	25 mg daily with a meal; Complera daily with a meal	200 mg twice daily as tablets or dissolved in water to form a slurry to drink; ETR effective in patients with resistance (K103N) to other NNRTIs

Table 35-3. Non-nucleoside Reverse Transcriptase Inhibitors *(Continued)*

	Efavirenz (EFV)	Nevirapine (NVP)	Rilpivirine (RPV)	Etravirine (ETR)
Food effect	Take on an empty stomach to reduce side effects.	Take without regard to meals.	Take with a meal.	Take following a meal.
Adverse events	Neuropsychiatric symptoms[a], rash, ↑ liver function tests (LFTs), false-positive results with some cannabinoid and benzodiazepine screening assays, teratogenic in monkeys	Rash (including Stevens–Johnson syndrome), symptomatic hepatitis (including fatal hepatic necrosis)	Rash, depression, insomnia, headache, ↑ QT interval; use caution in patients with baseline viral loads > 100,000 copies/mL due to increased failure rates and resistance.	Rash (including Stevens–Johnson syndrome); nausea; hypersensitivity reactions, characterized by rash, constitutional findings, and sometimes organ dysfunction, including hepatic failure, have been reported.
Drug interactions	Metabolized by CYP2B6 and CYP3A4	CYP450 substrate	CYP3A4 substrate	CYP3A4, CYP2C9, and CYP2C19 substrate
	CYP3A4 mixed inducer/inhibitor (more an inducer than an inhibitor)[c]	Inducer of CYP3A4 and CYP2B6[c]		CYP3A4 inducer; CYP2C9 and 2C19 inhibitor[c]
Monitoring[b]	CNS side effects, LFTs, rash	LFTs 2, 4, and 6 weeks, and then monthly for the first 18 weeks	LFTs, rash, depression, QT interval when given with medications that could increase RPV levels	LFTs, rash, nausea

CNS, central nervous system.
Boldface indicates one of top 100 drugs for 2012 by units sold at retail outlets, www.drugs.com/stats/top100/2012/units.
a. CNS side effects include dizziness, somnolence, insomnia, abnormal dreams, confusion, abnormal thinking, impaired concentration, amnesia, agitation, depersonalization, hallucinations, and euphoria. Use caution in patients with a psychiatric history or previous addictions.
b. Monitor all for signs and symptoms of NNRTI class toxicities, rash, and hepatic toxicity.
c. See Tables 35-4 and 35-5.

Table 35-4. Drugs That Should Not Be Used with NNRTIs

Drug category	Efavirenz	Nevirapine	Etravirine	Rilpivirine
Antimycobacterials	Rifapentine	Rifapentine	Rifampin, rifapentine	Rifampin, rifapentine, rifabutin
Gastrointestinal agents	Cisapride	None	None	Proton pump inhibitor drugs
Neuroleptics	Pimozide	None	None	None
Psychotropics	Midazolam, triazolam	None	None	None
Ergot alkaloids (vasoconstrictor)	Ergotamine derivatives	None	None	None
Herbs	St. John's wort	St. John's wort	St. John's wort	St. John's wort
Antiretroviral agents	Other NNRTIs	Atazanavir +/− ritonavir, other NNRTIs	Unboosted PIs, atazanavir/ritonavir, fosamprenavir/ritonavir, tipranavir/ritonavir, other NNRTIs	Other NNRTIs
Other	None	Ketoconazole	Carbamazepine, phenobarbital, phenytoin, clopidogrel	Carbamazepine, oxcarbazepine, phenobarbital, phenytoin

Table 35-5. Drug Interactions with NNRTIs Requiring Dose Modifications or Cautious Use

Concomitant drug class/name	NNRTI	Effect on NNRTI or concomitant drug concentrations	Dosing recommendations and clinical comments
Acid reducers			
Antacids	Rilpivirine (RPV)	↓ RPV expected when given simultaneously	Give antacids at least 2 hours before or at least 4 hours after RPV.
H$_2$-receptor antagonists	RPV	↓ RPV	Give H$_2$-receptor antagonists at least 12 hours before or at least 4 hours after RPV.
Proton pump inhibitors (PPIs)	RPV	↓ RPV	Contraindicated; do not co-administer.
Anticoagulants/antiplatelets			
Warfarin	Efavirenz (EFV), Nevirapine (NVP)	↑ or ↓ warfarin possible	Monitor INR, and adjust warfarin dose accordingly.
	Etravirine (ETR)	↑ warfarin possible	Monitor INR, and adjust warfarin dose accordingly.
Clopidogrel	ETR	↓ activation of clopidogrel possible	ETR may prevent metabolism of clopidogrel (inactive) to its active metabolite. Avoid co-administration, if possible.
Anticonvulsants			
Carbamazepine	EFV	Carbamazepine + EFV: carbamazepine AUC ↓ 27% and EFV AUC 36%	Monitor anticonvulsant and EFV levels, or, if possible, use alternative anticonvulsant to those listed.
Phenobarbital			
Phenytoin		Phenytoin + EFV: ↓ EFV and ↓ phenytoin possible	
	ETR	↓ anticonvulsant and ETR possible	Do not co-administer. Consider alternative anticonvulsant.
	NVP	↓ anticonvulsant and NVP possible	Monitor anticonvulsant and NVP levels and virologic responses, or consider alternative anticonvulsant.
	RPV	↓ RPV possible	Contraindicated; do not co-administer. Consider alternative anticonvulsant.
Antidepressants			
Bupropion	EFV	Bupropion AUC ↓ 55%	Titrate bupropion dose on the basis of clinical response.
Sertraline	EFV	Sertraline AUC ↓ 39%	Titrate sertraline dose on the basis of clinical response.
Antifungals			
Fluconazole	ETR	ETR AUC ↑ 86%	No dosage adjustment is necessary. Use with caution.
	NVP	NVP AUC ↑110%	Increased risk of hepatotoxicity is possible with this combination. Monitor NVP toxicity, or use alternative ARV agent.
	RPV	↑ RPV possible	No dosage adjustment is necessary. Clinically monitor for break-through fungal infection.

Drug	ARV	Effect	Recommendation
Itraconazole	EFV	Itraconazole and OH-itraconazole AUV, C_{max} and C_{min} ↓ 35–44%	Failure to achieve therapeutic itraconazole concentrations has been reported. Avoid this combination if possible. If co-administered, closely monitor itraconazole concentration and adjust dose accordingly.
	ETR	↓ itraconazole possible, ↑ ETR	Dose adjustments for itraconazole may be necessary. Monitor itraconazole level and antifungal response.
	NVP	↓ itraconazole possible, ↑ NVP possible	Avoid this combination if possible. If co-administered, closely monitor itraconazole concentration and adjust dose accordingly.
	RPV	↑ RPV possible	No dosage adjustment is necessary. Clinically monitor for break-through fungal infection.
Posaconazole	EFV	Posaconazole AUC ↓ 50%, ↔EFV	Avoid concomitant use unless the benefit outweighs the risk. If co-administered, monitor posaconazole concentration and adjust dose accordingly.
	RPV	↑ RPV possible	No dosage adjustment is necessary. Clinically monitor for break-through fungal infection.
Voriconazole	EFV	Voriconazole AUC ↓ 77%, EFV AUC ↑ 44%	Use is contraindicated at standard doses. Dose: Voriconazole 400 mg bid, EFV 300 mg daily.
	ETR	Voriconazole AUC ↑ 14%, ETR ↑ 36%	No dosage adjustment is necessary. Use with caution. Consider monitoring voriconazole level.
	NVP	↓ voriconazole possible, ↑ NVP possible	Monitor for toxicity and antifungal response.
	RPV	↑ RPV possible	No dosage adjustment is necessary. Clinically monitor for break-through fungal infection.
Antimycobacterials			
Clarithromycin	EFV	Clarithromycin AUC ↓ 39%	Monitor for effectiveness, or consider alternative agent, such as azithromycin, for *Mycobacterium avium* complex (MAC) disease prophylaxis and treatment.
	ETR	Clarithromycin AUC ↓ 39%, ETR AUC ↑ 42%	Consider alternative agent, such as azithromycin, for MAC prophylaxis and treatment.
	NVP	Clarithromycin AUC ↓ 31%	Monitor for effectiveness, or consider alternative agent, such as azithromycin, for MAC prophylaxis and treatment.
	RPV	↔ clarithromycin, expected ↑ RPV possible	Consider alternative macrolide, such as azithromycin, for MAC prophylaxis and treatment.
Rifabutin	EFV	Rifabutin ↓ 38%	Dose: Rifabutin 450–600 mg once daily or 600 mg three times a week if EFV is not co-administered with a PI.
	ETR	Rifabutin and metabolite AUC ↓ 17%, ETR AUC ↓ 37%	If ETR is used with an RTV-boosted PI, rifabutin should not be co-administered. If not, dose rifabutin 300 mg once daily.
	NVP	Rifabutin AUC ↑ 17% and metabolite AUC ↑ 24%, NVP C_{min} ↓ 16%	No dosage adjustment is necessary. Use with caution.
	RPV	RPV AUC ↓ 46%	Contraindicated; do not co-administer.

(continued)

Table 35-5. Drug Interactions with NNRTIs Requiring Dose Modifications or Cautious Use (*Continued*)

Concomitant drug class/name	NNRTI	Effect on NNRTI or concomitant drug concentrations	Dosing recommendations and clinical comments
Rifampin	EFV	EFV AUC ↓ 26%	Maintain EFV dose at 600 mg dose once daily, and monitor for virologic response. Consider therapeutic drug monitoring. Some clinicians suggest EFV 800 mg dose in patients who weigh > 60 kg.
	ETR	Significant ↓ ETR possible	Do not co-administer.
	NVP	NVP ↓ 20–58%	Do not co-administer.
	RPV	RPV AUC ↓ 80%	Contraindicated; do not co-administer.
Rifapentine	EFV, ETR, NVP, RPV	↓ NNRTI expected	Do not co-administer.
Benzodiazepines			
Alprazolam	EFV, ETR, NVP, RPV	No data	Monitor for therapeutic effectiveness of alprazolam.
Diazepam	ETR	↑ diazepam possible	Decreased dose of diazepam may be necessary.
Cardiac medications			
Dihydropyridine calcium channel blockers (CCBs)	EFV, NVP	↓ CCBs possible	Titrate CCB dose on the basis of clinical response.
Diltiazem	EFV	Diltiazem AUC ↓ 69% ↓ verapamil possible	Titrate diltiazem or verapamil dose on the basis of clinical response.
Verapamil	NVP	↓ diltiazem or verapamil possible	
Corticosteroids			
Dexamethasone	EFV, ETR, NVP	↓ EFV, ETR, NVP possible	Consider alternative corticosteroid for long-term use. If dexamethasone is used with NNRTI, monitor virologic response.
	RPV	Significant ↓ RPV possible	Use is contraindicated with more than a single dose of dexamethasone.
Hepatitis C NS3/4A–protease inhibitors			
Boceprevir	EFV	EFV AUC ↑ 20%, boceprevir AUC ↓ 19%, C_{min} ↓ 44%	Co-administration is not recommended.
Telaprevir	EFV	EFV AUC ↔, telaprevir AUV ↓ 26%, C_{min} ↓ 47%. With TDF: EFV AUC ↓ 15–18%, telaprevir AUC ↓ 18–20%	Increase telaprevir dose to 1,125 mg every 8 hours.

Herbal products

Drug	ARV	Effect	Recommendation
St. John's wort	EFV, ETR, NVP, RPV	↓ NNRTIs	Do not co-administer.

Hormonal Contraceptives

Drug	ARV	Effect	Recommendation
Hormonal contraceptives	EFV	Ethinyl estradiol ↔, levonorgestrel AUC ↓ 83%, norelgestromin AUC ↓ 64%, ↓ etonogestrel (implant) possible	Use alternative or additional contraceptive methods. Norelgestromin and levonorgestrel are active metabolites of norgestimate.
	ETR	Ethinyl estradiol AUC ↑ 22%; norethindrone: no significant effect	No dosage adjustment is necessary.
	NVP	Ethinyl estradiol AUC ↓ 20%, norethindrone AUC ↓ 19%	Use alternative or additional contraceptive methods.
	RPV	Ethinyl estradiol AUC ↑ 14%; norethindrone: no significant change	No dosage adjustment is necessary.
Levonorgestrel (for emergency contraception)	EFV	Levonorgestrel AUC ↓ 58%	Effectiveness of emergency postcoital contraception may be diminished.

HMG-CoA reductase inhibitors

Drug	ARV	Effect	Recommendation
Atorvastatin	EFV, ETR	**Atorvastatin** AUC ↓ 32–43%	Adjust **atorvastatin** according to lipid responses, not to exceed the maximum recommended dose.
	RPV	**Atorvastatin** AUC ↔, **atorvastatin** metabolites ↑	No dosage adjustment is necessary.
Fluvastatin	ETR	↑ fluvastatin possible	Dose adjustments for fluvastatin may be necessary.
Lovastatin	EFV	Simvastatin AUC ↓ 68%	Adjust simvastatin dose according to lipid responses, not to exceed the maximum recommended dose. If EFV is used with RTV-boosted PI, simvastatin and lovastatin should be avoided.
Simvastatin	ETR, NVP	↓ lovastatin possible, ↓ simvastatin possible	Adjust lovastatin and simvastatin dose according to lipid responses, not to exceed the maximum recommended dose. If ETR or NVP are used with RTV-boosted PI, simvastatin and lovastatin should be avoided.
Pitavastatin	EFV, ETR, NVP, RPV	No data	There is no dosage recommendation.
Pravastatin	EFV	Pravastatin AUC ↓ 44%	Adjust statin dose according to lipid responses, not to exceed the maximum recommended dose.
Rosuvastatin	ETR	Rosuvastatin: No data, No significant effect expected	No dosage adjustment is necessary.

(continued)

Table 35-5. Drug Interactions with NNRTIs Requiring Dose Modifications or Cautious Use *(Continued)*

Concomitant drug class/name	NNRTI	Effect on NNRTI or concomitant drug concentrations	Dosing recommendations and clinical comments
Narcotics/treatment for opioid dependence			
Buprenorphine	EFV	Buprenorphine AUC ↓ 50%, norbuprenorphine AUC ↓ 71%	No withdrawal symptoms have been reported. No dosage adjustment is recommended, but monitor for withdrawal symptoms.
	ETR	Buprenorphine AUC ↓ 25%	No dosage adjustment is necessary.
	NVP	No significant effect	No dosage adjustment is necessary.
Methadone	EFV	Methadone AUC ↓ 52%	Opioid withdrawal is common; increased methadone dose is often necessary.
	ETR	No significant effect	No dosage adjustment is necessary.
	NVP	Methadone AUC ↓ 37–51%: NVP; no significant effect	Opioid withdrawal is common; increased methadone dose is often necessary.
	RPV	R-methadone AUC ↓ 16%	No dosage adjustment is necessary, but monitor for withdrawal symptoms.
Phosphodiesterase type 5 (PDE5) inhibitors			
Sildenafil	ETR	Sildenafil AUC ↓ 57%	Sildenafil dose may need to be increased on the basis of clinical effect.
	RPV	Sildenafil ↔	No dosage adjustment is necessary.
Tadalafil	ETR	↓ tadalafil possible	May need to increase tadalafil dose based on clinical effect.
Vardenafil	ETR	↓ vardenafil possible	May need to increase vardenafil dose based on clinical effect.
Miscellaneous interactions			
Atovaquone/proguanil	EFV	↓ atovaquone AUC 75% ↓ proguanil AUC 43%	There is no dosage recommendation. Consider alternative drug for malaria prophylaxis, if possible.

ARV, antiretroviral; AUC, area under the curve; HMG-CoA, 3-hydroxy-3-methyl-glutaryl-coenzyme A; INR, international normalized ratio; RTV, ritonavir.

Table 35-6. Protease Inhibitors

Generic name (abbreviation)—trade name	Formulations	Dosing recommendations	Metabolism	Storage	Adverse events[a]
Atazanavir (ATV)—Reyataz	100, 150, 200, 300 mg capsules	ART-naïve: 400 mg once daily or ATV 300 mg + RTV 100 mg once daily; with TDF or in ART-experienced patients: ATV 300 mg + RTV 100 mg once daily With EFV in ART-naïve patients: ATV 400 mg + RTV 100 mg once daily Take with food.	CYP3A4[b] Dosage adjustment recommended in patients with hepatic insufficiency Normal GI acid concentrations needed for absorption; drug interactions with PPIs, histamine-2 blockers, and antacids	Room temperature	Indirect hyperbilirubinemia, prolonged PR interval (some patients experienced asymptomatic first-degree atrioventricular block); use with caution in patients with underlying conduction defects or on concomitant medications that can cause PR prolongation; nephrolithiasis; skin rash ↑ LFTs
Darunavir (DRV)—Prezista	75, 150, 300, 400, 600 mg tablets	ART-naïve or ART-experienced with no DRV mutations: DRV 800 mg + RTV 100 mg once daily; ART-experienced with at least one DRV mutation: DRV 600 mg + RTV 100 mg twice daily Take with food.	CYP3A4 inhibitor and substrate[b]	Room temperature	Rash (10%): DRV has a sulfonamide moiety; Stevens–Johnson syndrome and erythema multiforme have been reported; hepatotoxicity; GI intolerance; headache; ↑ LFTs
Fosamprenavir (FPV)—Lexiva (a pro-drug of amprenavir; APV)	700 mg tablet; 50 mg/mL oral suspension	ART-naïve: FPV 1,400 mg twice daily or FPV 1,400 mg + RTV 100–200 mg once daily or FPV 700 mg + RTV 100 mg twice daily PI-experienced patients: FPV 700 mg + RTV 100 mg twice daily With EFV: FPV 700 mg + RTV 100 mg twice daily or FPV 1,400 mg + RTV 300 mg once daily	CYP3A4 inhibitor, inducer, and substrate[b] Dosage adjustment recommended in patients with hepatic insufficiency	Room temperature	Skin rash (12–19%); FPV has a sulfonamide moiety; GI intolerance, headache, ↑ LFTs, nephrolithiasis

(continued)

Table 35-6. Protease Inhibitors *(Continued)*

Generic name (abbreviation)—trade name	Formulations	Dosing recommendations	Metabolism	Storage	Adverse events[a]
		Tablet: Take without regard to meals (if not boosted with RTV tablet). Suspension: Take without food. FPV with RTV tablet: Take with meals.			
Indinavir (IDV)—Crixivan	100, 200, 400 mg capsules	800 mg every 8 hours Take 1 hour before or 2 hours after meals; may take with skim milk or low-fat meal. IDV 800 mg + RTV 100–200 mg twice daily without regard to meals	CYP3A4 inhibitor and substrate Dosage adjustment recommended in patients with hepatic insufficiency	Room temperature	Nephrolithiasis: Drink 48 oz water daily to ↓ incidence. GI intolerance, hepatitis, indirect hyperbilirubinemia, headache, asthenia, blurred vision, dizziness, rash, metallic taste, thrombocytopenia, alopecia, hemolytic anemia
Lopinavir + ritonavir (LPV/r)—Kaletra	Tablets: LPV 200 mg + RTV 50 mg or LPV 100 mg + RTV 25 mg Oral solution: Each 5 mL contains LPV 400 mg + RTV 100 mg. Oral solution: 42% alcohol	LPV/r 400/100 mg twice daily or LPV/r 800/200 mg once daily Once-daily dosing is not recommended for patients with >3 LPV-associated mutations; pregnant women; or patients receiving EFV, NVP, FPV, NFV, carbamazepine, phenytoin, or phenobarbital. With EFV or NVP: LPV/r 500/125 mg tablet twice daily or LPV/r 533/133 mg oral solution twice daily Tablet: Take without regard to meals. Oral solution: Take with food.	CYP3A4 inhibitor and substrate	Tablet is stable at room temperature. Oral solution should be refrigerated and is stable for up to 2 months at room temperature.	GI intolerance, pancreatitis, asthenia, ↑ LFTs, PR interval prolongation, QT interval prolongation, and torsades de pointes have been reported; however, causality could not be established.

Drug	Dosage forms	Dosing recommendations	Metabolism	Storage	Adverse effects
Nelfinavir (NFV)—Viracept	250, 625 mg tablets; 50 mg/g oral powder	1,250 mg twice daily or 750 mg three times a day. Dissolve tablets in a small amount of water, mix well, and consume immediately. Take with food.	CYP2C19 and CYP3A4 substrate. Metabolized to active M8 metabolite; CYP3A4 inhibitor	Room temperature	Diarrhea, ↑ LFTs
Ritonavir (RTV)—Norvir	100 mg tablets; 100 mg soft gel capsules; 80 mg/mL oral solution. Oral solution: 43% alcohol	As pharmacokinetic booster for other PIs: 100–400 mg per day in one or two divided doses. Tablets: Take with food. Capsule and oral solution: To improve tolerability, take with food if possible.	CYP3A4 greater than 2D6 substrate; potent CYP3A4 and 2D6 inhibitor	Tablets: room temperature. Capsules: refrigeration, but can be left at room temperature up to 30 days. Oral solution: room temperature	GI intolerance, paresthesias (circumoral and extremities), hepatitis, asthenia, taste perversion
Saquinavir (SQV)—Invirase	500 mg tablets; 200 mg hard gel caps	SQV 1,000 mg + RTV 100 mg twice daily. Unboosted SQV is not recommended. Take with meals or within 2 hours after a meal.	CYP3A4 inhibitor and substrate	Room temperature	GI intolerance, headache, ↑ LFTs, PR interval prolongation, QT interval prolongation, and torsades de pointes have been reported. Patients with pre-SQV QT interval > 450 msec should not receive SQV.
Tipranavir (TPV)—Aptivus	250 mg capsules; 100 mg/mL oral solution	TPV 500 mg + RTV 200 mg twice daily. Unboosted TPV is not recommended. With RTV tablets: Take with meals. With RTV caps or solution: Take without regard to meals.	CYP3A4 inducer and substrate. Net effect when combined with RTV—CYP3A4, 2D6	Capsules: refrigeration; remain stable at room temperature for up to 60 days. Oral solution: room temperature; should be used within 60 days of opening bottle	Hepatotoxicity: clinical hepatitis (including hepatic decompensation and hepatitis-associated fatalities) has been reported. Skin rash has occurred (3–21%). TPV has a sulfonamide moiety; use with caution in patients with known allergy. Rare cases of fatal and nonfatal intracranial hemorrhages have been reported. Risks include brain lesion, head trauma, recent neurosurgery, coagulopathy, hypertension, alcoholism, use of anti-coagulant or antiplatelet agents including vitamin E.

GI, gastrointestinal; LFT, liver function test; PPI, proton pump inhibitor.
a. Class side effects of all PIs: hyperlipidemia, particularly hypertriglyceridemia, hyperglycemia, fat maldistribution, possible increased bleeding episodes in patients with hemophilia.
b. See Tables 35-7 and 35-8.

All should be dose adjusted for hepatic impairment. Most should be taken with food (except fosamprenavir, tipranavir, lopinavir/ritonavir tablets, and indinavir). Atazanavir and indinavir require normal acid levels in the stomach for absorption and are associated with kidney stone formation and increases in indirect bilirubin. Darunavir, fosamprenavir, and tipranavir contain sulfa. Caution is warranted for patients with a history of severe sulfa allergies.

Most PIs are CYP3A4 inhibitors. Ritonavir is the most potent inhibitor in the class and is primarily used for intensification of other PIs. See Tables 35-7 and 35-8 for more information about drug interactions.

Ritonavir capsules, lopinavir/ritonavir solution, and tipranavir should be refrigerated.

Goals of intensification are as follows:

- Decrease pill burden
- Decrease frequency of doses (i.e., decrease from q8h to q12h)
- Increase drug levels, resulting in decreased resistance

Class toxicities are as follows:

- Fat maldistribution
- Hyperglycemia
- Hyperlipidemia
- Possible increased bleeding episodes in patients with hemophilia

Baseline PI monitoring is done 4–6 weeks after starting the PI. Monitoring should then take place every 3–6 months thereafter. The following tests are required:

- Glucose test
- Liver function tests (LFTs)
- Total cholesterol panel (particularly triglycerides)
- Signs and symptoms of gastrointestinal (GI) side effects
- Signs and symptoms of fat redistribution

Usually, one PI (boosted PIs preferred) is used in combination with two NRTIs.

Entry inhibitors

Entry inhibitors include enfuvirtide (T20) and maraviroc. Enfuvirtide is a fusion inhibitor, whereas maraviroc is a CCR5 (chemokine [C-C motif] receptor 5) antagonist. See Table 35-9 for information.

Enfuvirtide (T20) (Fuzeon)

Enfuvirtide's mechanism of action is to bind to glycoprotein 41 on the HIV surface, thus inhibiting HIV binding to the CD4 cell.

The dose is 90 mg subcutaneous every 12 hours. Side effects include injection-site reactions, an increased rate of bacterial pneumonia, and hypersensitivity.

Enfuvirtide is generally reserved for deep salvage regimens. Preferably, it should be used with at least two other active drugs. Resistance develops quickly with less potent regimens and in cases of poor adherence.

No known significant drug interactions have been seen to date. Enfuvirtide can be taken without regard to meals. It should be stored at room temperature; the reconstituted form should be stored in the refrigerator, where it will be stable for 24 hours.

Maraviroc (Selzentry)

Maraviroc's mechanism of action is to bind to CCR5 receptors on the CD4 cell surface, which inhibits HIV binding and entry into the CD4 cell.

Perform Trofile testing before using maraviroc to determine the patient's tropism. The patient must be CCR5 tropic only.

Maraviroc is a CYP3A4 substrate. The dose depends on drug reactions:

- Use 150 mg po every 12 hours when giving maraviroc with strong CYP3A4 inhibitors (most PIs).
- Use 300 mg po every 12 hours when giving maraviroc with enfuvirtide, tipranavir/ritonavir, nevirapine, or weak CYP3A4 inhibitors.
- Use 600 mg po every 12 hours when giving with CYP3A4 inducers (efavirenz, rifampin, etc.).

Side effects include abdominal pain, cough, dizziness, musculoskeletal symptoms, pyrexia, rash, upper respiratory tract infections, hepatotoxicity, and orthostatic hypotension.

Preferably, use maraviroc with at least two other active drugs. Take it without regard to meals.

Integrase strand transfer inhibitors

INSTIs include raltegravir (Isentress), dolutegravir (Tivicay), and elvitegravir (available only in combination tablet Stribild) (Table 35-10). INSTIs block activity of the integrase enzyme, thereby preventing HIV DNA from meshing with the CD4 cell DNA. INSTIs chelate with cations and should be separated from medications that contain them.

Table 35-7. Drugs That Should Not Be Used with PIs

Drug category	Saquinavir + ritonavir	Darunavir + ritonavir	Tipranavir + ritonavir	Fosamprenavir +/− ritonavir	Lopinavir + ritonavir	Atazanavir +/− ritonavir
Antimycobacterials	Rifampin, rifapentine	Rifampin, rifapentine	Rifampin, rifapentine	Rifampin, rifapentine	Rifampin, rifapentine	Rifampin, rifapentine
Antiretrovirals	None	None	Etravirine	Etravirine	None	Etravirine, nevirapine
Cardiac agents	Amiodarone, dofetilide, flecainide, lidocaine, propafenone, quinidine	None	Amiodarone, flecainide, propafenone, quinidine	Flecainide, propafenone	None	None
Ergot alkaloids (vasoconstrictor)	Ergot derivatives	Ergot derivatives	Ergot derivatives	Ergot derivatives	Ergot derivatives	Ergot derivatives
GI drugs	Cisapride	Cisapride	Cisapride	Cisapride	Cisapride	Cisapride
Herbs	St. John's wort, garlic supplements	St. John's wort	St. John's wort	St. John's wort	St. John's wort	St. John's wort
Lipid-lowering agents	Simvastatin, lovastatin	Simvastatin, lovastatin	Simvastatin, lovastatin	Simvastatin, lovastatin	Simvastatin, lovastatin	Simvastatin, lovastatin
Neuroleptics	Pimozide	Pimozide	Pimozide	Pimozide	Pimozide	Pimozide
Psychotropics	Midazolam, triazolam, trazodone	Midazolam, triazolam	Midazolam, triazolam	Midazolam, triazolam	Midazolam, triazolam	Midazolam, triazolam
Other	Alfuzosin, salmeterol, sildenafil for pulmonary arterial hypertension	Alfuzosin, salmeterol, sildenafil for pulmonary arterial hypertension	Alfuzosin, salmeterol, sildenafil for pulmonary arterial hypertension	Alfuzosin, salmeterol, sildenafil for pulmonary arterial hypertension	Alfuzosin, salmeterol, sildenafil for pulmonary arterial hypertension	Alfuzosin, salmeterol, sildenafil for pulmonary arterial hypertension

Table 35-8. Drug Interactions with PIs Requiring Dose Modifications or Cautious Use

Concomitant drug	PI	Effect on PI or concomitant drug concentrations	Dosing recommendations and clinical comments
Acid reducers			
Antacids	ATV +/− RTV	When given simultaneously, ↓ ATV expected	Give ATV at least 2 hours before or 1 hour after antacids or buffered medications.
	FPV	APV AUC ↓ 18%; no significant change in APV C_{min}	Give FPV simultaneously with or at least 2 hours before or 1 hour after antacids.
	TPV/r	TPV AUC ↓ 27%	Give TPV at least 2 hours before or 1 hour after antacids.
H₂-receptor antagonists	RTV-boosted PIs		
	ATV/r	↓ ATV	H₂-receptor antagonist dose should not exceed a dose equivalent to famotidine 40 mg twice daily in ART-naïve patients or 20 mg twice daily in ART-experienced patients.
			Give ATV 300 mg + RTV 100 mg simultaneously with or more than 10 hours after the H₂-receptor antagonist.
	PIs without RTV		
	ATV	↓ ATV	H₂-receptor antagonist single dose should not exceed a dose equivalent of famotidine 20 mg or total daily dose equivalent of famotidine 20 mg twice daily in ART-naïve patients. Give ATV at least 2 hours before and at least 10 hours after the H₂-receptor antagonist.
	FPV	APV AUC ↓ 30%; no significant change in APV C_{min}	Give FPV at least 2 hours before H₂-receptor antagonist if concomitant use is necessary. Consider boosting with RTV.
Proton pump inhibitors (PPIs)	ATV	↓ ATV	PPIs are not recommended in patients receiving unboosted ATV.
	ATV/r	↓ ATV	PPIs should not exceed a dose equivalent to omeprazole 20 mg daily in PI-naïve patients. PPIs should be administered at least 12 hours before ATV/r. PPIs are not recommended in PI-experienced patients.
	TPV/r	↓ omeprazole	May need to ↑ omeprazole dose.
	SQV/r	SQV AUC ↑ 82%	Monitor for SQV toxicities.
Anticoagulants			
Warfarin	ATV +/− RTV, DRV/r, FPV +/− RTV, LPV/r, SQV/r, TPV/r	↑ or ↓ warfarin possible, DRV/r ↓ S-warfarin AUC 21%	Monitor INR closely when stopping or starting PI, and adjust warfarin dose accordingly.
Anticonvulsants			
Carbamazepine	RTV-boosted PIs		
	ATV/r, FPV/r, LPV/r, SQV/r, TPV/r	↑ carbamazepine possible, may ↓ PI levels substantially	Consider alternative anticonvulsant or monitor levels of both drugs, and assess virologic response. Do not co-administer with LPV/r once daily.
	DRV/r	Carbamazepine AUC ↑ 45%, no change in DRV levels	Monitor anticonvulsant level, and adjust dose accordingly.
	PIs without RTV		
	ATV, FPV	May ↓ PI levels substantially	Monitor anticonvulsant level and virologic response. Consider alternative anticonvulsant, RTV boosting for ATV and FPV, and/or monitoring of PI level.

Table 35-8. Drug Interactions with PIs Requiring Dose Modifications or Cautious Use *(Continued)*

Concomitant drug	PI	Effect on PI or concomitant drug concentrations	Dosing recommendations and clinical comments
Lamotrigine	LPV/r	Lamotrigine AUC ↓ 50%, LPV no significant change	Titrate lamotrigine dose to effect or consider alternative anticonvulsant. A similar interaction is possible with other RTV-boosted PIs.
Phenobarbital	All PIs	May ↓ PI levels substantially	Consider alternative anticonvulsant or monitor levels of both drugs, and assess virologic response. Do not co-administer with LPV/r once daily.
Phenytoin	RTV-boosted PIs		
	ATV/r, DRV/r, SQV/r, TPV/r, LPV/r	↓ phenytoin possible, ↓ PI possible	Consider alternative anticonvulsant or monitor levels of both drugs, and assess virologic response. Do not co-administer with LPV/r once daily
	FPV/r	Phenytoin AUC ↓ 22%, APV AUC ↑ 20%	Monitor phenytoin level, and adjust dose accordingly. No change to FPV/r dose recommended.
	PIs without RTV		
	ATV, FPV	May ↓ PI levels substantially	Consider alternative anticonvulsant, RTV boosting for ATV and FPV, and/or monitoring PI level. Monitor anticonvulsant level and virologic response.
Valproic acid (VPA)	LPV/r	↓ VPA possible, LPV AUC ↑ 75%	Monitor VPA levels and virologic response. Monitor for LPV-related toxicities.
Antidepressants			
Bupropion	LPV/r, TPV/r	↓ bupropion AUC	Titrate bupropion dose based on clinical response.
Paroxetine	DRV/r, FPV/r	↓ paroxetine AUC	Titrate paroxetine dose based on clinical response.
Sertraline	DRV/r	↓ sertraline AUC	Titrate sertraline dose based on clinical response.
Trazodone	ATV +/− RTV, DRV/r, FPV +/− RTV, LPV/r, TPV/r	RTV 200 mg bid (for 2 days), ↑ trazodone AUC 240%	Use lowest dose of trazodone, and monitor for CNS and cardiovascular adverse events.
	SQV/r	↑ trazodone expected	Contraindicated; do not co-administer.
Tricyclic anti-depressants (TCAs)	All RTV-boosted PIs	↑ TCA expected	Use lowest possible TCA dose, and titrate on the basis of clinical assessment and/or drug levels.
Antifungals			
Fluconazole	TPV/r	TPV AUC ↑ 50%	Fluconazole dose > 200 mg daily is not recommended. If high-dose fluconazole is indicated, consider alternative PI or another class of ARV drug.
Itraconazole	RTV-boosted PIs		
	ATV/r, DRV/r, FPV/r, TPV/r	↑ itraconazole possible, ↑ PI possible	Consider monitoring itraconazole level to guide dosage adjustments. High doses (> 200 mg/day) are not recommended unless dose is guided by itraconazole levels.
	LPV/r	↑ itraconazole	Consider not exceeding 200 mg itraconazole daily, or monitor itraconazole level.
	SQV/r	Bidirectional interaction has been observed.	Dose is not established, but decreased itraconazole dosage may be warranted. Consider monitoring itraconazole levels.
	PIs without RTV		
	ATV, FPV	↑ itraconazole possible, ↑ PI possible	Consider monitoring itraconazole level to guide dosage adjustments.
Posaconazole	ATV/r, ATV	ATV AUC ↑	Monitor for adverse effects of ATV.

(continued)

Table 35-8. Drug Interactions with PIs Requiring Dose Modifications or Cautious Use *(Continued)*

Concomitant drug	PI	Effect on PI or concomitant drug concentrations	Dosing recommendations and clinical comments
Voriconazole	ATV/r, DRV/r, FPV/r, LPV/r, SQV/r, TPV/r	RTV ↓ voriconazole AUC	Do not co-administer voriconazole and RTV unless benefit outweighs risk. If administered, consider monitoring voriconazole level, and adjust dose accordingly.
	ATV, FPV	↑ voriconazole possible, ↑ PI possible	Monitor for toxicities.
Clarithromycin	ATV +/− RTV	Clarithromycin AUC ↑ 94%	May cause QTc prolongation. Reduce clarithromycin dose by 50%. Consider alternative therapy.
	DRV/r, FPV/r, LPV/r, SQV/r, TPV/r	↑ clarithromycin AUC	Monitor for clarithromycin-related toxicities, or consider alternative macrolide. Reduce clarithromycin dose by 50% in patients with CrCl 30–60 mL/min. Reduce clarithromycin dose by 75% in patients with CrCl less than 30 mL/min.
Rifabutin	ATV +/− RTV, DRV/r, FPV +/− RTV, LPV/r, SQV/r, TPV/r	↑ rifabutin AUC	Administer rifabutin 150 mg once daily or 300 mg three times a week. Monitor for antimycobacterial activity, and consider therapeutic drug monitoring.
Benzodiazepines			
Alprazolam Diazepam	All PIs	↑ benzodiazepine possible	Consider alternative benzodiazepine, such as lorazepam, oxazepam, or temazepam.
Midazolam Triazolam	All PIs	↑ benzodiazepine expected	Do not co-administer with PIs. Parenteral midazolam can be used with caution as a single dose and can be given in a monitoring situation for procedural sedation.
Cardiac medications			
Bosentan	All PIs	LPV/r ↑ bosentan, ↓ ATV expected	Do not co-administer bosentan and ATV without RTV. Bosentan dose adjustments are required.
Digoxin	RTV, SQV/r	↑ digoxin levels	Use with caution. Monitor digoxin levels and for symptoms of toxicity.
Dihydropyridine calcium channel blockers (CCBs)	All PIs	↑ dihydropyridine possible	Use with caution. Titrate CCB dose, and monitor closely. ECG monitoring recommended if used with ATV.
Diltiazem	ATV +/− RTV	Diltiazem AUC ↑ 125%	Decrease diltiazem dose by 50%. ECG monitoring is recommended.
	DRV/r, FPV +/− RTV, LPV/R, SQV/r, TPV/r	↑ diltiazem possible	Use with caution. Adjust diltiazem according to clinical response and toxicities.
Corticosteroids			
Dexamethasone	All PIs	↓ PI levels possible	Use systemic dexamethasone with caution, or consider alternative corticosteroid for long-term use.
Fluticasone (inhaled or intranasal)	All RTV-boosted PIs	↑ fluticasone AUC and C_{max}	Co-administration can result in adrenal insufficiency, including Cushing's syndrome. Do not co-administer unless potential benefits of inhaled fluticasone outweigh the risks of systemic corticosteroid adverse effects.
Hepatitis C NS3/4A protease inhibitors			
Boceprevir	ATV/r, DRV/r, LPV/r	↓ ATV/r, DRV/r, LPV/r levels; DRV/r and LPV/r ↓ boceprevir levels	Co-administration is not recommended.
Telaprevir	DRV/r, FPV/r, LPV/r	↓ telaprevir levels ↓ DRV/r, FPV/r levels	Co-administration is not recommended.

Table 35-8. Drug Interactions with PIs Requiring Dose Modifications or Cautious Use *(Continued)*

Concomitant drug	PI	Effect on PI or concomitant drug concentrations	Dosing recommendations and clinical comments
Hormonal contraceptives			
Hormonal contraceptives	ATV/r	↓ ethinyl estradiol AUC and C_{min} ↑ norgestimate	Oral contraceptive should contain at least 35 mcg of ethinyl estradiol.
	DRV/r, FPV +/− RTV, LPV/r	↓ ethinyl estradiol ↓ norethindrone	Use alternative or additional contraceptive method.
	SQV/r, TPV/r	↓ ethinyl estradiol	
	ATV	↑ ethinyl estradiol ↑ norethindrone	Use oral contraceptive that contains no more than 30 mcg of ethinyl estradiol or use alternative contraceptive.
HMG-CoA reductase inhibitors			
Atorvastatin	ATV +/− RTV, LPV/r	↑ **atorvastatin**	Titrate **atorvastatin** dose carefully, and use lowest dose necessary.
	DRV/r, FPV +/− RTV, SQV/r	↑ **atorvastatin**	Titrate **atorvastatin** dose carefully, and use the lowest necessary dose. Do not exceed 20 mg **atorvastatin** daily.
	TPV/r	↑ **atorvastatin**	Do not co-administer
Pravastatin	DRV/r	↑ pravastatin AUC	Use lowest possible starting dose with careful monitoring.
Rosuvastatin	ATV/r, LPV/r	↑ rosuvastatin AUC and C_{max}	Titrate rosuvastatin dose carefully. Do not exceed 10 mg rosuvastatin daily.
	DRV/r, SQV/r	↑ rosuvastatin AUC and C_{max}	Titrate rosuvastatin dose carefully. Use the lowest necessary dose while monitoring for toxicities.
Narcotics/treatment for opioid dependence			
Buprenorphine	ATV	↑ buprenorphine AUC ↓ ATV levels	Do not co-administer buprenorphine with unboosted ATV.
	ATV/r, DRV/r	↑ buprenorphine AUC	Monitor for sedation. Buprenorphine dose reduction may be necessary.
	TPV/r	↓ buprenorphine ↓ TPV	Consider monitoring TPV levels.
Methadone	ATV/r, DRV/r, FPV +/− RTV, LPV/r, SQV/r, TPV/r	↓ methadone levels	Opioid withdrawal unlikely but may occur. No adjustment in methadone is usually required, but monitor for opioid withdrawal and increase methadone dose as clinically indicated.
Phosphodiesterase type 5 (PDE5) inhibitors			
Sildenafil	All PIs	↑ sildenafil levels	For treatment of ED: Start with sildenafil 25 mg every 48 hours, and monitor for adverse effects of sildenafil. For treatment of PAH: Contraindicated
Tadalafil	All PIs	↑ tadalafil	For treatment of ED: Start with tadalafil 5 mg dose, and do not exceed a single dose of 10 mg every 72 hours. Monitor for adverse effects of tadalafil. For treatment of PAH: If on a PI more than 7 days—start with tadalafil 20 mg daily and increase to 40 mg daily based on tolerability. If on tadalafil and require a PI—stop tadalafil 24 hours prior to PI initiation, and restart 7 days after PI initiation as above. For treatment of BPH: Maximum daily dose is 2.5 mg daily.

(continued)

Table 35-8. Drug Interactions with PIs Requiring Dose Modifications or Cautious Use *(Continued)*

Concomitant drug	PI	Effect on PI or concomitant drug concentrations	Dosing recommendations and clinical comments
Vardenafil	All PIs	↑ vardenafil levels	Start with vardenafil 2.5 mg every 72 hours, and monitor for adverse effects of vardenafil.
Miscellaneous interactions			
Colchicine	All PIs	↑ colchicine levels	For gout flares: Colchicine 0.6 mg × 1 dose, followed by 0.3 mg 1 hour later. Do not repeat dose for at least 3 days.
			For prophylaxis of gout flares: Colchicine 0.3 mg once daily or every other day.
			Do not co-administer in patients with hepatic or renal impairment.
Salmeterol	All PIs	↑ salmeterol possible	Do not co-administer.
Atovaquone/ proguanil	ATV/r, LPV/r	↓ atovaquone and proguanil	Consider alternative drug for malaria prophylaxis if possible.

BPH, benign prostatic hyperplasia; CrCl, creatinine clearance; ECG, electrocardiogram; ED, erectile dysfunction; PAH, pulmonary arterial hypertension.

Table 35-9. Entry Inhibitors

	Maraviroc (MVC)	Enfuvirtide (T20)
Trade name	Selzentry	Fuzeon
Classification	Entry inhibitor: CCR5 antagonist	Entry inhibitor: fusion inhibitor
Form	150, 300 mg tablets	Injectable, in lyophilized powder to be reconstituted with sterile water
Dosing recommendations	MVC 150 mg po every 12 hours when giving with strong CYP3A4 inhibitors (most PIs)	T20 90 mg/mL injected subcutaneously twice daily; powder should be reconstituted with 1.1 mL sterile water for injection.
	MCV 300 mg po every 12 hours when giving with enfuvirtide, tipranavir/ritonavir, nevirapine, or weak CYP3A4 inhibitors	
	MCV 600 mg po every 12 hours when giving with CYP3A4 inducers (efavirenz, rifampin, etc.)	
Food effect	Take with or without food.	Take with or without food.
Adverse events	Abdominal pain, cough, dizziness, musculoskeletal symptoms, pyrexia, rash, upper respiratory tract infections, hepatotoxicity, orthostatic hypotension	Local injection site reactions, increased bacterial pneumonia, hypersensitivity reactions
Drug interactions	CYP3A4 substrate. Do not use with St. John's wort. Dose adjustments are needed with itraconazole, ketoconazole, voriconazole, carbamazepine, phenobarbital, phenytoin, clarithromycin, rifabutin, rifampin.	Catabolism
Storage	Room temperature	Room temperature; reconstituted solution should be refrigerated and used within 24 hours.
Additional information	Trofile testing should be done before using maraviroc to determine patient's tropism—must be CCR5 tropic only.	

Table 35-10. Integrase Inhibitors

	Raltegravir (RAL)	Elvitegravir (EVG)	Dolutegravir (DTG)
Trade name	Isentress	Stribild	Tivicay
Classification	Integrase inhibitor	2 NRTIs 1 Integrase inhibitor	Integrase inhibitor
Form	400 mg tablets	Elvitegravir 150 mg Cobicistat (COBI) 150 mg Tenofovir 300 mg Emtricitabine 200 mg	50 mg tablets
Dosing recommendations	RAL 400 mg twice daily	One tablet daily	50 mg once daily (no resistance) 50 mg twice daily (certain resistance patterns)
Food effect	Take with or without food.	Take with food.	Take with or without food.
Adverse events	Nausea, headache, diarrhea, pyrexia, creatinine phosphokinase elevation	GI side effects, renal dysfunction, proteinuria (see tenofovir, emtricitabine)	Hypersensitivity, ↑ LFTs in patients with hepatitis C virus or hepatitis B virus, GI side effects, fatigue, hepatitis, myositis, renal impairment, pruritus
Drug interactions	UGT1A1-mediated glucuronidation occurs. Do not give with rifampin. Dose adjustments may be necessary with other medications metabolized by UGT1A1.	COBI: inhibits CYP3A and 2D6, p-glycoprotein, BCRP, OATP1B1, OATP1B3 EVG: modest inducer of CYP2C9 Separate from cations. Drug interactions[a]	Metabolized by UGT1A1 and, to a lesser extent, CYP3A Also blocks the OCT-2 renal transporter Do not give with etravirine, efavirenz, nevirapine, fosamprenavir/ritonavir, tipranavir/ritonavir, anticonvulsants, St. John's wort, or metformin. Separate from cations.
Storage	Room temperature	Room temperature	Room temperature
Additional information		Do not start if CrCl < 70 mL/min. Stop if CrCl < 50 mL/min while on treatment. ↑ SCr > 0.4 mg/dL should be closely monitored for renal safety.	

CrCl, creatinine clearance; SCr, serum creatinine.
a. See Table 35-7.

Raltegravir is metabolized through UDP-glucurono-syltransferase 1A1 (UGT1A1)-mediated glucuronidation. Drug interactions occur with rifampin and other drugs that affect UGT1A1. The dose is 400 mg po every 12 hours. Side effects include nausea, headache, diarrhea, pyrexia, and creatinine phosphokinase (CPK) elevation. Take it without regard to meals.

Dolutegravir is metabolized through UGT1A1 and, to a minor extent, CYP3A. It inhibits the OCT-2 renal transporter; therefore, mild elevations in serum creatinine may be seen. Drug interactions occur with metformin and other drugs that are eliminated through the OCT-2 renal transporter

and with medications that are strong inhibitors or inducers of UGT1A1 (rifampin) or CYP3A (nevirapine, fosamprenavir/ritonavir, tipranavir/ritonavir, anticonvulsants).

Elvitegravir is currently available only in the combination tablet Stribild (tenofovir 300 mg, emtricitabine 200 mg, elvitegravir 150 mg, cobicistat 150 mg) dosed once daily with food. Cobicistat is an inhibitor of CYP3A4 and is used to boost levels of elvitegravir. It has no antiretroviral activity. Cobicistat inhibits tubular secretion of creatinine by blocking the MATE-1 transporter, which increases serum creatinine and decreases creatinine clearance without affecting true glomerular filtration rates (GFRs). Serum creatinine, GFR, urine protein, and urine glucose should be monitored. Stribild should not be initiated in patients with GFR < 70 mL/min and should be discontinued if GFR declines below 50 mL/min after starting. Patients who experience a confirmed increase in serum creatinine of > 0.4 mg/dL from baseline should be closely monitored for renal safety. Do not give with other renally toxic medications. Use caution with other medications affecting or affected by CYP3A4.

Potential Benefits of Early Therapy

- Maintenance of a higher CD4 cell count and prevention of potentially irreversible damage to the immune system
- Decreased risk for HIV-associated complications that can sometimes occur at CD4 cell count > 350 cells/mm^3, including tuberculosis, non-Hodgkin's lymphoma, Kaposi's sarcoma, peripheral neuropathy, human papillomavirus–associated malignancies, and HIV-associated cognitive impairment
- Decreased risk of nonopportunistic conditions, including cardiovascular disease, renal disease, liver disease, and malignancies and infections that are not associated with AIDS
- Decreased risk of HIV transmission to others, which will have positive public health implications

Potential Risks of Early Therapy

- Development of treatment-related side effects and toxicities
- Development of drug resistance because of incomplete viral suppression, resulting in the loss of future treatment options
- Less time for the patient to learn about HIV and its treatment and less time to prepare for the need for adherence to therapy
- Increased total time on medication, with a greater chance of treatment fatigue
- Premature use of therapy before the development of more effective, less toxic, or better-studied combinations of antiretroviral drugs
- Transmission of drug-resistant virus in patients who do not maintain full virologic suppression

Counseling

All patients should be counseled on the importance of adherence. Greater than 95% adherence is necessary to decrease the incidence of resistance. Patients should be given tools to facilitate adherence to complicated regimens (e.g., pillboxes, calendars, pagers, etc.).

Patients should be counseled on class side effects, especially any that are unique or potentially serious. Patients should also be counseled concerning important drug interactions (prescription, over-the-counter, herbal, vitamin, and natural remedies) that could affect their regimen (e.g., proton pump inhibitors, H2 blockers, antacids with atazanavir and rilpivirine, and cations with dolutegravir and elvitegravir) and any food requirements or restrictions.

Antiretroviral Therapy in the HIV-Infected Pregnant Woman

All pregnant HIV-infected women should receive combination antiretroviral regimens to prevent perinatal transmission regardless of viral load or CD4 cell count. Preferred regimens include two nucleosides (abacavir/lamivudine, tenofovir and emtricitabine or lamivudine, or zidovudine/lamivudine) combined with a boosted PI (atazanavir/ritonavir or lopinavir/ritonavir) or NNRTI (efavirenz, which may be initiated after 8 weeks of pregnancy). Transmission rates can be reduced to less than 1% in women treated with combination therapy, and undetectable viral loads can be maintained for the majority of the pregnancy. If possible, regimens should be given during labor and delivery. IV zidovudine during labor is now recommended only if the viral load of the woman is above 1,000 copies/mL at delivery time. The 6-week neonatal component of the zidovudine chemoprophylaxis regimen is generally recommended for all HIV-exposed neonates to reduce perinatal transmission of HIV.

Guidelines for prevention of vertical transmission can be located as a living document at www.aidsinfo.nih.gov, which is updated regularly.

Postexposure Prophylaxis

General guidelines

Universal precautions should be taken. The most common infectious exposure is through needlesticks or cuts (1 in 300 risk). The risk with mucous membrane exposure is much lower (1 in 1,000 risk).

Postexposure prophylaxis (PEP) can reduce HIV infection by about 80%. Start therapy within 72 hours of exposure. The length of therapy is 4 weeks. The preferred treatment regimen is with tenofovir/emtricitabine and raltegravir.

Guidelines for PEP can be located as a living document at www.aidsinfo.nih.gov, which is updated regularly.

Nonoccupational PEP

Patients with exposure to HIV through a known positive source, such as sexual exposure or injection drug use, should receive nonoccupational PEP (nPEP) within 72 hours of the exposure. The length of therapy is 28 days. Figure 35-1 provides an algorithm for evaluation and treatment when nonoccupational exposure occurs. Table 35-11 describes nPEP antiretroviral regimens.

Opportunistic Infections

Only two opportunistic infections require primary prophylaxis:

- **Pneumocystis jiroveci *pneumonia (PCP)*:** Treatment is required when CD4 cell count falls below 200/mm^3. The treatment of choice is trimethoprim-sulfamethoxazole (TMP-SMX) DS po daily (see Table 35-12 for alternatives).
- **Mycobacterium avium *complex (MAC) bacteremia*:** Treatment is required when CD4 cell count falls below 50/mm^3. Azithromycin 1,200 mg po every week is the treatment of choice.

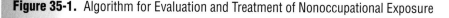

Figure 35-1. Algorithm for Evaluation and Treatment of Nonoccupational Exposure

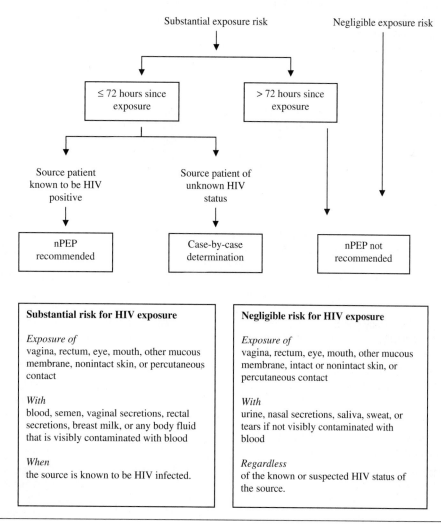

Table 35-11. nPEP Antiretroviral Regimens

Type of regimen	Substantial exposure risk	Negligible exposure risk
Preferred	Zidovudine + lamivudine or emtricitabine	Lopinavir/ritonavir
	Tenofovir + lamivudine or emtricitabine	Efavirenz
Alternative	Stavudine + lamivudine or emtricitabine	Atazanavir +/– ritonavir
	Didanosine + lamivudine or emtricitabine	Fosamprenavir +/– ritonavir
	Abacavir + lamivudine or emtricitabine	Indinavir +/– ritonavir
		Saquinavir/ritonavir
		Nelfinavir
Triple NRTI (only when other regimens cannot be used)	Abacavir + lamivudine + zidovudine	

Table 35-12. Opportunistic Infections

Pathogen	Indication	First choice	Alternative regimens	Comments
Pneumocystis jiroveci pneumonia	Prophylaxis: CD4 cell count < 200/mm^3; thrush; unexplained fever ≥ 2 weeks; history of PCP	TMP-SMX	Dapsone, atovaquone, or aerosolized pentamidine	Primary and secondary prophylaxis can be stopped for PCP on immune reconstitution (patients on HAART with CD4 cell count > 200/mm^3 for > 3 months).
	Acute infection	TMP 15–20 mg/kg/day + SMX 75–100 mg/kg/day po or IV × 21 days in 3–4 divided doses	Pentamidine IV, primaquine + clindamycin, dapsone + TMP, or atovaquone	Patients with PO$_2$ < 70 mm Hg or A-a gradient > 35 mm Hg should receive a corticosteroid taper; treatment is for 21 days.
Candida	Treatment	Fluconazole, clotrimazole troches, nystatin suspension, itraconazole, posaconazole, amphotericin B, anidulafungin, caspofungin, micafungin, or voriconazole	Any of the preferred regimens	*Thrush:* treat for 10–14 days; CD4 cell count. *Esophagitis:* treat for 2–3 weeks. Chronic use of azoles might promote development of resistance.
Cryptococcal meningitis	Induction therapy (for at least 2 weeks)	Amphotericin B or lipid formulation amphotericin + flucytosine	Amphotericin B + fluconazole, amphotericin B alone, or fluconazole	Condition is spread through inhalation of soil contaminated with bird droppings. It is very important to manage increased intracranial pressures.
	Consolidation therapy (for at least 8 weeks)	Fluconazole	Itraconazole	
	Maintenance therapy	Fluconazole	Itraconazole	Maintenance therapy is lifelong or until CD4 cell count ≥ 200/mm^3 for > 6 months as a result of ART.

Table 35-12. Opportunistic Infections *(Continued)*

Pathogen	Indication	First choice	Alternative regimens	Comments
Toxoplasmosis	Treatment (for at least 6 weeks)	Pyrimethamine + leucovorin + sulfadiazine	Pyrimethamine + leucovorin + clindamycin or atovaquone or azithromycin, TMP-SMX, atovaquone alone, or atovaquone + sulfadiazine	Condition is spread through raw or under-cooked meat (lamb, beef, pork) and by contact with infected cat feces.
				Dexamethasone may be required if significant cerebral edema is present.
Toxoplasmosis	Chronic maintenance therapy	Pyrimethamine + leucovorin + sulfadiazine	Pyrimethamine + leucovorin + clindamycin or atovaquone	Maintenance therapy is lifelong or until CD4 cell count ≥ 200/mm^3 for > 6 months as a result of ART and patient is free of signs and symptoms.
Histoplasmosis	Induction therapy (treat for at least 2 weeks)	Liposomal amphotericin B or itraconazole	Amphotericin B, amphotericin B lipid complex, or posaconazole	Condition is spread through inhalation of dust particles. Histoplasmosis is found in soils heavily contaminated by avian or bat feces. The Ohio and Mississippi River valleys are endemic areas in the United States.
	Maintenance therapy (for at least 12 months)	Itraconazole	Posaconazole	Maintenance therapy can be stopped after 12 months of treatment, CD4 cell count ≥ 150/mm^3, ART for > 6 months, and urine and serum antigen < 4.1 units.
Mycobacterium avium complex	Treatment and maintenance therapy	Clarithromycin + ethambutol +/− rifabutin	Azithromycin + ethambutol Alternative third drugs: amikacin, streptomycin, ciprofloxacin, levofloxacin, moxifloxacin	Maintenance therapy may be discontinued after 12 months of treatment, CD4 cell count > 100/mm^3 for 6 months on ART after treatment, and patient is asymptomatic.
Mycobacterium avium complex	Primary prophylaxis: generally recommended at CD4 cell count < 50/mm^3	Azithromycin or clarithromycin	Rifabutin or azithromycin + rifabutin	It may be possible to discontinue treatment when CD4 cell count > 100/mm^3 for > 6 months in patients on ART.
Cytomegalovirus retinitis	Treatment (for 21 days)	Intraocular ganciclovir, valganciclovir, foscarnet, or ganciclovir	Cidofovir	Oral ganciclovir should not be used as sole induction therapy.
				Optimization of ART is an important part of initial therapy.
	Maintenance	Valganciclovir or intraocular ganciclovir	Ganciclovir, foscarnet, or cidofovir	Maintenance therapy can be stopped with inactive disease, CD4 cell count > 100–150/mm^3 for 3–6 months in patients on ART.

HAART, highly active antiretroviral therapy.

All other primary prophylaxis occurs only if the patient is antigen-positive or at high risk of exposure to the causative factor. All other opportunistic infections are treated when the patient is diagnosed. After treatment, patients receive suppressive therapy.

Some primary and secondary prophylaxis could possibly be discontinued with immune reconstitution (undetectable viral load and an increase in CD4 cells in response to ART; see Table 35-12).

Immune reconstitution inflammatory syndrome in response to existing or indolent opportunistic infections can sometimes occur when ART is started.

Guidelines for prophylaxis and treatment of opportunistic infections can be located as a living document at www.aidsinfo.nih.gov, which is updated regularly.

35-5. Questions

Use the following case study to answer Questions 1–4:

C. T. is a 23-year-old HIV-positive female who presents to the emergency department with shortness of breath and a fever. Physical exam reveals a temperature of 102°F, heart rate of 100 bpm, and decreased breath sounds in the left lower lobe of lungs. Her chest x-ray is positive for infiltrates in the left lung. She is diagnosed with PCP. She has no previous history of opportunistic infections and is not on any medications at this time (she has not been seen by a health care provider in over a year). Her CD4 cell count is 13 cells/mm^3, and her viral load is 170,198 copies/mL.

1. What is the treatment of choice for C. T.'s PCP?

   A. TMP-SMX DS 2 tabs po q8h for 21 days, then 1 tab po daily
   B. Azithromycin 500 mg po on day 1, then 250 mg po daily indefinitely
   C. Doxycycline 100 mg po twice daily for 7 days, then 100 mg po daily
   D. Clarithromycin 500 mg po twice daily for 10 days, then 250 mg po daily
   E. Vancomycin 1 g IV q12h for 10 days, then TMP-SMX DS po daily

2. Should C. T. receive any other prophylaxis against opportunistic infections?

   A. Yes, against MAC: Zithromax 1,200 mg po weekly
   B. Yes, against thrush: Diflucan 100 mg po daily
   C. Yes, against toxoplasmosis: Bactrim DS 1 tab po every Monday, Wednesday, and Friday
   D. Yes, against CMV: Valcyte 450 mg po every Monday, Wednesday, and Friday
   E. No

3. Six weeks later, C. T. presents to the HIV clinic for follow-up. Her CD4 cell count is 12 cells/mm^3, and her viral load is 140,202 copies/mL. Should C. T. be started on HIV therapy?

   A. Yes; her CD4 cell count is < 200 cells/mm^3, and she has had an opportunistic infection.
   B. Yes; her viral load is > 100,000 copies/mL.
   C. Yes; her Western blot was positive for HIV.
   D. Yes; all patients with HIV should be treated as soon as the diagnosis is made.
   E. No

4. C. T. wishes to be started on HIV therapy. Which of the following would be an appropriate regimen?

   A. Zidovudine + efavirenz + nelfinavir
   B. Zidovudine + stavudine + indinavir
   C. Stavudine + didanosine + fosamprenavir
   D. Tenofovir/emtricitabine + atazanavir + ritonavir
   E. Nelfinavir + indinavir + fosamprenavir

5. HIV can be transmitted by

   A. unprotected sexual contact with an infected person.
   B. sharing of needles or syringes with an infected person.
   C. infected mother to infant (vertical transmission).
   D. transfusion of blood (before 1985).
   E. all of the above.

6. M. J. is 13 weeks pregnant and just tested positive for HIV. Her viral load is 22,434 copies/mL, and her CD4 cell count is 425 cells/mm^3. M. J. wishes to receive treatment for her HIV. Which of the following would be an appropriate regimen for M. J.?

   A. Zidovudine + stavudine + indinavir
   B. Tenofovir/emtricitabine + atazanavir + ritonavir

C. Zidovudine/lamivudine + nelfinavir
D. Stavudine + didanosine + nevirapine
E. No treatment is necessary.

7. Which of the following would be an important drug interaction with Isentress?

   A. Metoprolol
   B. Tums
   C. Citalopram
   D. Sulfamethoxazole/trimethoprim
   E. Truvada

8. R. C. is a nurse in the emergency department. She has just been stuck with a needle that was used for an HIV-positive patient with a known high viral load. Which of the following is true concerning postexposure prophylaxis?

   I.   The regimen should be started within 72 hours of exposure.
   II. R. C. will need to be treated only with zidovudine.
   III. R. C. will need to be treated with a combination of tenofovir/emtricitabine and raltegravir.
   IV. Treatment will continue for 4 weeks.

   A. I, III, and IV only
   B. II only
   C. II, III, and IV only
   D. I and IV only
   E. I, II, and IV only

9. The CD4 cell count relates to

   I.   the activity of the virus.
   II. the status of the immune system.
   III. how much a patient is at risk for acquiring an opportunistic infection.
   IV. when the patient was infected.
   V.   time to death in treated patients.

   A. IV and V only
   B. I, II, and III only
   C. II and III only
   D. II, III, and IV only
   E. I, II, and V only

10. The viral load relates to

    A. the activity of the virus and efficacy of antiretroviral therapy.
    B. the status of the immune system.
    C. when the patient was infected.

D. how much a patient is at risk for acquiring an opportunistic infection.
E. time to death in a treated patient.

11. S. J. presents to the emergency department with extreme flank pain with nausea and vomiting. He is diagnosed with a kidney stone. His past medical history is positive for HIV and diabetes. His medications include indinavir, lamivudine, didanosine, metformin, and dapsone. Which of his medications might have caused his kidney stone?

    A. Indinavir
    B. Lamivudine
    C. Didanosine
    D. Metformin
    E. Dapsone

12. L. L. comes to the clinic with a chief complaint of burning and tingling in his feet that started about 1 month ago. His current medications include nelfinavir, stavudine, lamivudine, sertraline, and gemfibrozil. Which medication might be causing this problem?

    A. Nelfinavir
    B. Stavudine
    C. Lamivudine
    D. Sertraline
    E. Gemfibrozil

13. S. E. presents to the emergency department with a 2-day history of extreme nausea, vomiting, and abdominal pain. Labs reveal elevations in amylase and lipase, and a diagnosis of pancreatitis is made. His medications include nevirapine, tenofovir, didanosine, and amitriptyline. Which of his medications could have caused his pancreatitis?

    A. Nevirapine
    B. Tenofovir
    C. Didanosine
    D. Amitriptyline
    E. All of the above

14. Which HIV medication should not be used until HLA-B*5701 testing has been performed to assess risk for hypersensitivity?

    A. Efavirenz
    B. Ritonavir

C. Zidovudine
D. Abacavir
E. Lamivudine

15. C.J. is starting efavirenz, tenofovir, lamivudine, and TMP-SMX. What should C.J. be counseled about concerning efavirenz?

A. Anemia
B. CNS side effects
C. Neutropenia
D. Renal toxicity
E. Kidney stones

16. Which of the following can cause hepatotoxicity and requires monitoring of liver enzymes at baseline, 2 weeks, 4 weeks, 6 weeks, and then monthly for the first 18 weeks of therapy?

A. Zidovudine
B. Zalcitabine
C. Lopinavir/ritonavir
D. Fosamprenavir
E. Nevirapine

17. Which of the following can cause hyperglycemia, hyperlipidemia (particularly elevations in triglycerides), and lipodystrophy?

A. Lopinavir/ritonavir
B. Delavirdine
C. Didanosine
D. Abacavir
E. Lamivudine

18. Lactic acidosis and hepatic steatosis have been reported with which of these antiretroviral medications?

A. Nevirapine
B. Efavirenz
C. Stavudine
D. Saquinavir
E. Nelfinavir

19. The mechanism of action of nucleoside reverse transcriptase inhibitors is to

A. directly inhibit reverse transcriptase.
B. prevent entry of the proviral DNA into the nucleus of the CD4 cell.
C. cause chain termination, resulting in a defective copy of proviral DNA.

D. prevent entry of HIV into the CD4 cell.
E. prevent cleavage of the newly formed polypeptide chains into viable HIV.

20. The mechanism of action of non-nucleoside reverse transcriptase inhibitors is to

A. prevent cleavage of the newly formed polypeptide chains into viable HIV.
B. prevent entry of HIV into the CD4 cell.
C. prevent entry of the proviral DNA into the nucleus of the CD4 cell.
D. directly inhibit reverse transcriptase.
E. cause chain termination, resulting in a defective copy of proviral DNA.

21. The mechanism of action of protease inhibitors is to

A. cause a defective copy of proviral DNA to be made.
B. prevent entry of the proviral DNA into the nucleus of the CD4 cell.
C. prevent cleavage of the newly formed polypeptide chains into viable HIV.
D. prevent entry of HIV into the CD4 cell.
E. directly inhibit reverse transcriptase.

22. Which of the following medications if used with atazanavir can result in decreased levels and effectiveness of atazanavir?

A. Loratadine
B. Tenofovir
C. Esomeprazole
D. Metoclopramide
E. Glipizide

23. Which of the following opportunistic infections are the only ones requiring primary prophylaxis?

A. PCP and MAC
B. PCP and toxoplasmosis
C. MAC and histoplasmosis
D. MAC and CMV
E. PCP and thrush

24. The antifungal of first choice for maintenance therapy after treatment of cryptococcal meningitis is

A. itraconazole.
B. fluconazole.
C. ketoconazole.
D. amphotericin B.
E. terbinafine.

25. The first-choice antifungal for treatment of histoplasmosis is

A. itraconazole.
B. fluconazole.
C. ketoconazole.
D. caspofungin.
E. terbinafine.

35-6. Answers

1. **A.** The treatment of choice for PCP is TMP-SMX in patients who are not allergic to sulfa medications. Duration of treatment is 21 days. Because this patient's CD4 cell count is < 200 cells/mm³ and she has had PCP, she will require secondary prophylaxis once treatment is completed. Preferred prophylaxis is once-daily TMP-SMX DS.

2. **A.** This patient's CD4 cell count is < 50 cells/mm³; therefore, she requires primary prophylaxis against MAC. Zithromax is the drug of choice. Prophylaxis against other opportunistic infections is generally not required.

3. **A.** Current guidelines state that any patient who has had an opportunistic infection or a CD4 cell count < 200 cells/mm³ should start treatment for HIV. This patient has had both.

4. **D.** Most regimens contain two NRTIs and either one PI or one NNRTI. Answer A includes one NRTI, one NNRTI, and one PI. Answer E includes three PIs. Zidovudine and stavudine competitively inhibit each other and would not be used in the same regimen (thus, Answer B is incorrect). Didanosine and stavudine should not be used together because of increased toxicity (which makes Answer C incorrect).

5. **E.** All items are important risk factors for transmission of HIV. Breast-feeding, history of sexually transmitted diseases, occupational exposure

to HIV-infected fluids (rare), and household exposure to HIV-infected fluids (rare) are also risk factors.

6. **B.** All HIV-positive pregnant women should receive treatment for HIV to decrease the risk of transmission to their offspring. Zidovudine and stavudine competitively inhibit each other and should not be used together. Nelfinavir is an unboosted PI and is not recommended in pregnancy. Stavudine and didanosine together are contraindicated in pregnancy because of increased risk of lactic acidosis and liver damage.

7. **B.** Integrase inhibitors chelate with cations and should be separated from medications that contain them.

8. **A.** The approved regimen for postexposure prophylaxis is tenofovir/emtricitabine and raltegravir. Treatment should continue for 4 weeks and should start within 72 hours of exposure.

9. **C.** CD4 cell count describes the status of the immune system (i.e., how much a patient is at risk for acquiring an opportunistic infection).

10. **A.** Viral load relates to the activity of the virus and efficacy of antiretroviral therapy. The goal of therapy is an undetectable viral load (< 50 copies/mL).

11. **A.** Indinavir can cause kidney stones. Patients should drink at least 48 oz of water a day to decrease the risk of developing a kidney stone.

12. **B.** The "D" drugs, d4T (stavudine) and ddI (didanosine), can cause peripheral neuropathy and pancreatitis.

13. **C.** The "D" drugs, d4T (stavudine) and ddI (didanosine), can cause peripheral neuropathy and pancreatitis.

14. **D.** HLA-B*5701 testing should be performed prior to use of abacavir to assess risk of hypersensitivity.

15. **B.** Efavirenz can cause central nervous system (CNS) side effects such as dizziness, trouble sleeping, drowsiness, trouble concentrating, and unusual dreams during the first 2–4 weeks of treatment.

16. **E.** All NNRTIs can cause hepatotoxicity. There have been rare reports of hepatotoxicity after just one dose of nevirapine. Liver enzymes should be monitored at baseline, 2 weeks, 4 weeks, 6 weeks, and then monthly for the first 18 weeks of therapy.

17. **A.** Class side effects of PIs include hyperglycemia, hyperlipidemia, fat maldistribution, and increased bleeding in hemophiliacs.

18. **C.** Class side effects of NRTIs include lactic acidosis and hepatic steatosis.

19. **C.** NRTIs affect reverse transcriptase by causing chain termination, resulting in a defective copy of proviral DNA.

20. **D.** NNRTIs affect reverse transcriptase by directly inhibiting reverse transcriptase, resulting in less proviral DNA being made.

21. **C.** PIs prevent cleavage of the newly formed polypeptide chains into viable HIV, resulting in an immature virus that is unable to infect other CD4 cells.

22. **C.** Atazanavir levels are decreased by proton pump inhibitors, H_2 blockers, and antacids.

23. **A.** PCP requires primary prophylaxis when the CD4 cell count falls below 200 cells/mm^3. The preferred medication is TMP-SMX. MAC requires primary prophylaxis when the CD4 cell count falls below 50 cells/mm^3. The preferred medication is azithromycin.

24. **B.** Generally, cryptococcal meningitis is initially treated with amphotericin B during the induction phase and then fluconazole for the consolidation phase and maintenance therapy.

25. **A.** Histoplasmosis is generally initially treated with amphotericin B or itraconazole for induction therapy and then itraconazole for maintenance therapy.

35-7. References

Bartlett JG, Gallant JE. 2003 *Medical Management of HIV Infection*. Baltimore, MD: Johns Hopkins University Press; 2008:357–60.

Carr A, Miller J, Law M, et al. A syndrome of lipoatrophy, lactic acidaemia, and liver dysfunction associated with HIV nucleoside analog therapy: Contribution to protease inhibitor–related lipodystrophy syndrome. *AIDS*. 2000;14:F25–32.

Carr A, Samars K, Thorisdottir A, et al. Diagnosis, prediction, and natural course of HIV-1 protease inhibitor associated lipodystrophy, hyperlipidaemia, and diabetes mellitus: A cohort study. *Lancet*. 1999;353:2093–99.

Centers for Disease Control and Prevention. 1993 revised classification system for HIV infection and expanded surveillance case definition for AIDS among adolescents and adults. *MMWR*. 1992;41:1–19.

Centers for Disease Control and Prevention, Perinatal HIV Guidelines Working Group. Public Health Service Task Force recommendations for the use of antiretroviral drugs in pregnant women infected with HIV-1 for maternal health and for reducing perinatal HIV-1 transmission in the United States. *MMWR*. 1998;47:1–30.

Chaisson RE, Keruly JC, Moore RD. Association of initial CD4 cell count and viral load with response to highly active antiretroviral therapy. *JAMA*. 2000;284:3128–29.

Chesney MA. Factors affecting adherence to antiretroviral therapy. *Clin Infect Dis*. 2000;30(suppl 2): S171–76.

Finzi D, Hermankova M, Pierson T, et al. Identification of a reservoir for HIV-1 in patients on highly active antiretroviral therapy. *Science*. 1997;278:1295–300.

Furret H, Egger M, Opravil M, et al. Discontinuation of primary prophylaxis against *Pneumocystis carinii* pneumonia in HIV-1 infected adults treated with combination antiretroviral therapy: Swiss HIV Cohort Study. *N Engl J Med*. 1999;340:1301–6.

Hoen B, Dumon B, Harzic M, et al. Highly active antiretroviral treatment initiated early in the course of symptomatic primary HIV-1 infections: Results of the ANRS 053 trial. *J Infect Dis*. 1999;180: 1342–46.

Mellors JW, Munoz A, Giorgi JV, et al. Plasma viral load and CD4 lymphocytes as prognostic markers of HIV-1 infections. *Ann Intern Med*. 1997;126:946–54.

National Institutes of Health. Report of the NIH panel to define principles of therapy of HIV infection. *MMWR*. 1998;47(RR-5):1–41.

Sperling RS, Shapiro DE, Coombs RW, et al. Maternal viral load, zidovudine treatment, and the risk of transmission of human immunodeficiency virus type 1 from mother to infant: Pediatric AIDS Clinical Trials Group Protocol 076 Study Group. *N Engl J Med*. 1996;335:1621–29.

U.S. Food and Drug Administration; Health Resources and Services Administration; National Institutes of Health; National Center for HIV, STD, and TB Prevention; National Institute for Occupational Safety and Health; and National Center for Infectious Diseases. Notice to readers update: Provisional Public Health Service recommendations for chemoprophylaxis after occupational exposure to HIV. *MMWR*. 1996;45:468–80.

U.S. Public Health Service and Infectious Diseases Society of America. 1999 USPHS/IDSA guidelines for the prevention of opportunistic infections in persons infected with human immunodeficiency virus. *MMWR*. 1999;48(RR-10):1–67.

Vittinghoff E, Scheer S, O'Malley P, et al. Combination antiretroviral therapy and recent declines in AIDS incidence and mortality. *J Infect Dis*. 1999;179:717–20.

Yeni PG, Hammer SM, Hirsch MS, et al. Treatment for adult HIV infection: 2004 recommendations of the International AIDS Society–USA Panel. *JAMA*. 2004;292:250–65.

Immunization

36

Stephan L. Foster

36-1. Key Points

- The two types of vaccine antigens are (1) live viruses and (2) inactivated viruses or bacterial components.
- There are two types of immunity: active and passive.
- Adverse effects of inactivated vaccines include pain at the injection site and mild systemic symptoms (mild fever). Adverse effects of live vaccines include local injection site reactions and may mimic a mild case of the disease.
- Live vaccines should be avoided during pregnancy and in immunosuppressed persons.
- Influenza viruses undergo shifts and drifts, which account for the need for yearly vaccine changes.
- Wound management must include evaluation for the need for tetanus toxoid and tetanus immune globulin.
- Diphtheria toxoid (DT) and tetanus toxoid should always be given together, unless a contraindication to one of the components exists. If there is a need for one, then there is a need for both.
- A combination vaccine of tetanus, diphtheria, and pertussis (Tdap) is available for use in children over 7 years of age, adolescents, and adults. Children under the age of 7 years receive the pediatric version of the diphtheria, tetanus, and pertussis (DTaP) or DT vaccine (if they are unable to tolerate the pertussis vaccine). Revaccination following the receipt of one dose of Tdap should occur every 10 years with Td.
- The hepatitis B vaccine is now recommended for all infants, starting at birth, as well as all adolescents. Other indications include adults with diabetes and high-risk occupations or behaviors.

- The hepatitis A vaccine is recommended for all children over the age of 1 year and for travel to most parts of the world.
- Inactivated polio vaccine is the only polio vaccine recommended for use in the United States. Oral polio vaccine is not recommended because of the high incidence of vaccine-associated paralytic poliomyelitis.
- A second dose of the measles, mumps, and rubella (MMR) vaccine and the varicella vaccine is recommended at 4–6 years of age.
- Combination vaccines are available to decrease the number of injections.

36-2. Study Guide Checklist

The following topics may guide your study of this topic area:

- Understanding of the immune system
- Type of vaccines
- Reading a vaccine schedule
- Timing and spacing issues
- Contraindications and precautions
- Storage and handling of vaccines
- Knowledge of vaccine-preventable disease
- Vaccine indications and dosages

36-3. Introduction

Definitions

- *Immunity:* A naturally or artificially acquired state resulting in an individual being resistant or relatively resistant to the occurrence or effects of a foreign substance. Immunity is the mechanism the body develops for protection from infectious disease. It is usually very specific to a single organism or to a group of closely related organisms.

- *Antigen:* A live or inactivated substance capable of evoking antibody production; antigens can be a live organism, such as bacteria or virus, or an inactivated or killed organism or portion of an organism. A live organism generally evokes the most effective immune response.
- *Antibody:* A protein evoked by an antigen that acts to eliminate that antigen.

Mechanisms for Acquiring Immunity

Active immunity

Active immunity is produced by an individual's own immune system. Immunity acquired in this manner has a delayed onset and is usually permanent. Active immunity may be acquired by having an active disease or by vaccination. B-lymphocytes (B cells) circulate in the blood and bone marrow for many years. Re-exposure to the antigen causes the cells to replicate and to produce antibody. These cells are also called *memory B cells.*

Passive immunity

Passive immunity is produced by an animal or human and transferred to another. Immunity acquired in this manner has a rapid onset and usually has a brief duration. An infant receives this type of immunity from his or her mother. All types of blood products contain varying amounts of antibody. Immune globulins and hyperimmune globulins are also used to induce passive immunity. One source of passive immunity is antitoxins, which contain antibodies against a known toxin.

36-4. Vaccines

Vaccination is the process of producing active immunity through the use of vaccines. The immunological response is similar to natural infection, with a lower risk than that of the disease itself.

Classification of Vaccines

Live attenuated vaccines

Live vaccines are produced by modifying a virus or bacteria to produce immunity. These vaccines usually do not produce disease, but they may. When disease occurs, it is usually much milder than the natural disease. These vaccines must replicate to be effective. They require special handling, such as protection from heat and light, to keep them alive. Circulating antibodies from another source may destroy the vaccine virus and cause vaccine failure.

The following live vaccines are available in the United States in 2014:

- Herpes zoster
- Influenza (live attenuated)
- Measles
- Mumps
- Rotavirus
- Rubella
- Typhoid oral
- Varicella
- Vaccinia (smallpox)
- Yellow fever

Inactivated vaccines

Inactivated vaccines are composed of all or a fraction of a virus or bacterium. These fractions include subunits (subvirions), bacterial cell wall polysaccharides, conjugated (attached to a protein carrier) bacteria cell wall polysaccharides, or inactivated toxins (toxoids). The bacteria or virus is inactivated using heat, chemicals, or both. Inactivated vaccines are not alive and cannot replicate; therefore, they are unable to induce disease. Inactivated antigens are not affected by circulating antibody.

The following inactivated vaccines are available in the United States in 2014:

- Anthrax
- Diphtheria
- *Haemophilus influenzae* type B
- Hepatitis A
- Hepatitis B
- Human papillomavirus
- Influenza (inactivated)
- Japanese encephalitis
- Meningococcal A, C, Y, W-135 polysaccharide
- Meningococcal A, C, Y, W-135 conjugate
- Pertussis, acellular
- Pneumococcal polysaccharide
- Pneumococcal conjugate
- Polio
- Rabies
- Tetanus toxoid
- Typhoid injectable

Vaccination Schedules

Vaccination schedules are available for children, adolescents, and adults from the U.S. Centers for Disease Control and Prevention (CDC). These schedules are updated yearly by the Advisory Committee on Immunization Practices (ACIP) and can be found at www.cdc.gov/vaccines/schedules/index.html. The schedules indicate the best times to administer vaccines. Additional catch-up schedules are available for children and adolescents who are behind in their vaccinations.

The CDC schedules describe intervals between doses of the same vaccine in a series. The minimum interval in a series for most vaccines is 4 weeks. Decreasing the interval may interfere with antibody response and protection. Increasing the interval does not affect vaccine effectiveness. It is never necessary to restart a series except for the oral typhoid vaccine.

Administration of Multiple Vaccines

There are no contraindications to the simultaneous administration of any vaccines. Inactivated and live vaccines may be given in any combination at the same time.

Most live vaccines must be separated from the administration of antibodies, such as blood products and immune globulins. Inactivated vaccines are not affected by circulating antibody.

If two live vaccines are not given at the same time, a 4-week minimal interval must be observed. The exception to this is oral live vaccines (oral typhoid and rotavirus vaccines), which can be administered simultaneously or at any interval with other live vaccines. No specific time interval is necessary between two inactivated vaccines or an inactivated plus a live vaccine.

Vaccine Adverse Reactions

Adverse reactions are any untoward side effects caused by a vaccine.

Local reactions are the most common type of adverse reaction. They include pain, swelling, and redness at the site of injection. They usually occur within minutes to hours of the injection and are usually mild and self-limiting. Systemic adverse reactions include fever, malaise, myalgias, and headache. Systemic adverse reactions are more common following live vaccines and are similar to a mild case of the disease.

Allergic reactions are reactions to the vaccine antigens or to some component of the vaccine. Although rare, these reactions may be life threatening.

Another potential problem is syncope; therefore, it is important to monitor patients for at least 15 minutes following vaccination.

The Vaccine Adverse Events Reporting System is a surveillance system monitored by the CDC, which should be notified within 30 days of an adverse event that requires medical attention.

Contraindications and Precautions

A *contraindication* is a condition that increases the risk of an adverse reaction or decreases the effect of a vaccine.

A *precaution* is a condition that *might* increase the risk of an adverse event or decrease the effect of a vaccine.

Contraindications include the following:

- An anaphylactic reaction to any previous dose of vaccine or to any of its components
- Pregnancy for live vaccines and selected inactivated vaccines
- Immunosuppression for live vaccines
- Active, untreated tuberculosis for live vaccines
- In the case of the diphtheria, tetanus, and acellular pertussis (diphtheria, tetanus, and pertussis [DTaP] or tetanus, diphtheria, and pertussis [Tdap]), encephalopathy that occurred within 7 days of a previous DTaP or Tdap vaccine

Precautions include the following:

- Acute moderate to severe illness
- Recent administration of antibody-containing blood products and live vaccines
- For the Tdap or DTaP vaccine, unstable or evolving neurological disorder
- For the measles, mumps, and rubella (MMR) vaccine, history of thrombocytopenia or thrombocytopenic purpura
- High fever, shock, persistent crying, or seizure caused by a previous dose of DTaP or Tdap
- Guillain–Barré syndrome within 6 weeks of a previous dose of a tetanus-containing vaccine or influenza vaccine

Vaccine Management

- Maintain cold chain from manufacturer until vaccine is administered.
- Follow manufacturers' recommendation for shipping.
- Keep nonfrozen vaccines from freezing during transport.
- Refrigerate or freeze depending on vaccine immediately on arrival.

- Use stand-alone refrigerators and freezers.
  - Monitor temperatures daily.
  - Do not store vaccines in refrigerator door.
  - Store vaccines in the middle of the refrigerator.
  - Stabilize temperature with water bottles in the refrigerator and frozen coolant packs in the freezer.
  - Use a calibrated thermometer in each storage unit, and monitor at least twice a day.
  - Keep a temperature log.
- Perform proper inventory management.
  - Maintain inventory log.
  - Rotate stock.
  - Follow manufacturer's guidelines for shelf life.
  - Check expiration dates.
  - Designate a person to be responsible for vaccines.
  - Train all staff members to recognize vaccine shipment arrivals.
- Follow manufacturers' directions for reconstitution.

36-5. Diseases and Vaccines

Pneumococcal Disease

There are 90 known serotypes of Gram-positive *Streptococcal pneumonia* bacteria with a polysaccharide capsule. Serious primary diseases associated with *S. pneumonia* include pneumonia, sepsis, and meningitis.

Rates of disease

Highest rates are seen in children less than 2 years of age. Other children at high risk include those with asplenia, patients with human immunodeficiency virus (HIV), American Indians and Alaskan Natives, African Americans, and day care attendees. Patients over the age of 50 have fatality rates of 30–60%.

Pneumococcal disease is one of the leading causes of vaccine-preventable diseases. Pneumococcal bacteria are common respiratory tract inhabitants, with estimated asymptomatic carriage rates varying from 5% to 70%. Transmission is through direct person-to-person droplet contamination or auto-inoculation by carriers.

Clinical features include abrupt onset, fever, otitis media, shaking, chills, productive cough, pleuritic chest pain, dyspnea, hypoxia, tachypnea, headaches, lethargy, vomiting, irritability, nuchal rigidity, seizures, coma, and death.

Resistance to antibiotics is up to 40% in some areas of the United States.

23-valent polysaccharide vaccine (Pneumovax-23 by Merck)

The vaccine's effectiveness has been reported to range from 50% to 80% for the prevention of invasive pneumococcal disease, although this rate varies greatly among trials. The vaccine is ineffective in children less than 2 years old.

Indications

- Adults over the age of 65
- Everyone over 2 years of age with certain chronic diseases
- Smokers 19–64 years of age

Dose

The dosage is 0.5 mL intramuscular (IM) or subcutaneous.

Revaccination is recommended in the following cases:

- Patients at high risk of disease if more than 5 years have passed since the previous dose
- Everyone 65 years and older who received an initial dose under the age of 65 and if more than 5 years have passed since the previous dose

Adverse reactions

Adverse reactions include pain, swelling, and redness at the injection site and slight to moderate systemic reactions such as fever and myalgias.

13-valent conjugated polysaccharide vaccine (Prevnar by Pfizer)

The 13-valent pneumococcal conjugate vaccine (PCV13) replaced the 7-valent vaccine in 2010. It contains the same serotypes included in the 7-valent vaccine and adds six additional serotypes.

Indications

- All children less than 2 years of age
- Children 24–59 months of age with high-risk medical conditions
- Approved by the U.S. Food and Drug Administration (FDA) for adults 50 years of age and older; however, it is not recommended by the ACIP for routine use in this age group.
- One dose for all adults who are immunocompromised (e.g., asplenia, cerebrospinal fluid leaks, cochlear implants)

Dose

The usual dose is 0.5 mL administered IM at 2, 4, 6, and 12–15 months of age (see schedules for catch-up recommendations).

Revaccination is not routinely recommended, but high-risk children should receive the 23-valent polysaccharide vaccine after 2 years of age.

Adverse reactions

Adverse reactions include pain, swelling, and redness at the injection site; difficulty moving the limb (rare); and slight to moderate systemic reactions such as fever and myalgias.

Influenza

Influenza is an RNA (ribonucleic acid) virus of the orthomyxovirus family.

Antigenic drift, which is frequent minor changes in the antigenic structure of the virus, can reach epidemic proportions, but not every year. For this reason, yearly adjustments in vaccine formulations are required. All three types (A, B, and C) can undergo drifts.

Antigenic shift, which is major changes in one or both of the major antigens in influenza A, resulting in a different subtype, can cause major pandemics.

Influenza A

Subtypes are based on two surface antigens: hemagglutinin and neuraminidase. Six types of hemagglutinin (H1, H2, H3, H5, H7, H9) cause disease in humans and cause virus attachment to cells. Two types of neuraminidase cause disease in humans (N1, N2) and have a role in viral release from cells.

Influenza A causes moderate to severe disease in all ages and can be transmitted in other animals.

Influenza B

Influenza B has no subgroups but has two distinct genetic lineages (Victoria and Yamagata). It causes milder disease and affects primarily children. It affects only humans.

Influenza C

Influenza C is rarely reported, and many cases are subclinical. No vaccine is available against type C infection.

Influenza disease

Major serious complications in all types include pneumonia, Reye's syndrome (progressive neuro-logical symptoms associated with aspirin use in children), myocarditis, worsening of chronic bronchitis, and death.

Influenza is one of the leading causes of vaccine-preventable disease, with 20,000–40,000 deaths during epidemics. Pandemics could result in the deaths of millions of people. Rates of disease are highest in the elderly (> 65 years of age), children less than 2 years of age, and persons of any age with medical conditions.

Influenza virus penetrates the respiratory epithelial cells and destroys the host. Virus is shed in respiratory secretions for 5–10 days, and transmission is through direct person-to-person droplet contamination or contact. The incubation period is approximately 2 days (range, 1–5 days).

Clinical features include abrupt onset, fever, myalgias, sore throat, nonproductive cough, and headache.

Disease peaks between December and March in the Northern Hemisphere but may occur earlier or later. Year-round cases may be seen in tropical climates.

Resistance to antivirals changes regularly.

Inactive influenza vaccine (Fluvirin and Flucelvax by Novartis; Fluzone, Fluzone High-Dose, and Fluzone Intradermal by Sanofi Pasteur; Fluarix and FluLaval by GlaxoSmithKline; Afluria by CSL, Flublok by Protein Sciences)

All are inactivated split-virus vaccines. They contain three antigens (two type A viruses and one type B virus—trivalent) or four antigens (two type A viruses and two type B viruses—quadrivalent).

Vaccines are named according to the virus type/geographic origin/strain sequence number/year of isolation (hemagglutinin neuraminidase for type A only): for example, A/California/7/2009-like (2009 H1N1) or B/Massachusetts/2/2012-like.

Vaccines are effective in up to 90% of healthy adults, 50–60% of the elderly, and 30–40% of the frail elderly.

Indications

Vaccination is indicated for all persons over 6 months of age unless contraindications exist.

Contraindications

Contraindications include severe allergic reactions to previous dose.

Precautions

Use precaution with moderate to severe illness or a history of Guillain-Barré syndrome within 6 weeks of receipt of a previous dose of influenza vaccine. Patients with egg allergy should be assessed for severity of allergy, and options should be discussed (see ACIP recommendations).

Dose

Normal doses are 6–35 months: 0.25 mL IM (repeat in 1 month if first time); 3–8 years: 0.5 mL (repeat in 1 month if first time); > 8 years: 0.5 mL.

Fluzone by Sanofi Pasteur is indicated for those ≥ 6 months of age. Fluvirin by Novartis is indicated for those ≥ 4 years of age. Fluarix and FluLaval by GlaxoSmithKline is indicated for those ≥ 3 years of age. Afluria by CSL is indicated for those ≥ 9 years of age. Fluzone High-Dose is indicated for adults ≥ 65 years of age, and Fluzone Intradermal is indicated for adults 18–64 years of age.

All influenza vaccines must be shaken prior to use. Revaccination yearly is needed.

Adverse reactions

Adverse reactions include pain, swelling, and redness at the injection site and slight to moderate systemic reactions such as fever, myalgias, chills, and malaise. Severe neurologic reactions are rare.

Intranasal live attenuated influenza vaccine (FluMist by MedImmune)

Intranasal live attenuated influenza vaccine (LAIV) is an attenuated, cold-adapted live influenza vaccine. It is a quadrivalent vaccine with the same antigens as inactivated influenza vaccine. Its efficacy is 86–93%. LAIV must be kept refrigerated. A new formulation of FluMist containing two type A and two type B antigens has been approved by the FDA.

Indications

Indications are similar to those of inactivated vaccine unless contraindications exist:

- Healthy persons 2–49 years of age

Contraindications

With the following contraindications, use inactivated influenza vaccine:

- Children 2–4 years of age with a history of wheezing or asthma
- Persons with chronic medical diseases
- Close contacts of severely immunocompromised persons who require a protective environment

- Pregnant women
- Children receiving aspirin therapy
- Persons with a history of Guillain–Barré syndrome within 6 weeks of a previous dose of influenza vaccine
- Persons with a history of egg allergy

Dose

The dose is 0.1 mL sprayed in each nostril (0.2 mL total). Children age 2–8 years who receive influenza vaccine for the first time need two doses 6–8 weeks apart.

Adverse reactions

Systemic adverse reactions are similar to those of the inactivated vaccine and include nasal congestion, headache, and vomiting.

Tetanus

Tetanus is caused by an exotoxin produced by *Clostridium tetani* and is characterized by generalized rigidity and convulsive spasms of skeletal muscles. It usually involves muscles of the face (lockjaw) and neck.

Complications include laryngospasm, fractures, hypertension, nosocomial infections, pulmonary embolism, aspiration, and death.

Tetanus toxoid vaccine

Tetanus toxoid is usually combined with diphtheria toxoid and pertussis vaccine.

Diphtheria

Diphtheria toxin is produced by *Corynebacterium diphtheriae* and presents with nonspecific upper respiratory infection symptoms that develop into pharyngitis. Two to three days later, a bluish-white membrane starts to form that can cover the entire soft palate. The membrane can turn dark if bleeding occurs, and manipulation of the membrane can result in bleeding. Airway obstruction may occur.

Other complications may include myocarditis, neuritis with paralysis, respiratory failure, and death.

Diphtheria toxoid vaccine

Diphtheria toxoid vaccine is combined with tetanus toxoid and pertussis vaccine. A single-toxoid antigen is not available.

Pertussis

Pertussis, or whooping cough, is caused by *Bordetella pertussis*, which produces a toxin that paralyzes the respiratory cilia and causes inflammation of the respiratory tract.

The presentation of pertussis is in three stages. The first stage is a catarrhal stage with nonspecific upper respiratory infection symptoms. After 1–2 weeks, the paroxysmal stage with the characteristic cough and inspiratory whoop begins and lasts up to 6 weeks. Recovery, the third stage, is gradual, and the cough usually resolves in 2–3 weeks. The presentation in older children and adults may be much milder. They may present with a persistent mild cough that lasts up to 7 days. The illness may appear to be similar to other upper respiratory infections.

Pertussis complications may include pneumonia, encephalopathy, seizures, and death. The overall case fatality rate is 0.2%. Pertussis is cyclical in nature with peaks every 3–5 years. The United States has been experiencing an increasing number of cases, with the latest peak in 2012 of more than 48,000 cases.

Pertussis vaccine

Pertussis vaccine is combined with tetanus toxoid and diphtheria toxoid for children. A single-toxoid antigen is not available. A whole-cell vaccine was developed in the 1930s but is no longer available in the United States. Acellular pertussis vaccine was first licensed in 1991 and has fewer side effects than the whole-cell vaccine. However, it appears to have a shorter duration of protection than the whole-cell vaccine.

Available vaccines

- DTaP (Tripedia and Daptacel by Sanofi Pasteur and Infanrix by GlaxoSmithKline) is indicated for children ages 2 months to 7 years.
- Diptheria toxoid (DT) is available for pediatric patients with a contraindication to pertussis vaccine.
- Tdap (Adacel by Sanofi Pasteur, FDA approved for ages 11–64, and Boostrix by GlaxoSmithKline, approved for > 10 years of age) is indicated for everyone over the age of 10.
- Td (various manufacturers) is recommended for everyone over the age of 7 years following one dose of Tdap.
- The ACIP recommends a single dose of Tdap dose in all children 7 years of age and older and all adults who have not received pertussis vaccination regardless of the interval since their

Table 36-1. Guidelines for Tetanus Wound Management

Vaccination history	Clean minor wounds		All other wounds	
	Td or Tdap[a]	TIG	Td or Tdap[a]	TIG
Unknown or < 3 years since last dose	Yes	No	Yes	Yes
Three or more years since last dose	No[b]	No	No[c]	No

Td, tetanus–diphtheria vaccine; Tdap, tetanus–diphtheria–pertussis vaccine; TIG, tetanus immune globulin.
a. dap should be used if the patient has not previously received Tdap and is 10 years of age or older.
b. Yes, if > 10 years since last dose.
c. Yes, if > 5 years since last dose.

last Td vaccination. Additional recommendations include vaccination of pregnant women during every pregnancy at 27–36 weeks gestation.
- Recommendations for wound management may or may not include Tdap, Td, or tetanus immune globulin (Table 36-1).

Dose

- ***Pediatric dose:*** A 0.5 mL IM dose of DTaP vaccine is given at 2, 4, 6, and 15–18 months of age. A booster dose should be given at 4–6 years.
- ***Adolescent dose:*** A 0.5 mL dose of Tdap of vaccine is given at 11–12 years.
- ***Adult dose:*** A 0.5 mL dose of Tdap is given one time only. It is to be administered regardless of the interval since a previous Td was administered. A booster dose of Td is recommended every 10 years following the single dose of Tdap.

Adverse reactions

Adverse reactions include pain, swelling (nodule may form), and redness at the injection site; systemic reactions are uncommon. An exaggerated (Arthus-type) reaction with extensive, painful swelling from shoulder to elbow can occur at the injection site and is thought to be caused by too-frequent injections of the tetanus antigen component of the combination vaccines.

Hepatitis B

Hepatitis B is caused by a DNA (deoxyribonucleic acid) virus. It is one of the most common infections worldwide.

Complications are usually related to chronic infections with hepatitis B virus and include chronic hepatitis, cirrhosis, liver failure, hepatocellular carcinoma, and death. Twenty-five percent of all carriers develop chronic, active hepatitis. The risk of becoming a carrier following infection ranges from 6% to 50%.

Hepatitis B vaccine

The first vaccine was a plasma-derived vaccine released in 1981, and it was removed from the market in 1992. The current vaccine is hepatitis B surface antigen, produced using recombinant-DNA technology. It was first released in 1986. Two products are currently marketed: Recombivax HB (Merck) and Engerix-B (GlaxoSmithKline). Although the antigen contents are different, the two vaccines are interchangeable.

Combination vaccines are available.

Dose

The usual pediatric dose is 0.5 mL IM given at birth, 2 months, and 6 months. The usual adult dose is 1 mL given at 0, 2, and 6 months. Indications include all infants, all adolescents, and high-risk adults (e.g., those with multiple sex partners or sexually transmitted diseases, injection drug abusers, patients on dialysis, patients with hemophilia, and patients with diabetes).

Adolescents 11–15 years of age may be given a two-dose series separated by 4 months. This dose is approved for only Recombivax HB.

Serological testing may not reflect immune status after 2 years following vaccination, but immunity continues. Booster doses should not be given.

Adverse reactions

Adverse reactions include pain, swelling (nodule may form), and redness at the injection site; systemic reactions are uncommon.

Hepatitis A

Hepatitis A is caused by an RNA virus and is the most common hepatitis infection in the United States. Although serious complications are not as common as with hepatitis B, morbidity and its associated costs (health care costs, lost work days) are significant. There is no risk of the patient becoming a chronic carrier. Transmission is human to human by the fecal–oral route of exposure. Exposure of an unimmunized person to hepatitis A requires the administering immune

globulin intramuscular (IGIM) as well as beginning the hepatitis A vaccine series, except for healthy persons 1–40 years of age, who may receive the vaccine only if administered within 2 weeks of exposure.

Hepatitis A vaccine

The available vaccines are Havrix by GlaxoSmithKline and VAQTA by Merck. These are inactivated whole-virus vaccines. Both vaccines are available in pediatric and adult formulations.

Hepatitis A vaccine is indicated for all high-risk patients and routinely for all children 1–2 years of age. Catch-up immunization should be given to all children up to 18 years of age. It is not indicated for children less than 1 year of age. The two vaccines use different potency measurements, but the volume and schedule of the dose is the same.

Dose

Children and adolescents over 1 year of age are given 0.5 mL, repeated in 6–12 months (Havrix) or 6–18 months (VAQTA), for two doses total.

Adults over 18 years of age are given 1 mL, repeated in 6–12 months, for two doses total.

Adverse reactions

Adverse reactions include pain, swelling, and redness at the injection site; systemic reactions are uncommon.

Combination vaccine

Twinrix, by GlaxoSmithKline, is a combination product with hepatitis B (adult dose) and hepatitis A (pediatric dose).

Dose

The usual dose is 1 mL, given at 0, 1, and 6–12 months. An accelerated schedule can be given at 0, 7 days, and 21–30 days, followed by a booster at 1 year, if protection is needed earlier.

The vaccine is indicated for persons 18 years of age and older.

Adverse reactions

Adverse reactions include pain, redness, and swelling at the injection site. Mild systemic reactions are rare.

Haemophilus Influenzae Type B

Haemophilus influenzae is a Gram-negative coccobacillus, whose outer shell consists of a polyribosylribitol phosphate (PRP) polysaccharide capsule. Six distinctly different types of *H. influenzae* exist, labeled a–f; however, *H. influenzae* type b (Hib) is responsible for 95% of human disease.

The organism enters through the nasopharynx and may cause disease or may colonize the nasopharynx, creating an asymptomatic carrier.

The most common clinical infections caused by Hib are meningitis, epiglottitis, pneumonia, arthritis, and cellulitis. Meningitis accounts for 50–65% of all clinical disease and results in a mortality rate of 2–5% and neurological sequelae in 15–30% of cases. Other diseases caused by *H. influenzae* include otitis, sinusitis, and bronchitis; however, these illnesses are usually caused by nontypeable (unencapsulated) strains.

Hib is primarily a disease of children, with a peak at age 6–7 months. It rarely attacks after the age of 5 years. Transmission is human to human by respiratory droplet spread to susceptible individuals.

Haemophilus influenzae vaccine

The incidence of Hib disease has decreased by more than 99% since the introduction of a vaccine. The first vaccine licensed (1985–88) was a pure polysaccharide vaccine that was ineffective in children less than 18 months of age. Current vaccines are polysaccharide vaccines conjugated to protein carriers. The specific carriers vary by manufacturer.

PRP-T (ActHIB by Sanofi Pasteur) and PRP-OMB (PedvaxHIB by Merck) are indicated for infants ≥ 6 weeks of age. Doses given before 6 weeks of age may inhibit the production of antibodies to subsequent doses; therefore, the vaccines are contraindicated in children less than 6 weeks of age. PRP-T (Hiberix by GlaxoSmithKline) is indicated only for the booster dose at 15 months to 4 years of age.

Dose
The usual dose for infants is 0.5 mL IM given at 2, 4, and 6 months. A booster dose is recommended for children 12–15 months of age. If PRP-OMB (PedvaxHIB) is used for the pediatric series, the 6-month dose should be omitted.

The catch-up series for Hib vaccine varies by age and manufacturer. Consult the package insert for complete dosing information.

Vaccination of children over 59 months of age is not indicated unless certain medical indications exist. These include persons with asplenia, those with immunodeficiency conditions, and those undergoing immunosuppressive therapy.

DTaP-Hib-IPV (Pentacel by Sanofi Pasteur) must not be used before the age of 6 weeks. MenHibrix by GlaxoSmithKline is a combination product with meningococcal conjugate type C and Y vaccine indicated for infants age 6 weeks to 18 months at high risk for meningococcal disease in the United States.

Adverse reactions
Adverse reactions include pain, swelling, and redness at the injection site; systemic reactions are uncommon.

Meningococcal Disease

Meningococcal disease is caused by *Neisseria meningitidis,* a Gram-negative bacteria with a polysaccharide capsule. The clinical diseases caused by *N. meningitidis* include meningitis, sepsis, pneumonia, myocarditis, and urethritis. *N. meningitidis* is one of the leading causes of meningitis in the United States. The types of *N. meningitidis* that cause over 95% of disease are serogroups A, B, C, W-135, and Y.

Approximately 800–1,200 cases occur per year, with an incidence rate of 0.4 case per 100,000 people.

Polysaccharide meningococcal vaccine (Menomune by Sanofi Pasteur)

This polysaccharide vaccine is effective against serogroups A, C, W-135, and Y. The vaccine does not protect against serogroup B, a common cause of infection.

The vaccine is FDA approved for persons over the age of 2 years. Those who should be vaccinated include military personnel, freshmen college students living in dormitories, those with anatomic or functional asplenia, anyone with potential exposure (such as laboratory workers), and travelers to the "meningitis belt" of Sub-Saharan Africa. Evidence of immunization is required for religious pilgrimages to Saudi Arabia for the Islamic Hajj. Vaccine may also be useful during an outbreak.

Dose
The dose is 0.5 mL given subcutaneously. A booster dose is needed after 3–5 years if the potential for reexposure continues.

Adverse reactions
Adverse reactions include pain, swelling (nodule may form), and redness at the injection site, as well as mild systemic reactions, such as fever, headaches, and malaise.

Conjugated polysaccharide meningococcal vaccine (Menactra by Sanofi Pasteur and Menveo by Novartis)

These polysaccharide vaccines are conjugated to a protein to increase efficacy. They are effective against serogroups A, C, W-135, and Y. The vaccines do not protect against serogroup B, a common cause of infection.

Indications

Menactra is approved for persons 2–55 years of age as a single dose and from 9 to 23 months as a 2 dose series. Menveo is FDA approved starting at age 2 months as a 4 dose series. The number of doses and the interval varies if the series is started at a later age. It is given as a single dose from 2 to 55 years of age and may be repeated after 2 months for select high-risk conditions. The ACIP does not recommend these vaccines for routine use in infants and children. The ACIP recommends routine vaccination for persons ages 11–12 years with a booster dose at age 16 (5 years after previous dose), and two doses given 2 months apart for persons ages 2 months through 54 years for certain chronic diseases (see ACIP recommendation).

Indications are the same as for the polysaccharide vaccine; however, revaccination is recommended for persons every 5 years who were previously vaccinated and who remain at high risk for the disease.

Dose

The dose is 0.5 mL given intramuscularly.

Adverse reactions

Adverse reactions include pain, swelling, and redness at the injection site, as well as mild systemic reactions, such as fever, headaches, and malaise.

Combination vaccine

MenHibrix by GlaxoSmithKline is a combination product with meningococcal conjugate type C and Y vaccine and Hib vaccine indicated for infants age 6 weeks to 18 months at high risk for meningococcal disease in the United States.

Polio

The three poliovirus types are identified as P1, P2, and P3. The virus enters the mouth and replicates in the gastrointestinal tract. From the gastrointestinal tract, the virus enters the bloodstream and infects the cells of the central nervous system.

Up to 95% of all infections are asymptomatic; however, these persons may transmit the infection to others. Approximately 4–8% of infections are mild with nonspecific upper respiratory infection, gastroenteritis, and influenza-like symptoms. Some 1–2% of infections present as nonparalytic aseptic meningitis, which typically resolves in 2–10 days. Flaccid paralysis occurs in less than 1% of those infected. Transmission is person to person by the fecal–oral route.

Polio vaccine (IPOL by Sanofi Pasteur)

The current vaccine available in the United States is an inactivated, trivalent injectable vaccine (IPV, or inactivated polio vaccine). Use of oral polio vaccine (OPV) was discontinued in the United States because of the elimination of wild-type polio disease and because yearly cases of vaccine-associated paralytic poliomyelitis were reported.

Dose

The pediatric dose is 0.5 mL IM given at 2, 4, 6–18 months, and 4–6 years of age. Routine vaccine or booster doses for adults are not recommended unless traveling to an endemic area.

Adverse reactions

Adverse reactions include minor pain, swelling, and redness at the injection site; systemic reactions are uncommon.

Measles, Mumps, and Rubella

Measles

Measles is a viral infection whose main presentation is a maculopapular rash. The virus is shed through the nasopharynx. Ten to 12 days after exposure, the prodromal phase begins, with progressive fever, cough, coryza, and conjunctivitis. Two to 4 days after the prodromal phase begins, a maculopapular rash begins on the face and head and gradually spreads throughout the body. The rash lasts 3–5 days, then gradually fades.

The incubation period is 10–12 days. Transmission is person to person through large respiratory droplets. Measles is highly contagious. There has been a recent surge in measles cases because of importation from other countries and increasing numbers of unvaccinated persons in the United States.

Complications may include pneumonia, otitis, encephalitis, and death.

Mumps

Mumps is a viral infection with a presentation of parotitis in 30–40% of cases. The virus is shed through the nasopharynx. Fourteen to 18 days after exposure, the prodromal phase begins, with headache, malaise, myalgias, and low-grade fever. Two days after the prodromal phase begins, the parotitis begins. Symptoms start to decrease after 1 week and disappear after 10 days.

The incubation period is 14–18 days (range, 14–25 days). Transmission is person to person through large respiratory droplets.

Complications can include orchitis, oophoritis, pancreatitis, and deafness.

Rubella

Rubella is a viral infection with up to 20–50% of cases subclinical and inapparent. The virus is shed through the nasopharynx. A prodromal phase of 1–5 days begins after incubation, with headache, malaise, myalgias, lymphadenopathy, low-grade fever, and upper respiratory infection symptoms. This phase is rare in children. Fourteen to 17 days after exposure, a maculopapular rash appears, first on the face and then descending to cover the rest of the body. The rash disappears after about 3 days.

The incubation period is 14 days (range, 12–23 days). Transmission is person to person through large respiratory droplets.

Complications may include arthritis, arthralgias, encephalitis, and hemorrhaging. The major complication is congenital rubella syndrome (CRS), which occurs in the offspring of a woman who had rubella during pregnancy. Babies born with CRS have major birth defects that can affect many organs.

Measles–mumps–rubella vaccine (MMRII by Merck)

The current vaccine available in the United States is a live attenuated vaccine against all three diseases.

Contraindications

This vaccine is contraindicated in pregnancy. Pregnancy should be avoided for 4 weeks following vaccination. Other contraindications include immunosuppressive disease or patients receiving immunosuppressive therapy, as well as those receiving antibody-containing blood products.

Dose

The usual pediatric dose is 0.5 mL IM given at 12 months of age. A second dose is recommended at 4–6 years of age to produce immunity in those who did not respond to the first dose.

Serologic testing may be necessary to document immunity.

Single-antigen vaccines are no longer available.

Adverse reactions

Adverse reactions include minor pain, swelling, and redness at the injection site and systemic reactions that mimic a mild case of the diseases.

Varicella (Chicken Pox)

Varicella is a viral infection caused by the herpes zoster virus. The primary infection is called *chicken pox*, and the recurrent disease is herpes zoster (called *shingles*).

The virus enters through the respiratory tract and replicates in the nasopharynx and regional lymph glands. The incubation period is 14–16 days (range, 10–21 days).

A prodromal phase may precede the rash with a slight fever and malaise. The rash progresses from a macule to a papule to a vesicle before it crusts over. The rash appears in several waves that last 2–3 days each. The rash first appears on the face and then the trunk (where most of the rash occurs) and the extremities.

Recurrent disease (herpes zoster) appears to be related to aging and immunosuppression. Recurrent disease usually presents as an outbreak of lesions along a dermatome and is usually unilateral. Neuralgia and intense pain may be present.

Transmission of varicella is person to person by infected respiratory secretions. Transmission by patients with herpes zoster is by direct contact with a nonimmune person.

Complications may include pneumonia, secondary bacterial infections, central nervous system infections, and sepsis.

Varicella vaccine (Varivax by Merck)

The current vaccine available in the United States is a live attenuated vaccine.

Contraindications

This vaccine is contraindicated in pregnancy, and pregnancy should be avoided for 4 weeks following vaccination. Other contraindications include immunosuppressive disease or patients receiving immunosuppressive therapy, as well as those receiving antibody-containing blood products. Guidelines for use in HIV patients are available (http://cid.oxford journals.org/content/early/2013/11/26/cid.cit684.full .pdf+html).

Dose

The pediatric dose is 0.5 mL IM, given at 12–18 months of age. A second dose is recommended at 4–6 years of age.

The adult dose (age > 13 years) is two doses of 0.5 mL, each separated by 4–8 weeks.

The vaccine must be stored frozen at +5°F (−15°C) or colder. The diluent used to reconstitute the vaccine should be stored at room temperature or refrigerated.

Adverse reactions

Adverse reactions include minor pain, swelling, and redness at the injection site and systemic reactions that mimic a mild case of the disease, including a mild generalized rash.

Herpes zoster vaccine (Zostavax by Merck)

This vaccine is the same strain of virus as in Varivax but 14 times the dose. It is a live attenuated vaccine that is approximately 50% effective in preventing herpes zoster.

Indication

It is indicated for all adults over the age of 60 years, regardless of previous zoster disease.

Contraindications

Contraindications include immunosuppression, both disease and medically induced.

Dose

The usual dose is 0.65 mL subcutaneous (must be reconstituted).

The vaccine must be stored frozen at +5°F (−15°C) or colder. The diluent used to reconstitute the vaccine should be stored at room temperature or refrigerated.

Adverse reactions

Adverse reactions include pain, redness, and swelling at the injection site and an increased incidence of headache.

Rotavirus

Rotavirus is the most common cause of severe gastroenteritis in infants and small children. Symptoms range from mild, watery diarrhea of limited duration to severe diarrhea with vomiting and fever that can result in dehydration.

In the United States, prior to a vaccine, approximately 27 million episodes, 205,000–272,000 emergency visits, 410,000 outpatient visits, 55,000–70,000 hospitalizations, and 20–60 deaths occurred each year because of rotavirus infection. Significant reductions in clinical disease and hospitalization rates have occurred since the introduction of the vaccine.

Rotavirus is transmitted by the fecal–oral route by close person-to-person contact through contaminated objects, food, and water.

Rotavirus vaccines

Two rotavirus vaccines are available:

- Pentavalent human–bovine reassortant rotavirus vaccine (RotaTeq [RV5] by Merck)
- Monovalent human rotavirus vaccine (Rotarix [RV1] by GlaxoSmithKline)

RV5 is a live oral vaccine that contains five reassortant rotaviruses and is available as a liquid that requires no reconstitution. RV1 is a live oral vaccine that contains one human rotavirus strain and is a lyophilized powder that must be reconstituted prior to administration.

Dose

Both vaccines are administered orally. RV5 contains 2 mL per dose, and RV1 contains 1 mL per dose.

RV5 is a three-dose series given at 2, 4, and 6 months of age. RV1 is a two-dose series given at 2 and 4 months of age. The rotavirus series should be started no sooner than 6 weeks of age and must be completed by 8 months, 0 days of age.

The rotavirus vaccine can be administered simultaneously with all other pediatric vaccines indicated at the same age. It should not be given to infants who had a severe reaction to a previous dose.

Precautions include altered immunocompetence, acute gastroenteritis, moderate or severe acute illness, preexisting chronic gastrointestinal disease, and a previous history of intussusception.

Adverse effects

A previous rotavirus vaccine (RotaShield) was removed from the market in 1999 because of an increased incidence of intussusception. Adverse effects may include diarrhea and vomiting.

Human Papillomavirus

Human papillomavirus (HPV) is the most common sexually transmitted disease in the United States. Although most HPV infections are asymptomatic and self-limiting, persistent infection can cause cervical cancer and genital warts.

Approximately 100 HPV types exist, with 40 types affecting the genital area and the remainder associated with skin warts. High-risk viruses can cause low- and high-grade cervical cell abnormalities and anogenital cancers. Approximately 70% of cervical cancers are caused by HPV types 16 and 18. HPV types 6 and 11 cause 90% of all genital warts.

HPV vaccines

Two HPV vaccines are available:

- Quadrivalent human papillomavirus vaccine (Gardasil by Merck) protects against HPV types 6, 11, 16, and 18 (HPV4).
- Bivalent human papillomavirus vaccine (Cervarix by GlaxoSmithKline) protects against HPV types 16 and 18 (HPV2).

Indications
Both vaccines are indicated for the prevention of disease caused by the types of HPV in the specific vaccine; they are not used for the treatment of HPV infection.

The HPV vaccines are indicated for all women 9–26 years of age and should be given routinely to all 11- to 12-year-old girls. One vaccine (HPV4) is recommended by the ACIP for the prevention of HPV disease in males 9–21 years of age. Although the ACIP does not recommend routine vaccination of males 22–26 years of age, the vaccine may be given at the discretion of the provider and patient.

Contraindications
HPV vaccine is contraindicated in persons who had a reaction to a previous dose.

Dose
The HPV vaccine is inactivated and administered as a three-dose series given at 0, 2, and 6 months. The vaccine must be shaken, and 0.5 mL is administered intramuscularly in the deltoid area.

The HPV vaccine may be given simultaneously with other recommended vaccines.

Adverse reactions
Adverse reactions are primarily local and include pain, redness, and swelling at the injection site. A systemic reaction of fever may occur.

Combination Vaccines

As mentioned in previous sections, several vaccination combinations are on the market:

- Tetanus, diphtheria, and pertussis combinations (various manufacturers): DTaP, DT, Td, Tdap

- Twinrix by GlaxoSmithKline: a combination product with hepatitis B (adult dose) and hepatitis A (pediatric dose)
- Pediarix (GlaxoSmithKline)
  - DTaP + hepatitis B + inactivated polio
  - Indicated when all vaccine components indicated
  - Not approved for < 6 weeks or > 7 years of age
  - Efficacy, contraindications, and adverse reactions similar to those of the vaccine components given separately
  - Dose: 0.5 mL IM given at 2, 4, and 6 months of age
  - Must be shaken vigorously prior to drawing up in syringe
  - Can be given even if infant receives birth dose of hepatitis B vaccine
- Pentacel (Sanofi Pasteur)
  - DTaP + Hib + inactivated polio
  - Indicated when all vaccine components indicated
  - Not approved for < 6 weeks or > 4 years of age
  - Efficacy, contraindications, and adverse reactions similar to those of the vaccine components given separately
  - Dose: 0.5 mL IM given at 2, 4, and 6 months of age
  - Must be shaken vigorously prior to drawing up in syringe
  - Can be given even if infant receives birth dose of hepatitis B vaccine
- ProQuad by Merck: a combination vaccine of measles, mumps, rubella, and varicella vaccine
- Kinrix by GlaxoSmithKline: a combination of DTaP and IPV to be given at 4–6 years of age
- MenHibrix by GlaxoSmithKline: a combination of meningococcal types CY and Hib vaccine

36-6. Questions

Use the following case study to answer Questions 1 and 2:

A 67-year-old patient presents to your pharmacy for a refill of his blood pressure medication. It is June, and he asks you to review his immunization status with him.

1. About which adult vaccine do you need to ask his status?

   A. Influenza vaccine
   B. Pneumococcal vaccine
   C. Meningococcal vaccine
   D. Hepatitis A vaccine
   E. Hepatitis B vaccine

2. The patient states that he received his pneumococcal vaccine 4 years ago. When should he receive another?

   A. Never
   B. Every year
   C. In 5 years
   D. When he reaches the age of 68
   E. When he reaches the age of 72

3. Which of the following describes the current injectable influenza vaccine used in the United States?

   A. Inactivated virus
   B. Live attenuated virus
   C. Conjugated vaccine
   D. Toxoid
   E. Toxin

4. Which one of the following is an indication for meningococcal conjugate vaccine?

   I. All adolescents 11–12 years of age, with a booster at age 16 or 5 years after last dose
   II. All infants
   III. Patients with liver disease
   IV. An adult backpacking in Europe
   V. College graduate students

   A. I only
   B. II, III, and V only
   C. I, II, and III only
   D. II, III, IV, and V only
   E. All of the above

5. At what age does one switch from DTaP to Tdap?

   A. 2 years
   B. 5 years
   C. 7 years
   D. 10 years
   E. DTaP can be used in all age groups.

6. Which of the following vaccines has *both* a polysaccharide and a conjugated vaccine on the U.S. market?

   A. Influenza
   B. Hepatitis A vaccine
   C. *Haemophilus influenzae* type B vaccine
   D. Pneumococcal vaccine
   E. MMR vaccine

7. Which polio vaccine schedule is recommended in the United States?

   A. Four doses of IPV
   B. Four doses of OPV
   C. Four doses of IPV plus a booster at 18 years of age
   D. Two doses of OPV and 2 doses of IPV
   E. Polio vaccine is no longer recommended in the United States.

8. Hepatitis B vaccine is a

   A. polysaccharide vaccine.
   B. recombinant hepatitis B surface antigen vaccine.
   C. live vaccine.
   D. conjugate vaccine.
   E. toxoid.

Use the following case study to answer Questions 9 and 10:

An 18-year-old healthy student is told that she needs to come to the pharmacy for her routine vaccinations prior to starting college. She will be living in the dormitory at school. She has not received any vaccines since grade school.

9. Which of the following vaccines are indicated for this patient?

   A. Hepatitis B vaccine
   B. Hepatitis A vaccine
   C. Meningococcal vaccine
   D. Pneumococcal vaccine
   E. Herpes zoster vaccine

10. The patient is exposed to a patient with hepatitis A 1 month later. She should receive which of the following vaccines?

   A. Hepatitis A vaccine series only
   B. Hepatitis B vaccine series only
   C. Hepatitis A vaccine series plus IGIM

D. Hepatitis A vaccine plus hepatitis B vaccine series

E. IGIM only

11. Which of the following is a high-risk group that should be targeted for pneumococcal vaccination?

A. Persons 6 months to 49 years of age
B. Persons with diabetes
C. Patients 21–49 years of age with hypertension
D. 35-year-old construction worker
E. 40-year-old health care worker

12. Which complication of rubella infection is the most significant health problem?

A. Congenital rubella syndrome
B. Secondary infection
C. Patent ductus arteriosus
D. Diarrhea
E. Arthritis

13. Which of the following is a valid contra-indication to the receipt of an injectable live-virus vaccine?

A. Current administration of antibiotics
B. Recent administration of antibody-containing blood products
C. Age over 12 months
D. Allergies to penicillin
E. A parent or sibling with a cold who is living in the same household

14. The most common adverse reaction to an inactivated vaccine is

A. rash.
B. severe headache.
C. injection-site reaction.
D. rhinorrhea.
E. stomach pain.

15. The only vaccine recommended at birth is

A. DTaP.
B. IPV.
C. Hib.
D. pneumococcal conjugate vaccine.
E. hepatitis B.

16. A 32-year-old female is injured in an automobile accident, and her spleen is removed. Which of the following vaccines is recommended for asplenic adult patients and is to be repeated every 5 years?

A. Pneumococcal vaccine
B. Meningococcal vaccine
C. IPV
D. *Haemophilus influenzae* type B vaccine
E. Influenza vaccine

17. If a second dose of a vaccine were given too soon (before the minimal interval time has passed), the correct course of action would be

A. restarting the entire series.
B. not counting that dose and repeating it after the minimal time has passed since the incorrect dose.
C. not worrying about it and continuing with the next dose as scheduled.
D. drawing antibody titers to confirm immunity.
E. doubling the next dose.

18. Which of the following groups of children are at increased risk for pneumococcal disease and should be vaccinated?

A. All adolescents at age 11–12 years
B. Adults of Native Alaskan descent
C. Teenagers of African American descent
D. Obese children
E. Children infected with HIV

19. Which of the following statements are true concerning Hib vaccine?

A. One dose of Hib is recommended for all children over the age of 5 years if they have not received a previous dose.
B. Standard dosing for Hib vaccine is 2, 4, 6, and 12–15 months of age.
C. The 6-month dose is omitted if ActHIB is used for the first two doses.
D. Hib vaccine is not routinely recommended for children 12–15 months of age.
E. Hib vaccine is given only to high-risk infants.

20. Which of the following vaccines available in the United States is a live, attenuated virus vaccine?

A. Polio (IPV)
B. *Haemophilus influenzae* vaccine (Hib)
C. DTaP
D. Varicella vaccine
E. Pneumococcal vaccine

36-7. Answers

1. **B.** Routine vaccinations in an adult are a yearly influenza vaccine (if in season), Tdap vaccine if not previously vaccinated, and a single pneumococcal vaccine for patients over the age of 65 or younger with select chronic illnesses (such as diabetes). June is too early in the season to indicate the influenza vaccine. Meningococcal and hepatitis vaccines are recommended only for certain indications.

2. **D.** Routine revaccination with pneumococcal vaccine is not recommended. Revaccination is recommended for select high-risk groups and everyone age 65 years and older who received an initial dose under the age of 65 and if more than 5 years have elapsed since the previous dose.

3. **A.** Injected influenza vaccine is an inactivated, split-virus vaccine. The LAIV is administered intranasally.

4. **A.** The ACIP recommends including all adolescents age 11–12 years with a booster at age 16 (or 5 years since last dose) among the other high-risk recommendations (asplenia, travel to endemic areas, meningococcal outbreaks).

5. **C.** DTaP is indicated for children under the age of 7 years. Because of adverse effects of DTaP in children 7 years of age and older, Tdap is used.

6. **D.** Polysaccharide pneumococcal vaccine (23-valent) is indicated for those over the age of 2 years, and conjugated polysaccharide vaccine (13-valent) is approved for ages 2 months to 7 years (FDA approved for over age 50 years but not ACIP recommended). Also there are two meningococcal conjugate vaccines and a meningococcal polysaccharide vaccine.

7. **A.** OPV is no longer recommended in the United States, and vaccination with IPV will continue until poliovirus is eradicated worldwide.

8. **B.** Hepatitis B vaccine is a recombinant hepatitis B surface antigen vaccine.

9. **C.** Meningococcal vaccine is routine for adolescents, and catch-up is recommended if they missed it at a younger age.

10. **A.** The hepatitis A vaccine alone will protect a healthy individual between 1 and 40 years of age who has previously been exposed to the virus.

11. **B.** All persons over the age of 65 years and patients with certain chronic diseases are in need of pneumococcal vaccination.

12. **A.** Complications of rubella may include arthritis, arthralgias, encephalitis, and hemorrhaging; however, the major complication is congenital rubella syndrome, which occurs in the offspring of a woman who had rubella during pregnancy. Babies born with CRS have major birth defects that can affect many organs.

13. **B.** Live-virus vaccines will be killed if antibodies have been administered recently. The length of time that must separate these two products depends on the dose and type of antibody-containing blood product being used.

14. **C.** Local reactions are the most common type of adverse reaction and include pain, swelling, and redness at the site of injection. These reactions usually occur within minutes to hours of the injection and are usually mild and self-limiting. Systemic adverse reactions include fever, malaise, myalgias, and headache and are more common following live vaccines.

15. **E.** All the other listed vaccines are first given at 2 months of age. Hepatitis B vaccine is recommended at birth to decrease the incidence of hepatitis B in infants of hepatitis B–infected mothers.

16. **B.** Asplenic patients require protection against the encapsulated bacteria (pneumococcus, meningococcus, and *Haemophilus*), as well as common viral infections. The meningococcal vaccine is to be repeated every 5 years. Previous series completions of routine vaccines, such as measles, varicella, and polio, are adequate for protection. Td vaccines should be repeated every 10 years following a single dose of Tdap, and influenza vaccine should be administered yearly.

17. **B.** The minimal interval in a series for most vaccines is 4 weeks. Decreasing the interval may interfere with antibody response and protection. Usually, the last dose in a series is separated from the previous dose by 4–6 months. Increasing the interval does not affect vaccine effectiveness. You never need to restart a series except for oral typhoid vaccine.

18. **E.** Rates of pneumococcal disease are highest in children < 2 years of age (vaccination is routine in all infants), those with asplenia, patients with HIV, and patients with certain chronic conditions. Obesity is not considered a high-risk disease for pneumococcal infection.

19. **B.** Hib vaccine is routinely administered to all infants and may be indicated for children over the age of 5 with certain chronic conditions. This vaccine is relatively complicated to use because recommendations vary among manufacturers (PedvaxHIB or Comvax do not require the 6 month dose). Please consult package inserts before administering.

20. **D.** Varicella vaccine, LAIV, measles–mumps–rubella vaccines, and rotavirus vaccines are the only live vaccines routinely administered in the United States. Other nonroutinely administered live vaccines include oral typhoid vaccine, vaccinia (smallpox) vaccine, and yellow fever vaccine. The majority of vaccines are inactivated or killed vaccines.

36-8. References

Advisory Committee on Immunization Practices. A comprehensive immunization strategy to eliminate transmission of hepatitis B virus infection in the United States (Part 1). *MMWR*. 2005;54(RR-16): 1–23.

Advisory Committee on Immunization Practices. A comprehensive immunization strategy to eliminate transmission of hepatitis B virus infection in the United States (Part 2). *MMWR*. 2006;55(RR-16): 1–25.

Advisory Committee on Immunization Practices. Bivalent human papillomavirus vaccine (HPV2, Cervarix) for use in females and updated HPV vaccination recommendations from the ACIP. *MMWR*. 2010;59(20):626–29.

Advisory Committee on Immunization Practices. FDA licensure for quadrivalent human papillomavirus vaccine (HPV4, Gardasil) for use in males and guidance from ACIP. *MMWR* 2010;59(20): 630–32.

Advisory Committee on Immunization Practices. General recommendations on immunizations. *MMWR*. 2011;60(RR-02):1–60.

Advisory Committee on Immunization Practices. Preventing tetanus, diphtheria, and pertussis among adults: Use of tetanus, reduced diphtheria toxoid, and acellular pertussis vaccine. *MMWR*. 2006;55 (RR-17):1–33.

Advisory Committee on Immunization Practices. Prevention and control of *Haemophilus influenzae* type b disease: Recommendations of the ACIP. *MMWR* 2014;63(RR-1):1–14.

Advisory Committee on Immunization Practices. Prevention and control of meningococcal disease. *MMWR*. 2013;62(RR-2):1–32.

Advisory Committee on Immunization Practices. Prevention and control of seasonal influenza with vaccines: Recommendations of the ACIP—United States, 2013–2014. *MMWR*. 2013;62(RR-07): 1–43.

Advisory Committee on Immunization Practices. Prevention of hepatitis A through active or passive immunization. *MMWR*. 2006;55(RR-7):1–23.

Advisory Committee on Immunization Practices. Prevention of herpes zoster. *MMWR*. 2008;57(5): 1–30.

Advisory Committee on Immunization Practices. Prevention of measles, rubella, congenital rubella syndrome, and mumps, 2013. *MMWR* 2013;62 (RR-4):1–40.

Advisory Committee on Immunization Practices. Prevention of pneumococcal disease among infants and children: Use of PCV13 and PPSV23. *MMWR*. 2010;59(RR-11):1–18.

Advisory Committee on Immunization Practices. Prevention of rotavirus gastroenteritis among infants and children. *MMWR*. 2009;58(RR-2):1–24.

Advisory Committee on Immunization Practices. Prevention of varicella. *MMWR*. 2007;56 (RR-4): 1–40.

Advisory Committee on Immunization Practices. Quadrivalent human papillomavirus vaccine. *MMWR*. 2007;56(RR-2):1–24.

Advisory Committee on Immunization Practices. Update on herpes zoster vaccine: Licensure for persons aged 50–59 years. *MMWR* 2011:60(44):1528.

Advisory Committee on Immunization Practices. Updated recommendations for prevention of invasive pneumococcal disease among adults using the 23-valent pneumococcal polysaccharide vaccine (PPSV23). *MMWR*. 2010;59(34):1102–6.

Advisory Committee on Immunization Practices. Updated recommendations for the use of tetanus toxoid, reduced diphtheria toxoid, and acellular pertussis (Tdap) vaccine from the Advisory Committee on Immunization Practices. *MMWR*. 2011; 60(RR-01):13–15.

Advisory Committee on Immunization Practices. Updated recommendations of the ACIP regarding routine poliovirus vaccination. *MMWR*. 2009;58 (30);829–30.

Advisory Committee on Immunization Practices. Use of hepatitis B vaccination for adults with diabetes mellitus. *MMWR*. 2011;60(50):1709–11.

Advisory Committee on Immunization Practices. Use of PCV13 and PPSV23 vaccine for adults with immunocompromising conditions. *MMWR* 2012; 61(40):816–19.

Centers for Disease Control and Prevention. *Epidemiology and Prevention of Vaccine: Preventable Diseases*. 12th ed. Atlanta, GA: CDC; 2011.

Centers for Disease Control and Prevention. Vaccines and immunizations Web site. Available at: http://www.cdc.gov/vaccines.

Grabenstein JD. *ImmunoFacts: Vaccines and Immunologic Drugs 2013*. St. Louis, MO: Facts and Comparisons; 2013.

Plotkin SA, Orenstein WA, Offitt P, eds. *Vaccines*. 6th ed. Philadelphia, PA: WB Saunders; 2013.

Pediatrics 37

Catherine M. Crill

37-1. Key Points

- The pharmacokinetics and pharmacodynamics of medications are altered by developmental differences in absorption, distribution, metabolism, and elimination in pediatric patients.
- Pharmacotherapy should be adjusted according to the developmental differences to optimize therapeutic efficacy while minimizing the risk of toxicity.
- Although spontaneous resolution does occur in many cases of acute otitis media, antibiotic therapy is initiated to prevent complications such as meningitis and mastoiditis. The observation option is an acceptable initial treatment for select patients.
- The incidence of drug-resistant *Streptococcus pneumoniae* is increasing. Because of its safety profile, cost, and excellent pharmacodynamic profile against sensitive and drug-resistant *S. pneumoniae*, high-dose amoxicillin remains the drug of choice for uncomplicated acute otitis media.
- Therapy for cystic fibrosis should focus on halting the progression of the disease and maintaining pulmonary function. Appropriate therapies decrease mucus viscosity and increase clearance of secretions; manage acute infectious exacerbations; and, by using appropriate pancreatic enzyme supplementation, maintain normal growth and development.
- Pharmacokinetics of medications in cystic fibrosis patients may be altered; therapeutic drug monitoring and dose alterations should be conducted to ensure efficacy and decrease toxicity.

- An accurate diagnosis of attention-deficit/hyperactivity disorder (ADHD) should be obtained prior to initiating drug therapy.
- Pharmacotherapy for ADHD is stimulants (first line). Second-line agents are atomoxetine, followed by extended-release guanfacine and clonidine.
- ADHD pharmacotherapy should be titrated to the desired functional effect without increasing the risk of side effects.
- ADHD therapy should include behavioral modification. Monitoring of drug and nondrug therapy should include input from different environments (e.g., parents, teachers).
- Bacterial and viral conjunctivitis may occur in the first month of life. Antimicrobial ointment administration should be instituted after delivery for prophylaxis.
- Bacterial, viral, and allergic conjunctivitis should be treated with antimicrobial therapy (bacterial); symptomatic therapy (bacterial, viral, allergic); and ocular antihistamines, decongestants, mast cell stabilizers, or combination products (allergic).

37-2. Study Guide Checklist

The following topics may guide your study of this subject area:
- Developmental considerations in pediatric patients with respect to drug absorption, distribution, metabolism, and excretion
- Differentiation between acute otitis media, otitis media with effusion, and recurrent otitis media
- Common bacterial organisms associated with acute otitis media and their resistance patterns

- Recommended treatment regimens for an initial episode of acute otitis media and for patients unresponsive to initial therapy or observation therapy
- Administration techniques for otic and ophthalmic medications
- Recommended drug therapies for cystic fibrosis
- Recommended drug therapies for ADHD
- Considerations for conjunctivitis management based on patient age and whether the cause is bacterial, viral, or allergic

37-3. Special Drug Therapy Considerations in Pediatric Patients

Pediatric Age Definitions

- *Preterm:* < 37 weeks gestation
- *Term:* ≥ 37 weeks gestation
- *Neonate:* < 1 month
- *Infant:* 1 month to < 1 year
- *Child:* 1–11 years
- *Adolescent:* 12–16 years

Absorption

Gastric pH

Infants may be considered to be in a relative state of achlorhydria (because of decreased basal acid secretion and total volume of secretions). However, they are capable of producing sufficient gastric acid with stimuli (e.g., in response to histamine or pentagastrin challenge, enteral feeding, or stress).

Gastric acid production reaches adult values by approximately 3 years of age.

Implications for drug therapy
- Increased bioavailability of basic drugs
- Decreased bioavailability of acidic drugs
- Increased bioavailability of acid-labile drugs (e.g., penicillin G)

Gastric emptying time in pediatric patients

Gastric emptying time (GET) is longer for pediatric patients than for adults. GET is inversely related to postconceptional age.

GET is characterized by irregular and unpredictable peristalsis and decreased motility. Premature neonates have longer GET than term neonates and have a greater incidence of gastroesophageal reflux. GET is related to the type of feeding. Formula-fed infants exhibit longer transit time than do breast-fed infants.

Pediatric GET approaches adult function by 7–9 months. Stomach muscles are mature at 7 months. Stomach muscles are completely innervated at 9 months.

Implications for drug therapy
Absorption of sustained-release products (e.g., theophylline) is erratic. The rate of absorption in the small intestine, where most drugs are absorbed, is slower; peak drug concentrations are lower for children than for adults.

Pancreatic enzymes and bile salts

- Low levels of amylase and lipase
- Low intraluminal bile acid concentrations and synthesis
- Decreased proteolytic ability

Implications for drug therapy
- Erratic absorption of drugs requiring pancreatic enzymes for hydrolysis (e.g., chloramphenicol)
- Decreased absorption of lipid-soluble drugs
- Decreased fat absorption from enteral feedings
- Decreased absorption of fat-soluble vitamins

Gastrointestinal mucosa

- Functional integrity of intestinal mucosa is decreased.
- The surface area of the gastric mucosa is small compared to that of intestinal mucosa (most drugs are absorbed from the small intestine).
- Changes in splanchnic blood flow in the neonatal period may alter the concentration gradient across the intestinal mucosa.

Other absorption routes

Skin
Absorption through the skin is inversely related to the thickness of the stratum corneum and directly related to hydration of the skin. Neonates (particularly premature) have increased skin hydration. The stratum corneum of preterm infants is immature and ineffective as an epidermal barrier.

Premature neonates may develop drug toxicity if a drug is administered through the dermal route.

Intramuscular route
Drug delivery is restricted by volume of medication and the pain associated with administration. Results are

variable in premature neonates because of (1) blood flow and vasomotor instabilities; and (2) insufficient muscle mass and tone, contraction, and oxygenation.

Rectal administration

Rectal administration is effective for drug delivery in older infants and children.

Administration through intraosseous route

This vessel-rich marrow (in children up to 5 years of age) is a great site for drug delivery to the systemic circulation. It may be an acceptable route in emergency situations for children over 5 years of age (vessel-rich marrow is then replaced by yellow marrow).

Distribution

Protein binding

- Decreased albumin and α_1-acid glycoprotein concentrations
- Lower binding capacity
- Qualitative differences in neonatal plasma proteins
- Competitive binding by endogenous substances (unconjugated bilirubin, free fatty acids)
- Risk of kernicterus (hypoalbuminemia, unconjugated hyperbilirubinemia, displacement by highly protein-bound drugs or free fatty acids)
- Exhibition of adult-like binding by 3–6 months of age; adult concentrations of albumin and α_1-acid glycoprotein at 10–12 months of age

Differences in body composition

- Vascular and tissue perfusion are altered.
- The brain and liver are the largest organs in children.
- Total body water is greater in neonates and infants.
- Extracellular fluid volume is greater in neonates and infants.
- There is a relative lack of adipose tissue in neonates and infants (adipose tissue level increases into adulthood).

Implications for drug therapy in neonates and infants

- Increased free fraction of drugs can occur.
- Increased potential of drug displacement by endogenous substances is present.
- Potential risk of kernicterus with physiologic jaundice (unconjugated hyperbilirubinemia) is present.

- Hydrophilic drugs, which parallel water volume in the body (e.g., aminoglycosides), exhibit greater volume of distribution (V_d).
- Lipophilic drugs (e.g., diazepam) parallel body fat and will exhibit a smaller V_d.

Liver Metabolism

Phase I reactions (nonsynthetic): Oxidation, reduction, hydrolysis, and hydroxylation

- The hepatic cytochrome P450 (CYP450) enzyme system is responsible for most phase I reactions.
- The capacity of isoenzymes in the CYP450 system at birth is 20–70% of adult capacity and increases with postnatal age.
- Full capacity for reduction is present at birth.
- Hydrolysis is most developed at birth, followed by the processes of oxidation and hydroxylation.
- Benzyl alcohol, a preservative present in certain medications, can accumulate in neonates because of underdeveloped alcohol dehydrogenase. Gasping syndrome (i.e., metabolic acidosis, respiratory failure, seizures, neurologic deterioration, cardiovascular collapse) can result.

Phase II reactions (synthetic): Conjugation with glycine or glutathione, glucuronidation, sulfation, methylation, and acetylation

- The sulfation pathway is the most developed pathway at birth.
- Glucuronidation (i.e., UDP-glucuronosyltransferase [UGT] activity) begins around 2 months of age. It reaches adult capacity by 2 years of age.
- Assumptions about substances primarily metabolized by glucuronidation (e.g., morphine, bilirubin, chloramphenicol) are as follows:
  - They are potentially toxic in neonates.
  - They may exhibit long half-lives (e.g., toxicity with chloramphenicol).
  - They may require greater dosing in infants (e.g., morphine conjugated to its more active metabolite).
  - They may be metabolized by another pathway in infants (e.g., acetaminophen is primarily metabolized through sulfation in infants).
- Methylation is functional in infants but is not significantly expressed in adults. (Methylation is responsible for the conversion of theophylline to caffeine.)

Implications for drug therapy

- For drugs undergoing phase I and II reactions, the metabolism is reduced and the half-life is prolonged in infants and neonates.
- Insufficiency of one pathway may lead to metabolism through another.
- Adverse drug reactions are more likely in younger children (i.e., five times more likely in children under 1 year of age and three and one-half times more likely in children 1–4 years of age).
- Drug metabolism, which is slower in the neonate, increases between 1 and 5 years of age and is similar to that in adults after puberty.

Renal Elimination

- Renal blood flow is only 5–6% of cardiac output at birth, compared with 15–25% in adults.
- Glomerular filtration rate (GFR) is lower at birth and reaches adult values by 1–5 months of age in term infants.
- Tubular secretion is low at birth and reaches adult values by 7 months of age in term infants.
- Renal elimination is affected by prematurity and postconceptional age. It increases with maturity.

Estimation of GFR or creatinine clearance in pediatric patients

- The average creatinine clearance (CrCl) values (normal renal function) are shown in Table 37-1.
- The estimation of CrCl is altered by differences in renal blood flow, glomerular filtration, tubular secretion, and muscle mass.

- It may be affected by the presence of maternal serum creatinine (SCr) over the first week of life (i.e., false underestimation of CrCl).
- The Schwartz equation may be used for estimating GFR in pediatric patients:

$$\text{GFR}\left(\text{mL/min/1.73 m}^2\right) = k \times (\text{length in cm})/\text{SCr}$$

where k = proportionality constant that changes with age and sex (Table 37-2).

Alternately, the Bedside Chronic Kidney Disease in Children (CKiD) equation, also referred to as the updated or modified Schwartz equation, may be a better estimate of GFR in pediatric patients with moderate to severe kidney disease:

$$\text{GFR}\left(\text{mL/min/1.73 m}^2\right) = 0.413 \times \left(\text{height in cm}\right)/\text{SCr}$$

Other Pediatric Drug Issues

- Digoxin-like immunoreactive substance (DLIS) is produced in infants. DLIS may interfere with digoxin assays and falsely elevate concentrations.
- Di(2-ethylhexyl)phthalate (DEHP), a plasticizer contained in intravenous (IV) bags, is shown to have an effect on the male reproductive system. Pediatric patients at highest risk of DEHP exposure are neonates on extracorporeal membrane oxygenation, those receiving parenteral and enteral nutrition, and those receiving plasma exchange transfusions.
- Propylene glycol, an additive used to promote stability in certain IV medications, can cause hyperosmolarity in infants.
- Potentially fatal central nervous system and respiratory depression because of morphine

Table 37-1. Average CrCl Values (Normal Renal Function)

Age (term)	Value (ml/min/1.73 m²)
5–7 days	50.6 ± 5.8
1–2 months	64.6 ± 5.8
5–8 months	87.7 ± 11.9
9–12 months	86.9 ± 8.4
> 18 months (male)	124 ± 26
> 18 months (female)	109 ± 13.5
Adult (male)	105 ± 14
Adult (female)	95 ± 18

Table 37-2. Proportionality Constant for Calculation of CrCl Using the Schwartz Equation[a]

Age	k
Low birth weight ≤ 1 year	0.33
Full term ≤ 1 year	0.45
1–12 years	0.55
14–21 years (female)	0.55
14–21 years (male)	0.70

a. Schwartz, Brion, Spitzer, 1987.

accumulation may occur in neonates of mothers who are CYP2D6 ultrarapid metabolizers and are taking codeine for postpartum pain.

37-4. Specific Infections and Disease States in the Pediatric Population

Otitis Media

Otitis media is an inflammatory process of the middle ear.

Classification

- *Acute otitis media* is the rapid onset of signs and symptoms of inflammation in the middle ear. Uncomplicated acute otitis media is not accompanied by otorrhea (discharge from the ear).
  - *Nonsevere:* Mild otalgia (ear pain) for < 48 hours and temperature < 39°C or 102.2°F
  - *Severe:* Moderate to severe otalgia, otalgia for at least 48 hours, or fever ≥ 39°C or 102.2°F
- *Recurrent otitis media* is the diagnosis of three or more separate episodes of acute otitis media within a 6-month period or four episodes within a year (with at least one episode in the past 6 months).
- *Otitis media with effusion* is inflammation of the middle ear with the presence of fluid in the middle ear (effusion) without the associated signs or symptoms of acute infection.

Clinical presentation

Signs and symptoms include fever, otalgia (often manifested as ear tugging or pulling), otorrhea, changes in balance or hearing, irritability, difficulty sleeping, lethargy, anorexia, vomiting, and diarrhea. Associated findings may be runny nose, congestion, or cough.

Pathophysiology

Eustachian tube dysfunction

The infant's eustachian tube is shorter and more horizontal than that of the adult, thus preventing drainage of middle ear secretions into the nasopharynx and promoting pooling of secretions in the middle ear. Anatomic abnormalities increase risk (e.g., cleft palate, adenoid hypertrophy). An immature immune system or altered host defenses also increase risk, as do viral infections and allergies.

Risk factors include male gender; Native American, Canadian Eskimo, or Alaskan descent; family history of acute otitis media or respiratory tract infection; early age of first episode (earlier age is associated with greater severity and recurrence); day care environment; parental smoking; lack of breast-feeding in infancy; and pacifier use.

Complications include mastoiditis, meningitis, subdural empyema, hearing loss, and delayed speech and language development.

Microbial pathogens

Historically, up to 50% of cases of otitis media were thought to be viral in origin. However, with accurate diagnosis of acute otitis media (i.e., differentiating between acute disease and otitis media with effusion), the majority of cases are bacterial with or without a viral component. The primary bacteria responsible for acute otitis media are discussed below.

- *Streptococcus pneumoniae* has been responsible over time for the majority of bacterial otitis media cases. Bacterial resistance, which occurs primarily through alteration in penicillin-binding protein (decreased affinity for binding sites), is common.
- *Haemophilus influenzae* (primarily nonencapsulated or nontypeable strains) has been considered the second-most-common organism responsible for bacterial otitis media cases. Bacterial resistance occurs through β-lactamase production.
- *Moraxella catarrhalis* is the third-most-common organism responsible for bacterial otitis media cases. Almost all strains are β-lactamase producing.

With the advent of the pneumococcal 7-valent (PCV7) and 13-valent (PCV13) vaccines, the otopathogens responsible for acute otitis media are changing. The incidence of acute otitis media because of *S. pneumoniae* and *H. influenzae* strains are now approximately equal. With respect to *S. pneumoniae*, the majority of strains identified in acute otitis media cases are those that are not represented in the vaccine.

Diagnosis

In 2004, the American Academy of Pediatrics (AAP) and the American Academy of Family Physicians (AAFP) published clinical practice guidelines on the diagnosis and management of acute otitis media.

These guidelines established diagnostic criteria and the use of pneumatic otoscope or tympanometry to differentiate between episodes of acute otitis media and otitis media with effusion. The guidelines were also the first official support in North America for an observation therapy option in acute otitis media for select patients. In 2013, these guidelines were revised to further strengthen the diagnostic criteria. It is important to note that the 2013 guidelines apply to the diagnosis and management of uncomplicated acute otitis media in infants and children 6 months to 12 years of age. For management in infants less than 6 months of age, the earlier guidelines may still be used.

When middle ear disease is present, otoscopic examination determines color, translucency, and position. Redness or opacity of membrane, absence of light reflection, or bulging membrane will be observed.

Pneumatic otoscopic examination determines mobility of the tympanic membrane (i.e., presence or absence of effusion). The membrane will not move briskly with positive and negative pressure if effusion is present. Tympanometry may also be used to determine the presence of middle ear effusion.

Tympanocentesis (i.e., a needle is inserted through the tympanic membrane to withdraw fluid) allows for culture and identification of the pathogen.

According to the 2013 guidelines, middle ear effusion on examination with pneumatic otoscope or with tympanometry must be present to diagnose acute otitis media. In addition, acute otitis media should be diagnosed with moderate to severe bulging of the tympanic membrane or new onset of otorrhea. Alternately, acute otitis media may be diagnosed with mild bulging of the tympanic membrane and recent onset (< 48 hours) of ear pain or intense erythema of the tympanic membrane.

Treatment principles and goals

- Assess and control pain.
- Eradicate infection.
- Prevent complications.
- Avoid unnecessary antibiotic therapy.
- Improve compliance.
- Eliminate presence of effusion.
- Prevent recurrence.

Drug therapy

Many episodes of otitis media will have spontaneous resolution; however, because of a risk of complications from untreated otitis media, antimicrobials remain the mainstay of therapy. Observation therapy may be appropriate in select patients.

First-line therapy

High-dose amoxicillin (Amoxil) is the recommended first-line treatment for acute otitis media. Amoxicillin has excellent in vitro activity against *S. pneumoniae* and most *H. influenzae*. It has the optimal pharmacodynamic profile of the available agents and reaches good concentrations in middle ear fluid. Amoxicillin has an excellent safety and efficacy profile with a narrow spectrum of activity. It is palatable and inexpensive. It may overcome drug-resistant *S. pneumoniae* with higher doses (i.e., achieves greater concentrations in middle ear fluid). It does not eradicate β-lactamase–producing organisms.

For penicillin-allergic patients, cefdinir (Omnicef), cefpodoxime (Vantin), cefuroxime (Ceftin), or ceftriaxone (Rocephin) may be used.

Amoxicillin-clavulanate (Augmentin) should be used as first-line therapy in patients who have received amoxicillin in the past 30 days, those with conjunctivitis, or those in whom β-lactamase-positive *H. influenzae* or *M. catarrhalis* is indicated.

Dosing issues and drug resistance

Antimicrobial treatment options are described in Table 37-3.

Dosages are as follows:

- **Amoxicillin (Amoxil):** A high dose is recommended (80–90 mg/kg/day).
- **Amoxicillin-clavulanate (Augmentin):** A high dose is recommended (90 mg/kg/day of amoxicillin with 6.4 mg/kg/day of clavulanate). Maintain daily clavulanate dose < 10 mg/kg/day to prevent diarrhea.
- **Ceftriaxone (Rocephin):** An intramuscular (IM) dose of 50 mg/kg/dose (single dose versus three daily doses) is recommended. More than a single dose may be necessary to prevent recurrence within 5–7 days of the initial dose.

Duration of therapy

Two courses of therapy are possible:

- Standard course (10-days)
- Shorter course (1–7 days)

Advantages of the shorter course are improved compliance, decreased adverse effects of drug therapy, decreased risk of bacterial resistance, and lower costs. Disadvantages are delayed or no cure, increased risk of complications from untreated acute otitis media, and greater risk of recurrence.

Table 37-3. Antimicrobial Therapy for Acute Otitis Media

Initial antibiotics or after treatment failure with observation		Treatment failure after 48–72 hours of antibiotics	
First line	**Alternative**	**First line**	**Alternative**
Amoxicillin (Amoxil) 80–90 mg/kg/day or Amoxicillin-clavulanate (Augmentin)[a] 90 mg/kg/day amoxicillin + 6.4 mg/kg/day clavulanate	Cefdinir (Omnicef) 14 mg/kg/day in 1 or 2 doses or Cefuroxime (Ceftin) 30 mg/kg/day in 2 doses or Cefpodoxime (Vantin) 10 mg/kg/day in 2 doses or Ceftriaxone (Rocephin) 50 mg/kg/day IM or IV for 1–3 days[b]	Amoxicillin-clavulanate (Augmentin) 90 mg/kg/day amoxicillin + 6.4 mg/kg/day clavulanate or Ceftriaxone (Rocephin) 50 mg/kg/day IM or IV for 3 days[b]	Ceftriaxone (Rocephin) 50 mg/kg/day for 3 days[b] or Clindamycin[c] (Cleocin) 30–40 mg/kg/day in 3 doses ± 2nd- or 3rd-generation cephalosporin or Clindamycin[c] (Cleocin) + 2nd- or 3rd-generation cephalosporin or Tympanocentesis Consult specialist

a. Amoxicillin-clavulanate is first-line therapy in patients who have received amoxicillin in the past 30 days, those with conjunctivitis, those with a history of recurrent otitis media unresponsive to amoxicillin, or those in whom β-lactamase activity for *H. influenzae* or *M. catarrhalis* is indicated.
b. More than 1 ceftriaxone dose may be needed to prevent recurrence.
c. Clindamycin does not have activity against *H. influenzae*. It should be used when penicillin-resistant *S. pneumoniae* is suspected.

The 2013 guidelines recommend the standard 10-day course in children < 2 years of age or severe symptoms at any age. A 7-day course may be used in children 2–5 years of age (and a 5–7 day course in children 6 years and older) with mild to moderate acute otitis media.

Other therapy

Antipyretics (acetaminophen [Tylenol] and ibuprofen [Motrin]) or analgesics may be used. Use acetaminophen with caution in high doses to avoid hepatotoxicity. Use ibuprofen with caution in patients with vomiting, diarrhea, and poor fluid intake, because dehydration predisposes them to ibuprofen-induced renal insufficiency. Avoid alternating antipyretic therapy. Encourage parents to choose one agent, inform them of any adverse effects, and educate them about symptoms of these effects (e.g., hepatotoxicity or renal insufficiency).

Narcotic analgesics may be used for moderate to severe pain not controlled with acetaminophen or ibuprofen.

Topical analgesics include otic solutions, such as antipyrine-benzocaine (Auralgan, Americaine Otic), and naturopathic otic solutions.

Topical antimicrobials may have a place in therapy, particularly with ruptured tympanic membranes (fluoroquinolone or fluoroquinolone and steroid combination otic suspensions [Floxin, Cipro HC, Ciprodex]).

Antihistamines and decongestants are ineffective at eliminating effusion or relieving symptoms. Use them only if indicated for other signs or symptoms.

Patient instructions and counseling

- Complete the entire course of prescribed antibiotics.
- Shake bottle well before administering dose. Follow labeling regarding temperature for storage of medication.
- Contact the health care provider if patient develops a rash or has difficulty breathing, or if symptoms persist after 72 hours of initiating therapy.

Adverse drug events

- *Gastrointestinal effects:* Nausea and diarrhea; discoloration of stools (with cefdinir [Omnicef])
- *Hypersensitivity:* Rash, anaphylaxis

Nondrug therapy

Local heat or cold therapy may be used (counsel the caregiver on appropriate use and technique to prevent burn injury).

Tympanostomy tubes decrease recurrent episodes, restore hearing, and relieve discomfort. Risks include anesthesia and permanent tympanic membrane scarring.

Observation therapy

Observation therapy is appropriate only when follow-up at 48–72 hours can be ensured and antimicrobials initiated if symptoms persist or worsen. This therapy is *not* appropriate for the following patients:

- Infants < 6 months of age
- Infants and children between 6 months and 2 years of age with otorrhea, severe symptoms (toxic-appearing child, otalgia > 48 hours, or temperature ≥39°C or 102.2°F), or bilateral disease
- Children ≥ 2 years of age with otorrhea or severe symptoms as described above

Immunization and immunoprophylaxis

Pneumococcal conjugate vaccination should provide some protection against strains responsible for a majority of bacterial otitis media.

H. influenzae type B vaccination is of no benefit in otitis media. Most strains causing otitis media are nontypeable and not prevented by vaccination.

Killed and live-attenuated intranasal influenza vaccine may decrease episodes of acute otitis media during the respiratory illness season. Annual influenza vaccination is recommended for infants and children age 6 months and older as part of the childhood immunization schedule.

Risk reduction

- Encourage exclusive breast-feeding for 6 months.
- Eliminate passive exposure to tobacco smoke.
- Avoid supine bottle feeding.
- Reduce or eliminate pacifier use after 6 months of age.
- Reduce incidence of upper respiratory infections by altering day care attendance (when possible).

Recurrent otitis media

The use of antimicrobials for otitis media prophylaxis is not recommended. Risk factor reduction in this group of patients is important. Tympanostomy tubes may be recommended with recurrent otitis media.

Otitis media with effusion

In 2004, the AAP, AAFP, and the American Academy of Otolaryngology–Head and Neck Surgery published a clinical practice guideline on otitis media with effusion. It applies to infants and children (2 months to 12 years of age) with or without developmental disabilities or underlying conditions that predispose patients to otitis media with effusion. Recommendations include the following:

- Use pneumatic otoscopy as the primary diagnostic method.
- Distinguish otitis media with effusion from acute otitis media.
- Determine the risk of speech, language, and learning problems.
  - *At-risk children:* More rapid evaluation and intervention
  - *Children not at risk:* Watchful waiting for 3 months from date of onset or diagnosis
- No role exists for antihistamines, decongestants, antimicrobials, or corticosteroids.
- Hearing testing is recommended with effusion lasting ≥ 3 months or when language delay, learning problems, or hearing loss occur.
- For persistent otitis media with effusion (not at risk), perform evaluations every 3–6 months until effusion is resolved, hearing loss is identified, structural abnormalities are suspected, or the child becomes a surgical candidate (tympanostomy tube insertion is preferred).

Otitis Externa

Otitis externa is an inflammation of the outer ear canal, also referred to as *swimmer's ear.*

Clinical presentation

Patients present with itching, pain, otic exudate, and hearing impairment.

Pathophysiology

Moisture is present in the ear canal, and the integrity of the ear canal is disrupted. The most common organisms are *Pseudomonas aeruginosa* and *Staphylococcus aureus.* Other pathogens include fungi and *Bacillus* and *Proteus* species.

Therapy consists of antibiotic or steroid otic preparations such as neomycin, polymyxin B, and hydrocortisone (Cortisporin Otic), or neomycin, colistin, and hydrocortisone (Coly-Mycin S Otic). Fluoroquinolone otic preparations such as ciprofloxacin (Cipro HC) and ofloxacin (Floxin) can also be used, as well as acetic acid and hydrocortisone otic preparations (VoSol HC Otic) or oral analgesics.

Preventive measures include drying ears after exposure to moisture; using drops containing isopropyl alcohol, with or without acetic acid to reduce pH; and avoiding cotton swabs.

Otic drops should be administered to a pediatric patient as follows:

1. Wash hands before and after administration.
2. Warm otic drops to room temperature by holding bottle in hands for several minutes. Avoid instilling cold or hot drops into the ear canal.
3. Shake the bottle if indicated on the label.
4. Tilt the child's head to the side, or have the child lie down.
5. Pull the child's ear backward and upward (for children < 3 years, pull ear backward and downward), and instill the drops in the ear canal. Do not put the dropper bottle inside the ear canal. To remain free from contamination, it should not come into contact with the ear.
6. Press gently on the small flap over the ear to push the drops into the canal.
7. Have the child remain in the same position for the period of time indicated in the labeling. If this is not possible, place a cotton ball gently into the ear to prevent the drops from draining out of the ear canal.
8. Wipe excess medication from the outside of the ear.

Cystic Fibrosis

Cystic fibrosis is an autosomal recessive disease of exocrine gland function resulting in abnormal mucus production.

Genetic classification

Cystic fibrosis is the result of a gene mutation on the long arm of chromosome 7. The protein encoded by this gene, the cystic fibrosis transmembrane conductance regulator (CFTR), is a channel involved in the transport of water and electrolytes.

Defects in processing

The most common genetic mutation involves a 3-base-pair deletion at position 508 (ΔF508). Patients homozygous for ΔF508 are pancreatic insufficient.

Prognosis is not as good as that for patients who are pancreatic sufficient. Defects exist in protein production, regulation, and conduction.

Clinical presentation

Pulmonary complications
Initial manifestations include chronic cough, wheezing, hyperinflation of lungs, or lower respiratory tract infections. Patients present with hypoxia, clubbing, labored breathing, and acute respiratory exacerbations (fever, sputum production, increased oxygen requirements, dyspnea); changes in forced vital capacity (FVC), forced expiratory volume in 1 second (FEV_1), and residual volume; and the development of a chronic obstructive picture as the disease progresses.

Gastrointestinal complications
Gastrointestinal complications include poor digestion of proteins and fats, resulting in foul-smelling steatorrhea, and distal intestinal obstruction (commonly manifested as vomiting of bilious material, abdominal distension, and pain).

Infants may have meconium ileus and gastroesophageal reflux.

Other complications
Patients may also have the following complications:

- Cirrhosis, cholelithiasis
- Problems with pancreatic function
- Insulin insufficiency, diabetes mellitus
- Malnutrition
- Nasal polyps and sinusitis, anemia, arthritis, osteopenia, osteoporosis

Pathophysiology

A defect exists in the chloride transport channel in secretory epithelial cells. Normally, chloride is transported out of blood followed by sodium and water. However, with cystic fibrosis, decreased chloride and water secretion and increased sodium absorption lead to thick, dehydrated secretions and mucus. Exocrine gland involvement includes pancreas, hepatobiliary ducts, gastrointestinal tract, and the lungs (secretions build up and block airways and pancreatic and hepatobiliary exocrine flow).

Pulmonary system

Initial obstruction of small airways with mucus plugging results in bronchiolitis and persistence of bacteria, as follows:

- *Early bacterial pathogens: S. aureus* is the primary pathogen in younger patients.
- *Later bacterial pathogens: P. aeruginosa* is the primary pathogen in late childhood.
- *Other bacterial pathogens: Alcaligenes, Stenotrophomonas, Mycobacteria, Aspergillus,* and *Burkholderia* can be present.

Viral pathogens can also be present.

Chronic pulmonary infection and inflammation progress to large airway and eventual chronic obstructive disease.

Pancreatic system

Pancreatic enzyme insufficiency (trypsin, chymotrypsin, lipases, amylase) and decreased bicarbonate secretion (necessary for optimal pancreatic enzyme activity) can occur. Thus, maldigestion of fats and proteins and fat-soluble vitamin deficiency may develop.

Insulin insufficiency (resistance and decreased secretion) leads to glucose intolerance and the development of diabetes mellitus (occurs later in the disease process and may be associated with increased morbidity and mortality).

Biliary system

Biliary cirrhosis or fatty infiltration may lead to portal hypertension, development of bleeding varices, hypersplenism, and cholelithiasis.

Sweat glands

A high concentration of sodium and chloride exists in sweat (representing the failure of sweat glands to reabsorb sodium and chloride).

Reproductive system

Male infertility is common because of bilateral absence of vas deferens. Female infertility is due to abnormal cervical mucus.

Diagnostic criteria

Testing for cystic fibrosis is required in all states as part of the newborn screen. Laboratory confirmation of CFTR dysfunction should be obtained through sweat chloride analysis (i.e., administration of pilocarpine):

- Sweat is collected, and electrolytes are measured.

- Chloride of 60 mEq/L or more is diagnostic.
- Chloride of 40–59 mEq/L is indeterminate, and tests may need to be repeated.

Treatment goals

- Halt or decrease disease progression.
- Maintain normal growth and development and nutrition status.
- Maintain pulmonary function.
- Optimize drug therapy for pharmacokinetic differences in cystic fibrosis patients.

Drug therapy

Drug therapy for cystic fibrosis is described in Table 37-4.

Pancreatic enzyme replacement products have historically been marketed in the United States as unapproved products. Because of variability in the amount of enzymes in these products, the U.S. Food and Drug Administration (FDA) mandated, effective April 2010, that all manufacturers of pancreatic enzyme replacement products submit a new drug application with the FDA to continue to market their products in the United States. As a result of this mandate, many existing products have been removed from the market. As of May 2014, only six FDA-approved pancreatic enzyme replacement products are available in the United States (see Table 37-4).

Antibiotic therapy in acute exacerbations

Empiric therapy should be used initially. The patient should then be treated on the basis of sputum culture and sensitivity. Administer intravenously two antibiotics for 14–21 days in combination with aggressive therapy for clearance of secretions. Provide coverage for *S. aureus* and *P. aeruginosa*.

Double coverage of antibiotics is recommended when *Pseudomonas* species are suspected, so typically use an antipseudomonal penicillin (piperacillin [Pipracil], mezlocillin [Mezlin], piperacillin-tazobactam [Zosyn], ticarcillin-clavulanate [Timentin], ticarcillin [Ticar], aztreonam [Azactam]) or cephalosporin (ceftazidime [Fortaz]), a carbapenem (meropenem [Merrem], imipenem-cilastatin [Primaxin]), or a quinolone (ciprofloxacin [Cipro]) plus an aminoglycoside (tobramycin [Nebcin]).

Most *S. aureus* are β-lactamase producers, so use an extended spectrum penicillin–β-lactamase inhibitor combination (e.g., ticarcillin-clavulanate [Timentin]). Use vancomycin (Vancocin) for methicillin-resistant *S. aureus*.

Table 37-4. Drug Therapy for Cystic Fibrosis

Therapeutic category	Indication and mechanism of action	Comments
Nutrition therapy		
Pancreatic enzymes: Delayed-release capsule with enteric-coated microspheres (Creon, Pertzye) or beads (Zenpep); capsule with enteric-coated micro-tablets (Pancreaze, Ultresa); tablet (Viokace)	Supplementation or replacement of pancreatic enzymes (treatment of malabsorption syndrome); aid in digestion of proteins, carbohydrates, and fats	Primary enzyme component is lipase. Products are not interchangeable. Dose is typically whole dose with meals and half dose with snacks. Capsule formulations may be opened and contents sprinkled on soft acidic food (e.g., applesauce); contents of capsules must not be crushed or chewed. New dosage strengths for Creon and Zenpep allow for dosing in infants; can give 1 capsule (3,000 units lipase) per 120 mL formula. Adequate replacement decreases bowel movements and improves stool consistency. Viokace is the only nonenteric-coated FDA-approved pancreatic enzyme product and must be taken with a proton pump inhibitor. It is approved for use in adults with chronic pancreatitis or after pancreatectomy. It is not approved for use in cystic fibrosis patients.
Fat-soluble vitamins	Supplementation of fat-soluble vitamins A, D, E, and K	Vitamins may be dosed individually, through the use of 1 or 2 multivitamins daily, or with a water-miscible combination preparation.
Antibiotics		
Parenteral antibiotics	Eradication or suppression of acute infection and pulmonary exacerbations	Altered pharmacokinetics may affect and complicate therapy. Appropriate duration of parenteral therapy has not been determined. Combination therapy is standard of care for *Pseudomonas* infection. Monotherapy may have advantages (decreased toxicity, resistance, cost), though it is not currently recommended.
Inhaled tobramycin (TOBI)	Eradication of initial infection and suppression of chronic infection	Use results in significant improvement in FEV_1, decreased hospitalizations, and decreased need for IV antibiotics. Product is recommended for chronic therapy in both mild and moderate to severe disease.
Azithromycin (Zithromax)	Antimicrobial and anti-inflammatory properties	Chronic oral therapy is recommended to improve lung function and reduce pulmonary exacerbations in patients colonized with *P. aeruginosa* and should be considered in patients not colonized with *P. aeruginosa* to reduce pulmonary exacerbations.
Inhaled aztreonam (Cayston)	Suppression of chronic infection	Product is recommended for chronic therapy in both mild and moderate to severe disease in patients colonized with *P. aeruginosa* to improve lung function and quality of life.
Antistaphylococcal antibiotics	Antimicrobial properties and suppression of chronic infection	Product is not recommended for prophylaxis in cystic fibrosis patients. Evidence is insufficient to recommend for or against chronic oral use in patients colonized with *Staphylococcus aureus*.
Antipseudomonal antibiotics	Suppression of chronic infection	Evidence is insufficient to recommend for or against chronic oral use in patients colonized with *P. aeruginosa*.

(continued)

Table 37-4. Drug Therapy for Cystic Fibrosis *(Continued)*

Therapeutic category	Indication and mechanism of action	Comments
Inhalation therapy		
Hypertonic saline inhalation	Liquefaction of pulmonary secretions	Nebulization therapy can be accomplished with hypertonic saline with or without other therapies.[a]
		For chronic therapy, 6–7% hypertonic saline given via nebulization therapy twice daily is recommended to improve lung function and quality of life and reduce exacerbations.
		A recent trial found no benefit of inhaled hypertonic saline in children < 6 years of age and infants.
Bronchodilators (β_2-agonists)	Bronchodilator in reversible or obstructive airway disease	Evidence is insufficient to recommend for or against chronic use of inhaled β_2-agonists.
Inhaled aztreonam and tobramycin	See "Antibiotics" above.	See "Antibiotics" above.
Recombinant human DNase (dornase alfa, Pulmozyme)	Contribution of DNA in mucus to viscosity; mechanism of action through cleavage of DNA (thereby decreasing mucus viscosity)	Chronic therapy is recommended in patients with asymptomatic or mild disease and with moderate to severe disease.
		Product improves pulmonary function and decreases pulmonary exacerbations.
N-acetylcysteine (Mucomyst)	Lowered mucus viscosity through sulfhydryl group, which opens the disulfide bond in mucoproteins	Bad taste and odor are present.
		Significant efficacy has not been documented.
Inhaled anticholinergics	Bronchodilation	Evidence is insufficient to recommend for or against chronic use.
Inhaled cromolyn	Bronchodilation	Evidence is insufficient to recommend for or against chronic use.
Inhaled other antibiotics (carbenicillin, ceftazidime, colistin, gentamicin)	Bronchodilation	Evidence is insufficient to recommend for or against chronic use.
Other therapy		
Ivacaftor (Kalydeco)	Lowered mucus viscosity through direct effects on the defective CFTR protein (CFTR potentiator); improves chloride transport through CFTR channels with the G551D mutation (4% of cystic fibrosis population)	In patients ≤ 6 years with the G551D mutation, chronic therapy resulted in improved pulmonary function, lower sweat chloride levels, and weight gain.
		Chronic therapy is recommended for patients with at least 1 G551D CFTR mutation to improve lung function, quality of life, and reduce exacerbations.
Ursodeoxycholic acid (ursodiol, Actigall)	Bile acid that suppresses hepatic synthesis and secretion of cholesterol; inhibits intestinal cholesterol absorption; solubilizes cholesterol	Product aids in dissolution of stones with cholelithiasis.
Ibuprofen (Motrin)	Nonsteroidal anti-inflammatory; controls airway inflammation	For individuals 6 to 17 years of age with an $FEV_1 \geq 60\%$ predicted, the chronic use of oral ibuprofen is recommended (peak plasma concentration 50–100 µg/mL) to slow loss of pulmonary function.
		For individuals ≥ 18 years, evidence is insufficient to recommend for or against the chronic use of oral ibuprofen.
		High dosages are needed to achieve good concentrations (requires therapeutic drug monitoring).
Corticosteroids	Anti-inflammatory	Corticosteroids (inhaled or oral) are not used routinely and not recommended for chronic therapy. They have positive effects on pulmonary function but negative effects on growth and development, glucose sensitivity, and bone health.
Leukotriene modifiers	Decreased pulmonary inflammation	Evidence is insufficient to recommend for or against chronic use.

DNA, deoxyribonucleic acid.

a. Other therapies include bronchodilators, inhaled tobramycin, recombinant human DNase, and N-acetylcysteine.

Burkholderia and *Stenotrophomonas* species are commonly resistant. Follow culture and sensitivity results. Antibiotics that may be effective include trimethoprim-sulfamethoxazole (Septra, Bactrim), chloramphenicol, ceftazidime [Fortaz] (*B. cepacia*), doxycycline (Vibramycin), and piperacillin [Pipracil] (*S. maltophilia*).

Patient instructions and counseling

Compliance with therapeutic regimens is important.

Pancreatic enzyme supplementation
- Give immediately before or during snacks and meals.
- Capsule may be opened and contents sprinkled on applesauce or other acidic carrier.
- Contents should not be crushed or chewed.

Aminoglycosides
- Monitor urine output.
- Use ibuprofen with caution if dehydration, diarrhea, or decreased oral intake is present.

Ivacaftor (Kalydeco)
- Take with fat-containing food.
- Monitor liver function at baseline, every 3 months during first year, and annually thereafter. Interrupt therapy if liver function tests are greater than five times the upper limit of normal.

Adverse drug events

- ***Aminoglycosides:*** Nephrotoxicity, ototoxicity
- ***Ibuprofen (Motrin):*** Renal insufficiency
- ***Fluoroquinolones:*** Arthropathy
- ***Ivacaftor (Kalydeco):*** Elevated liver enzymes

Drug interactions

Pancreatic enzymes and acid suppression therapy may decrease inactivation of enzymes by gastric acid, thereby reducing dose requirement.

Ivacaftor use with CYP3A inhibitors or grapefruit or Seville oranges requires ivacaftor dose reduction. Use with CYP3A4 inducers decreases effectiveness of ivacaftor.

Monitoring parameters

Clinical status should be monitored:

- Fever and activity level
- Pulmonary function (as indicated by FEV_1, FVC, residual volume, and chest radiography)

Pharmacokinetic considerations

Aminoglycosides
- Increased clearance and larger V_d, necessitating greater dosing
- Concentration-dependent killing
- Postantibiotic effect against Gram-negative organisms
- Higher dosing (10 mg/kg/day tobramycin [Nebcin])
  - Once-daily dosing preferred over conventional three-times-daily dosing
- Conventional dosing:
  - Peak concentrations of 8–12 mcg/mL
  - Trough concentrations of < 2 mcg/mL

β-Lactams
- No change or increased clearance
- No change or increased V_d
- No postantibiotic effect or concentration-dependent killing

Fluoroquinolones
- Concentration-dependent killing
- Postantibiotic effect against Gram-negative organisms

Nondrug therapy

Pulmonary percussion therapy and postural drainage
The purpose of this therapy is to clear mucus and secretions from the pulmonary system. Therapy is initiated once or twice per day and can be conducted more often based on disease severity. Percussion is usually conducted after nebulization therapy with or without bronchodilator or mucolytic. Therapy with handheld devices or oscillatory vests can be done.

Transplantation
Lung transplantation is an option. Liver–lung transplantation can be done if the liver is involved.

Attention-Deficit/Hyperactivity Disorder

According to the American Psychiatric Association's *Diagnostic and Statistical Manual of Mental Disorders*, 5th edition (DSM-5) attention-deficit/hyperactivity disorder (ADHD) is a persistent pattern of inattention, hyperactivity/impulsivity, or both that interferes with development; has symptoms presenting in two or more settings; and negatively impacts directly on social, academic, or occupational functioning.

Classification

DSM-5 makes the following classifications:

- *Combined presentation:* Enough symptoms of inattention and hyperactivity/impulsivity are present for the past 6 months.
- *Predominantly inattentive presentation:* Enough symptoms of inattention, but not hyperactivity/impulsivity, are present for the past 6 months.
- *Predominantly hyperactive-impulsive presentation:* Enough symptoms of hyperactivity/impulsivity, but not inattention, are present for the past 6 months.

Clinical presentation

- *Inattention:* Symptoms include a lack of attention to detail, careless mistakes, difficulty paying attention, tendency not to listen, difficulty following through on instructions, loss of focus, distraction and disorganization, difficulty organizing tasks, avoidance of tasks that require a lot of mental effort, forgetfulness, and frequent misplacement of items.
- *Hyperactivity and impulsivity:* Symptoms include fidgeting or squirming in seat, difficulty staying seated, inappropriate running or climbing (restlessness in adolescents and adults), tendency to behave as if driven by a motor, inability to play quietly, overly talkative, speaking or acting out without thinking, difficulty waiting one's turn, and frequent interruption of others.

Pathophysiology

ADHD results from an imbalance in catecholamine neurotransmission (specifically between dopamine and norepinephrine).

Genetic basis

Genetic studies have primarily evaluated genes involved in neurotransmission. ADHD is likely due to the interaction of many genes. Most evidence currently indicates that dopamine active transporter 1 (DAT1) and dopamine D_2 and D_4 receptors are responsible (dopamine and norepinephrine are potent agonists of the D_4 receptor).

Diagnostic criteria

Children must have six or more symptoms of inattention, hyperactivity/impulsivity, or both for at least 6 months.

- Symptoms must be present prior to 12 years of age.
- Impairment must present in two or more settings (e.g., home and school).
- Clinically significant impairment occurs in social, academic, or occupational environments.
- Symptoms do not occur exclusively during another psychotic or mental illness (e.g., schizophrenia, mood disorder).

Treatment goals

- Educate the patient and family.
- Improve functioning and behavior.
- Achieve effective drug therapy with minimal side effects.

Drug therapy

Table 37-5 describes drug therapy for ADHD.

The AAP released an updated clinical practice guideline for the diagnosis, evaluation, and treatment of ADHD in 2011. Recommendations for treatment vary on the basis of patient age as follows:

- Preschool-age children (4–5 years of age): First-line therapy is behavior therapy. Methylphenidate (see Table 37-5 for brand names) may be added to behavior therapy if there is not significant improvement in the child's functioning.
- Elementary school–age children (6–11 years of age): First-line therapy should be drug therapy in combination with behavior therapy.
- Adolescents (12–18 years of age): Drug therapy should be used with the assent of the patient and preferably in combination with behavior therapy.

Stimulants are recommended as first-line drug therapy. Second-line drugs, in descending order, include atomoxetine (Strattera), extended-release guanfacine (Intuniv), and extended-release clonidine (Kapvay). Before the release of the 2011 guidelines, antidepressants (tricyclics, bupropion [Wellbutrin]) had been considered second-line drug therapy after stimulants; however, they are no longer recommended for ADHD management.

Patient counseling

Advise patients and caregivers of the need to store medications away from other children or siblings because of the potential for lethal overdose (tricyclic antidepressants) and for abuse (stimulants).

Table 37-5. Drug Therapy for Attention-Deficit/Hyperactivity Disorder

Therapeutic category	Indication and mechanism of action	Comments
Stimulants (first-line therapy)		
Mixed amphetamine salts (amphetamine/dextroamphetamine): Intermediate-acting (**amphetamine/ dextroamphetamine**, Adderall) Long-acting (**Adderall XR**) *Dextroamphetamine:* Short-acting (Dexedrine, DextroStat) Intermediate-acting (Dexedrine Spansule) *Lisdexamfetamine dimesylate:* Long-acting (**Vyvanse**) *Methylphenidate:* Short-acting (**methylphenidate**, Methylin, Ritalin) Intermediate-acting (Metadate ER, Methylin ER, Ritalin SR) Long-acting (Concerta, Daytrana, Metadate CD, Ritalin LA) *Dexmethylphenidate:* Short-acting (Focalin) Long-acting (Focalin XR)	Reuptake blockade of catecholamines (norepinephrine and dopamine) in pre-synaptic nerve endings	Products are classified as C-IIs with the potential for drug dependency. Do not give after 4:00 pm because later doses may cause insomnia. Amphetamines are not labeled for use in children < 3 years of age. Lisdexamfetamine is the pro-drug of dextroamphetamine; it was developed to discourage the potential for drug abuse. **Methylphenidate** is not labeled for use in children < 6 years of age. Daytrana is a transdermal patch and should be applied every morning to alternating hips and worn for 9 hours. Dexmethylphenidate, the d-threo-enantiomer of racemic methyl-phenidate, is thought to be the more active enantiomer. Methylin is available as a chewable tablet and an oral solution. Short-acting Adderall and Ritalin tablets may be crushed or chewed. The labeling for the following intermediate- or long-acting products allows for opening the capsule and sprinkling contents on applesauce: **Adderall XR**, Focalin XR, Metadate CD, Ritalin LA. Drug holidays may be recommended to determine if need for stimulant is still present and to minimize side effects (e.g., summer is a good time to see if patient is outgrowing disease).
Second-line therapy		
Atomoxetine (Strattera)	Noradrenergic-specific reuptake inhibitor	Atomoxetine is a nonstimulant, noncontrolled agent. It may take up to 4–6 weeks to see maximum effects. Discontinue in patients who develop jaundice or laboratory evidence of liver injury. Capsule should not be opened.
Guanfacine (extended-release; Intuniv)	α_2-receptor agonist	Guanfacine was previously marketed under brand name Connexyn. It is FDA approved for use as monotherapy or as adjunctive therapy with stimulants. Maximum effects may take 2–4 weeks. Tablet must be swallowed whole; do not crush or chew. Label recommends taking with a high-fat meal.
Clonidine (extended-release; Kapvay)	α_2-receptor agonist	Clonidine is FDA approved for use as monotherapy or as adjunctive therapy with stimulants. Maximum effects may take 2–4 weeks. Clonidine is a good option to use for ADHD and coexisting conditions such as sleep disturbances or tics. Tablet must be swallowed whole; do not crush or chew.

Boldface indicates one of top 100 drugs for 2012 by units sold at retail outlets, www.drugs.com/stats/top100/2012/units.

Adverse drug events

Stimulants may cause appetite suppression, abdominal pain, headache, insomnia, jitteriness, and weight loss (not height dependent). Stimulants may also lower the seizure threshold. Methylphenidate (see Table 37-5 for brand names) is contraindicated in patients with motor tics and Tourette syndrome.

Labeling for all the stimulants and for atomoxetine (Strattera) includes warnings for an increased risk of psychosis or mania, aggression or violent behavior, and anxiety or panic attacks.

In addition, atomoxetine (Strattera) labeling includes warnings for increased risk of suicidal ideation in children and adolescents and for the potential for severe liver injury. It is also contraindicated in patients with pheochromocytoma or a history of pheochromocytoma because of serious reactions (hypertension, tachyarrhythmia).

In December 2011, the FDA released a safety announcement regarding the use of stimulants (amphetamine and methylphenidate products) and atomoxetine (Strattera) in pediatric and adult patients. The announcement summarized current evidence that has failed to demonstrate an association between the use of stimulants or atomoxetine (Strattera) and adverse cardiovascular events (myocardial infarction, stroke, sudden cardiac death). The FDA continues to recommend the avoidance of stimulants and atomoxetine (Strattera) in patients with a history of cardiovascular disease, structural cardiac abnormalities, or both or in those patients for whom an increase in blood pressure would be undesirable.

Atomoxetine (Strattera) has been associated with gastrointestinal symptoms and sedation early in therapy; these side effects can be offset by starting with half the therapeutic dose for the first week of therapy. Appetite suppression can also occur.

α_2-adrenergic agonists (guanfacine [Intuniv], clonidine [Kapvay]) may cause hypotension, bradycardia, syncope, and sedation, especially within the first month of therapy. Somnolence is a common effect with these agents. Rebound hypertension is also possible with abrupt withdrawal; thus, tapering is recommended when discontinuing these products.

Drug interactions

Methylphenidate (see Table 37-5 for brand names)

- Methylphenidate should not be given with monoamine oxidase (MAO) inhibitors (severe hypertension has occurred).
- Caffeine may enhance stimulant effects.
- Methylphenidate may inhibit metabolism of phenytoin (Dilantin), phenobarbital (Luminal, Solfoton), warfarin (Coumadin), and tricyclics.

Atomoxetine (Strattera)

- Atomoxetine should not be given with MAO inhibitors (serious, sometimes fatal reactions have occurred).
- Atomoxetine is a substrate for CYP2D6; dosing should be titrated more slowly with concomitant use of strong CYP2D6 inhibitors (e.g., fluoxetine [Prozac], paroxetine [Paxil], quinidine [Quinidex]).

Guanfacine (Intuniv)

- Guanfacine is a substrate for CYP3A4; dosing should be adjusted accordingly when given concomitantly with strong CYP3A4 inhibitors (e.g., ketoconazole [Nizoral]) or inducers (e.g., rifampin [Rifadin, Rimactane]).
- Co-administration with valproic acid (Depakene, Stavzor) results in increased valproic acid concentrations; therapeutic drug monitoring of valproic acid should be conducted and dose adjustments made (if necessary) when using these agents together.

Tricyclics

- Multiple pharmacodynamic and pharmacokinetic drug interactions exist.
- Increased plasma concentrations of tricyclics could result in potential toxicity when certain antidepressants are added to the regimen (fluoxetine [Prozac], sertraline [Zoloft], fluvoxamine [Luvox], paroxetine [Paxil]) as well as with cimetidine [Tagamet], methylphenidate (see Table 37-5 for brand names), diltiazem [Cardizem], quinidine [Quinidex], and verapamil (Calan, Verelan, Isoptin).
- Decreased concentrations of tricyclic antidepressants may be seen with concomitant administration of carbamazepine and phenytoin.
- Increased therapeutic effect and potential toxicity may occur with MAO inhibitors.
- Increased central nervous system (CNS)-depressant effects occur with alcohol and sedatives.

Recommendations for therapy and monitoring

The efficacy of therapy should be monitored. Assess behavior changes, and evaluate feedback from teachers and parents.

Monitor patients periodically for changes in blood pressure and heart rate. The American Heart Association also recommends that all children be screened for cardiovascular disease risk factors prior to initiating therapy. An electrocardiogram (ECG) is warranted only prior to initiation of stimulant or atomoxetine

(Strattera) therapy in patients with risk factors for cardiovascular disease.

Stimulants

Begin with a low dose, and titrate upward to optimal functioning ability. The patient may need a decreased dose if side effects occur or if no further improvement is seen with the larger dose. If one stimulant fails, try another stimulant for the patient. For children who fail two stimulants, second-line therapy includes atomoxetine (Strattera) or an α_2-adrenergic agonist.

Atomoxetine (Strattera)

Because of the boxed warning for suicidal ideation when initiating therapy, patients should be monitored for any changes in behavior that necessitate referral to a mental health clinician.

Tricyclics

Initial and periodic ECGs are needed.

Pharmacokinetic considerations

Methylphenidate (see Table 37-5 for brand names) does not distribute well into adipose tissue (dose on milligram basis instead of milligrams per kilogram).

Nondrug therapy

- Behavioral techniques (e.g., positive reinforcement, time out, response cost, token economy)
- Environmental modifications
- Classroom management

Conjunctivitis

Conjunctivitis is an inflammation of the conjunctiva of the eye.

Classification

Conjunctivitis may be bacterial, viral, or allergic.

Clinical presentation

Conjunctivitis is characterized by redness of the eye, itching, ocular discharge, foreign body sensation, and crusting of the eye and eyelid. The patient may have altered vision because of the presence of discharge.

Pathophysiology

Conjunctivitis of the newborn

Inflammation of the conjunctiva often occurs in the first month of life. Causative agents include topical antimicrobial agents; bacteria (primarily *Neisseria gonorrhoeae, Chlamydia trachomatis, Staphylococcus aureus, Staphylococcus epidermidis, Streptococcus pneumoniae, Escherichia coli*, and other Gram-negative bacteria); and viruses (primarily herpes simplex).

Bacterial conjunctivitis (beyond first month of life)

The most common bacteria are *Staphylococcus aureus, Staphylococcus epidermidis, Streptococcus pneumoniae*, and *Haemophilus influenzae* (also gonococcal and chlamydial). Treat bacterial conjunctivitis with antibiotic therapy.

Viral conjunctivitis

Viral conjunctivitis, also known as pink eye, is contagious. Adenovirus is the most common causative agent.

This condition is commonly preceded by a cold or sore throat or exposure to another person with viral conjunctivitis.

Herpes simplex is another cause of viral conjunctivitis. Corneal involvement may lead to permanent visual damage.

Allergic conjunctivitis

Allergic conjunctivitis is caused by exposure to dander, pollen, or topical eye preparation. Most patients will exhibit itching of the eye.

Diagnostic criteria

Diagnosis is based on the patient's symptoms.

Treatment goals

- Eliminate or avoid the allergen (allergic conjunctivitis).
- Treat the underlying infection (bacterial conjunctivitis).
- Decrease severity, and provide symptomatic relief (all forms).

Drug therapy

Neonatal

Preventive medicine includes prophylaxis after delivery with erythromycin ophthalmic ointment (generic):

- **Onset day 1:** No treatment (secondary to prophylaxis after delivery)
- **Onset days 2–4 (Neisseria gonorrhoeae):** Penicillin G (Pfizerpen) or ceftriaxone (Rocephin) for 7 days

- *Onset days 3–10 (Chlamydia trachomatis):* Oral erythromycin (Erythrocin) + erythromycin ointment (generic) for 14 days
- *Onset days 2–16 (herpes simplex):* Possibly IV acyclovir (Zovirax)

Bacterial (beyond first month of life)

Ophthalmic antibiotic drops (bacitracin-polymyxin B [generic], trimethoprim-polymyxin B [generic], erythromycin [generic], or fluoroquinolone [ciprofloxacin (Ciloxan), gentamicin (Garamycin), or tobramycin (Tobrex)]) should be used in combination with an ophthalmic antibiotic ointment (erythromycin [generic] or bacitracin [generic]) at bedtime for 5–7 days.

Gonococcal

Ceftriaxone (Rocephin) should be used for one dose. With corneal ulceration, use systemic IV ceftriaxone therapy. Also treat for *Chlamydia* species.

Chlamydial

Administer a single dose of azithromycin (Zithromax) to children.

Viral

Ocular lubricant (e.g., artificial tears product) should be administered every 3–4 hours while the patient is awake.

Allergic

Remove allergen. Use ocular lubricant (e.g., artificial tears product); ocular decongestants (phenylephrine [Relief], naphazoline [Naphcon, All Clear, All Clear AR, Allerest, Clear Eyes, Clear Eyes ACR], tetrahydrozoline [most Visine products, Murine Tears Plus, Opti-Clear, Tetrasine Extra], oxymetazoline: α-adrenergic activity [Visine LR], ketotifen [Alaway, Zaditor]); antihistamines (olopatadine [Patanol]); antihistamine–decongestant combination products (pheniramine and naphazoline [Naphcon-A, Opcon-A, Visine-A], antazoline and naphazoline [Vasocon-A]); topical mast cell stabilizer (cromolyn sodium [Crolom]); combination mast cell stabilizer and antihistamine; or oral antihistamine therapy.

Adverse drug events

Ocular decongestants can cause rebound congestion of the conjunctiva. This reaction is less common with naphazoline (multiple products) and tetrahydrozoline (multiple products).

Instilling of eye drops and ointment

Wash hands before and after administration. Tilt head back, grasp lower eyelid and pull away from eye, place dropper or ointment tube over eye, and have the patient look up immediately before instilling the drop or ointment.

For ointment, use a sweeping motion and instill 0.25 to 0.5 inch of ointment inside eyelid. Close eye after instillation, and wait 1–2 minutes. Blot excess ointment or solution away from around the eye. Vision may be temporarily blurred with ointment administration.

Wait 5 minutes between drops for multiple drop therapy. For suspension, place that drop in the eye last. For use of both ointment and drops, instill drops first and wait 10 minutes before applying ointment.

Patient instructions and counseling

- Wash hands before and after administration.
- Do not share towels or linens.
- Store products according to labeling instructions.

Nondrug therapy

Cold compresses are a helpful nondrug therapy.

Select Medication Issues, Drug Contraindications, Boxed Warnings, and Labeling Changes Specific to Pediatric Patients

- Sulfonamides should not be used in neonates and infants ≤ 2 months of age because of risk of kernicterus.
- Ceftriaxone (Rocephin) should not be used in neonates ≤ 28 days of age because of the risk of kernicterus.
- Use of fluoroquinolones in patients ≤ 18 years of age may cause arthropathy and cartilage lesions while growth plate is open. They are used in a few conditions as second-line agents.
- Tetracyclines are contraindicated in children ≤ 8 years of age because of drug deposition into developing teeth and bone.
- Aspirin is contraindicated because of risk of Reye's syndrome. It is used in certain conditions (e.g., Kawasaki disease).
- Isotretinoin (Accutane) is contraindicated in adolescents because of risk of birth defects, mental problems, and suicide. Birth control is required for females taking isotretinoin.
- Promethazine (Phenergan) is contraindicated for children ≤ 2 years of age because of respiratory depression and death.
- All antidepressants carry a warning about the potential for increased suicidal behavior in children and adolescents.

- Fentanyl (Duragesic) is contraindicated for children ≤ 2 years of age and should be used in children ≥ 2 years of age only if they are already using other opioid pain medications (i.e., they are opioid tolerant).
- The use of Elidel cream (pimecrolimus) and Protopic ointment (tacrolimus) in children ≤ 2 years of age is not recommended because of possible cancer risk.
- There is a risk of ceftriaxone and calcium precipitation with the concomitant use of ceftriaxone (Rocephin) and IV calcium-containing products. Deaths attributable to intravascular and pulmonary precipitates have occurred in neonates. Ceftriaxone (Rocephin) should not be used in neonates (≤ 28 days of age) if they are receiving or are expected to receive IV calcium-containing products. In all other patients, the lines may be flushed well with a compatible fluid between the use of ceftriaxone (Rocephin) and an IV calcium-containing product.
- Over-the-counter cough and cold medicines are not to be used in infants and children ≤ 4 years of age because of the risk of serious and potentially life-threatening side effects. Combination products are not recommended in pediatric patients.
- Antiepileptic agents include a warning about the risk of suicidal thoughts or actions.
- The infant formulation of acetaminophen [Tylenol] (80 mg/0.8 mL) has been removed from the market. Only a single acetaminophen liquid concentration (160 mg/5 mL) is now commercially available.
- There have been postmarketing reports of sudden death in children and adults receiving stimulants or atomoxetine (Strattera) for ADHD (see section on ADHD).
- Heparin carries warnings for the potential for dosing errors and deaths in neonates.
- Tumor necrosis factor (TNF)-α blocking agents carry warnings for the risk of lymphoma and malignancy in children and adolescents with autoimmune disorders.
- Codeine-containing products carry warnings for the risk of respiratory depression and death in children who are CYP2D6-ultrarapid metabolizers receiving codeine after tonsillectomy, adenoidectomy, or both.
- Kaletra (lopinavir/ritonavir) carries a warning for propylene glycol accumulation and toxicity (cardiac toxicity, lactic acidosis, acute renal failure, CNS depression, respiratory complications, death) in preterm neonates.

- IV magnesium sulfate products carry a warning that use in pregnant women for preterm labor beyond 5–7 days can lead to hypocalcemia and bone abnormalities in the developing fetus.
- In addition to warnings regarding birth defects, particularly neural tube defects, in children born to women taking valproate sodium (Depacon), valproic acid (Depakene, Stavzor), and divalproex sodium (Depakote), these products now carry an additional warning regarding impaired cognitive development and lower IQ scores in children born to women taking the drug. These products should not be used in women of childbearing age (e.g., for migraine prevention) unless the drug is essential to medical management.
- The FDA released a safety announcement in August 2011 regarding the potential for a small increased risk of death in individuals taking recombinant human growth hormone (somatropin [Nutropin, Humatrope, Norditropin, Saizen, Genotropin, others]). The FDA is reviewing information regarding this risk, which stemmed from the results of the Santé Adulte Gh Enfant (SAGhE) Study conducted in France, and at this time does not recommend discontinuing treatment.

37-5. Questions

Use the following case study to answer Questions 1 and 2:

A 4-day-old male infant (37 weeks' gestation, birth weight 3.2 kg, length 50 cm) has been admitted to the hospital secondary to spiking temperatures. He has demonstrated decreased oral intake and irritability since being discharged from the newborn nursery 2 days ago. He is started on IV fluid at maintenance volume and antimicrobial therapy with ampicillin 165 mg IV q6h and gentamicin 14 mg IV once daily. Cultures have been obtained from blood, urine, and cerebrospinal fluid and are pending. Laboratory assessment includes the following: Na 142 mEq/L, K 3.5 mEq/L, Cl 108 mEq/L, HCO$_3$ 22 mEq/L, BUN 15 mg/dL, SCr 0.9 mg/dL, and Glc 88 mg/dL.

1. What is the patient's estimated creatinine clearance (mL/min/1.73 m²)?

A. 100
B. 75
C. 60
D. 50
E. 25

2. Which of the following is the most accurate reason for this patient's creatinine clearance estimate?

   A. Presence of maternal serum creatinine
   B. Increased water loss via postdelivery diuresis
   C. Increased glomerular filtration rate
   D. Increased tubular secretion rate
   E. Aminoglycoside-induced nephrotoxicity

3. Aminoglycosides are hydrophilic compounds. Which of the following is true regarding aminoglycoside pharmacokinetic parameters in neonates compared with those in adults?

   A. Decreased clearance
   B. Increased V_d
   C. Decreased half-life
   D. Unchanged elimination
   E. Increased liver metabolism

4. Which of the following is most likely to complicate phenytoin therapy in a 2-day-old breast-fed neonate with new-onset seizures?

   A. Decreased renal elimination
   B. Altered liver metabolism
   C. Increased albumin stores
   D. Decreased triglycerides
   E. Physiological jaundice

5. A drug metabolized through which of the following reactions is a concern in the neonatal population?

   A. Hydrolysis
   B. Reduction
   C. Sulfation
   D. Glucuronidation
   E. Methylation

Use the following case study to answer Questions 6 through 8:

A 7-month-old formula-fed female is brought to your pharmacy by her mother, who describes the infant as having new onset of fever (102.5°F) and increased irritability in the past 24 hours. The mother states that she stayed home with the infant today instead of sending her to day care. Family history is significant for an older sibling with a recent upper respiratory tract infection. Examination of the infant's ear canal using a pneumatic otoscope reveals a bulging, red

tympanic membrane with no mobility on negative or positive pressure. Computer records reveal that she was treated for acute otitis media at 3 months of age.

6. Decisions for antimicrobial therapy in this patient should be based on coverage for which of the following pathogens?

   A. *Staphylococcus epidermidis, Streptococcus pneumoniae,* and *Pseudomonas aeruginosa*
   B. *Streptococcus pneumoniae, Haemophilus influenzae,* and *Moraxella catarrhalis*
   C. *Haemophilus influenzae, Streptococcus pyogenes,* and *Pseudomonas aeruginosa*
   D. *Streptococcus pneumoniae, Staphylococcus aureus,* and *Moraxella catarrhalis*
   E. *Staphylococcus epidermidis, Pseudomonas aeruginosa,* and *Burkholderia cepacia*

7. The drug of choice for this patient's current episode of acute otitis media is

   A. amoxicillin.
   B. amoxicillin-clavulanate.
   C. IM ceftriaxone.
   D. cefixime.
   E. trimethoprim-sulfamethoxazole.

8. When the pharmacist is counseling the patient's mother about the antibiotic suspension prescribed by the patient's health care provider, which of the following should be discussed?

   I. Risk factors for otitis media
   II. Whether the suspension should be refrigerated
   III. The need to shake the suspension vigorously prior to administration

   A. I only
   B. III only
   C. I and II only
   D. II and III only
   E. I, II, and III

9. Which of the following is a common side effect of amoxicillin-clavulanate therapy?

   A. Hemolytic anemia
   B. Liver function test abnormalities
   C. Pancreatitis
   D. Diarrhea
   E. Headache

10. Which of the following is a side effect that should be a concern in a child with acute otitis media, nausea, and vomiting who is receiving ibuprofen for fever?

    A. Stevens–Johnson syndrome
    B. Renal insufficiency
    C. Hyponatremia
    D. Oral candidiasis
    E. Liver failure

11. How is otitis externa, or swimmer's ear, best treated?

    A. Instill an antimicrobial and steroid solution into the ear canal.
    B. Apply antimicrobial ointment into the ear canal with a cotton swab.
    C. Instill an antihistamine solution into the ear canal.
    D. Increase pH of the ear canal with administration of Burow's solution.
    E. Decrease pH of ear canal with administration of dilute HCl solution.

Use the following case study to answer Questions 12 and 13:

A 15-year-old patient (40 kg) with cystic fibrosis is admitted to the hospital secondary to an acute pulmonary exacerbation. Home medications include Creon as directed, TOBI nebulization, ADEK once daily, and dornase alfa (once daily via nebulization). She is started on ceftazidime 2 g IV q8h and tobramycin 130 mg IV q8h.

12. Which of the following should be ordered in this patient?

    A. Serum tobramycin peak concentration
    B. Serum tobramycin trough concentration
    C. Serum tobramycin peak and trough concentrations
    D. Sputum ceftazidime concentration
    E. Sputum ceftazidime and tobramycin concentrations

13. Sputum cultures taken from this patient shortly after hospital admission are positive for *Staphylococcus aureus* (non–methicillin sensitive). Which of the following agents should be initiated at this time?

    A. Oxacillin
    B. Ticarcillin
    C. Piperacillin
    D. Vancomycin
    E. Amikacin

14. Which of the following is a pancreatic enzyme supplement?

    A. Actigall
    B. Beractant
    C. Pulmozyme
    D. Vyvanse
    E. Zenpep

15. Which of the following can be used to decrease the viscosity of pulmonary secretions?

    A. Exosurf
    B. Mucomyst
    C. Protilase
    D. Liquaemin
    E. Serevent

16. Counseling a patient on the use of pancreatic enzyme supplementation should include which of the following?

    A. Capsules may be opened and sprinkled over any food.
    B. Capsule contents should not be crushed or chewed.
    C. The total daily dose may be given at one time in the evening.
    D. Adequate supplementation will increase bowel movement frequency.
    E. The supplementation dose should not change with diet changes.

17. An 8-year-old patient is newly diagnosed with attention-deficit/hyperactivity disorder. Which of the following is considered first-line therapy for this patient?

    A. Intuniv
    B. Kapvay
    C. Strattera
    D. Vyvanse
    E. Wellbutrin

18. Atomoxetine is associated with which of the following serious adverse effects?

    A. Hepatic injury
    B. Renal failure
    C. Cardiovascular collapse
    D. Anaphylaxis
    E. Toxic epidermal necrolysis

19. A 9-year-old male patient is being started on imipramine therapy after failing therapy for ADHD with stimulants or second-line agents. This patient has two siblings, a 15-year-old brother and a 3-year-old sister. The pharmacist instructs the parents to keep the medicine away from siblings and in a safe place. What is the most likely reason for the pharmacist's concern regarding imipramine?

    A. Toxicity with overdose
    B. Abuse potential
    C. Stability of product
    D. Increased suicide risk
    E. Appetite suppression

20. A decrease in seizure threshold is a side effect of which of the following agents used for ADHD?

    A. Atomoxetine
    B. Clonidine
    C. Guanfacine
    D. Imipramine
    E. Methylphenidate

Use the following case study to answer Questions 21 and 22:

A patient comes in to your pharmacy and describes the development of itchy, red eyes, which are often swollen and draining. The patient says these symptoms occur every spring.

21. Which of the following is the most likely cause of this patient's ocular disorder?

    A. Viral conjunctivitis
    B. Bacterial conjunctivitis
    C. Allergic conjunctivitis
    D. Blepharitis
    E. Episcleritis

22. Which of the following therapies is the most appropriate recommendation for this patient's symptoms?

    A. Intranasal steroid
    B. Pseudoephedrine
    C. Bacitracin ointment
    D. Ocular phenylephrine
    E. Ocular olopatadine

23. Which of the following is most commonly associated with bacterial conjunctivitis beyond the first month of life?

A. *Chlamydia*
B. *Clostridium*
C. *E. coli*
D. *Neisseria*
E. *Staphylococcus*

24. Which of the following is a side effect of the prolonged use of ocular decongestants?

    A. Peripheral vasodilation
    B. Rebound conjunctival congestion
    C. Development of arrhythmias
    D. Development of tolerance
    E. Development of allergy to product

37-6. Answers

1. E. Using the Schwartz equation, this patient's estimated creatinine clearance is 25 mL/min/1.73 m² ($CrCl = 0.45 \times 50/0.9$).

2. A. The presence of maternal SCr that decreases in neonates over the first week of life may cause a false underestimate of calculated CrCl during this time. If one assumes that by the end of the first week of life, this patient's SCr has decreased to a more typical SCr of 0.4 mg/dL for a normal infant, the estimated CrCl would be 59 mL/min/1.73 m² ($CrCl = 0.45 \times 52/0.4$). Although infants do experience postdelivery diuresis, it should not decrease creatinine clearance. Other factors that affect CrCl in the neonate and infant include a decreased glomerular filtration rate and a decreased tubular secretion rate. Finally, this infant has been started on a standard, once-daily aminoglycoside dose with no indications of renal insufficiency or drug-induced nephrotoxicity at this time.

3. B. Aminoglycosides are hydrophilic compounds; they will exhibit larger volumes of distribution in patients with greater total body water. Neonates and infants have greater total body water, greater extracellular fluid volume, and a relative lack of adipose tissue. With aminoglycosides, when the extracellular fluid volume decreases, the volume of distribution decreases, elimination rate increases, and the half-life decreases. In general, the elimination and clearance of aminoglycosides decreases with increasing age.

4. E. Phenytoin is a highly plasma protein–bound drug. The total and free concentrations of highly

protein-bound drugs may be altered because of developmental differences in protein binding (decreased protein concentrations and altered binding capacity) and displacement by endogenous substances (e.g., free fatty acids and unconjugated bilirubin). Physiological jaundice, as exhibited by increasing total and unconjugated bilirubin concentrations, may occur in the neonatal period. Unconjugated bilirubin may displace drugs from albumin-binding sites. Additionally, one of the by-products of lipid metabolism, free fatty acids, may also displace drugs from albumin-binding sites (thereby increasing the free drug concentration). Kernicterus (also known as *yellow brain*) may occur when unconjugated bilirubin displaced by drugs or other endogenous substances (e.g., free fatty acids) crosses the blood–brain barrier, where it can deposit in the brain and cause neurologic complications. Because free fatty acids are not included in routine laboratory panels, serum triglycerides may serve as a surrogate marker of serum free fatty acid status.

5. **D.** UDPG (uridine diphosphoglucose)–glucuronyl transferase is responsible for conjugation of endogenous substances (bilirubin) and medications (morphine and chloramphenicol). The capacity for glucuronidation metabolism does not begin until around 2 months of age and reaches adult capacity by 2 years of age. Medications metabolized through this system are potential toxins in the neonatal population. An example would be the use of chloramphenicol in neonates and the development of "gray-baby syndrome" because of drug accumulation. Hydrolysis, reduction, sulfation, and methylation are functional in the neonatal period and should not pose drug therapy complications in this population.

6. **B.** The most common bacterial pathogens in acute otitis media are *Streptococcus pneumoniae, Haemophilus influenzae,* and *Moraxella catarrhalis.*

7. **A.** Despite the emergence of drug-resistant *Streptococcus pneumoniae,* high-dose amoxicillin (90 mg/kg/day)—because of its excellent pharmacodynamic profile, side effect profile, and cost—remains the drug of choice in uncomplicated acute otitis media. Amoxicillin-clavulanate is considered first-line therapy in patients who have received amoxicillin in the past 30 days, those with conjunctivitis, those

with recurrent otitis media unresponsive to amoxicillin, or those in whom β-lactamase coverage for *H. influenzae* or *M. catarrhalis* is indicated. IM ceftriaxone is an acceptable alternative or second-line agent, whereas cefixime and trimethoprim-sulfamethoxazole are not included in the AAP/AAFP guidelines as recommended therapies for acute otitis media.

8. **E.** Counseling should include specific information about the antibiotic, its side effect profile, storage information, information about administering the medicine, dosage instructions, the importance of taking the full course, and the need to shake the bottle prior to administering the dose. In addition, a discussion of risk factors for acute otitis media and preventive measures (pneumococcal and flu immunization) is appropriate in a counseling session.

9. **D.** The most common side effects with amoxicillin-clavulanate therapy include rash, urticaria, nausea, vomiting, and diarrhea. Although the other listed side effects may be seen with other antibiotic therapies, they do not typically occur with amoxicillin-clavulanate therapy.

10. **B.** Dehydration, which may develop in a child who is vomiting, is a risk factor for ibuprofen-induced renal insufficiency. If ibuprofen is used as an antipyretic or analgesic in pediatric patients, the parents or caregivers should be counseled regarding this risk and the need to follow intakes and outputs during the period of acute illness (i.e., gastroenteritis) when the child may be receiving ibuprofen therapy.

11. **A.** The treatment of otitis externa includes the instillation of an antimicrobial and steroid otic solution into the ear canal. Cotton swabs should be avoided to prevent otitis externa. Antihistamine solutions are not indicated in the treatment of otitis externa. Otic solutions containing acetic acid may also be of benefit in otitis externa by decreasing (not increasing) the pH of the ear canal and lowering its bacteria-harboring potential. Hydrochloric acid in any form should not be used in the ear canal.

12. **C.** Therapeutic drug monitoring is a critical part of the overall therapeutic plan in patients with cystic fibrosis. Patients with cystic fibrosis exhibit altered pharmacokinetic parameters of aminoglycosides, primarily increased clearance and greater volumes of distribution. When using conventional (rather than once daily) dosing,

tobramycin peak concentrations should be obtained to make sure the dose being given is sufficient to reach concentrations of 8–12 mcg/mL, and trough concentrations should be obtained to ensure adequate renal clearance (cystic fibrosis patients receive higher mg/kg doses).

13. **D.** *S. aureus* is a common pathogen in cystic fibrosis patients. Methicillin-sensitive *S. aureus* may be treated with a number of agents (e.g., oxacillin); however, methicillin-resistant *S. aureus* should be treated with vancomycin.

14. **E.** Zenpep is the brand name for a pancreatic enzyme supplement. It is available as a delayed-release capsule with enteric-coated beads.

15. **B.** Mucomyst is the brand name for N-acetylcysteine, which lowers mucus viscosity (the sulfhydryl group opens the disulfide bond in mucoproteins).

16. **B.** Pancreatic enzyme products are available in various formulations (powder, tablet, and capsule with enteric-coated microspheres, beads, or microtablets). The capsule formulations may be opened and the contents sprinkled over acidic foods (e.g., applesauce). Contents should not be crushed or chewed. Additionally, the dose should be based on the amount and type of food (i.e., full doses with meals or half doses with snacks and light meals). Adequate replacement will actually decrease bowel movements and improve stool consistency (i.e., decrease steatorrhea).

17. **D.** Stimulants are considered first-line therapy for ADHD. Vyvanse (lisdexamfetamine dimesylate) is the only stimulant listed. Intuniv (guanfacine) and Kapvay (clonidine) are α_2-receptor agonists, and Strattera (atomoxetine) is a noradrenergic-specific reuptake inhibitor; both classes of drugs are considered second-line therapy for ADHD. Wellbutrin is an antidepressant, and although antidepressants were previously recommended as potential second-line therapy in ADHD management, they are no longer recommended per the 2011 ADHD guidelines.

18. **A.** Atomoxetine's labeling has a boxed warning about the potential for severe liver injury. Atomoxetine should be discontinued in any patient who develops jaundice or laboratory evidence of liver injury.

19. **A.** Overdose of tricyclic antidepressants may be fatal because of the development of arrhythmias. Because this patient has a younger sibling in the house, there is a potential for the child to get into her older brother's medicine. Stimulants may have the potential for abuse in patients who do not have ADHD (i.e., the 15-year-old brother), but tricyclic antidepressants are not associated with a high abuse potential. There are no stability issues with imipramine. Atomoxetine (Strattera) carries a warning for suicide risk, and appetite suppression can be seen with stimulants.

20. **E.** Stimulants (methylphenidate) may lower the seizure threshold. The other agents listed are not associated with seizure occurrence.

21. **C.** Allergic conjunctivitis occurs after exposure to allergens, primarily dander or pollen. Patients suffering from allergic conjunctivitis will typically complain of eye itching.

22. **E.** Antimicrobial therapy (bacitracin ointment) has no place in therapy for allergic conjunctivitis. Ocular lubricants, decongestants, antihistamines (olopatadine), mast cell stabilizers, or combinations of these products are appropriate options for allergic conjunctivitis. Intranasal steroids may be used for allergic rhinitis, not conjunctivitis. Oral decongestants (pseudoephedrine) are not recommended for allergic conjunctivitis. Although ocular decongestants (phenylephrine) are recommended for allergic conjunctivitis, naphazoline or tetrahydrozoline products are preferred because of decreased rebound conjunctival congestion.

23. **E.** The most common pathogens in neonatal bacterial conjunctivitis are *Neisseria gonorrhoeae*, *Chlamydia trachomatis*, *Staphylococcus aureus*, *Staphylococcus epidermidis*, *Streptococcus pneumoniae*, and *Escherichia coli*. Bacterial conjunctivitis beyond the first month of life is most commonly caused by *Staphylococcus aureus*, *Staphylococcus epidermidis*, *Streptococcus pneumoniae*, and *Haemophilus influenzae*. *Clostridium*, an anaerobe, is not a common bacterial pathogen in conjunctivitis.

24. **B.** Not unlike reactions from prolonged use of nasal decongestants, prolonged use of ocular decongestants may cause rebound congestion of the conjunctiva. This effect is less pronounced with naphazoline and tetrahydrozoline.

37-7. References

American Academy of Family Physicians, American Academy of Otolaryngology–Head and Neck Surgery, American Academy of Pediatrics Subcommittee on Otitis Media with Effusion. Otitis media with effusion. *Pediatrics.* 2004;113:1412–29.

American Academy of Pediatrics, Subcommittee on Attention-Deficit/Hyperactivity Disorder and Steering Committee on Quality Improvement and Management. ADHD: Clinical practice guideline for the diagnosis, evaluation, and treatment of attention-deficit/hyperactivity disorder in children and adolescents. *Pediatrics.* 2011;128:1007–22.

American Pharmaceutical Association. *Special Report: Medication Administration Problem-Solving in Ambulatory Care.* Washington, DC: American Pharmaceutical Association; 1994:9.

American Psychiatric Association. *Diagnostic and Statistical Manual of Mental Disorders* (DSM-5), 5th ed. Washington, DC: American Psychiatric Association; 2013.

Cooper WO, Habel LA, Sox CM, et al. ADHD drugs and serious cardiovascular events in children and young adults. *N Engl J Med.* 2011;365:1896–904.

Fiscella RG, Jensen MK. Ophthalmic disorders. In: Krinsky DL, Berardi RR, Ferreri SP, et al., eds. *Handbook of Nonprescription Drugs: An Interactive Approach to Self-Care.* 17th ed. Washington, DC: American Pharmacists Association; 2012: 509–30.

Flume PA, Mogayzel PJ, Robinson KA, et al. Cystic fibrosis pulmonary guidelines: Treatment of pulmonary exacerbations. *Am J Respir Crit Care Med.* 2009;180:802–8.

Kearns GL, Abdel-Rahman SM, Alander SW, et al. Developmental pharmacology: Drug disposition, action, and therapy in infants and children. *N Engl J Med.* 2003;349:1157–67.

Krypel L. Otic disorders. In: Krinsky DL, Berardi RR, Ferreri SP, et al., eds. *Handbook of Nonprescription Drugs: An Interactive Approach to Self-Care.* 17th ed. Washington, DC: American Pharmacists Association; 2012:557–69.

Leeder JS, Kearns GL. Pharmacogenetics in pediatrics: Implications for practice. *Pediatr Clin North Am.* 1998;44:55–77.

Lieberthal AS, Carroll AE, Chonmaitree T, et al. The diagnosis and management of acute otitis media. *Pediatrics.* 2013;131:e964–99.

Miyagi SJ, Collier AC. Pediatric development of glucuronidation: The ontogeny of hepatic UGT1A4. *Drug Metab Dispos.* 2007;35:1587–92.

Mogayzel PJ Jr, Naureckas ET, Robinson KA, et al. Cystic fibrosis pulmonary guidelines. Chronic medications for maintenance of lung health. *Am J Respir Crit Care Med.* 2013;187:680–9.

Oszko MA. Common ear disorders. In: Herfindal ET, Gourley DR, eds. *Textbook of Therapeutics: Drug and Disease Management.* 7th ed. Baltimore, MD: Lippincott Williams & Wilkins; 2000:1049–56.

Rosenfeld M, Ratjen F, Brumback L, et al. Inhaled hypertonic saline in infants and children younger than 6 years with cystic fibrosis: The ISIS randomized controlled trial. *JAMA.* 2012;307(21):2269–77.

Schwartz GJ, Brion LP, Spitzer A. The use of plasma creatinine concentration for estimating glomerular filtration rate in infants, children, and adolescents. *Pediatr Clin North Am.* 1987;34:571–90.

Schwartz GJ, Haycock GB, Edelmann CM, et al. A simple estimate of glomerular filtration rate in children derived from body length and plasma creatinine. *Pediatrics.* 1976;58(2):259–63.

Schwartz GJ, Muñoz A, Schneider MF, et al. New equations to estimate GFR in children with CKD. *J Am Soc Nephrol.* 2009;20:627–37.

Solomon SD. Common eye disorders. In: Herfindal ET, Gourley DR, eds. *Textbook of Therapeutics: Drug and Disease Management.* 7th ed. Baltimore, MD: Lippincott Williams & Wilkins; 2000:1037–48.

Stewart CF, Hampton EM. Effects of maturation on drug disposition in pediatric patients. *Clin Pharmacol.* 1987;6:548–64.

U.S. Food and Drug Administration. Drug safety communication: Safety review update of medications used to treat attention-deficit/hyperactivity disorder (ADHD) in adults. Web page: http://www.fda.gov/Drugs/DrugSafety/ucm279858.htm.

U.S. Food and Drug Administration. Updated questions and answers for healthcare professionals and the public: Use an approved pancreatic enzyme product (PEP). Web page: http://www.fda.gov/Drugs/DrugSafety/PostmarketDrugSafetyInformation forPatientsandProviders/ucm204745.htm.

Wright CC, Vera YY. Cystic fibrosis. In: DiPiro JT, Talbert RL, Yee GC, et al., eds. *Pharmacotherapy: A Pathophysiologic Approach.* 8th ed. New York, NY: McGraw-Hill; 2011:525–37.

Yaffe SJ, Aranda JV. *Pediatric Pharmacology: Therapeutic Principles in Practice.* 2nd ed. Philadelphia, PA: WB Saunders; 1992.

Geriatrics and Gerontology

38

William Nathan Rawls

38-1. Key Points

Alzheimer's Disease

- Alzheimer's disease is a progressive neurologic disease that results in impaired memory, intellectual functioning, and behavior.
- Alzheimer's disease has no cure, but therapies exist to decrease memory impairment as well as improve behavior and patient functioning.
- Other forms of dementia that are potentially reversible should be identified and treated accordingly.
- New drug therapies may slow the progression of Alzheimer's disease and allow patients to remain in the least restrictive environment possible.
- Caregiver support and education are important measures to ensure patient safety and well-being.

Parkinson's Disease

- Parkinson's disease is a chronic, progressive neurologic disease for which no cure exists; medications are available to slow the progression of symptoms.
- The etiology of Parkinson's disease is unknown but may involve genetic susceptibility combined with environmental toxins and age-related changes in the brain.
- Dopamine, the central neurotransmitter, is decreased in Parkinson's disease, and current drug therapy is primarily directed at increasing dopamine levels.
- Drug therapy monitoring in Parkinson's disease requires an understanding of a variety of different medications that may cause significant adverse effects.
- Physical therapy, occupational therapy, dietary considerations, and support counseling for caregivers are necessary components of treating Parkinson's disease.

Glaucoma

- Glaucoma, a group of eye diseases, is characterized by increased intraocular pressure resulting in damage to the optic nerve and possible blindness.
- Open-angle glaucoma is the most common form of this disease; angle-closure glaucoma can be a medical emergency.
- The goal of therapy is to reduce intraocular pressure with the simplest medication regimen possible.
- Drug therapy for glaucoma usually begins with a topical β-adrenergic antagonist; patients often require combination therapy.
- Medication compliance is essential in the control of glaucoma. Education of the patient and the caregiver is required to overcome treatment barriers.

Urinary Incontinence

- Urinary incontinence is a significant issue with social and functional implications for geriatric patients.
- Urge incontinence is the most common complaint in older women whereas overflow incontinence is the most frequent issue for geriatric men.

- Drug therapy can improve symptoms but may not completely resolve urinary incontinence.
- Correctly identifying the type of urinary incontinence is important because the drug therapy for one type can worsen another type of incontinence.

38-2. Study Guide Checklist

The following topics may guide your study of this subject area:

- Risks associated with taking multiple medications
- Changes in pharmacokinetics associated with aging
- Basic steps in evaluating medication regimens in older adults
- Proposed mechanism of action for drugs used to treat Alzheimer's disease
- Trade names and available dosage forms of drugs used to treat Alzheimer's disease
- Significant drug interactions of drugs used to treat Alzheimer's disease
- Symptoms of Parkinson's disease
- Actions of various categories of drugs used to treat Parkinson's disease
- Considerations for selection of medications to treat Parkinson's disease
- The role of medications in treating glaucoma
- Actions of each category of medications used to treat glaucoma
- Trade names and available dosage forms of medications used to treat glaucoma
- Patient instructions for the use of medications to treat glaucoma
- Types of urinary incontinence as it relates to medication treatment selection
- Actions of various categories of drugs used to treat urinary incontinence
- Trade names and available dosage forms of drugs used to treat urinary incontinence
- Drug interactions that can worsen urinary incontinence

38-3. Overview

Gerontology is the study of the problems of aging and all its aspects. *Geriatrics* focuses on the diseases associated with aging and the treatments for those conditions. Geriatrics is of particular concern for pharmacists.

More than 12% of the U.S. population is older than 65 years of age. By 2050, the percentage is expected to increase to over 20%.

Persons older than 65 years of age have more chronic illnesses and take more prescription and nonprescription drugs than persons in younger age groups. The use of herbal or dietary supplements by older adults has increased significantly in the past 10 years, with the increased risk of adverse events and drug interactions.

Age-related physiologic changes and increased medication use contribute to a greater risk of adverse drug events. Changes in vision, hearing, and mental functioning can result in increased problems with medication compliance.

The ability of aging individuals to live independently is closely tied to the following three functions: bowel and bladder control, ambulation, and cognitive functioning. Impairment of any one of these areas can result in loss of independence and increased health care costs. Medication review and consultation can ensure maximal benefit from drug therapies while identifying medications that can negatively affect these critical functions.

Adverse Drug Events in the Older Adult

Drug-related hospitalizations occur four times more often for older adults than for younger adults. Nearly 100,000 older adults are hospitalized each year because of adverse drug effects; insulin, oral hypoglycemic agents, and warfarin are the most often implicated medications.

Older adults receiving multiple medications are at risk of a "prescribing cascade" that occurs when an unrecognized adverse effect of a medication is treated as a new illness and additional medications are prescribed.

Older adults are at increased risk of drug–drug interactions when taking multiple medications, and this potential is decreased by medication simplification.

The possibility that a newly developed medical condition or worsening of an existing illness is related to an older adult's medication or herbal use should be considered when a pharmacist is making medication recommendations.

Changes in Pharmacokinetics Associated with Aging

Decreased absorption of various drugs occurs secondary to decreased stomach acidity and changes in blood flow to the stomach (the least altered by aging). Absorption is also altered by co-administration of medications that either bind or compete for absorption. For example, antacids can decrease the absorption of drugs such as digoxin, iron, and phenytoin, thereby reducing their clinical benefit.

Altered drug distribution is caused by a decrease in total body water, increased lipid storage, and decreased serum albumin in malnourished elderly persons. These factors can contribute to increased serum levels of drugs. With increased body fat as seen in many older adults, greater storage of lipid-soluble drugs occurs. Benzodiazepines such as diazepam will accumulate with repeated doses and have a prolonged effect; they should therefore be avoided in the elderly population. Hydrophilic drugs are distributed in lean body mass and can accumulate in older persons with increased blood levels that can prove excessive. Digoxin and ethanol are examples of hydrophilic drugs that may cause toxicity when taken by the elderly.

The body's goal is to remove foreign substances from the blood, and this action includes medications. Drug metabolism is necessary to allow the elimination of most drugs. However, decreased hepatic blood flow and reduced hepatic enzyme activity cause slower drug metabolism. Increased levels of drugs require increased metabolism by the liver, but a decrease in liver size and function is associated with aging. The resulting increase in drug levels can produce adverse effects.

Elimination of drugs by the kidneys is slowed because of decreased renal blood flow and lowered glomerular filtration. Thus, drug accumulation develops.

The Cockcroft–Gault formula for estimating creatinine clearance (CrCl) can be used to predict renal function in the elderly:

$$CrCl(mL/min) = \frac{(140 - age) \times weight\ in\ kg}{72 \times Cr}$$

Note: Use ideal body weight. The equation above is for males. For females, multiply the result by 0.85. The use of any formula for predicting renal clearance of drugs is limited by patient variability, general health, and concurrent medical conditions.

In dosing the elderly, the general rule is to start with doses lower than those used in younger patients and to increase doses at a slower rate.

38-4. Drugs of Concern

The following drugs most often cause adverse events among the elderly, resulting in hospitalization:

- Warfarin
- Insulin
- Oral hypoglycemic agents
- Oral antiplatelet agents

The following drugs can cause psychiatric symptoms:

- Anticholinergics
- Narcotics
- Tricyclic antidepressants
- Central nervous system stimulants
- Antiparkinson drugs

The following drugs can produce anxiety symptoms:

- Theophylline
- Nasal decongestants
- β-agonists
- Antiparkinson drugs
- Appetite suppressants

The following drugs can contribute to nutritional deficiencies:

- Diuretics
- Digoxin, digitalis
- Laxatives (overuse)
- Sedatives (overuse)

38-5. Medication Compliance and the Older Adult

Types of noncompliant behavior in the elderly include the following:

- Failure to take medications
- Premature discontinuation of a medication
- Excessive consumption of a medication
- Use of medications not currently prescribed

Several strategies can improve patient medication compliance:

- Limit the number of different medications, and decrease the dose frequency.
- Simplify dosage instructions.
- Tailor the regimen to the patient's schedule.
- Use compliance aids and telephone reminders.
- Enlist the assistance of family members and friends.

38-6. Basic Components of Evaluating Drug Therapy in Older Adults

These questions should be answered in an evaluation of drug therapy:

- Why is the drug being used? A diagnosis or reason should be given.
- Is the drug being given correctly? The dosage, form, and schedule of administration should be analyzed.
- Are any symptoms or complaints related to drug therapy?
- Is monitoring of treatment ongoing?
- What is the endpoint of therapy?

Suggestions on how to review a geriatric patient's medications include the following:

- Consider all medications (not just the obvious), but focus first on the most likely to cause issues.
- Consider length of therapy, including when a drug was added or a dosage was increased or decreased.
- Remember basic mechanisms of action.
- Try to match reported symptoms with possible medication side effects.
- Consider that lack of response to treatment may be related to drug therapy (for example, interactions).
- Review lab results, if available, and recommend additional tests only if necessary.
- Simplify medications in a manner that will aid in identifying which change caused a specific result.

38-7. Alzheimer's Disease and Related Dementias

Dementia is the decline in intellectual abilities (e.g., impairment of memory, judgment, abstract thinking) coupled with changes in personality. Dementia patients tend to be described as cognitively impaired.

Cognition is the mental process by which people become aware of objects of thought and perception, including all aspects of thinking and remembering. Impairment of cognition significantly affects the life of the dementia patient, his or her family members, and the community in general.

Types of Dementia

Alzheimer's disease accounts for approximately 70% of dementias. Vascular dementias account for approximately 15% of dementias. Patients may have both Alzheimer's disease and vascular dementia.

Other Causes of Dementia

- Vascular disease and cerebrovascular accidents (strokes)
- Neurologic disorders such as Parkinson's disease, frontotemporal dementia, dementia with Lewy bodies, and Huntington's chorea
- Metabolic disorders such as hypothyroidism, alcoholism, and anemia
- Infectious diseases such as meningitis, syphilis, and acquired immune deficiency syndrome

Clinical Presentation

Alzheimer's disease is a progressive neurologic disease that results in impaired memory and intellectual functioning and altered behavior. Alzheimer's disease is characterized by the slow onset of symptoms leading to loss of ability to function independently. Symptoms may include psychoses with hallucinations, illusions, and delusional thinking. As Alzheimer's disease progresses, the brain continues to deteriorate.

Depression can cause cognitive impairment similar to that of Alzheimer's disease and should be identified and treated.

Pathophysiology

Hallmark pathologic changes in the brain are linked to Alzheimer's disease (i.e., neuritic plaques and neurofibrillary tangles increase). Neuritic plaques are composed of amyloid proteins deposited on neurons. Neurofibrillary tangles exist within neurons and disrupt normal function.

Neurotransmitters are also altered in Alzheimer's disease. Acetylcholine concentrations decrease significantly.

Diagnostic Criteria

Diagnosis of Alzheimer's disease requires the presence of memory impairment and one or more of the following:

- Aphasia (language disturbance)
- Apraxia (impaired motor abilities)

- Agnosia (failure to recognize objects)
- Disturbance of executive function (e.g., planning, organizing)

Treatment Principles

When evaluating a patient for treatment of dementia and Alzheimer's disease, review the patient's medications and consider any that might cause mental confusion or worsen underlying disease states. Drugs that block activity of acetylcholine can worsen dementia and decrease the effectiveness of medications used to treat Alzheimer's disease.

Anticholinergic drugs are used for a variety of conditions, ranging from depression to incontinence. Indications should be identified before treating Alzheimer's disease. Anticholinergic effects can be additive (i.e., a combination of anticholinergic drugs can result in toxicity even when each is given at low doses; see Table 38-1).

Provide support to caregivers, and treat the patient's behavioral and mood symptoms.

Consider a trial of a cholinesterase inhibitor, and monitor for benefits to memory and cognitive functioning.

Monitoring

Monitor memory and cognitive functions every 6–12 months.

Routinely assess behaviors and ability to perform activities of daily living (e.g., bathing, feeding, toileting, dressing).

Monitor for focal neurologic signs and symptoms that may suggest other causes of changes in cognitive function.

Drug Therapy

The pharmacologic approach to treatment falls into two categories:

- Medications used to control behavioral and emotional symptoms
- Medications used to slow or reverse the disease process

Symptomatic therapy

Medications used to control behavioral and emotional symptoms are used to provide symptomatic improvement and do not affect the outcome of the disease.

Anxiolytics are used to decrease anxiety and possibly agitation, motor restlessness, and insomnia. Such medications include lorazepam (Ativan), oxazepam (Serax), and buspirone (Buspar). The benzodiazepines can increase the risk of falls and injury.

Antidepressants improve depression, which can worsen the cognitive functioning of a patient with

Table 38-1. Anticholinergic Drugs That Can Worsen Alzheimer's Disease

Class	Drugs
Antidepressants	*Highest effects:* amitriptyline, amoxapine, clomipramine, protriptyline
	Moderate effects: bupropion, doxepin, imipramine, maprotiline, trimipramine
Antiparkinsonian agents	Benztropine, trihexyphenidyl
Antipsychotics	*Highest effects:* clozapine, mesoridazine, olanzapine, promazine, triflupromazine, thioridazine
	Moderate effects: chlorpromazine, chlorprothixene, pimozide
Antispasmodics	Atropine, belladonna alkaloids, dicyclomine, glycopyrrolate, hyoscyamine, methscopolamine, oxyphencyclimine, propantheline, oxybutynin, flavoxate, terodiline
Antihistamines	*Highest effects:* carbinoxamine, clemastine, diphenhydramine, promethazine
	Moderate effects: azatadine, brompheniramine, chlorpheniramine, cyproheptadine, dexchlorpheniramine, triprolidine, hydroxyzine
Antiemetic–antivertigo agents	Meclizine, scopolamine, dimenhydrinate, trimethobenzamide, prochlorperazine
Other agents with some anticholinergic activity	Paroxetine

Alzheimer's disease. Antidepressants include sertraline (Zoloft) and citalopram (Celexa).

Antipsychotics are used to decrease psychotic symptoms such as hallucinations and delusions. Antipsychotics such as haloperidol (Haldol), risperidone (Risperdal), and aripiprazole (Abilify) may reduce agitation and aggressiveness in dementia patients. A U.S. Food and Drug Administration (FDA) black box warning concerning the risk of increased mortality (cardiac events and infections) is associated with the use of antipsychotics in demented elderly patients.

Sedative-hypnotics are used for short-term treatment of insomnia but can increase confusion and memory impairment. These medications include trazodone (Desyrel), zolpidem (Ambien), and temazepam (Restoril).

Cholinesterase inhibitors

Medications used to slow or reverse the symptoms of Alzheimer's (see Table 38-2) affect acetylcholine activity in the brain. Acetylcholine levels may be decreased by as much as 90% in Alzheimer's disease. These levels can be increased by inhibiting the enzyme acetylcholinesterase.

Acetylcholinesterase inhibitors increase acetylcholine but do not replace lost cholinergic neurons or change the underlying pathology. This class of medications is used to prevent or slow deterioration in cognitive functioning.

The first cholinesterase inhibitor approved to treat Alzheimer's disease was tacrine (Cognex), which proved beneficial but caused hepatotoxicity (damage to the liver).

Safer cholinesterase inhibitors include the following:

- Donepezil (Aricept) is selective for acetylcholinesterase in the brain (i.e., not in peripheral tissues) and is approved for mild to moderate and moderate to severe dementia. A 23 mg tablet is now approved for moderate to severe dementia, but additional benefits of this higher dose are modest at best, and it has an increased incidence of adverse effects.
- Rivastigmine (Exelon), a nonselective cholinesterase inhibitor, decreases acetylcholinesterase. It is approved for mild to moderate Alzheimer's disease and dementia associated with Parkinson's disease.
- Galantamine (Razadyne) is a selective acetylcholinesterase inhibitor that activates nicotinic receptors, which may increase acetylcholine. It is approved for mild to moderate Alzheimer's disease dementia.

Patient instructions and counseling
Donepezil (Aricept)
Give orally, 5 mg daily for 4–6 weeks. Increase dosage to 10 mg daily at bedtime. Take with or without food. A 23 mg dose is available that has shown statistical significance but less clear observable benefits. This higher dose causes increased adverse effects, and there is limited research to support clinical benefits.

Rivastigmine (Exelon)
Oral doses are given with a gradual dosage increase. Begin at 1.5 mg twice daily and then 3 mg twice

Table 38-2. Drugs Used to Treat Alzheimer's Disease

Generic name	Trade name	Usual dosage	Dosage forms	Adverse effects
Donepezil	Aricept	5, 10, 23 mg at bedtime	5, 10, 23 mg tablets; 5 mg/5mL oral solution; 5, 10 mg disintegrating tablets	Nausea and vomiting
Rivastigmine	Exelon	1.5–6 mg bid	1.5, 3, 4.5, 6 mg capsules; 4.6 mg/24 h, 9.5 mg/24 h, 13.3mg/24 h transdermal patches; 2 mg/mL oral solution	Nausea and vomiting, anorexia, weight loss
Galantamine	Razadyne	4–12 mg bid	4, 8, 12 mg tablets; 8, 16, 24 mg extended-release capsules; 4mg/mL oral solution	Nausea and vomiting
Memantine	**Namenda**	5-10mg bid 7–28 mg daily	5, 10 mg tablets 7, 14, 21, 28 mg extended-release capsules; 5, 10 mg tablets; 2 mg/mL oral solution	Headache, constipation, dizziness, hypertension

Boldface indicates one of top 100 drugs for 2012 by units sold at retail outlets, www.drugs.com/stats/top100/2012/units.

daily, 4.5 mg twice daily, and 6 mg twice daily, with a minimum of 2 weeks between dose increases. If rivastigmine is discontinued because of adverse effects, restart at beginning dose. Take with meals in divided doses. Transdermal patch dosing begins with 4.6 mg every 24 hours, once daily for 4 weeks. It then increases to 9.5 mg every 24 hours, once daily.

Galantamine (Razadyne)

Doses begin with 4 mg twice daily for 4 weeks, 8 mg twice daily for 4 weeks, and then 12 mg twice daily. If galantamine is discontinued for more than a few days, restart at the beginning dose. In hepatic or renal dysfunction, doses should not exceed 16 mg/day. Do not use in instances of severe dysfunction. Take with meals in divided doses. Initiate therapy with extended-release capsules at 8 mg daily with a morning meal for 4 weeks. Increase the dose to 16 mg daily for 4 weeks and then 24 mg daily.

Adverse drug events

- **Donepezil:** Side effects include nausea, vomiting, and gastrointestinal (GI) symptoms. These side effects may be minimized by increasing the dose at 6 weeks.
- **Rivastigmine:** Side effects include nausea, vomiting, GI upset, and possibly significant weight loss. Adverse effects are dose related and may be lessened by increasing the dose at a slower rate.
- **Galantamine:** Adverse effects include nausea, vomiting, and GI upset. Slow dose titration will decrease side effects.

N-methyl-D-aspartate–receptor antagonists

Blocking the excitotoxicity effects of the neurotransmitter glutamate at N-methyl-D-aspartate (NMDA) receptors has been reported to be beneficial in Alzheimer's disease. Memantine (Namenda) is an NMDA-receptor antagonist used for moderate to severe Alzheimer's disease dementia. There is no evidence to support memantine use in mild Alzheimer's disease, and efficacy is modest at best in moderate Alzheimer's dementia. Immediate-release tablets have been discontinued, and now doses begin with 7 mg daily for 1 week, with weekly increases to 28 mg daily, if tolerated.

The dose should be reduced to 14 mg daily in patients with renal impairment (CrCl less than 30 mL/min).

Side effects include drowsiness, dizziness, headache, blood pressure elevations, and motor restlessness.

Drug–drug interactions

Anticholinergic drugs will reduce the effectiveness of cholinesterase inhibitors and cause dry mouth, blurred vision, constipation, and mental confusion (i.e., conditions that are more problematic in the elderly).

Cytochrome P450 enzyme inhibitors of 2D6 and 3A4 increase levels of galantamine and donepezil by inhibiting their metabolism.

Dextromethorphan (Robitussin DM), a potent NMDA-receptor antagonist, should be used cautiously with memantine. This caution also includes co-administration with amantadine and ketamine. Smoking and nicotine products may alter levels of memantine. Concurrent use of amantadine increases the potential for adverse effects.

Parameters to monitor

- Monitor cognitive function (e.g., poor results on mini–mental state exam, decline in performance of activities of daily living, incidence of behaviors that indicate cognitive decline).
- Watch for signs and symptoms of toxicity.
- Discontinue treatment with active peptic ulcer disease, severe bradycardia, and acute medical illness.
- Perform periodic complete blood cell count and basic chemistries.
- Look for expected benefits with the use of cholinesterase inhibitors and NMDA-receptor antagonists. Such benefits include improvement in memory, some stabilization of behaviors or mood, and possible slowing of the progression of the disease.

Nonprescription agents

High-dose vitamin E (2,000 units daily) has been recommended as an antioxidant to slow progression of Alzheimer's disease. Vitamin E may interfere with vitamin K absorption and result in increased risk of bleeding. Increased mortality has been reported with high-dose vitamin E. The potential toxicity of high-dose vitamin E may outweigh the benefits.

Ginkgo biloba, an herb, has been used to treat symptoms of Alzheimer's disease with reports of modest benefits. Ginkgo biloba is associated with increased risk of bleeding and hemorrhage, especially when combined with daily aspirin use, and is not recommended. There is growing evidence that ginkgo biloba does not provide any benefits over a placebo.

Observational studies of vitamin D (ergocalciferol) have shown a slowing of cognitive decline in Alzheimer's disease. Clear benefits and dosage considerations will require further research.

Nondrug Therapy

The treatment of Alzheimer's disease includes nonpharmacologic and pharmacologic therapies. Patients need to live in an environment that permits safe activities while minimizing risk.

Caregivers need training and support to deal with the behavioral and functional issues associated with this disease. Caregivers are at risk for depression and stress-related medical illnesses. Caregivers may also neglect their own health care needs and should be encouraged to maintain a healthy lifestyle.

38-8. Parkinson's Disease

Parkinson's disease (PD) is a chronic progressive neurologic disorder with symptoms that present as a variable combination of rigidity, tremor, bradykinesia, and changes in posture and ambulation. An estimated 1 million persons in the United States suffer from PD. Approximately 60,000 new cases are diagnosed each year.

The risk of developing PD increases with age, and a substantial increase in the U.S. population of persons over 60 years of age is predicted.

Because medications are the primary treatment for PD, pharmacists play an important role in the care of these patients.

Classification

The two classes of PD are primary parkinsonism and secondary parkinsonism. Primary parkinsonism has no identified cause. Secondary parkinsonism can be the result of drug use (e.g., reserpine, metoclopramide, antipsychotics); infections; trauma; or toxins.

Clinical Presentation

Clinical signs and symptoms of PD develop insidiously, progress slowly, may fluctuate, and worsen with time despite pharmacologic therapy.

Symptoms

Tremors at rest may begin unilaterally and are present in 70% of PD patients. Tremors that do not occur during sleep may worsen with stress.

Rigidity of limbs and trunk may develop. The face may have a masklike expression. Patients may have difficulty dressing or standing from a seated position.

Akinesia (the absence of movement) and bradykinesia (slowed movements) can occur. Postural instability with abnormal gait and an increased risk of falls are often experienced.

Depression and possibly dementia are possible nonmotor symptoms of PD.

Other symptoms include micrographia (small writing), drooling, decreased blinking, constipation, and incontinence. Patients may develop dysphagia (difficulty swallowing) and dysarthia (difficulty with speech).

Pathophysiology

PD involves a progressive degeneration of the substantia nigra in the brain with a decrease in dopaminergic cells (more than the typical decrease that accompanies normal aging). The most significant neurotransmitter in PD is dopamine, but other neurotransmitters may play a role (e.g., acetylcholine, glutamate, GABA [γ-aminobutyric acid], serotonin, norepinephrine).

The etiology is unknown, but genetic susceptibility is possible. Environmental toxins combined with aging may also be responsible for the development of PD.

Diagnostic Criteria

Clinical diagnosis is based on the presence of bradykinesia and either rest tremor or rigidity. The stages of the disease are described in Table 38-3.

Treatment Principles and Goals

The goal for treating PD is to relieve symptoms and maintain or improve quality of life for the patient. Treatment should be initiated when functional impairment and discomfort for the patient or caregiver occurs.

A safe environment and caregiver support programs in addition to medications will often allow patients to remain in the community.

Table 38-3. The Stages of Parkinson's Disease

Stage	Characteristics
1	Only unilateral involvement, with minimal or no functional impairment
2	Bilateral involvement without impairment of balance
3	Mild to moderate bilateral disease, with some postural instability (patient can maintain independence)
4	Severe disability (patient is unable to live alone independently)
5	Inability to walk or stand without assistance

Drug Therapy

Mechanism of action

Medications increase dopamine or dopamine activity by directly stimulating dopamine receptors or by blocking acetylcholine activity, which results in increased dopamine effects (Table 38-4).

Selection of an initial medication to treat PD may vary with the prescriber. Most therapy will begin with levodopa or with a direct dopamine agonist. Some experts will initiate therapy with a dopamine agonist in patients younger than 60 years of age. All medications that increase dopamine activity should not be discontinued abruptly because of the risk of sudden onset of Parkinson's symptoms.

Levodopa (Sinemet when combined with carbidopa)

Levodopa is the most effective drug in the treatment of PD and is converted to dopamine in the body. It is given with carbidopa, a decarboxylase inhibitor that prevents the peripheral conversion of levodopa to dopamine, thereby reducing nausea and vomiting while allowing more drug to pass through the blood–brain barrier.

Generally, doses are increased gradually to minimize the risk of side effects with the goal of improving symptoms with the lowest dose possible. In maintenance therapy or advanced disease, doses are given before meals to facilitate absorption. Carbidopa effectively inhibits peripheral conversion of levodopa at doses of 100 mg/day.

Levodopa provides benefits to all stages of PD, but chronic use is associated with adverse effects. Patients may have periods of good mobility alternating with periods of impaired motor function.

Dopamine agonists

Dopamine agonists work directly on dopamine receptors and do not require metabolic conversion. They may be used as monotherapy or as adjunctive therapy, allowing lower doses of carbidopa-levodopa. Some clinicians will initiate therapy with a direct dopamine agonist in younger newly diagnosed patients. Pramipexole (Mirapex), bromocriptine (Parlodel), and ropinirole (Requip) are available orally, and rotigotine is administered as a transdermal patch.

Apomorphine (Apokyn) is a direct-acting dopamine agonist that is administered by subcutaneous injection. It causes significant nausea and vomiting, and an antiemetic (e.g., trimethobenzamide) is given concurrently. Apomorphine is reserved for the treatment of "off" episodes associated with advanced disease. Monitor for orthostatic hypotension after initial doses and with dose escalation.

Selective monoamine oxidase type B inhibitors

Monoamine oxidase (MAO)-B inhibitors may be used as initial therapy in early PD and as adjunct treatment for more advanced disease. Although neuroprotective properties have been seen in animal models, benefits as monotherapy are modest.

With doses used for PD, adverse effects from consuming tyramine-containing foods would not be expected.

Catechol-O-methyl transferase inhibitors

Catechol-O-methyl transferase (COMT) inhibitors impair the secondary pathway that is responsible for the peripheral conversion of levodopa to dopamine and are ineffective when given alone. These medications should always be prescribed in conjunction with carbidopa-levodopa (Sinemet). They are most often used to treat patients during end-of-dose wearing-off periods and patients experiencing motor fluctuations.

Treatment complications and strategies for improving patient response include the following:

- *No initial response:* If the patient does not initially respond to levodopa (carbidopa-levodopa combination), gradually increase the dose to at least 1,000–1,500 mg of levodopa.
- *Suboptimal response:* After increasing levodopa, add another drug (e.g., a dopamine agonist, selegiline [Eldepryl], or a COMT inhibitor).
- *"On and off" phenomenon:* This type of response is associated with advancing disease and loss of

Table 38-4. Drugs for Treating Parkinson's Disease

Generic name	Trade name	Mechanism of action	Dosage and available strengths and forms
Carbidopa-levodopa	Sinemet	Increases dopamine (levodopa); prevents metabolism (carbidopa)	Give 25/100 mg/day at breakfast; increase to 25/100 mg tid. Dosage may be increased to 25/250 mg qid. Sustained-release 25/100 mg and 50/200 mg tablets are available. Oral disintegrating tablets (Parcopa) 10/100, 25/100, and 25/250 mg are available.
Bromocriptine	Parlodel	Directly stimulates dopamine receptors	Give 1.25 mg bid with meals; increase by 2.5 mg/day every day, up to 100 mg/day; 2.5 and 5 mg tablets are available.
Pramipexole	Mirapex	Directly stimulates dopamine receptors	Give 0.125 mg tid; increase weekly to 0.5–1.5 mg tid; 0.125, 0.25, 1, and 1.5 mg tablets are available.
Ropinirole	Requip	Directly stimulates dopamine receptors	Give 0.25 mg tid; increase gradually to a maximum of 24 mg/day; 0.25, 0.5, 1, 2, 4, and 5 mg tablets are available. Extended-release 2, 3, 4, 6, and 8 mg tablets are available.
Rotigotine	Neupro	Directly stimulates dopamine receptors	Apply transdermal patch 2 mg/24 h daily; increase weekly by 2 mg/24 h. 1 mg/24 h, 2 mg/24 h, 3 mg/24 h, 4 mg/24 h, 6 mg/24 h, and 8 mg/24 h patches are available.
Apomorphine	Apokyn	Directly stimulates dopamine receptors	Give 0.2–0.6 mL (2–6 mg) subcutaneous for acute attacks. Oral antiemetic (trimethobenzamide) is given concurrently.
Selegiline	Eldepryl, Carbex, Atapryl, Zelapar	Inhibits monoamine oxidase B; increases dopamine and serotonin	Initially give 5 mg at breakfast; increase to 5 mg at breakfast and lunch. 5 mg capsules, 5 mg tablets, and 1.25 mg oral disintegrating tablets (Zelapar) are available.
Rasagiline	Azilect	Inhibits monoamine oxidase B; increases dopamine and serotonin	Initial monotherapy is 1 mg once daily, as adjunct to levodopa 0.5–1 mg daily. 0.5 and 1 mg tablets are available.
Entacapone	Comtan	Inhibits catechol-O-methyl transferase (COMT), increasing dopamine	Give 200 mg with each dose of carbidopa-levodopa; maximum is 1,600 mg/day. 200 mg tablets are available.
Tolcapone	Tasmar	Inhibits COMT, increasing dopamine	Give 100 mg tid; discontinue if no benefits in 3 weeks. 100 and 200 mg tablets are available.
Amantadine	Symmetrel	May increase presynaptic release of dopamine; blocks reuptake	Give 100 mg bid; maximum is 400 mg/day. 100 mg tablets, 100 mg capsules, and 50 mg/5 mL syrup are available.
Benztropine	Cogentin	Blocks acetylcholine; may balance dopamine	Give 1–2 mg po, IM, or IV at bedtime or 0.5–6 mg/day in divided doses. 0.5, 1, and 2 mg tablets and 1 mg/mL injection are available.
Trihexyphenidyl	Artane	Blocks acetylcholine; may balance dopamine	Give 1 mg/day up to 5 mg/day (divided doses); 2 and 5 mg tablets and 2 mg/5 mL elixir are available.
Carbidopa-levodopa-entacapone	Stalevo	Combined effects of all three agents	Dosage is individualized, up to 8 tablets per day. Six dosage combinations are available.

IM, intramuscular; IV, intravenous.

benefits from a dose of medication. Use more frequent doses or sustained-release levodopa.

- *Acute intermittent hypomobility "off" episodes:* Such episodes are seen in advanced disease. They can be treated with subcutaneous injections of apomorphine, a direct-acting dopamine agonist.
- *End-of-dose or "wearing-off" period:* A decreased duration of benefit after a dose is experienced during a wearing-off period. Levodopa wanes after less than 4 hours; therefore, use combination therapy (two or more drugs), give levodopa more frequently, or use sustained-release carbidopa-levodopa (Sinemet CR).

Patient instructions and counseling

- Usually take medications on an empty stomach. Eat shortly afterward to avoid upset stomach.
- Take a missed dose as soon as possible. Skip the missed dose if the next scheduled dose is within 2 hours. Parkinson medications should not be abruptly discontinued because of the risk of rapid worsening of symptoms.
- Dizziness, drowsiness, and stomach upset may occur and make operating equipment dangerous.
- Report any confusion, mood changes, and uncontrolled movements to the prescriber as soon as possible.
- If taking a sustained-release product, do not crush.

Adverse effects and drug–drug interactions

Adverse effects of medications used to treat PD are described in Table 38-5. See Table 38-6 for information concerning drug–drug interactions.

As PD progresses, increasing dopamine levels can result in hallucinations and delusions. Psychotic symptoms can also be associated with advanced PD. Treatment of psychoses with antipsychotic medications can result in worsening motor symptoms secondary to dopamine D_2 receptor antagonism. Clozapine (Clozaril) has proven effective in decreasing hallucinations and delusions, but its use is complicated by the need for frequent blood monitoring to detect possible blood dyscrasias. Low doses of other antipsychotics are sometimes used with the goal of titrating between worsening motor function and improvement of psychotic symptoms.

Parameters to monitor

- Liver function, complete blood count, basic chemistries (periodically)
- Blood pressure, pulse, electrocardiogram (periodically)
- Reduction of rigidity, tremor, slowed movements
- Examination for mental confusion, mood changes, psychotic thinking

Nondrug Therapy

Educate the patient and caregiver about the benefits and side effects of PD medications. Provide aids for

Table 38-5. Adverse Effects of Medications Used to Treat Parkinson's Disease

Drug	Adverse effects
Dopaminergics	
Levodopa, pramipexole, bromocriptine, ropinirole, amantadine	Nausea and vomiting, agitation, confusion, depression, psychoses, orthostatic hypotension, dyskinetic movements, "sleep attacks," "pathologic gambling" (dopamine agonists), possible heart failure (pramipexole)
MAO-B inhibitors	
Selegiline, rasagiline	Nausea and vomiting, insomnia, dizziness, agitation, confusion, dyskinetic movements, anorexia
Amantadine	Confusion, dizziness, depression, anxiety, psychoses, insomnia
COMT inhibitors	
Tolcapone, entacapone	Nausea and vomiting, diarrhea, dyskinesia, urine coloration, possible liver toxicity (tolcapone)
Anticholinergics	
Benztropine, trihexyphenidyl	Dry mouth, blurred vision, constipation, urinary retention, confusion, agitation, psychoses

Table 38-6. Drug–Drug Interactions with Medications Used to Treat Parkinson's Disease

Medication	Interacting drug	Outcome
Dopamine agonists (e.g., bromocriptine, ropinirole)	Dopamine antagonists (e.g., haloperidol, metoclopramide)	Inhibition of benefits with worsening parkinsonism
Levodopa	Dopamine antagonists	Inhibition of benefits with worsening parkinsonism
Apomorphine	Ondansetron, other serotonin-receptor antagonists, dopamine antagonists	Severe hypotension and loss of consciousness Inhibition of benefits with worsening parkinsonism
Selegiline	Serotonergics, selective serotonin reuptake inhibitors, buspirone, mirtazapine	Serotonin syndrome (confusion, agitation, tremor, seizures, coma)
COMT inhibitors	Nonselective MAO inhibitors: phenelzine	Serotonin syndrome; hypertensive crisis secondary to increased catecholamines

compliance to enable the patient to participate in medication use as long as he or she is physically capable.

Physical therapy or occupational therapy may be important in maintaining physical activity and improving safety of working and living quarters. As PD progresses, speech therapy may be necessary to maintain the ability to communicate.

Dietary consultation may assist the patient in nutritional concerns related to swallowing difficulties and food selections.

38-9. Glaucoma

Glaucoma is a group of eye diseases characterized by an increase in intraocular pressure (IOP), which causes pathologic changes in the optic nerve and typical visual-field defects. Glaucoma affects more than 4 million Americans, and as many as 15 million more people may have increased IOP but no clinical signs and symptoms of glaucoma.

The prevalence of glaucoma increases with age and is most often seen in those 65 years of age or older. The number of persons with glaucoma is expected to increase with the aging U.S. population. With improved screening programs to identify those with increased IOP, an increase in the number of those diagnosed with glaucoma is expected.

Classification

Open-angle glaucoma is a form of primary glaucoma. The angle of the anterior chamber remains open in an eye, but filtration of aqueous humor is gradually diminished because of the tissues of the angle. Open-angle glaucoma accounts for approximately 80–90% of cases.

Angle-closure (narrow-angle) glaucoma is a form of primary glaucoma in an eye characterized by a shallow anterior chamber and a narrow angle. The filtration of aqueous humor is compromised because of the iris blocking the angle.

Congenital glaucoma results from defective development of the structures in and around the anterior chamber of the eye and results in impairment of aqueous humor.

Clinical Presentation

Clinical signs and symptoms of open-angle glaucoma develop slowly and may present with only minor symptoms, such as headache and mild eye pain. Optic nerve damage results from chronic elevations in IOP. Hence, early and consistent treatment is important to prevent loss of vision.

Acute angle-closure glaucoma presents with blurred vision, severe ocular pain, and possible nausea and vomiting. It should be considered a medical emergency, and immediate care should be recommended.

Chronic angle-closure glaucoma may have symptoms similar to those of open-angle glaucoma.

Tonometry is used to screen for IOP, but direct ophthalmoscopy (slit-lamp examination) is necessary to accurately evaluate the eye for changes in the optic nerve.

Pathophysiology

The pathogenesis of glaucoma results from changes in aqueous humor (the fluid filling the eye and in front of the lens) outflow that result in increased IOP. This increase in pressure leads to optic nerve atrophy and progressive loss of vision.

Increased IOP can result from decreased elimination or increased production of aqueous humor. Aqueous humor is secreted by the ciliary processes into the posterior chamber of the eye. It then flows through the trabecular meshwork and the canal of Schlemm.

Open-angle glaucoma is the result of decreased elimination of aqueous humor as it passes through the trabecular meshwork, thereby resulting in elevated IOP.

Angle-closure glaucoma is caused by papillary blockage of aqueous humor outflow. This blockage can result when a patient has a narrow anterior chamber in the eye or a dilated pupil where the iris comes into greater contact with the lens. With the blocking of outflow, aqueous humor accumulates in the posterior chamber, presses the lens forward, and further decreases drainage, with possible complete blockage as the outcome.

Diagnostic Criteria

- Elevated IOP as determined by tonometry
- Funduscopic assessment to identify characteristic changes in the optic disc and retina

Treatment Principles

Figure 38-1 illustrates the treatment of open-angle glaucoma. Treatment principles of glaucoma are as follows:

- Reduce IOP to prevent optic nerve damage and visual field loss.
- Use topical medications as first-line treatment.
- Consider acute angle-closure glaucoma as a medical emergency.

Monitoring

Periodic screening for increased IOP should be done, with yearly examinations for those over 65 years of age and as part of a routine eye examination.

Drug Therapy

Mechanism of action

Medications are considered the mainstay of therapy for the treatment of glaucoma (Table 38-7). Topical medications treat glaucoma by increasing aqueous humor

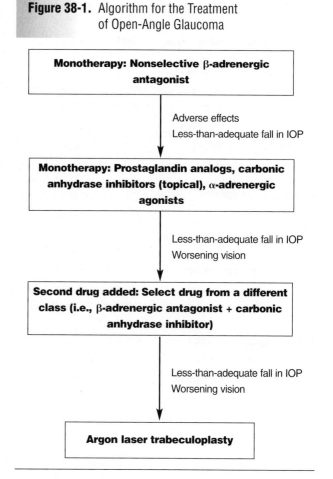

Figure 38-1. Algorithm for the Treatment of Open-Angle Glaucoma

outflow or by decreasing aqueous humor production. Prostaglandins, α-adrenergic agonists, and cholinergics all reduce IOP by increasing aqueous humor outflow. β-adrenergic antagonists, α-adrenergic agonists, and carbonic anhydrase inhibitors decrease aqueous humor formation (Table 38-8).

Prostaglandins

Prostaglandin analogs are used as first-line treatment (or in combination with β-blockers).

Prostaglandins are dosed once daily, which is a significant advantage in managing glaucoma.

β-adrenergic antagonists

β-adrenergic antagonists are also used as initial therapy and can be nonselective (i.e., they block both β_1 and β_2 receptors) or selective (i.e., they block only β_1 receptors). Drugs that block only β_1 receptors are considered cardioselective and cause less decrease in blood pressure and heart rate. Nonselective

Table 38-7. Medications for the Treatment of Glaucoma

Generic name	Trade name	Form	Usual dosage	Comments
Nonselective β antagonists				
Timolol	Timoptic	0.25, 0.50% solution and gel-forming solution	1 drop twice daily; gel solution used once daily	
Carteolol	Ocupress	1% ophthalmic solution	1 drop twice daily	
Levobunolol	Betagan	0.25, 0.50% solution	1 or 2 drops 1–4 times daily	
Metipranolol	Optipranolol	0.3% solution	1 drop twice daily	
Selective β₁ antagonists				
Betaxolol	Betoptic	0.25, 0.50% solution	1 or 2 drops twice daily	Drug is cardioselective. It has less effect on heart rate and blood pressure.
Carbonic anhydrase inhibitors				
Acetazolamide	Diamox	125, 250 mg tablets; 500 mg extended-release capsules	250 mg 1–4 times daily; extended-release 1 or 2 times daily	Do not use with sulfa allergy.
Dorzolamide	Trusopt	2% solution	1 drop 3 times daily	Do not use with sulfa allergy.
Brinzolamide	Azopt	1% solution	1 drop 3 times daily	Do not use with sulfa allergy.
Methazolamide	Neptazane	25, 50 mg tablets	15–50 mg 1–3 times daily	Do not use with sulfa allergy.
Prostaglandin analogs				Often chosen as initial therapy because of once daily dosing and few side effects
Latanoprost	Xalatan	0.005% solution, refrigerated	1 drop at bedtime	Drug can change blue eyes to brown.
Bimatoprost	Lumigan	0.03% solution	1 drop at bedtime	Drug can cause darkening of eyelids and eyelashes.
Travoprost	Travatan	0.004% solution	1 drop at bedtime	Ocular hyperemia frequently occurs.
Unoprostone	Rescula	0.15% solution	1 drop twice daily	If used with another drop, wait 5 minutes.
α₂-adrenergic agonists				
Brimonidine	Alphagan	0.15% solution	1 drop 3 times daily	Wait at least 15 minutes after using before placing soft contacts.
Dipivefrin	Propine	0.1% solution	1 drop twice daily	Dipivefrin is a prodrug of epinephrine.
Cholinergics (miotics)				
Pilocarpine	Pilocar	0.5, 1, 2, 3, 4, 6, 8% solution; 4% gel	1 or 2 drops 3–4 times daily; ½ inch gel at bedtime	A once weekly dose form (Ocuserts) is available.

Table 38-8. Classification, Mechanism of Action, and Adverse Effects of Glaucoma Medications

Medication class	Mechanism of action	Adverse effects
β-adrenergic antagonists (timolol, metipranolol, carteolol, levobunolol, etc.)	Decrease in aqueous humor formation with slight increase in outflow (β selective)	Adverse cardiac effects, worsening pulmonary disease, depression, dizziness
Miotics (cholinergics) (pilocarpine, carbachol)	Increase in aqueous humor outflow	Miosis, brow ache, dizziness, nausea, flushing, itching, sweating, confusion
Carbonic anhydrase inhibitors (dorzolamide, brinzolamide)	Decrease in aqueous humor formation	Lethargy, decreased appetite, GI upset, urinary frequency
Prostaglandin analogs (latanoprost, travoprost, bimatoprost)	Increased uveoscleral outflow without effect on aqueous humor formation	Iris pigmentation, eyelid darkening, macular edema
α_2-adrenergic agonists (apraclonidine, brimonidine)	Decrease in aqueous humor formation	Tachycardia, dry mouth, eyelid elevation, central nervous system effects in elderly and very young persons
Other α-adrenergic agonists (epinephrine, dipivefrin)	Increase in aqueous humor outflow	Tachycardia, increased blood pressure, allergic responses

β antagonists include timolol (Timoptic), carteolol (Ocupress), levobunolol (Betagan), and metipranolol (Optipranolol). β_1-selective antagonists include betaxolol (Betoptic) and levobetaxolol (Betaxon).

Therapy is initiated with a single topical ophthalmic solution, and additional agents are added if the decrease in IOP is less than acceptable. The effects of therapy on IOP should be apparent after a week of treatment.

Topical carbonic anhydrase inhibitors and α_2 agonists may be used in treatment.

Medications such as epinephrine, pilocarpine, and oral carbonic anhydrase inhibitors are prescribed less often, but they are considered to be effective adjunctive drugs.

Patient instructions and counseling

Multiple factors present obstacles that can interfere with good compliance. Patients are often asymptomatic and do not feel treatment is necessary. Because decreased vision is associated with glaucoma, patients may have difficulty with written instructions.

Adequate glaucoma therapy often requires two or more types of eye drops that may have to be given more than once daily. Correct administration of eye drops requires coordination and reasonable cognitive functioning.

Glaucoma is more common in the elderly, who may have more difficulty complying with prescribed medications.

Patient guidelines concerning the use of eye drops to treat glaucoma follow:

- Wash hands before administering eye drops, and avoid touching the dropper tip.
- Confirm that the medication is not outdated and has been stored properly.
- Looking upward, pull the lower lid down and instill the correct number of drops.
- Close the eye to allow the medication to have maximal effect.
- In most cases, wait 5 or more minutes between different medications.

Adverse drug events

Table 38-8 describes the adverse effects that may be seen with glaucoma medications.

Drug–drug interactions

Drug interactions between topical medications and systemic drugs are unlikely.

Acetazolamide interacts with the following:

- Aspirin to cause increased aspirin levels and possible toxicity
- Cyclosporine to cause increased cyclosporine levels
- Lithium to cause either increased or decreased lithium levels
- Phenytoin to cause an increased risk of osteomalacia

Parameters to monitor

Medication use is critical to the successful treatment of glaucoma and should be monitored by the health professional.

Other aspects

Combination products are available: timolol 0.5% and dorzolamide 2% (Cosopt), and brimonidine 0.2% and timolol 0.5% (Combigan). These combinations effectively lower IOP and require only twice-daily doses. This simplified dosing should improve compliance with treatment. Combinations (i.e., using two drugs from different categories) represent a sound treatment approach. Poor response to therapy may result in the prescribing of multiple medications, which may negatively affect the patient's ability to successfully use the more complex regimen.

Nondrug Therapy

Laser surgery

Argon laser (trabeculoplasty) has proven effective as adjunctive therapy that increases the flow of aqueous humor.

Surgery

A surgical procedure involves creating new means of drainage for aqueous humor to leave the anterior chamber.

38-10. Urinary Incontinence

Urinary incontinence in older adults often results in functional limitations and medical complications; it negatively affects social activities. Urinary incontinence is more common in elderly women than men and more common in institutionalized patients.

Types of Urinary Incontinence

Transient incontinence is common in elderly adults and can be the result of a variety of causes such as infections, delirium, stool impaction, restricted mobility, and pharmaceuticals. Medications prescribed for other conditions can cause urinary incontinence (Table 38-9). Sedative-hypnotic and opioid use may result in decreased alertness and inability to respond in a timely manner to the urge to urinate. Diuretics

Table 38-9. Medications That Can Worsen or Cause Urinary Incontinence

Class	Effect
Diuretics	Increased urine output
Sedative hypnotics	Sedation interfering with response to body's signal
Anticholinergics	Altered alertness, decreased bladder contractility
Opiates	Sedation, decreased bladder contractility
α-adrenergic receptor agonists	Excessive internal urethral sphincter tone
α-adrenergic receptor blocking agents	Decreased internal urethral sphincter tone
Combination OTC products containing antihistamine/ decongestants	Combined effect with decreased urine flow (in males)

OTC, over-the-counter.

increase urine flow and increase urinary frequency and challenge older adults in reaching the toilet in a timely manner. Anti-cholinergic drugs, used to treat certain types of urinary incontinence, can impair the bladder's contractility and result in incomplete voiding. α-adrenergic receptor agonists can result in urinary retention by increasing internal urethral sphincter tone.

Urge incontinence (detrusor hyperactivity) is more common in older women than men and is the result of a sudden bladder contraction that often results in complete bladder emptying prior to reaching a toilet.

Overflow incontinence is more common in elderly men and often relates to prostatic enlargement. Common symptoms include frequent urinations of small amounts, and this frequency may interfere with sleep.

Stress incontinence is more common in women and may be caused by pelvic floor laxity and inadequate sphincter contractility.

Functional incontinence in elderly persons is the result of decreased mobility and decreased manual dexterity, environmental barriers, and lack of motivation to remain continent of urine.

Pathophysiology

In simple terms, urination takes place when the detrusor muscle contracts the bladder and the internal and external urethral sphincters relax. Urinary incontinence in older adults may be the result of a variety of factors. The prevalence of uninhibited detrusor contractions may increase with age, and urethral closure pressure may decrease. In males, prostate enlargement may obstruct urine flow and result in residual urine remaining in the bladder, which can result in urinary tract infections. In addition, the ability to be able to successfully control urination requires adequate cognitive functioning so that there is proper response to the urge to urinate. Patients with dementia or delirium may not be able to control bowel and bladder functions.

Clinical Presentation

The classic presentation of urinary incontinence is either sudden, uncontrolled release of large amounts of urine (urge incontinence) or the frequent release of small amounts of urine ("dribbling" associated with overflow incontinence). Stress incontinence is the loss of bladder control associated with physical stresses such as coughing or sneezing. Treatment is complicated by the fact that older adults may present with mixed incontinence, as seen when an older woman may have stress incontinence while developing urge incontinence.

Diagnostic Criteria

An accurate history of urinary frequency and the amount voided is critical to determining the most likely type of urinary incontinence. In addition, to determine the extent of overflow incontinence, the amount of urine remaining in the bladder after voiding can be evaluated by the use of a catheter or ultrasound. More than 100–120 mL of urine remaining in the bladder would indicate abnormal urinary retention. A urinalysis also provides information to determine whether a urinary tract infection is present.

Treatment Principles

When evaluating a patient for treatment of urinary incontinence, review the patient's prescription and over-the-counter and herbal medications for agents that could cause or worsen urinary incontinence. Be prepared to suggest alternative medications that would be less likely to worsen incontinence and would not interact with potential drug therapies. Although symptoms should improve with treatment, complete resolution may not be achieved.

Drug Therapy

The pharmacologic approach to treatment is based on the type of incontinence and the patient's other medical conditions (see Table 38-10). Treatment is complicated by the fact that the treatment for one type of urinary incontinence may worsen symptoms in other types.

Urge incontinence

Anticholinergic drugs are prescribed to decrease detrusor hyperactivity. A variety of agents are available that decrease urinary frequency and improve control. Sustained-release oxybutynin (Ditropan) is effective and produces fewer adverse effects than immediate-release oxybutynin. Newer agents such as tolterodine (Detrol) and solifenacin (VESIcare) are reported to be more selective for the bladder, but all can cause anticholinergic adverse effects similar to those of oxybutynin and other first-generation anticholinergics. Mirabegron (Myrbetriq) is a selective β(3)-adrenergic agonist that causes bladder relaxation and provides modest benefit for urge incontinence. It may be an alternative for patients who cannot tolerate anticholinergic therapy.

Overflow incontinence

α-adrenergic receptor-blocking agents improve symptoms of overflow incontinence by decreasing internal urethral sphincter contractility. The internal sphincter is controlled by α-adrenergic receptors; stimulation causes contraction, and α-blocking agents allow this sphincter to remain open longer during urination with more complete voiding. Newer α-adrenergic receptor blockers such as tamsulosin (Flomax) are more selective for bladder function and may have less risk of adverse effects but have the potential to cause similar events as seen with earlier drugs such as terazosin (Hytrin). All α-receptor blocking agents have similar efficacy.

In older males, overflow incontinence is usually associated with prostate enlargement, and the addition of a 5-α-reductase inhibitor may be necessary. Drugs such as finasteride (Proscar) and dutasteride (Avodart) inhibit the conversion of testosterone to a more active form and treat benign prostatic hyperplasia (BPH) by reducing prostate enlargement. This in combination with an α-blocking agent improves urine flow to a greater extent than either drug used alone. 5-α-reductase inhibitors are usually added if a trial of an α-blocker is not successful because the

Table 38-10. Medications Used to Treat Urinary Incontinence

Generic name	Trade name	Used to treat	Dosage and available strengths and forms
α-adrenergic receptor blockers			
Terazosin	Hytrin	Overflow	1 mg at bedtime, slow increase up to 10 mg; 1, 2, 5, 10 mg tablets
Doxazosin	Cardura	Overflow	Immediate release: 1 mg daily, titrate up to 8 mg if needed; 1, 2, 4, and 8 mg tablets
	Cardura XL		Extended release: 4 mg daily, increase to 8 mg daily after 3–4 weeks; 4, 8 mg tablets
Prazosin	Minipress	Overflow	2 mg twice daily; 1, 2, 5 mg capsules
Tamsulosin	Flomax	Overflow	0.4 mg daily before a meal, increase to 0.8 mg daily after 2–4 weeks if needed; 0.4 mg tablets
Alfuzosin	Uroxatral	Overflow	Extended release: 10 mg daily; 10 mg tablets
5-α-reductase inhibitors			
Finasteride	Proscar	Overflow	5 mg daily with up to 6 months for response; 5 mg tablets
Dutasteride	Avodart	Overflow	0.5 mg daily with up to 6 months for response; 0.5 mg gel capsules
Anticholinergics			
Oxybutynin	Ditropan	Urge	Immediate release: 2.5 mg 2–3 times daily, increase to 5 mg 2–3 times daily; 5 mg tablets, 5 mg/5 mL syrup
	Ditropan XL		Extended release: 5–10 mg daily, increase weekly by 5 mg to maximum 30 mg daily; 5, 10, 15 mg tablets
	Oxytrol	Urge	Transdermal patch, 1 patch q 3 days (3.9 mg/day)
	Gelnique	Urge	Transdermal gel once daily; 3% gel, 100 mg/g gel packets
Tolterodine	Detrol	Urge	Immediate release: 1–2 mg twice daily; 1, 2 mg tablets
			Extended release: 2–4 mg once daily; 2, 4 mg tablets
Trospium	Sanctura	Urge	Immediate release: 20 mg twice daily (once daily for age > 75 years); 20 mg tablets
	Sanctura XR		Extended release: 60 mg daily; 60 mg capsules
Darifenacin	Enablex	Urge	Extended release: 7.5 mg once daily, after 2 weeks may increase to 15 mg daily; 7.5, 15 mg tablets
Solifenacin	**VESIcare**	Urge	5 mg daily, may increase to 10 mg daily; 5, 10 mg tablets
Fesoterodine	Toviaz	Urge	Extended release: 4 mg daily, may increase to 8 mg daily; 4 mg tablets
β₃ adrenergic agonist			
Mirabegron	Myrbetriq	Urge	Extended release: 25 mg once daily, may increase to 50 mg once daily; 25–50 mg tablets

Boldface indicates one of top 100 drugs for 2012 by units sold at retail outlets, www.drugs.com/stats/top100/2012/units.

reduction of testosterone activity can negatively affect libido and cause impotence. The use of the herbal product saw palmetto for BPH-related urinary incontinence was systematically reviewed and found to be no better than a placebo.

Stress incontinence

Several nonpharmacologic approaches are used to treat stress incontinence, but if not contraindicated, α-adrenergic agonists are often prescribed. The use of drugs such as pseudoephedrine, ephedrine, and midodrine (ProAmatine, Orvaten) stimulate the urethral sphincter and may improve bladder control. These drugs are associated with the risk of hypertension, anxiety, and insomnia and should be used with caution. The antidepressant duloxetine (Cymbalta) has been shown to be more effective than a placebo for stress incontinence, but its usefulness is limited because of frequent adverse effects.

Patient Instructions and Counseling

Adverse drug effects should be reviewed with the patient or caregiver with instructions to communicate with the prescriber or pharmacist for possible dosage adjustment or medication change. Patients should be advised to keep a record of changes in urination patterns, such as frequency of loss of control, as well as how often they need to urinate during the night.

Adverse Drug Events

- *Anticholinergics:* All agents can cause anticholinergic adverse effects such as dizziness, dry mouth, blurred vision, and confusion. There is a significant risk of falls associated with anticholinergics as well as a risk of worsening dementia.
- *α-adrenergic receptor blocking agents:* Side effects include lower blood pressure, orthostatic hypotension, dizziness, headache, and somnolence.
- *α-adrenergic receptor agonists:* Hypertension, anxiety, and insomnia are side effects.

Drug Interactions

Anticholinergics can worsen overflow incontinence by weakening bladder contractions and decreasing urine flow while α-adrenergic receptor agonists can cause increased internal urethral sphincter pressure and further decrease flow. Antihistamine–decongestant combinations have the ability to significantly decrease urine flow in older males.

The concurrent use of α-adrenergic receptor agonists and α-adrenergic blockers should be avoided.

Nondrug Therapy

Pelvic-floor muscle exercises are used to improve urine control but require motivation to commit to daily practice. Increased physical activity and weight loss in obese patients may improve urine control. Timed voiding is a useful behavioral technique where patients attempt to urinate at regular intervals and have decreased risk of sudden urine loss. Pessaries are devices that may benefit women by supporting pelvic organ prolapse and reducing urinary urgency. Surgical procedures are sometimes indicated to correct anatomical issues or to remove structural impediments to urine flow.

38-11. Questions

1. Of the following pharmacokinetic processes, which is the least altered by aging?

   A. Absorption
   B. Distribution
   C. Metabolism
   D. Elimination
   E. Excretion

2. Based on pharmacokinetic changes associated with aging, which of the following medications would be most likely to accumulate with repeated doses?

   A. Alprazolam
   B. Diazepam
   C. Donepezil
   D. Penicillin
   E. Selegiline

3. Galantamine increases levels of which neurotransmitter?

   A. Acetylcholine
   B. Dopamine
   C. Melatonin
   D. Norepinephrine
   E. Serotonin

4. Weight loss is most often associated with which of the following?

   A. Donepezil
   B. Galantamine
   C. Mirtazapine
   D. Rivastigmine
   E. Memantine

5. Of the following medications, which has FDA approval only for moderate to severe Alzheimer's disease?

   A. Donepezil
   B. Exelon
   C. Galantamine
   D. Namenda
   E. Aricept

6. Of the following medications used to treat behavioral and emotional symptoms in Alzheimer's patients, which has an FDA black box warning of increased mortality?

   A. Buspirone
   B. Citalopram

C. Lorazepam

D. Risperidone

E. Zolpidem

7. The maximum daily dose of galantamine in patients with renal impairment is

A. 8 mg/day.

B. 12 mg/day.

C. 16 mg/day.

D. 24 mg/day.

E. 32 mg/day.

8. All of the following could worsen cognition in Alzheimer's disease patients *except*

A. dicyclomine.

B. dimenhydrinate.

C. meclizine.

D. trazodone.

E. trihexyphenidyl.

9. Memantine's reported benefit in treating the symptoms of Alzheimer's disease is thought to be the result of

A. increasing serotonin receptor activity.

B. blocking the effect of glutamate on receptors.

C. directly blocking acetylcholine receptors.

D. decreasing intracellular dopamine activity.

E. decreasing amyloid deposits in the brain.

10. Which of the following works by direct stimulation of dopamine receptors?

A. Amantadine

B. Benztropine

C. Entacapone

D. Ropinirole

E. Selegiline

11. Urge urinary incontinence secondary to detrusor hyperactivity is most effectively treated with which of the following medications?

A. Avodart

B. Sanctura

C. Tamsulosin

D. Midodrine

E. Proscar

12. What would be the most likely outcome if a Parkinson's patient on levodopa were also prescribed haloperidol?

A. Excessive nausea and vomiting

B. Hypertensive crisis

C. Tachycardia and possible chest pain

D. Worsening symptoms of Parkinson's disease

E. Excessive somnolence

13. Which of the following inhibits MAO?

A. Benztropine

B. Bromocriptine

C. Pramipexole

D. Rasagiline

E. Tolcapone

14. How does carbidopa affect levodopa?

A. It slows the release from presynaptic neurons.

B. It prevents the excretion of dopamine.

C. It increases stimulation of dopamine receptors.

D. It decreases tolerance to normal doses.

E. It inhibits the peripheral conversion to dopamine.

15. C.H. is an 82-year-old male with a history of falls related to low blood pressure and now reports urinary incontinence. Which of the following would have the greatest potential for worsening his orthostatic hypotension?

A. Alfuzosin

B. Darifenacin

C. Doxazosin

D. Dutasteride

E. Tamsulosin

16. Which of the following statements are true concerning the treatment of Parkinson's disease?

I. Entacapone is not used as monotherapy except for patients with end-of-dose wearing-off periods and for those experiencing motor fluctuations.

II. Pramipexole has been reported to cause "sleep attacks."

III. Food–drug interactions would not be expected with selegiline when given at doses of 10 mg daily.

A. I only

B. III only

C. I and II only

D. II and III only

E. I, II, and III

17. Timolol ophthalmic drops would be more likely to cause which adverse effect as compared to levobetaxolol ophthalmic drops?

    A. Agitation and restlessness
    B. Nausea and vomiting
    C. Confusion
    D. Change in heart rate and blood pressure
    E. Altered intraocular pressure

18. Which of the following would *not* be considered for monotherapy of glaucoma?

    A. Latanoprost
    B. Dorzolamide
    C. Carteolol
    D. Methazolamide
    E. Brimonidine

19. Which of the following can cause iris pigmentation changes?

    A. Acetazolamide
    B. Betaxolol
    C. Brimonidine
    D. Latanoprost
    E. Pilocarpine

20. Which of the following is available as a fixed combination product?

    A. Dorzolamide and timolol
    B. Betaxolol and bimatoprost
    C. Bimatoprost and levobunolol
    D. Latanoprost and timolol
    E. Methazolamide and latanoprost

21. All of the following are available as an ophthalmic solution *except*

    A. brimonidine.
    B. dipivefrin.
    C. dorzolamide.
    D. methazolamide.
    E. metipranolol.

22. Which of the following should *not* be used if a patient has a sulfa allergy?

    A. Betaxolol
    B. Bimatoprost
    C. Brimonidine
    D. Brinzolamide
    E. Unoprostone

23. Which of the following is true about prostaglandin analogs?

    A. They cause an increase in aqueous humor synthesis.
    B. They cause a decrease in aqueous humor formation.
    C. They cause an increase in uveoscleral outflow without effect on aqueous humor formation.
    D. They cause pupil contraction resulting in aqueous humor outflow.
    E. They cause a decrease in uveoscleral outflow.

24. During a recent visit to his pharmacy, 79-year-old R. H. is recommended a combination antihistamine/decongestant for his runny nose and congestion. He says he is currently taking Proscar and Flomax. What would be the potential effect of taking these medications?

    A. Increased drowsiness when combining Flomax with an antihistamine/decongestant
    B. Decreased urine output and more frequent urinations
    C. Decreased absorption of Proscar, resulting in fewer benefits
    D. Increase in bladder spasms and sudden discharge of urine
    E. Dry mouth and blurred vision secondary to taking Proscar with a decongestant

38-12. Answers

1. **A.** Of all the age-related changes of the pharmacokinetic process, absorption is the least altered, perhaps because most drugs are passively absorbed.

2. **B.** Diazepam is a lipid-soluble drug and will accumulate in older adults secondary to increased storage in body fat. The potential for accumulation is much less with the other medications listed.

3. **A.** Galantamine is a cholinesterase inhibitor, and all cholinesterase inhibitors increase levels of acetylcholine, the neurotransmitter that appears to be involved with memory function.

4. **D.** Weight loss, probably because of nausea and vomiting, is a warning for rivastigmine. In

controlled trials, approximately 26% of women on doses of 9 mg/day or greater had weight loss of equal to or greater than 7% of their baseline weight. There is less reported weight loss with donepezil, galantamine, and memantine. The antidepressant mirtazapine is associated with weight gain in the elderly.

5. **D.** Namenda did not show benefit in mild to moderate Alzheimer's disease and is only FDA approved for moderate to severe disease. The others listed are all acetylcholinesterase inhibitors and are approved for mild to moderate Alzheimer's disease. Donepezil is also approved for moderate to severe disease.

6. **D.** Risperidone, as well as other atypical antipsychotics, increases mortality risk when given to dementia patients with agitation or aggressive behaviors. This is probably a class effect, and any antipsychotic should be used only if no alternative medication is effective.

7. **C.** With renal or hepatic dysfunction, galantamine doses should not exceed 16 mg/day. With severe renal or hepatic dysfunction, galantamine should not be used.

8. **D.** All of the drugs listed—with the exception of trazodone—have anticholinergic activity. Decreasing the activity of acetylcholine could worsen dementia and block benefits of cholinesterase inhibitors. Trazodone is an antidepressant with sedating properties but little anticholinergic activity. It may be given at bedtime to help with sleep. Trazodone has a side effect of orthostatic hypotension.

9. **B.** Glutamate is the main excitatory neurotransmitter in the central nervous system, and one theory states that blocking the effects of glutamate on NMDA receptors will block neurotoxic effects and decrease symptoms of Alzheimer's disease.

10. **D.** Ropinirole directly stimulates dopamine receptors; the other drugs treat Parkinson's disease by different mechanisms.

11. **B.** Sanctura (trospium) is an anticholinergic that decreases acetylcholine-mediated contractions of the detrusor muscle. This improves bladder control in urge incontinence. Avodart (dutasteride) and Proscar (finasteride) are used to treat overflow incontinence by reducing prostate enlargement. Tamsulosin, an α-adrenergic

antagonist, would decrease bladder control in urge incontinence. Midodrine, an α-adrenergic agonist, is used for stress incontinence and is less beneficial for urge incontinence than the use of an anticholinergic.

12. **D.** Haloperidol and other antipsychotics block dopamine activity and can worsen PD. They can also block the benefits of PD medications, which increase dopamine activity.

13. **D.** Rasagiline is an MAO inhibitor that is selective for MAO-B, which decreases the potential for drug–drug and drug–food interactions. At higher doses, this selectivity lessens.

14. **E.** Carbidopa inhibits the peripheral conversion of levodopa to dopamine, thus allowing more levodopa to cross the blood–brain barrier, and decreases adverse effects from dopamine.

15. **C.** Doxazosin, an α-adrenergic antagonist, could improve urine flow but has the potential to induce orthostatic hypotension and falls with geriatric patients being at greater risk. Alfuzosin and tamsulosin have a similar mechanism of action but may produce less orthostatic hypotension because of greater selectivity to bladder function.

16. **D.** Entacapone should always be given with carbidopa-levodopa because benefits depend on carbidopa inhibiting the peripheral conversion of levodopa.

17. **D.** Timolol is a nonselective β-adrenergic antagonist that causes a reduction in heart rate and blood pressure. There is enough absorption from eye drops to produce cardiac effects.

18. **D.** All of the other choices could be considered as monotherapy for glaucoma. Methazolamide is an oral carbonic anhydrase inhibitor and is used in conjunction with ophthalmic drops.

19. **D.** Latanoprost, a prostaglandin analog, is known to change iris pigmentation and to darken eyelashes.

20. **A.** Dorzolamide plus timolol is a combination ophthalmic solution for treating glaucoma. An advantage for using a combination product would be increased compliance.

21. **D.** Methazolamide and acetazolamide are both available only as oral tablets or capsules. Topical carbonic anhydrase inhibitors are brinzolamide and dorzolamide.

22. D. Patients with sulfa allergy should not be given a carbonic anhydrase inhibitor.

23. C. Prostaglandin analogs increase outflow without changing aqueous humor formation. β-adrenergic antagonists decrease formation with only a slight increase in outflow.

24. B. R.H.'s current medications indicate that he has overflow incontinence and that a decongestant would counter the benefits of tamsulosin and an antihistamine could decrease bladder contractions. The result would be urinary retention and more frequent release of small amounts of urine.

38-13. References

American Geriatrics Society 2012 Beers Update Expert Panel. American Geriatrics Society updated Beers Criteria for potentially inappropriate medication use in older adults. *J Am Geriatr Soc.* 2012;60(4): 616–31.

Boland MV, Ervin AM, Friedman DS, et al. Comparative effectiveness of treatments for open-angle glaucoma: A systematic review for the U.S. Preventive Services Task Force. *Ann Intern Med.* 2013; 158(4):271–79.

Cho S, Lau SW, Tandon V, et al. Geriatric drug evaluation: where we are now and where should we be in the future? *Arch Intern Med.* 2011;171(10): 937–40.

Farlow MR, Cummings JL. Effective pharmacologic management of Alzheimer's disease. *Am J Med.* 2007;120(5):388–97.

Fernandez HH. Updates in the medical management of Parkinson disease. *Cleve Clin J Med.* 2012;79(1): 28–35.

Griebling TL. *Urinary incontinence in the elderly.* *Clin Geriatr Med.* 2009;25(3):445–57.

Kwon YH, Fingert JH, Kuehn MH, et al. Primary open-angle glaucoma. *N Engl J Med.* 2009;360: 1113–24.

Qato DM, Alexander GC, Conti RM, et al. Use of prescription and over-the-counter medications and dietary supplements among older adults in the United States. *JAMA.* 2008;300(24):2867–78.

Rawls WN. Alzheimer's disease. In: Herfindal ET, Gourley DR, eds. *Textbook of Therapeutics.* 8th ed. Philadelphia, PA: WB Saunders; 2006:1811–28.

Stacy M. Medical treatment of Parkinson disease. *Neurol Clin.* 2009;27(3):605–31.

Toxicology and Chem-Bioterrorism

Peter A. Chyka

39-1. Key Points

- Medications are the most common cause of poisoning morbidity and mortality. Any chemical can become toxic if too much is taken in relation to body weight and physiologic capacity. A large number of poisonings occur in young children, but most fatalities occur in adults.

- Several approaches can minimize the risk of unintentional childhood poisonings (e.g., use of safety latches, proper storage of poisonous substances, adherence to label instructions), but the proper use of child-resistant containers (safety caps) is one of the most effective means.

- As part of the Poison Prevention Packaging Act of 1970, pharmacists are required to dispense oral prescription drugs (with certain exceptions such as nitroglycerin and oral contraceptives) in child-resistant containers unless the patient or prescriber indicates the desire for a nonsafety cap.

- Immediate first aid for a poison exposure can minimize potential toxic effects and involves water and fresh air, depending on the route of exposure. Contact a poison control center immediately through the nationwide access number (1-800-222-1222) to determine whether first aid should be administered or whether a poisoning emergency exists.

- Ipecac syrup—an orally administered emetic—has questionable effectiveness, and its use is now generally avoided.

- Activated charcoal—an orally administered adsorbent—is often the only treatment necessary if the toxin can be adsorbed and it is used within 1–2 hours of ingestion. It should be avoided in ingestions of aliphatic hydrocarbons and caustics and in patients with absent bowel sounds, and it is not useful with ingestion of heavy metals (sodium, lithium, iron, lead) or simple alcohols.

- Other hospital-based therapies include supportive and symptomatic care, multiple doses of activated charcoal (to enhance systemic elimination when appropriate), whole bowel irrigation with products such as CoLyte and GoLYTELY (to evacuate the intestinal tract), hemodialysis (to enhance systemic elimination), and use of antidotes (to antagonize or reverse toxic effects).

- Substance abuse often leads to acute and chronic toxicity from a variety of medications, commercial products, and illicit agents. The management of acute toxicity from substance abuse typically follows the same general approaches as those for poisoning and overdose. A challenge faced in many acute drug overdose episodes is determining the agents taken and possible adulterants or contaminants. Chronic abuse can lead to dependence, tolerance, and withdrawal.

- Few antidotes are available relative to the large number of potential poisons. The use of an antidote is usually an adjunct to conventional and supportive therapies.

- Acetylcysteine is a glutathione substitute in the metabolism of the acetaminophen-toxic reactive metabolite. It is most effective in preventing hepatotoxicity if given within 10 hours of an acetaminophen overdose, and it may also help later to minimize hepatic injury once it has begun. Oral (Mucomyst) and intravenous (Acetadote) preparations are available.

- Atropine is used to treat the muscarinic effects (bronchorrhea, bradycardia, etc.) produced by organophosphate and carbamate insecticides and anticholinesterase nerve gas agents by competing with acetylcholine for binding at muscarinic receptors in the nervous system.

■ Pralidoxime (Protopam) reactivates the enzyme acetylcholinesterase by dephosphorylation and allows metabolism of accumulated amounts of acetylcholine produced by enzyme inhibition from exposures to anticholinesterase nerve gas agents and organophosphate and carbamate insecticides.

■ Digoxin immune Fab (Digibind, DigiFab) is a specific antibody for digoxin, but it exhibits some cross-reactivity with other digoxin-like compounds. It is a sheep-derived antigen-binding fragment reserved for the treatment of life-threatening symptoms of digoxin overdose (e.g., bradycardia, ventricular arrhythmias, second- and third-degree heart block, hyperkalemia).

■ Flumazenil (Romazicon) is a competitive antagonist of benzodiazepines at the benzodiazepine receptor in the central nervous system (CNS). It is used in the treatment of severe CNS and respiratory depression that may occur when benzodiazepines are used as an anesthetic or taken as an overdose. Seizures may occur when flumazenil is administered to patients with co-ingestants of tricyclic antidepressants—drugs that lower the seizure threshold—and to patients requiring benzodiazepines for seizure control.

■ Administration of naloxone (Narcan), a competitive antagonist of opiate binding at the opioid receptors in the CNS, reverses the CNS and respiratory depression of opioid toxicity. Naloxone may precipitate withdrawal symptoms in opioid-dependent patients.

■ Bioterrorism is the deliberate use of infectious biological agents to cause illness such as smallpox (*variola* virus), anthrax (*Bacillus anthracis*), plague (*Yersinia pestis*), botulism (*Clostridium botulinum*), tularemia (*Francisella tularensis*), and viral hemorrhagic fevers (e.g., Ebola, Marburg, Lassa, Machupo).

■ The following chemicals can be used in warfare and may be used in a terrorist attack:
  • Substances that act on nerves (e.g., anticholinesterase agents such as sarin)
  • Substances that are blistering or vesicant agents (e.g., mustard agents, lewisites)
  • Substances that act on blood (e.g., arsine, cyanide)
  • Substances that act on the pulmonary system (e.g., phosgene, chlorine, ammonia)
  • Substances that are incapacitating (e.g., fast-acting CNS depressants or hallucinogens)
  • Substances that can also be used in riot control (e.g., various lacrimating agents such as chloroacetophenone and vomiting agents such as adamsite)

■ The U.S. Centers for Disease Control and Prevention maintains the Strategic National Stockpile that can be rapidly deployed to communities for life-saving medicines, supplies, and equipment necessary to counter chemical and biological threats.

39-2. Study Guide Checklist

The following topics may guide your study of this subject area:

■ Basic first-aid and general treatment measures for a poison exposure
■ Poison prevention measures for patient counseling
■ Matching of antidotes with the toxic agent
■ The mechanism of action of common antidotes
■ The route of administration of common antidotes
■ Recognition of typical toxic effects of common serious poisonings and drug overdoses
■ General categories of potential chemical and biological terrorist threats

39-3. Overview of Poisoning and Toxicology

Poisoning in America

Poisoning exposures and overdoses affect more than 2.5 million people annually, and more than 43,000 deaths occur yearly, of which drugs cause nearly 90%. A large number of poisonings occur in young children (< 1% of deaths are in preschool-age children), but most fatalities occur in adults. In 2008, poisoning became the leading cause of injury-related death in the United States.

Any chemical can become toxic if the exposure is too great in relation to body weight and physiologic capacity. Medications are the most common cause of poisoning morbidity and mortality.

Most poisonings in preschool-age children are unintentional or accidental. Unintentional poisonings can also occur in adolescents and adults; however, intentional (suicide and drug abuse) poisonings and overdoses are common.

Toxicology is the study of the adverse effects of chemicals and other xenobiotics on living organisms. There are several specialized areas of toxicology, including basic science and clinical, analytical, forensic, regulatory, and occupational settings, that have a unique focus and purpose.

In general, toxicity occurs when too much of a substance is taken in relation to a normally tolerable dose. Different mechanisms by which a chemical can produce toxicity include the following:

- Exaggeration of pharmacologic effects
- Formation of reactive toxic metabolites
- Formation of intracellular free radicals
- Interference with enzyme action
- Interference with DNA (deoxyribonucleic acid) or RNA (ribonucleic acid) synthesis
- Inactivation of biochemical cofactors
- Initiation of premature cell aging (apoptosis)
- Tissue destruction on contact

Poison Prevention Approaches and Pharmacy

Poison Prevention Packaging Act of 1970: Safety caps

This law was enacted to prevent preschool-age children from opening and ingesting harmful substances or to delay the opening of packaging containing such substances (to limit the amount of harmful substance that may be ingested within a reasonable amount of time).

Drugs requiring safety caps include aspirin, ibuprofen, acetaminophen, and oral prescription drugs with certain exceptions (e.g., birth control pills and nitroglycerin).

Use of poison control centers

A poison control center determines if a true poisoning exists, recommends first aid, refers poisoning victims to health care facilities for further evaluation and treatment, monitors the progress and outcome of each poisoning case, and documents poisoning experiences. Programs and materials on poison prevention are also available.

Nationwide access is available by calling 1-800-222-1222 for 24-hour poison control center services for the area from which the call is placed in the United States.

Poison prevention tips for consumers

- Store all drugs and chemicals out of the reach of children.

- Never put chemicals in food containers.
- Choose products with safety caps when there is a choice, and use them properly.
- Read and follow all label directions carefully.
- Never call medicine "candy."
- Use safety latches.

Pharmacy Requirements of the Joint Commission on Accreditation of Healthcare Organizations

- Maintain and keep available the medical staff–approved stock of antidotes and other emergency drugs in both the pharmacy and the patient care areas.
- Maintain authoritative and current antidote information.
- Keep the phone number of the poison control center readily available in areas outside the pharmacy where drugs are stored.

Emergency Actions

First aid should be administered, if applicable. Table 39-1 describes first-aid techniques.

Other considerations

- Avoid wasting time looking for an "antidote" at home.

Table 39-1. First Aid for Poisoning Emergencies

Type of emergency	First-aid response
Inhaled poison	Immediately get the person to fresh air. Avoid breathing fumes. Open doors and windows wide.
Poison on the skin	Remove any contaminated clothing. Flood skin with water for at least 15 minutes.
Poison in the eye	Remove contact lenses. Flood the eye with water, pouring it from a large glass 2–3 inches from the eye. Repeat for a total of 15–30 minutes. Do not force the eyelid open.
Swallowed poison	Unless the victim is unconscious, is having convulsions, or cannot swallow, give a small glassful (2–4 oz) of water immediately. Call a poison control center for advice about whether other actions are needed.

- Do not use home remedies such as saltwater, mustard powder, raw eggs, hydrogen peroxide, cooking grease, or gagging.
- Immediately call 911 or an ambulance if the person is not breathing, has had a seizure, or is unresponsive.
- For other situations, contact a poison control center immediately to determine whether first aid should be used or whether a poisoning emergency exists.

Decontamination of the Gastrointestinal Tract

The practice of using drugs to decrease the absorption of other drugs from the gastrointestinal tract is in a state of change. For example, ipecac syrup is being abandoned by many as a home- or hospital-based therapy, and its use is primarily at the preference of the consulting poison control center or health care professional. Current recommendations, as well as basic information about the drugs in case they are encountered, are described in this section.

Current recommendations

Ipecac syrup has questionable effectiveness, and its use is generally avoided.

Gastric lavage involves placing a tube into the stomach through a nostril or the mouth and repetitively washing out the stomach contents with water or a saline solution. This method of gastric decontamination is of questionable effectiveness, particularly if it is performed more than 1 hour after ingestion of toxin.

Cathartics such as magnesium citrate are no longer routinely used.

Activated charcoal given orally is often the only treatment necessary if the toxin is adsorbed and the activated charcoal is used within 1–2 hours of ingestion of the toxin.

Whole bowel irrigation can be considered if the toxin is poorly or slowly adsorbed and its presence in the gastrointestinal tract is likely.

Ipecac syrup

Indications and dosage
Ipecac syrup was previously used for general prophylaxis of selected poisonings of expected minor or moderate severity in alert patients. Many clinicians have abandoned it as a prehospital or hospital treatment. In 2003, the American Academy of Pediatrics recommended that ipecac syrup no longer be used routinely as a home treatment for poisoning.

Contraindications
- The patient is experiencing pronounced sleepiness, coma, or seizures.
- The patient has ingested caustics, aliphatic hydrocarbons, and fast-acting agents that produce coma or seizures (e.g., tricyclic antidepressants, clonidine, calcium channel blockers, β-blockers, and hypoglycemic agents).
- Time since ingestion is believed to be 1 hour or more.

Adverse effects
- *Common:* Diarrhea, sleepiness, protracted vomiting
- *Uncommon:* Mallory–Weiss (esophageal) tears, tracheal aspiration into the lungs

Disadvantage
A disadvantage of ipecac syrup is that emesis and the drug's relative lack of efficacy complicate administration of other oral therapies.

Activated charcoal

Indications and dosage
This agent is occasionally used to adsorb poisons in an alert or comatose patient. Administer as a slurry by mouth in alert patients or through a lavage tube:

- *Children:* 25–50 g
- *Adults:* 25–100 g

Contraindications
- Ingestions of aliphatic hydrocarbons and caustics
- Absence of patient's bowel sounds
- Ingestions of heavy metals (sodium, lithium, iron, or lead) or simple alcohols

Adverse effects
- *Uncommon:* Tracheal aspiration, pneumonitis
- *Common:* Emesis, soiling of clothes and furnishings

Advantages and disadvantages
- *Advantages:* Rapid onset of action, nonspecific action for a wide variety of chemicals, reasonable effectiveness within 1 hour of ingestion
- *Disadvantages:* Messy and difficult administration, possible removal of beneficial drugs together with the toxin

Cathartics

Cathartics were previously used as an adjunct to activated charcoal administration to decrease gastrointestinal transit time. Their efficacy is unproved. Fluid and electrolyte disturbances are possible with repeated doses.

Cathartics may contribute to emesis following activated charcoal use.

Agents previously used include magnesium citrate, magnesium sulfate, sodium sulfate, and sorbitol. Some activated charcoal products contain sorbitol mixed in the preparation. The sorbitol concentration varies from brand to brand.

Whole bowel irrigation

Indications and technique

Whole bowel irrigation is generally used to wash out the gastrointestinal tract when using charcoal may be inappropriate (e.g., if iron or lithium was ingested) and the toxin is suspected to be present in the gastrointestinal tract (e.g., when drugs are sustained-release formulations or when the patient ingested illicit drugs packed in condoms). It is not routinely used to treat poisonings except in these unique circumstances.

Use larger volumes of polyethylene glycol electrolyte solutions (e.g., CoLyte, GoLYTELY) than the amounts conventionally used for bowel preparation. Administer by mouth or through a gastric or duodenal tube for treatment of poisoning:

- **Children:** 25 mL/kg/h (approximately 500 mL/h) up to 2–5 L
- **Adults:** 2 L/h up to 5–10 L

Contraindications

- Ingestion of caustics or aliphatic hydrocarbons
- Patients with absent bowel sounds or gastrointestinal tract obstruction

Adverse effects

Few adverse effects have been reported, but limited results are available from which to draw conclusions. Some nausea and vomiting have been reported.

Advantages and disadvantages

- **Advantages:** Prompt whole bowel evacuation within 2 hours
- **Disadvantages:** Messy procedure because of rectal effluent

Other hospital-based therapies

These therapies include supportive and symptomatic care, multiple doses of activated charcoal (to enhance systemic elimination when appropriate), hemodialysis (to enhance systemic elimination when appropriate), and use of antidotes (to antagonize or reverse toxic effects when indicated).

39-4. Substance Abuse and Toxicology

Substance abuse often leads to acute and chronic toxicity. Table 39-2 describes selected drugs of abuse.

During 2012, 41.5 million Americans age 12 and older (16% of the population) admitted using an

Table 39-2. Selected Drugs and Substances of Abuse

Substance (slang names)	Methods of abuse	Major or unique health effects
Androgenic anabolic steroids (roids), Drug Enforcement Administration (DEA) Schedule III	These drugs are taken orally, injected, or applied topically, typically in cycles of weeks or months ("cycling"). Users often combine several different types of steroids ("stacking").	Anabolic steroids are synthetic derivatives of testosterone. Abuse can lead to serious health problems, some irreversible. *Men:* Shrinking of the testicles, reduced sperm count, infertility, baldness, gynecomastia, and increased risk for prostate cancer can occur. *Women:* Growth of facial hair, male-pattern baldness, changes in or cessation of the menstrual cycle, enlargement of the clitoris, and deepened voice can occur. *Adolescents:* Stunted growth by premature skeletal maturation and accelerated puberty changes can occur. Other major side effects include jaundice, fluid retention, high blood pressure, and severe acne. Extreme mood swings, including manic-like symptoms leading to violence and depression, are often experienced when drugs are stopped, and such symptoms may contribute to dependence.

(continued)

Table 39-2. Selected Drugs and Substances of Abuse *(Continued)*

Substance (slang names)	Methods of abuse	Major or unique health effects
Barbiturates (barbs, downers); DEA Schedule II, III, IV	Barbiturates can be ingested or injected.	Barbiturates are central nervous system (CNS) depressants that at high doses can become general anesthetics.
		With high doses, coma, ataxia, depressed reflexes, hypotension, and respiratory depression can occur.
		CNS depressants should not be combined with any medication or substance that causes sedation, including prescription pain medicines, certain over-the-counter cold and allergy medications, or alcoholic drinks. The effects of the drugs can combine to slow breathing or to slow both the heart and respiration, which can be fatal.
		Discontinuing prolonged use of high doses of barbiturates can lead to withdrawal.
Cocaine (snow, crack [street name given to cocaine that has been processed from cocaine hydrochloride to the freebase for smoking], rock), DEA Schedule II	Cocaine can be sniffed or snorted, injected, or smoked (freebase and crack cocaine). It is poorly absorbed orally.	Cocaine is a CNS stimulant that produces euphoric effects and hyperstimulation such as dilated pupils, increased temperature, tachycardia, and hypertension.
		Prolonged cocaine snorting can result in ulceration of the mucous membranes of the nose and can damage the nasal septum enough to cause it to collapse.
		Cocaine-related deaths are often a result of cardiac arrest or seizures followed by respiratory arrest.
		Tolerance to the euphoric effects develops.
		When addicted individuals stop using cocaine, they often become depressed.
Dextromethorphan (DXM, DM, robo, velvet, rojo)	This drug is taken orally by drinking dextromethorphan-containing cough syrups. Availability of the powdered form has led to repackaging as capsules or tablets and to snorting.	Dextromethorphan is the dextro isomer of levomethorphan. It has no analgesic, opiate-like, dependence-producing properties. A behaviorally active metabolite, dextrorphan is structurally related to PCP (phencyclidine) and ketamine and may contribute to its abuse potential.
		The typical clinical presentation of intoxication involves hyperexcitability, lethargy, ataxia, slurred speech, sweating, hypertension, and nystagmus. Abusers report a heightened sense of perceptual awareness, altered time perception, and visual hallucinations.
		The majority of abuse occurs among teenagers and young adults who use dextromethorphan alone or mixed with other drugs. It has been sold as "ecstasy." It has been identified as a filler in confiscated samples of bogus heroin and bogus ketamine.
		Procedures to extract dextromethorphan from cough syrups are described on the Internet, which has led to the availability of powdered forms.
Ethanol (various names and alcoholic drinks)	Ethanol is typically ingested.	Ethanol is a CNS depressant that at high doses can lead to hypotension, hypoglycemia, respiratory depression, and death. Acute intoxication leads to ataxia, sedation, emesis, and slurred speech.
		Chronic abuse leads to many medical complications such as esophageal varices, hepatic failure with ascites, and malnutrition.
		Tolerance, dependence, and withdrawal develop with chronic abuse.
Gamma-hydroxybutyrate, or GHB (liquid ecstasy, soap, easy lay, Georgia home boy, somatomax, scoop, grievous bodily harm), DEA Schedule I	GHB is ingested.	GHB is a CNS depressant abused for euphoric, sedative, and anabolic (body-building) effects.
		Coma and seizures are likely; increased risk of seizures occurs when combined with methamphetamine.
		Use with alcohol causes nausea and difficulty breathing.

Table 39-2. Selected Drugs and Substances of Abuse *(Continued)*

Substance (slang names)	Methods of abuse	Major or unique health effects
		GHB and two of its precursors, gamma-butyrolactone and 1,4-butanedio, have been involved in poisonings, overdoses, date rapes, and deaths. They are produced by illicit laboratories.
		GHB may produce withdrawal effects.
Heroin (smack, H, skag, junk), DEA Schedule I	Heroin can be injected, snorted, or smoked.	Abuse is associated with fatal overdose, spontaneous abortion, collapsed veins, and infectious diseases, including HIV/AIDS and hepatitis.
		Effects include euphoria ("rush") followed by an alternately wakeful and drowsy state ("on the nod").
		CNS depression, respiratory depression, miosis (pinpoint pupils), and pulmonary edema can occur.
		Heroin may have unknown additives and contaminants.
		With regular use, tolerance develops and withdrawal is possible.
Inhalants (various names)	Inhalants are sniffed or huffed.	Inhalants include a variety of breathable chemical vapors that produce psychoactive effects. They are found in industrial or household solvents or solvent-containing products, including paint thinners or solvents, degreasers, dry-cleaning fluids, gasoline, and glues.
		Nearly all abused inhalants produce short-term intoxicating and CNS depressant effects similar to anesthetics.
		Intoxication usually lasts only a few minutes. Successive inhalations lead to loss of inhibition and control. Continued use can lead to coma.
		In some cases, heart failure and death occur within minutes of a session of prolonged use ("sudden sniffing death").
Injected drugs (various names)	Such drugs are injected, which is referred to as "shooting up" or "mainlining."	Injecting drug users are at risk for transmitting or acquiring HIV/AIDS, hepatitis, bacterial infections, and fungal infections if needles or other injection equipment are shared. Chronic users may develop collapsed veins, infection of the heart lining and valves, skin abscesses, cellulitis, and liver disease.
		Because some abusers dissolve the tablets in water and inject the mixture, emboli can form from the insoluble materials in the tablets.
Ketamine (K, special K, cat Valium, vitamin K), DEA Schedule III	Ketamine is injected or snorted.	Ketamine is an anesthetic that has been approved for human and veterinary use.
		Certain doses can cause dream-like states and hallucinations.
		At high doses, ketamine can cause delirium, amnesia, impaired motor function, hypertension, depression, and potentially fatal respiratory depression.
Lysergic acid diethylamide, or LSD (acid, L, blotter, cubes, sugar, dots), DEA Schedule I	LSD is ingested. It is often added to absorbent paper, such as blotter paper, and divided into small decorated squares ("blotter acid") or placed on dot-like candy ("dots") or sugar cubes ("cubes," "sugar").	LSD is a hallucinogen sold on the street in tablets, capsules, and liquid form.
		Effects are unpredictable. Physical effects include mydriasis (dilated pupils), elevated temperature, tachycardia, hypertension, sweating, loss of appetite, sleeplessness, dry mouth, and tremors.
		Sensations and feelings change more dramatically than do the physical signs. In sufficient doses, the drug produces delusions and visual hallucinations.
		Some users experience severe, terrifying thoughts and feelings; fear of losing control; fear of insanity and death; and despair. Fatal accidents have occurred during intoxication. Many users experience flashbacks.

(continued)

Table 39-2. Selected Drugs and Substances of Abuse *(Continued)*

Substance (slang names)	Methods of abuse	Major or unique health effects
Marijuana (pot; herb; weed; grass; widow; ganja; hash; and trademarked varieties of cannabis, such as Bubble Gum, Northern Lights, Juicy Fruit, Afghani #1, and a number of Skunk varieties), DEA Schedule I	Marijuana is smoked as a cigarette ("joint," "nail"), in a pipe ("bong"), or in blunts (cigars that have been emptied of tobacco and refilled with marijuana, often in combination with another drug). It is also ingested when mixed in food or brewed as a tea.	Main active chemical in marijuana is THC (delta-9-tetrahydrocannabinol). Delirium, conjunctivitis, and food craving are typical. Short-term effects include problems with memory and learning, distorted perception, difficulty in thinking and problem solving, loss of coordination, and tachycardia. Risk of heart attack more than quadruples in the first hour after smoking marijuana in people with cardiovascular risk. Users experience the same respiratory problems as cigarette smokers (see nicotine); burning and stinging of the mouth and throat, often accompanied by a heavy cough, can occur. Drug craving and withdrawal effects can occur.
3-4,-methylenedioxy-methamphetamine, or MDMA (ecstasy, Adam, XTC, hug, beans, love drug), DEA Schedule I	MDMA is ingested, snorted, injected, or used in suppository form.	MDMA is a synthetic, psychoactive drug with both stimulant and hallucinogenic properties. It increases pulse and blood pressure. In high doses, it can cause malignant hyperthermia leading to rhabdomyolysis (muscle breakdown with kidney and cardiovascular system failure). Psychological difficulties, which include confusion, depression, sleep problems, drug craving, severe anxiety, and paranoia, occur during use and sometimes for weeks afterward. Physical symptoms include muscle tension, involuntary teeth clenching, nausea, blurred vision, nystagmus, faintness, chills, and sweating. Content of the MDMA pills also varies widely and may include caffeine, dextromethorphan, heroin, and mescaline. In some areas, the MDMA-like substance paramethoxyamphetamine has led to death when mistaken for true MDMA; deaths were due to complications from hyperthermia.
Methamphetamine (crank, meth, speed, chalk, ice, crystal, glass), DEA Schedule II	Methamphetamine can be ingested, snorted in the powder form, or injected. The clear, chunky crystals resembling ice can be smoked and are referred to as "ice," "crystal," and "glass."	Methamphetamine is an addictive stimulant chemically related to amphetamine. It produces euphoria, irritability, insomnia, confusion, tremors, convulsions, anxiety, paranoia, and aggressiveness. Higher doses lead to hypertension, tachycardia, stroke, arrhythmias, cardiovascular collapse, and death. Hyperthermia and convulsions can result in death. Prolonged use leads to extreme anorexia and is associated with tooth decay and skin lesions. Methamphetamine is made in illegal laboratories and may contain contaminants and by-products. The potential for abuse and dependence is high.
Nicotine (various names and products)	Nicotine is smoked with tobacco in cigarettes, cigars, and pipes. It also is in chewing tobacco, nicotine gum, nicotine patches, and electronic cigarettes.	Nicotine is a highly addictive CNS stimulant and sedative. Stimulation is followed by depression and fatigue, leading the user to seek more nicotine. Women who smoke and take oral contraceptives are more prone to cardiovascular and cerebrovascular diseases, especially those older than 30 years of age. Pregnant women have an increased risk of having stillborn or premature infants or infants with low birth weight. Respiratory problems include daily cough and phlegm production, more frequent acute respiratory illness, a heightened risk of lung infections, and a greater tendency toward obstructed airways and cancer of the respiratory tract and lungs. Tar in cigarettes is associated with a higher rate of lung cancer, emphysema, and bronchial disorders.

Table 39-2. Selected Drugs and Substances of Abuse *(Continued)*

Substance (slang names)	Methods of abuse	Major or unique health effects
		Carbon monoxide in the smoke increases the chance of cardiovascular diseases.
		Nicotine tolerance, dependence, and withdrawal symptoms occur.
Opioids (various names), DEA Schedule II, III, IV	Opioids are ingested or injected; powder may be snorted.	Opioids include morphine; codeine; oxycodone (Oxycontin, MS Contin); hydrocodone (Vicodin); hydromorphone (Dilaudid); and meperidine (Demerol).
		They cause drowsiness and constipation. Large single doses cause coma, hypotension, respiratory depression, and, in some cases, seizures and death. Mixing with alcohol and other CNS depressants increases the risk of coma and death.
		Chronic use of opioids produces tolerance, physical dependence, and withdrawal symptoms.
Phencyclidine, or PCP (angel dust, ozone, wack, rocket fuel; killer joints or crystal supergrass when combined with marijuana), DEA Schedule I, II	PCP is snorted, smoked, or eaten. For smoking, PCP is often applied to a leafy material such as mint, parsley, oregano, or marijuana.	PCP is an addictive hallucinogen and sedative that often leads to psychological dependence, craving, and compulsive PCP-seeking behavior. Users often become violent or suicidal and are very dangerous to themselves and others.
		At low to moderate doses, effects include slight tachypnea, more pronounced tachycardia and hypertension, shallow respirations, and profuse sweating. Generalized numbness of the extremities and muscular lack of coordination also may occur. Psychological effects include distinct changes in body awareness, similar to those associated with alcohol intoxication.
		At high doses, effects include decreased blood pressure, pulse, and respirations; nausea and vomiting; blurred vision and nystagmus; drooling; ataxia; and seizures, coma, and death (though death more often results from accidental injury or suicide during PCP intoxication). Psychological effects at high doses include illusions, hallucinations, and effects that mimic the full range of symptoms of schizophrenia.
		Interactions with other CNS depressants, such as alcohol and benzodiazepines, can lead to coma.
		PCP is illegally manufactured in illicit laboratories.
Flunitrazepam, or Rohypnol (rophie, roofies, roche, roach, rope, the date rape drug, forget-me), DEA Schedule IV	Flunitrazepam is ingested as a tablet or mixed in an alcoholic drink.	Rohypnol, a trade name for flunitrazepam, is a benzodiazepine that is not sold in the United States but is smuggled in. It produces sedative-hypnotic effects, including muscle relaxation and amnesia. It can also produce physical and psychological dependence.
		When mixed with alcohol, flunitrazepam can incapacitate victims, prevent them from resisting sexual assault, and produce anterograde amnesia. It may also be lethal when mixed with alcohol or other CNS depressants.
		Clonazepam (Klonopin) and alprazolam (Xanax) are being abused like flunitrazepam.
Stimulants, amphetamines, and related compounds (speed, dexies, uppers), DEA Schedule II	These drugs are ingested. Tablets can also be crushed and snorted or injected.	These substances are CNS stimulants that increase alertness, attention, and energy, as well as increase blood pressure, pulse, and respiration.
		High doses can lead to arrhythmias; hypertension; hyperthermia; and potential for cardiovascular failure, stroke, or lethal seizures.
		Taking high doses of some stimulants repeatedly over a short period of time can lead to hostility or feelings of paranoia in some individuals.
		Stimulants such as dextroamphetamine (Dexedrine) and methylphenidate (Ritalin) can be addictive when misused.

DrugFacts, National Institute on Drug Abuse, National Institutes of Health, 2012; Drug fact sheets, Diversion Control Program, Drug Enforcement Administration, U.S. Department of Justice Web site.

illicit drug in the past year, and 2.9 million started using illicit drugs.

During 2011, 5 million adults were treated in emergency departments for drug-related episodes, with 2.3 million for adverse drug reactions, 2.5 million for drug and substance abuse, and 77,000 children for unintentional poisonings.

Management of the acute condition generally follows the same guidelines as those for management of poisonings and overdoses. A challenge in treating patients during acute drug overdose is determining the possible agents taken and possible adulterants (e.g., talc, strychnine, other drugs) or contaminants.

Chronic abuse can foster dependence, which often leads to withdrawal symptoms when the patient stops using the drugs. Detoxification programs, long-term behavioral counseling, and drugs to produce aversion or substitution to drug-taking behaviors are often needed.

39-5. Antidotes

Role of Antidotes

An antidote counteracts or changes the nature of a poison. Few antidotes are available relative to the large number of potential poisons. Table 39-3 lists antidotes that are commonly used in the treatment of a patient with a poisoning or an overdose.

Many hospitals have an insufficient stock of antidotes. The pharmacy and therapeutics committee of a hospital should regularly review the inventory of antidotes that are stocked at the hospital.

Selected Antidotes

Acetylcysteine

Acetylcysteine is available under the trade names Mucomyst (10, 20% oral solution) and Acetadote (20% for injection).

Uses
Acetylcysteine is used to treat acute acetaminophen overdose. An unapproved indication is to treat adverse reactions to drugs and diagnostic agents that may produce free radicals as part of the adverse reaction; the dosage regimen is unique to the particular application.

Mechanism of action
Acetylcysteine protects the liver from the toxic effects of an acetaminophen metabolite by supplying a surrogate for glutathione to aid in metabolism of the reactive metabolite. Other mechanisms are also proposed, which include providing sulfate for acetaminophen metabolism and minimizing the formation of free radicals.

This agent may be useful in minimizing hepatotoxic injury once it has begun. It also may aid in cases of fulminant hepatic failure.

Indications
Acute overdoses of acetaminophen produce a reactive metabolite that leads to hepatotoxicity (jaundice, coagulopathy, hypoglycemia, hepatic failure, hepatic encephalopathy, hepatorenal failure). Symptoms become evident 1–2 days after ingestion.

Acetylcysteine can prevent or minimize hepatic injury if given early. For best results, administer within 10 hours of ingestion of acetaminophen overdose. It is minimally effective when started 24 hours after ingestion.

The need for therapy is determined by obtaining a serum concentration of acetaminophen at least 4 hours after ingestion (and within 24 hours) and plotting it on the acetaminophen nomogram to determine whether there is a risk for hepatotoxicity.

Contraindications
Use of acetylcysteine is contraindicated if there is a known hypersensitivity to the drug.

Adverse effects
With oral administration, nausea and vomiting are common.

With intravenous (IV) administration, anaphylactoid reactions (rash, hypotension, wheezing, dyspnea) have been reported. Acute flushing and erythema may occur during the first hour of infusion and typically resolve spontaneously.

Dosage
Table 39-3 gives dosage information on drug products for oral or IV administration available in the United States.

Atropine

Uses
Atropine is used in cases of organophosphate (including chemical terrorism nerve agents) and carbamate anticholinesterase insecticide poisoning.

Mechanism of action
Atropine is an anticholinergic agent that competitively inhibits acetylcholine at muscarinic receptors.

Table 39-3. Commonly Used Antidotes[a]

Toxin	Antidote (trade name)	Adult dose	Pediatric dose
Acetaminophen	Acetylcysteine (Mucomyst)	Oral loading dose: 140 mg/kg; maintenance dose: 70 mg/kg every 4 hours for 17 doses	Same as adult dose regimen
	Acetylcysteine (Acetadote)	IV infusion: 150 mg/kg in 200 mL 5% dextrose in water (D_5W) over 1 hour, then 50 mg/kg in 500 mL D_5W over 4 hours, followed by 100 mg/kg in 1,000 mL D_5W over 16 hours	Same as adult dose regimen
Anticholinergic compounds	Physostigmine salicylate (Antilirium)	1–2 mg slow IV infusion over 3–5 minutes titrated to effect	0.02 mg/kg slow IV infusion over 3–5 minutes titrated to effect
Arsenic	Succimer (Chemet)	10 mg/kg orally 3 times per day	Same as adult dose regimen
	Dimercaprol, also called British antilewisite (BAL in Oil), only if unable to tolerate oral succimer	3–5 mg/kg IM every 4–6 hours	Same as adult dose regimen
Benzodiazepines	Flumazenil (Romazicon)[b]	0.2 mg IV bolus titrated to effect or total dose of 3 mg	0.01 mg/kg IV bolus titrated to effect or total dose of 1–3 mg
β-blockers	Glucagon (GlucaGen)[c]	5–10 mg IV bolus, followed by 5–10 mg/h IV infusion titrated to effect	0.15 mg/kg mg IV bolus, followed by 0.1 mg/h IV infusion titrated to effect
Calcium channel blockers	Calcium chloride 10%	10–20 mL IV bolus; repeat doses and IV infusions common	0.1–0.2 mL/kg IV bolus; repeat doses and IV infusions common
	Glucagon (GlucaGen)[c]	5–10 mg IV bolus, followed by 5–10 mg/h IV	0.15 mg IV bolus, followed by 0.1 mg/h IV infusion titrated to effect
Carbamates	Atropine	2–4 mg IV bolus, repeat doses titrated to effect	1 mg/kg IV bolus, repeat doses titrated to effect
Cyanide	Sodium nitrite 3% and sodium thiosulfate 25% (Nithiodote)[d]	Sodium nitrite: 300 mg slow IV infusion; sodium thiosulfate: 12.5 g IV infusion	Sodium nitrite: 0.2 mL/kg to maximum of 300 mg slow IV infusion; sodium thiosulfate: 1 mL/kg up to 12.5 g IV infusion
	Hydroxocobalamin (CyanoKit)[d]	5 g IV infusion over 15 min; up to 5 g more based on response	70 mg/kg IV infusion
Digoxin	Digoxin immune Fab (Digibind, DigiFab)	Empiric dosing: 10–20 vials IV bolus for life-threatening toxicity (see package insert for other dosing regimens)	Empiric dosing: same as adult dose regimen (see package insert for other dosing regimens)
Ethylene glycol, methanol	Ethanol 10%[c]	Loading dose 10 mL/kg IV or orally, followed by maintenance dose 1–2 mL/kg/h IV infusion or oral dose	Same as adult dose regimen
	Fomepizole (Antizol)	15 mg/kg IV bolus; smaller repeat doses may be necessary	Same as adult dose regimen
Iron	Deferoxamine (Desferal)	5–15 mg/kg/h IV infusion titrated to effect	Same as adult dose regimen

(continued)

Table 39-3. Commonly Used Antidotes[a] *(Continued)*

Toxin	Antidote (trade name)	Adult dose	Pediatric dose
Isoniazid	Pyridoxine (vitamin B_6) for injection[c]	1 g per gram ingested or empiric dosing of 5 g IV bolus	1 g per gram ingested or empiric dosing of 75 mg/kg IV bolus up to 5 g
Lead	Succimer (Chemet)	10 mg/kg orally 3 times per day; repeat doses common	Same as adult dose regimen
	Dimercaprol, also called British antilewisite (BAL), only for lead encephalopathy (BAL in Oil)	3–5 mg/kg IM or 50–75 mg/m² IM	Same as adult dose regimen
	Calcium disodium ethylenediaminetetraacetic acid (Calcium Disodium Versenate)	20–30 mg/kg diluted in 250 mL IV infusion over 12–24 hours (start 4 hours after BAL administration)	Same as adult dose regimen
Methemoglobinemia	Methylene blue	1–2 mg/kg slow IV infusion; repeat doses common	Same as adult dose regimen
Opioids	Naloxone (Narcan)	0.4–2 mg IV titrated to effect	Same as adult dose regimen
Organophosphates	Atropine	2–4 mg IV bolus; repeat doses titrated to effect	0.1 mg/kg IV bolus; repeat doses titrated to effect
	Pralidoxime (Protopam)	1–2 g slow IV infusion, followed by 500 mg/h continuous infusion or 1 g every 4 hours	20–40 mg/kg slow IV infusion, followed by 5–10 mg/kg/h continuous infusion or 20 mg/kg every 4 hours
Salicylate	Sodium bicarbonate	150 mEq with 40 mEq KCl in 1 L of D_5W infused to maintain urine output at 1–2 mL/kg/h and a urine pH approximately 7.5	Same as adult dose regimen
Snake envenomation, crotaline[b] (rattlesnakes, cottonmouth, copperhead)	Crotalidae polyvalent immune Fab, ovine (CroFab)	Empiric dose: 4–6 vials IV infusion over 1 hour; additional doses depend on patient response (see package insert for dosing)	Same as adult dose regimen
Tricyclic antidepressants, agents with type 1a antiarrhythmic effects	Sodium bicarbonate	1–2 mEq/kg IV bolus; repeat boluses titrated to QRS duration (do not exceed arterial pH of 7.55)	Same as adult dose regimen
Warfarin, superwarfarin rodenticides	Fresh-frozen plasma	Fresh-frozen plasma for life-threatening hemorrhage	Same as adult indication
	Vitamin K_1 (Mephyton, AquaMEPHYTON)	10–50 mg slow IV infusion or taken subcutaneously or orally	0.6 mg/kg slow IV infusion or taken subcutaneously or orally

Based on American College of Emergency Physicians, 1999.

IM, intramuscular.

a. The table lists common antidotes that may need to be used emergently for patients presenting with acute toxic ingestion or dermal or inhalation exposure. Dosages are derived from standard texts and references and are given as convenience references. These should not be considered specific treatment guidelines; consult appropriate resources.

b. Potential risks may exceed the benefits because of precipitation of intractable seizures.

c. Off-label indication for use.

d. Information updated by author.

It has little effect on nicotinic receptors in cases of organophosphate insecticide poisoning.

Indications

- For control of pulmonary hypersecretion, atropine is given in repeated doses intravenously until secretions have decreased. Atropinization may have to be maintained for hours to days.
- For control of bradycardia, atropine is given until the heart rate increases to an acceptable rate or until a need for alternatives is indicated.
- Nontoxicologic indications for atropine include premedication to anesthesia induction (for antisecretory effects) and ophthalmic mydriasis and cycloplegia.

Contraindications

There are no contraindications in cases of insecticide poisoning. Contraindications for other indications include the following:

- Hypersensitivity to atropine or anticholinergics
- Narrow-angle glaucoma
- Reflux esophagitis
- Obstructive gastrointestinal disease
- Ulcerative colitis or toxic megacolon
- Obstructive uropathy
- Unstable cardiovascular status in acute hemorrhage or thyrotoxicosis
- Paralytic ileus or intestinal atony
- Myasthenia gravis

Adverse effects

Exaggeration of anticholinergic effects (e.g., tachycardia, hypertension, sedation, hallucinations, mydriasis, changes in intraocular pressure, warm red skin, dry mouth, urinary retention, ileus, dysrhythmias, seizures) can occur.

When large doses of atropine are used, the agent should be free of preservatives because agents such as benzyl alcohol or chlorobutanol can produce their own toxicity.

Dosage

For bronchorrhea and bronchospasm from organophosphates or carbamates, the adult dose is 2–5 mg (pediatric dose is 0.05 mg/kg) slowly administered intravenously. This dose is repeated at 10- to 30-minute intervals until bronchial hypersecretion is resolved. Severe poisonings may require up to 100 mg over a few hours to several grams over several weeks. If atropinization is required for several days, continuous atropine infusion may be used (rates of 0.02–0.08 mg/kg/h are recommended).

For symptomatic bradycardia from mild poisonings, the adult dose is 1 mg (pediatric dose is 0.01 mg/kg) intravenously. For moderate to severe poisonings, adult doses increase to 2–5 mg (pediatric doses are 0.02–0.05 mg/kg) and should be repeated every few minutes until the heart rate increases.

These doses for atropine are higher than those routinely used for indications not related to organophosphate poisoning, such as bradycardia after a myocardial infarction.

Digoxin immune Fab (Digibind, DigiFab)

Uses

Digoxin immune Fab is used to treat life-threatening acute or chronic digoxin poisoning.

Some cross-reactivity with digitoxin and other digoxin-like compounds (digitalis, foxglove, lily of the valley, and bufadienolide from cane frogs) can occur.

Mechanism of action

Digoxin immune Fab binds digoxin in plasma, promotes redistribution from tissues, and enhances elimination in the urine. The digoxin bound to digoxin immune Fab is inactive. Each 40 mg (1 vial) binds 0.6 mg of digoxin.

Digoxin immune Fab is a monovalent, digoxin-specific, antigen-binding fragment (Fab) that is produced in healthy sheep.

Indications

Chronic digoxin toxicity typically begins with nausea, vomiting, diarrhea, fatigue, confusion, blurred vision, diplopia, and the observation of white borders or halos around dark objects. Deterioration of renal function, hypokalemia, or drug interactions often leads to toxicity.

Acute digoxin poisoning has early symptoms similar to those of chronic poisoning, but the onset is more abrupt. Nausea and vomiting are common, and the serum potassium concentration is typically normal or dangerously elevated.

A wide variety of arrhythmias occur with acute or chronic digoxin poisoning.

Digoxin immune Fab is reserved for life-threatening symptoms such as bradycardia, second- and third-degree heart block that is unresponsive to atropine, ventricular arrhythmias, and hyperkalemia (typically in excess of 5 mEq/L).

Contraindications

Digoxin immune Fab is relatively contraindicated in patients with hypersensitivity to sheep.

Adverse effects

Common adverse effects include hypokalemia, allergic reactions (1% of patients), and hypotension. For patients on maintenance digoxin therapy, the abrupt binding of digoxin will lead to loss of therapeutic effect and a prompt decrease in potassium concentrations.

Dosage

Digoxin immune Fab is administered by IV infusion or rapid IV bolus (Table 39-3).

Dosage is determined by one of several approaches, depending on available information, as follows: empiric dosage of 10–20 vials (Table 39-3), dosing based on the dose of digoxin ingested, or dosing based on the serum digoxin concentration.

Flumazenil (Romazicon)

Uses

Flumazenil is used in cases of benzodiazepine overdose and in reversal of conscious sedation and general anesthesia from benzodiazepines.

Mechanism of action

Flumazenil is a competitive antagonist of the benzodiazepine receptor in the central nervous system (CNS).

Indications

Flumazenil should be used adjunctively with supportive care. Sedation can recur following ingestion of a benzodiazepine with a long half-life, requiring additional doses of flumazenil. In a suicidal overdose, it is rarely used because of the risk of potential co-ingestants. If no response occurs to a 5 mg cumulative dose, the sedation is probably not related to a benzodiazepine.

Contraindications

Flumazenil is contraindicated in patients with known hypersensitivity to it.

Co-ingestion of tricyclic antidepressants may precipitate ventricular dysrhythmias or seizures. Other mixed overdoses can decrease the seizure threshold (i.e., haloperidol, bupropion, lithium).

Abrupt benzodiazepine withdrawal following flumazenil use in patients on maintenance benzodiazepine therapy, such as for treatment of epilepsy, can precipitate seizures.

Flumazenil is contraindicated in patients with increased intracranial pressure because the antidote may potentially alter cerebral blood flow.

It can produce withdrawal in the benzodiazepine-dependent patient.

Adverse effects

Flumazenil has a wide margin of safety when not contraindicated.

Side effects include agitation, sweating, headache, abnormal vision, dizziness, and pain at the administration site. Rarely reported side effects include bradycardia, tachycardia, hypotension, and hypertension.

Dosage

Table 39-3 gives dosage information for IV administration.

Naloxone (Narcan)

Uses

Naloxone is used in the following cases:

- Reversal of opioid anesthesia
- Respiratory or CNS depression related to opioid toxicity
- Empiric administration in patients with altered mental status of unknown etiology

Mechanism of action

Naloxone is an opioid antagonist. It competes at three CNS opioid receptors (mu, kappa, delta) and leads to reversal of the depressive opioid effects.

Indications

Opioids cause sedation, respiratory depression, hypotension, miosis, and analgesia. Because it has no agonist activity, naloxone will not worsen respiratory depression. The goal of therapy is to restore adequate spontaneous respirations.

When administering naloxone, monitor a patient for respiratory rate changes and for opiate withdrawal symptoms (anxiety, hypertension, tachycardia, diarrhea, seizure). To avoid withdrawal, use the lowest possible dose that maintains proper spontaneous ventilation. The patient should be observed for respiratory depression once naloxone therapy is discontinued because the half-life of naloxone may be shorter than that of the opioid. If a patient is not responsive to 15 mg of naloxone, it is doubtful that an opioid is causing the respiratory depression.

Contraindications
■ Avoid in patients with a known hypersensitivity to the drug.
■ Use with caution in the opiate-dependent patient.
■ Use with caution in patients with preexisting cardiovascular disease or those receiving cardio-toxic drugs.

Adverse effects
Use in an opiate-dependent patient can precipitate withdrawal. Withdrawal convulsions in a neonate can be life threatening.

Hypertension and dysrhythmias occur more often with opioid reversal in postoperative patients who have underlying cardiac and pulmonary complications.

Dosage
The IV route is preferred in emergency situations because of the rapid onset of action within 1–2 minutes (Table 39-3).

The intramuscular and subcutaneous routes have erratic and slower absorption.

Naloxone has poor oral bioavailability.

Pralidoxime (Protopam)

Uses
Pralidoxime is used in cases of severe poisoning by an organophosphate anticholinesterase insecticide or chemical terrorism nerve agent.

Mechanism of action
Pralidoxime dephosphorylates acetylcholinesterase and regenerates acetylcholinesterase activity.

Indications
Pralidoxime is indicated in severe organophosphate or nerve agent poisoning, in combination with atropine, to resolve nicotinic (muscle and diaphragmatic weakness, fasciculations, muscle cramps) and central (coma, seizures) cholinergic manifestations. It is ineffective for organophosphates without anticholinesterase activity.

Pralidoxime use in cases of carbamate poisoning is controversial, but some sources recommend it for severe cases.

Contraindications
Pralidoxime should not be used in patients who are hypersensitive to the drug.

Adverse effects
■ Tachycardia, dizziness, hyperventilation, and laryngospasm associated with rapid IV infusion
■ Nausea, vomiting, diarrhea, bitter aftertaste, and rash after oral doses
■ Blurred vision and diplopia
■ Possible neuromuscular blockade (weakness) with high levels or in patients with myasthenia gravis

Dosage
See Table 39-3 for IV doses.

39-6. Terrorism and Disaster Preparedness

The world continues to face the threat of attacks with biological, chemical, explosive, and radiological weapons. Health care professionals should have an awareness of the potential for biological terrorism, an appreciation for epidemiologic clues of a chem-bioterrorist event, and a basic understanding of the classes of agents that can be weaponized and their effects.

Biological Threats

Bioterrorism is the deliberate use of infectious biological agents to cause illness and is categorized for risk by the U.S. Centers for Disease Control and Prevention (CDC) as follows:

■ *Category A* agents are high-priority agents that can be easily transmitted, can result in high mortality rates, and have the potential for major public health impact. They include smallpox, anthrax, plague, botulism, tularemia, and viral hemorrhagic fevers (filoviruses [e.g., Ebola, Marburg] and arenaviruses [e.g., Lassa, Machupo]).
■ *Category B* agents include brucellosis; epsilon toxin of *Clostridium perfringens;* food safety threats (e.g., *Salmonella* species, *Escherichia coli* O157:H7, *Shigella*); glanders (*Burkholderia mallei*); melioidosis (*B. pseudomallei*); psittacosis (*Chlamydia psittaci*); Q fever (*Coxiella burnetii*); ricin; staphylococcal enterotoxin B; typhus fever;

viral encephalitis (alphaviruses such as Venezuelan equine encephalitis, eastern equine encephalitis, and western equine encephalitis); and water safety threats (e.g., *Vibrio cholerae, Cryptosporidium parvum*).

■ *Category C* agents include emerging infectious disease threats such as Nipah virus and hantavirus.

See Table 39-4 for clinical features and suggested treatment for likely forms of category A threats and

for ricin, a category B agent that has been weaponized and used in terrorism.

The mode of transmission for many biological agents is similar to that of other infectious diseases:

■ Aerosol (most common form for biological weapons)
■ Dermal contact
■ Injection
■ Food
■ Water

Table 39-4. Biological Agents That May Be Used in a Terrorist Attack

Biological agent and description	Clinical features	Treatment
Smallpox is caused by the *variola* virus and may be spread by aerosol or direct contact with infected persons or fluids.	Early symptoms resemble a mild viral illness, with a 2- to 4-day nonspecific prodrome of fever and myalgia before rash onset. Pustules form, and then scabs form and fall off, leaving pitted scars. When all the scabs have fallen off (in about 3 weeks), patients are no longer contagious. Smallpox rash is typically most prominent on the face and extremities, and lesions form at the same time.[a]	No specific treatment exists. A live-virus vaccine of *vaccinia* virus (Dryvax) is primarily preventive for close contacts, but vaccination within 4 days of exposure *may* prevent or lessen disease.
Anthrax is caused by *Bacillus anthracis*, a Gram-positive spore-forming rod. It has three major forms (cutaneous, inhalation, gastrointestinal), and none are contagious.	*Cutaneous:* This form begins as a small papule and progresses to a vesicle in 1–2 days, followed by a necrotic, normally painless ulcer. Victim may have fever, malaise, headache, and regional lymphadenopathy. *Inhalation:* This form initially resembles a viral illness with sore throat, mild fever, muscle aches, and malaise. It often has minimally productive cough, nausea or vomiting, and chest discomfort, which may progress to respiratory failure and shock, with meningitis frequently developing.[b] *Gastrointestinal:* This form causes severe abdominal or oropharyngeal distress, followed by fever and signs of septicemia, bloody vomit, and diarrhea.	Based on 2014 CDC recommendations, ciprofloxacin and doxycycline are the preferred antibiotics for postexposure prophylaxis (PEP) of children and adults, while levofloxacin is preferred for adults 18 years of age and older. A selection of several intravenous antibiotics are recommended for systemic symptoms; see the CDC Web site (www.bt.cdc.gov) for specific indications. Persons at risk for inhalation anthrax need 60 days of prophylactic antibiotics. Oral ciprofloxacin, doxycycline, levofloxacin, or moxifloxacin is preferred for cutaneous anthrax. Anthrax Vaccine Adsorbed (BioThrax) given intramuscularly is indicated for active immunization for the prevention of disease caused by *B. anthracis* in persons age 18–65 years at high risk of exposure. Raxibacumab (available since 2013 from the CDC) is an antitoxin that blocks the activity of the anthrax toxin. It is used in combination with antibiotics that target the bacteria.
Plague, caused by *Yersinia pestis*, has several forms, with pneumonic plague being the most virulent.	Clinical features of aerosolized pneumonic plague include fever, cough with mucopurulent sputum, hemoptysis, and chest pain with signs consistent with severe pneumonia 1–6 days after exposure. Septic shock and high mortality can occur within 2–4 days of symptom onset without early treatment. *Y. pestis*–caused bubonic plague is less likely to be weaponized.	Early treatment for pneumonic plague with streptomycin or gentamicin is advised. Levofloxacin is also indicated (2012) for the prevention and treatment of *Y. pestis* infections. Other antibiotics may also be effective. A vaccine is no longer manufactured.

Table 39-4. Biological Agents That May Be Used in a Terrorist Attack *(Continued)*

Biological agent and description	Clinical features	Treatment
Botulism, caused by *Clostridium botulinum,* may be foodborne or airborne.	Clinical features include acute symmetric descending paralysis in a proximal to distal pattern; prominent bulbar palsies such as diplopia, dysarthria, dysphonia, and dysphagia that typically present 12–72 hours post-exposure; and respiratory dysfunction from respiratory muscle paralysis or upper airway obstruction without sensory deficits.	Antitoxin (most effective within 24 hours of exposure) is maintained and dispensed by the CDC. Most patients recover after supportive care, often with mechanical ventilation for weeks to months.
Tularemia, caused by *Francisella tularensis,* is one of the most infectious bacteria known.	Inhalation exposure causes an abrupt onset of a nonspecific febrile illness beginning 3–5 days postexposure, with incipient pneumonia, pleuritis, and hilar lymphadenopathy. Without treatment, respiratory failure, shock, and death are possible. Like botulism and anthrax, tularemia is not contagious, so patients who have tularemia do not need to be isolated.	Prompt treatment with streptomycin, gentamicin, chloramphenicol, doxycycline, or ciprofloxacin is advised, as is early PEP use of doxycycline or ciprofloxacin.
Viral hemorrhagic fevers (VHFs) include filoviruses, arenaviruses, bunyaviruses, and flaviviruses. (Other VHFs exist but are not considered a serious bioterrorism risk.) Filoviruses and arenaviruses are most virulent, but all viruses listed here are considered serious biological threats; exposure is by all routes, including direct and aerosol.	With filoviruses (Ebola and Marburg types), an abrupt onset of an undifferentiated febrile illness with high fever occurs 2–21 days after exposure. A maculopapular rash, prominent on the trunk, develops about 5 days later, with progressive bleeding symptoms such as petechiae, ecchymosis, disseminated intravascular coagulation, and hemorrhages. With arenaviruses (Lassa and multiple New World arenaviruses, including Machupo, which causes Bolivian hemorrhagic fever), symptoms and onset are similar to filoviruses, but with a gradual onset of rash, hemorrhagic diathesis, and shock. Bunyaviruses cause Rift Valley fever (< 1% develop hemorrhagic fever). Flaviviruses cause yellow fever, Omsk hemorrhagic fever, and Kyasanur Forest disease.	The mainstay of treatment is supportive to maintain fluid and electrolyte balance, circulatory volume, and blood pressure. There are no FDA-approved antiviral drugs or vaccines.
Ricin, from castor beans, is cytotoxic through inhibition of protein synthesis; abrin is a similar toxalbumin agent.	Within a few hours of inhalation, victims develop cough and dyspnea, with the lungs rapidly becoming severely inflamed and filled with fluid. Skin might turn blue from cyanosis or flush red. Ingestion causes internal bleeding of the stomach and intestines. Injection kills the closest muscles and lymph nodes before spreading to other organs. Death can occur within 36–48 hours of all types of exposure from multiple organ failure.	No antidote is available. The mainstay of treatment is supportive, varying with the route of exposure. If victims survive more than 5 days, survival is likely.

FDA, Food and Drug Administration.

a. In contrast, chicken pox rash is prominent on the trunk and develops in groups of lesions over several days.

b. In contrast, influenza patients rarely have a runny nose and usually have an abnormal chest x-ray and a high white blood cell count.

Chemical Threats

Toxic chemicals that may be used in warfare and in a chemical terrorism attack include nerve, vesicant or blister, blood, choking or pulmonary, incapacitating, and tear- and vomit-inducing (riot control) agents. See Table 39-5 for descriptions and symptoms of chemicals most likely to be used, together with treatments.

Normally, toxic chemicals used for these purposes are liquids or solids. Often they are dispersed in the air in aerosols.

The CDC also considers several commonly available agents to be threats, including hydrofluoric acid; benzene; ethylene glycol (antifreeze); and various metals such as arsenic, mercury, and thallium.

Radiological Threats

Radiological weapons involve nuclear radiation or radioactive materials with various radionucleotides. Radionucleotides can produce topical and systemic effects that may be immediate or delayed, depending on the agent, route of exposure, and extent of exposure.

Medical management of radiological emergencies and terrorist attacks is specific for radionucleotides. Guidance on treatment is available from the Radiation Emergency Assistance Center/Training Site (REAC/TS) at the Oak Ridge Institute for Science and Education (Oak Ridge, Tennessee). The emergency response phone number is 1-865-576-1005; ask for REAC/TS. For program information, see www.orise.orau.gov/reacts.

Table 39-5. Chemical Agents That May Be Used in a Terrorist Attack[a]

Chemical agents	Clinical features	Treatment
Nerve agents: G agents: sarin (GB), soman (GD), tabun (GA), cyclohexyl sarin (GF) V agents: VX	These nerve agents are organophosphates that attach to and inhibit acetylcholinesterase at muscarinic and nicotinic receptors, causing cholinergic crisis with miosis; vomiting; diarrhea; excessive bronchial, lacrimal, dermal, nasal, and salivary secretions; bradycardia or tachycardia; skeletal muscle fasciculations; paralysis; seizures; and respiratory failure. They are well absorbed through all routes of exposure. Symptoms occur within minutes after significant exposure and up to 18 hours after liquid exposure.	Rapid, thorough decontamination is needed. Antidotes include atropine to reverse muscarinic symptoms and pralidoxime early to restore acetylcholinesterase before permanent deactivation (aging) of the enzyme. Also give diazepam or lorazepam for seizures.
Blister agents: Mustards and nitrogen mustards Lewisites Chloroarsines Mustard–lewisite combinations Phosgene oxime (CX)	Vesicants cause blistering of the skin and mucous membranes on contact, damaging skin, eyes, and lungs. Damage is immediate, but significant symptoms can be delayed by 2–24 hours. Liquid forms are more likely to cause dermal burns and scarring than will gas. Mustards are absorbed through the skin, distributed systemically, and can cause bone marrow suppression in 3–5 days. Lewisites and chloroarsines are arsenical vesicants that can also cause increased capillary permeability leading to hypovolemia, shock, and organ damage. Phosgene oxime is readily absorbed by inhalation and causes immediate, painful corrosive and necrotic tissue damage on contact.	Sulfur and nitrogen mustards (thought to be alkylating agents that cross-link DNA strands) have no antidote. Avoidance of contact or rapid, thorough decontamination is the only prevention. Treatment is supportive. Exposure is not usually fatal (sulfur type < 5% fatal in World War I). No mustard is in tissue or blister fluids. British antilewisite is a specific antidote for lewisite, used intramuscularly for systemic effects or topically as skin or eye ointment. Chloroarsine treatment is similar, except atropine sulfate ointment is used for eyes. No antidote exists for phosgene oxime. Rapid decontamination and supportive treatment are used, as for any corrosive agent.

Table 39-5. Chemical Agents That May Be Used in a Terrorist Attack[a] *(Continued)*

Chemical agents	Clinical features	Treatment

Blood agents:
 	
  Arsine (SA)
 	
  Cyanide gases: hydrogen cyanide (AC), cyanogen chloride (CK)
 	
  Cyanide solids: potassium (KCN), sodium (NaCN) cyanide
	Arsine is a gas that causes nausea, vomiting, hemolysis, and secondary renal failure in 1–2 hours to 11 days.
	
	Inhalation of highly concentrated cyanide causes an increased rate and depth of breathing in 15 seconds, convulsions in 30 seconds, cessation of respiration in 2–4 minutes, and cessation of heartbeat in 4–8 minutes. Progress and severity of symptoms after ingestion or inhalation of lower gas concentrations are slower and dose dependent. Gas may have irritating, lacrimating properties like riot control agents (CK).
		For arsines, use symptomatic management of hemolysis, normally without chelation.
		
		Cyanides bind to cytochrome oxidase. Two antidote kits are available. Nithiodote has a methemoglobin-forming agent (sodium nitrite) that binds cyanide and a sulfur donor to convert it to excretable sodium thiocyanate (sodium thiosulfate). CyanoKit combines hydroxocobalamin with cyanide to form nontoxic cyanocobalamin (vitamin B_{12}). Fresh air, oxygen, and supportive treatment are essential.

Choking and pulmonary agents:
 	
  Phosgene (CG)
 	
  Diphosgene (DP)
 	
  Ammonia
 	
  Chlorine (CL)
 	
  Hydrogen chloride
 	
  Nitrogen oxide (NO)
 	
  Perfluoroisobutylene (PHIB)
 	
  Red phosphorous (RP)
 	
  White phosphorous
 	
  Others
	Phosgene gas causes eye, nose, throat, and pulmonary irritation, with serious pulmonary injury and edema delayed up to 48 hours, because it hydrolyzes to hydrochloric acid in moist conditions. Phosgene is the prototype agent in the group. Other agents cause immediate irritation with potential for more severe delayed effects.	Phosgene has no antidote. Good decontamination and symptomatic treatment are needed.
		
		Treatment of other agents is similar because all agents in this class are gases with no antidotes. Thorough, rapid decontamination with fresh air is the best initial management, with thorough flushing of exposed eyes and skin and symptomatic treatment.

Incapacitating agents	These agents contain a variety of fast-acting central nervous system and respiratory depressants, often with hallucinogenic properties. The CDC list includes BZ/agent 15 (glycolate anticholinergic), cannabinoids, fentanyls and other opioids, LSD, and phenothiazines.	Management is decontamination with supportive treatment, and antidotes should be used when they exist (physostigmine for anticholinergics; naloxone for opioids).
Riot control and tear gases	Lacrimators include chloroacetophenone (CN) in several solvents and chloropicrin (PS), bromobenzylcyanide (CA), dibenzoxazepine (CR), and 2-chlorobenzalmalononitrile (CS) gases.	Treatment is symptomatic after decontamination. No antidotes are available.
Vomiting agents	These agents include adamsite (DM), diphenylchloroarsine (DA), and diphenylcyanoarsine (DC). They are rapidly incapacitating, irritant gases.	Symptomatic measures are used for sneezing, coughing, and vomiting (e.g., antiemetics).

a. Military names are in parentheses.

The early use of stable iodine, taken as potassium iodide or sodium iodide tablets, can reduce the uptake of radioiodine by the thyroid. Many individuals near nuclear reactors will maintain a stock of stable iodine tablets in the event of a radioactive accident. Ingestion of stable iodine is of little value for other radionucleotide exposures unless the radioactive constituents are unknown, as in a "dirty bomb."

Prussian blue 500 mg capsules are approved for the treatment of patients with exposures to radioactive cesium (Cs-137) and thallium (Tl-201). Prussian blue absorbs the radioactivity that is recirculated in the intestines and thereby enhances its elimination in the stool. The drug is available from the CDC.

Calcium and zinc salts of diethylene triamine pentaacetic acid for IV infusion and aerosol nebulization are approved to treat patients who have been exposed to radionucleotides that may be found in a "dirty bomb" such as plutonium, americium, and curium. The drugs form chelates with the radionucleotides that are excreted in the urine. The drugs are available from the CDC.

Emergency Preparedness

Pharmacists are in a unique position to quickly recognize communitywide patterns of symptoms, illness, and mortality in humans and animals that can be important clues to terrorist events.

The CDC advises that if citizens believe that they have been exposed to a biological or chemical agent, or if they believe an intentional biological threat will occur or is occurring, they should contact their local health or police department or another law enforcement agency (e.g., the Federal Bureau of Investigation). These agencies will notify the state health department and other response partners through a preestablished notification list that channels to the CDC.

The CDC maintains the Strategic National Stockpile (SNS) to ensure the availability and rapid deployment of life-saving pharmaceuticals, antidotes, and other medical supplies and equipment necessary to counter nerve agents, biological pathogens, and chemical agents. The SNS program stands ready for immediate deployment to any U.S. location in the event of a terrorist attack using a biological toxin or chemical agent directed against a civilian population. A limited stock of drugs to treat nerve agents (CHEMPACK) has been deployed to emergency medical services and hospital sites throughout the United States and is maintained by the CDC. For further information, see the CDC Web site at www.bt.cdc.gov.

Pharmacists should consider volunteering in their communities to assist with emergency preparedness. Roles in mass dispensing and vaccination clinics, SNS deployment, and general disaster medical relief are possible opportunities. Contact the local health department or emergency medical services agency.

Essential steps to volunteering for emergency preparedness include reaching an understanding with one's family and employer, registering as a volunteer and identifying skills to contribute, obtaining security credentials, participating in training, and doing whatever it takes when needed.

39-7. Questions

1. Flumazenil is contraindicated in which of the following?

    I.   A patient with QRS widening with a known ingestion of Elavil (amitriptyline)
    II. A patient who was previously given flumazenil and who now complains of abnormal vision and dizziness
    III. A patient with known use of cocaine

    A. I only
    B. II only
    C. I and II only
    D. I and III only

2. A patient is brought to the emergency department. She is experiencing CNS and respiratory depression, which are suspected to be related to ingestion of her sister's MS Contin (morphine). You recommend supportive care and the administration of which of the following?

    A. Flumazenil
    B. Naloxone
    C. Lorazepam
    D. Flumazenil and Narcan

3. A police officer presents to the emergency room with a rash. He fears that he was exposed to a biological weapon several days before the rash appeared. You notice the rash is forming pustules and is most prominent on the face and extremities. The patient says the rash developed all at once. He has possibly contracted which of the following?

    A. Smallpox
    B. Chicken pox

C. Anthrax
D. Tularemia

4. What is the recommended treatment for smallpox?

   I. Supportive, because there is no specific treatment
   II. Ciprofloxacin
   III. Doxycycline

   A. II or III only
   B. II and III only
   C. I only
   D. II only

5. Which of the following is the currently available prevention for smallpox?

   I. Dryvax
   II. A live-virus preparation of the vaccinia virus
   III. Avoidance of direct contact with infected persons and their body fluids

   A. I only
   B. I and II only
   C. II and III only
   D. I, II, and III

6. A patient presents with a black, necrotic, painless skin lesion on her arm. She also complains of fever, malaise, headache, and swelling of her underarm lymph nodes. Which of the following is the possible biological agent responsible for these symptoms?

   A. Hemorrhagic fever virus
   B. Anthrax
   C. Botulism
   D. Arsine

7. The recommended antibiotic treatment for anthrax may include which of the following?

   A. Ciprofloxacin
   B. Doxycycline
   C. Amoxicillin
   D. Any of the above

8. Inhalation exposure to anthrax requires which of the following?

   A. Postexposure prophylaxis with ciprofloxacin, doxycycline, or levofloxacin for 60 days

   B. Immediate vaccination of civilian personnel
   C. Early treatment with streptomycin or gentamicin
   D. Early treatment with ribavirin

9. A cab driver presents to the emergency department with vomiting, diarrhea, sweating, salivation, moist rales, bradycardia, muscle tremor, and weakness. He reports inhaling a mist dropped from a low-flying plane several hours earlier. You also note that he has miosis and his respiratory difficulty is increasing rapidly. Which of the following is the likely mechanism of toxicity of the poison?

   A. Inhibition of protein synthesis
   B. Binding of the agent to cytochrome oxidase
   C. Inhibition of acetylcholinesterase
   D. An alkylating agent that cross-links DNA strands

10. The recommended initial management of muscarinic symptoms from an organophosphate poisoning includes all *except* which of the following?

    A. Immediate decontamination of skin and eyes
    B. Atropine
    C. British antilewisite
    D. Pralidoxime

11. A patient with initially mild symptoms of organophosphate poisoning deteriorates and develops seizures. Which of the following would be indicated?

    A. Phenytoin
    B. Diazepam
    C. Lithium
    D. Dryvax

12. Which of the following conditions or situations is *not* a contraindication to the use of ipecac syrup?

    A. High blood pressure controlled with drug therapy
    B. Seizures shortly before administration
    C. Unresponsiveness to verbal commands
    D. Ingestion of a corrosive agent

13. Which of the following is an effect of activated charcoal?

    A. Minimizes drug absorption from the gastrointestinal tract
    B. Increases urinary flow
    C. Enhances systemic elimination of certain drugs
    D. A and C

14. Which of the following is useful in the treatment of acetaminophen poisoning?

    A. Acetylcysteine
    B. Dimercaprol
    C. Pralidoxime
    D. Atropine

15. Digoxin immune Fab is used to treat which of the following signs or symptoms of digoxin poisoning?

    A. Hypokalemia
    B. Ventricular tachycardia
    C. Second-degree heart block unresponsive to atropine
    D. B and C

16. How does crack cocaine differ from pharmaceutical cocaine?

    A. Crack cocaine is more stable under heat and can be smoked.
    B. Pharmaceutical cocaine is the hydrochloride salt.
    C. Crack cocaine is the freebase form of cocaine and may be contaminated with other substances.
    D. All of the above

17. Which of the following mechanisms is associated with the production of hepatic injury from an acute overdose of acetaminophen?

    A. Interference with RNA synthesis
    B. Interference with transaminase enzyme activity
    C. Direct toxicity of acetaminophen
    D. Formation of a toxic metabolite

18. Which of the following signs or symptoms is characteristic of an acute exposure to an organophosphate as an insecticide or terrorist weapon?

    A. Dry mouth and mucous membranes
    B. Excessive bronchial secretions
    C. Muscle rigidity
    D. Urinary retention

39-8. Answers

1. **D.** Flumazenil is contraindicated in all patients who have ingested a tricyclic antidepressant and have cardiac symptoms because its use could cause ventricular dysrhythmias. It is not recommended in mixed overdose where the co-ingested drug can cause a seizure (i.e., cocaine). Statement II describes associated adverse effects that may occur with the administration of flumazenil; they are not contraindications.

2. **B.** Naloxone is an opioid antagonist.

3. **A.** Smallpox is the most likely agent. The agent causes formation of a pustular rash that is typically most prominent on the face and extremities. Lesions form at the same time. Chicken pox rash is most prominent on the trunk and develops in successive groups of lesions over several days. Anthrax forms painless necrotic lesions. Tularemia causes a nonspecific febrile illness that rapidly develops into pneumonia.

4. **C.** Smallpox has no specific treatment, but the live-vaccine (Dryvax) *may* lessen the disease if given within 4 days of the exposure. Ciprofloxacin and doxycycline are used in the management of anthrax, plague, and tularemia.

5. **D.** All options are correct.

6. **B.** Anthrax forms a painless, necrotic ulcer. Hemorrhagic fever viruses cause a rash that develops into petechiae, ecchymosis, hemorrhages, and other bleeding symptoms. Botulism causes a symmetric descending paralysis. Tularemia causes a nonspecific febrile illness that rapidly develops into pneumonia. Arsine is a chemical agent that causes nausea, vomiting, hemolysis, and secondary renal failure. Arsine is produced when water comes into contact with metallic arsenide or when acids come into contact with metallic arsenic or arsenical compounds. The mechanism of hemolysis is not specifically known, but the most recent mechanism postulated involves a direct arsine–hemoglobin interaction that forms arsenic metabolites, causing direct alteration of the erythrocyte cell membrane.

7. **D.** Ciprofloxacin, levofloxacin, and doxycycline are approved by the FDA for treatment of

anthrax, while amoxicillin can be used when the other drugs are not tolerated or pose patient-specific risks. These agents can be used separately or in combination, depending on the symptoms and the patient's sensitivity to the agents. Antimicrobial resistance to ciprofloxacin has been growing rapidly because of widespread overuse after the anthrax-contaminated mail episodes in 2002.

8. **A.** Persons at risk for inhalational anthrax need 60 days of prophylactic antibiotics. Ciprofloxacin and doxycycline are FDA approved for postexposure prophylaxis in adults and children; levofloxacin is used in adults 18 years of age and older. If these drugs are not tolerated, amoxicillin can be used. In 2009, a vaccine (BioThrax) became available that can be given postexposure in conjunction with antibiotics or as a vaccination for high-risk personnel (e.g., military or lab personnel likely to be in contact with the bacteria). Streptomycin and gentamicin are among the suggested treatments for pneumonic plague. Ribavirin is a potential treatment for some hemorrhagic fever viruses.

9. **C.** The symptoms exhibited are classically cholinergic, and the likely chemical agents causing these symptoms are organophosphates such as nerve agents or possibly organophosphate pesticides. Both can be spread by low-flying planes. Inhibition of protein synthesis is the mechanism of toxicity of ricin. Cyanides bind to cytochrome oxidase, thereby interrupting normal cellular respiration and causing rapid convulsions. Blister agents such as sulfur and nitrogen mustards are thought to be alkylating agents that cross-link DNA strands, thereby separating dermal layers in the skin and causing fluid-filled blisters to form.

10. **C.** British antilewisite is a specific antidote for lewisite. It also is used as a chelator for treatment of acute arsenic, inorganic or elemental mercury, gold, and other heavy metal poisonings. The other measures are treatments for organophosphate agents. Good decontamination and disposal of contaminated clothes (especially leather) are needed because organophosphates are well absorbed across the skin, through the lungs, and through ingestion—essentially all possible routes of exposure. Atropine is used for muscarinic symptoms (miosis; nausea and vomiting; diarrhea; urination; bradycardia; excessive bronchial, lacrimal, dermal, nasal, and salivary

secretions). Pralidoxime is used with atropine to resolve severe organophosphate symptoms (such as those from exposure to nerve agents), including nicotinic symptoms of muscle weakness and cramps, fasciculations, and tachycardia and CNS symptoms such as coma and seizures.

11. **B.** Recommended treatment for seizures attributable to organophosphate agents is either diazepam or lorazepam. Phenytoin is a seizure medication, but benzodiazepines (then barbiturates if benzodiazepines fail) are generally preferred over phenytoin for the control of overdose- or withdrawal-related seizures. Lithium is not a seizure medicine and, in fact, may cause seizures with elevated blood concentrations. Dryvax is a vaccine for smallpox.

12. **A.** Controlled high blood pressure is not a problem with the use of ipecac syrup, but the other situations are clear contraindications because of potential aspiration (seizures and unresponsiveness) and additional esophageal burns on vomiting up gastric contents (corrosive).

13. **D.** Activated charcoal adsorbs chemicals on contact and prevents their absorption into the bloodstream. For certain drugs (e.g., phenobarbital, theophylline), multiple doses of activated charcoal can promote the back diffusion of drugs across the intestinal capillary bed into the lumen of the gut, trap it there, and promote its elimination. The elimination half-life can be decreased by as much as one-half.

14. **A.** Acetylcysteine prevents the development of liver injury from acetaminophen if given early after ingestion and, in some cases, may help minimize the effects of hepatotoxicity after it has occurred.

15. **D.** Digoxin immune Fab is reserved for life-threatening symptoms because of its profound effects, scarcity, and high cost. Most serious cases of digoxin poisoning have normal or high potassium concentrations because of the digoxin's interference with the sodium-potassium ATPase pump.

16. **D.** All are differences between the two forms of cocaine.

17. **D.** Acetaminophen forms a toxic metabolite that has a direct toxic effect within the hepatocyte. It has other proposed mechanisms, but this mechanism is thought to be the inciting event.

18. **B.** Excessive bronchial secretions are one of the principal causes of death from exposure to organophosphates. The other symptoms are not observed.

39-9. References

General Toxicology

American College of Emergency Physicians. Clinical policy for the initial approach to patients presenting with acute toxic ingestion or dermal or inhalation exposure. *Ann Emerg Med.* 1999;33: 735–61.

Chyka PA. Clinical toxicology. In: Dipiro JT, Talbert RL, Yee GC, et al., eds. *Pharmacotherapy: A Pathophysiologic Approach.* 9th ed. New York, NY: McGraw-Hill; 2014:133–58.

DrugFacts. National Institute on Drug Abuse, National Institutes of Health Web site. http://www.drugabuse.gov/publications/term/160/drugfacts. Accessed August 18, 2014.

Drug fact sheets. Drug Enforcement Administration, U.S. Department of Justice Web site. http://www.justice.gov/dea/druginfo/factsheets.shtml. Accessed August 18, 2014.

Nelson LS, Lewin NA, Howland MA, et al., eds. *Goldfrank's Toxicologic Emergencies.* 9th ed. New York, NY: McGraw-Hill; 2011.

Olson KR, ed. *Poisoning & Drug Overdose.* 6th ed. New York, NY: Lange/McGraw-Hill; 2012.

Osterhoudt KC, Penning TM. Drug toxicity and poisoning. In: Brunton LL, Chabner BA, Knollmann BC, eds. *Goodman and Gilman's The Pharmacological Basis of Therapeutics.* 12th ed. New York, NY: McGraw-Hill; 2011:73–87.

Terrorist Threats

Abramowicz M, ed. Prevention and treatment of injury from chemical warfare agents. *Med Letter.* 2002;44:1–4.

Emergency preparedness and response. U.S. Centers for Disease Control and Prevention Web site. http://www.bt.cdc.gov.

Kales SN, Christiani DC. Acute chemical emergencies. *N Engl J Med.* 2004;350:800–8.

Managing radiation emergencies: Guidance for hospital medical management. Oak Ridge Institute for Science and Education Web site. http://www.orise.orau.gov/reacts/guide/care.htm. Accessed August 18, 2014.

Setlak P. Bioterrorism preparedness and response: Emerging role for health-system pharmacists. *Am J Health-Syst Pharm.* 2004;61:1167–75.

Shepherd G, Schwartz RB. Emergency preparedness: Identification and management of chemical and radiological exposures. In: Dipiro JT, Talbert RL, Yee GC, et al., eds. *Pharmacotherapy: A Pathophysiologic Approach.* 9th ed. New York, NY: McGraw-Hill; 2014:17–97.

Terriff CM, Brouillard JE, Costanigro LT. Emergency preparedness: Identification and management of biological exposures. In: Dipiro JT, Talbert RL, Yee GC, et al., eds. *Pharmacotherapy: A Pathophysiologic Approach.* 9th ed. New York, NY: McGraw-Hill; 2014:159–78.

Anemias

40

Jessica N. Lee

40-1. Key Points

- Anemia is a reduction in red cell mass, which decreases the blood's oxygen-carrying capacity.
- Iron deficiency anemia (IDA) is the most common anemia, accounting for 25% of all cases. IDA presents as a microcytic, hypochromic anemia.
- Iron preparations are best absorbed on an empty stomach but usually are not tolerated without the co-administration of food.
- Megaloblastic anemias are macrocytic and result from folic acid or vitamin B_{12} deficiency.
- It is essential to determine if the megaloblastic anemia is due to either folate or vitamin B_{12} deficiency because folate therapy can mask the hematopoietic features of vitamin B_{12} deficiency while allowing the sometimes irreversible neurologic sequelae to progress.
- Vitamin B_{12} requires intrinsic factor to be optimally absorbed.
- Patients with chronic kidney disease typically are anemic because of the lack of erythropoietin production.
- Anemia of chronic kidney disease is treated with subcutaneous or intravenous (IV) epoetin and IV iron therapy.
- Patients receiving epoetin must have routine monitoring of hematocrit, hemoglobin, and blood pressure.
- Darbepoetin has the same mechanism of action as epoetin, but it is longer acting and can be administered less frequently.

40-2. Study Guide Checklist

The following topics may guide your study of this subject area:

- Diagnostic criteria for anemia
- Various types of anemia and potential causes of each
- Presenting symptoms that could lead to suspicion of anemia
- Different available dosage forms of both oral and IV iron preparations and when to recommend each
- Drug interactions that could affect oral iron administration
- Indications for drugs other than iron preparations (i.e., folic acid, vitamin B_{12}, epoetin alfa, darbepoetin alfa)
- Monitoring parameters for patient response to treatment
- Possible nondrug treatment options
- Unique patient counseling points to maximize response to treatment while minimizing potential adverse effects

40-3. Disease Overview

Anemia is a reduction in red cell mass that decreases the oxygen-carrying capacity of the blood. The World Health Organization guidelines suggest a plasma

---

Editor's Note: This chapter is based on the 10th edition chapter written by Roland N. Dickerson.

hemoglobin (Hgb) concentration < 12 mg/dL for nonpregnant females, < 11 mg/dL for pregnant females, and < 13 mg/dL for males as diagnostic for anemia. This chapter will focus on iron deficiency anemia (IDA), megaloblastic anemia, and anemia of chronic kidney disease.

Epidemiology

Approximately 3.4 million Americans have anemia. Anemia is more common in menstruating and pregnant women than in men. Seventy-five percent of all anemias result from iron deficiency, anemia of chronic disease, and acute bleeding. The remaining 25% of anemia cases are due to bone marrow damage, decreased erythropoiesis, and hemolysis. IDA is the single most common form of anemia, accounting for 25% of all cases.

Kinetic Approach to Anemia

Using the kinetic methodology, one can classify anemia by three major mechanisms: decreased red blood cell (RBC) production (due to lack of nutrients, bone marrow disorders, or suppression), increased RBC destruction (e.g., hemolytic anemia), or blood loss. It includes evaluation of parameters such as reticulocyte count and reticulocyte production index, which are more tedious and costly than the conventional morphological approach to evaluating anemia.

Classification by Morphology

The most common way to classify an anemia is by the morphology (shape and structure) of the RBCs.

Macrocytic (large-sized cell) morphology (RBC size > 100 fL)

Anemias in this class include megaloblastic (oval cells often with hypersegmented neutrophils) and normoblastic (round cells) and may result from the following:

- Megaloblastic
  - Folic acid deficiency
  - Vitamin B_{12} deficiency or pernicious anemia (lack of intrinsic factor)
- Normoblastic
  - Alcohol
  - Liver disease

- Hypothyroidism
- Nucleoside reverse transcriptase inhibitors
- Valproic acid

Normocytic (normal-sized cell) morphology (RBC size 80–100 fL)

Anemias in this class may result from the following:

- Acute blood loss
- Bone marrow failure (decreased RBC production)
- Hemolysis (increased RBC destruction)
- Immunologic destruction, such as occurs in autoimmune diseases
- Anemia of chronic disease or chronic inflammation (early onset)

Microcytic (small-sized cell) morphology (RBC size < 80 fL)

Anemias in this class include the following:

- Hypochromic (pale RBCs lacking hemoglobin with decreased mean corpuscular Hgb and mean corpuscular Hgb concentration)
  - IDA
  - Anemia of chronic disease or chronic inflammation (late onset)
- Normochromic (normal color RBCs)
  - Certain genetic anomalies, such as thalassemia

Clinical Presentation

The signs and symptoms of anemia depend on the amount of time during which the anemia has developed and the severity of RBC depletion. An anemia that has developed over a long period of time may be asymptomatic in the beginning stages and then progress to fatigue, malaise, headache, exertional dyspnea, angina, pallor, or loss of skin tone. A patient with acute anemia (from recent blood loss, for example) may present with tachycardia, shortness of breath, or lightheadedness. Many of the signs and symptoms of anemia are secondary to tissue hypoxia. In the case of hypoxia, blood supply is shunted to life-sustaining organs (brain, heart, kidney) and away from nonvital organs (e.g., extremities, nail beds), which results in pallor of the skin. The various types of anemia have additional signs and symptoms that will be discussed in further detail elsewhere in the chapter.

Pathophysiology

Iron deficiency anemia

IDA is the most common anemia, accounting for one-fourth of all anemia cases. It is caused by iron store depletion resulting from

- Inadequate oral intake of iron (especially animal protein)
- Increased iron demands, such as those found in
  - Pregnant or lactating women
  - Infants and adolescents who experience periods of rapid growth
  - The elderly
- Blood loss as a result of
  - Menstruation or postpartum blood loss
  - Trauma
  - Gastrointestinal (GI) ulcers
- Inadequate absorption as a result of
  - Medications (e.g., tetracyclines, antacids, histamine-2 [H2] antagonists, proton-pump inhibitors)
  - Gastrectomy
  - Enteritis or malabsorption syndrome
  - Ingestion of large amounts of tannins (tea) or phytates (brans, grains)
- Disease states, such as
  - Carcinomas
  - Rheumatoid arthritis

Hemoglobin is composed of iron (heme) and proteins (globin). Lack of iron results in reduced hemoglobin synthesis. The RBCs produced under those conditions are

- Hypochromic (decreased concentration of hemoglobin)
- Microcytic (smaller-sized cells)

Megaloblastic anemias

Megaloblastic anemias are caused by either a deficiency in or an inability to use vitamin B_{12} (cobalamin) or folic acid.

Vitamin B_{12} deficiency can result from

- **Decreased intake:** This problem may occur with patients who are strict vegetarians (e.g., ovo-lacto vegetarians) or in alcoholics with a poor diet.
- **Decreased absorption:** For vitamin B_{12} to be absorbed at the terminal ileum, intragastric intrinsic factor must be attached to it. The lack of production of intrinsic factor results in pernicious anemia, which can be inherited or acquired by gastrectomy. Malabsorption can also occur in patients with gastric bypass surgery, chronic pancreatitis, and chronic diarrhea (e.g., celiac disease, short bowel syndrome, regional enteritis, inflammatory bowel disease, HIV enteropathy, *Helicobacter pylori* infections), or it can result from metformin therapy (calcium-dependent ileal membrane antagonism).
- **Achlorhydria:** Vitamin B_{12} requires an acidic environment to be absorbed. Chronic therapy with proton pump inhibitors and H2 antagonists may contribute to vitamin B_{12} deficiency; those with atrophic gastritis may be vitamin B_{12} deficient as well.

Folic acid deficiency can result from

- **Decreased intake:** This problem is found especially in patients who are alcoholic, indigent, or elderly.
- **Decreased absorption:** This problem occurs in patients with inflammatory bowel disease or malabsorption disorders.
- **Increased demands:** For example, deficiencies may occur during pregnancy or growth spurts or could accompany malignancy or long-term hemodialysis.
- **Use of certain drugs:** Such drugs include trimethoprim, sulfasalazine, pyrimethamine, triamterene, methotrexate, cyclophosphamide, hydroxyurea, mercaptopurine, 5-fluorouracil, and phenytoin.

Anemia of Chronic Kidney Disease

The primary reason patients with chronic kidney disease are anemic is because of the lack of erythropoietin (EPO) production. EPO is a hormone produced primarily (90%) in the kidneys that stimulates the synthesis and differentiation of erythroid progenitor cells (precursors to RBCs). The uremic environment in patients with chronic kidney disease decreases the lifespan of RBCs.

Folic acid deficiency also can develop as a result of increased folic acid demands during synthesis of RBCs. Additionally, folic acid can be removed during hemodialysis. Patients with chronic kidney disease become iron deficient as a result of iron and blood loss during dialysis and the diseased kidneys' impaired ability to manufacture EPO in response to that loss.

Diagnostic Criteria

If anemia is suspected, a complete blood cell count (CBC) should be performed, which includes the following:

- Hgb
- Hct (hematocrit)
- RBC count
- Red cell indices: The three major indices include mean corpuscular volume (MCV), which is a measure of the size of RBCs; mean corpuscular hemoglobin (MCH), which represents the percent volume of hemoglobin in RBCs; and mean corpuscular hemoglobin concentration (MCHC), which is a measure of the weight of hemoglobin. It is more useful than MCH because it is independent of cell size. A low MCHC often is reflective of iron deficiency anemia.
- Platelets
- Reticulocyte count (the amount of immature nucleated RBCs or pre-RBCs)
- RBC distribution width (RDW), which indicates the variability of RBC size. A high RDW may indicate a mixed anemia, particularly in the case of a normal MCV. RDW alone is not sensitive enough to detect mixed anemias and must be followed up with more specific diagnostic studies.
- Red cell morphology
- Serum iron, total iron binding capacity (TIBC), transferrin saturation, and ferritin
- Indirect (unconjugated) bilirubin concentration, which is a by-product of RBC destruction

Other tests include the following:

- Stool test for presence of blood
- Peripheral blood smear
- Thorough history and physical examination

Iron deficiency anemia

Blood work

Serum iron, transferrin, and TIBC historically have been used to confirm IDA. Serum transferrin concentration (one of the major transport proteins for iron) and TIBC (the amount of binding space left for iron on the transferrin protein) increase with iron deficiency, whereas transferrin saturation will decrease to < 15%. Transferrin saturation is the amount of iron that is bound to transferrin; the normal range is ~20–50%. It is calculated by the following formula: transferrin saturation = (serum iron concentration/ TIBC) × 100. Unfortunately, serum iron is not very sensitive and may be a misleading marker of total body iron stores. A variety of conditions such as infection, stress, and inflammation may cause hypoferremia, because serum iron is an acute phase reactant that decreases during these conditions. These inflammatory conditions result in the sequestration of iron into the reticuloendothelial system as well as an increase in the hepatic production of hepcidin, which decreases intestinal iron absorption. Serum transferrin also is an acute phase reactant protein that decreases during these conditions.

Serum ferritin (the storage form of iron) is now considered the best and most reliable initial marker of choice for assessing iron status. A patient with a serum ferritin concentration < 45 ng/mL has a significant potential for iron deficiency; a concentration < 25 ng/mL indicates a very high probability of iron deficiency. Unfortunately, serum ferritin also is influenced by stress, inflammation, and neoplasia, because serum ferritin concentration is increased under these conditions. As the iron deficiency progresses, Hgb will decrease, because iron is a component of Hgb. As a result, the RBCs will become paler in color (MCH and MCHC will be decreased), and the RBCs will become smaller in size (decreased MCV), indicating a microcytosis. The blood smear will reflect a microcytic, hypochromic cell.

Specific signs and symptoms

In addition to the general signs and symptoms listed previously for anemia, the following additional symptoms may be present in severe IDA:

- Koilonychia (spoon-shaped nails)
- Angular stomatitis or glossitis
- Pica (appetite for nonfood substances such as chalk, soil, ice, or clay)

Megaloblastic anemias (macrocytic anemias due to vitamin B_{12} or folate deficiency)

Blood work

Blood work should show the following:

- Decreased Hct and Hgb
- Decreased RBC count
- Elevated MCV, which indicates a macrocytosis
- Abnormalities in serum homocysteine, methylmalonic acid, or both
- Normal ferritin

Because of the lack of sensitivity and specificity of serum vitamin B_{12} (cobalamin) and folate concentrations, many clinicians now use serum homocysteine or methylmalonic acid to ascertain if a patient has a vitamin B_{12} or folate deficiency. Those compounds are used because vitamin B_{12} or folate must be present for either their synthesis or their metabolism. For example, the normal metabolism of methylmalonic acid to succinyl-coenzyme A requires the presence of vitamin B_{12} (cobalamin). Without sufficient amounts of vitamin B_{12}, serum methylmalonic acid concentration is elevated. Without sufficient folate intake, serum homocysteine is elevated (and methylmalonic acid is normal). Because cobalamin also is required for the metabolism of homocysteine, a patient with elevated serum concentrations of both homocysteine and methylmalonic acid likely would have a vitamin B_{12} deficiency, although a combined vitamin B_{12} and folate deficiency is possible. A patient with a macrocytic anemia and normal concentrations of homocysteine and methylmalonic acid likely has a non-vitamin deficiency macrocytic anemia from liver disease, alcohol abuse, treatment with valproic acid, nucleoside reverse transcriptase inhibitors, or hypothyroidism or from increased reticulocytosis. The diagnostic utility of these metabolites is given in Table 40-1. The clinician must appropriately diagnose whether the megaloblastic anemia is due to folate or vitamin B_{12} depletion. An incorrect diagnosis may lead to permanent neurologic sequelae if a vitamin B_{12} deficiency is misdiagnosed and treated as a folate deficiency without appropriate vitamin B_{12} supplementation.

Vitamin B_{12} deficiency

Because of the large amount of vitamin B_{12} stored in the liver, it generally takes 3–5 years of prevalence of the etiology (e.g., malabsorption, drug therapy, etc.) before the deficiency is manifested. If the etiology for the megaloblastic anemia is vitamin B_{12} deficiency,

serum methylmalonic acid concentration definitely will be elevated, and serum homocysteine concentration also likely will be elevated.

Additional signs and symptoms include the following:

- Loss of vibratory sensation in lower extremities
- Ataxia or vertigo
- Glossitis
- Muscle weakness
- Neuropsychiatric abnormalities (e.g., irritability or emotional instability, dementia, psychosis)

Folic acid deficiency

Folic acid deficiency results in an increased serum homocysteine concentration with a normal serum methylmalonic acid concentration. Folate deficiency can occur sooner than vitamin B_{12} deficiency, with signs and symptoms of deficiency appearing within 6 months of folate depletion. Overall, signs and symptoms of folic acid deficiency anemia are very similar to vitamin B_{12} deficiency anemia, except that the neurological symptoms that may be present with vitamin B_{12} deficiency anemia are absent. Folic acid supplementation is given to pregnant women preemptively, because folate depletion can lead to neural tube birth defects (e.g., spina bifida) during fetal development.

Anemia of chronic kidney disease

As the name implies, this anemia occurs in patients with chronic kidney disease who require maintenance hemodialysis. The etiology for this type of anemia is multifactorial, including the effects of hemodialysis itself, which can lead to hemolysis, the removal of water-soluble vitamins (e.g., vitamin B_{12} and folate), and iron deficiency. Lack of EPO production also is a major factor. EPO is a hormone released from the kidney that stimulates the bone marrow to make new RBCs. Before diagnosis, other causes must be ruled out. A CBC usually will reveal a normochromic, normocytic anemia.

Bone marrow failure

In aplastic anemia, the bone marrow fails to produce multiple types of blood cells, resulting in anemia, neutropenia (decreased neutrophils), and thrombocytopenia (decreased platelets). About half of aplastic anemia cases are believed to be caused by drugs or chemicals. Drugs that cause aplastic anemia include chloramphenicol, felbamate, carbamazepine, and phenytoin.

Table 40-1. Vitamin-Dependent Metabolites in Patients with Vitamin B_{12} or Folate Deficiency

Serum metabolite concentrations	Vitamin deficiency
Elevated HCY, normal MMA	Folate deficiency
Elevated HCY, elevated MMA	Vitamin B_{12} deficiency or possibly a combined vitamin B_{12}/folate deficiency
Normal HCY, elevated MMA	Vitamin B_{12} deficiency
Normal HCY, normal MMA	Macrocytic anemia not due to a folate or vitamin B_{12} deficiency

HCY, homocysteine; MMA, methylmalonic acid.

Hemolysis

Hemolysis may be due to genetically inherited enzyme deficiencies. One common example is glucose-6-phosphate dehydrogenase (G6PD) deficiency. G6PD deficiency can lead to hemolysis, because RBCs deficient in G6PD are susceptible to hemolysis when exposed to certain oxidant drugs such as dapsone, sulfamethoxazole, and nitrofurantoin.

Treatment Principles and Goals

Iron deficiency anemia

In IDA treatment, the first goal is to normalize Hgb and Hct:

- Hgb should increase 2 g/dL in 3 weeks.
- Hct should increase 6% in 3 weeks.
- Reticulocytosis usually will occur within 1 week.

If those indices do not improve within their respective time frames, the diagnosis should be reevaluated, and compliance with therapy should be confirmed. A second goal is to replenish iron stores. Although Hgb and Hct will return to normal within 1–2 months, iron therapy should be continued for 3–6 months after Hgb is normalized to replenish total body iron stores.

Megaloblastic anemias

Goals of vitamin B₁₂ replacement

Hgb should increase within 1 week. If neurologic symptoms were present, they should improve within 24–72 hours. However, if vitamin B_{12} deficiency is longstanding, symptoms may not be relieved for several months. In some cases, some residual neurologic signs and symptoms may not resolve completely. Maintenance administration of vitamin B_{12} should continue for as long as nutritional intake, increased losses, or malabsorption is a problem.

Goals of folic acid replacement

RBC morphology will correct within a few days. Hgb will start to normalize within 10 days. Hct will return to normal levels within 2 months. Maintenance administration of folic acid should continue for as long as nutritional intake, increased losses, or malabsorption is a problem.

40-4. Drug Therapy

Iron Deficiency Anemia

Treatment consists of iron supplementation to achieve a total elemental iron dose of about 200 mg per day (Table 40-2). The total daily dose usually is divided into 2–3 dosing intervals throughout the day. The ferrous sulfate salt, which is 20% elemental iron, is the most commonly used and inexpensive salt form for iron therapy. Treatment of IDA with ferrous sulfate 325 mg three times daily for 3–6 months will be adequate for many patients.

Iron is best absorbed in the reduced (ferrous) form. Iron is maximally absorbed in the duodenum, primarily because of the acidic nature of the stomach. Vitamin C (ascorbic acid) may facilitate increased absorption of iron, although its clinical relevancy has been questioned. Additionally, orange juice may improve absorption. High-fiber foods, tea (rich in iron-binding tannins), coffee, and milk should be avoided during the administration of iron preparations. It is recommended that the iron product be taken on an empty stomach; however, most patients experience significant adverse GI effects necessitating that the drug be taken with either a snack or food. Some patients can tolerate only a product with a low elemental iron content (e.g., ferrous gluconate), a slow-release/sustained release preparation, or an enteric-coated iron product. However, the sustained release and enteric-coated products are

Table 40-2. Common Oral Iron Preparations Used To Treat IDA

Generic name	Trade name	Elemental Fe (%)	Dose (mg)	Fe content (mg)
Ferrous sulfate	Feosol, Fer-in-Sol	20	325	65
Ferrous gluconate	Fergon	12	300	35
Ferrous fumarate	Femiron, Fumerin, Feostat	33	300	99
Polysaccharide iron complex	Niferex, Ferrex	100	150	150
Carbonyl iron	Feosol Carbonyl Iron	100	45	45

less effective, because absorption is delayed because of slower dissolution, and iron is not available for absorption until the product has reached the jejunum or ileum, where iron absorption is decreased. If the patient is selected for one of these latter therapeutic options, then clinical recovery from the IDA would be expected to occur at a slower rate, and increased duration of therapy from 3–6 months to 6–12 months would be expected.

Once the iron deficiency has been adequately treated, maintenance therapy may consist of a lower dose (e.g., ferrous sulfate 325 mg once daily or a multivitamin product that is enriched with iron) if the precipitating cause for the IDA is still evident (e.g., menses). Additionally, dietary intake of meat, fish, and poultry may be encouraged, because iron from vegetable, grain, and dairy sources is poorly absorbed.

Patient instructions (for oral supplementation)

- Take iron supplementation 1–2 hours prior to a meal (on an empty stomach if tolerable).
- If iron is intolerable on an empty stomach, take it with a small snack, but try to avoid dairy products or tea. Food can decrease the absorption of iron by 50%. Iron may be taken with an acidic fruit beverage such as orange juice to improve absorption.
- Keep out of reach of children. Iron is a major cause of ingestion deaths in children.
- Take iron 1 hour before or 3 hours after any antacids.
- Some medications interact with iron. Please ask your health care provider or pharmacist before taking any new medications in combination with iron.
- If constipation occurs, you may take over-the-counter docusate.

Adverse drug effects

The oral formulation primarily has GI effects:

- Dark-colored stools
- Constipation or diarrhea
- Nausea or vomiting

Drug interactions

- *Antibiotics (tetracycline and quinolones):* Iron binds to these antibiotics, preventing absorption.
- *Antacids:* Iron needs an acidic environment for optimal absorption.

Intravenous (IV) iron preparations should be used only in the following cases:

- Iron malabsorption with the inability to overcome the malabsorption with enteral iron supplementation
- Oral noncompliance with severe anemia
- Refusal of blood transfusion for severe anemia
- Chronic kidney disease patients or cancer patients receiving human recombinant erythropoiesis stimulating agents

Patients with an active infection should not receive IV iron therapy. When iron is given intravenously, free iron concentration can easily exceed maximum transferrin saturation (unlike when given orally). The abundant free iron is then available to be used by various microorganisms for proliferation and may actually increase the virulence of the offending organisms.

Five IV iron products are available in the United States:

- Iron dextran (INFeD and Dexferrum)
- Ferric gluconate (Ferrlecit)
- Iron sucrose (Venofer)
- Ferumoxytol (Feraheme)
- Ferric carboxymaltose (Injectafer)

Ferumoxytol was approved in 2009 for IDA in adult patients with chronic kidney disease. Ferric carboxymaltose was approved in 2013 for IDA of various etiologies in adult patients who cannot tolerate or who have not responded well to oral iron products.

Mechanism of action

Iron supplementation corrects the iron deficiency and enables Hgb to be synthesized at normal levels.

Published methods for calculating the parenteral dose or iron deficit differ. One method follows:

$$\text{iron deficit}(mg) = \left[0.3 \times \text{weight}(lb)\right]$$
$$\times \left[\left(\text{target Hgb} - \text{current Hgb}\right)/\text{target Hgb} * 100\right]$$

Iron dextran may be given intravenously in intermittent doses (e.g., 100 mg daily) or as a total dose infusion mixed in 250–1,000 mL of normal saline (0.9% NaCl) over 4–6 hours. Iron dextran formulations carry a black box warning about fatal anaphylactic reactions. A 25 mg test dose must be administered by slow IV push or intermittent infusion, and the patient must be observed for any adverse or allergic reactions for up to 1 hour after administration. This test dose is required before the patient can receive a larger therapeutic dose of iron dextran. The other IV iron products do not contain dextran and have a better safety profile; therefore, they do not require a test dose. Iron dextran is the only IV iron product approved for total dose infusion. Iron dextran also may be given intramuscularly (by Z-track injection to prevent potential skin staining) at doses up to 100 mg per injection. Iron dextran can be added to lipid-free parenteral nutrition solutions; however, it cannot be added to lipid-containing parenteral nutrition solutions, because iron is a trivalent cation and can disrupt the emulsification of lipids, resulting in *oiling out* or coalescence of lipid particles.

Ferumoxytol does not require dilution, and doses of 510 mg may be given as a rapid IV push at a rate of 1 mL/second (30 mg/second). It should not be given intramuscularly or subcutaneously. Ferumoxytol is approved to deliver 1,000 mg of IV iron in two doses. The second dose should be administered 5–8 days after the first dose. The IV iron formulations may have the following adverse effects:

- Immediate reaction (within minutes of infusion)
  - Malaise, urticaria, nausea, diaphoresis, headache
  - Anaphylactic: Anaphylactoid reaction, hypotension, circulatory collapse. Premedication with antihistamines and corticosteroids may prevent anaphylaxis but is rarely done because of the low incidence of these reactions.
- Delayed reaction (within 1–2 days after infusion)
  - Myalgias, arthralgias, fever, flu-like symptoms

Monitoring parameters

- Have reticulocytes, Hgb, and Hct increased?
- Is the iron tolerable? (Tolerance will influence compliance.)
- Is the patient improving symptomatically?

Kinetics

Bioavailability of oral iron preparations is increased in an acidic environment and is decreased by food.

Megaloblastic Anemias

Treatment of an existing vitamin B_{12} deficiency usually is done by the parenteral route; however, some clinicians have been successful with sublingual, intranasal, or high-dose oral therapy. Early and aggressive treatment is warranted, particularly if the patient has any neurologic signs and symptoms, because these adverse effects may not be completely reversible if the anemia has been allowed to persist for a substantial time.

A severe vitamin B_{12} deficiency (e.g., neurologic signs or symptoms) usually is corrected through intramuscular (IM) or subcutaneous vitamin B_{12} (cyanocobalamin) injection, although IV administration, if available, also is an option. Multiple dosing schemes are published in the literature. Some typical methods are as follows:

- Initially 1,000 mcg IM, IV, or subcutaneous every day for 1 week, then 1,000 mcg IM, IV, or subcutaneous every week for 4–6 weeks
- 1,000 mcg IM, IV, or subcutaneous every week for 4–6 weeks
- 500 mcg intranasally or sublingually daily for 4–6 weeks (for less severe deficiency)

Once the deficiency has been corrected, various maintenance methods for prevention of recurrence exist depending on the etiology for the deficiency. If the etiology is low dietary intake such as with vegans (particularly ovo lacto-vegetarians), one simple maintenance solution is daily ingestion of a multivitamin that meets the Dietary Reference Intake for vitamin B_{12}. If the etiology is malabsorption due to achlorhydria, pernicious anemia, chronic pancreatitis, drug-induced malabsorption, or gastric bypass therapy, either sublingual or intranasal administration (500 mcg weekly) is reasonable. Hot liquids or foods should be avoided for 1 hour before and after intranasal administration in an effort to avoid rhinorrhea and potentially reduce absorption. High oral doses of vitamin B_{12} may be used as maintenance therapy for some patients (e.g., 1,000–2,000 mcg daily is necessary to benefit from passive absorption). For patients with short bowel syndrome or severe malabsorption, the oral route should be avoided. The parenteral route also is an option (e.g., 1,000 mcg IM, IV, or subcutaneous every 1–3 months), although most patients would prefer sublingual or nasal administration.

Mechanism of action

Vitamin B_{12} supplementation allows for normal synthesis of the RNA involved in RBC synthesis.

Patient instructions

If injections are given at home, the patient or caregiver should be counseled on sterile injection techniques and proper needle disposal.

Adverse drug effects

Vitamin B_{12} supplementation can cause the following adverse effects:

- Hyperuricemia or hypokalemia caused by increased synthesis of reticulocytes
- Sodium retention
- An expansion of the intravascular volume as a result of increased RBC synthesis, which can increase cardiac output and cause angina or dyspnea
- Itching in 1–10% of patients
- Diarrhea in 1–10% of patients
- Anaphylaxis in < 1% of patients

Monitoring parameters

- Monitor CBC. Is there an increase in Hgb? The hemoglobin should improve within 2 weeks. The anemia should correct within 1–2 months, although abnormalities in the blood smear may persist for several months.
- Is the patient improving symptomatically (especially neurologic symptoms, if present)?
- Methylmalonic acid concentrations should normalize within 1 month depending on the intensity of the repletion therapy.

Kinetics

Intrinsic factor is necessary for vitamin B_{12} absorption. It must be present for vitamin B_{12} to be transported optimally across the GI mucosa. Also, a small amount of passive diffusive absorption (about 1%) of vitamin B_{12} occurs, which is independent of intrinsic factor.

Vitamin B_{12} is bound in blood to transcobalamin II and converted in tissues to active coenzymes methylcobalamin and deoxyadenosylcobalamin.

Folic Acid Deficiency Anemia

Folic acid deficiency is corrected by administering 1 mg folic acid daily for 4 months. Five mg daily may be given if the patient has severe malabsorption. Once the underlying cause of the deficiency is corrected, folic acid supplementation may be discontinued. Long-term folate administration is necessary if the cause is not corrected, such as in hemodialysis, chronic drug therapy with sulfasalazine, or alcoholism.

Mechanism of action

Folic acid supplementation allows for normal RNA synthesis, which is involved in the synthesis of RBCs.

Patient instructions

- Stress the importance of compliance with the regimen.
- Women of childbearing age should be counseled to take a multivitamin containing folic acid, regardless of whether an anemia is present, to prevent neural tube birth defects.

Adverse drug effects

Fewer than 1% of patients have allergic reactions to folic acid.

Drug interactions

Folic acid may increase phenytoin metabolism.

Phenytoin, primidone, sulfasalazine, para-aminosalicylic acid, and oral contraceptives may decrease folic acid concentrations.

Chloramphenicol may blunt the response to folic acid.

Monitoring parameters

- Is the RBC morphology normalizing?
- Are the Hgb and Hct normalizing? An improvement in Hgb should occur within 2 weeks. The anemia should be corrected within 1–2 months.
- Homocysteine concentrations should normalize within 1 month.
- Is the patient complying?

Kinetics

Folic acid is a water-soluble B vitamin absorbed in the small intestine with peak concentrations occurring at 30 minutes to 1 hour.

Anemia of Chronic Kidney Disease
Recombinant human erythropoietin

The primary cause of anemia in chronic kidney disease is decreased EPO synthesis; therefore, the optimal drug for this type of anemia is an erythropoiesis stimulating agent (ESA). Epoetin alfa (Procrit, Epogen) and darbepoetin alfa (Aranesp) are ESAs with similar mechanisms of action, but darbepoetin alfa has a longer half-life.

An ESA is indicated in the treatment of anemia associated with chronic kidney disease, including dialysis and nondialysis patients. ESAs are indicated to elevate or maintain the RBCs and to decrease the need for transfusions in these patients. The goal of combined iron therapy and ESAs for anemia of chronic kidney disease is to reach a target Hgb ≥ 10 g/dL through a slow, steady increase (usually within 2–4 months). Rapid increases in or overcorrection of Hgb concentrations as a result of ESA use has led to increased thrombotic vascular events, congestive heart failure, and cardiac ischemia. The U.S. Food and Drug Administration has removed the labeling for a specific Hgb or Hct target range because of those safety concerns. The National Kidney Foundation–Kidney Disease Outcomes Quality Initiative (NKF-KDOQI) guidelines recommend that epoetin be administered subcutaneously, because that route of administration is as effective as, or better than, IV administration. However, epoetin often is administered intravenously in patients receiving hemodialysis, because the dialysis port offers easy IV access. Concurrent IV iron therapy

also is recommended for effective erythropoiesis during therapy with ESAs.

Mechanism of action
Human recombinant EPO stimulates erythropoiesis (increased RBC production).

Patient instructions
Epoetin alfa is available in preservative-free single dose vials, multidose vials, and predrawn syringes. All dosage forms should be stored at 36–46°F (2–8°C) until ready for use.

Adverse drug effects
Table 40-3 shows adverse effects of epoetin alfa and the percentage of patients reporting them. The most common adverse effect is elevated blood pressure and is associated with the rate of rise in Hgb concentration. Increased thromboembolic complications, cardiac failure, and cardiac ischemia have been asso-

Table 40-3. Percentage of Patients Reporting Adverse Effects of Epoetin Alfa

Event	Patients treated with epoetin alfa ($n = 200$)	Patients on placebo ($n = 135$)
Hypertension	24%	19%
Headache	16%	12%
Arthralgias	11%	6%
Nausea	11%	9%
Edema	9%	10%
Fatigue	9%	14%
Vomiting	8%	5%
Chest pain	7%	9%
Skin reaction at site of administration	7%	12%
Asthenia	7%	12%
Dizziness	7%	13%
Clotted access	7%	2%
Significant adverse events[a]		
Seizure	1.1%	1.1%
Cerebrovascular accident—transient ischemic attack	0.4%	0.6%
Myocardial infarction	0.4%	1.1%
Death	0.0%	1.7%

Reproduced from Procrit package insert with permission of Ortho Biotech Products.
a. Significant adverse events of concern in patients with chronic kidney disease treated in double-blind, placebo-controlled trials occurred in the percentages of patients shown during the blinded phase of the studies.

ciated with a rapid rise in Hgb (e.g., > 1 g/dL within 2 weeks). ESAs are contraindicated in patients with uncontrolled hypertension. Pure red cell aplasia (PRCA), in association with neutralizing antibodies to native EPO, has been reported rarely in the literature. If PRCA is suspected, discontinue epoetin immediately.

Drug interactions
No drug interactions have been reported.

Monitoring parameters
Prior to initiation of therapy, the patient's iron stores should be evaluated. Transferrin saturation should be at least 20% and ferritin at least 100 ng/mL. Monitor Hgb very closely. The dose should be titrated to maintain the lowest hemoglobin concentration sufficient to avoid an RBC transfusion. Once the Hct approaches the target Hgb concentration (e.g., 10 g/dL per the NKF-KDOQI guidelines), the dose of epoetin should be decreased. If Hgb increases more than 1 g/dL within 2 weeks, the dose should be decreased. The dose should be increased if Hgb has not increased 1 g/dL in 8 weeks.

Blood pressure should be adequately controlled prior to initiation of ESA therapy. Blood pressure must be closely monitored and controlled during therapy.

Monitor serum chemistries.

Kinetics
The half-life of epoetin is approximately 4–13 hours. The half-life of epoetin in patients not on dialysis with serum creatinine > 3 is no different than in patients requiring dialysis.

Darbepoetin

Mechanism of action
Darbepoetin has the same mechanism of action as epoetin.

Patient instructions
Counseling points are very similar for both darbepoetin and epoetin, except that all darbepoetin vials are single-use only; therefore, the patient should dispose of the vial as instructed after each dose. Darbepoetin is also available in predrawn syringes.

Adverse drug effects
The most common adverse effects are

- *Cardiovascular:* Hypertension, hypotension, edema, arrhythmia

- *GI:* Nausea, vomiting, diarrhea, constipation
- *Central nervous system:* Fatigue, fever, headache
- *Neuromuscular or skeletal:* Myalgia, arthralgia, limb pain
- *Respiratory:* Infection, dyspnea, cough

Drug interactions
No drug interactions have been reported.

Monitoring parameters
- Monitor patient's iron stores prior to and during therapy.
- Monitor patient's blood pressure.
- Adjust dose by closely monitoring Hgb every week until a maintenance dose is established. Target Hgb is ≥ 10 g/dL. Increase dose if Hgb increases more than 1 g/dL over a 4-week period. Decrease dose by 25% if Hgb increases more than 1 g/dL over a 2-week period.

Kinetics
Darbepoetin's half-life is 21 hours when administered intravenously and 49 hours when administered subcutaneously. Its half-life is approximately three times longer than epoetin's half-life. Because of its longer half-life, less frequent dosing options are available with darbepoetin.

40-5. Nondrug Therapy

Iron Deficiency Anemia

Dietary supplementation plays an important role in IDA treatment:

- Increase intake of iron-rich foods, such as meat, fish, and poultry.
- Orange juice may improve iron absorption.
- Avoid tea or milk with concurrent iron administration.

Folic Acid Deficiency Anemia

Dietary supplementation also is important in treating folic acid deficiency:

- To get as much dietary folate as possible, do not overcook vegetables. Eat them raw, microwaved, or steamed.
- Eat a wide variety of properly prepared vegetables and fruits.

40-6. Questions

Use Patient Profile 40-1 to answer Questions 1–5.

1. Which of the following medications could present a problem with this patient's iron supplement?

   A. Acetaminophen
   B. Ranitidine
   C. Maalox
   D. Docusate
   E. Ranitidine and Maalox

2. The patient admits to you that he is not able to take his iron tablet because it makes him nauseated. What advice can you give him?

   A. Take your iron with some crackers and milk.
   B. Take your iron with some crackers and water.
   C. Don't worry about it. It's only a vitamin.
   D. Start taking iron with the largest meal of the day.
   E. Take iron after breakfast.

3. If the patient's anemia progresses to severe stages, what effects may he experience?

   A. Koilonychia (spooning of the nails)
   B. Pica (e.g., craving ice, clay, chalk)
   C. Glossitis (sore, beefy red tongue)
   D. Extreme fatigue
   E. All of the above

4. If you were to examine the patient's peripheral blood smear, you would find cells that are

   A. microcytic and hypochromic.
   B. macrocytic and hypochromic.
   C. macrocytic and normochromic.
   D. microcytic and normochromic.

5. When one is examining this patient's iron study results, which of the following would be consistent with IDA?

   A. Elevated TIBC
   B. Elevated ferritin
   C. Elevated MCV
   D. Elevated Hgb
   E. Elevated Hct

6. Which iron preparation is most likely to cause an anaphylactic reaction?

   A. IV iron dextran
   B. IV iron sucrose
   C. IV sodium ferric gluconate
   D. Extended-release ferrous sulfate po
   E. Immediate-release ferrous sulfate po

7. Why are sustained-release (SR) preparations of iron *not* the ideal formulation?

   A. The incidence of nausea is higher with SR formulations.
   B. They are dosed only once daily, and goal Hgb levels are not attained.
   C. Because SR preparations are dissolved in the small intestines, the alkaline environment results in a lower bioavailability than the acidic environment of the stomach.
   D. Dissolution in the small intestines is not bioavailable, because intrinsic factor is not present in the small intestines.
   E. SR preparations require dosing with food.

Patient Profile 40-1—SuperPrice Drug Store

Patient: 62-year-old male

Weight: 193 lb

Problem list:

Gastroesophageal reflux disease

Iron deficiency anemia

Hypertension

Medication record:

Ferrous sulfate 325 mg tid

Hydrochlorothiazide 25 mg daily

Allergies: NKDA

OTC recommendations:

Maalox 1 tbsp q2h prn for "indigestion"

Acetaminophen 325 mg q4–6h prn for headache

Ranitidine 75 mg daily prn for "heartburn"

Docusate 100 mg daily for constipation

8. Which of the following options would you advise a patient to drink with meals to optimize iron absorption from meals?

   A. Orange juice
   B. Coffee
   C. Tea
   D. Milk
   E. Wine

9. The most likely regimen to supplement vitamin B_{12} is

   A. 1,000 mcg po every month.
   B. 1,000 mcg IV every month.
   C. 1,000 mcg IM every month.
   D. 1,000 mcg IM every day.
   E. 1,000 mcg SQ every 2 months.

10. To be absorbed, vitamin B_{12} requires which of the following?

    A. Pernicious factor
    B. Transcobalamin II
    C. Intrinsic factor
    D. Vitamin B_{12} absorption factor
    E. Hydrochloric acid

11. Which of the following patients probably has a diet that prevents folic acid deficiency?

    A. Strict vegetarians
    B. Alcoholics
    C. The indigent
    D. People who routinely overcook their vegetables
    E. A college student whose diet consists of burgers and potato chips

12. Folic acid may interact with which of the following medications?

    A. Propranolol
    B. Propoxyphene
    C. Piroxicam
    D. Phenytoin
    E. Prednisone

13. The two macrocytic anemias are

    A. vitamin B_{12} deficiency and iron deficiency anemias.
    B. vitamin B_{12} deficiency and folic acid deficiency anemias.
    C. iron deficiency and folic acid deficiency anemias.

    D. sickle cell anemia and anemia of chronic kidney disease.
    E. iron deficiency and pernicious anemias.

14. The best regimen to replace folic acid is

    A. folic acid 1 mg po every day for 3–4 months.
    B. folic acid 10 mg po every day for 3–4 months.
    C. folic acid 10 mg IV for 2 weeks, then 1 mg po every day for 2 months.
    D. folic acid 1 mg po three times weekly for 3–4 months.
    E. folic acid 1 mg po once monthly for 6 months.

15. The most common medication given to treat anemia of chronic kidney disease is

    A. vitamin B_{12}.
    B. a solution of citric acid in combination with sodium acetate.
    C. epoetin alfa.
    D. ferrous sulfate po.
    E. folic acid po.

16. What advantage does darbepoetin have over epoetin?

    A. Lower incidence of hypertension
    B. Fewer drug interactions
    C. Lower cost
    D. Longer half-life and less frequent administration
    E. Improved tolerability

17. The most common side effect of epoetin is

    A. anaphylaxis.
    B. hypertension.
    C. pure red cell aplasia.
    D. injection site reaction.
    E. weight gain.

18. Prior to initiation of epoetin therapy, which of the following should be evaluated?

    A. Folic acid and vitamin B_{12} levels
    B. Transferrin and ferritin levels
    C. EPO receptor level
    D. Presence or absence of intrinsic factor
    E. Stomach acid pH

Patient Profile 40-2—Central Dialysis Center

Patient: 44-year-old female

Weight: 148 lb

Diagnosis:

Hypertension

Diabetes mellitus

End-stage renal disease

Hyperlipidemia

Labs:

Ferritin: 80 ng/mL (normal)

Transferrin saturation: 15% (low)

Hct: 32% (low)

Hgb: 8.6 g/dL (low)

Allergies: Penicillin (rash)

Dialysis schedule: Monday, Wednesday, Friday

Medications:

Insulin NPH 30 U bid

Simvastatin 20 mg nightly

Atenolol 25 mg after dialysis

Nephrocaps 1 capsule daily

---

19. In which of the following patients would it be possible to teach self-administration of epoetin at home?

    I. A patient on home hemodialysis taking epoetin via IV administration
    II. A patient on home peritoneal dialysis taking epoetin via subcutaneous administration
    III. A patient on home hemodialysis taking epoetin via subcutaneous administration

    A. II only
    B. II and III only
    C. III only
    D. I, II, and III
    E. I only

Use Patient Profile 40-2 to answer Questions 20–23.

20. Which of the following will be monitored when the patient starts epoetin therapy?

    A. Blood pressure
    B. Hematocrit
    C. Serum chemistries
    D. Iron profile
    E. All of the above

21. The target Hgb range for the patient is

    A. 11–12 g/dL.
    B. 9–11 g/dL.
    C. 11–13 g/dL.
    D. 12–13 g/dL.
    E. 9–14 g/dL.

22. Which of the patient's medications will interact with epoetin?

    A. Insulin
    B. Simvastatin
    C. Atenolol
    D. Nephrocaps
    E. No medications are known to interact with epoetin.

23. What medication should be added to the patient's regimen?

    A. Oral propranolol
    B. IV iron
    C. Oral levothyroxine
    D. IM vitamin B_{12}
    E. Oral vitamin B_6

40-7. Answers

1. **E.** Iron is best absorbed in an acidic environment. Therefore, antacids dramatically decrease the absorption of iron. Iron supplements should be taken 1 hour before or 3 hours after antacids.

2. **B.** Many patients are not able to tolerate iron on an empty stomach. Those patients should

take iron with a small snack. Milk would not be acceptable in this case, because dairy products decrease the absorption of iron.

3. **E.** Koilonychia, pica, extreme fatigue, and glossitis all are symptoms of severe iron deficiency anemia.

4. **A.** Iron deficiency produces a hypochromic (low-Hgb) anemia, given that iron is a component of the Hgb molecule. The cells also are microcytic (meaning "small cell"), because they spend a longer time in the marrow awaiting proper Hgb synthesis and therefore divide more.

5. **A.** TIBC is elevated in IDA. TIBC is a measure of the amount of binding space left on transferrin (the transport protein of iron). Less iron in the blood means that more space is available on the transferrin molecule.

6. **A.** IV iron dextran has the highest incidence of anaphylaxis among the four IV iron preparations available.

7. **C.** SR preparations are left intact in the stomach and are dissolved in the small intestine. The alkaline environment of the small intestine tends to form insoluble iron complexes that cannot be absorbed.

8. **A.** Tea and milk can decrease the absorption of iron from a meal by more than 50%. Orange juice, however, can double the absorption of iron from food.

9. **C.** The most common IM dose of vitamin B_{12} is 1,000 mcg per month. However, vitamin B_{12} may be supplemented by the oral route if absorption is not impaired. Additionally, it may be supplemented in very high doses, such as 1,000–2,000 mcg per day, in pernicious anemia.

10. **C.** Vitamin B_{12} requires intrinsic factor for absorption.

11. **A.** Folic acid deficiency is found in alcoholics, the indigent, and—rarely—in people who routinely overcook their vegetables. Strict vegetarians do not develop folic acid deficiency because a folate-rich diet includes various types of vegetables.

12. **D.** Phenytoin increases the metabolism of folate, thereby decreasing the effectiveness of folic acid.

13. **B.** Both vitamin B_{12} deficiency anemia and folic acid deficiency anemia are macrocytic (large cell) anemias. Both iron deficiency anemia and sickle cell anemia are microcytic and hypochromic anemias.

14. **A.** Folic acid is administered po because it is absorbed easily. The proper dose is 1 mg folic acid po every day, and the deficiency should be corrected after 3–4 months.

15. **C.** Epoetin is the most common medication used to treat anemia of chronic kidney disease, because it stimulates erythropoiesis. The lack of EPO production is the primary cause of anemia of chronic kidney disease.

16. **D.** Darbepoetin is very similar to epoetin because it has the same mechanism of action and similar side effects. However, it has a longer half-life and can be administered less frequently.

17. **B.** Hypertension is the most common adverse drug effect from epoetin.

18. **B.** Transferrin and ferritin levels should be evaluated prior to epoetin therapy. IDA is a common problem in patients with end-stage renal disease. The patient's transferrin should be at least 20% and ferritin should be at least 100 ng/mL before epoetin therapy is initiated.

19. **D.** Patients on home peritoneal dialysis or hemodialysis can be taught to self-administer subcutaneous injections. Additionally, if patients are receiving home hemodialysis, they can be taught to take their epoetin intravenously through the dialysis venous port.

20. **E.** Iron profiles need to be monitored prior to starting epoetin and periodically during therapy because IDA is very common in dialysis patients. Blood pressure needs to be monitored because increased blood pressure is the most common adverse effect of epoetin. Hct levels need to be checked as a measure of response to epoetin, and levels should be maintained at 30–36%. Serum chemistries need to be monitored regularly in any patient with end-stage renal disease, because most electrolytes are regulated by the kidneys.

21. **A.** The target range of Hgb for patients receiving epoetin is 11–12 g/dL.

22. **E.** No medications are known to interact with epoetin.

23. **B.** The patient's ferritin is < 100 ng/mL, and her transferring saturation is less than 20%. Most hemodialysis patients receiving epoetin will need iron therapy at some point during their treatment.

40-8. References

Alleyne M, Horne MK, Miller JL. Individualized treatment for iron deficiency anemia in adults. *Am J Med.* 2008;121(11):943–48.

Aranesp [package insert]. Thousand Oaks, CA: Amgen Biotech Company; December 2013.

Aslinia F, Mazza JJ, Yale SH. Megaloblastic anemia and other causes of macrocytosis. *Clin Med Res.* 2006;4:236–41.

Cook K, Ineck B, Lyons W. Anemias. In: Dipiro JT, Talbert RL, Yee GC, et al., eds. *Pharmacotherapy: A Pathophysiologic Approach.* 8th ed. New York, NY: McGraw-Hill; 2011:1718–40.

Feraheme [package insert]. Waltham, MA: AMAG Pharmaceuticals; 2014.

Goodnough LT, Nemeth E, Ganz T. Detection, evaluation, and management of iron-restricted erythropoiesis. *Blood.* 2010;116(23):4754–61.

Injectafer [package insert]. Shirley, NY: American Regent Inc.; July 2013.

Kidney Disease: Improving Global Outcomes (KDIGO) Anemia Work Group. KDIGO clinical practice guidelines for anemia in chronic kidney disease. *Kidney Int Suppl.* 2012;2(4):279–335.

Killip S, Bennett JM, Chambers MD. Iron deficiency anemia. *Am Fam Physician.* 2007;75:671–8.

Krikorian S, Shafai G, Shamim K. Managing iron deficiency anemia of CKD with IV iron. *US Pharmacist.* 2013;38(8):22–26.

Kumpf VJ. Update on parenteral iron therapy. *Nutr Clin Pract.* 2003;18:318–26.

National Kidney Foundation. KDOQI clinical practice guidelines and clinical practice recommendations for anemia in chronic kidney disease: 2007 update of hemoglobin target. *Am J Kidney Dis.* 2007;50:471–530.

National Kidney Foundation. KDOQI clinical practice guidelines and clinical practice recommendations for anemia in chronic kidney disease. *Am J Kidney Dis.* 2006;47(suppl 3):S11–15.

Pieracci FM, Barie PS. Diagnosis and management of iron-related anemias in critical illness. *Crit Care Med.* 2006;34(7):1898–905.

Procrit [package insert]. Horsham, PA: Janssen Products; December 2013.

Procrit [package insert]. Raritan, NJ: Ortho Biotech Products; 2000.

Schwenk MH. Ferumoxytol: A new intravenous iron preparation for the treatment of iron deficiency anemia in patients with chronic kidney disease. *Pharmacotherapy.* 2010;30(1):70–79.

Snow CF. Laboratory diagnosis of vitamin B_{12} and folate deficiency. *Arch Intern Med.* 1999;159:1289–98.

Unger EF, Thompson AM, Blank MJ, Temple R. Erythropoiesis-stimulating agents: Time for a re-evaluation. *New Engl J Med.* 2010;362:189–92.

Weiss G, Goodnough LT. Anemia of chronic disease. *New Engl J Med.* 2005;352:1011–23.

Thromboembolic Disease

Gale L. Hamann

41-1. Key Points

- Appropriate *venous thromboembolism* (VTE) prophylaxis should be used with all patients who have risk factors for its development. *ACCP Evidence-Based Clinical Practice Guidelines* (9th edition) has guidelines for VTE prophylaxis specific for at-risk patient populations.

- Unfractionated heparin (UFH) should be administered as a bolus of 80 IU/kg intravenous (IV), then a maintenance infusion of 18 IU/kg/h. Heparin is monitored by activated partial thromboplastin time (aPTT) levels. A therapeutic aPTT range should be determined for each hospital or laboratory that corresponds to an antifactor Xa concentration of 0.3–0.7 IU/mL.

- Low molecular weight heparin (LMWH) offers a more predictable response at lower doses without the need to monitor levels, except in patients with severe renal impairment or in obesity. It has a lower incidence of osteoporosis and heparin-induced thrombocytopenia. It can also be administered once or twice daily by subcutaneous injection, which allows care to shift from the hospital to the outpatient arena.

- An acute VTE should be treated with IV UFH, LMWH, or fondaparinux to provide immediate anticoagulation, followed by the initiation of warfarin therapy. Warfarin should be initiated at 5–7.5 mg daily for most patients. Patients with malnutrition, liver disease, or heart failure; patients who are taking drugs known to increase the responsiveness to warfarin; patients who have a high risk for bleeding; or elderly patients may be started at a lower dose. UFH, LMWH, or fondaparinux should be overlapped with warfarin for at least 4–5 days or until two consecutive international normalized ratios (INRs) are within the therapeutic range.

- Patients with a single VTE with reversible, time-limited risk factors should be anticoagulated for 3 months. Patients with a single idiopathic VTE should be anticoagulated for at least 3 months, but consider long-term therapy depending on the risk–benefit ratio. Patients with a recurrent VTE should be anticoagulated long term.

- Rivaroxaban is an oral factor Xa inhibitor used for the treatment of an acute deep venous thrombosis (DVT) or pulmonary embolism (PE) at a dose of 15 mg bid with food for 21 days followed by 20 mg daily with food. It can also be used to reduce the risk of recurrence of a DVT or PE at a dose of 20 mg daily with food. Rivaroxaban is also indicated for DVT prophylaxis in patients undergoing hip replacement surgery at a dose of 10 mg daily for 35 days or for knee replacement surgery at a dose of 10 mg daily for 12 days. Unlike warfarin therapy, no blood monitoring is necessary with rivaroxaban.

41.2. Study Guide Checklist

The following topics may guide your study of this subject area:

- Definition and epidemiology of venous thromboembolic disease
- Clinical presentation of thromboembolic disease
- Pathophysiology of thromboembolic disease
- Risk factors associated with thromboembolic disease

- Diagnosis of thromboembolic disease
- Prophylactic therapies for the prevention of thromboembolic disease
- Treatment of thromboembolic disease
- Mechanism of actions of the various anticoagulants
- Pharmacokinetic considerations of the various anticoagulants
- Indications for the various anticoagulants
- Trade names and available dosage forms of the various anticoagulants
- Frequency of dosing regimen
- Major adverse drug reactions of the various anticoagulants
- Significant drug interactions of the various anticoagulants
- Patient counseling points for the various anticoagulants

41-3. Venous Thromboembolic Disease

Definition and Epidemiology

Venous thromboembolism (VTE) is a disease process that involves the development of a deep venous thrombosis, a pulmonary embolism, or both.

A *pulmonary embolism* (PE) is a thrombus or foreign substance from the systemic circulation that lodges in the pulmonary artery or its branches and causes a complete or partial occlusion of pulmonary blood flow.

A *deep venous thrombosis* (DVT) is a thrombus that forms most commonly in the popliteal or femoral veins, the veins of the calf, or the iliac veins of the upper leg. Veins of the upper extremities are less commonly involved.

Approximately 2 million Americans develop VTE each year; 600,000 people in this group have VTE manifested as a PE, and of these, 200,000 die. An estimated 1 million people in the United States will develop a clinically silent PE that goes undiagnosed.

Complications of VTE are postthrombotic syndrome and pulmonary hypertension. *Postthrombotic syndrome* is characterized as swelling in the affected lower extremity after a DVT. *Pulmonary hypertension* is a complication that can occur after a PE and is characterized by elevated arterial pressures in the pulmonary vasculature.

The incidence of VTE increases with age and doubles in each decade of life after age 50. VTE costs an estimated $1.5 billion annually.

Clinical Presentation

The most common symptoms of a PE are dyspnea, cough, hemoptysis, tachypnea, tachycardia, pleuritic chest pain, diaphoresis, and overwhelming anxiety. The patient may be cyanotic and hypoxemic secondary to having a reduced ability to oxygenate the blood. Patients with a massive PE may present with syncope. The mortality rate of a PE ranges from 2.3% to 17%.

The most common symptoms of a DVT are pain, tenderness, edema, and erythema of the affected extremity. Other symptoms may include dilation of the superficial veins, a palpable cord, and a positive Homans' sign.

Pathophysiology

Venous thrombi generally form in areas of the veins where blood flow is slowed or disrupted. Often they begin as small thrombi in the large venous sinuses of a valve cusp pocket in the veins of the calf or thigh. Trauma to vessels causes the release of tissue factor. Tissue factor, in turn, activates the coagulation cascade. This activity results in the formation of thrombin and ultimately the formation of fibrin to form clots. Other common factors that can precipitate the development of a thrombus include disrupted blood flow from immobility or hypercoagulability.

Risk factors for VTE include the following:

- Age over 40 years
- Prolonged immobility
- Major surgery involving the abdomen, pelvis, and lower extremities
- Trauma, especially fractures of the hips, pelvis, and lower extremities
- Malignancy
- Pregnancy
- Previous VTE
- Congestive heart failure or cardiomyopathy
- Stroke
- Acute myocardial infarction
- Indwelling central venous catheter
- Hypercoagulability
- Estrogen therapy
- Varicose veins
- Obesity
- Inflammatory bowel disease
- Nephrotic syndrome
- Myeloproliferative disease

A PE is the result of a dislodged thrombus that is embolized from a thrombus in the deep venous structures of the legs, pelvis, or arms. The embolus travels to the lungs, where it is trapped in the pulmonary arterial microvasculature. Blood flow is obstructed by the PE, which leads to lung edema and reduced pulmonary compliance. This condition results in inadequate oxygen exchange, leading to hypoxemia. Blood flow in the pulmonary artery increases right ventricular afterload, which may lead to right ventricular dilation, dysfunction, and ischemia.

Diagnosis

A DVT is diagnosed on the basis of a detailed history and clinical symptoms. A duplex ultrasound, which measures both blood flow and compressibility of the affected vessel, confirms the diagnosis.

A PE is diagnosed on the basis of a detailed history and clinical symptoms. A spiral CT (computed tomography) scan or a ventilation-perfusion scan confirms the diagnosis.

VTE Prophylaxis

Table 41-1 shows recommendations for VTE prophylaxis.

VTE Treatment

VTE treatment success with unfractionated heparin (UFH) is related to obtaining therapeutic activated partial thromboplastin time (aPTT) levels as rapidly as possible (Table 41-2). Studies have indicated that the VTE recurrence risk is 20–25% higher if aPTT levels are not within the therapeutic range at 24 hours. The therapeutic range for an aPTT is determined by an antifactor Xa chromogenic assay of 0.3–0.7 IU/mL.

The use of low molecular weight heparin (LMWH) has enabled treatment of a DVT to move from a hospitalization of 5–7 days to either a hospital stay of 1–2 days or outpatient management (Table 41-3).

Table 41-1. Recommendations for VTE Prophylaxis

Medical condition	Recommended therapy
General medical	
General medical patients with risk factors	LMWH, LDUH bid or tid, or fondaparinux; if at risk for bleeding, GCS, or IPC
General and abdominal-pelvic surgery	
Low risk for VTE:	
Patients undergoing minor procedures with no additional VTE risk factors	Early and frequent ambulation
Moderate risk for VTE:	
Not at high risk for major bleeding	LMWH, LDUH, or mechanical prophylaxis preferably with IPC
At high risk for major bleeding	Mechanical prophylaxis preferably with IPC
Higher risk for VTE:	
Not at high risk for major bleeding	LMWH, LDUH combined with ES or IPC; if LMWH or LDUH contraindicated, then use fondaparinux, low-dose aspirin, or mechanical prophylaxis preferably with IPC
Surgery for cancer, not at high risk for major bleeding	Extended-duration prophylaxis for 4 weeks with LMWH
At high risk for major bleeding	Mechanical prophylaxis with IPC until bleeding risk decreases, then use appropriate pharmacologic thromboprophylaxis
Orthopedic Surgery	
Elective total hip or knee replacement	LMWH, fondaparinux, rivaroxaban, LDUH, warfarin, aspirin, or IPC for a minimum of 10–14 days and up to 35 days
Hip fracture surgery	LMWH, fondaparinux, warfarin, aspirin, or IPC for at least 10 days and up to 35 days

Ageno, Gallus, Wittkowsky, et al., 2012.
LMWH, low molecular weight heparin: enoxaparin 30 mg subcutaneous q12h, enoxaparin 40 mg subcutaneous q24h, dalteparin 5,000 units subcutaneous q24h; LDUH, low-dose unfractionated heparin, 5,000 units subcutaneous q8–12h; fondaparinux 2.5 mg subcutaneous q24h; GCS, graduated compression stocking; IPC, intermittent pneumatic compression device; ES, elastic stocking; warfarin, target INR (international normalized ratio) 2.5, range 2.0–3.0.

Table 41-2. Guidelines for Anticoagulation: IV Unfractionated Heparin

Indication	Guidelines
VTE suspected	Obtain baseline aPTT, PT, and CBC count.
	Check for contraindications to heparin therapy.
	Order imaging study; administer IV bolus of heparin 80 IU/kg or 5,000 IU.
VTE confirmed	Rebolus with IV heparin 80 IU/kg, and start maintenance infusion at 18 IU/kg/h.
	Check aPTT at 6 hours to keep aPTT in a range that corresponds to a therapeutic blood heparin level.
	Check platelet count between days 1 and 3.
	Start warfarin therapy on day 1 at 5 mg, and adjust subsequent daily dose according to INR.
	Stop heparin after at least 4–5 days of combined therapy when INR is ≥ 2.0 for 24 hours.
	Anticoagulate with warfarin for at least 3 months at an INR of 2.5; range of 2.0–3.0.

Adapted with permission from Kearon, Kahn, Agnelli, et al., 2008.
CBC, complete blood count; IV, intravenous; INR, international normalized ratio; PT, prothrombin time.
For treatment with subcutaneous UFH, give 250 IU/kg subcutaneous q12h to obtain a therapeutic aPTT in 6 hours.

Table 41-3. Guidelines for Anticoagulation: LMWH or Fondaparinux

Indication	Guidelines
VTE suspected	Obtain baseline aPTT, PT, and CBC.
	Check for contraindications to LMWH or fondaparinux therapy.
	Order imaging study; administer LMWH or fondaparinux.
VTE confirmed	Continue LMWH or fondaparinux.
	Check platelet count between days 3 and 5.
	Start warfarin therapy on day 1 at 5 mg, and adjust subsequent daily dose according to INR.
	Stop LMWH or fondaparinux after at least 4–5 days of combined therapy when INR is ≥ 2.0 for 24 hours.
	Continue warfarin for at least 3 months at an INR of 2.5; range of 2.0–3.0.

Adapted with permission from Kearon, Kahn, Agnelli, et al., 2008.
CBC, complete blood count; INR, international normalized ratio; PT, prothrombin time.
Dalteparin sodium 200 anti Xa IU/kg per day subcutaneous; single dose should not exceed 18,000 IU. Enoxaparin 1 mg/kg subcutaneous q12h or 1.5 mg/kg subcutaneous q24h; single dose should not exceed 180 mg. Fondaparinux 5 mg for < 50 kg; 7.5 mg for 50–100 kg; 10 mg for > 100 kg subcutaneous q24h.

With outpatient DVT treatment, the diagnosis may take place in either a physician's office or the emergency department. After a Doppler ultrasound confirms the diagnosis of a DVT, the patient is educated on administration of LMWH and receives the first dose of LMWH at that time. LMWH and warfarin are then administered on an outpatient basis. Warfarin is monitored with an international normalized ratio (INR) at 1- or 3-day intervals. After two therapeutic INRs, the LMWH may be discontinued; warfarin is continued for at least 3 months, and the patient is evaluated for long-term anticoagulation or as indicated (Table 41-4). Another therapy is rivaroxaban, an oral factor Xa inhibitor. Rivaroxaban is effective within 2–4 hours, so no other therapies such as LMWH or heparin are necessary. For acute DVT or PE, rivaroxaban is administered 15 mg bid with food for 21 days followed by 20 mg daily with food.

Drug Therapy

Unfractionated heparin

Mechanism of action
UFH binds to antithrombin (AT) and converts it from a slow progressive thrombin inhibitor to a rapid thrombin inhibitor. This, in turn, catalyzes inactivation of factors XIIa, XIa, IXa, Xa, and IIa (thrombin).

Therapeutic use
- Prevention and treatment of VTE
- Prevention of VTE in patients with a previous VTE or a known hypercoagulability
- Prophylaxis for VTE in high-risk populations
- Prevention of a mural thrombosis after myocardial infarction (MI)

Table 41-4. Duration of Anticoagulation Therapy

Indication	Duration of anticoagulation
VTE secondary to transient risk factor	Warfarin therapy for 3 months
First unprovoked VTE	Warfarin therapy for at least 3 months, but consider long-term therapy based on risk–benefit ratio
Second unprovoked VTE	Warfarin therapy long term
VTE and cancer	LMWH for the first 3–6 months of long-term anticoagulation therapy, followed by anticoagulation with LMWH or warfarin therapy long term or until cancer resolves

Adapted with permission from Kearon, Kahn, Agnelli, et al., 2008.

- Treatment of patients with unstable angina and MI
- Prevention of acute thrombosis after coronary thrombolysis

Patient counseling

Patients need to monitor for signs and symptoms of bleeding or bruising, especially at surgical sites.

Parameters to monitor

Heparin is monitored by an aPTT, which is sensitive to the inhibitory effects of heparin on factors IIa (thrombin), IXa, and Xa.

The College of American Pathologists and the American College of Chest Physicians (ACCP) recommend against the use of a fixed aPTT therapeutic range of 1.5–2.5 times a control aPTT. They do recommend that a therapeutic aPTT range be established on the basis of an antifactor Xa concentration of 0.3–0.7 units/mL.

An aPTT should be measured 6 hours after a bolus dose of heparin or after any dosage change and then every 6 hours until a therapeutic aPTT is reached. Once a therapeutic aPTT is achieved, an aPTT may be evaluated every 24 hours.

Platelet count and hematocrit should be evaluated at baseline and every 1–3 days.

Pharmacokinetics

The pharmacokinetics of heparin differ depending on whether an intravenous (IV) or subcutaneous route of administration is used.

Heparin is cleared from the body by a rapid saturable mechanism that occurs at therapeutic doses. A second, slower unsaturable first-order clearance that is largely by renal means occurs at high doses.

The half-life of heparin varies from approximately 30 minutes after an IV bolus of 25 IU/kg to 60 minutes after an IV bolus at 100 IU/kg.

Dosing

Heparin should be dosed using a weight-based nomogram. A therapeutic range for heparin is determined by an antifactor Xa chromogenic assay of 0.3–0.7 IU/mL. Weight-based dosing nomograms are effective in achieving a therapeutic aPTT, although they are not universally transferable to every hospital. Published nomograms are specific only for the reagent and instrument used to validate that nomogram.

Determining a therapeutic range by using the calculation of 1.5–2.5 times the mean control aPTT may be erroneous. Previous weight-based nomograms, which used a therapeutic range based on the calculation of 1.5–2.5 times the control aPTT, have been recognized to be accurate only for that aPTT

reagent used. Table 41-5 is an example of a weight-based dosing nomogram. Each hospital should develop its own nomogram based on its therapeutic range.

Another approach to heparin therapy is to administer an IV bolus of 5,000 IU followed by a continuous infusion of at least 30,000–35,000 IU over 24 hours. The infusion rate is adjusted to maintain a therapeutic aPTT.

UFH may be administered subcutaneously every 12 hours. The patient should receive an initial dose of 17,500 IU or 250 IU/kg subcutaneous q12h. The dose should be adjusted to an aPTT that corresponds to a plasma heparin level of antifactor Xa chromogenic assay of 0.3–0.7 IU/mL. This level should be measured 6 hours after the injection.

Alternatively, UFH may be administered as a fixed dose that is unmonitored. An initial dose of 333 IU/kg is administered, followed by 250 IU/kg subcutaneous every 12 hours.

Adverse effects

The most common adverse effects are minor bleeding in the form of gingival bleeding, epistaxis, and ecchymosis. The most common serious adverse effects of heparin are gastrointestinal or urogenital bleeding.

Fatal or life-threatening adverse effects often result from intracranial or retroperitoneal bleeding.

Transient thrombocytopenia may occur within the first 2–4 days of therapy, which will resolve with continued therapy. Heparin-induced thrombocytopenia may also occur, which requires discontinuation of the heparin.

Osteoporosis is a risk with chronic use.

Table 41-5. Body Weight–Based Dosing of IV Heparin

aPTT	Dose
Initial dose	80 IU/kg bolus, then 18 IU/kg/h
< 35	80 IU/kg bolus, then 4 IU/kg/h
35–45	80 IU/kg bolus, then 2 IU/kg/h
46–70[a]	No change
71–90	Decrease infusion rate by 2 IU/kg/h
> 90	Hold infusion 1 hour, then decrease infusion rate by 3 IU/kg/h

Adapted from Raschke, Gollihare, Peirce, 1996.
a. The therapeutic aPTT range of 46–70 seconds corresponded to antifactor Xa activity of 0.3–0.7 IU/mL at the time this study was performed. The therapeutic range at any institution should be established by correlation with antifactor Xa levels in this range.

Table 41-6. LMWH and Pentasaccharide Dosage Forms

Generic name	Trade name	Form and dose
LMWH		
Dalteparin	Fragmin	2,500, 5,000, 7,500, 10,000, 12,500, 15,000, 17,500, 18,000 unit syringe
Enoxaparin	**Lovenox**	30, 40, 60, 80, 100, 120, 150 mg syringe
Tinzaparin	Innohep	20,000 anti Xa IU/mL per 2 mL vial
Pentasaccharide		
Fondaparinux	Arixtra	2.5, 5, 7.5, 10 mg syringe

Boldface indicates one of top 100 drugs for 2012 by units sold at retail outlets, www.drugs.com/stats/top100/2012/units.

Contraindications

Contraindications include the following:

- Active bleeding
- Severely uncontrolled hypertension
- History of heparin-induced thrombocytopenia

Use epidural or spinal anesthesia with caution because patients are at risk of developing an epidural or spinal hematoma, which can result in long-term or permanent paralysis.

LMWHs and pentasaccharide

Table 41-6 describes LMWH and pentasaccharide dosage forms. The pharmacokinetics of LMWHs and pentasaccharides are described in Table 41-7.

Mechanism of action

LMWHs inhibit factor Xa and, to a much lesser extent, factor IIa.

Table 41-7. Pharmacokinetics of LMWHs and Pentasaccharides

Drug	Bioavailability (%)	Half-life (hours)	Xa:IIa binding ratio
Enoxaparin	92	3–6	1.9:1
Dalteparin	87	3–5	2.7:1
Tinzaparin	90	2–6	2:1
Fondaparinux	100	17–21	Only Xa binding

Boldface indicates one of top 100 drugs for 2012 by units sold at retail outlets, www.drugs.com/stats/top100/2012/units.

Fondaparinux is a pentasaccharide. It binds selectively to AT, which potentiates the inactivation of factor Xa in the coagulation cascades, thus inhibiting the formation of thrombin.

Advantages of LMWH and fondaparinux over UFH

- LMWHs and fondaparinux have fewer interactions with plasma proteins; thus, they have a more predictable response at lower doses.
- LMWHs have a much longer half-life, which allows them to be administered subcutaneously every 12–24 hours.
- Fondaparinux has a half-life of 17–21 hours, which allows dosing every 24 hours.
- LMWHs have a lower incidence of osteoporosis and heparin-induced thrombocytopenia. Fondaparinux does not cause heparin-induced thrombocytopenia and can be used as an anticoagulant to treat heparin-induced thrombocytopenia.

Therapeutic use

- Prevention and treatment of VTE
- Prevention of VTE in patients with a previous VTE or a known hypercoagulability
- Prophylaxis for VTE in high-risk populations
- Arterial embolism prevention in patients with mechanical or tissue prosthetic heart valve replacement
- Arterial embolism prevention in patients with atrial fibrillation or atrial flutter
- Arterial embolism prevention in patients with an acute cardioembolic stroke

Patient counseling

- Strict compliance is necessary to ensure a consistent level of anticoagulation.
- Notify a health care provider if bruising, hematuria, melena, hemoptysis, epistaxis, gingival bleeding, or any other abnormal bleeding occurs.
- Consult a health care provider or pharmacist before taking any over-the-counter medications.
- Avoid aspirin or nonsteroidal anti-inflammatory drugs (NSAIDs).
- The air bubble in the LMWH or fondaparinux syringe should be near the plunger before injection. This method ensures that all of the drug is expelled from the syringe and helps minimize the amount of bleeding, bruising, and hematoma formation from the injection site.

Parameters to monitor

Monitor platelet counts, hematocrit and hemoglobin, and signs and symptoms of bleeding. Bone mineral density should be monitored with long-term use.

Anti Xa heparin levels can be monitored in obese patients or in patients receiving LMWH who have significant renal impairment. Anti Xa levels should be drawn 4 hours after a dose. Therapeutic levels are 0.6–1 IU/mL for twice-daily dosing and 1–2 IU/mL for once-daily dosing. The therapeutic range for dalteparin is 0.5–1.5 IU/mL 4–6 hours after receiving 3–4 doses.

Prothrombin time (PT)/INR and aPTT are not useful in monitoring LMWH.

Currently, fondaparinux has no direct monitoring parameters.

Dosing LMWH and fondaparinux
See Tables 41-8 and 41-9 for dosage requirements.

Adverse effects
The most common adverse effects are minor bleeding in the form of gingival bleeding, epistaxis, and ecchy-mosis. The most common serious adverse effects of heparin are gastrointestinal or urogenital bleeding.

Fatal or life-threatening adverse effects often result from intracranial or retroperitoneal bleeding.

Heparin-induced thrombocytopenia can occur with LMWH, but its incidence is greater with UFH.

Osteoporosis can occur with chronic use.

Direct thrombin inhibitors

Argatroban
Mechanism of action
Argatroban is a synthetic molecule that reversibly binds to thrombin.

Therapeutic use
Argatroban is used for prophylaxis and treatment of thrombosis associated with heparin-induced thrombocytopenia and percutaneous coronary intervention.

Table 41-8. Indications and Recommended Doses of LMWH and Fondaparinux

Indication	Enoxaparin	Dalteparin	Tinzaparin	Fondaparinux
Total hip replacement	30 mg subcutaneous q12h *or* 40 mg subcutaneous q24h	5,000 units subcutaneous 0–14 hours before surgery, then q24h *or* 2,500 units subcutaneous 2 hours before surgery, then 5,000 units q24h *or* 2,500 units subcutaneous 2 hours before surgery and 4–8 hours after, then 5,000 units q24h		2.5 mg subcutaneous q24h starting 6–8 hours after surgery
Total knee replacement	30 mg subcutaneous q12h			2.5 mg subcutaneous q24h starting 6–8 hours after surgery
Abdominal surgery	40 mg subcutaneous q24h	2,500 units subcutaneous 1–2 hours before surgery, then 5,000 units q24h		2.5 mg subcutaneous q24h starting 6–8 hours after surgery
Hip fracture				2.5 mg subcutaneous q24h starting 6–8 hours after surgery
Acute medical illness	40 mg subcutaneous q24h	5,000 units subcutaneous q24h		
Trauma	30 mg subcutaneous q12h			
DVT treatment with or without PE	1 mg/kg subcutaneous q12h *or* 1.5 mg/kg subcutaneous q24h		175 units/kg subcutaneous q24h	5 mg for < 50 kg; 7.5 mg for 50–100 kg; 10 mg for > 100 kg subcutaneous q24h
VTE in patients with cancer		200 IU/kg subcutaneous daily for 1 month, followed by 150 IU/kg for 5 months		
Unstable angina	1 mg/kg subcutaneous q12h	120 units/kg subcutaneous q12h		

Enoxaparin is one of top 100 drugs for 2012 by units sold at retail outlets, www.drugs.com/stats/top100/2012/units.

Table 41-9. Enoxaparin Dosage Regimens for Patients with Severe Renal Impairment (Creatinine Clearance < 30 mL/min)

Indication	Dosage regimen
Prophylaxis in abdominal surgery	30 mg subcutaneous once daily
Prophylaxis in hip or knee replacement surgery	30 mg subcutaneous once daily
Prophylaxis in medical patients during acute illness	30 mg subcutaneous once daily
Prophylaxis of ischemic complications of unstable angina and non-Q-wave myocardial infarction, when concurrently administered with aspirin	1 mg/kg subcutaneous once daily
Inpatient treatment of acute DVT with or without PE, when administered in conjunction with warfarin sodium	1 mg/kg subcutaneous once daily
Outpatient treatment of acute DVT without PE, when administered in conjunction with warfarin sodium	1 mg/kg subcutaneous once daily

Enoxaparin is one of top 100 drugs for 2012 by units sold at retail outlets, www.drugs.com/stats/top100/2012/units.

Patient counseling

Monitor symptoms of bruising and bleeding, and report them to a health care provider immediately.

Parameters to monitor

Monitor complete blood count (CBC) and signs and symptoms of bleeding. The aPTT is used to monitor and to adjust argatroban therapy. The aPTT should be drawn 2 hours after an infusion is started and after each dosage change.

Argatroban will also elevate a PT/INR. For patients on concomitant warfarin therapy, this effect may impede monitoring and make proper assessment of the INR difficult. For combination therapy, argatroban may be discontinued after an INR is > 4. An INR should be drawn after 4–6 hours. If the INR is in the therapeutic range, continue with warfarin only. If the INR is below the therapeutic range, restart argatroban and increase the dose of warfarin. Repeat this procedure until the INR is within the therapeutic range.

Pharmacokinetics

Argatroban is metabolized in the liver to inactive metabolites. The half-life is 0.5–1 hour.

Dosing

Administer a continuous IV infusion at the rate of 2 mcg/kg/min. Adjust infusion rate to maintain an aPTT ratio of 1.5–2.5. The usual dose is 2–10 mcg/kg/min.

The dose should be reduced in moderate hepatic insufficiency. A continuous IV infusion should begin at a rate of 0.5 mcg/kg/min. Because of the prolonged elimination half-life, measure the aPTT 4 hours after initiation or a dosage change.

Adverse effects

The most common adverse effects are minor bleeding in the form of gingival bleeding, epistaxis, and ecchymosis. The most common serious adverse effects are gastrointestinal or urogenital bleeding.

Fatal or life-threatening adverse effects often result from intracranial or retroperitoneal bleeding.

There is no known antidote for argatroban. The anticoagulant effect declines rapidly after discontinuation of the drug.

Nonhemorrhagic effects such as fever, nausea, vomiting, and allergic reactions rarely occur.

Warfarin (Coumadin)

Dosage forms
- **Tablets:** 1 mg (pink), 2 mg (lavender), 2.5 mg (green), 3 mg (tan), 4 mg (blue), 5 mg (peach), 6 mg (teal), 7.5 mg (yellow), 10 mg (white)
- **Injections (IV):** 5 mg powder for reconstitution (2 mg/mL)

Mechanism of action

Warfarin is a vitamin K antagonist that produces its pharmacologic effect by interfering with the interconversion of vitamin K and its 2,3-epoxide (vitamin K epoxide). Warfarin leads to the depletion or reduction in activity of vitamin K–dependent coagulation proteins (factors II, VII, IX, and X) produced in the liver. The level and activity of the vitamin K–dependent clotting factors decline over 6–96 hours. At least 4–5 days of warfarin therapy are necessary before a patient is completely anticoagulated.

Therapeutic use
- Prevention and treatment of VTE
- Prevention of VTE in patients with a previous VTE or a known hypercoagulability
- Prophylaxis for VTE in high-risk populations
- Prevention of arterial embolism in patients with mechanical or tissue prosthetic heart valve replacement

- Prevention of arterial embolism in patients with atrial fibrillation or atrial flutter
- Prevention of arterial embolism in patients with a previous cardioembolic stroke
- Prevention of acute MI in patients with peripheral arterial disease

Patient counseling
- Warfarin should be taken at the same time every day.
- Strict compliance is necessary to ensure a consistent level of anticoagulation.
- Strict compliance with a consistent vitamin K diet is necessary to ensure a consistent level of anticoagulation.
- Notify the health care provider in the event of hematuria, melena, epistaxis, hemoptysis, increased bruising, or any abnormal bleeding.
- Notify all health care providers, including dentists, of warfarin therapy.
- Blood monitoring to determine an adequate level of anticoagulation and compliance is necessary at regular intervals.
- Consult a health care provider or pharmacist before taking any new prescription or over-the-counter medications.
- Avoid aspirin or NSAIDs unless instructed otherwise by a health care provider.
- Women of childbearing age should use an effective form of birth control because warfarin has teratogenic effects.

Parameters to monitor
Warfarin therapy is monitored by a PT. The PT responds to a reduction in factors II, VII, and X. The INR is used to standardize the responsiveness of thromboplastin to the anticoagulant effects of warfarin. The INR is calculated by the following equation:

$$INR = (observed\ PT/mean\ normal\ PT)^{ISI}$$

where ISI = International Sensitivity Index, which is a measure of thromboplastin sensitivity. The lower the ISI, the more responsive the thromboplastin is to the anticoagulant effects of warfarin.

The *ACCP Evidence-Based Clinical Practice Guidelines* (9th edition) recommends two intensities of anticoagulation: a less intense level with a target INR of 2.5 and a range of 2.0–3.0 and a high-intensity level of anticoagulation with a target INR of 3.0 and a range of 2.5–3.5 (Table 41-10).

Upon initiation of warfarin therapy, the INR should be evaluated daily if the patient is in the hospital and every 2–3 days if the patient is not hospitalized.

Table 41-10. Recommended Therapeutic Ranges for Warfarin

Indication	Target INR (INR range)
Prophylaxis of VTE (high-risk surgery)	2.5 (2.0–3.0)
Treatment of VTE	2.5 (2.0–3.0)
Prevention of thromboembolic events in patients with antiphospholipid syndrome with a lupus inhibitor	2.5 (2.0–3.0)
Prevention of arterial embolism in atrial fibrillation	2.5 (2.0–3.0)
Prevention of arterial embolism with a mechanical prosthetic heart valve in the aortic position	2.5 (2.0–3.0)
Prevention of arterial embolism with a mechanical prosthetic heart valve in the mitral position	3.0 (2.5–3.5)
In patients with a mechanical mitral or aortic valve at low risk of bleeding, suggest adding an antiplatelet agent such as low-dose aspirin (50–100 mg/day) to the VKA therapy.	

Ageno, Gallus, Wittkowsky, et al., 2012.
VKA, vitamin K antagonist.

Pharmacokinetics
Warfarin is a racemic mixture of two optically active isomers, warfarin S and warfarin R, in roughly equal amounts. The S isomer is three to four times more potent than the R isomer.

Warfarin is rapidly and completely absorbed from the gastrointestinal tract with peak concentration in approximately 90 minutes. Warfarin is 99% protein bound with a half-life of 36–42 hours.

The onset of anticoagulation occurs after 4–5 days of therapy and is caused by the depletion of the clotting factors rather than steady-state concentrations of warfarin. Thus, the onset of action is based on the half-life of the clotting factors II, VII, IX, and X. The S isomer of warfarin is metabolized by cytochrome (CYP) 2C9 and, to a lesser extent, by CYP3A4. The R isomer is metabolized by CYP1A2 and CYP3A4 and, to a lesser extent, by CYP2C19.

Dosing
Time in the therapeutic range and intensity of anticoagulation are critical for optimizing the therapeutic efficacy of warfarin and minimizing the risk of hemorrhage.

Warfarin initiation does not require loading. Loading doses can result in an inappropriate increase in the INR, which is not reflective of an anticoagulant effect.

Initiating warfarin at 5 mg daily should result in an INR around 2.0 in 4–5 days for most patients. An alternative method is to administer between 5 and 10 mg for the first 1–2 days and then adjust the dose depending on the INR response.

Initiating warfarin at a dose of ≤ 5 mg daily may be appropriate in the elderly; in patients with liver disease, heart failure, or malnutrition; in patients taking drugs known to increase the responsiveness to warfarin; or in patients with a high risk of bleeding.

Initiating warfarin at a dose of 7.5–10 mg daily may be appropriate for young, healthy, or obese patients.

If a rapid anticoagulant effect is indicated, IV heparin, LMWH, or fondaparinux should be administered along with warfarin for at least 4–5 days until a therapeutic INR is reached. Heparin, LMWH, or fondaparinux may be discontinued when the INR is within the therapeutic range on two consecutive occasions.

Disease state interaction
Disease states that can increase the response to warfarin are hyperthyroidism, congestive heart failure, liver disease, fever, and genetic increased warfarin sensitivity.

Disease states that can decrease the response to warfarin are hypothyroidism and genetic warfarin resistance. Patient nonadherence can also result in a reduced warfarin response.

Drug–drug interactions
Warfarin is a drug with a narrow therapeutic index. Numerous drugs interact with warfarin. Drugs that either inhibit or induce CYP2C9 or 3A4 and, to a lesser extent, CYP1A2 or 2C19, potentiate or reduce the anticoagulant effect. The S isomer is more active than the R isomer; thus, drugs that inhibit or induce the S isomer will have a more significant effect on warfarin than drugs that inhibit or induce the R isomer (Table 41-11).

Drug–food interactions
Foods that contain high amounts of vitamin K can reduce the anticoagulant effect of warfarin (Table 41-11). It is important that patients be consistent in their consumption of these foods and that they evenly space their consumption over a 7-day period. If a patient suddenly stops eating these foods, the INR may dramatically increase.

Adverse effects
The most common adverse effect is minor bleeding in the form of gingival bleeding, epistaxis, and ecchymosis. The most common serious adverse effects of warfarin are either gastrointestinal or urogenital bleeding.

Table 41-11. Drugs and Foods That Can Interact with Warfarin

Type of interaction	Interacting substance
Potentiation of anticoagulant effect	Acetaminophen, alcohol (acute use), anabolic steroids, cimetidine, clofibrate, disulfiram, piroxicam, omeprazole, simvastatin, sulfinpyrazone
Highly significant potentiation of anticoagulant effect	Amiodarone, ciprofloxacin, erythromycin, fluconazole, isoniazid, itraconazole, ketoconazole, levothyroxine, metronidazole, phenytoin, trimethoprim-sulfamethoxazole, vitamin E (high doses)
Reduction of anticoagulation effect	Alcohol (chronic use), dicloxacillin, griseofulvin
Highly significant reduction of anticoagulation effect	Barbiturates, carbamazepine, cholestyramine, enteral feeding, nafcillin, rifampin, vitamin K–containing foods (broccoli, brussels sprouts, cabbage, canola oil, cauliflower, coleslaw, collard greens, endive, green kale, lettuce, mayonnaise, mustard greens, soybean oil, spinach)

Warfarin-induced skin necrosis is a rare, but serious adverse effect. Skin necrosis begins within 10 days of warfarin initiation. It is characterized by painful, erythematous lesions on breast, thighs, and buttocks, which may progress to hemorrhagic lesions. It may be associated with protein C deficiency and, to a lesser effect, protein S deficiency. The concomitant use of UFH, LMWH, or fondaparinux with initiation of warfarin can prevent its occurrence.

Purple toe syndrome is a dark blue-tinged discoloration of the feet that occurs rarely 3–8 weeks after warfarin initiation.

Fatal or life-threatening adverse effects are related to intracranial or retroperitoneal bleeding.

Several treatment options are available for the reversal of anticoagulation. Treatment may be necessary for a supratherapeutic INR or before an invasive procedure. Simply withholding warfarin will reduce the level of anticoagulation. For an INR of 6 to 10, an estimated 2.5 days may be needed for an INR to be reduced below 4. Phytonadione, which is also referred to as vitamin K, will reverse the effects of warfarin. Phytonadione may be administered orally or IV. If phytonadione is administered IV, it should be diluted in at least 50 mL of IV fluid and administered over 20 minutes to minimize the risk of anaphylactic reactions. It should not be administered intramuscularly because of hematoma formation or subcutaneously because of erratic absorption. Administration of oral phytonadione together with withholding of warfarin therapy may result in a reduction in an INR of 6–10 to an INR of < 4 in approximately 1.4 days. IV phytonadione begins reversing an INR within 2 hours. Other treatment options for reversing an INR include fresh frozen plasma, nonactivated prothrombin complex concentrate (PCC), or recombinant factor VII. PCC is available as a three factor or four factor concentrate. Three factor PCC contains factors II, IX, and X, whereas four factor concentrate contains factors II, VII, IX, and X.

Special precautions must be taken for patients undergoing invasive procedures. Table 41-12 outlines the risk stratifications for perioperative arterial or venous thromboembolism. Box 41-1 outlines the recommendations for managing anticoagulation in these patients.

Rivaroxaban (Xarelto)

Dosage forms
- Tablets: 10, 15, 20 mg

Mechanism of action
Rivaroxaban is a factor Xa inhibitor and does not require cofactors such as antithrombin for activity. Factor Xa is involved in both the intrinsic and the extrinsic coagulation pathways.

Therapeutic use
- DVT/PE treatment
- Reduction in the risk of recurrence of DVT/PE
- Reduction of the risk of stroke and systemic embolism in patients with nonvalvular atrial fibrillation
- DVT prophylaxis in patients undergoing hip or knee replacement surgery

Patient counseling
- Rivaroxaban is used for the treatment of a DVT or PE or to reduce the risk of the recurrence of a DVT or PE.
- Rivaroxaban lowers the risk of developing a blood clot after hip or knee replacement surgery.
- Rivaroxaban should be taken daily with food in patients with a DVT or PE or once daily at the same time of the day with or without food for prevention of a blood clot after hip or knee replacement surgery.
- Failure to take rivaroxaban on a consistent basis greatly increases the chance of developing a blood clot.
- Strict compliance is necessary to ensure a consistent level of anticoagulation.
- If you forget to take the medication, take it as soon as you remember the same day. Do not take two doses to make up for the missed dose.

Table 41-12. Suggested Patient Risk Stratification for Perioperative Arterial or Venous Thromboembolism

Risk	Mechanical heart valve	Atrial fibrillation	VTE
High	Any mitral valve prosthesis	CHADS$_2$ score of 5 or 6	Recent (within 3 months) VTE
	Older (caged ball or tilting disc) aortic valve prosthesis	Recent (within 3 months) stroke or transient ischemic attack	Severe thrombophilia (e.g., deficiency of protein C, protein S, or antithrombin; antiphospholipid antibodies; or multiple abnormities)
	Recent (within 6 months) stroke or transient ischemic attack	Rheumatic valvular heart disease	
Moderate	Bileaflet aortic valve prosthesis and one of the following: atrial fibrillation, prior stroke or transient ischemic attack, hypertension, diabetes, congestive heart failure, age > 75 years	CHADS$_2$ score of 3 or 4	VTE within the past 3 to 12 months
			Nonsevere thrombophilic conditions (e.g., heterozygous factor V Leiden mutation, heterozygous factor II mutation)
			Recurrent VTE
			Active cancer (treated within 6 months) or palliative
Low	Bileaflet aortic valve prosthesis without atrial fibrillation and no other risk factors for stroke	CHADS$_2$ score of 0 or 2 (and no prior stroke or transient ischemic attack)	Single VTE occurred > 12 months ago and no other risk factors

Gage, Waterman, Shannon, et al. 2001.
CHADS$_2$, congestive heart failure (1 point), hypertension (1 point), age (1 point), diabetes (1 point), stroke (2 points).

Box 41-1. Recommendations for Managing Anticoagulation Therapy in Patients Requiring Invasive Procedures

---

Patients with Low Risk of Thromboembolism

- Discontinue warfarin 5 days before procedure.
- Consider bridging with low-dose subcutaneous LMWH.
- Suggest therapeutic-dose subcutaneous LMWH over other management options.

Patients with Moderate Risk of Thromboembolism

- Discontinue warfarin 5 days before procedure.
- Consider bridging with therapeutic-dose subcutaneous LMWH or IV UFH or with low-dose subcutaneous LMWH over not bridging during interruption of warfarin therapy.
- Suggest therapeutic-dose subcutaneous LMWH over other management options.

Patients with High Risk of Thromboembolism

- Discontinue warfarin 5 days before procedure.
- Bridge with therapeutic-dose subcutaneous LMWH or IV UFH during interruption of warfarin therapy.
- In patients whose INR is still elevated (> 1.5) 1 to 2 days before surgery, administer 1 to 2 mg oral vitamin K to normalize INR.
- Discontinue therapeutic-dose LMWH 24 hours before procedure, and administer half the total daily dose as the last preoperative dose.
- Discontinue UFH approximately 4–6 hours before a procedure.
- Suggest LMWH over IV UFH.
- Restart warfarin 12–24 hours after procedure or when hemostasis is adequate.
- Resume therapeutic-dose LMWH approximately 24 hours after the procedure or when hemostasis is adequate.
- In patients at high bleeding risk, delay therapeutic-dose LMWH or UFH for 48–72 hours or administer low-dose LMWH or UFH when hemostasis is secured, or completely avoid LMWH or UFH.
- Individualize treatment plans based on postoperative hemostasis and bleeding risk.

Patients Undergoing Minor Dental or Dermatologic Procedure or Cataract Removal

- Continue warfarin therapy around the time of the procedure.
- Co-administer an oral prohemostatic agent such as tranexamic acid or epsilon amino caproic acid mouthwash for dental procedures.

Adapted with permission from Douketis, Berger, Dunn, et al., 2008.

- Do not stop taking rivaroxaban without talking to your health care provider.
- Notify your health care provider in the event of hematuria, melena, epistaxis, hemoptysis, increased bruising, or any abnormal bleeding.
- Notify all health care providers, including dentists, of rivaroxaban therapy.
- Avoid aspirin or NSAIDs unless instructed otherwise by a physician.

Parameters to monitor
- No routine blood monitoring is necessary.
- Creatinine clearance (CrCl) should be calculated before beginning drug therapy and used to determine the dosing regimen.
- Hematocrit and hemoglobin as well as signs and symptoms of bleeding should be continuously monitored.

Pharmacokinetics
Bioavailability of rivaroxaban is dose dependent. The 10 mg dose is estimated to be 80–100% bioavailable, which is not affected by food. The 15 mg and 20 mg doses administered with food increase the bioavailability, and thus, it is recommended that these tablets be taken with the evening meal.

Rivaroxaban is renally excreted, and dosage adjustment is necessary for patients with renal insufficiencies. The elimination half-life is 5–9 hours for patients ages 20–45 and 11–13 hours for patients older than age 65.

Dosing
Treatment of a DVT/PE:

- 15 mg bid with food for 21 days followed by 20 mg daily with food

Reduction of the risk of recurrent DVT or PE:

- 20 mg daily with food

DVT prophylaxis in patients undergoing hip replacement surgery:

- 10 mg daily with or without meals for CrCl > 30 mL/min for 35 days
- Use with caution for CrCl 30–50 mL/min.

DVT prophylaxis in patients undergoing knee replacement surgery:

- 10 mg daily with or without meals for CrCl > 30 mL/min for 12 days
- Use with caution for CrCl 30–50 mL/min.

Drug–drug interactions

Concomitant use of drugs that are P-glycoprotein and CYP3A4 inhibitors or inducers can interact with rivaroxaban. Ketoconazole, itraconazole, lopinavir, ritonavir, indinavir, and conivaptan can increase rivaroxaban exposure and increase bleeding risk and should be avoided.

Rifampin, carbamazepine, phenytoin, and St. John's wort can decrease the exposure of rivaroxaban, thus decreasing its effectiveness, and should be avoided.

NSAIDs and antiplatelet agents such as aspirin, clopidogrel, dipyridamole/aspirin, ticagrelor, and prasugrel can increase the risk of bleeding and should be used with caution.

Adverse effects

The most common adverse effects are related to bleeding. Minor bleeding includes gingival bleeding, epistaxis, or ecchymosis. Major bleeding is most often gastrointestinal or urogenital; involves the surgical site; or is intracranial, which can be fatal or life threatening. Unlike warfarin, no reversal agent for rivaroxaban is known.

Contraindications

- For nonvalvular atrial fibrillation, avoid use in patients with CrCl < 15 mL/min.
- For DVT prophylaxis, avoid use in patients with CrCl < 30 mL/min.
- Active bleeding

41-4. Questions

Use the following case study to answer Questions 1 and 2:

A 24-year-old female presents to the emergency department with complaints of severe shortness of breath, dyspnea, and chest pain. She is also experiencing tachycardia and tachypnea. Two days earlier she noticed pain and swelling in her left lower extremity. Her medical history is negative for thrombosis. Her current medications include Tri-Levlen daily and ibuprofen 600 mg q6h prn for pain. A duplex ultrasound of the left lower extremity revealed a DVT. Her vital signs are T, 98.4°F; P, 124/min; R, 36/min; BP, 162/100 mm Hg; Wt, 220 lb (100 kg); Ht, 5" 4'.

1. The most likely cause of her shortness of breath, dyspnea, and chest pain is

   A. bronchitis.
   B. asthma exacerbation.
   C. pulmonary embolism.
   D. heart failure exacerbation.
   E. atrial fibrillation.

2. This patient is started on heparin therapy. Which dosage regimen is most appropriate?

   A. IV heparin 20,000 IU bolus, then 5,000 IU/h
   B. IV heparin 8,000 IU bolus, then 1,800 IU/h
   C. IV heparin 5,000 IU bolus, then 500 IU/h
   D. IV heparin 5,000 IU q12h
   E. Subcutaneous heparin 5,000 IU q12h

3. All of the following are risk factors for a DVT *except*

   A. hip replacement surgery.
   B. knee replacement surgery.
   C. hernia repair surgery.
   D. hip fracture surgery.
   E. abdominal surgery.

4. Which diagnostic test would be most helpful with the diagnosis of a pulmonary embolism?

   A. Chest x-ray
   B. Electrocardiogram
   C. Spiral CT of the chest
   D. Bronchoscopy
   E. Echocardiogram

5. A 25-year-old patient is started on warfarin for an acute DVT. What is an appropriate starting dose of warfarin?

   A. 1 mg daily
   B. 7.5 mg daily
   C. 15 mg daily
   D. 20 mg daily
   E. 25 mg daily

6. Which laboratory test is used to monitor heparin therapy?

   A. aPTT
   B. PT
   C. INR
   D. Clotting time
   E. Factor XIa

7. A 47-year-old patient is diagnosed with a lower-extremity DVT. The patient's height is 6 feet and weight is 220 lb (100 kg). The

physician would like to treat this patient as an outpatient with warfarin and LMWH. Which dose would be the most appropriate?

A. Enoxaparin 30 mg subcutaneous q12h
B. Enoxaparin 40 mg subcutaneous q24h
C. Enoxaparin 100 mg subcutaneous q12h
D. Enoxaparin 200 mg subcutaneous q12h
E. Enoxaparin 220 mg subcutaneous q12h

8. How long should enoxaparin be continued in a patient with an acute DVT?

A. At least 4–5 days until the INR is > 2.0 for 24 hours
B. At least 4–5 days until the INR is > 3.0 for 24 hours
C. At least 24 hours until the INR is > 4.0 for 24 hours
D. At least 48 hours until the INR is > 4.0 for 24 hours
E. At least 7–10 days until the INR is > 3.5 for 24 hours

9. All of the following statements are important information to communicate to a patient on warfarin therapy *except*

A. take warfarin every day without missing any doses.
B. eat a consistent amount of vitamin K–rich foods per week.
C. report any symptoms of bleeding to your physician.
D. take warfarin with meals and remain standing for 30 minutes.
E. do not take aspirin-containing products unless directed to do so by your physician.

10. Which of the following is an example of a vitamin K–rich food that can lower an INR?

A. Green beans
B. Spinach
C. Lima beans
D. Sweet peas
E. Green peppers

11. Which of the following cardiovascular drugs is most likely to affect an INR?

A. Sotalol
B. Eprosartan
C. Amiodarone
D. Disopyramide
E. Dofetilide

12. Which of the following drugs used to treat seizures is the most likely to interact with warfarin therapy?

A. Lamotrigine
B. Carbamazepine
C. Topiramate
D. Levetiracetam
E. Tiagabine

Use the following case study to answer Questions 13 and 14:

A 58-year-old male is scheduled for a total knee replacement tomorrow. He has a medical history of hypertension for which he is treated with amlodipine 5 mg daily. His height is 6" 2′, and his weight is 176 lb (80 kg).

13. Which of the following is the best DVT prophylaxis therapy for this patient?

A. Fondaparinux 7.5 mg subcutaneous q12h
B. Lovenox 80 mg subcutaneous q12h
C. Rivaroxaban 10 mg daily
D. Xarelto 20 mg daily
E. Dabigatran 150 mg bid

14. Which of the following is the best answer for the duration of therapy for this patient?

A. 7 days
B. 12 days
C. 14 days
D. 17 days
E. 21 days

15. Fondaparinux is an anticoagulant that inhibits which clotting factor?

A. IIa
B. IXa
C. Xa
D. XIa
E. VIIa

16. A 47-year-old patient is receiving argatroban for a pulmonary embolism. What is the most common reason for use of argatroban in this patient?

A. Heparin-induced thrombocytopenia
B. Heparin-induced thrombocytosis
C. Heparin-induced neutropenia
D. Heparin-associated thrombocytosis
E. Heparin-associated thrombocytopenia

17. A 68-year-old male presents to the emergency department with complaints of epistaxis as well as bruising on his arms and legs. He has been taking warfarin 8 mg daily. His INR is 10.2. What is the most appropriate therapy to reverse his warfarin toxicity?

    A. Hold warfarin for 4 days; restart warfarin at a lower dose when his INR is < 3.0.
    B. Hold warfarin and administer vitamin K 0.5 mg IV; restart warfarin at a lower dose when his INR is < 3.0.
    C. Hold warfarin and administer tranexamic acid 10 mg IV; restart warfarin at a lower dose when his INR is < 3.0.
    D. Hold warfarin and administer vitamin K 5 mg po; restart warfarin at a lower dose when his INR is < 3.0.
    E. Hold warfarin and administer prothrombin complex 5 mg po; restart warfarin at a lower dose when his INR is < 3.0.

18. A 63-year-old patient is receiving warfarin 7.5 mg daily for a PE. What therapeutic INR range is indicated for this patient?

    A. 1.0–2.0
    B. 1.5–2.5
    C. 2.0–3.0
    D. 2.0–3.5
    E. 2.5–3.5

19. A 56-year-old female presents to the emergency department with complaints of flank pain, dysuria, and increased urinary frequency. She is diagnosed with a urinary tract infection. Her past medical history includes type 2 diabetes mellitus, hypertension, and recurrent DVTs. Her medications include metformin 1 g bid, quinapril 40 mg daily, and warfarin 5 mg daily. What would be the most appropriate antibiotic to treat this patient's UTI?

    A. Septra DS bid
    B. Ciprofloxacin 500 mg bid
    C. Rifampin 300 mg qid
    D. Doxycycline 100 mg bid
    E. Erythromycin 500 mg qid

20. A 45-year-old patient comes into the pharmacy with a prescription for warfarin 7.5 mg daily that was written 5 months ago. Which of the following is the best action to take?

    A. Fill the prescription because it is a valid prescription.
    B. Fill only half of the prescription, and ask the patient to contact his or her doctor.
    C. Call the physician to verify that the warfarin dose is correct.
    D. Ask the patient to return tomorrow so you can ask the managing pharmacist.
    E. Refuse to fill the prescription because it is legally too old to process.

21. What color is warfarin 7.5 mg?

    A. White
    B. Blue
    C. Yellow
    D. Pink
    E. Green

22. Which of the following is a common side effect associated with unfractionated heparin?

    A. Hypokalemia
    B. Hypoglycemia
    C. Ecchymosis
    D. Nausea
    E. Hyponatremia

23. What is the length of anticoagulation therapy for an acute DVT associated with a hospitalization for surgery?

    A. 3 months
    B. 6 months
    C. 9 months
    D. 12 months
    E. Long term

24. Advantages of LMWH over UFH include all of the following *except*

    A. subcutaneous administration.
    B. no dosage adjustment needed with renal insufficiency.
    C. once- or twice-daily dosing.
    D. predictable response at lower doses.
    E. lower incidence of heparin-induced thrombocytopenia.

41-5. Answers

1. **C.** Symptoms of shortness of breath, dyspnea, chest pain, tachycardia, and tachypnea, along with a recent history of a DVT, are indications

of a pulmonary embolism. A ventilation-perfusion scan or a spiral CT of the chest would confirm the diagnosis.

2. **B.** Several studies have indicated that weight-based dosing of heparin is more effective in obtaining therapeutic aPTT than standard heparin titration. A weight-based protocol with an 80 IU/kg IV bolus followed by an infusion of 18 IU/kg per hour should produce aPTTs close to the therapeutic range. The other doses are not appropriate.

3. **C.** High-risk surgeries involve the abdomen and lower extremities; thus, hip and knee replacements as well as hip fracture surgery are major risk factors for the development of a VTE. Hernia repair surgery is considered minor surgery and, unless the patient has other risk factors, would not require DVT prophylaxis other than early ambulation.

4. **C.** A spiral CT of the chest or a ventilation-perfusion scan would be necessary to confirm the diagnosis of a PE. Chest x-ray, electrocardiogram, echocardiogram, or bronchoscopy would not assist with the diagnosis.

5. **B.** Warfarin 7.5 mg daily should result in an INR around 2.0 within 4–5 days. The other doses are either extremely low or high for the majority of patients. Higher doses of warfarin may elevate an INR, but this increase may not be associated with a level of anticoagulation. A rapid increase in INR is due to depletion of factor VII rather than the anticoagulant effect that is associated with depletion of factors II and X.

6. **A.** The aPTT is a laboratory test used to monitor heparin therapy. The aPTT should be checked 6 hours after a dosage change and every 24 hours if it is within the therapeutic range. A PT/INR is used to monitor warfarin therapy.

7. **C.** Enoxaparin 100 mg subcutaneous q12h or 1 mg/kg subcutaneous q12h is the dose for treatment of an acute DVT. Enoxaparin 30 mg subcutaneous q12h and 40 mg subcutaneous q24h are doses used for DVT prophylaxis. Enoxaparin 200 mg subcutaneous q12h and 220 mg subcutaneous q12h are extremely high doses.

8. **A.** For the treatment of an active DVT or PE, at least 4–5 days of heparin or LMWH overlap with warfarin is needed before an anticoagulant effect is produced by warfarin. Heparin or LMWH should be discontinued after an INR is > 2.0 for 24 hours.

9. **D.** Statements A, B, C, and E are important to discuss with patients on warfarin. Patients should follow strict compliance with warfarin. They should eat vitamin K–rich foods consistently over the course of a week and report any symptoms of bleeding to their health care provider.

10. **B.** Green, leafy vegetables contain higher amounts of vitamin K; thus, spinach can reduce an INR. Although lima beans, sweet peas, green peppers, and green beans are the color green, they do not have a large amount of vitamin K.

11. **C.** Amiodarone can cause a dose-dependent increase in an INR by inhibiting CYP2C9. The dose of warfarin may need to be reduced by 35–50% when amiodarone is added to warfarin therapy.

12. **B.** Carbamazepine induces the cytochrome P450 isozymes 1A2, 2C9, and 3A4. Warfarin is a substrate for the isozymes 1A2, 2C9, and 3A4, and thus carbamazepine induces the metabolism of warfarin. This results in the need for larger-than-normal doses of warfarin to achieve a therapeutic INR.

13. **C.** Rivaroxaban 10 mg daily is the correct dose for DVT prophylaxis associated with a knee replacement. Fondaparinux 7.5 mg subcutaneous daily, Lovenox 80 mg subcutaneous q12 h, and Xarelto 20 mg daily are all treatment doses, and dabigatran is not indicated for DVT prophylaxis associated with a knee replacement.

14. **B.** 12 days is the recommended treatment duration for prophylaxis associated with a knee replacement.

15. **C.** Fondaparinux inhibits factor Xa.

16. **A.** Heparin-induced thrombocytopenia is a very serious adverse reaction associated with heparin therapy that results in a dramatic reduction of platelets. This reaction is associated with potentially life- or limb-threating thrombotic events. If heparin-induced thrombocytopenia is suspected, all forms of heparin or LMWH need

to be discontinued immediately. Argatroban is a direct thrombin inhibitor that does not cause heparin-induced thrombocytopenia and is an alternative anticoagulant therapy for patients with heparin-induced thrombocytopenia.

17. **D.** Warfarin toxicity with an INR of 10.2 can be effectively reversed by holding the dose of warfarin and administering vitamin K 5 mg orally. Warfarin should be restarted when the INR is < 3.0. The IV route is used only in emergency situations because anaphylactic reactions are possible. Prothrombin complex is administered IV only for severe bleeding situations.

18. **C.** The therapeutic range for oral anticoagulation is an INR of 2.0–3.0, with a target of 2.5. Increased bleeding is associated with an INR > 4.0, and embolic events are more common with an INR < 1.5.

19. **D.** Doxycycline 100 mg bid would be the most appropriate therapy for a UTI. Septra DS, erythromycin, and ciprofloxacin will interact with warfarin to elevate the INR.

20. **C.** Warfarin is a drug that requires continuous blood monitoring to ensure that a therapeutic INR is maintained. It is recommended that an INR is evaluated monthly. A prescription written for warfarin 5 months ago may indicate that a patient is not being monitored appropriately. Therefore, it would be appropriate to contact the prescriber to verify the warfarin prescription and to ensure the patient is being monitored.

21. **C.** Warfarin 7.5 mg is yellow, 1 mg is pink, 10 mg is white, and 4 mg is blue.

22. **C.** Minor bleeding and bruising are common side effects of heparin therapy. Other common areas for bleeding are the urogenital and gastrointestinal tracts.

23. **A.** The duration of anticoagulation therapy for patients with an acute DVT associated with a hospitalization for surgery is 3 months. The hospitalization, immobilization, and surgery are reversible risk factors for the development of a DVT. Studies have demonstrated that 3 months of anticoagulation are adequate in this setting. Longer durations of therapy are not necessary.

24. **B.** Because LMWHs are renally eliminated, their doses must be adjusted for creatinine clearance < 30 mL/min. Guidelines have recently been released for enoxaparin dosing in renal impairment. For DVT prophylaxis, enoxaparin should be administered 30 mg subcutaneous q24h rather than q12h. For DVT treatment, enoxaparin should be administered 1 mg/kg subcutaneous q24h rather than q12h.

41-6. References

Ageno W, Gallus A, Wittkowsky A, et al. Oral anticoagulant therapy: Antithrombotic therapy and prevention of thrombosis, 9th ed: American College of Chest Physicians Evidence-Based Clinical Practice Guidelines. *Chest.* 2012;141(suppl 2):e44S–e88S.

Douketis JD, Berger PB, Dunn AS, et al. The perioperative management of antithrombotic therapy: American College of Chest Physicians Evidence-Based Clinical Practice Guidelines. 8th ed. *Chest.* 2008;133(suppl 6):299S–339S.

Falck-Ytter Y, Francis C, Johanson N, et al. Prevention of VTE in orthopedic surgery patients: Antithrombotic therapy and prevention of thrombosis, 9th ed: American College of Chest Physicians Evidence-Based Clinical Practice Guidelines. *Chest.* 2012;141(suppl 2):e278S–e325S.

Gage BF, Waterman AD, Shannon W, et al. Validation of clinical classification schemes for predicting stroke: Results from the National Registry of Atrial Fibrillation. *JAMA.* 2001;285(22):2864–70.

Geerts WH, Bergqvist D, Pineo GF, et al. Prevention of venous thromboembolism: American College of Chest Physicians Evidence-Based Clinical Practice Guidelines. 8th ed. *Chest.* 2008;133(suppl 6):381S–453S.

Gould M, Garcia D, Wren S, et al. Prevention of VTE in nonorthopedic surgical patients: Antithrombotic therapy and prevention of thrombosis, 9th ed: American College of Chest Physicians Evidence-Based Clinical Practice Guidelines. *Chest.* 2012;141(suppl 2):e227S–e277S.

Guyatt G, Akl E, Crowther D, et al. Executive summary: Antithrombotic therapy and prevention of thrombosis panel, 9th ed: American College of Chest Physicians Evidence-Based Clinical Practice Guidelines. *Chest.* 2012;141(suppl 2):e7S–e47S.

Hirsh J, Bauer KA, Donati MB, et al. Parenteral anticoagulants: American College of Chest Physicians Evidence-Based Clinical Practice Guidelines. 8th ed. *Chest.* 2008;133(suppl 6):141S–59S.

Hirsh J, Guyatt G, Albers, GW, et al. Executive summary: American College of Chest Physicians Evidence-Based Clinical Practice Guidelines. 8th ed. *Chest.* 2008;133(suppl 6):71S–105S.

Kahn S, Lim W, Dunn A, et al. Prevention of VTE in nonsurgical patients: Antithrombotic therapy and prevention of thrombosis, 9th ed: American College of Chest Physicians Evidence-Based Clinical Practice Guidelines. *Chest.* 2012;141(suppl 2):e195S–e226S.

Kearon C, Akl E, Comerota A, et al. Antithrombotic therapy for VTE disease: Antithrombotic therapy and prevention of thrombosis, 9th ed: American College of Chest Physicians Evidence-Based Clinical Practice Guidelines. *Chest.* 2012;141(suppl 2): e419S–e494S.

Kearon C, Kahn SR, Agnelli G, et al. Antithrombotic therapy for venous thromboembolic disease: American College of Chest Physicians Evidence-Based Clinical Practice Guidelines. 8th ed. *Chest.* 2008;133(suppl 6):454S–545S.

Raschke RA, Gollihare B, Peirce JC. The effectiveness of implementing the weight-based heparin nomogram as a practice guideline. *Arch Intern Med.* 1996;156:1645–49.

Federal Pharmacy Law

42

Carol A. Schwab

42-1. Study Guide Checklist

The following topics may guide your study of this subject area:

- Legal responsibilities of the pharmacist and other pharmacy personnel
- Requirements for acquiring and distributing pharmaceutical products
- Legal requirements that must be followed in issuing and dispensing a prescription or drug order
- Conditions for making an offer to counsel and counseling patients, including proper documentation
- Requirements for distributing and dispensing nonprescription pharmaceutical products, including controlled substances
- Proper procedures for recordkeeping related to pharmacy practice, pharmaceutical products, and patients, including requirements for protecting patient confidentiality
- Qualifications, application procedures, required examinations, and internship requirements for licensure, registration, or certification of individuals engaged in the storage, distribution, and dispensing of pharmaceutical prescription and nonprescription products
- Requirements and application procedures for the registration, licensure, and certification for a practice setting or business entity
- Operational requirements for a registered, licensed, certified, or permitted practice setting
- Regulatory structure and terms found in the laws and rules that regulate or affect the manufacture, storage, distribution, and dispensing of pharmaceutical products, both prescription, nonprescription, and controlled substances
- The authority, responsibilities, and operation of the agencies that enforce the laws and rules that regulate or affect the manufacture, storage, distribution, and dispensing of pharmaceutical products (Multistate Pharmacy Jurisprudence Examination Blueprint Competency Statements, National Association of Boards of Pharmacy, www.nabp.net/programs/examination/mpje/mpje-blueprint, accessed March 31, 2014)

42-2. Federal Regulation of Drug Development, Production, and Marketing

Overview of the Federal Food, Drug, and Cosmetic Act and Other Significant Legislation

The text of the federal Food, Drug, and Cosmetic Act (FDCA) is under title 21 of the U.S. Code and can be found at the U.S. Food and Drug Administration (FDA) Web page (www.fda.gov/RegulatoryInformation/

Chapter 42 covers the basics of federal pharmacy law. It is not intended to be a comprehensive review of the law. Although the language of the statutes and regulations has been closely followed throughout Chapter 42, the language has been paraphrased or summarized in many instances for simplicity and clarity. For complete details of the rules, please refer to the cited statutes and regulations. Chapter 42 has been written for educational purposes only. It is not intended as legal advice, nor should it be relied on as such. Laws change frequently and without notice, and a change in the law could make the information in Chapter 42 inaccurate. For specific legal questions, please consult an attorney.

Legislation/FederalFoodDrugandCosmeticAct
FDCAct/default.htm).

Pure Food and Drug Act of 1906

This law prohibited misbranded and adulterated foods and drugs from being distributed through interstate commerce. The misbranding provision prevented false claims about the drug's strength, quality, and purity. It did not protect consumers against false claims about the drug's efficacy. Congress amended the law in 1912 to prohibit false efficacy claims, but the law was difficult to enforce.

Food, Drug, and Cosmetic Act of 1938

This law forms the nucleus of today's FDCA, although it has been amended many times by the laws that are subsequently discussed in this section. It required that any new drug could not be marketed until the drug had been proved safe when used according to directions on the label. In addition, the law expanded the definition of adulterated and misbranded, and required drug labels to include adequate directions for use and warnings about habit-forming drugs contained in the product. The law applied to food, drugs, cosmetics, and medical devices. Drugs marketed prior to 1938 were grandfathered in and exempted from the requirement that they be proved safe before being marketed.

Durham-Humphrey Amendment of 1951

This amendment to the FDCA is also known as the Prescription Drug Amendment, and it established two classes of drugs: prescription and over-the-counter (OTC). A drug classified as a prescription drug did not have to include "adequate directions for use" as long as the labeling contained the legend: "Caution: Federal law prohibits dispensing without a prescription." The pharmacist dispensing the drug pursuant to a prescription met the "adequate directions for use" requirement by including the directions from the prescriber on the label. This amendment also authorized oral prescriptions and refills on prescription drugs.

Food Additives Amendment of 1958

This amendment was passed in response to concerns that food additives could cause cancer. It required that components added to food must receive pre-

market approval for safety. The Delaney Clause, also known as the anticancer clause, prohibits approval of any food additive that might cause cancer.

Color Additives Amendment of 1960

This amendment requires manufacturers to establish the safety of color additives in foods, drugs, and cosmetics. This amendment also contains an anticancer clause that prohibits the approval of any color additive that might cause cancer.

Kefauver-Harris Amendment of 1962

This amendment is also known as the Drug Efficacy Amendment. It requires new drugs to be proved effective as well as safe. The requirement was retroactive to apply to all drugs marketed between 1938 and 1962. The retroactive provision was a huge burden on the FDA, and the Drug Efficacy Study Implementation was not completed until the 1970s. The law also transferred jurisdiction of prescription drug advertising from the Federal Trade Commission (FTC) to the FDA and required that all advertising carry labeling on possible side effects (jurisdiction of OTC drug advertising remains with the FTC). The amendment established the requirement for good manufacturing practices (GMPs), registration with the FDA by drug manufacturers, recordkeeping requirements, and regular inspections. It also requires animal testing before testing on humans, informed consent of research subjects before participating in a clinical trial, and reporting of adverse drug events.

Medical Device Amendment Act of 1976

This amendment was designed to protect consumers against potentially dangerous or useless medical devices. It provides for the classification of medical devices according to their function and requires premarket approval that parallels premarket approval for new drugs. It established (1) performance standards and conformance with GMP regulations and (2) recordkeeping and reporting requirements.

Federal Anti-Tampering Act of 1982

This law made it a federal crime to tamper with OTC products and required tamper-resistant packaging. This law is discussed in more detail later in Chapter 42.

Orphan Drug Act of 1983

This law (21 USC 360bb) was passed to create tax and exclusive licensing incentives for manufacturers to develop and market drugs or biological products for the treatment of rare diseases or conditions that affect fewer than 200,000 Americans.

Drug Price Competition and Patent-Term Restoration Act of 1984

Also known as the Hatch-Waxman Amendment, this law was intended to make generic drugs more readily available while at the same time providing incentives to drug manufacturers to develop new drugs. It achieved both purposes by streamlining the generic drug approval process and by giving patent extensions to new, innovative drugs.

Prescription Drug Marketing Act of 1987

This law addressed the problem of drug diversion by placing more stringent controls on the distribution of prescription drug products and samples, as follows:

- Limiting the distribution of drugs beyond conventional retail sale
- Banning the diversion of drugs from legitimate channels of distribution
- Specifying precise storage, handling, and record-keeping requirements for prescription drug samples
- Banning the sale, trade, or purchase of prescription drug samples and making it illegal for a pharmacy to possess prescription drug samples
- Prohibiting, with some exceptions, hospitals and other health care entities from reselling their pharmaceuticals to other businesses
- Requiring state licensing of prescription drug wholesalers under federal guidelines
- Banning reimportation of prescription drugs produced in the United States

Safe Medical Devices Act of 1990

This law amended the Medical Device Amendment Act of 1976 by giving the FDA additional authority over medical devices. It expedited the premarket device approval process and added postmarketing approval requirements. It required health care facilities that use medical devices to report problems to the FDA, and it gave the FDA new authority over recalls for medical devices.

Nutrition Labeling and Education Act of 1990

This law mandated nutrition labeling on food products and authorized health claims on product labeling as long as the claims conformed to FDA regulations. It standardized the use of labeling terms with health implications, such as "light" or "low fat."

Generic Drug Enforcement Act of 1992

This law was motivated by a scandal involving bribery of FDA staff to facilitate the approval process for generic drug products. This act makes false statements, bribes, failure to disclose material-related facts, and other related offenses felonies.

Prescription Drug User Fee Act of 1992

This law requires manufacturers to pay fees for applications and supplements when the FDA must review clinical studies. The fees were intended to provide revenues to hire additional reviewers to speed up the new drug application (NDA) reviews.

Dietary Supplement Health and Education Act of 1994

This law created a special regulatory structure for dietary supplements that is more stringent than that for foods but less stringent than that for drugs. Manufacturers must follow GMPs, but no premarket approval by the FDA is required. The law defines dietary supplements and permits manufacturers to make certain structure or function claims that do not need preapproval from the FDA. For example, claiming that a dietary supplement "maintains a healthy circulatory system" is acceptable without prior FDA approval. However, claims that indicate the dietary supplement is intended to "diagnose, treat, cure, or prevent any disease" require FDA approval because only a drug can make those claims. The FDA aggressively polices manufacturers who make unapproved health claims that are false or misleading (www.fda.gov/Food/IngredientsPackagingLabeling/LabelingNutrition/ucm2006881.htm, accessed April 2, 2014).

FDA Modernization Act of 1997

This law made significant changes that affected every aspect of the FDA's activities. The highlights of this law include the following:

- Streamlined regulatory procedures to ensure the expedited availability of safe and effective drugs and devices
- Increased public accountability of the FDA

- Required a compliance plan developed in consultation with industry representatives, scientific experts, health care professionals, and consumers
- Created a fast-track approval process for drugs intended for serious or life-threatening diseases
- Replaced the legend "Caution: Federal law prohibits dispensing without a prescription" with the legend "Rx only"
- Clarified conditions under which pharmacists may perform extemporaneous compounding of prescriptions
- Exempted pharmacists from the strict regulatory federal GMP standards and requirements for NDAs
- Created a data bank for information on clinical trials
- Authorized scientific panels to review clinical investigations
- Expanded the rights of manufacturers to disseminate unlabeled use information and required specification that such use is not FDA approved
- Encouraged manufacturers to conduct research for new uses of approved drugs and to submit supplemental NDAs (SNDAs) for these uses
- Eliminated the manufacturers' requirement that certain substances must carry the label: "Warning—May be habit forming"
- Expanded the FDA's authority over OTC drugs by establishing ingredient labeling requirements for inactive ingredients and preempted states from establishing labeling requirements for OTC drugs and cosmetics when federal requirements exist
- Mandated priority review for breakthrough technologies for medical devices
- Allowed the FDA to contract with outside scientific experts for review of medical device applications

Best Pharmaceuticals for Children Act of 2002

This law provided mechanisms for studying on- and off-patent drugs in children. The act extended the provision from the 1997 Food and Drug Administration Modernization Act that offered an additional 6 months of patent exclusivity for on-patent drugs being tested for pediatric use.

Medicare Prescription Drug Improvement and Modernization Act of 2003

This law added prescription drug and preventive health care benefits to the Medicare program. The law also provides extra help for persons with low incomes. The prescription drug benefits became available in 2006. All people with Medicare are able to enroll in plans that cover prescription drugs, although plans may vary. The "donut hole" limited benefits for many Medicare beneficiaries. Seniors had to pay 100% of the drug costs above $2,250 until they reached $3,600 in out-of-pocket spending. At that point, Medicare would pay about 95% of drug costs. The Affordable Care Act has minimized the impact of the "donut hole." In 2013, covered participants received a 50% discount when buying Part D–covered brand-name prescription drugs. By 2020, the donut hole will be phased out completely.

Dietary Supplement and Nonprescription Drug Consumer Protection Act of 2006

This law established two parallel, mandatory reporting systems for serious adverse events: one for OTC drugs and the other for dietary supplements.

FDA Amendments Act of 2007

The act greatly increased the responsibilities and authority of the FDA, as well as reauthorized several critical FDA programs. It gave the FDA additional authority and requirements with regard to premarketing and postmarketing safety, including the authority to require postmarketing studies and clinical trials, safety labeling changes, and Risk Evaluation and Mitigation Strategies (REMS). It required the "side effects" statement that notifies patients to report adverse drug events (this statement is discussed in more detail later in Chapter 42). It also made changes in the rules regarding direct-to-consumer advertising by allowing the FDA to pre-review direct-to-consumer ads. Because censorship is unconstitutional, the law allows the FDA only to make recommendations about the ad. The FDA may require a change in the ad only if the change addresses serious risks associated with the drug's use.

Family Smoking Prevention and Tobacco Control Act of 2009

This law, commonly referred to as the Tobacco Control Act, gives the FDA authority to regulate the manufacture, distribution, and marketing of tobacco products to protect public health.

FDA Food Safety Modernization Act of 2011

The act is the most sweeping reform of U.S. food safety laws in more than 70 years. It aims to ensure that the U.S. food supply is safe by shifting the focus from responding to contamination to preventing it.

Drug Quality and Security Act of 2013 (DQSA)

The DQSA creates a voluntary registration process whereby facilities that compound drugs outside the traditional practice of pharmacy may register with the FDA as an outsourcing facility that is exempt from FDA requirements, such as the FDCA's adequate directions for use requirements, the new drug provisions, and the drug tracing provisions. Registered facilities must pay fees, be subject to inspections, and comply with labeling requirements. This law was passed in response to the events involving numerous deaths from meningitis and compounded drugs in 2012.

Drug Supply Chain Security Act

This law, title II of the DQSA, establishes requirements for tracing prescription drug products through the pharmaceutical supply distribution chain. The purpose of this law is to protect consumers from exposure to drugs that may be counterfeit, stolen, contaminated, or otherwise harmful.

Definitions

Drug

The definition of a drug is divided into four parts (21 USC 321(g)).

Part A
Article recognized in the official *United States Pharmacopoeia/National Formulary* (USP/NF, U.S. Pharmacopeial Convention, www.usp.org), or the official *Homeopathic Pharmacopoeia of the United States* (HPUS, Homeopathic Pharmacopoeia Convention of the United States, www.hpus.com), or any supplements of these references

Part B
Article intended for use in the diagnosis, cure, mitigation, treatment, or prevention of disease in humans or other animals

Part C
Article (other than food) intended to affect the structure or any function of the body of humans or other animals

Part D
Article intended for use as a component of any articles specified in the above but not including devices or their components, parts, or accessories

Food

The term *food* means articles used for food or drink for humans or other animals, chewing gum, and articles used for components of any such article (21 USC 321(f)). Special categories of food have been recognized to avoid regulating these foods as drugs.

Special dietary foods supply a special dietary need that exists by reason of a physical, physiological, pathological, or other condition, including conditions of disease, convalescence, pregnancy, lactation, infancy, allergic hypersensitivity to food, underweight, overweight, or the need to control the intake of sodium.

Medical foods are foods that are formulated to be consumed or administered enterally under the supervision of a physician and that are intended for the specific dietary management of a disease or condition for which distinctive nutritional requirements, based on recognized scientific principles, are established by medical evaluation (21 USC 360ee).

Cosmetic

The term *cosmetic* means articles intended to be rubbed, poured, sprinkled, or sprayed on; introduced into; or otherwise applied to the human body or any part thereof for cleansing, beautifying, promoting attractiveness, or altering the appearance. The term also includes articles intended for use as a component of any such articles. The term does not include soap (21 USC 321(i)). The FDA does not have premarket approval for cosmetics, and manufacturers are not required to register with the FDA or to follow GMPs. Cosmetics must list the ingredients on the label in descending order of predominance. Warnings regarding the following are also required: (1) inhaling contents under pressure may be harmful or fatal; (2) the safety of the product has not been determined; and (3) the presence of coal tar in hair dye. The FDA may remove a cosmetic from the market if it is misbranded or adulterated or is a health hazard. Cosmetics must conform to the Poison Prevention Packaging Act (PPPA), or they are considered misbranded. A cosmetic may be considered a drug if it claims to treat a condition. For example, a shampoo that treats dandruff is considered to be both a cosmetic and a drug.

Dietary supplement

A *dietary supplement* is a product that is intended for ingestion, intended to supplement the diet, and contains any one or more of the following: a vitamin; a mineral; an herb or other botanical; an amino acid; a dietary substance for use by humans to supplement the diet by increasing the total dietary intake; or a concentrate, metabolite, constituent, extract, or combination of the above (21 USC 321(ff)). The FDA regulates dietary supplements less stringently than drugs, but claims by the manufacturer that the dietary supplement treats a disease (rather than maintaining health) may bring the product under FDA regulation as if it were a drug.

Medical device

The term *device* means an instrument, apparatus, implement, machine, contrivance, implant, in vitro reagent, or other similar or related article, including any component, part, or accessory that is (1) recognized in the USP/NF or any supplement to it; (2) intended for use in the diagnosis of disease or other conditions, or in the cure, mitigation, treatment, or prevention of disease, in humans or other animals; or (3) intended to affect the structure or any function of the body of humans or other animals, and that does not achieve its primary intended purposes through chemical action within or on the body of humans or other animals and that is not dependent upon being metabolized for the achievement of its primary intended purposes (21 USC 321(h)). Questions arise when a drug is used with a medical device—is it a drug or a medical device? For example, an intrauterine device that delivers hormones would be treated as a drug.

Registration

Each year, every person who owns or operates any establishment in any state engaged in the manufacture, preparation, propagation, compounding, or processing of a drug or drugs must register with the Secretary of Health and Human Services (HHS) his or her name, places of business, and all such establishments. Registration must occur before engaging in any of the listed activities, and a separate registration must be made for each establishment that engages in the activities. Pharmacists who compound are exempt from registering as manufacturers if they "do not manufacture, prepare, propagate, compound, or process drugs or devices for sale other than in the regular course of their business of dispensing or selling drugs or devices at retail." Compounding "in the regular course of business" means to compound a drug pursuant to a prescription or in reasonable anticipation of receiving a prescription (anticipatory compounding). If a pharmacist compounds a drug product outside the regular course of business, the FDA will deem that pharmacist a manufacturer and all the requirements that apply to manufacturers will apply to that pharmacist, including registration, GMPs, labeling and packaging requirements, NDA requirements, and so on. Under the DQSA, facilities that compound outside the regular course of business may voluntarily register with the FDA as an outsourcing facility to avoid these FDCA requirements.

Development and Approval of New Drugs

Legend drugs versus over-the-counter drugs

Legend drugs are prescription-only drugs, and federal law requires the legend "Rx only" on the labeling of these products. The FDA classifies drugs as prescription drugs when the supervision of a physician is required for its safe use. OTC drugs do not require either the supervision of a physician for their safe use or a prescription. Federal law requires that these drugs be labeled with adequate directions for use that inform the consumer of what type of ailments the drug is designed to help and how to safely use the product. "Behind-the-counter" drugs are not officially recognized as a third classification, but, in reality, these are drugs that may be sold only by pharmacists.

Investigational new drug

Before a new drug can be marketed, the manufacturer or other sponsor must complete an extensive testing process to ensure that the new drug is safe and effective for its proposed use. The first step in this process is to submit an investigational NDA to the FDA. The application must include any animal studies that reflect on the safety of the drug and the proposed clinical protocols to be used in testing the drug on humans. Within 30 days, the FDA determines whether the investigational new drug is suitable for testing.

Phase 1

Phase 1 clinical trials are designed to test the safety of the new drug and to assess its toxicological, pharmacokinetic, and pharmacological properties. In a

Phase 1 trial, a small group of healthy individuals is given the drug.

Phase 2

Phase 2 clinical trials are designed to test the effectiveness of the drug. Investigators give the drug to a larger group of human subjects (100 or more) who have the disease or symptoms of the condition to be treated by the new drug. This stage of the research not only tests the effectiveness of the new drug, but also provides information about dosage, relative safety, and adverse effects.

Phase 3

Phase 3 is the final phase of a clinical trial before FDA approval. This phase involves thousands of patients and multiple clinical research sites that are part of a controlled clinical study. Usually, an experimental group is given the drug being tested, and a control group is given a placebo. The studies are "double blinded," meaning that neither the patient nor the investigator knows to which group the patient has been randomly assigned. This phase provides data about the drug's effectiveness compared to the control group receiving the placebo. If the drug satisfactorily completes each of the three phases, the manufacturer or sponsor files an NDA with the FDA for marketing approval.

Phase 4

Phase 4 is the postmarketing surveillance of an approved drug. Health professionals are encouraged to report any problems with the drug, and manufacturers submit yearly reports on new information about the drug. The FDA uses Phase 4 to determine whether the drug should stay on the market.

Exception for immediate and life-threatening diseases

The Food and Drug Administration Modernization Act modified the FDCA to allow an investigational new drug to be accessible outside a clinical trial to treat patients with immediate or life-threatening diseases for which no satisfactory alternative treatment is available if there is reasonable basis to conclude that the drug may be effective and would not expose patients to unreasonable and significant risk.

New drug application

An NDA is submitted to the FDA by the manufacturer or sponsor after Phases 1, 2, and 3 of the clinical trials have been successfully completed. The FDA has at least 6 months to review the application, and experts and others have an opportunity to comment on the submission. If the FDA approves the application, the manufacturer may begin to market the drug.

Risk Evaluation and Mitigation Strategy

The FDA Amendments Act of 2007 authorized the FDA to require sponsors to include an REMS in a pending NDA when the FDA believes that it is necessary to ensure that the benefits of the drug outweigh the risks (21 USC 355-1). The FDA may also mandate a postmarket REMS when it believes an approved drug may have a patient safety issue. An REMS may require one or more methods for protecting the consumer from potentially dangerous drugs. For example, an REMS might require distribution of medication guides, a patient package insert, a communication plan aimed at health care professionals, specialized training for prescribers, or restrictions on the type of health care setting from which the drug may be dispensed.

Expedited approval (fast track)

The FDA may grant a new drug "fast track" status if it is intended for treatment of a serious or life-threatening condition and addresses an unmet medical need. The sponsor must agree to conduct postapproval studies to validate the product's use.

Drug classifications

During the approval process, the FDA classifies new drugs based on their chemical and therapeutic characteristics.

Review classifications

- Type P classification means that the new drug is given priority review either because no other effective drugs are available to treat a particular illness or because the new drug has a significant advantage over currently marketed drugs.
- Type S classification means a standard review because the new drug is similar to other drugs currently on the market.
- Type O classification indicates the drug under review treats a rare disease affecting fewer than 200,000 Americans.

Chemical classifications

- Type 1 classification indicates a new molecular structure from existing drugs used for the therapeutic purpose. This classification indicates a new and unique drug.

- Type 2 classification indicates a new derivative of a molecular structure already approved in the United States.
- Type 3 classification indicates a new formulation of a drug already marketed in the United States.
- Type 4 classification indicates a new combination of two or more drugs.
- Type 5 classification indicates a drug being manufactured by a new company.
- Type 6 classification means a new therapeutic indication for a drug that is already approved.
- Type 7 classification indicates that the drug is already marketed without an approved NDA.
- Type 8 classification indicates that the product is an over-the-counter switch.
- Type 10 classification indicates that the product is a new indication submitted as a distinct NDA, not consolidated.

There is no type 9 classification. For more information, see www.fda.gov/Drugs/InformationOnDrugs/ucm075234.htm.

Drugs for rare diseases or conditions

The FDA may authorize an investigational new drug or device, prior to FDA approval of the drug or device, to be used for the diagnosis, monitoring, or treatment of a serious disease or condition in emergency situations. For an individual patient to obtain a new drug or device in this situation, the following conditions must be met (21 USC 360bbb):

- A licensed physician must determine that the person has no comparable or satisfactory alternative therapy available to diagnose, monitor, or treat the disease or condition involved and that the probable risk to the person from the investigational drug or investigational device is not greater than the probable risk from the disease or condition.
- The FDA determines that there is sufficient evidence of safety and effectiveness to support the use of the investigational drug or device.
- The FDA determines that provision of the investigational drug or investigational device will not interfere with the initiation, conduct, or completion of clinical investigations to support marketing approval.
- The sponsor, or clinical investigator, of the investigational drug or investigational device submits to the Secretary of HHS a clinical protocol describing the use of the investigational drug or investigational device in a single patient or a small group of patients.

Naming new drugs

The responsibility for designating the generic name for a new drug is held by the United States Adopted Names Council (USANC). The Secretary of HHS gives final approval. The name must be short, distinctive, and not likely to be confused with other existing names. The name should also provide some indications of the therapeutic or chemical class to which the drug belongs.

National Drug Code

The Drug Listing Act of 1972 requires registered drug establishments to provide the FDA with a current list of all drugs manufactured, prepared, propagated, compounded, or processed by them for commercial distribution (see section 510 of the FDCA [21 USC 360]). Drug products are identified and reported using a unique, three-segment number, called the National Drug Code (NDC), which serves as a universal product identifier for human drugs (FDA Web site, www.fda.gov/drugs/informationondrugs/ucm142438.htm). If a prescription drug product has an NDC of "0137-0145-10," the "0137" is assigned by the FDA and identifies the manufacturer or distributor (known as the "labeler's code"). The "0145" is assigned by the manufacturer and identifies a specific strength, dosage form, and formulation for that particular manufacturer. The "10" is also assigned by the manufacturer and identifies the trade package size and characteristics, such as blister pack or bottle of 100 tablets. An NDC does not denote FDA approval of a drug. (Note: The FDA's standard 10-digit number conflicts with HIPAA's 11-digit standard for NDC. The FDA suggests adding an asterisk to the product code or the package code, instead of 0, to comply with both HIPAA and the FDA standard. For more information, see www.fda.gov/drugs/developmentapprovalprocess/ucm070829).

Brand-name or proprietary drugs

A *brand name* is the name assigned to the drug by the manufacturer. If the drug is a proprietary drug, the manufacturer is the innovator company to first market the drug and holds a patent on the drug, giving the manufacturer exclusive rights to market the drug.

Patent issues
Without patents, manufacturers would have little financial incentive to research and develop a new

drug because nothing would prevent other companies from marketing generic versions of the drug after it has been approved by the FDA. Patents prevent this situation by giving the innovator company the exclusive rights to market the drug for a period of years. However, generic drugs keep the cost of pharmaceuticals down. The laws try to balance the two competing interests by extending certain patent rights of innovator companies to encourage research and development of new drugs and by streamlining the approval process for generic drugs.

Supplemental new drug application

An innovator company submits an SNDA when it wants to make changes in an approved drug product.

Generic drugs

Definition

When a patent for a proprietary drug expires, generic versions of the drug may be marketed by other companies. The generic version is usually cheaper than the proprietary drug.

Abbreviated new drug application

An abbreviated new drug application (ANDA) is submitted by a company that wants to market a drug after the innovator company's patent expires. Compared to an NDA, this process is streamlined and requires proof that the new drug product is similar to the innovator's drug product in pharmacokinetic properties, bioavailability, and clinical activity. An easy way to distinguish this application from an SNDA is to remember that an ANDA is submitted by *another* company, while an SNDA is submitted by the *same* company that first marketed the drug.

Drug recalls

If a marketed drug is determined to have problems, the FDA encourages the manufacturer to issue a drug recall notice. A pharmacy that sells a recalled drug product is probably violating the FDCA because the product is most likely to be considered adulterated or misbranded. It is the manufacturer's responsibility to send wholesalers and pharmacies written recall notices of Class I and Class II recalls.

Drug recalls fall into three classes:

- Class I recalls are the most significant and mean that the drug product may cause serious adverse health consequences including death. This recall should include stocks in pharmacies and notice to patients to whom the drug has been dispensed.
- Class II recalls mean that the drug product may cause temporary or reversible effects, but the probability of serious adverse effects is remote. This type of recall usually involves only stocks in pharmacies.
- Class III recalls mean that the drug is unlikely to cause any adverse health consequences.

Unapproved Drugs

In 2006, the FDA estimated that thousands of prescription and OTC drug products that have never been approved by the FDA are being marketed illegally. Pharmacists should use professional judgment before dispensing or selling an unapproved drug. (Note: Distinguish between an unapproved *drug* and an unapproved or off-label *use* of an approved drug.)

Current Good Manufacturing Practice

GMP is a set of regulations that specify the minimum standards required to manufacture pharmaceutical products in the United States. A manufacturer must be registered with the FDA and must describe its manufacturing and production processes as part of the NDA process.

Labeling Requirements

Definitions

The term *label* is defined as a display of written, printed, or graphic matter on the immediate container of any article. The label must appear on the outside container or wrapper of a retail package, or it must be easily legible through the outside container or wrapper.

The term *labeling* is defined to include all labels and other written, printed, or graphic matter on any article or its containers or wrappers, or accompanying such article. For example, a package insert is considered part of a drug's labeling.

Labeling requirements for the manufacturer

Extensive regulations control what a manufacturer must put on the product's labeling. To avoid having the product deemed misbranded, a manufacturer must include the following on the product's labeling (21 CFR 201.1, 201.55, 201.100):

- Name or address of the manufacturer, packer, or distributor
- Established name of the drug or drug product

- Ingredient information, including quantity and proportion of each active ingredient
- Names of inactive ingredients if not for oral use (with some exceptions)
- Generic and proprietary names
- Quantity in terms of weight measure (e.g., 100 mg)
- Net quantity of the container (e.g., 100 tablets)
- Statement of the recommended or usual dosage or reference to the package insert
- Identifying lot or control number
- Legend "Rx only"
- Specific route or routes of administration (e.g., oral, subcutaneous injection)
- Special storage instructions, if appropriate (e.g., refrigeration)
- Expiration date established by the manufacturer

Unit-dose packaging and labeling

Unit-dose packaging is more cost effective for health care facilities because it cuts down on wasted drugs prescribed for inpatient use. To meet this need, manufacturers provide their products in single-dose or unit-dose packaging that is too small to contain the required labeling information. The FDA has issued guidelines about what information should be contained on each unit-dose package:

- Generic name and trade name, if appropriate
- Quantity of active drug or drugs present
- Name of manufacturer, packer, or distributor
- Repackager's lot number
- Expiration date
- Any other appropriate information

Adequate information for use

Prescription drug labeling must contain "adequate information for use" as opposed to "adequate directions for use" that is required for OTC drug labeling (21 CFR 201.100(c)(1)). This information is designed for the health care provider—not the patient. To meet this requirement, the labeling must include the following:

- The drug's indications
- Side effects
- Dosages
- Routes, methods, frequency, and duration of administration
- Contraindications
- Other warnings and precautions that enable a practitioner to administer, prescribe, or dispense the drug safely

Exemptions from labeling requirements

Some products are exempt from the FDCA labeling or packaging requirements (21 USC 353).

Drugs or devices are exempt from the labeling and packaging requirements if, in accordance with the practice of the trade, they are to be processed, labeled, or repacked in substantial quantities at establishments other than those where originally processed or packed, on condition that such drugs and devices are not adulterated or misbranded under the provisions of chapter 9 of title 21 upon removal from such processing, labeling, or repacking establishment (21 USC 353(a)).

Prescription drugs are exempt from the labeling and packaging requirements if the drugs are dispensed pursuant to a legitimate prescription issued by a practitioner who is licensed to administer the drug. If a pharmacist dispenses a prescription drug contrary to these rules, the drug is deemed to be misbranded. The drug may be dispensed only (1) upon a written prescription of a practitioner licensed by law to administer such drug, (2) upon an oral prescription of such practitioner that is reduced promptly to writing and filed by the pharmacist, or (3) by refilling any such written or oral prescription if such refilling is authorized by the prescriber either in the original prescription or by oral order that is reduced promptly to writing and filed by the pharmacist (21 USC 353(b)).

Labeling requirements for the pharmacist

Although prescription drugs dispensed by a pharmacist to a patient are exempt from most of the labeling and packaging requirements of the FDCA, some requirements must be met to avoid a charge of misbranding.

A dispensed prescription is exempt from the labeling and package rules of the FDCA if the drug bears a label containing the following:

- Name and address of the dispenser
- Serial number and date of the prescription or of its filling
- Name of the prescriber
- If stated in the prescription, the name of the patient, the directions for use, and cautionary statements, if any, contained in such prescription

This exemption does not apply to any drug dispensed pursuant to diagnosis by mail or to any drug dispensed without a legitimate prescription issued by a practitioner licensed to administer the drug (21 USC 353(b)(2)).

The exemption also does not apply to any drug

- That is dispensed with a false or misleading label
- That is an imitation of another drug
- That is offered for sale under the name of another drug
- That is subject to the packaging requirements of the USP or the HPUS
- That must be packaged to prevent deterioration
- That must be packaged in conformity with the PPPA (21 USC 353(b)(2))

Package inserts

Manufacturers' package inserts are for informational use only and are intended for the health care provider. They are not for promotional use. The information in the package insert must be approved by the FDA in the premarketing approval process.

Information contained in a package insert includes the following:

- Description of the drug
- Clinical pharmacology
- Indications and usage
- Contraindications
- Warnings
- Precautions
- Adverse reactions
- Potential for abuse or patient dependence
- Symptoms and treatment of overdose
- Dosage and administration
- Available dosage forms of the product
- Date of the most recent revision of the labeling
- Recommended or usual dosage

In 2006, the FDA designed a new format for package inserts to improve patient safety. The 2006 changes included the following:

- A highlights section providing
  - Immediate access to information about drug benefits and risks
  - Boxed warnings
  - Indications for use
  - Dosage and administration information
- A table of contents section to facilitate easy access to detailed information about safety and efficacy
- The date of initial product approval
- A toll-free number and Internet reporting information to encourage reporting of side effects
- A section on "patient counseling information" designed to encourage communication between health professionals and patients

Black box warnings may be required when the use of a high-risk drug may lead to death or serious injury.

Pregnancy warnings must be included in package inserts and fall into five categories:

- Category A (clear evidence of no risk to fetus)
- Category B (animal studies failed to show risk to fetus)
- Category C (risk to fetus is undetermined)
- Category D (positive evidence of risk to fetus)
- Category E (risk to fetus outweighs any possible benefit)

Over-the-Counter Drugs

Nonprescription drug labeling

Nonprescription drugs (OTC) have been approved by the FDA as safe and effective for self-medication by consumers without the guidance of a physician. However, the labeling of these products must conform to the regulations or be deemed misbranded. Labeling requirements for OTC drugs are as follows:

- A statement of the identity of the product
- Name and address of manufacturer, packer, or distributor
- Net quantity of the contents of the package
- Cautions and warnings needed to protect the consumer
- Adequate directions for use (sufficient information so that a layperson can use the product safely) that include the following:
  - Statement of all conditions, uses, and purposes
  - Quantity or dosage for each intended use and for persons of different ages and physical conditions
  - Frequency of administration or application
  - Duration of administration or application
  - Time of administration or application (e.g., meals, onset of symptoms)
  - Route or method of administration or application
  - Preparation necessary for use (e.g., shaking, dilution)
- A drug facts panel that includes the following information:
  - Active ingredients
  - Purpose
  - Uses
  - Warnings
  - Directions
  - Other information as required
  - Inactive ingredients in alphabetical order
  - A section for "Questions?" and "Comments?" with a telephone number

Federal Anti-Tampering Act

In response to the 1982 Tylenol murders, Congress passed this law (18 USC 1365) to require tamper-evident packaging on selected OTC drug products and cosmetics that are accessible to the public while held for sale.

Tamper-evident packaging is required on selected OTC drug products and cosmetics, particularly those that are taken orally. The requirements are twofold (21 CFR 211.132):

- Some type of barrier that will provide visible evidence of entry if disturbed
- Directions to the consumer on how to determine if tampering has occurred

Dermatological, dentifrice, insulin, and lozenge products are exempted from this requirement.

The following acts constitute a violation of this law:

- Tampering with consumer products is malicious mischief and may result in fines, imprisonment (up to life if death resulted from the tampering), or both.
- False communications that a consumer product has been tainted may result in fines, imprisonment for not more than 5 years, or both.
- Threats that can be reasonably believed about violating this law may result in fines, imprisonment for not more than 5 years, or both.
- Conspiracy of two or more persons to commit a crime under this law may result in fines, imprisonment for not more than 10 years, or both.

Prohibited Acts under the FDCA

Section 301 of the FDCA prohibits more than 50 different acts, including the following that may be of particular interest to pharmacists (21 USC 301):

- The introduction or delivery for introduction into interstate commerce of any food, drug, device, tobacco product, or cosmetic that is adulterated or misbranded
- The adulteration or misbranding of any food, drug, device, tobacco product, or cosmetic in interstate commerce
- The receipt in interstate commerce of any food, drug, device, tobacco product, or cosmetic that is adulterated or misbranded, and the delivery or proffered delivery of such items for pay or otherwise

- The introduction or delivery for introduction into interstate commerce of any article in violation of 21 USC 344 (emergency permit control), 350d (registration of food facilities), 355 (new drugs), or 360bbb-3 (authorization of medical products for use in emergencies)
- The refusal to permit access to or copying of any record to be kept as required by the FDCA; the failure to establish or maintain any record or make any report required under the FDCA; the refusal to permit access to or verification or copying of any such required record; or the violation of any recordkeeping requirement
- The refusal to permit entry or inspection as authorized by the FDCA
- The manufacture of any food, drug, device, tobacco product, or cosmetic that is adulterated or misbranded
- Forging, counterfeiting, simulating, or falsely representing, or without proper authority using any mark, stamp, tag, label, or other identification device authorized or required by regulation under the FDCA
- Any act that causes a drug to be a counterfeit drug, or the sale or dispensing, or the holding for sale or dispensing, of a counterfeit drug
- The alteration, mutilation, destruction, obliteration, or removal of the whole or any part of the labeling of or the doing of any other act with respect to a food, drug, device, tobacco product, or cosmetic, if such act is done while such article is held for sale after shipment in interstate commerce and results in such article being adulterated or misbranded
- The failure of the manufacturer, packer, or distributor to provide all printed matter that is required to be included in any package in which a prescription drug is to be sold to any licensed, authorized practitioner who makes a written request for such information
- The failure to register in accordance with the requirements of the FDCA
- The introduction or delivery into interstate commerce of a dietary supplement that is unsafe under the provisions of the FDCA
- The importation of a drug in violation of the FDCA; the sale, purchase, or trade of a drug sample in violation of the FDCA; and the sale, purchase, trade, or counterfeiting of any coupon in violation of the FDCA
- The importation of a prescription drug in violation of the FDCA
- The falsification of a report of a serious adverse event

Misbranding and Adulteration

The manufacture, sale or delivery, holding, or offering for sale of any food, drug, device, tobacco product, or cosmetic that is adulterated or misbranded is illegal (21 USC 331).

Adulteration

Adulteration refers to the composition of a product. Note in the definition that a drug may be adulterated even if it is proved to be "pure." A product is adulterated if it

- Contains, in whole or part, any filthy, putrid, or decomposed substance
- Has been prepared, packaged, or held under unsanitary conditions where it may have been contaminated
- Has been manufactured under conditions that do not meet the GMP standards
- Contains an unapproved color additive
- Contains a drug recognized in official compendia, but its strength, purity, or quality is lower than the official standards, unless plainly stated on its label
- Has a container composed of a poisonous or deleterious substance that may leach into the product contents
- Contains a drug not recognized in official compendia, but its strength, quality, or purity is lower than that listed on the label
- Contains any ingredient as a substitute for the active drug

Misbranding

Misbranding refers to the labeling of a product. The FDA must approve the exact wording of a drug's label as part of the NDA process. A drug is misbranded if the labeling

- Is false or misleading
- Is missing either the name or the location of the manufacturer, packer, or distributor
- Does not contain a word, statement, or other information required by law displayed in a prominent, readable manner
- Does not include the established name of the active drug
- Does not have each active drug ingredient and its quantity identified (unless prescription is not for human use)
- Does not have each inactive ingredient listed in alphabetical order (except prescriptions not for human use or nonprescription cosmetics)
- Does not state "Rx only" if the drug is available only by prescription (unless prescription is dispensed to consumers)
- Does not contain a precautionary statement concerning a drug that is subject to deterioration
- Is missing an accurate statement of the quantity of the contents in terms of weight, measure, or numerical count (reasonable variations are permitted, and exemptions exist for small packages)
- Has inadequate directions for use of nonprescription drugs or does not include appropriate warnings required to protect those using the medication or packaging
- Has inadequate information for use (prescription drugs)
- Does not conform to the requirements as prescribed in the official compendium (if listed in the compendium)
- Offers the sale of a drug under the name of another drug
- Offers the sale of an imitation of another drug
- Prescribes, recommends, or suggests a dosage dangerous to health
- Does not conform to the requirements for packaging and labeling of color additives
- Does not include all advertisements and other descriptive material required for prescription drugs (information for use)

Additionally, a drug is misbranded if one of the following occurs:

- The container is misbranded.
- It was manufactured, prepared, propagated, compounded, or processed in an establishment not duly registered under applicable law.
- It was not manufactured using tamper-evident or tamper-resistant packaging as required by law.
- It does not conform to the PPPA of 1970 (child-resistant packaging, discussed in more detail later in Chapter 42).
- A pharmacy dispenses a prescription-only drug without a legal prescription or an authorized refill.

Inspections

Authorized agents of the FDA, upon presenting appropriate credentials and a written notice to the owner, operator, or agent in charge, may enter, at reasonable times, any factory, warehouse, or establishment in which food, drugs, devices, tobacco products, or cosmetics are manufactured, processed, packed, or held for introduction into interstate commerce

(21 USC 374). They also may enter any vehicle being used to transport or hold such food, drugs, devices, tobacco products, or cosmetics in interstate commerce. They may inspect, at reasonable times, within reasonable limits, and in a reasonable manner, such factory, warehouse, establishment, or vehicle and all pertinent equipment, finished and unfinished materials, containers, and labeling therein. A warrant is not required.

FDA inspectors may enter and inspect pharmacies to determine whether they are engaged in the manufacture of drug products (e.g., compounding outside the scope of their professional practice). Pharmacies are *not* engaged in manufacturing if they do not, either through a subsidiary or otherwise, manufacture, prepare, propagate, compound, or process drugs or devices for sale other than in the regular course of their business of dispensing or selling drugs or devices at retail. For example, a pharmacy is not engaged in manufacturing if it compounds drug products only in response to receiving a legitimate prescription issued by an authorized prescriber in the usual course of its professional practice.

In the event that the FDA inspectors find that a pharmacy is engaged in manufacturing, the scope of the inspection extends to include records, files, papers, processes, controls, and facilities that bear on whether prescription drugs, nonprescription drugs intended for human use, restricted devices, or tobacco products are adulterated or misbranded or otherwise in violation of the FDCA.

Unless the owner, operator, or agent in charge gives consent, the inspection does not include financial data, sales data other than shipment data, pricing data, personnel data (other than data as to qualification of technical and professional personnel performing functions subject to the FDCA), and research data (other than data relating to new drugs, antibiotic drugs, devices, and tobacco products that are subject to reporting and inspection regulations under the FDCA).

Under the DQSA, registered outsourcing facilities are subject to a risk-based inspection schedule.

Drug Samples

A drug sample is not intended to be sold (21 CFR 203.31). It is usually intended to acquaint a prescriber with a drug product by providing several doses for short-term or initial therapy. It is illegal for a retail pharmacy to obtain, possess, or distribute drug samples. Institutional pharmacy practice sites may possess drug samples under specified conditions.

Manufacturers, through their representatives, may distribute drug samples to a practitioner licensed to prescribe the drug to be sampled or, at the written request of such a licensed practitioner, to the pharmacy of a hospital or other health care entity. In either case, the following requirements must be met:

- The manufacturer or authorized distributor of record must receive from the licensed practitioner a written request signed by the licensed practitioner before the delivery of the drug sample.
- The manufacturer or authorized distributor of record must verify with the appropriate state authority that the practitioner requesting the drug sample is licensed or authorized under state law to prescribe the drug product.
- A receipt must be signed by the recipient when the drug sample is delivered.
- The receipt must be returned to the manufacturer or distributor.
- Required inventories must be kept.

Medical Devices

Examples of devices include infusion pumps, cardiac pacemakers, and heart monitors.

Definition

The term *device* (21 USC 321(h)) means an instrument, apparatus, implement, machine, contrivance, implant, in vitro reagent, or other similar or related article, including any component, part, or accessory, that

- Is recognized in the USP/NF, or any supplement to them
- Is intended for use in the diagnosis of disease or other conditions, or in the cure, mitigation, treatment, or prevention of disease, in man or other animals
- Is intended to affect the structure or any function of the body of humans or other animals
- Does not achieve its primary intended purposes through chemical action within or on the body of humans or other animals and is not dependent upon being metabolized for the achievement of its primary intended purposes (This part of the definition distinguishes it from a drug.)

The legal distinction between a drug and a device becomes less clear when a drug is used in conjunction with a device. For example, an intrauterine device that releases hormones would likely be classified as a drug rather than a device.

Classes

The classes of medical devices (21 CFR 860.3) are as follows:

- Class I medical devices pose the least potential harm to users. Examples include needles, scissors, and latex gloves.
- Class II medical devices require more regulation than Class I devices to ensure safety and effectiveness. Examples include insulin syringes, infusion pumps, thermometers, and electric heating pads.
- Class III medical devices are often life-sustaining devices, pose a potential or unreasonable risk of injury or illness, or do both. Class III devices require premarket approval. Examples include pacemakers, soft contact lenses, and replacement heart valves.

Tracking

A manufacturer of any Class II or Class III device that fits within one of the three criteria listed below must track that device if the FDA issues a tracking order to that manufacturer (21 CFR 821.20). The three criteria (21 CFR 821.1(a)) are as follows:

- The failure of the device would be reasonably likely to have serious adverse health consequences.
- The device is intended to be implanted in the human body for more than 1 year.
- The device is a life-sustaining or life-supporting device used outside a device user facility.

Reports

Device user facilities, manufacturers, importers, and distributors are required to keep records and make reports of adverse events resulting from the use of medical devices (21 CFR 803.1). These reports help ensure that devices are not adulterated or misbranded and are safe and effective for their intended use:

- A device user facility must report deaths and serious injuries that a device has or may have caused or contributed to, establish and maintain adverse event files, and submit summary annual reports.
- A manufacturer or importer must report deaths and serious injuries that a device has or may have caused or contributed to, must report certain device malfunctions, and must establish and maintain adverse event files. A manufacturer must also submit specified follow-up reports.

- A medical device distributor must maintain records (files) of incidents but is not required to report these incidents.

42-3. Dispensing Prescription Drugs

Written, Oral, or Electronic Prescriptions

A written prescription must be signed by the prescriber on the date it is issued.

Oral prescriptions were authorized under the Durham-Humphrey Amendment of 1951. An oral prescription must be promptly reduced to writing by the pharmacist and filed. There are limitations on oral prescriptions for schedule II drugs, discussed later in Chapter 42.

Electronic records, signatures, and contracts in interstate commerce were recognized as legally valid under the Electronic Signatures in Global and National Commerce Act of 2000 (E-Sign) (PL 106-229). Electronic prescriptions were authorized under the Medicare Prescription Drug, Improvement, and Modernization Act of 2003 (known as Medicare Part D) (70 Fed. Reg. 13397 (2005) and 73 Fed. Reg. 18918 (2008)). The e-prescribing provision preempts any state law that limits a prescriber's ability to transmit electronic prescriptions for Medicare patients. Most states have laws that permit the electronic transmission of prescriptions, both by fax (image transmission) and electronically (data transmission). Note the special rules that apply to e-prescriptions for controlled substances discussed later in Chapter 42.

Refills

Refills of prescription drugs were authorized under the Durham-Humphrey Amendment of 1951. Pharmacists should note the refills on the back of the written prescription or by other recording method, such as a computer system.

A pharmacist may not refill a prescription unless there is specific authorization, either oral or written, from an authorized prescriber. A secretary can communicate the refill (or new prescription) authorization, but the pharmacist should confirm that someone who has prescribing authority has actually authorized the refill (or new prescription).

Prescribers may limit the number of refills for prescription drugs, and the pharmacist must comply with the prescriber's directions. However, controlled substances have strict limits on refills imposed by law, which must be followed by both the prescriber and the dispenser, as discussed later in Chapter 42.

Prescription Drug Labeling

When filling a prescription by an authorized prescriber, pharmacists are not required to comply with the stringent labeling requirements imposed on manufacturers of prescription drugs (21 USC 353(b)(2)). (Note: This exemption does not apply when the prescription is written pursuant to a diagnosis by mail.) However, to avoid a charge of misbranding, a pharmacist must comply with certain labeling requirements for a prescription drug.

Under federal law (21 USC 353(b)(2)), the label of a dispensed prescription drug must contain the following:

- Name and address of the dispenser
- Serial number of the prescription
- Date of the prescription or of its filling
- Name of the prescriber
- Name of the patient, if stated in the prescription
- Directions for use
- Cautionary statements, if any, contained in such prescription

In addition, the label must comply with the following requirements:

- The label must not be false or misleading (21 USC 352(a)).
- The drug dispensed must not be an imitation drug (21 USC 352(i)(2)).
- The drug must not be sold under the name of another drug (21 USC 352(i)(3)).
- The packaging and labeling must conform to official compendia standards (21 USC 352(g)).
- If it is a drug susceptible to deterioration, it must be packaged and labeled appropriately (21 USC 352(h)).
- The drug must be packaged in conformance with the PPPA (21 USC 352(p)).

Tamper-Resistant Prescription Paper

Effective October 1, 2008, federal law (Tamper-Resistant Prescription Law [Section 7002(b) of the U.S. Troop Readiness, Veterans' Care, Katrina Recovery, and Iraq Accountability Appropriations Act of 2007]) requires that written prescriptions (excluding electronic, oral, or faxed) for Medicaid-covered outpatient drugs must be issued on a tamper-resistant paper. To meet this requirement, the prescription form must be designed to prevent (1) unauthorized copying of a completed or blank prescription pad, (2) erasure or modifications of information written on the prescription pad by the prescriber, and (3) use of counterfeit prescription forms. The law applies whenever Medicaid pays any portion of the prescription. If the prescription form does not comply with the law, the pharmacist may fill the prescription on an emergency basis (note special rules for emergency oral prescriptions of schedule II drugs discussed later in Chapter 42), provided that the pharmacy obtains a compliant prescription within 72 hours after the fill date. The compliant prescription may be in the form of a written prescription on tamper-resistant paper or may be obtained by verbal communication with the prescriber, by fax, or by e-prescription.

Side Effects Statement

Effective July 1, 2009, dispensers are required to distribute a side effects statement on all new and refill prescriptions (21 CFR 209.1).

The rule applies to pharmacists and all authorized dispensers. The rule does not apply to authorized dispensers dispensing or administering prescription drug products to patients in a hospital or health care facility under an order of a licensed practitioner, or as part of supervised home health care. The rule also does not apply to a physician who provides drug samples as a precursor to issuing a new prescription.

The purpose of providing the side effects statement is to enable consumers to report side effects of prescription drug products to the FDA.

The side effects statement provided with each prescription drug product must read: "Call your doctor for medical advice about side effects. You may report side effects to FDA at 1-800-FDA-1088" (21 CFR 209.10).

An authorized dispenser or pharmacy must choose one or more of the following options to distribute the side effects statement (21 CFR 209.11):

- Distribute the side effects statement on a sticker attached to the unit package, vial, or container of the drug product.
- Distribute the side effects statement on a preprinted pharmacy prescription vial cap.
- Distribute the side effects statement on a separate sheet of paper.
- Distribute the side effects statement in consumer medication information.
- Distribute the appropriate FDA-approved Medication Guide that contains the side effects statement.

Product Information for Prescription Drugs

The different types of product information are considered part of a drug's labeling, and they must be approved by the FDA.

Manufacturer's insert

This information is intended for the prescriber, who is considered the "learned intermediary" and is charged with giving the appropriate information and warnings to the patient. The "learned intermediary" doctrine has served to insulate manufacturers from liability for failure to warn patients of the potential risks associated with using the drug. However, when manufacturers engage in direct-to-consumer advertising, manufacturers have a legal duty to properly warn consumers of the potential risks associated with the marketed drug. Historically, manufacturers' package inserts were difficult to read, but recent regulations have required manufacturers to put the information in easier-to-read formats, including table of contents, black box warnings, and so forth.

Patient package insert

Many potentially dangerous drugs must be dispensed with a patient package insert (PPI). The requirement applies to potentially dangerous drugs such as

- Accutane (brand name removed from the market in 2009)
- Statin drugs
- Oral contraceptives (21 CFR 310.501)
- Drug products containing estrogen (21 CFR 310.515)

PPIs must be written in language that a layperson can understand. They are intended to educate the patient about the proper use of the drug and the potential risks inherent in using the drug.

All dispensers (including prescribers who dispense from their offices) are required to distribute PPIs. The manufacturer of the drug is required to provide dispensers with a sufficient number of PPIs. Failure to include a PPI when it is required is misbranding.

The rule applies to pharmacy practice sites located in hospitals and long-term care facilities. Pharmacists in these practice sites must distribute PPIs to both outpatients and inpatients. For inpatients, the PPI must be distributed before the initial dose of the drug and then again every 30 days thereafter, as long as the therapy continues.

A pharmacist does not meet the legal obligations by distributing PPIs to the prescriber. Dispensers must give a PPI to the patient—not the prescriber.

Medication guides

Except as required by law, medication guides (MedGuides) are prepared by manufacturers on a voluntary basis in language easily understood by laypeople (63 Fed. Reg. 66378).

The FDA can mandate a MedGuide for drugs posing a "serious and significant public health concern." MedGuides are required under the following circumstances:

- Patient labeling could prevent serious adverse effects.
- The product has serious risks relative to benefits.
- Patient adherence to directions is crucial.

If a MedGuide is required for a specific drug, it is required for new and refill prescriptions, and the requirement applies only to dispensers who dispense on an outpatient basis. The manufacturer is responsible for providing the MedGuides to dispensers.

Hundreds of prescription drugs require the dispenser to distribute a MedGuide. The list of drugs may be accessed on the FDA Web site at www.fda.gov/Drugs/DrugSafety/ucm085729.htm.

Poison Prevention Packaging Act of 1970

The purpose of this law is to protect children under 5 years of age from accidental poisoning (16 CFR Part 1700; see also U.S. Consumer Product Safety Commission, *Poison Prevention Packaging: A Guide for Healthcare Professionals,* www.cpsc.gov/cpscpub/pubs/384.pdf [accessed June 1, 2012]). The U.S. Consumer Product Safety Commission (CPSC) has had the responsibility for overseeing the enforcement of this law since 1973 (16 CFR 1700.2). (Note: Do not confuse the PPPA with the Anti-Tampering Act, which is designed to protect all consumers by requiring tamper-evident packaging.) For a list of substances covered under the PPPA, see 16 CFR 1700.14.

Requirements

The PPPA requires child-resistant closures that prevent access by young children to almost all prescription drugs dispensed directly to consumers, nonprescription drugs, and hazardous household products.

To pass the child-resistant test, 80% of children under 5 years of age in a test panel should not be able to open the package within 10 minutes.

To make sure the packaging can be opened by older adults, 90% of adults between 50 and 70 years of age in a test panel should be able to open the package within 5 minutes, and then do so a second time within 1 minute.

Rules for pharmacies

All new and refill prescriptions must be dispensed with child-resistant safety closures, except under the following circumstances (16 CFR 1701.1(b), (d)):

- The prescriber specifies that safety closures should not be used.
- The patient indicates that he or she does not want a safety closure used.
- The container is being used in a facility in which drugs remain under the control of health care professionals, such as in a hospital or nursing home. (Note: Pharmacies providing drugs to patients in assisted-living facilities still need to use child-resistant safety closures.)

Waivers

Either the patient or the prescriber can request that the pharmacist dispense a prescription drug without a child safety closure.

The prescriber may waive the safety closure for that prescription and any refills, but he or she may not request a blanket waiver for all future prescriptions for that patient.

The patient may request a blanket waiver for all prescriptions. The pharmacist should obtain the patient's written waiver and periodically check with the patient to ensure that a blanket waiver remains appropriate for the patient.

Reuse of containers

As a general rule, child safety closures should not be reused because continued use compromises the closure's effectiveness. For a refill, all plastic parts (both the closure and the container) should be replaced. If the container is glass or threaded plastic, the container may be reused as long as the closure is replaced.

A pharmacist may dispense a drug in a reversible container (child resistant if one side is used and not child resistant if the other side is used) as long as it is dispensed in the child-resistant mode. However, the CPSC discourages this practice.

The CPSC requires all dispensers (including prescribers who dispense prescription drugs or drug samples from their offices) to use child-resistant safety closures (U.S. Consumer Product Safety Commission, *Poison Prevention Packaging: A Guide for Healthcare Professionals*, www.cpsc.gov/cpscpub/pubs/384.pdf [accessed June 1, 2012]).

Manufacturer's packaging

Manufacturers of prescription drugs may package them for distribution to pharmacies in different types of packages, depending on whether the package will be the one in which the drug is ultimately given to the consumer or whether the pharmacist will repackage the drug before it is dispensed to the consumer. If the package is to be given directly to the consumer, the manufacturer must use special packaging. Examples of packages intended to be given directly to the consumer include mnemonic dispensing devices; dropper bottles; packages with "tear-off" labels; packages that incorporate ancillary instructions for consumer handling, storage, or use on permanently affixed portions of their labels; and products intended to be reconstituted in their original containers. If the drug is supplied in a bulk package from which individual prescriptions are intended to be repackaged by the pharmacist, the manufacturer does not need to use special packaging (16 CFR 1701.1(b)).

Exemptions for easy access

To make drugs and hazardous household products readily available to elderly or handicapped persons who are unable to use those substances in special packaging, manufacturers and packers are permitted to package such substances in noncomplying packaging of a single size, provided that complying packaging is also supplied and the noncomplying packages are conspicuously labeled to indicate that they should not be used in households where young children are present (16 CFR 1700.5).

Exemptions from the PPPA

Manufacturers or packers may apply for an exemption (16 CFR Part 1702) from these rules for their products if they make an appropriate application and explain the reason for the exemption based on one or more of the following grounds (16 CFR 1702.7):

- If the justification is based on a lack of need for special packaging to protect young children from serious injury or illness from the substance, the justification shall state how the lack of toxicity and lack of adverse human experience for the substance clearly supports granting the exemption.
- If the exemption is requested because special packaging is not technologically feasible, practicable, or appropriate for the substance, the justification shall explain why.
- If the exemption is requested because special packaging is incompatible with the particular substance, the justification shall explain why.

Generic Substitution

To encourage generic substitution for more expensive brand-name drugs, the Medicaid Maximum Allowable Cost Program was implemented in 1974. By setting an upper limit on what Medicaid would reimburse for certain multisource drugs, this law encouraged states to allow generic substitution and encouraged pharmacists to substitute generic drugs when appropriate. The primary purpose of the law was to lower Medicaid costs.

Definitions

- The *generic name* is the single specific name assigned to a drug by the USANC.
- The *trade* or *brand name* is the unique name selected by the drug's manufacturer.
- A *single-source product* is manufactured by only one manufacturer.
- A *multisource product* is manufactured by more than one manufacturer.
- A *reference listed drug* (RLD) is the brand-name drug to which generic drugs are rated for bioequivalency.

Mandatory and permissive substitution

Drug product selection laws vary from state to state.

In mandatory substitution states, the pharmacist is required to substitute a less expensive generic drug for a brand-name drug unless the prescriber has indicated to "Dispense as written" or a similar notation.

In permissive substitution states, a pharmacist may choose to substitute a less expensive generic drug for the brand-name drug, but only if the prescriber writes the prescription in a way that permits substitution.

If a prescription is written generically (no brand name indicated), the pharmacist may dispense any product in the generic class, subject to professional judgment.

Labeling a generic drug with the brand-name drug is considered misbranding and may open a pharmacist to a criminal charge of deceptive business practices.

Drug product substitution

Pharmacists are responsible for ensuring that the substituted drug is bioequivalent to the prescribed brand-name drug.

The FDA publishes the *Orange Book* to help pharmacists and prescribers determine the bioequivalence of generic drugs (U.S. Food and Drug Administration, *Orange Book: Approved Drug Products with Therapeutic Equivalence Evaluations*, www.accessdata.fda.gov/scripts/cder/ob/default.cfm). Generic drugs are rated to denote bioequivalence:

- "A" rated products are bioequivalent and therapeutically equivalent to the brand-name (RLD) drug product. Substitutions of the same strength and dosage forms are permitted.
- "B" rated products are not bioequivalent, and substitutions are not permitted.
- "AB" rated products have had problems with bioequivalence, but the problems have been resolved and substitutions of the same strength and dosage forms are permitted.

Pharmacy Compounding versus Manufacturing

Before the proliferation of pharmaceutical companies, pharmacists compounded drugs to meet the critical needs of patients. Although pharmaceutical companies have made pharmacy compounding less critical, pharmacists compound a significant number of chemotherapeutic agents, intravenous products, radiopharmaceuticals, topical preparations, and tablets and capsules. As long as pharmacists compound within the usual course of their professional practice, they do not need to meet the extensive legal requirements imposed on manufacturers (e.g., current GMP, registration, records and inventories, investigational new drug (IND) applications, clinical trials, patent issues, inspections). To avoid enforcement procedures for failing to register as a manufacturer, a pharmacy does not want to engage in any activity that would cross the line between practicing in the regular course of pharmacy business and manufacturing. The following rules apply.

Pharmacy exemptions

Pharmacies are exempt from registering as manufacturers if they do not manufacture, prepare, propagate, compound, or process drugs or devices for sale other than in the regular course of their business of dispensing or selling drugs or devices at retail (21 USC 360(g)(1)). Generally, state law determines whether a pharmacy falls within this definition. A pharmacy that compounds only in response to legitimate prescriptions issued by authorized prescribers would not need to register as a manufacturer (21 USC 353a(a)).

A pharmacy or other facility that is registered with the FDA as an outsourcing facility under the DQSA is exempt from registering as a manufacturer and is exempt from many of the FDCA requirements that apply to manufacturers.

A pharmacy may not advertise or promote a particular drug that it compounds, but it may advertise and promote the compounding service (21 USC 353a(c)).

A pharmacy that repackages OTC products or in any way changes the container, wrapper, or labeling of these products for resale must register as a manufacturer (21 USC 360(a)(1)). A pharmacy that is in the business of repackaging prescription drug products for sale to other health care providers must register as a manufacturer (21 USC 360(a)(1)).

FDA 2002 Compliance Policy Guide (CPG)

CPG 460.200 Pharmacy Compounding (Reissued 05/29/2002), www.fda.gov/ICECI/Compliance Manuals/CompliancePolicyGuidanceManual/ucm 074398.htm, is obsolete and was withdrawn on December 4, 2013.

Patent issues

Pharmacies that compound drugs that are commercially available run the risk of violating patent rights, in addition to being considered a manufacturer.

Compounding and new drug issues

A drug that has not been approved by the FDA is a *new drug* within the meaning of the FDCA (21 USC 321(p) and 21 CFR 310.3). Drugs compounded by pharmacies fall within the definition of a "new drug" but are exempt from new drug requirements (e.g., IND applications, clinical trials, FDA approval) only if they are compounded in the regular course of pharmacy practice and comply with the prescription labeling requirements discussed previously.

Off-Label Uses of Approved Drugs

Once a drug has been approved by the FDA and introduced into the market, health professionals may find new therapeutic uses of the drug that have not been approved by the FDA and are not included in the drug's product insert. Authorized prescribers may legally prescribe off-label uses of FDA-approved drugs, and pharmacists may legally dispense them, subject to their professional judgment.

Before dispensing a drug for an off-label use, a pharmacist should use professional judgment in determining the risk to the patient, as follows:

- If there is no unreasonable risk to the patient, the pharmacist should dispense the drug.
- If there is an unreasonable risk of harm to the patient, the pharmacist should confirm with the prescriber that the prescription is the proper drug and dosage.
- If there is a significant risk of harm to the patient, the pharmacist may ask the prescriber to justify the prescription.

Manufacturers cannot advertise off-label uses of an approved drug to consumers. However, manufacturers may distribute peer-reviewed research papers that describe off-label uses of their drugs.

A good source for off-label uses of drugs is the AHFS Drug Information database published by the American Society of Health-System Pharmacists (www .ahfsdruginformation.com).

Mailing Medications through the United States Postal Service

The outside packaging of any drugs that are mailed should not have any markings that would indicate the nature of the contents (USPS Publication 52, § 474). In addition, the following restrictions apply to the mailing of drugs through the United States Postal Service (USPS).

Prescription and nonprescription drugs that are not controlled substances may be mailed under the following rules (USPS Publication 52, § 473.2):

- For prescription medicines containing a non-narcotic drug(s), only a pharmacist or medical practitioner who dispenses the medicine may mail such substances to the patients under their care.
- For nonprescription medicines, the mailer must meet all applicable federal, state, or local laws that may apply (such as the PPPA of 1970 and the CPSC requirements).

Poisonous drugs and medicines may be sent only from the manufacturer or dealer to licensed physicians, surgeons, dentists, pharmacists, druggists, cosmetologists, barbers, and veterinarians. Some poisonous drugs are subject to the requirements for mailing hazardous materials (USPS Publication 52, § 473.3).

Controlled substances and drugs containing controlled substances may be mailed under the following rules (USPS Publication 52, § 473.1):

- If the distribution of the controlled substance is illegal under the Controlled Substances Act, it is illegal to mail it.
- For mailable controlled substances, generally both the mailer and the addressee must meet either of the following conditions:
  - Be registered with the Drug Enforcement Administration (DEA)
  - Be exempted from DEA registration, such as military, civil defense, and law enforcement personnel, in performing official duties
- For prescription medicines containing mailable narcotic drugs (controlled substances), only pharmacists or medical practitioners who dispense the medicine may mail such substances to the patients under their care.

42-4. Importation and Exportation

Drugs manufactured in other countries are often much less expensive than drugs manufactured in the United States. Consequently, some U.S. citizens prefer to purchase their medications from other countries, primarily Canada or Mexico. Generally, importing drugs from other countries into the United States is illegal because the FDA either has not approved the drug or has not approved the manufacturer to manufacture the drug. The FDA views this problem as a consumer safety issue because unapproved drugs from unapproved manufacturers are more likely to be adulterated, misbranded, counterfeit, or unsafe. By 2023, the FDA, under the Drug Supply Chain Security Act, will have developed a system to determine at the individual package level where a drug has been in the supply chain. The following general rules apply.

Exportation

When a manufacturer ships drug products from the United States to a foreign country, it is called exportation. Exportation is a legal practice when it is done by the original manufacturer or licensed wholesaler and there is no intention to reimport the drug products.

Importation

When someone brings drug products into the United States that were obtained in a foreign country, it is called importation. As a general rule, importing drugs into the United States from a foreign country is illegal. Personal use exceptions to this rule are discussed later in Chapter 42.

Reimportation

Reimportation describes the situation when the drug products have been manufactured within the United States meeting all FDA requirements, shipped to a foreign country, and then shipped back to the United States. The FDA considers this illegal unless it is done by the original manufacturer for emergency use.

Personal Use Exceptions

If a U.S. resident reenters the United States from a foreign country with drugs obtained in the foreign country, he or she is illegally importing drugs unless one of the following exceptions apply.

Compassionate use policy

Under this policy, the FDA permits the personal importation of small amounts of drugs under the following conditions:

- The drug is not approved for use in this country.
- The drug is used for treatment of a serious condition for which no satisfactory treatment is available in the United States.
- The drug does not pose an unreasonable risk.
- The patient seeking to import the drug must provide the name of a U.S. physician who is treating the patient with the unapproved drug.

Medicare Prescription Drug, Improvement, and Modernization Act of 2003

Provisions in this law permit the Secretary of HHS to allow the wholesale importation of drugs from Canada, but only if the Secretary certifies that the program would pose no additional risk to public health and safety and would significantly reduce prescription drug costs. To date, the Secretary has not certified any such program.

Canadian personal use exemption

This exemption was created by the Department of Homeland Security Appropriations Act of 2007 (PL 109-295). It applies to individual patients who are transporting from Canada into the United States:

- FDA-approved prescription drugs
- On their person
- In a quantity not to exceed a 90-day supply
- That are not a controlled substance or a biological product

Personal use exemption under the Controlled Substances Act

Any individual who has in his or her possession a controlled substance listed in schedules II, III, IV, or V, which he or she has lawfully obtained for his or her personal medical use or for administration to an animal accompanying him or her, may enter or depart the United States with such substance provided the following conditions are met (21 CFR 1301.26):

- The controlled substance is in the original container in which it was dispensed to the individual.
- The individual makes a declaration to an appropriate official of the Bureau of Customs and Border protection stating
  - that the controlled substance is possessed for his or her personal use, or for an animal accompanying him or her.
  - the trade or chemical name and the symbol designating the schedule of the controlled substance if it appears on the container label, or, if such name does not appear on the label, the name and address of the pharmacy or practitioner who dispensed the substance and the prescription number.
- In addition, a U.S. resident may import into the United States no more than 50 dosage units combined of all such controlled substances in the individual's possession that were obtained abroad for personal medical use. This 50-dosage-unit limitation does not apply to controlled substances lawfully obtained in the United States pursuant to a prescription issued by a DEA registrant.

42-5. Regulation of Pharmacy Practice

Omnibus Budget Reconciliation Act of 1990 (OBRA '90)

The Medicaid Prudent Pharmaceutical Purchasing Program provisions of OBRA '90 (PL 101-508) had a tremendous effect on pharmacy law. They mandated national standards of pharmacy practice by requiring states, as a condition for participating in Medicaid, to establish expanded standards of practice for pharmacists. Although the applicable provisions of OBRA '90 specifically applied only to Medicaid patients, most states passed regulations that applied to all patients. The primary purpose of the pharmacy provisions of OBRA '90 was to save the federal government money on the theory that improving the quality of drug therapy would reduce the costs of health care. One of the primary mechanisms for accomplishing this goal is drug use review (DUR), which consists of retrospective review (42 USC 1396r-8(g)(2)(B)), educational programs (42 USC 1396r-8(g)(2)(D)), and prospective review (42 USC 1396r-8(g)(2)(A)).

Retrospective review

This requirement applies to states, not pharmacists. Each state must establish a committee (DUR board) consisting of physicians, pharmacists, and other health care professionals to review the use of drugs over a specified period of time to identify patterns of fraud, abuse, gross overuse, or inappropriate or medically unnecessary care among physicians, pharmacists, and individuals receiving Medicaid benefits, or associated with specific drugs or groups of drugs. The committee may suggest changes to prescribing habits and may initiate educational programs for prescribers and pharmacists.

Educational programs

State DUR boards, either directly or through qualified health care organizations, must provide active and ongoing educational outreach programs to educate practitioners on common drug therapy problems with the aim of improving prescribing or dispensing practices.

Prospective review

Whereas retrospective review occurs after drugs have been dispensed, prospective review occurs at the point of dispensing. It is a comprehensive review of the patient's prescription order before the prescription is dispensed. The process includes screening of prescriptions, patient counseling by the pharmacist, and pharmacist documentation of relevant patient information.

Screening

A pharmacist must conduct a review of drug therapy before each prescription is filled or delivered to a patient or a patient's caregiver, typically at the point of sale or point of distribution (42 USC 1396r–8(g)(2)(A)(i)). The review includes screening for potential drug therapy problems caused by

- Therapeutic duplication
- Drug–disease contraindications
- Drug–drug interactions (including serious interactions with nonprescription or OTC drugs)
- Incorrect drug dosage or duration of drug treatment
- Drug–allergy interactions
- Clinical abuse and misuse

Patient counseling

The pharmacist must offer to counsel each patient or the patient's caregiver who presents a prescription (42 USC 1396r-8(g)(2)(A)(ii)(I)). Counseling must be conducted in person, whenever practicable, or through access to a telephone service that is toll-free for long-distance calls. Counseling should include matters that the pharmacist deems significant about the following:

- The name and description of the medication
- The route, dosage form, dosage, route of administration, and duration of drug therapy
- Special directions and precautions for preparation, administration, and use by the patient
- Common severe side or adverse effects or interactions and therapeutic contraindications that may be encountered, including their avoidance, and the action required if they occur
- Techniques for self-monitoring drug therapy
- Proper storage
- Prescription refill information
- Action to be taken in the event of a missed dose

The law does not require a pharmacist to provide counseling when a patient or patient's caregiver refuses counseling. The pharmacist is not required to verify the offer to provide counseling or a refusal of the offer.

Patient profile

A pharmacist must make a reasonable effort to obtain, record, and maintain, at a minimum, the following information about patients (42 USC 1396r-8(g)(2)(A)(ii)(II)):

- Name, address, telephone number, date of birth (or age), and gender
- Individual history, where significant, including disease state or states, known allergies and drug reactions, and a comprehensive list of medications and relevant devices
- Pharmacist comments relevant to the individual's drug therapy

State law

Because the federal government has no power to directly regulate professional practice, state law is required to implement the OBRA '90 rules. State laws differ, and pharmacists must know the specific state laws and regulations that apply to prospective drug review for their state. A few states limit these rules for patients who receive Medicaid benefits. Most states apply the rules to all patients. Some states mandate counseling only for new prescriptions, while other states also require counseling (or an offer to counsel) for refills. Most states require face-to-face counseling, but a few states do not. Most states mandate patient medication records, but a few states do not.

Health Insurance Portability and Accountability Act (HIPAA)

HIPAA protects a patient's private health information, defined as protected health information (PHI), and imposes penalties on covered entities that make unauthorized disclosures of PHI. Covered entities include health plans, health care clearinghouses, and health care providers that conduct financial or administrative transactions electronically (45 CFR 164.104).

A pharmacy, as a covered entity, is subject to HIPAA, most significantly the privacy and security rules. The privacy rules protect a patient's rights to access their health records, maintain confidentiality of PHI, and authorize its disclosure. The privacy rules also control how, when, and to whom PHI may be disclosed without patient authorization. The security rules protect the confidentiality, integrity, and availability of electronic health information.

The privacy rules cover prescriptions, patient records systems, patient prescription profiles, recorded pharmacist comments relevant to the patient therapy, and payment records.

Notice of privacy practices

An individual has a right to adequate notice of the uses and disclosures of PHI that may be made by the covered entity and of the individual's rights and the covered entity's legal duties with respect to PHI (45 CFR 164.520(a)(1)).

"Notice of Privacy Practices"

Pharmacies must provide a "Notice of Privacy Practices" to each patient on the day the pharmacy first provides service or, in an emergency, as soon as reasonably practicable after the emergency treatment situation (45 CFR 164.520(c)(2)(i)). The notice must include the following (45 CFR 164.520(b)):

- The way the pharmacy intends to use and disclose the PHI
- The legal duties of the pharmacy to protect the confidentiality of the PHI
- A statement of the patient's rights and how the patient can exercise those rights
- An explanation of how the patient may complain of violations and how to file a complaint
- The contact person for dealing with a patient's privacy concerns

If the pharmacy has a Web site, the notice must be posted prominently on the Web site (45 CFR 164.520(c)(3)). The pharmacist may e-mail the notice to the patient, if the patient agrees to the electronic notice (45 CFR 164.520(c)(3)(ii)).

Patient acknowledgment

Except in an emergency treatment situation, a pharmacist must make a good faith effort to obtain from the patient a written acknowledgment of receipt of the "Notice of Privacy Practices" (45 CFR 164.520(c)(2)(ii)).

If the pharmacist cannot obtain the acknowledgment, he or she must document good faith efforts to obtain the acknowledgment and the reason that the acknowledgment was not obtained. A pharmacist may not refuse to treat a patient who refuses to sign the acknowledgment. The patient or the patient's personal representative may sign the acknowledgment.

Retention of documentation

A covered entity must retain copies of the notices issued by the covered entity and, if applicable, any written acknowledgments of receipt of the notice or documentation of good faith efforts to obtain such written acknowledgment for 6 years from the date of its creation or the date when it last was in effect, whichever is later (45 CFR 164.520(e) and 45 CFR 164.530(j)(2)).

General rule

A covered entity cannot use or disclose PHI without written patient authorization unless permitted by law.

Use and disclosure of PHI

Permissible uses and disclosures of PHI without written patient authorization include the following (45 CFR 164.502(a) and 45 CFR 164.506).

Treatment

The term *treatment* means the provision, coordination, or management of health care and related services by one or more health care providers, including the coordination or management of health care by a health care provider with a third party; consultation between health care providers relating to a patient; or the referral of a patient for health care from one health care provider to another (45 CFR 164.501). For a pharmacist, treatment includes dispensing medications, counseling patients, developing and maintaining patient profiles, consulting with a patient's other health care providers, and providing refill reminder services.

Payment

The term *payment* includes submitting claims for reimbursement, determining patient eligibility and extent of coverage, and sending bills to patients (45 CFR 164.501).

Health care operations

For pharmacists, the term *health care operations* includes activities necessary to operate a pharmacy, such as quality assessment, fraud detection, audits, certifications, and business management (45 CFR 164.501).

Other

Other permitted uses and disclosures of PHI without written patient authorization include the following (45 CFR 164.512):

- Disclosures to the patient or to his or her personal representative

- Public health activities (e.g., reporting of communicable disease)
- Judicial and administrative proceedings
- Law enforcement purposes
- Serious threats to health and safety
- Disclosures that are required by law (e.g., child abuse reports)

Minimum necessary standard

When using or disclosing PHI or when requesting PHI from another covered entity, a pharmacy must make reasonable efforts to disclose the minimum necessary amount of PHI to accomplish the intended purpose of the use, disclosure, or request (45 CFR 164.502(b)). This requirement does not apply to

- Disclosures to or requests by a health care provider for treatment
- Uses or disclosures made to the individual patient or his or her personal representative
- Uses or disclosures authorized by the patient or personal representative
- Disclosures made to the Department of HHS for compliance and enforcement purposes
- Uses or disclosures that are required by law

Incidental use and disclosure

PHI that is incidentally disclosed to a permitted use or disclosure is not a violation of HIPAA if reasonable safeguards have been taken to protect the PHI (45 CFR 164.502(a)(1)(iii)). To determine whether a disclosure is incidental, a pharmacy should ask three questions:

- Is there a permissible use?
- Is the disclosure incidental to this permissible use?
- Were appropriate safeguards taken to protect the PHI?

De-identified information

Information that cannot be identified as belonging to any particular individual is not considered individually identifiable health information and is not subject to the HIPAA rules, and it may be used or disclosed without patient authorization (45 CFR 164.502(d)(2)).

Disclosures to business associates

A covered entity may disclose PHI to a business associate and may allow a business associate to create or receive PHI on its behalf, if the covered entity obtains satisfactory assurance that the business associate will appropriately safeguard the information (45 CFR 164.502(e)(1)). A refill reminder service is an example of a business associate of a pharmacy. Under recent law, business associates are now subject to the same penalties for violating HIPAA as a covered entity.

Right of access

With a few exceptions, an individual has a right of access to inspect and obtain a copy of PHI about the individual (45 CFR 164.524).

Right to request amendment

An individual has the right to have a covered entity amend PHI (45 CFR 164.526). A covered entity may deny an individual's request for amendment, if it determines that the PHI was not created by the covered entity or if the PHI is accurate and complete.

Rights of parents and minor children

If a parent or guardian has authority to act on behalf of an unemancipated minor in making decisions related to health care, a covered entity must treat him or her as a personal representative, and the parent or guardian has access to the minor's PHI (45 CFR 164.502(g)(3)). (An unemancipated minor is someone younger than 18 years old who is dependent upon parental support and subject to parental control. The definition depends on state law.) A parent or guardian would not have access to a minor's PHI under the following conditions:

- Under state law, the minor has the right to consent to the health care service.
- A court or another person authorized by law consents to the health care service.
- A parent or guardian agrees to the confidentiality between a covered health care provider and the minor with respect to the health care service.

Written authorization

Other uses and disclosures of PHI that are not for a permissible use or disclosure require written authorization from the patient (45 CFR 164.508).

Written authorizations must be detailed and customized for the particular use or disclosure intended. Blanket authorizations are not permitted.

The authorization must contain an expiration date, although if the authorization is for research, language to the effect that the expiration date is "none" or until "end of research study" is acceptable. The authorization must be signed by the patient, and the patient must receive a copy of the signed authorization.

Uses or disclosures that require a patient's written authorization include the following:

- Marketing
- Research
- Employment applications
- Applications for insurance coverage

Marketing

The term *marketing* (45 CFR 164.501) means to make a communication about a product or service that encourages others to purchase or use the product or service, unless the communication is made for one of the following purposes:

- For description of a health-related product or service of the covered entity
- For treatment of the individual (includes information about general health)
- For case management or care coordination for the individual, or to direct or recommend alternative treatments, therapies, health care providers, or settings of care to the individual. (Note: Pharmacists must beware of taking payment for recommending alternative treatments to patients because this activity could violate the Anti-Kickback Statute.)

Marketing also includes the situation in which a covered entity sells PHI to another entity to enable that entity to communicate information about its own product or service that encourages recipients of the communication to purchase or use that product or service.

It is not marketing and no patient authorization is required if the communication is in the form of a face-to-face communication made by a covered entity to an individual or a promotional gift of nominal value provided by the covered entity (45 CFR 164.508(a)(3)).

If the marketing involves direct or indirect remuneration to the covered entity from a third party, the authorization must state that such remuneration is involved (45 CFR 164.508(a)(3)).

HIPAA policies and procedures

Pharmacies must develop policies and procedures to implement HIPAA privacy standards and identify a privacy officer to oversee the pharmacy's compliance programs. The pharmacy must train its personnel about its HIPAA policies and procedures. A pharmacy must provide and enforce sanctions against an employee who violates the pharmacy's policies and procedures (45 CFR 164.530).

Breach of unsecured PHI

A pharmacy must report breaches of unsecured PHI for breaches occurring on or after September 23, 2009 (45 CFR 164.400–414). Depending on the seriousness of the breach, notifications must be made to the individual (45 CFR 164.404), the media (45 CFR 164.406), and the Secretary of HHS (45 CFR 164.408).

Penalties

- For unintentional violations of HIPAA, a covered entity may be assessed civil penalties of up to $1.5 million in a calendar year (45 CFR 160.404).
- For intentional violations of HIPAA, a person who uses or discloses PHI obtained from a covered entity without authorization may be assessed monetary penalties ranging from $50,000 to $250,000 and sentenced to prison from 1 to 10 years, depending on the seriousness of the violation (42 USC 1320d–6).

Fraud and Abuse Statutes

Medicare and Medicaid Fraud and Abuse Statute

The Part D program requires pharmacies to have a comprehensive program to prevent and correct waste, fraud, and abuse (42 USC 1320a–7b(a)). It is illegal to knowingly make a false statement or representation of a material fact in any application for a benefit or payment. Examples of violations include billing for nonexistent prescriptions, billing for the brand drug when a generic was dispensed, billing for prescriptions that were filled but never picked up, and inappropriate use of dispense-as-written codes.

Anti-Kickback Statute

This statute prohibits anyone from knowingly and willfully soliciting, receiving, offering, or paying any remuneration in exchange for inducing referrals or furnishing any goods or services paid for by Medicare or Medicaid (42 USC 1320a–7b(b)).

Violation of this statute is a felony, punishable by a maximum fine of $25,000 per violation, 5 years' imprisonment, or both. An example of a violation would be a pharmaceutical company that pays a pharmacist to recommend its product as an alternative treatment instead of the one prescribed by the physician.

False Claims Act

This statute prohibits a person from knowingly presenting a false or fraudulent claim to the federal government for payment (31 USC 3729). It also prohibits making or using a false record or statement to get a false claim submitted to the federal government paid or approved. Violation of this law results in the imposition of civil monetary penalties.

Federal Antitrust Laws

Antitrust law prevents individual competitors from entering into agreements that reduce competition and adversely affect the consumers' interest in cost containment. For example, if two pharmacies agree not to underprice the other, it is considered price fixing and a violation of the antitrust laws because it deprives the consumer of the benefits of competition.

42-6. The Closed System of Controlled Substance Distribution

The Comprehensive Drug Abuse Prevention and Control Act (DEA Web site, www.deadiversion.usdoj.gov/21cfr/21usc/index.html), more commonly known as the Controlled Substances Act (CSA), establishes a "closed system" for distribution of drugs that are *controlled substances*. The term *closed system* means that only those persons or entities registered with the DEA may legally engage in manufacturing, distributing, and dispensing of controlled substances.

State versus Federal Authority

Controlled substances may be regulated under both federal and state law. Although federal law does not preempt state law in the regulation of controlled substances, state law cannot conflict with federal law. Generally, the following rules apply in deter-mining whether federal or state law applies to a given situation:

- If a person can comply with one law without violating the other law, the person must comply with the stricter law. For example, if state law prohibits the use of certain drugs for weight control, but federal law has no such prohibition, state law should be followed because it is the stricter law and it does not violate federal law to comply with the state law.
- If a person cannot comply with one law without violating the other law, the person must comply with federal law. For example, if state law legalizes a drug that is a schedule I drug under federal law, a person cannot comply with state law without violating federal law. A positive conflict exists between federal and state law, and federal law must be followed.

Classification of Controlled Substances

Five schedules of controlled substances are currently established (21 USC 812).

Schedule I

- The drug or other substance has a high potential for abuse.
- The drug or other substance has no currently accepted medical use in treatment in the United States.
- There is a lack of accepted safety for use of the drug or other substance under medical supervision.

Schedule II

- The drug or other substance has a high potential for abuse.
- The drug or other substance has a currently accepted medical use in treatment in the United States or a currently accepted medical use with severe restrictions.
- Abuse of the drug or other substances may lead to severe psychological or physical dependence.

Schedule III

- The drug or other substance has a potential for abuse less than the drugs or other substances in schedules I and II.
- The drug or other substance has a currently accepted medical use in treatment in the United States.

■ Abuse of the drug or other substance may lead to moderate or low physical dependence or high psychological dependence.

Schedule IV

■ The drug or other substance has a low potential for abuse relative to the drugs or other substances in schedule III.
■ The drug or other substance has a currently accepted medical use in treatment in the United States.
■ Abuse of the drug or other substance may lead to limited physical or psychological dependence relative to the drugs or other substances in schedule III.

Schedule V

■ The drug or other substance has a low potential for abuse relative to the drugs or other substances in schedule IV.
■ The drug or other substance has a currently accepted medical use in treatment in the United States.
■ Abuse of the drug or other substance may lead to limited physical or psychological dependence relative to the drugs or other substances in schedule IV.

Scheduled Listed Chemical Products

To fight the illegal manufacture and use of methamphetamine, Congress created a new category of drugs under the CSA: "scheduled listed chemical products." The law regulates OTC sales of any product containing ephedrine, pseudoephedrine, or phenylpropanolamine, which are precursor chemicals to the manufacture of methamphetamine. The rules regulating OTC sales of these drugs are discussed later in Chapter 42.

Authority for Scheduling

The U.S. Attorney General has the authority to add a drug to a schedule, transfer a drug between schedules, and remove a drug from a schedule (21 USC 811). Before adding, transferring, or removing a drug, the Attorney General must request a scientific and medical evaluation from the Secretary of HHS. The Attorney General is bound by the recommendation of the Secretary.

In cases in which the Attorney General finds that the scheduling of a substance in schedule I is necessary to avoid an imminent hazard to the public safety, the Attorney General may by order, on a temporary basis and without regard to the requirements of obtaining a recommendation from the Secretary of HHS, schedule the substance in schedule I.

This section also allows exclusion of a nonnarcotic substance from a schedule if the substance may be lawfully sold, under the FDCA, without a prescription.

Manufacturing, Packaging, and Labeling

Every commercial container of a controlled substance (except for nonnarcotic controlled substances that have been exempted by application (21 CFR 1308.31)) must have printed on the label a symbol designating the schedule in which it is listed (21 CFR 1302.03). The word *schedule* need not be used. For example, the symbol for a schedule III drug would be either CIII or C-III. If the commercial container is too small to accommodate a label, the symbol is not required as long as the symbol is printed on the box or package from which the container is removed when dispensing to an ultimate user. The symbol is not required on a commercial container or its labeling if the controlled substance is being used in clinical research involving blind or double-blind studies.

The label of a drug listed in schedule II, III, or IV shall, when dispensed to or for a patient, contain a clear, concise warning that it is a crime to transfer the drug to any person other than the patient (21 USC 825(c)).

Registration

General requirements

Every person who manufactures or distributes any controlled substance or list I chemical, or who proposes to engage in the manufacture or distribution of any controlled substance or list I chemical, must register annually with the Attorney General (DEA registration) (21 USC 822).

Every person who dispenses, or who proposes to dispense, any controlled substance, must register with the Attorney General every 3 years. (Note: The term *dispense* for these purposes includes the act of prescribing controlled substances.)

Registered persons are authorized to possess, manufacture, distribute, or dispense such substances or chemicals (including any such activity in the conduct of research) only to the extent authorized by their registration.

Activities considered "coincident" to the registration are also permitted.

Registration as a dispenser allows a registrant to engage in the following activities as coincident to his or her registration (21 CFR 1301.13(e)):

- A registered dispenser may conduct research and instructional activities with those substances for which registration was granted, except that a midlevel practitioner may conduct such research only to the extent expressly authorized under state statute.
- A pharmacist may manufacture an aqueous or oleaginous solution or solid dosage form containing a narcotic controlled substance in schedules II–V in a proportion not exceeding 20% of the complete solution, compound, or mixture. (Note: Even though the pharmacy would not have to register under the CSA as a manufacturer in this scenario, the pharmacy may need to register as a manufacturer under the FDCA. State law also needs to be considered.)
- A retail pharmacy may perform central fill pharmacy activities.

Any person who engages in more than one group of independent activities must obtain a separate registration for each group of activities (e.g., dispensing, distributing, or manufacturing) (21 CFR 1301.13).

A separate registration is required for each principal place of business or professional practice at one general physical location where controlled substances are manufactured, distributed, imported, exported, or dispensed by a person (21 CFR 1301.12). This rule excludes the following places:

- Warehouses where controlled substances are stored but not distributed
- An office used by agents for sales, but not to store or distribute controlled substances
- An office used by a practitioner (who is registered at another location) to prescribe, but not to store, administer, or dispense controlled substances
- Freight-forwarding facilities

The certificate of registration must be conspicuously displayed at a pharmacy or other location registered with the DEA.

Registration of online pharmacies (Ryan Haight Online Pharmacy Consumer Protection Act of 2008)

An online pharmacy must first be registered with the DEA as a pharmacy. After it is registered as a phar-

macy, the online pharmacy must apply for a modification of registration to operate as an online pharmacy.

The term *online pharmacy* means a person, entity, or Internet site, whether in the United States or abroad, that knowingly or intentionally delivers, distributes, or dispenses, or offers or attempts to deliver, distribute, or dispense, a controlled substance by means of the Internet (21 USC 802(52)).

A pharmacy Web site is exempted from the definition of an *online pharmacy* if its Internet-related activity regarding controlled substances is limited to filling new prescriptions for controlled substances in schedules III, IV, or V; refilling those prescriptions; or both (21 USC 802(52), (55), (56)). For this purpose, filling new prescriptions means that the pharmacy has previously dispensed the controlled substance to the patient by means other than the Internet and pursuant to a valid prescription issued by an authorized prescriber. The pharmacy has contacted the prescriber who issued the original prescription at the request of the patient to determine if the prescriber will authorize the issuance of a new prescription after determining that there is a legitimate medical purpose for the issuance of the new prescription. If the pharmacy is exempted from the definition, it is not required to obtain a modification of its registration authorizing it to operate as an online pharmacy.

Registration of Opioid Treatment Programs

Practitioners who dispense narcotic drugs to individuals for maintenance treatment or detoxification treatment must obtain annually a separate registration for that purpose (21 USC 823(g)). This registration is in addition to DEA registration as a dispenser.

This additional registration requirement is waived for practitioners who qualify under the Drug Addiction Treatment Act (DATA) to treat addiction in an office-based practice (21 USC 823(g)(2)).

A registered practitioner who qualifies under DATA may dispense and prescribe narcotic drugs in schedules III, IV, or V. Before the initial dispensing of narcotic drugs in schedules III, IV, or V to patients for maintenance or detoxification treatment, the practitioner must submit to the Secretary of HHS a notification of the intent of the practitioner to begin dispensing the drugs for such purpose. The notification must contain the following certifications by the practitioner:

- The practitioner is a qualifying physician (e.g., holds a subspecialty certification in the treatment of addiction) (21 USC 823(g)(2)(G)).

- The practitioner has the capacity to refer the patients for appropriate counseling and other appropriate ancillary services.
- The total number of such patients of the practitioner at any one time will not exceed 30 for the first year. After the first year, the practitioner may submit a second application to treat up to 100 patients with approval of the Secretary.

Within 45 days of receiving the notification, the Secretary determines whether the applicant meets the requirements under DATA. If so, the Attorney General assigns an identification number to the practitioner that is included in his or her registration as a dispenser.

If the Secretary fails to determine whether the applicant qualifies under DATA within the 45-day period, the Attorney General must assign the applicant an identification number.

The practitioner may begin to prescribe or dispense the FDA-approved narcotic drugs for such purposes prior to the expiration of the 45-day period if it facilitates the treatment of an individual patient and the practitioner notifies both the Secretary and the Attorney General of the intent to begin prescribing or dispensing the FDA-approved narcotic drugs (21 USC 823(g)(2)(E)(ii)(I)).

Exceptions to the registration requirements

The following persons are not required to register individually with the DEA (21 USC 822(c)):

- An agent or employee of any registered manufacturer, distributor, or dispenser of any controlled substance or list I chemical if such agent or employee is acting in the usual course of his or her business or employment. The registered facility must assign identification numbers for each employee or agent who handles or prescribes controlled substances using the facility's DEA number.
  - For example, a pharmacist who is employed by a registered pharmacy does not need to apply for an individual DEA registration.
  - For example, a physician employee of a hospital may issue prescriptions for controlled substances using the hospital's DEA registration number and prescription forms. He or she must add his or her assigned hospital internal code number and must stamp, type, or handprint her name on each prescription issued (21 CFR 1306.05(g)).

- A common or contract carrier or warehouseman, or an employee thereof, whose possession of the controlled substance or list I chemical is in the usual course of his or her business or employment. For example, FedEx does not need to register with the DEA before shipping a controlled substance.
- An ultimate user who lawfully possesses the controlled substance.

(Note: Individual states may require registration under state law that does not exempt agents or employees of registered entities, and the individual practitioner must register under state law, even if he or she is exempt from DEA registration under federal law.)

Denial, revocation, or suspension of a registration

The Attorney General may deny, revoke, or suspend a registration. A suspension or revocation may be limited to a particular schedule or schedules.

Generally, the Attorney General issues an order to show why the registration should not be revoked or suspended. The registration can be revoked simultaneously with initiation of proceedings (issuing an order to show cause) if an imminent danger exists to public health or safety.

The Attorney General may suspend or revoke a registration to manufacture, distribute, or dispense upon finding that the registrant

- Has materially falsified any application required to be filed under the CSA
- Has been convicted of a felony under any law of the United States, or of any state, relating to any substance defined as a controlled substance or a list I chemical
- Has had his or her state license or registration suspended, revoked, or denied by competent state authority and is no longer authorized by state law to engage in the manufacturing, distribution, or dispensing of controlled substances or list I chemicals or has had the suspension, revocation, or denial of his or her registration recommended by competent state authority
- Has committed such acts as would render his or her registration inconsistent with the public interest
- Has been excluded (or directed to be excluded) from participation in a state or federal health care plan (such as Medicare or Medicaid) as a result of submitting false claims to the federal government for reimbursement

Inventories

General requirements

A registrant is required to make an initial inventory as soon as the registrant first engages in the manufacture, distribution, or dispensing of controlled substances (21 USC 827).

Every registrant must maintain a complete and accurate record of each controlled substance received, sold, delivered, or otherwise disposed of (although a perpetual inventory is not required).

Each inventory must contain a complete and accurate record of all controlled substances on hand on the date the inventory is taken (21 CFR 1304.11). Controlled substances are *on hand* if they are in the possession of or under the control of the registrant, including substances returned by a customer, ordered by a customer but not yet invoiced, stored in a warehouse on behalf of the registrant, and in the possession of employees of the registrant and intended for distribution as complimentary samples.

A separate inventory must be taken for each registered location and each independent activity registered.

The registrant must take an inventory every 2 years. After the initial inventory, the biennial inventory may be prepared on the registrant's general inventory date as long as this date is within 6 months of the biennial inventory date that would otherwise apply. For example, assume that the initial inventory date for controlled substances is April 1, 2012, and the registrant's usual inventory date is on December 31 of each year. The biennial inventory date for controlled substances would be April 1, 2014. However, the registrant could prepare this inventory during its usual inventory date of December 31, 2013 (within 6 months of the biennial inventory date.) The registrant could not wait until its regular inventory date of December 31, 2014, to prepare the biennial inventory for controlled substances because it would be outside the 6-month window.

An inventory for a newly scheduled drug must be taken on the effective date of the regulation that makes it a controlled substance.

All records required by law must be maintained separately from all other records of the registrant, or alternatively, in the case of nonnarcotic controlled substances, the information must be readily retrievable from ordinary business records.

Inventories must be kept and be available for at least 2 years for inspection and copying by authorized personnel.

The inventory requirements do not apply to the following situations:

- Prescribing of controlled substances in schedule II, III, IV, or V by practitioners acting in the lawful course of their professional practice unless such substance is prescribed in the course of maintenance or detoxification treatment of an individual
- Administering of a controlled substance in schedule II, III, IV, or V unless the practitioner regularly engages in the dispensing or administering of controlled substances and charges his or her patients, either separately or together with charges for other professional services, for substances so dispensed or administered or unless such substance is administered in the course of maintenance treatment or detoxification treatment of an individual
- Use of controlled substances at registered establishments that qualify for a drug research exemption
- Use of controlled substances at registered establishments that keep records with respect to such substances in preclinical research or in teaching
- Any exemption granted to any person by the Attorney General upon a finding that the record requirement is not necessary for carrying out the purposes of the law

Inventorying open containers

In determining the number of units of each finished form of a controlled substance in a commercial container that has been opened, the dispenser must inventory the substances as follows (21 CFR 1304.11(e)(3)):

- If the substance is listed in schedule I or II, the registrant must make an exact count or measure of the contents.
- If the substance is listed in schedule III, IV, or V, the registrant may make an estimated count or measure of the contents, unless the container holds more than 1,000 tablets or capsules, in which case he or she must make an exact count of the contents. (Note: An estimated count of an open bottle should be consistent with the records of dispersal, such as the amount of the substance that has been dispensed pursuant to legitimate prescription orders.)

Periodic reports

The Attorney General may require certain registrants to make periodic reports of sales, deliveries, or any other disposal of a controlled substance:

- Manufacturers of any controlled substance
- Distributors of narcotic controlled substances: the report must include the registration number of the person or entity to whom the sale, delivery, or other disposal was made
- Pharmacies that dispense controlled substances by means of the Internet: They must report the total quantity of each controlled substance that the pharmacy has dispensed each month. No reporting is required unless the pharmacy has met one of the following thresholds in the month for which the reporting is required:
  - 100 or more prescriptions have been dispensed.
  - 5,000 or more dosage units of all controlled substances combined have been dispensed.

If an online pharmacy does not meet the reporting thresholds for a reporting period, it must file a report stating that it did not meet the reporting thresholds.

Ordering Controlled Substances

DEA Form 222

Procedures governing the issuance, use, and preservation of orders for schedule I and II controlled substances are set forth generally by 21 USC 828 and specifically by 21 CFR Part 1305. It is unlawful to distribute a schedule I or II drug except pursuant to a written order on DEA Form 222 or pursuant to the Controlled Substance Ordering System (CSOS) (21 CFR 1305.21), with the following exceptions:

- Lawful exportation
- Delivery to a common carrier in the lawful and usual course of business, or to or by a warehouseman for storage in the lawful and usual course of business

Executed DEA Form 222 must be kept for at least 2 years for inspection and copying by authorized agents. DEA Form 222 is available through the Attorney General.

Only registrants may use DEA Form 222 to order controlled substances in schedule I (for approved research) or schedule II (21 CFR 1305.04).

A registrant may authorize one or more individuals, whether or not located at his or her registered location, to issue orders for schedule I and II controlled substances on the registrant's behalf by executing a power of attorney for each individual (21 CFR 1305.05) with the following conditions:

- The power of attorney must be retained in the files, with executed DEA Form 222 bearing the signature of the attorney.
- The power of attorney must be available for inspection together with other order records.
- A registrant may revoke any power of attorney at any time by executing a notice of revocation.
- A registrant that grants power of attorney must report to the DEA Certification Authority within 6 hours of either of the following (advance notice may be provided, where applicable) (21 CFR 1311.45):
  - The person with power of attorney has left the employ of the institution.
  - The person with power of attorney has had his or her privileges revoked.
- A registrant must maintain a record that lists each person who has been granted power of attorney to sign controlled substances orders.

A registrant obtains DEA Form 222 by submitting an order form requisition with his or her application for DEA registration (DEA Form 222a). To obtain forms subsequently, the registrant must request them in writing from the local DEA office (21 CFR 1305.11).

The purchaser must prepare and execute all three copies of each DEA Form 222 simultaneously, using a typewriter, pen, or indelible pencil (21 CFR 1305.12). The purchaser retains copy 3 and sends copies 1 and 2 to the supplier. The supplier retains copy 1 and sends copy 2 to the DEA. The DEA retains copy 2 (21 CFR 1305.13).

When the purchaser receives the order, he or she must record on copy 3 the number of containers received of each item and the date received. There are 10 numbered lines on each DEA Form 222, and only one item may be entered on each line (multiple units of each item may be ordered).

Order forms for carfentanil, etorphine hydrochloride, and diprenorphine must contain only these substances (21 CFR 1305.12(b)).

A DEA Form 222 may not be filled if the order is not complete; legible; or properly prepared, executed, or endorsed. It may not be filled if the order shows any alteration, erasure, or change of any description (21 CFR 1305.15).

Executed order forms must be maintained separately from all other records and retained by the purchaser and supplier for at least 2 years at the registered location printed on the form (21 CFR 1305.17).

Controlled Substance Ordering System (CSOS)

The CSOS is the electronic equivalent to DEA Form 222 (21 CFR 1305.21).

General requirements

A registrant may use the CSOS to purchase controlled substances listed in schedule I (for approved research), II, III, IV, or V, and may also use it to order noncontrolled substances (21 CFR 1305.21(c)).

Before filling an order submitted via the CSOS, the supplier must do the following:

- Verify the integrity of the signature and the order by using software that complies with Part 1311 of chapter 11 of title 21 to validate the order.
- Verify that the digital certificate has not expired.
- Check the validity of the certificate holder's certificate by checking the Certificate Revocation List. The supplier may cache the Certificate Revocation List until it expires.
- Verify the registrant's eligibility to order the controlled substances by checking the certificate extension data.

A supplier may not endorse an electronic order to another supplier to fill (21 CFR 1305.23). A written DEA Form 222 may be endorsed to another supplier if the original supplier cannot fill the order.

A supplier may not fill an electronic order if the required data fields have not been completed; the order is not signed using a digital certificate issued by the DEA; the digital certificate used has expired or has been revoked prior to signature; the purchaser's public key will not validate the digital signature; or the validation of the order shows that the order is invalid for any reason (21 CFR 1305.25).

Preservation of electronic records

A purchaser must, for each order filled, retain the original signed order and all linked records for that order for 2 years (21 CFR 1305.27). The purchaser must also retain all copies of each unaccepted or defective order and each linked statement.

A supplier must retain each original order filled and the linked records for 2 years.

If electronic order records are maintained on a central server, the records must be readily retrievable at the registered location.

A supplier must, for each electronic order filled, forward either a copy of the electronic order or an electronic report of the order to the DEA within 2 business days (21 CFR 1305.29).

Security Requirements

Registrants must provide effective controls and procedures to guard against theft and diversion of controlled substances (21 CFR 1301.71). The extent of the security required depends on whether the registrant is a practitioner (e.g., pharmacy, physician) or nonpractitioner (e.g., manufacturer, distributor). More stringent controls are placed on nonpractitioners.

Physical security controls for practitioners

- Controlled substances listed in schedule I must be stored in a securely locked, substantially constructed cabinet (21 CFR 1301.75).
- Controlled substances listed in schedules II, III, IV, and V must be stored in a securely locked, substantially constructed cabinet. However, pharmacies and institutional practitioners may disperse such substances throughout the stock of noncontrolled substances in such a manner as to obstruct the theft or diversion of the controlled substances.
- This rule also applies to nonpractitioners authorized to conduct research or chemical analysis under another registration.
- Carfentanil, etorphine hydrochloride, and diprenorphine must be stored in a safe or steel cabinet equivalent to a U.S. government Class V security container.

Other security controls for practitioners

- The registrant shall not employ any person who has access to controlled substances, and who has been convicted of a felony offense relating to controlled substances or who, at any time, had an application for registration with the DEA denied, or had a registration revoked or surrendered for cause (21 CFR 1301.76).
- The registrant must notify the local DEA, in writing, of the theft or significant loss of any controlled substances within 1 business day of discovery of such loss or theft. The registrant must complete and submit DEA Form 106 regarding the loss or theft.
- Central fill pharmacies, when selecting private, common, or contract carriers to transport filled prescriptions to a retail pharmacy for delivery to the ultimate user, must select carriers that provide adequate security to guard against in-transit losses. When central fill pharmacies contract

with private, common, or contract carriers to transport filled prescriptions to a retail pharmacy, the central fill pharmacy is responsible for reporting in-transit losses upon discovery of such loss by use of DEA Form 106.

- Retail pharmacies, when selecting private, common, or contract carriers to retrieve filled prescriptions from a central fill pharmacy, must select carriers that provide adequate security to guard against in-transit losses. When retail pharmacies contract with private, common, or contract carriers to retrieve filled prescriptions from a central fill pharmacy, the retail pharmacy is responsible for reporting in-transit losses upon discovery of such loss by use of DEA Form 106.
- The registrant must take precautions (e.g., ensuring that shipping containers do not indicate that contents are controlled substances) to guard against storage or in-transit losses (21 CFR 1301.74(e)).

Offenses and Penalties

Violations of the CSA carry severe penalties, including heavy fines and imprisonment.

Prohibited acts A

Except as authorized by the CSA, it is unlawful for any person knowingly or intentionally (21 USC 841)

- To manufacture, distribute, or dispense, or possess with intent to manufacture, distribute, or dispense, a controlled substance
- To create, distribute, or dispense, or possess with intent to distribute or dispense, a counterfeit substance

Note that this section makes everything involving a controlled substance illegal unless it is specifically authorized by law. Also note that this section applies to any person—not just registrants.

Penalties for prohibited acts A

Depending on the amount of illegal drugs involved, a person who is convicted of committing an act under this section will be sentenced to a term of imprisonment that may be at least 5 but not more than 40 years (21 USC 841(b)). If death or serious bodily injury results from the use of such substance, the term of imprisonment shall be at least 20 years or more than life. A fine of up to $2,000,000 may also be imposed if the defendant is an individual or

up to $5,000,000 if the defendant is other than an individual. Subsequent offenses incur more serious penalties.

Prohibited acts B

It is unlawful (21 USC 842) for any person

- Who is subject to the registration requirements to distribute or dispense a controlled substance in violation of the prescription requirements
- Who is a registrant to manufacture, distribute, or dispense a controlled substance not authorized by his or her registration
- Who is a registrant to distribute a controlled substance in violation of the packaging and labeling requirements
- To remove, alter, or obliterate a symbol or label required by the packaging and labeling requirements
- To refuse or negligently fail to make, keep, or furnish any record, report, notification, declaration, order or order form, statement, invoice, or information required by law
- To refuse any entry into any premises or inspection authorized by this subchapter or subchapter ii of chapter 13 of title 21
- To remove, break, injure, or deface a seal placed on controlled substances because of the suspension or revocation of a registration or because of forfeiture or to remove or dispose of substances so placed under seal
- To use, to his or her own advantage, or to reveal any information acquired in the course of an inspection authorized by this subchapter concerning any method or process that is a trade secret or is otherwise confidential, unless the disclosure is authorized by law
- Who is a regulated person to engage in a regulated transaction without obtaining the purchaser's identification
- Negligently to fail to keep a record or make a report required for transactions involving listed chemicals
- To distribute a laboratory supply to a person who uses, or attempts to use, that laboratory supply to illegally manufacture a controlled substance or a listed chemical, with reckless disregard for the illegal uses to which such a laboratory supply will be put
- Who is a regulated seller
  - To sell at retail a scheduled listed chemical product in excess of 3.6 grams per day per purchaser, knowing at the time of the transaction

(independent of consulting the logbook) that the transaction is a violation

- To knowingly or recklessly sell at retail such a product in nonliquid form (including gel caps) that is not in blister packs (each blister pack containing not more than two doses) or, if blister packs are not feasible, in unit dose packets or pouches
- To knowingly or recklessly sell at retail a scheduled listed chemical product in violation of the requirements for behind-the-counter access, maintenance of a logbook, and personnel training

■ Who is a regulated seller or an employee or agent of such seller to disclose confidential information maintained in logbooks, or to refuse to provide such a logbook to federal, state, or local law enforcement authorities

■ Who is a registrant to manufacture a controlled substance in schedule I or II; ephedrine, pseudoephedrine, or phenylpropanolamine; or any of the salts, optical isomers, or salts of optical isomers of such chemical, which is one of the following:

- Not expressly authorized by his or her registration and by a quota assigned to him or her
- In excess of a quota assigned to him or her

Penalties for prohibited acts B

Any person who violates this section shall be subject to a civil penalty of not more than $25,000, except the penalty for negligently keeping records (violations of 21 USC 842(a)(5) and (10)) is $10,000 (section (c)).

Prohibited acts C

It is unlawful (21 USC 843) for any person knowingly or intentionally

■ Who is a registrant to distribute a controlled substance classified in schedule I or II in the course of his or her legitimate business, except pursuant to DEA Form 222.

■ To use a registration number that is fictitious, revoked, suspended, expired, or issued to another person

■ To acquire or obtain possession of a controlled substance by misrepresentation, fraud, forgery, deception, or subterfuge

■ To furnish false or fraudulent material information in, or omit any material information from, any application, report, record, or other document required by law to be made, kept, or filed, or to present false or fraudulent identification

where the person is receiving or purchasing a listed chemical and the person is required to present identification

■ To make, distribute, or possess any punch, die, plate, stone, or other thing designed to print, imprint, or reproduce the trademark, trade name, or other identifying mark, imprint, or device of another or any likeness of any of the foregoing upon any drug or container or labeling thereof so as to render such drug a counterfeit substance

■ To possess any three-neck round-bottom flask, tableting machine, encapsulating machine, or gelatin capsule, or any equipment, chemical, product, or material that may be used to manufacture a controlled substance or listed chemical, knowing, intending, or having reasonable cause to believe that it will be used to manufacture a controlled substance or listed chemical in violation of this subchapter or subchapter II of chapter 13 of title 21

■ To manufacture, distribute, export, or import any three-neck round-bottom flask, tableting machine, encapsulating machine, or gelatin capsule, or any equipment, chemical, product, or material that may be used to manufacture a controlled substance or listed chemical, knowing, intending, or having reasonable cause to believe that it will be used to manufacture a controlled substance or listed chemical in violation of this subchapter or subchapter II of chapter 13 of title 21 or, in the case of an exportation, in violation of this subchapter or subchapter II of chapter 13 of title 21 or of the laws of the country to which it is exported

■ To create a chemical mixture for the purpose of evading a requirement regarding listed chemicals or to receive a chemical mixture created for that purpose

■ To distribute, import, or export a list I chemical without the registration required by law

■ To place in any newspaper, magazine, handbill, or other publications any written advertisement knowing that it has the purpose of seeking or offering illegally to receive, buy, or distribute a schedule I controlled substance

Penalties for prohibited acts C

Any person who violates this section shall be sentenced to imprisonment for a term of not more than 4 years (not more than 8 years if there are prior offenses) (21 USC 843(d)).

Any person with the intent to manufacture or facilitate the manufacture of methamphetamine violates paragraphs regarding three-neck round-bottom flasks and shall be sentenced to a term of imprisonment of not more than 10 years (not more than 20 years if there are prior offenses).

In addition, fines may be assessed, and the person convicted may be enjoined from engaging in any transaction involving a listed chemical for not more than 10 years.

Penalties for simple possession

Possession by any person (including a registrant) of a controlled substance or listed chemical is unlawful unless allowed under the CSA (21 USC 844).

It is unlawful for any person knowingly or intentionally to possess a controlled substance unless such substance was obtained directly, or pursuant to a valid prescription or order, from a practitioner, while acting in the course of his or her professional practice, or except as otherwise authorized by law.

It is unlawful for any person knowingly or intentionally to possess any list I chemical obtained pursuant to or under authority of a registration issued to that person if that registration has been revoked or suspended, if that registration has expired, or if the registrant has ceased to do business in the manner contemplated by his or her registration.

It is unlawful for any person to knowingly or intentionally purchase at retail during a 30-day period more than 9 grams of ephedrine base, pseudoephedrine base, or phenylpropanolamine base in a scheduled listed chemical product, except that, of such 9 grams, not more than 7.5 grams may be imported by means of shipping through any private or commercial carrier or the USPS.

Any person who violates this subsection may be sentenced to a term of imprisonment of not more than 1 year and shall be fined a minimum of $1,000, or both. For a second offense, he or she shall be sentenced to a term of imprisonment for at least 15 days but not more than 2 years and shall be fined a minimum of $2,500. For third and subsequent offenses, he or she shall be sentenced to a term of imprisonment for at least 90 days but not more than 3 years and shall be fined a minimum of $5,000.

A person convicted under this subsection for the possession of a mixture or substance that contains cocaine base shall be imprisoned at least 5 but not more than 20 years and fined a minimum of $1,000. The severity of the penalty depends on the amount of cocaine in the possession of the individual and whether he or she has prior convictions.

Any person convicted under this subsection for the possession of flunitrazepam shall be imprisoned for not more than 3 years, shall be fined as otherwise provided in this section, or both.

The imposition or execution of a minimum sentence required to be imposed under this subsection shall not be suspended or deferred. Further, upon conviction, a person who violates this subsection shall be fined the reasonable costs of the investigation and prosecution of the offense, unless the court determines that the defendant lacks the ability to pay.

As used in this section, the term *drug, narcotic, or chemical offense* means any offense that proscribes the possession, distribution, manufacture, cultivation, sale, transfer, or the attempt or conspiracy to possess, distribute, manufacture, cultivate, sell, or transfer any substance the possession of which is prohibited under this subchapter.

Civil penalty for possession of small amounts of certain controlled substances

This section provides penalties for any person (including a registrant) for unlawful possession of *personal use amounts*, as specified by the Attorney General by regulation (21 USC 844a) as follows:

- Any individual who knowingly possesses a controlled substance in an amount that, as specified by regulation of the Attorney General, is a personal use amount shall be liable to the United States for a civil penalty in an amount not to exceed $10,000 for each such violation.
- The income and net assets of an individual shall not be relevant to the determination whether to assess a civil penalty under this section or to prosecute the individual criminally.
- However, in determining the amount of a penalty under this section, the income and net assets of an individual shall be considered.
- A civil penalty may not be assessed under this section if the individual previously was convicted of a federal or state offense relating to a controlled substance. A civil penalty may not be assessed on an individual under this section on more than two separate occasions.

Criminal forfeitures

Persons convicted of controlled substance offenses punishable by imprisonment for more than 1 year shall forfeit to the United States all real and personal property constituting or derived from any proceeds the person obtained, directly or indirectly, as the result of the offense and any of the person's property used, or intended to be used, in any manner or part, to commit or to facilitate the commission of the offense (21 USC 853). The following property is subject to forfeiture to the United States (21 USC 881):

- All controlled substances that have been manufactured, distributed, dispensed, or acquired in violation of the law
- All raw materials, products, and equipment of any kind that are used, or intended for use, in manufacturing, compounding, processing, delivering, importing, or exporting any controlled substance or listed chemical in violation of this subchapter
- All property that is used, or intended for use, as a container for property described in paragraph (a), (b), or (i)
- All conveyances, including aircraft, vehicles, or vessels, that are used, or are intended for use, to transport, or in any manner to facilitate the transportation, sale, receipt, possession, or concealment of property described in paragraph (a), (b), or (i)
- All books, records, and research, including formulas, microfilm, tapes, and data that are used, or intended for use, in violation of this subchapter
- All moneys, negotiable instruments, securities, or other things of value furnished or intended to be furnished by any person in exchange for a controlled substance or listed chemical in violation of this subchapter, all proceeds traceable to such an exchange, and all moneys, negotiable instruments, and securities used or intended to be used to facilitate any violation of this subchapter
- All real property, including any right, title, and interest (including any leasehold interest) in the whole of any lot or tract of land and any appurtenances or improvements that is used, or intended to be used, in any manner or part to commit, or to facilitate the commission of, a violation of this subchapter punishable by more than 1 year's imprisonment
- All controlled substances that have been possessed in violation of the law
- All listed chemicals, all drug manufacturing equipment, all tableting machines, all encapsulating machines, and all gelatin capsules that have been imported, exported, manufactured, possessed, distributed, dispensed, acquired, or intended to be distributed, dispensed, acquired, imported, or exported, in violation of the law
- Any drug paraphernalia
- Any firearm used or intended to be used to facilitate the transportation, sale, receipt, possession, or concealment of property described in paragraph (a) or (b) and any proceeds traceable to such property

Pharmacy Inspections

Inspector

A DEA inspector is authorized to enter a pharmacy (controlled premises) to conduct an administrative inspection under the following circumstances (21 USC 880):

- The inspector must state his or her purpose and present to the owner, operator, or agent in charge of the premises appropriate credentials and written notice of his or her inspection authority (an administrative inspection warrant [AIW]).
- The inspector has the right
  - To inspect and copy records, reports, and other documents required to be kept or made under this subchapter
  - To inspect, within reasonable limits and in a reasonable manner, controlled premises and all pertinent equipment, finished and unfinished drugs, listed chemicals, and other substances or materials, containers, and labeling found therein, and all relevant records, files, papers, processes, controls, and facilities
  - To inventory any stock of any controlled substance or listed chemical and obtain samples of any such substance or chemical

Limits on the inspector's authority

Unless the owner, operator, or agent in charge consents in writing, the inspector is not authorized to inspect financial data, sales data other than shipment data, or pricing data (21 USC 880(b)(3)).

Warrants

An AIW is issued by a federal judge upon a showing of probable cause. For these purposes, the term *probable cause* means a valid public interest (21 USC 880(d)(1)). The warrant must be served during normal business hours (21 USC 880(d)(2)). (Note: The requirements for obtaining an AIW are much less than the requirements for obtaining a search warrant under the Fourth Amendment.)

Situations not requiring warrants

An AIW is not required under the following conditions (21 USC 880(c)):

- With the informed and voluntary consent of the owner, operator, or agent in charge of the controlled premises
- With the presentation of an administrative subpoena issued under the CSA (21 USC 876)
- In situations presenting imminent danger to health or safety
- In situations involving inspections of conveyances where there is a reasonable cause to believe that the mobility of the conveyance makes it impracticable to obtain a warrant
- In any other exceptional or emergency circumstance where time or opportunity to apply for a warrant is lacking
- In any other situation where a warrant is not constitutionally required (e.g., evidence is in plain view or obtained incidentally to a lawful arrest)

A registrant who is presented with an AIW by a DEA inspector may not refuse to consent to the inspection. Refusal under these circumstances is unlawful and carries a maximum penalty of $25,000 fine and up to a year in prison, or both.

Laws Related to the Controlled Substances Act

The Controlled Substance Registrant Protection Act of 1984

To combat the constant threat of robberies, burglaries, and other violent crimes, this law mandates a federal investigation under the following circumstances:

- The replacement cost of the controlled substances taken is $500 or greater.
- A registrant or other person is killed or suffers significant injury as a result of the crime.
- Interstate or foreign commerce is involved in the planning or execution of the crime.

Penalties under this law include the following:

- A prison sentence of up to 20 years, a fine of up to $25,000, or both, for robbery or burglary
- A prison sentence of up to 25 years, a fine of up to $35,000, or both, if a dangerous weapon was used in the commission of the crime

- A prison sentence of up to life, a fine of up to $50,000, or both, if death results from the crime

The Chemical Diversion and Trafficking Act of 1988

This law placed under federal control precursor chemicals, essential chemicals, tableting machines, and encapsulating machines commonly used in the illegal manufacture of controlled substances by imposing recordkeeping and import/export reporting requirements on transactions involving these materials.

The Anabolic Steroid Control Act of 2004

This law includes anabolic steroids in schedule III and provides for the automatic scheduling of anabolic steroids and their salts, esters, and ethers without the need to prove they promote muscle growth. Anabolic steroids have not been found to have moderate or low physical dependence, or high psychological dependence, as required for other drugs in schedule III.

The Combat Methamphetamine Epidemic Act of 2005

This law regulates the OTC sale of any product containing precursors to the manufacture of methamphetamine (ephedrine, pseudoephedrine, or phenylpropanolamine) by placing them into a new category of the CSA known as the *scheduled listed chemical products*.

The Methamphetamine Production Prevention Act of 2008

To discourage *smurfing* (purchasing products containing ephedrine, pseudoephedrine, or phenylpropanolamine from many different pharmacies that maintain only written logbooks), this law encourages and facilitates the use of electronic logbooks. Federal grants are provided to states to develop electronic logbook systems to prevent smurfing across state lines.

Ryan Haight Online Pharmacy Consumer Protection Act of 2008

This law amends the CSA by adding new regulatory requirements and criminal provisions designed to curtail the proliferation of rogue Internet sites that unlawfully dispense controlled substances via the Internet.

42-7. Dispensing Controlled Substances

Definitions

Dispense

The term *dispense* means to deliver a controlled substance to an ultimate user or research subject by, or pursuant to the lawful order of, a practitioner. The definition of *dispense* includes the prescribing and administering of a controlled substance and the packaging, labeling, or compounding necessary to prepare the substance for delivery to the ultimate user. The term *dispenser* means a practitioner who so delivers a controlled substance to an ultimate user or research subject (21 USC 802(10)).

Administer

The term *administer* refers to the direct application of a controlled substance to the body of a patient or research subject by

- A practitioner (or, in his or her presence, by his or her authorized agent)
- The patient or research subject at the direction and in the presence of the practitioner, whether such application be by injection, inhalation, ingestion, or any other means (21 USC 802(2))

Distribute

The term *distribute* means to deliver (other than by administering or dispensing) a controlled substance or a listed chemical. The term *distributor* means a person who so delivers a controlled substance or a listed chemical (21 USC 802(11)).

Ultimate user

The term *ultimate user* means a person who has lawfully obtained, and who possesses, a controlled substance for his or her own use or for the use of a member of his or her household or for an animal owned by him or her or by a member of his or her household (21 USC 802(27)). (Note: The DEA takes the position that if a pharmacist delivers a prescription for a controlled substance to someone other than the ultimate user or a member of his or her household, the pharmacist is engaging in an act of distributing, not dispensing. The act of distributing requires a different DEA registration from the act of dispensing.)

Practitioner

The term *practitioner* means a physician, dentist, veterinarian, scientific investigator, pharmacy, hospital, or other person licensed, registered, or otherwise permitted by the United States or the jurisdiction in which he or she practices or does research, to distribute, dispense, conduct research with respect to, administer, or use in teaching or chemical analysis a controlled substance in the course of professional practice or research (21 USC 802(21)).

Central fill pharmacy

The term *central fill pharmacy* refers to a pharmacy that is permitted by law in the state in which it is located to prepare valid prescription orders for controlled substances that are transmitted to it from a registered retail pharmacy, and to return the labeled, filled prescriptions to the retail pharmacy for delivery to the ultimate user. A central fill pharmacy is authorized to fill prescriptions on behalf of a retail pharmacy only if the retail pharmacy and central fill pharmacy have a contractual relationship providing for such activities or share a common owner (21 CFR 1300.01).

Reverse distributor

The term *reverse distributor* is a DEA registrant to whom a pharmacy can return unwanted, unusable, or outdated controlled substances (21 CFR 1300.01).

Prescriptions for Controlled Substances

Manner of issuance

All prescriptions for controlled substances must be dated and signed on the day issued, and include the following information (21 CFR 1306.05):

- Full name and address of the patient
- Drug name
- Strength
- Dosage form
- Quantity prescribed
- Directions for use
- Name, address, and registration number of the practitioner

Responsibility of prescriber and dispenser

- The prescriptions may be prepared by a secretary or agent for the signature of the prescriber, but the prescribing practitioner is responsible if the prescription does not conform in all essential respects to the law and regulations (21 CFR 1306.05(a)).
- A corresponding liability rests upon the pharmacist, including a pharmacist employed by a central fill pharmacy, who fills a prescription not prepared in conformance with the DEA regulations.

Purpose of the prescription

To be effective, a prescription for a controlled substance must be issued for a legitimate medical purpose by an individual practitioner acting in the usual course of his or her professional practice (21 CFR 1306.04(a)). Prescriptions that exceed a practitioner's prescribing authority are not legal prescriptions. For example, a dentist may not legally write a prescription for a controlled substance to treat a patient's back pain, but could legitimately write a prescription for the same drug to treat a patient's jaw pain.

Corresponding responsibility

The responsibility for the proper prescribing and dispensing of controlled substances rests with the prescriber, but a corresponding responsibility also rests upon the pharmacist who fills the prescription. A pharmacist who knowingly fills a prescription that is not issued in the usual course of professional treatment or in legitimate and authorized research is subject to the penalties provided for violations of the CSA (21 CFR 1306.04(a)). Courts have defined the term *knowingly* to mean what the pharmacist should have known based on obvious facts—not what the pharmacist actually knew (see, e.g., *United States v. Lawson*, 682 F.2d 480 (4th Cir. 1982)).

Prohibition of general dispensing

A practitioner may not obtain a supply of controlled substances by issuing a prescription for general dispensing to patients (21 CFR 1306.04(b)). This prescription is illegal. To obtain a supply of controlled substances for general dispensing to patients, the practitioner should purchase them from a pharmacy, manufacturer, or wholesaler using an invoice and receipt method.

Detoxification and/or maintenance treatment

A prescription may not be issued for maintenance or detoxification treatment unless the prescription is issued by a qualifying prescriber under DATA for an FDA-approved drug for that purpose (21 CFR 1306.04(c)). In this case, the prescriber also must provide his or her identification number issued by the DEA, or if within the 45-day application period, a written statement that the prescriber is acting under a good faith belief that the prescriber qualifies under DATA (21 CFR 1306.05(b)).

Miscellaneous

If the prescription is for gamma-hydroxybutyric acid (GHB), the practitioner must note on the face of the prescription the medical need of the patient for the prescription (21 CFR 1306.05(a)). GHB is a schedule III drug for FDA-approved uses and is available only through a single centralized pharmacy as part of a restricted distribution program.

Prescriptions for schedule II drugs

Written prescriptions

A pharmacist may dispense a schedule II drug only after receiving a written prescription by an authorized prescriber, except in emergency situations. A written prescription is not required when the schedule II drug is dispensed directly to the ultimate user by a practitioner other than a pharmacist (21 USC 829(a)). Written prescriptions include paper prescriptions and electronic prescriptions, and each prescription for a schedule II drug must be a separate prescription.

Oral prescriptions

Oral prescriptions for a schedule II drug are not permitted except in an emergency situation (21 CFR 1306.11(d)).

In the case of an emergency situation, a pharmacist may dispense a controlled substance listed in schedule II upon receiving oral authorization of a prescribing individual practitioner, provided that the following conditions are met:

- The quantity prescribed and dispensed is limited to the amount adequate to treat the patient during the emergency period (dispensing beyond the emergency period must be pursuant to a paper or electronic prescription signed by the prescribing individual practitioner).
- The prescription must be immediately reduced to writing by the pharmacist and must contain all required information, except for the signature of the prescribing individual practitioner.
- If the prescribing individual practitioner is not known to the pharmacist, he or she must make

a reasonable effort to determine that the oral authorization came from a registered individual practitioner, which may include a call to the prescribing individual practitioner using his or her phone number as listed in the telephone directory and/or other good faith efforts to ensure his or her identity.

■ Within 7 days after authorizing an emergency oral prescription, the dispensing pharmacist must receive from the prescribing individual practitioner a written prescription for the emergency quantity prescribed, as follows:

• In addition to all other requirements, the prescription must have written on its face "Authorization for Emergency Dispensing" and the date of the oral order.

• The paper prescription may be delivered to the pharmacist in person or by mail, but if delivered by mail, it must be postmarked within the 7-day period.

• Upon receipt, the dispensing pharmacist must attach this paper prescription to the oral emergency prescription that had earlier been reduced to writing.

• For electronic prescriptions, the pharmacist must annotate the record of the electronic prescription with the original authorization and date of the oral order.

• The pharmacist must notify the nearest DEA office if the prescribing individual practitioner fails to deliver a written prescription to him or her. Failure of the pharmacist to do so shall void the pharmacist's authority to dispense without a written prescription of a prescribing individual practitioner.

Central fill pharmacies are not authorized to prepare prescriptions for a controlled substance listed in schedule II upon receiving an oral authorization from a retail pharmacist or an individual practitioner.

For the purposes of authorizing an oral prescription of a controlled substance listed in schedule II of the Federal Controlled Substances Act, the term *emergency situation* (21 CFR 290.10) means those situations in which the prescribing practitioner determines

■ That immediate administration of the controlled substance is necessary, for proper treatment of the intended ultimate user

■ That no appropriate alternative treatment is available, including administration of a drug that is not a controlled substance under schedule II of the act

■ That it is not reasonably possible for the prescribing practitioner to provide a written prescription to be presented to the person dispensing the substance, prior to the dispensing

Electronic prescriptions for controlled substances

Effective June 1, 2010, the DEA rules (75 Fed. Reg. 16236 (2010), Electronic Prescriptions for Controlled Substances, or EPCS) modified the regulations to give practitioners the option of electronically writing prescriptions for controlled substances. The regulations also allow pharmacies to receive, dispense, and archive electronic prescriptions. However, stringent rules must be followed by both the prescriber and the pharmacy to prevent illegal diversion of controlled substances (21 CFR 1306.08(a)). The detailed regulations are set forth under 21 CFR Part 1311 and are beyond the scope of this review. The legal requirements have limited the use of EPCS, and some commentators predict that it may take several years before EPCS are in common use.

Under prior law, the DEA regulations did not permit EPCS, and electronic prescriptions were treated as oral prescriptions. State law may restrict the use of electronic prescriptions for controlled substances.

A practitioner may issue an electronic prescription for a schedule II, III, IV, or V controlled substance if the following conditions have been met (21 CFR 1311.100(b)):

■ The practitioner is registered as an individual practitioner or exempt from registration.

■ The practitioner uses an electronic prescription application that either a third-party auditor or a certification organization has found to be consistent with the regulations (e.g., processing integrity, security). The practitioner must also obtain a two-factor authentication credential from either an approved credential service provider or, for a digital certificate, a certified certification authority (21 CFR 1311.105(a)).

■ The prescription conforms to all other requirements under the law.

Before a pharmacy may dispense controlled substances pursuant to an electronic prescription, the pharmacy application must be approved by either a third-party auditor or a certification organization that has found that the pharmacy application conforms to the regulations (21 CFR 1311.200(a)).

When a pharmacist fills an EPCS in a manner that would require the pharmacist to make a written notation on the prescription if the prescription were a paper prescription, the pharmacist must make the same notation electronically when filling an electronic prescription and keep the annotation electronically in the prescription record or in linked files (21 CFR 1311.200(f)).

Recordkeeping requirements are as follows (21 CFR 1311.305):

- If a prescription is created, signed, transmitted, and received electronically, all records relating to that prescription must be retained electronically.
- Electronic records regarding controlled substance prescriptions must be maintained electronically for 2 years from the date of their creation or receipt (unless federal or state law requires a longer period).
- Electronic records regarding controlled substance prescriptions must be readily retrievable from all other records. They must be easily readable or easily converted into a format that a person can read.
- Digitally signed prescription records must be transferred or migrated with the digital signature.

Faxed prescriptions

A schedule II prescription may be transmitted by fax, if the original written (paper or electronic) signed prescription is presented to the pharmacist for review prior to the actual dispensing of the controlled substance (21 CFR 1306.11(a)). Several exceptions to this rule exist, and a faxed schedule II prescription may be used as the original prescription without a follow-up written prescription when the prescription is written for any of the following:

- A schedule II narcotic substance to be compounded for direct administration to a patient by parenteral, intravenous, intramuscular, subcutaneous, or intraspinal infusion (21 CFR 1306.11(e))
- A schedule II substance for a resident of a long-term care facility (21 CFR 1306.11(f))
- A schedule II narcotic substance for a patient enrolled in a hospice care program certified and/or paid for by Medicare, or a hospice program that is licensed by the state (21 CFR 1306.11(g))

Labeling

The pharmacist filling a written or emergency oral prescription for a controlled substance listed in schedule II must label the container or package showing the following information (21 CFR 1306.14(a)):

- Date of filling
- Pharmacy name and address
- Serial number of the prescription

- Name of the patient
- Name of the prescribing practitioner
- Directions for use and cautionary statements, if any, contained in the prescription or required by law, such as "Caution: Federal law prohibits the transfer of this drug to any person other than the patient for whom it was prescribed" (21 CFR 290.5)

If the prescription is filled at a central fill pharmacy, the central fill pharmacy must affix to the package a label showing the retail pharmacy name and address and a unique identifier (i.e., the central fill pharmacy's DEA registration number) indicating that the prescription was filled at the central fill pharmacy in addition to the other required information (21 CFR 1306.14(b)).

Prescriptions for institutionalized patients

The labeling requirements do not apply if the ultimate user is institutionalized and the following conditions are met (21 CFR 1306.14(c)):

- Not more than a 7-day supply of the controlled substance is dispensed at one time.
- The controlled substance is not in the possession of the ultimate user prior to its administration.
- The institution maintains appropriate safeguards and records regarding the proper administration, control, dispensing, and storage of the controlled substance.
- The system used by the pharmacist in filling a prescription is adequate to identify the supplier, the product, and the patient, and to provide the directions for use and cautionary statements.

Refills

No refills are permitted for schedule II drugs (21 USC 829(a)).

Multiple prescriptions

An individual practitioner may issue multiple prescriptions authorizing the patient to receive a total of up to a 90-day supply of a schedule II controlled substance if the following conditions are met (21 CFR 1306.12(b)):

- Each separate prescription is issued for a legitimate medical purpose by an individual practitioner acting in the usual course of his or her professional practice.
- The individual practitioner provides written instructions on each prescription indicating the earliest date on which a pharmacy may fill each prescription. No pharmacist may fill the prescription before that date (21 CFR 1306.14(e)).

- The individual practitioner concludes that providing the patient with multiple prescriptions in this manner does not create an undue risk of diversion or abuse.
- The issuance of multiple prescriptions is permissible under applicable state laws.
- The individual practitioner complies fully with all other laws and requirements.

Partial fills

The partial filling of a prescription for a schedule II controlled substance is permissible under the following conditions (21 CFR 1306.13(a)):

- The pharmacist is unable to supply the full quantity called for in a written or emergency oral prescription.
- The pharmacist makes a notation of the quantity supplied on the face of the written prescription (or written record of the emergency oral prescription) or in the electronic prescription record. The following information should be noted in the record for each partial fill:
  - Date
  - Quantity dispensed
  - Remaining quantity authorized to be dispensed
  - Identity of the dispensing pharmacist
- The remaining portion of the prescription may be filled within 72 hours of the first partial filling (21 CFR 1306.13(a)). The total quantity of schedule II controlled substances dispensed in all partial fillings must not exceed the total quantity prescribed.
- If the remaining portion is not or cannot be filled within the 72-hour period, the pharmacist must notify the prescriber.
- No further quantity may be supplied beyond the 72 hours without a new prescription.
- Schedule II drugs may be partially filled to permit dispensing of individual dosage units to patients in long-term care facilities and to patients who are terminally ill (21 CFR 1306.13(b)).
  - If there is any question whether a patient may be classified as having a terminal illness, the pharmacist must contact the practitioner prior to partially filling the prescription. Both the pharmacist and the prescribing practitioner have a corresponding responsibility to assure that the controlled substance is for a terminally ill patient.
  - The pharmacist must record on the prescription whether the patient is "terminally ill" or an "LTCF [long-term care facility] patient."

A prescription that is partially filled and does not contain the notation "terminally ill" or "LTCF patient" shall be deemed to have been filled in violation of the CSA.

- The total quantity of schedule II controlled substances dispensed in all partial fillings must not exceed the total quantity prescribed.
- Schedule II prescriptions for patients in an LTCF or patients with a medical diagnosis documenting a terminal illness are valid for a period not to exceed 60 days from the issue date unless they are terminated sooner by the discontinuance of medication.

Prescriptions for schedule III, IV, and V drugs

A pharmacist may dispense a controlled substance listed in schedule III, IV, or V that is a prescription drug under the FDCA only pursuant to the following (21 CFR 1306.21(a)):

- A paper prescription signed by a practitioner
- A facsimile of a signed paper prescription transmitted by the practitioner or the practitioner's agent to the pharmacy
- An electronic prescription that meets the requirements of law
- An oral prescription made by an individual practitioner and promptly reduced to writing by the pharmacist containing the required information except for the signature of the practitioner

Refills

No prescription for a controlled substance listed in schedule III or IV can be filled or refilled more than 6 months after the date on which the prescription was issued (21 CFR 1306.22(a)). (Note: This rule does not apply to schedule V drugs.) A prescription for a controlled substance listed in schedule III or IV cannot be refilled more than five times within the 6-month period. After the expiration of 6 months or five refills, whichever comes first, the prescriber must issue a new prescription.

The pharmacist must enter each refill of a prescription on the back of the prescription or on another appropriate document or electronic prescription record. If entered on another document, such as a medication record or electronic prescription record, the document or record must be uniformly maintained and readily retrievable (21 CFR 1306.22(b)).

The following information must be retrievable by the prescription number (21 CFR 1306.22(c)):

- Name and address of the person to whom it was dispensed
- Name and dosage form of the controlled substance

- Date filled or refilled
- Quantity dispensed
- Written or typewritten name or initials of the dispensing pharmacist for each refill
- Total number of refills for that prescription

If the pharmacist merely initials and dates the back of the prescription or annotates the electronic prescription record, it is deemed that the pharmacist has dispensed the full face amount of the prescription (21 CFR 1306.22(d)).

The prescribing practitioner may authorize additional refills of schedule III or IV controlled substances on the original prescription through an oral refill authorization transmitted to the pharmacist provided that the following conditions are met (21 CFR 1306.22(e)):

- The total quantity authorized, including the amount of the original prescription, does not exceed five refills nor extend beyond 6 months from the date of issue of the original prescription.
- The pharmacist obtaining the oral authorization must record on the reverse of the original paper prescription or must annotate the electronic prescription record with the date, quantity of refill, and number of additional refills authorized.
- The pharmacist must initial the paper prescription or annotate the electronic prescription record showing who received the refill authorization from the prescribing practitioner who issued the original prescription.
- The quantity of each additional refill authorized is equal to or less than the quantity authorized for the initial filling of the original prescription.
- The prescribing practitioner must execute a new and separate prescription for any additional quantities beyond the five-refill, 6-month limitation.

A computer application may be used as an alternative for the storage and retrieval of refill information for original paper prescription orders for controlled substances in schedules III and IV, if the following conditions are met (21 CFR 1306.22(f)):

- A computerized application must provide online retrieval (via computer monitor or hard-copy printout) of the original prescription order information for those prescription orders that are currently authorized for refilling.
- A computerized application must also provide online retrieval (via computer monitor or hard-

copy printout) of the current refill history for schedule III or IV controlled substance prescription orders (those authorized for refill during the past 6 months).

- The pharmacist must document that the refill information entered into the computer is correct.
- If the computer application provides a hard-copy printout of each day's controlled substance prescription order refill data, that printout must be verified, dated, and signed by the individual pharmacist who refilled the prescription order.
- This document must be maintained in a separate file at that pharmacy for a period of 2 years from the dispensing date.
- In lieu of a printout, the pharmacy must maintain a bound logbook, or separate file, in which each individual pharmacist involved in such dispensing must sign a statement each day, attesting to the fact that the refill information entered into the computer that day has been reviewed by him or her and is correct as shown. This book or file must be maintained at the pharmacy for a period of 2 years after the date of dispensing the appropriately authorized refill.
- In the event that a pharmacy's computerized application experiences system downtime, the pharmacy must have an auxiliary procedure that can be used for documentation of refills of schedule III and IV controlled substance prescription orders.

Partial fills

The partial filling of a prescription for a controlled substance listed in schedule III, IV, or V is permissible if the following conditions are met (21 CFR 1306.23):

- Each partial filling is recorded in the same manner as a refill.
- The total quantity dispensed in all partial fillings does not exceed the total quantity prescribed.
- No dispensing occurs after 6 months after the date on which the prescription was issued.

Labeling

The pharmacist filling a prescription for a controlled substance listed in schedule III, IV, or V must label the package with the following information (21 CFR 1306.24(a)):

- Pharmacy name and address
- Serial number of the prescription
- Date of initial filling (plus the date of the refill to comply with the FDCA)

- Name of the patient
- Name of the practitioner issuing the prescription
- Directions for use and cautionary statements, if any, contained in such prescription as required by law, such as "Caution: Federal law prohibits the transfer of this drug to any person other than the patient for whom it was prescribed" (21 CFR 290.5)

If the prescription is filled at a central fill pharmacy, the central fill pharmacy shall label the package to show the retail pharmacy name and address and a unique identifier (i.e., the central fill pharmacy's DEA registration number) indicating that the prescription was filled at the central fill pharmacy, in addition to the other required information (21 CFR 1306.24(b)).

Prescriptions for institutionalized patients

The labeling requirements do not apply when a controlled substance listed in schedule III, IV, or V is prescribed for administration to an ultimate user who is institutionalized, provided the following conditions are met (21 CFR 1306.24(c)):

- Not more than a 34-day supply or 100 dosage units, whichever is less, of the controlled substance listed in schedule III, IV, or V is dispensed at one time.
- The controlled substance listed in schedule III, IV, or V is not in the possession of the ultimate user prior to administration.
- The institution maintains appropriate safeguards and records the proper administration, control, dispensing, and storage of the controlled substance listed in schedule III, IV, or V.
- The system used by the pharmacist in filling a prescription is adequate to identify the supplier, the product, and the patient and to set forth the directions for use and cautionary statements, if any, contained in the prescription or required by law.

Transferred prescriptions

Pharmacies may transfer refill information among themselves under the following conditions (21 CFR 1306.25):

- The practice must be permitted by state law.
- It must be on a one-time basis only, unless the pharmacies share a real-time, online database. If so, they may transfer refill information back and forth up to the maximum number of refills permitted by the prescription or by law.

- The transfer may take place only by direct communication between two licensed pharmacists.
- The transferring pharmacist must
  - Write the word "Void" on the face of the invalidated prescription, or add the transfer information to the prescription record for electronic prescriptions
  - Record on the reverse of the invalidated prescription the name, address, and DEA registration number of the pharmacy to which it was transferred and the name of the pharmacist receiving the prescription information, or add this information to the prescription record for electronic prescriptions
  - Record the date of the transfer and the name of the pharmacist transferring the information
- The pharmacist receiving the information must write the word "transfer" on the face of the transferred prescription, reduce to writing all information required to be on a prescription, and include the following:
  - Date of issuance of original prescription
  - Original number of refills authorized on original prescription
  - Date of original dispensing
  - Number of valid refills remaining and date(s) and locations of previous refill(s)
  - Pharmacy's name, address, DEA registration number, and prescription number from which the prescription information was transferred
  - Name of pharmacist who transferred the prescription
  - Pharmacy's name, address, DEA registration number, and prescription number from which the prescription was originally filled
- For electronic prescriptions being transferred electronically, the transferring pharmacist must provide the receiving pharmacist with the following information in addition to the original electronic prescription data:
  - Date of the original dispensing
  - Number of refills remaining and the date(s) and locations of previous refill(s)
  - Transferring pharmacy's name, address, DEA registration number, and prescription number for each dispensing
  - Name of the pharmacist transferring the prescription
  - Name, address, DEA registration number, and prescription number from the pharmacy that originally filled the prescription, if different

- The pharmacist receiving a transferred electronic prescription must create an electronic record for the prescription that includes the receiving pharmacist's name and all the information transferred with the prescription.
- The original and transferred prescription(s) must be maintained for a period of 2 years from the date of last refill.

Controlled Substances Dispensed by Means of the Internet

No controlled substance that is a prescription drug may be delivered, distributed, or dispensed by means of the Internet without a valid prescription (21 USC 829(e)). For purposes of this rule, the term *valid prescription* means a prescription that is issued for a legitimate medical purpose in the usual course of professional practice by a practitioner who has conducted at least one in-person medical evaluation of the patient or by a covering practitioner.

The term *in-person medical evaluation* means a medical evaluation that is conducted with the patient in the physical presence of the practitioner, without regard to whether portions of the evaluation are conducted by other health professionals. This rule does not imply that one in-person medical evaluation demonstrates that a prescription has been issued for a legitimate medical purpose within the usual course of professional practice.

The term *covering practitioner* means, with respect to a patient, a practitioner who conducts a medical evaluation (other than an in-person medical evaluation) at the request of a practitioner who

- Has conducted at least one in-person medical evaluation of the patient or an evaluation of the patient through the practice of telemedicine, within the previous 24 months
- Is temporarily unavailable to conduct the evaluation of the patient

These rules do not apply to the delivery, distribution, or dispensing of a controlled substance by a practitioner engaged in the practice of telemedicine, or other practices approved by the Attorney General to be consistent with effective controls against diversion.

Opioid Treatment Programs (Formerly Known as Narcotic Treatment Programs)

Unless specifically allowed by law, it is illegal to prescribe or dispense narcotic drugs for the purpose of maintaining an addict's addiction or detoxifying an addict (21 CFR 1306.04(c)). The rule's intent is to ensure that addicts are treated for their addiction either in registered opioid treatment programs (OTPs) or by qualifying practitioners under DATA.

Definitions

The term *maintenance treatment* means the dispensing for a period in excess of 21 days of a narcotic drug or narcotic drugs in the treatment of an individual for dependence upon heroin or other morphine-like drugs (21 CFR 1300.01(26)).

The term *detoxification treatment* means the dispensing, for a specified period of time, of a narcotic drug or narcotic drugs in decreasing doses to an individual to alleviate adverse physiological or psychological effects incident to withdrawal from the continuous or sustained use of a narcotic drug and as a method of bringing the individual to a narcotic drug–free state within such period of time. There are two types of detoxification treatments: short-term detoxification treatment and long-term detoxification treatment (21 CFR 1300.01(10)).

- *Short-term detoxification treatment* is for a period not in excess of 30 days.
- *Long-term detoxification treatment* is for a period more than 30 days but not in excess of 180 days.

Opioid Treatment Programs

A practitioner may administer or dispense directly (but not prescribe) a narcotic drug listed in any schedule to a narcotic-dependent person for the purpose of maintenance or detoxification treatment if the practitioner meets both of the following requirements (21 CFR 1306.07):

- The practitioner is separately registered with DEA as an OTP.
- The practitioner is in compliance with DEA regulations regarding treatment qualifications, security, records, and unsupervised use of the drugs as required by the CSA.

In addition to registering every 3 years as a dispenser, a practitioner must register with the DEA annually to treat addicts in an OTP (21 CFR 1301.13(e)).

Only drugs approved by the FDA for this purpose may be administered or dispensed. Currently, the following drugs are approved by the FDA for this purpose:

- Methadone
- Levo-alpha-acetyl-methadol (LAAM)

Important: These drugs may not be prescribed for the purpose of maintenance or detoxification treatment nor dispensed by a pharmacist for that purpose.

Drug Addiction Treatment Act (Office-Based Treatment)

An individual practitioner may dispense or prescribe schedule III, IV, or V narcotic controlled drugs or combinations of narcotic controlled drugs that have been approved by the FDA specifically for use in maintenance or detoxification treatment without obtaining the separate registration as an OTP if the practitioner has met the requirements under DATA as discussed in a previous section (21 CFR 1301.28).

A prescription for a schedule III, IV, or V narcotic drug approved by the FDA specifically for detoxification or maintenance treatment must include the identification number issued by the Attorney General after certification by the Secretary of HHS (21 CFR 1301.28(b) and (d)) or a written notice stating that the practitioner is acting under the good faith belief that the practitioner qualifies under DATA, that the practitioner has applied for the number, that the Secretary will certify the practitioner, and that an identification number will be issued (21 CFR 1306.05).

The drugs that are currently approved by the FDA for this purpose are

- Buprenorphine sublingual tablets (Subutex)
- Buprenorphine/naloxone tablets (Suboxone)

(Note: The Substance Abuse and Mental Health Services Administration certifies qualifying practitioners under DATA rather than the DEA.)

A physician, or authorized hospital staff, may administer or dispense narcotic drugs in a hospital to maintain or detoxify a patient under the following conditions (21 CFR 1306.07(c)):

- The treatment is incidental to other medical or surgical treatment of conditions other than addiction.
- The treatment is to relieve intractable pain for which no relief or cure is possible or none has been found after reasonable efforts.

A physician who is not specifically registered to conduct a narcotic treatment program may administer (but not prescribe) narcotic drugs to a person for the purpose of relieving acute withdrawal symptoms when necessary while arrangements are being made for referral for treatment. Not more than 1 day's medication may be administered to the person or for the person's use at one time. Such emergency treatment may be carried out for a maximum of 3 days (21 CFR 1306.07(b)).

Dispensing of Nonprescription Controlled Substances

A controlled substance listed in schedules II, III, IV, or V that is not a prescription drug as determined under the FDCA may be dispensed by a pharmacist without a prescription to a purchaser at retail, provided that the following conditions are met (21 CFR 1306.26):

- A pharmacist dispenses the drug. A nonpharmacist employee may not dispense the drug even under the supervision of a pharmacist. After the pharmacist has fulfilled his or her professional and legal responsibilities, the actual cash or credit transaction or delivery may be completed by a nonpharmacist.
- Not more than 240 cc (8 oz) of any such controlled substance containing opium, nor more than 120 cc (4 oz) of any other such controlled substance, nor more than 48 dosage units of any such controlled substance containing opium, nor more than 24 dosage units of any other such controlled substance may be dispensed at retail to the same purchaser in any given 48-hour period.
- The purchaser is at least 18 years of age.
- The pharmacist requires every purchaser of a controlled substance under this section not known to him or her to furnish suitable identification (including proof of age where appropriate).
- The pharmacist must maintain a bound record book for dispensing nonprescription controlled substances. The book must contain the name and address of the purchaser, the name and quantity of controlled substance purchased, the date of each purchase, and the name or initials of the pharmacist who dispensed the substance to the purchaser.
- A prescription is not required for distribution or dispensing of the substance pursuant to any other federal, state, or local law.
- Central fill pharmacies may not dispense controlled substances to a purchaser at retail pursuant to this section.

DEA Registration Numbers

Although not included specifically in the DEA regulations, the method for determining the legitimacy of a DEA registration number is important for the pharmacist to know:

- Before October 1, 1985, DEA Certificate of Registration numbers for practitioners began with the letter "A." Since that date, the DEA Certificate of Registration numbers for practitioners begin with the letter "B." Further, a DEA Certificate of Registration number issued to a midlevel practitioner begins with the letter "M."
- Following the first letter is a second letter, which is the first letter of the registrant's last name. If the registrant's name begins with a number, the second letter may be a number rather than a letter. For example, 1st Street Pharmacy's DEA Certificate of Registration number would begin with B1, rather than BF.
- Following the two letters is a seven-digit computer-generated sequential number. The number is constructed so that it can be tested for verification by using the following formula:
  - Step 1: Determine the sum of the first, third, and fifth digits.
  - Step 2: Determine the sum of the second, fourth, and sixth digits, and then multiply the sum by two.
  - Step 3: Determine the sum of the two numbers determined in steps 1 and 2.
  - Step 4: The last digit of this third sum should be the same as the last digit of the seven-digit DEA Certificate of Registration number.
- Example: Dr. Jones' number could be: BJ3598123. [3 + 9 + 1 = 13; 5 + 8 + 2 = 15; 15 × 2 = 30; 13 + 30 = 43].

Disposal of Controlled Substances

Any person who needs to dispose of a controlled substance may request assistance from the Special Agent in Charge of the local DEA office for authority and instructions on how to dispose of the substance (21 CFR 1307.21).

The request should be made as follows:

- If the person is a registrant, he or she must list the controlled substance or substances that he or she desires to dispose of on DEA Form 41 and submit three copies of that form to the local DEA office.

- If the person is not a registrant, he or she must submit a letter stating the following:
  - Name and address of the person
  - Name and quantity of each controlled substance to be disposed of
  - How the applicant obtained the substance, if known
  - Name, address, and registration number, if known, of the person who possessed the controlled substances prior to the applicant, if known

The Special Agent in Charge will authorize and instruct the applicant to dispose of the controlled substance in one of the following ways:

- By transfer to a person registered under the act and authorized to possess the substance
- By delivery to an agent of the DEA or to the nearest office of the DEA
- By destruction in the presence of an agent of the DEA or other authorized person
- By such other means as the Special Agent in Charge may determine to ensure that the substance does not become available to unauthorized persons

If a registrant is required to dispose of controlled substances on a regular basis, the Special Agent in Charge may authorize the registrant to dispose of such substances without prior approval of the DEA in each instance. The registrant must keep records of each disposal and file periodic reports with the Special Agent in Charge summarizing the disposals made by the registrant. The Special Agent in Charge may place conditions on the disposal of controlled substances, including the method of disposal and the frequency and detail of reports.

Note: In December 2012, the DEA issued a notice of proposed rulemaking with regard to the disposal of controlled substances. Those proposed regulations implement the Secure and Responsible Drug Disposal Act of 2010 (the Disposal Act, Pub. L. 111-273, 124 Stat. 2858), which authorized the DEA to develop methods for the disposal of controlled substances that have been dispensed to an ultimate user. The proposed rule deletes the rules discussed in this section and creates a comprehensive set of regulations on controlled substance disposal. The proposed regulations create three additional voluntary disposal options available to ultimate users: take-back events, mail-back programs, and collection receptacle programs.

Recordkeeping

Registrants must keep a complete and accurate record of all controlled substances (21 USC 827(a)). For a pharmacy, a complete and accurate record includes the following documentation:

- Records of inventory
- Records of drugs received
- Records of drugs dispensed

To determine the amount of controlled substances that a pharmacy should have on hand, an inspector looks at the beginning (or most recent) inventory, adds the drugs purchased or received, and subtracts the drugs dispensed. Any discrepancy could result in charges of drug diversion or negligent recordkeeping.

Controlled substance records must be kept for at least 2 years at the place of registration (21 CFR 1304.21(b), 1304.04(a); 21 USC 827). Records that must be kept at the registered location include prescription records, inventories, and executed order forms (DEA Form 222 or electronic orders). Financial and shipping records (such as invoices and packing slips) may be kept at a central location rather than the registered location if the registrant has notified the DEA of his or her intention to keep central records (21 CFR 1304.04(a)(1)).

Records of inventory

Before a pharmacy can begin business, an initial inventory of controlled substances must be taken and again every 2 years thereafter (21 CFR 1304.11). This topic is discussed in more detail in a previous section.

Records of drugs received

Records of receipt must contain the following information: the name of the substance; the dosage form; the strength of the substance; the number of dosage units or volume in the container; the number of commercial containers received; the date of receipt; and the name, address, and registration number of the supplier (21 CFR 1304.22 (a)(2) and (c)).

Invoices are appropriate records of receipt for controlled substances listed in schedule III, IV, or V.

DEA Form 222 (or the CSOS) is required for the distribution of a schedule I or II controlled substance.

Records of drugs dispensed

Records of drugs dispensed include the following types of records:

- Prescription orders
- Nonprescription schedule V sales
- Distributions from a pharmacy to another practitioner
- Institutional medication orders
- Reports of disposal or destruction of controlled substances (DEA Form 41)
- Reports of theft or loss (DEA Form 106)

General requirements

A pharmacy that is registered to dispense a controlled substance may distribute (without being registered to distribute) a quantity of controlled substances (21 CFR 1307.11). Distribution may be made to another practitioner for the purpose of general dispensing by the practitioner to patients, provided the following conditions are met:

- The practitioner to whom the controlled substance is to be distributed is registered to dispense that controlled substance.
- The distribution is recorded by the distributing practitioner and by the receiving practitioner in accordance with law.
- If the substance is listed in schedule I or II, DEA Form 222 (or the CSOS) is used.
- The total number of dosage units of all controlled substances distributed by the pharmacy during each calendar year does not exceed 5% of the total number of dosage units of all controlled substances distributed and dispensed by the pharmacy during the same calendar year.

Each registered pharmacy must maintain the inventories and records of controlled substances as follows (21 CFR 1304.04(h)):

- Inventories and records of all controlled substances listed in schedules I and II must be maintained separately from all other records of the pharmacy.
- Paper prescriptions for schedule II controlled substances must be maintained at the registered location in a separate prescription file.
- Inventories and records of schedules III, IV, and V controlled substances must be maintained either separately from all other records of the pharmacy or in such form that the information required is readily retrievable from ordinary business records of the pharmacy.

Paper prescriptions for schedules III, IV, and V controlled substances must be maintained at the registered location either in a separate prescription file only for schedules III, IV, and V controlled substances or in such form that they are readily retrievable from the other prescription records of the pharmacy:

- Prescriptions are *readily retrievable* if, at the time they are initially filed, the face of the prescription is stamped in red ink in the lower right corner with the letter "C" no less than 1 inch high and filed either in the prescription file for controlled substances listed in schedules I and II or in the usual consecutively numbered prescription file for noncontrolled substances.
- The requirement to mark the hard copy prescription with a red "C" is waived if a pharmacy uses a computer application for prescriptions that permits identification by prescription number and retrieval of original documents by prescriber name, patient's name, drug dispensed, and date filled.

Records of electronic prescriptions for controlled substances must be maintained in an application that meets the requirements of law. The computers on which the records are maintained may be located at another location, but the records must be readily retrievable at the registered location if requested by the DEA or other law enforcement agent. The electronic application must be capable of printing out or transferring the records in a format that is readily understandable at the registered location. Electronic copies of prescription records must be sortable by prescriber name, patient name, drug dispensed, and date filled.

Sales of Scheduled Listed Chemical Products

These rules outline the requirements for retail sales of scheduled listed chemical products for personal use (21 CFR 1314.01). These products are nonprescription products under federal law and in most states, but some states have laws that require a prescription for these products.

Applicability of rules

The rules apply to regulated persons who sell listed chemical products to nonregulated persons for personal use in the following situations (21 CFR 1314.02):

- The products are sold at retail for personal use through face-to-face sales at stores or mobile retail vendors (e.g., farmers' markets, kiosks).

- The products are sold and shipped through the USPS or through private or common carriers (mail-order sales).

The term *mail-order sale* means a retail sale of scheduled listed chemical products for personal use in which a regulated person uses or attempts to use the USPS or any private or commercial carrier to deliver the product to the customer. Mail-order sale includes purchase orders submitted by phone, mail, fax, Internet, or any method other than face-to-face transaction (21 CFR 1314.03).

Packaging requirements

A regulated seller or mail-order distributor may not sell a scheduled listed chemical product in nonliquid form (including gel caps) unless the product is packaged either in blister packs, with each blister containing no more than two dosage units or, if blister packs are technically infeasible, in unit dose packets or pouches (21 CFR 1314.05).

Effect on state law

States may pass legislation regulating these products that differs from federal legislation unless a positive conflict exists between state law and federal law so that the two cannot consistently be enforced together (21 CFR 1314.10). It is important for the pharmacist to know the laws in the state in which he or she practices and to understand how state law works with federal law.

Loss reporting

A pharmacist (regulated seller) must report to the DEA any unusual or excessive loss or disappearance of a scheduled listed chemical product. The report must, if possible, be made orally as soon as practicable, and a written report must be filed within 15 days after the pharmacist becomes aware of the loss (21 CFR 1314.15).

Restrictions on sales quantity

Without regard to the number of transactions, a regulated seller (including a mobile retail vendor) may not in a single calendar day sell any purchaser more than 3.6 grams of ephedrine base, 3.6 grams of pseudoephedrine base, or 3.6 grams of phenylpropanolamine base in scheduled listed chemical products (21 CFR 1314.20). This daily limit also applies to mail-order sales (21 CFR 1314.100). (Note: phenylpropanolamine has been withdrawn from the market.)

A regulated seller may not sell to the same person more than 9 grams of a listed chemical product within a 30-day period (except for sales through mobile retail vendors and mail-order sales, which are limited to no more than 7.5 grams per 30-day period) (21 USC 844).

A mobile retail vendor may not in any 30-day period sell an individual purchaser more than 7.5 grams of ephedrine base, 7.5 grams of pseudoephedrine base, or 7.5 grams of phenylpropanolamine base in scheduled listed chemical products (21 CFR 1314.20). This 30-day limit also applies to mail-order sales (21 CFR 1314.100).

Thus, a person may not purchase more than 3.6 grams of these products per day, and no more than 9 grams during a 30-day period (this is a rolling 30-day period, not a calendar month) and no more than 7.5 grams of the 9 grams may be purchased from a mobile retail vendor or by mail order.

Storage

The regulated seller must place listed chemical products "behind the counter" and deliver the product directly into the custody of the purchaser (21 CFR 1314.25). A behind-the-counter placement of a product includes the product being stored in a locked cabinet that is located in an area of the facility where customers do not have direct access. Mobile retail vendors must store the products in a locked cabinet.

Recordkeeping for retail transactions

Except for purchase by an individual of a single sales package containing not more than 60 milligrams of pseudoephedrine, the regulated seller must maintain a written or electronic list of each scheduled listed chemical product sale that identifies the products by name, the quantity sold, the names and addresses of the purchasers, and the dates and times of the sales (referred to as the "logbook") (21 CFR 1314.30).

Retail procedure
The regulated seller must comply with the following procedure before completing a retail sale of a scheduled listed chemical product:

- The purchaser must present an identification card that provides a photograph and is issued by a state or the federal government, or a document that is considered acceptable for purposes of employment.
- The purchaser must sign the logbook as follows:
  - For written logbooks, the purchaser enters in the logbook his or her name, address, and the date and time of the sale.
  - For electronic logbooks, the purchaser provides a signature using a device that captures signatures in an electronic format or signs a bound paper book. If the purchaser signs a bound paper book, it must include the name of each product sold, the quantity sold, the name and address of the purchaser, and the date and time of the sale, or a unique identifier that can be linked to that electronic information.
- The logbook maintained by the seller must include the prospective purchaser's name, address, and the date and time of the sale. If the purchaser enters the information, the seller must determine that the name entered in the logbook corresponds to the name provided on the identification and that the date and time entered are correct. If the seller enters the information, the prospective purchaser must verify that the information is correct.
- The regulated seller must enter into the logbook the name of the product and the quantity sold. For electronic records, the seller may use a point-of-sale and bar-code reader.
- The regulated seller must include in the written or electronic logbook or display by the logbook, the following notice: "WARNING: Section 1001 of Title 18, United States Code, states that whoever, with respect to the logbook, knowingly and willfully falsifies, conceals, or covers up by any trick, scheme, or device a material fact, or makes any materially false, fictitious, or fraudulent statement or representation, or makes or uses any false writing or document knowing the same to contain any materially false, fictitious, or fraudulent statement or entry, shall be fined not more than $250,000 if an individual or $500,000 if an organization, imprisoned not more than five years, or both."

General procedure
The regulated seller must maintain each entry in the written or electronic logbook for not fewer than 2 years after the date on which the entry is made (21 CFR 1314.30(e)).

A record under this section must be kept at the regulated seller's place of business where the transaction occurred, except that records may be kept at a single, central location of the regulated seller if the regulated seller has notified the DEA of the intention to do so (21 CFR 1314.30(f)).

The records required to be kept under this section must be readily retrievable and available for inspection and copying by authorized employees of the DEA (21 CFR 1314.30(g)).

A record developed and maintained to comply with a state law may be used to meet the requirements of this section if the record includes the information specified in this section (21 CFR 1314.30(h)).

Training of sales personnel

Each regulated seller must ensure that all individuals who are responsible for delivering the products into the custody of purchasers or who deal directly with purchasers by obtaining payments for the products are trained in the regulations governing the sale of scheduled listed chemical products (21 CFR 1314.35).

The regulated seller must submit to the DEA a self-certification that all such individuals have undergone training provided by the regulated seller to ensure that the individuals understand the requirements that apply to the sale of these products.

The regulated seller must maintain a copy of each self-certification and all records demonstrating that all individuals involved in the sale of these products have undergone the training.

Verification of identity for mail-order sales

Each regulated person who makes a mail-order sale at retail of a scheduled listed chemical product must, prior to shipping the product, receive from the purchaser a copy of an identification card that provides a photograph and is issued by a state or the federal government, or a document that is considered acceptable for purposes of employment (21 CFR 1314.105).

Prior to shipping the product, the regulated person must determine that the name and address on the identification correspond to the name and address provided by the purchaser as part of the sales transaction. If the regulated person cannot verify the identities of both the purchaser and the recipient, the person may not ship the scheduled listed chemical product.

If the product is being shipped to a third party, the regulated person must verify that both the purchaser and the person to whom the product is being shipped live at the addresses provided. If the regulated person cannot verify the identities of both the purchaser and the recipient, the person may not ship the scheduled listed chemical product.

Reports for mail-order sales

Each regulated person required to report mail-order sales of scheduled listed chemical products must either submit a written report containing details of the sale on or before the 15th day of each month following the month in which the distributions took place, or upon request of and approval by the DEA, submit the report in electronic form, either via computer disk or direct electronic data transmission (21 CFR 1314.110).

If the DEA determines that a regulated seller or distributor required to submit reports has sold a scheduled listed chemical product in violation of the law, the DEA will serve upon the regulated seller or distributor an order to show cause why he or she should not be prohibited from selling scheduled listed chemical products (21 CFR 1314.150). The DEA may suspend, pending a final order, the right to sell scheduled listed chemical products if there is an imminent danger to the public health or safety (21 CFR 1314.155(a)).

42-8. Questions

1. Pharmacist Betty Jones decides to open her own community pharmacy. Which of the following DEA forms will she use to apply for a DEA Certificate of Registration for the new pharmacy?

   A. DEA Form 106
   B. DEA Form 222
   C. DEA Form 223
   D. DEA Form 224
   E. DEA Form 224a

2. You arrive at your community pharmacy one morning and discover that during the night, someone broke into the pharmacy and stole several commercial containers of controlled substances. Within how many business days must this theft of controlled substances be

reported to the field division office of the DEA in your area?

A. 1
B. 3
C. 7
D. 10
E. 30

3. As the owner of a community pharmacy, you recently employed a staff pharmacist and granted the pharmacist a power of attorney to order controlled substances. In addition to physically signing the DEA order form for schedule II controlled substances, the staff pharmacist completed the steps necessary to obtain authority from the DEA to place electronic orders for all schedules of controlled substances. Today, this pharmacist resigned from your employment. The pharmacist's resignation must be communicated to the DEA Certification Authority within what period of time?

A. 6 hours
B. 24 hours
C. 3 days
D. 7 days
E. 30 days

4. Which of the following is the federal agency that certifies private practice physicians to prescribe schedule III, IV, or V narcotic controlled substances for detoxification and maintenance treatment of opioid dependency?

A. Drug Enforcement Administration
B. U.S. Food and Drug Administration
C. Office of Inspector General
D. Substance Abuse and Mental Health Services Administration
E. Federal Trade Commission

5. Frank Wilson, a U.S. citizen, recently traveled outside the United States on business. While outside the country, he became very ill with a gastrointestinal infection and suffered severe nausea, vomiting, diarrhea, and dehydration. A physician in the town where he was located prescribed medications consisting of an antibiotic and two controlled substances. A local pharmacy dispensed the prescriptions, which were packaged, labeled, and dispensed in much the same manner as if dispensed in the United States. On returning to the United States 2 days after receiving the prescriptions, he proceeded to U.S. Customs, where he was asked if he was bringing any drugs into the country. He responded "yes" and handed the Customs officer the prescriptions. Regarding the controlled substance prescriptions, which of the following is true?

A. If either or both of the prescriptions are for a schedule II controlled substance, they will be seized by the Customs officer because federal law prohibits importation of a schedule II controlled substance.
B. Mr. Wilson can legally bring a maximum of 50 dosage units of each of the two controlled substances into the United States.
C. Mr. Wilson can legally bring a maximum of 50 dosage units combined of the two controlled substances into the United States.
D. Mr. Wilson can bring the antibiotic prescription into the United States but not the prescriptions for controlled substances.
E. Both A and D

6. A life-supporting or life-sustaining device that requires FDA approval before it can be marketed in interstate commerce in the United States is a

A. class I device.
B. class II device.
C. class III device.
D. class IV device.
E. class V device.

7. For purposes of classifying a drug as an *orphan drug*, a rare disease or condition is defined as follows: a disease or condition that affects (a) fewer than _____ persons in the United States or (b) more than _____ persons in the United States provided that there is no reasonable expectation that the cost of developing and making the drug available will be recovered.

A. 100,000
B. 200,000
C. 250,000
D. 500,000
E. 1,000,000

8. Which of the following is an unofficial compendia not included in the Official Compendia in the federal FDCA?

    A. *United States Pharmacopeia*
    B. *Homeopathic Pharmacopeia of the United States*
    C. *National Formulary*
    D. *Orange Book: Approved Drug Products with Therapeutic Equivalence Evaluations*
    E. Both B and C

9. When a pharmacy orders schedule II controlled substances using the DEA official triplicate order form, which copy (copies) of the form is (are) sent by the pharmacy to the supplier?

    A. Copy 1
    B. Copy 2
    C. Copy 3
    D. Copies 1 and 2
    E. Copies 2 and 3

10. A quality control manager at Widget Pharmaceuticals has just discovered that the manufacturing process has failed to follow Good Manufacturing Practices. A batch sample of a Widget Pharmaceuticals' intravenous solution has tested pure. If, in fact, the intravenous solution is pure, the solution would be

    A. adulterated.
    B. misbranded.
    C. both misbranded and adulterated.
    D. neither misbranded nor adulterated.
    E. nonsterile.

11. Pharmacies registered under the federal CSA are required to take a complete inventory of all controlled substances every _____ months.

    A. 6
    B. 12
    C. 18
    D. 24
    E. 36

12. Dr. Marcia Wilson is a neurologist treating attention deficit disorder (ADD) and attention deficit hyperactivity disorder (ADHD) patients. Among her treatments for these patients, she prescribes Ritalin, Concerta, and Adderall. Her general policy is that patients using these medications must be seen in her office every 3 months for evaluation. Because most of her patients prefer to obtain their prescriptions locally and third-party prescription drug plans will reimburse only for a 30-day supply, Dr. Wilson is forced to issue three prescriptions to provide adequate medication between office visits. According to the applicable DEA regulation on issuing multiple prescriptions for a schedule II controlled substance, for how many total days' supply of a schedule II controlled substance may Dr. Wilson issue multiple prescriptions to a patient?

    A. 60
    B. 90
    C. 120
    D. 150
    E. 180

13. According to the federal FDCA, which of the following may *not* legally receive and possess prescription drug samples from a manufacturer or authorized distributor of record?

    A. Freestanding retail pharmacies
    B. Pharmacies located within a hospital or other health care entity, at the written request of a licensed practitioner
    C. Osteopathic doctors
    D. Dentists
    E. Physician assistants

14. One of your regular patients comes into your pharmacy and reports that he developed a dry, hacking cough 2 days ago, and although he has been taking a nonprescription liquid cough suppressant, it has been ineffective in controlling the cough. He says that not too long ago, another pharmacy sold him a nonprescription cough suppressant containing codeine that was very effective. He asks if you have such a product, and you reply that you do and agree to sell him the product. Assuming that state law permits selling such a product without a prescription, you may sell not more than 240 cc (8 oz) of a controlled substance containing opium, nor more than 120 cc (4 oz) of any other controlled substance, nor more than 48 dosage units of a controlled substance containing opium, nor more than 24 dosage units of

any other controlled substance in any given period of how many hours?

A. 24
B. 36
C. 48
D. 60
E. 72

15. According to the federal FDCA, which of the following is exempt from registration with the FDA as a manufacturer?

A. A manufacturer of generic drug products
B. A manufacturer of brand-name drug products
C. A pharmacy compounding a product pursuant to a lawful prescription order
D. A pharmacy compounding a product to supply a physician for that physician to use in dispensing prescription orders
E. A pharmacy compounding nonsterile products for distribution to other pharmacies

16. "The rate and extent to which the active ingredient or therapeutic ingredient is absorbed from a drug and becomes available at the site of drug action" is the federal FDCA definition of which of the following?

A. Bioavailability
B. Bioequivalency
C. Dissolution
D. Area under the curve
E. Absorption

17. Under federal law, the daily sales limit of ephedrine base, pseudoephedrine base, or phenylpropanolamine base is _____ grams per purchaser, regardless of the number of transactions.

A. 1.8
B. 3.6
C. 7.2
D. 9.0
E. 14.4

18. At least how many days before introducing or delivering for introduction into interstate commerce a dietary supplement that contains a new dietary ingredient that has not been present in the food supply as an article used for food in a form in which the food has not been chemically altered must the manufac-

turer or distributor of that supplement, or of the new dietary ingredient, submit to the FDA information, including any citations to published articles, on which basis the manufacturer or distributor has concluded that the dietary supplement can reasonably be expected to be safe?

A. 30
B. 60
C. 75
D. 90
E. 120

19. Which of the following choices is an inappropriate method for a pharmacist to distribute the "side effects" statement?

A. A sticker attached to the prescription vial
B. A statement on a preprinted prescription vial cap
C. A statement in a consumer medication guide
D. A statement on a separate sheet of paper
E. A statement on a refrigerator magnet included in the prescription bag

20. The federal FDCA prohibits the selling, purchasing, or trading of a prescription drug that was purchased by a public or private hospital or other health care entity or donated or supplied at a reduced price to a charitable organization. Which of the following situations is covered by this prohibition?

A. The purchase or other acquisition by a hospital or other health care entity that is a member of a group-purchasing organization of a drug for its own use from the group-purchasing organization or from other hospitals or health care entities that are members of such an organization
B. A sale, purchase, or trade of a drug or an offer to sell, purchase, or trade a drug among hospitals or other health care entities that are under common control
C. A sale, purchase, or trade of a drug; an offer to sell, purchase, or trade a drug; or the dispensing of a drug pursuant to a prescription
D. The sale, purchase, or trade of a drug or an offer to sell, purchase, or trade a drug by a charitable organization to a nonprofit affiliate of the organization
E. A sale to a community pharmacy for non-emergency dispensing needs

21. A maximum of how many times may a prescription for a schedule III or IV controlled substance be refilled within 6 months of the date on which the prescription was issued?

    A. 1
    B. 2
    C. 3
    D. 4
    E. 5

22. Approximately 30 minutes ago, your community pharmacy received a prescription for a schedule II controlled substance by facsimile transmission. The patient for whom the prescription was issued has just arrived for the prescription. You may dispense the prescription solely on the basis of the facsimile prescription and use the facsimile prescription as the original prescription for purposes of recordkeeping.

    A. True
    B. False

23. With respect to a prescription for a controlled substance, which of the following may be maintained in an electronic database used for prescription dispensing rather than having to be placed on the actual prescription form maintained in the pharmacy's prescription files?

    A. Physician's DEA number
    B. Record of refills
    C. Patient address
    D. The word *void* or the word *transfer* required on issuing or receiving, respectively, a transferred prescription for a controlled substance
    E. Patient name

24. William Wilson has just presented you two empty prescription vials and requests that each be refilled. Both of the prescriptions are for solid, oral dosage formulations. When dispensing the refills (and assuming that neither Mr. Wilson nor the prescriber has requested non-child-resistant packaging), you may reuse the prescription vials and closures when dispensing the refills.

    A. True
    B. False

25. The FDA regulations regarding medication guides provide that where a medication guide is required for a particular prescription drug product, the medication guide must be provided to the patient on the initial dispensing of the drug but not on any refills thereafter.

    A. True
    B. False

42-9. Answers

1. **D.** DEA Form 224 is the application form for a new DEA Certificate of Registration. DEA Form 224a is the renewal application form that DEA mails to registrants approximately 60 days before the expiration of a DEA Certificate of Registration. DEA Form 106 is used to report theft or loss of controlled substances. DEA Form 222 is used to order schedule II controlled substances. DEA Form 223 is the number of the DEA Certificate of Registration that is displayed at the registrant's location. The applicable DEA regulation is 21 CFR 1301.13.

2. **A.** Although notification is required within one business day, completion and submission of DEA Form 106 is not required within one business day, but the form should be completed and submitted promptly. The applicable DEA regulation is 21 CFR 1301.76.

3. **A.** Recognize that before electronic ordering of controlled substances was permitted, notifying the DEA if a pharmacist with a power of attorney resigned or was terminated was not necessary. The power of attorney was useless without physical access to DEA Form 222. But with electronic ordering of controlled substances, a DEA Form 222 is not needed, so notification must be provided if the pharmacist had obtained the authority from DEA to submit electronic orders. The applicable DEA regulation is 21 CFR 1311.45.

4. **D.** The Substance Abuse and Mental Health Services Administration (SAMHSA), not the DEA, certifies physicians to prescribe schedule III, IV, and V narcotic controlled substances for detoxification and maintenance treatment of opioid dependency. Prescriptions for the currently approved products Suboxone and

Subutex for treatment of opioid dependency must include the physician's DEA number and the physician's "X" number signifying certification to treat opioid dependency. Also, only physicians may be approved to treat opioid dependency. Information about the medication-assisted treatment of opioid dependency is available on the SAMHSA Web site at www.dpt.samhsa.gov. The applicable DEA regulation is 21 CFR 1301.28.

5. **C.** The limitation associated with the exemption from import and export requirements for personal medical use is a combined 50 dosage units and not 50 dosage units of each controlled substance. The applicable DEA regulation is 21 CFR 1301.26.

6. **C.** The federal FDCA provides for three classes of medical devices: class I, class II, and class III. Generally, class I devices are not subject to premarket approval, and class II devices are subject to performance standards. Class III devices are life-supporting or life-sustaining devices and require premarket approval by FDA. The applicable section of the federal FDCA is 21 USC 360c.

7. **B.** The applicable section of the federal FDCA is 21 USC 360bb.

8. **D.** Although the *Orange Book: Approved Drug Products with Therapeutic Equivalence Evaluations* (FDA Orange Book) is an important publication for pharmacies, it is not one of the official compendia. The official compendia are established by the federal FDCA at 21 USC 321.

9. **D.** The pharmacy keeps copy 3 and sends copies 1 and 2 to the supplier. The applicable DEA regulation is 21 CFR 1305.12.

10. **A.** The applicable section of the federal FDCA is 21 USC 351.

11. **D.** Pharmacies are required to conduct a biennial inventory of all controlled substances. The applicable DEA regulation is 21 CFR 1304.11.

12. **B.** The applicable DEA regulation is 21 CFR 1306.12.

13. **A.** The applicable section of the federal FDCA is 21 USC 353.

14. **C.** The applicable DEA regulation is 21 CFR 1306.26.

15. **C.** Pharmacies are exempt from registration, provided that the compounding is "in the regular course of their business of dispensing or selling drugs or devices at retail." The applicable section of the federal FDCA is 21 USC 360. The DQSA also exempts compounded drugs from new drug requirements, labeling requirements, and track-and-trace requirements if the drug is compounded by or under the direct supervision of a licensed pharmacist in a registered outsourcing facility and meets other requirements.

16. **A.** The applicable section of the federal FDCA is 21 USC 355.

17. **B.** The applicable DEA regulation is 21 CFR 1314.20.

18. **C.** The applicable section of the federal FDCA is 21 USC 350b.

19. **E.** The applicable DEA regulation is 21 CFR 209.11.

20. **E.** The applicable section of the federal FDCA is 21 USC 353.

21. **E.** As provided in the DEA regulations, "No prescription for a controlled substance listed in schedule III or IV shall be filled or refilled more than 6 months after the date on which such prescription was issued and no such prescription authorized to be refilled may be refilled more than five times." The applicable DEA regulation is 21 CFR 1306.22.

22. **B.** Although in some situations a facsimile prescription for a schedule II controlled substance can be dispensed and can be used as the original prescription for recordkeeping, it cannot be in this situation of an ambulatory patient. The applicable DEA regulation is 21 CFR 1306.11.

23. **B.** All information required to be placed on a prescription for a controlled substance by either the CSA or the DEA regulations must be placed on the prescription. The only exemption is the record of refills. The applicable DEA regulation is 21 CFR 1306.22.

24. **B.** As stated by the CPSC in response to whether pharmacists may reuse prescription vials, "As a general rule, no. This prohibition is based on the wear associated with a plastic vial, which could compromise the package's

effectiveness. Since such wear or undetected damage with a glass container is negligible, the CPSC staff has indicated that it would have no objection to the reuse of a glass container, provided a new closure is used. This same consideration would be given to any other package type that is not prone to wear." See CPSC, "Poison Prevention Packaging: A Guide for Healthcare Professionals," available at www.cpsc.gov/CPSCPUB/PUBS/384.pdf.

25. **B.** Medication guides must be provided on each dispensing. The applicable FDA regulation is 21 CFR 208.24.

42-10. References

Electronic *Code of Federal Regulations* (CFR). Available at: www.ecfr.gov.

Federal Register (Fed. Reg.). Available at: www.gpo.gov/fdsys/browse/collection.action?collectionCode=FR.

United States Code (USC). Available at: uscode.house.gov/search/criteria.shtml.

U.S. Drug Enforcement Administration (DEA). *Pharmacist's Manual: An Information Outline of the Controlled Substances Act*. Washington, D.C.: U.S. Drug Enforcement Administration; 2010. Available at: www.deadiversion.usdoj.gov/pubs/manuals/pharm2/pharm_manual.pdf.

U.S. Drug Enforcement Administration, Office of DEA Diversion Control. Manuals. Available at: www.deadiversion.usdoj.gov/pubs/manuals/index.html.

U.S. Food and Drug Administration (FDA). National drug code directory. Available at: www.fda.gov/drugs/informationondrugs/ucm142438.htm.

U.S. Food and Drug Administration. Newly added guidance documents. Available at: www.fda.gov/Drugs/GuidanceComplianceRegulatoryInformation/Guidances/ucm121568.htm.

U.S. Food and Drug Administration. *Orange Book: Approved Drug Products with Therapeutic Equivalence Evaluations*. 32nd ed. Silver Spring, Md.: U.S. Food and Drug Administration; 2012. Available at: www.accessdata.fda.gov/scripts/cder/ob/default.cfm.

U.S. Postal Service. Publication 52, Hazardous, restricted, and perishable mail. Washington, D.C.: U.S. Postal Service; 2011. Available at: pe.usps.com/text/pub52/pub52c4_026.htm.

Index

Note: Page numbers followed by *b*, *f*, or *t* indicated material in boxes, figures, or tables, respectively.

A

A$_{1C}$, in diabetes mellitus, 316, 316*b*, 333
  alpha-glucosidase inhibitors and, 322
  amylin mimetics and, 328
  biguanides (metformin) and, 319
  colesevelam and, 324
  dipeptidyl peptidase-4 (DPP-4) inhibitors and, 323
  dopamine agonists and, 324
  incretin mimetics and, 328
  insulin and, 327
  secretagogues and, 320
  sodium-glucose co-transporter 2 inhibitors and, 323, 323*t*
  thiazolidinediones and, 321
AACE. *See* American Association of Clinical Endocrinologists
AADs. *See* antiarrhythmic drugs
AAFP. *See* American Academy of Family Physicians
AAP. *See* American Academy of Pediatrics
abacavir, 37, 757–762, 759*t*–761*t*
abatacept, 506*t*, 514
abbreviated new drug application (ANDA), 925
abciximab, 140*t*, 146, 152, 277, 287–288, 287*t*
Abilify. *See* aripiprazole
abiraterone acetate, 440*t*
"AB" rated products, for generic substitutions, 935
absence seizures, 561, 562
absolute bioavailability *(F)*, 111, 112, 118
absolute refractory period, 242
absorption, 112, 113. *See also specific drugs*
  clinical examples of, 124–127
  drug, disease, and dietary influences on, 121–123
  first-order, 113
  in older adults, 836–837, 855
  in pediatric patients, 810–811
  pH partition theory of, 28, 50
  questions and answers on, 127–135
  rate and extent of. *See* bioavailability
  route of administration and, 113
  of tablets, 37–38

absorption bases, 43, 62
ABW. *See* actual body weight
acarbose, 321–322, 322*t*
accreditation, of compounding pharmacy, 64
Accutane. *See* isotretinoin
ACE. *See* angiotensin-converting enzyme
acebutolol, 211*t*
ACE inhibitors (ACEIs). *See* angiotensin-converting enzyme inhibitors
Acetadote. *See* acetylcysteine
acetaminophen
  adverse reactions to, 517–518, 659
  asthma induced by, 678
  for cough, cold, and allergies, 653
  for critically ill patients, 401*t*
  dosage of, 674
  drug–drug interactions of, 659
  for fever, 659, 659*t*
  infant formulation of, 827
  intravenous formulations of, 402
  maximum daily dose of, 674
  mechanism of action, 517, 674
  for migraine, 549
  for osteoarthritis, 503, 517–518, 528
  for otitis media, 815
  overdose of, 859, 868, 869*t*, 881
  for pain, 535, 535*t*, 659, 659*t*
  patient instructions and counseling on, 517
  pediatric dosage of, 675
  product labeling for, 659
acetazolamide, 848*t*, 849
acetic acids, for rheumatoid arthritis, 509*t*
acetohexamide, 319–320, 320*t*
acetylation, in pediatric patients, 811
acetylcysteine
  for acetaminophen overdose, 859, 868, 869*t*, 881
  for cystic fibrosis, 820*t*, 832
ACG. *See* American College of Gastroenterology
achlorhydria
  in infants, 810
  in megaloblastic anemia, 885
acid(s), concentrated, 15

acid–base disorders
  in acute kidney disease, 371, 374, 395
  in chronic kidney disease, 369, 378, 379, 381, 385, 390–391
  nausea/vomiting and, 658
  in nutrition support therapy, 422
acid–base reactions, in incompatibility, 81–83
α_1-acid glycoprotein, 117
ACIP. *See* Advisory Committee on Immunization Practices
acitretin, for psoriasis, 637
aclidinium, for COPD, 692
acne (acne vulgaris), 624–628
  classification of, 624
  clinical presentation of, 624
  drug therapy for, 623, 644
  key points on, 623
  pathophysiology of, 624–625
  questions and answers on, 644
  systemic therapy for, 627–628
    antimicrobials in, 627, 627*t*
    corticosteroids in, 628
    isotretinoin in, 623, 627–628
  topical therapy for, 625–626
    antimicrobial agents in, 625–626, 625*t*
    azelaic acid 2% in, 626
    dapsone 5%, 626
    nonprescription agents in, 625
    retinoids in, 626, 626*t*
    treatment principles in, 625
  type I (comedonal), 624–625
  type II (papular), 624–625
  type III (pustular), 624–625
  type IV (nodulocystic), 624–625
ACP (American College of Physicians) Journal Club, 177
acquired immune deficiency syndrome (AIDS), 755–789. *See also* human immunodeficiency virus (HIV) infection
  definition of, 755
  drug therapy for, 755
  key points on, 755